MAGILL'S
MEDICAL
GUIDE

MAGILL'S MEDICAL GUIDE

Revised Edition
1998

Volume I
Abdomen — Fetal tissue transplantation

Medical Consultants

Culley C. Carson III, M.D.
University of North Carolina School of Medicine

Karen E. Kalumuck, Ph.D.
The Exploratorium, San Francisco

L. Fleming Fallon, Jr., M.D., M.P.H.
Bowling Green State University

Nancy A. Piotrowski, Ph.D.
University of California, Berkeley

Connie Rizzo, M.D.
Pace University

Project Editor
Tracy Irons-Georges

SALEM PRESS, INC.
Pasadena, California   Englewood Cliffs, New Jersey

Editor in Chief: Dawn P. Dawson
Project Editor: Tracy Irons-Georges
Research Supervisor: Jeffry Jensen
Photograph Editor: Karrie Hyatt
Production Editors: Janet Long, Joyce I. Buchea, Cynthia Beres
Proofreading Supervisor: Yasmine A. Cordoba
Page Layout and Design: James Hutson

Illustrations: Hans & Cassady, Inc., Westerville, Ohio

Note to Readers

The material presented in *Magill's Medical Guide: Revised Edition, 1998*, is intended for broad informational and educational purposes. Readers who suspect that they suffer from any of the physical or psychological disorders, diseases, or conditions described in this set should contact a physician without delay; this work should not be used as a substitute for professional medical diagnosis or treatment. This set is not to be considered definitive on the covered topics, and readers should remember that the field of health care is characterized by a diversity of medical opinions and constant expansion in knowledge and understanding.

Library of Congress Cataloging-in-Publication Data

Magill's medical guide / medical consultants, Culley C. Carson III . . . [et al.] : project editor, Tracy Irons-Georges. – Rev. ed. 1998.
    p. cm.
 Includes bibliographical references and index.
 1. Medicine—Encyclopedias. I. Carson, Culley C. II. Irons-Georges, Tracy.
 [DNLM: 1. Medicine encyclopedias.   W 13M194   1998]
 RC41.M34 1998
 610'.3—dc21   98-27251
 DNLM/DLC for Library of Congress   CIP
 ISBN 0-89356-937-2 (set)
 ISBN 0-89356-938-0 (vol 1)

First Printing

PRINTED IN THE UNITED STATES OF AMERICA

PUBLISHER'S NOTE

Magill's Medical Guide, Revised Edition 1998 does much more than simply combine the six volumes of the *Magill's Medical Guide, Health and Illness* (1995) and its *Supplement* (1996) into three handy volumes. In addition to format changes to reconcile the two sets, textual changes were made to bring the medical information up to date, both within the text and in the bibliographic sources that follow longer entries. A panel of five medical experts reviewed every entry in the original *Magill's Medical Guide* sets for accuracy, currency, and completeness, with an eye toward the latest breakthroughs in genetic and pharmacological research, surgical techniques, and public health concerns. They made both general and specific suggestions about which entries needed new material and which titles should be added to the list of contents. The result is an illustrated encyclopedia that constitutes a comprehensive survey of the state of medical science.

No articles from the original sets have been dropped, and 65 entries have been revised to address the latest breakthroughs. In addition, 22 new articles cover recent research and trends in medicine, including *Attention-deficit disorder*, *Cloning*, *Drug resistance*, *Ebola virus*, *Health maintenance organizations (HMOs)*, and *Lactose intolerance*. Shaded 500-word or 750-word boxes within 15 entries highlight such current topics as *New research and treatments* for addiction, AIDS, Alzheimer's disease, and Parkinson's disease; *The isolation of BRCA1 and BRCA2*, the genes responsible for a hereditary form of breast cancer; the use of *DNA testing* in forensic pathology; outbreaks of the condition commonly known as *"Flesh-eating" bacteria*; the use of vitamin and mineral *Supplements* for both general health and specific treatment for disease; and the health risks involved with some *Weight-loss medications*. The ready-reference top matter and cross-references for every article have been revised, and all bibliographies have been updated to list the latest sources and editions. In addition, 47 photographs have been added to the 329 medical drawings. Found throughout the encyclopedia, these illustrations provide invaluable visual context for entries about diseases, research, surgery, and human anatomy.

The 740 entries in this encyclopedia describe major diseases and disorders of the human body, the basics of human anatomy and physiology, specializations in medical practice, and common surgical and nonsurgical procedures. The *Revised Edition* offers entries by 176 writers from the fields of life science and medicine. Every article is now signed by the original author, including any medical or advanced degrees, and each revised article is also signed by the revising author. These writers examine various diseases and disorders, both genetic and acquired, the detailed knowledge of human bodily systems and structures that medical practice requires, and the medical professions and procedures that apply this knowledge.

Readers will find articles that focus both on specific disorders, such as *Heartburn* and *Crohn's disease*, and articles that survey the range of afflictions attacking a particular system, such as *Gastrointestinal disorders* and *Liver disorders*. The majority of articles treat physical disorders—from bacterial and viral infections (such as *Chickenpox*, *Rabies*, and *Strep throat*) to various types of cancer (*Breast cancer*, *Leukemia*, and *Prostate cancer*), genetic defects (*Down syndrome* and *Sickle-cell anemia*), and heart and circulatory disorders (*Angina* and *Arteriosclerosis*). Entries also appear on abdominal and gastrointestinal disorders, defects of bone and muscle, brain and nervous system problems, dental diseases, eating and nutritional disorders, endocrine disorders, conditions and disorders of the male and female reproductive systems, immune disorders, problems of the kidneys and urinary system, liver disorders, respiratory diseases, sexually transmitted diseases, skin disorders, sleep disorders, trauma-related disorders, vector-borne diseases, and visual disorders. Other entries consider psychic-emotional and learning disorders that originate in or have significant impact on the physical health of the body, such as *Schizophrenia* and *Dyslexia*. Some basic conditions that are often the object of medical attention are covered, including *Aging*, *Pregnancy and gestation*, *Childbirth* and its complications, *Puberty and adolescence*, *Menopause*, and *Sexuality*.

Entries on anatomy and biology include overviews of anatomical features and regions (such as *Glands*, *Reproductive system*, and *Skin*) and of biological components and processes (*DNA and RNA*, *Glycolysis*, and *Metabolism*). A broad view of medical practice—its areas of specialization and health care provision—is offered by entries on such topics as *Emergency medicine*, *Nursing*, and *Orthopedics*. Diagnostic and imaging techniques (*Angiography*, *Endoscopy*, and *Laboratory tests*), nonsurgical treatment options (*Antibiotics*), and surgical procedures, both major (*Amputation* and *Heart transplantation*) and minor (*Nasal polyp removal* and *Root canal treatment*), are covered.

In addition, other areas of medical science are represented: alternative medicine (such as *Acupuncture* and *Homeopathy*); ethical issues (*Abortion* and *Euthanasia*); genetics (*Genetic counseling* and *Mutation*); health care providers (*Allied health* and *Paramedics*); microbiology and cellular biology, (*Bacteriology* and *Enzymes*); organizations (the *American Medical Association*); plastic, cosmetic, and reconstructive surgery (*Grafts and Grafting*, *Liposuction*, and *Varicose vein removal*); procedures in the field of psychiatry (*Electroconvulsive therapy*); general surgical procedures (*Anesthesia* and *Laser use in surgery*); testing and examinations (*Blood testing* and *Electrocardiography*); and various types of transplantation (*Bone marrow transplantation* and *Liver transplantation*).

The articles in the *Revised Edition* are arranged in an encyclopedic format—alphabetically from *Abdomen* through *Zoonoses*. The lengths of the entries vary from brief definitions of 100 to 350 words (238 entries) to medium-length entries of 1,000 words (133 entries) to full, essay-length treatments of 2,500 to 3,500 words (369 entries). All entries begin with standard information about the type of article, the anatomy or bodily system affected, the specialties involved, and a brief definition of the topic. For articles of 1,000 words or more, next comes a list of key terms with brief definitions. For articles of 350 words or more, several main subsections of text follow.

In entries on diseases or disorders, the subsection "Causes and Symptoms" defines the condition and describes its cause and its possible manifestations in patients, and the subsection "Treatment and Therapy" explores the various treatments available to alleviate symptoms or effect a cure. In entries on anatomy or biology, "Structure and Functions" defines the physiological or biological system, including its components and role, and "Disorders and Diseases" describes the medical conditions that can result from malfunction of and injury to this physiological system. In entries on procedures, "Indications and Procedures" relates the circumstances under which the procedure is usually performed, identifying the condition it is intended to correct and detailing the basic steps involved, and "Uses and Complications" discusses the various applications and possible risks and complicating factors. In entries on specialties, "Science and Profession" addresses the training and responsibilities of various specialists and "Diagnostic and Treatment Techniques" outlines the means by which they counsel patients, diagnose conditions, perform operations or procedures, and otherwise treat medical problems. Topics that do not fall into these categories depart from these standard subheadings but follow a similar format style.

The last section of all longer entries is "Perspective and Prospects," which places the topic in a larger context within medicine—past, present, and future. For example, an entry on a disease may cover the earliest known investigation into the condition, the evolution of its treatment over time, and promising areas of research for a greater understanding of its causes and cure. An entry on a procedure may address the innovations that led to contemporary technology, improvements or changes that have been made in the procedure, and where this medical technique may be headed. Every entry ends with the author's byline and a listing of cross-references to other entries of interest in the encyclopedia. Articles of 1,000 words or more conclude with the section "For Further Information," which lists general bibliographic works for the reader to consult; bibliographies for entries of 2,500 or 3,500 words provide brief annotations evaluating the features, contents, and value of the sources.

Several special features assist readers in locating articles of interest. The "Alphabetical List of Contents" allows the scope of the encyclopedia to be seen in its entirety. In addition, the lists "Entries by Specialties and Related Fields" and "Entries by Anatomy or System Affected" direct the reader to articles; for example, a reader looking up "Oncology" on the specialty list will find entries on diseases (such as *Cancer*, *Malignancy and Metastasis*, and *Sarcoma*), specialties (such as *Cytology* and *Pathology*), diagnostic procedures (such as *Mammography* and *Screening*), and treatments (such as *Chemotherapy*, *Radiation Therapy*, and *Tumor Removal*). These three lists can be found at the end of each volume of the *Revised Edition*. In addition, Volume III contains an appendix detailing the training and duties of various health care providers, a Glossary of medical terms, and a comprehensive subject Index.

The contributors to this work are academicians from a variety of disciplines in the life sciences, as well as health care professionals and faculty members at medical teaching institutions; their names, degrees, and affiliations are listed in the front matter to Volume I. We thank them for generously sharing their expertise. Special acknowledgment is extended to the panel of Medical Consultants: Culley C. Carson III, M.D., from the University of North Carolina School of Medicine; L. Fleming Fallon, Jr., M.D., M.P.H., from Bowling Green State University; Karen E. Kalumuck, Ph.D., from The Exploratorium, San Francisco; Nancy A. Piotrowski, Ph.D., from the University of California, Berkeley; and Connie Rizzo, M.D., from Pace University. Finally, the editors acknowledge the fine work of the artists at Hans & Cassady, Inc., of Westerville, Ohio, who supplied all the medical illustrations that appear in the encyclopedia.

LIST OF CONTRIBUTORS

Richard Adler, Ph.D.
University of Michigan, Dearborn

E. Victor Adlin, M.D.
Temple University School of Medicine

Patricia Ainsa, M.P.H., Ph.D.
University of Texas, El Paso

Saeed Akhter, M.D.
*Texas Technological University
    Health Science Center*

Bruce Ambuel, Ph.D.
Medical College of Wisconsin

Walter Appleton
Independent Scholar

Pamela J. Baker, Ph.D.
Bates College

Iona C. Baldridge
Lubbock Christian University

Lawrence W. Bassett, M.D.
*Iris Cantor Professor of Radiology
University of California, Los Angeles,
    School of Medicine*

John A. Bavaro, Ed.D., R.N.
Slippery Rock University

Paul F. Bell, Ph.D.
*The Medical Center, Beaver,
    Pennsylvania*

Alvin K. Benson, Ph.D.
Brigham Young University

Matthew Berria, Ph.D.
Weber State University

Silvia M. Berry, M.Sc., R.V.T.
*Englewood Hospital and Medical
    Center, New Jersey*

Robert W. Block, M.D.
University of Oklahoma

Paul R. Boehlke, Ph.D.
*Wisconsin Lutheran College
Dr. Martin Luther College*

Barbara Brennessel, Ph.D.
Wheaton College

Peter N. Bretan, M.D.
*University of California Medical Center,
    San Francisco*

Kenneth H. Brown, Ph.D.
Northwestern Oklahoma State University

Edmund C. Burke, M.D.
*University of California Medical Center,
    San Francisco*

John T. Burns, Ph.D.
Bethany College

Lauren M. Cagen, Ph.D.
University of Tennessee, Memphis

Louis A. Cancellaro, M.D.
*Veterans Affairs Medical Center,
    Mountain Home, Tennessee*

Byron D. Cannon, Ph.D.
University of Utah

Culley C. Carson III, M.D.
*University of North Carolina
    School of Medicine*

Kathleen A. Chara, M.S.
Independent Scholar

Paul J. Chara, Jr., Ph.D.
Loras College

David L. Chesemore, Ph.D.
California State University, Fresno

Leland J. Chinn, Ph.D.
Biola University

Nancy Handshaw Clark, Ph.D.
AUC/Kingston Hospital

Arlene R. Courtney, Ph.D.
Western Oregon State College

Roy L. DeHart, M.D., M.P.H.
University of Oklahoma

Patrick J. DeLuca, Ph.D.
Mount St. Mary College

Katherine Hoffman Doman
Independent Scholar

Mark R. Doman, M.D.
*Veterans Affairs Medical Center,
    Mountain Home, Tennessee*

Miriam Ehrenberg, Ph.D.
*City University of New York,
    John Jay College*

C. Richard Falcon
*Roberts and Raymond Associates,
    Philadelphia*

L. Fleming Fallon, Jr., M.D., M.P.H.
Bowling Green State University

Frank J. Fedel
Henry Ford Hospital, Detroit

Mary C. Fields
Collin County Community College

K. Thomas Finley, Ph.D.
State University of New York, Brockport

Ronald B. France, Ph.D.
LDS Hospital, Salt Lake City, Utah

Katherine B. Frederich, Ph.D.
Eastern Nazarene College

Paul Freudigman, Jr., M.D.
*Pennsylvania State University,
    Hershey Medical Center*

C. George Fry, Ph.D.
Lutheran College of Health Professions

Jason Georges
Independent Scholar

Soraya Ghayourmanesh, Ph.D.
City University of New York

Douglas Gomery, Ph.D.
University of Maryland

Daniel G. Graetzer, Ph.D.
University of Montana

Hans G. Graetzer, Ph.D.
South Dakota State University

Frank Guerra, M.D.
*University of Colorado
    School of Medicine*

Lonnie J. Guralnick, Ph.D.
Western Oregon State College

Stephen J. Hage
Cedars-Sinai Medical Center

L. Kevin Hamberger, Ph.D.
Medical College of Wisconsin

Ronald C. Hamdy, M.D.
James H. Quillen College of Medicine

Linda Hart
Independent Scholar

Peter M. Hartmann, M.D.
York Hospital, Pennsylvania

H. Bradford Hawley, M.D.
Wright State University

Robert M. Hawthorne, Jr., Ph.D.
Independent Scholar

Martha M. Henze, R.D.
Boulder Community Hospital, Colorado

Carl W. Hoagstrom, Ph.D.
Ohio Northern University

David Wason Hollar, Jr., Ph.D.
Rockingham Community College

Carol A. Holloway
Independent Scholar

Ryan C. Horst
Eastern Mennonite University

Howard L. Hosick, Ph.D.
Washington State University

Katherine H. Houp, Ph.D.
Midway College

Shih-Wen Huang, M.D.
University of Florida

Larry Hudgins, M.D.
*Veterans Affairs Medical Center,
   Mountain Home, Tennessee*

Tracy Irons-Georges
Independent Scholar

Vicki J. Isola, Ph.D.
Independent Scholar

Louis B. Jacques, M.D.
*Wayne State University
   School of Medicine*

Thomas C. Jefferson, M.D.
*University of Arkansas for
   Medical Sciences*

Albert C. Jensen
Central Florida Community College

Karen E. Kalumuck, Ph.D.
The Exploratorium, San Francisco

Armand M. Karow, Ph.D.
Xytex Corporation

Cassandra Kircher
Elon College

Vernon N. Kisling, Jr., Ph.D.
University of Florida

Hillar Klandorf, Ph.D.
West Virginia University

Robert Klose, Ph.D.
University of Maine

Craig B. Lagrone, Ph.D.
Birmingham-Southern College

Victor R. Lavis, M.D.
University of Texas, Houston

Charles T. Leonard, Ph.D., P.T.
The University of Montana

Gary J. Lindquester, Ph.D.
Rhodes College

Stan Liu, M.D.
*University of California, Los Angeles,
   School of Medicine*

Maura S. McAuliffe
Independent Scholar

John Arthur McClung, M.D.
New York Medical College

Jeffrey A. McGowan
West Virginia University

Mary Beth McGranaghan
Chestnut Hill College

Wayne R. McKinny, M.D.
University of Hawaii School of Medicine

Laura Gray Malloy, Ph.D.
Bates College

Nancy Farm Manniko, Ph.D.
Michigan Technological University

Charles C. Marsh, Pharm.D.
*University of Arkansas for
   Medical Sciences*

Karen A. Mattern
*Visiting Nurse Association
   Home Health Services*

Grace D. Matzen
Molloy College

Robert D. Meyer, Ph.D.
Chestnut Hill College

Elva B. Miller, O.D.
Independent Scholar

Roman J. Miller, Ph.D.
Eastern Mennonite College

Randall L. Milstein, Ph.D.
Oregon State University

Eli C. Minkoff, Ph.D.
Bates College

Paul Moglia, Ph.D.
*St. Joseph's Hospital and Medical
   Center, Paterson, New Jersey*

Susan Mole
Siena Heights College

Sharon Moore, M.D.
*Veterans Affairs Medical Center,
   Mountain Home, Tennessee*

Rodney C. Mowbray, Ph.D.
University of Wisconsin, LaCrosse

William L. Muhlach, Ph.D.
Southern Illinois University

John Panos Najarian, Ph.D.
William Paterson College

Victor H. Nassar, M.D.
Emory University

Cindy Nesci, D.C.
Independent Scholar

Marsha M. Neumyer
*Pennsylvannia State University
   College of Medicine*

William D. Niemi, Ph.D.
Russell Sage College

Kathleen O'Boyle
Wayne State University

Annette O'Connor, Ph.D.
La Salle University

Sylvia Adams Oliver, Ph.D.
Washington State University

J. Timothy O'Neill, Ph.D.
*Uniformed Services University of the
   Health Sciences*

Janet Rose Osuch, M.D.
Michigan State University

Oliver Oyama, Ph.D.
*Duke/Fayetteville Area Health
   Education Center*

Maria Pacheco, Ph.D.
Buffalo State College

RoseMarie Pasmantier, M.D.
*State University of New York Health
   Science Center at Brooklyn*

Paul M. Paulman, M.D.
University of Nebraska Medical Center

Joseph G. Pelliccia, Ph.D.
Bates College

Carol Moore Pfaffly, Ph.D.
Fort Collins Family Medicine Center

Kenneth A. Pidcock, Ph.D.
Wilkes University

Nancy A. Piotrowski, Ph.D.
University of California, Berkeley

George R. Plitnik, Ph.D.
Frostburg State University

Layne A. Prest, Ph.D.
University of Nebraska Medical Center

Dandamudi V. Rao, Ph.D.
University of Medicine and Dentistry of New Jersey

C. Mervyn Rasmussen, M.D.
Bremerton Naval Hospital, Bremerton, Washington

Douglas Reinhart, M.D.
University of Utah

Wendy E. S. Repovich, Ph.D.
Eastern Washington University

John L. Rittenhouse
Eastern Mennonite College

Connie Rizzo, M.D.
Pace University

Larry M. Roberts
Independent Scholar

Eugene J. Rogers, M.D.
Chicago Medical School

John Alan Ross
Eastern Washington University

Lynne T. Roy
Cedars-Sinai Medical Center

John G. Ryan, Dr.P.H.
University of Texas, Houston

Virginia L. Salmon
Northeast State Technical Community College

Robert Sandlin, Ph.D.
San Diego State University

David K. Saunders, Ph.D.
Emporia State University

Rosemary Scheirer, Ed.D.
Chestnut Hill College

Steven A. Schonefeld, Ph.D.
Tri-State University

Rebecca Lovell Scott, Ph.D.
College of Health Sciences

John Richard Schrock, Ph.D.
Emporia State University

Rose Secrest
Independent Scholar

John J. Seidl, M.D.
Medical College of Wisconsin

John M. Shaw
Education Systems

Martha Sherwood-Pike, Ph.D.
University of Oregon

George C. Shields, Ph.D.
Lake Forest College

R. Baird Shuman, Ph.D.
University of Illinois, Urbana-Champaign

Sanford S. Singer, Ph.D.
University of Dayton

Jane A. Slezak, Ph.D.
Fulton Montgomery Community College

Genevieve Slomski, Ph.D.
Independent Scholar

Roger Smith, Ph.D.
Linfield College

Lisa Levin Sobczak, R.N.C.
Independent Scholar

William D. Stark, D.D.S.
Independent Scholar

James R. Stubbs, M.D.
University of South Alabama

Wendy L. Stuhldreher, Ph.D., R.D.
Slippery Rock University

Pavel Svilenov
Wisconsin Lutheran College

Steven R. Talbot
Independent Scholar

William F. Taylor
Independent Scholar

Gerald T. Terlep, Ph.D.
Bon Secours Hospital System

Leslie V. Tischauser, Ph.D.
Prairie State College

Mary S. Tyler, Ph.D.
University of Maine

John V. Urbas, Ph.D.
Kennesaw State College

Maxine Urton, Ph.D.
Xavier University

James Waddell, Ph.D.
University of Minnesota

Anthony J. Wagner, Ph.D.
Medical University of South Carolina

Edith K. Wallace, Ph.D.
Heartland Community College

Peter J. Walsh, Ph.D.
Fairleigh Dickinson University

Marc H. Walters, M.D.
Portland Community College

Marcia Watson-Whitmyre, Ph.D.
University of Delaware

Barry A. Weissman, O.D., Ph.D.
University of California, Los Angeles, School of Medicine

David J. Wells, Jr., Ph.D.
University of South Alabama Medical Center

Mark Wengrovitz, M.D.
Hershey Medical Center

Russell Williams, M.S.W.
University of Arkansas for Medical Sciences

Bradley R. A. Wilson, Ph.D.
University of Cincinnati

Stephen L. Wolfe, Ph.D.
University of California, Davis

Bonnie L. Wolff
Pacific Coast Cardiac and Vascular Surgeons

CONTENTS

MAGILL'S
MEDICAL
GUIDE

ABDOMEN

ANATOMY

ANATOMY OR SYSTEM AFFECTED: Bladder, gastrointestinal system, intestines, kidneys, liver, reproductive system, stomach, urinary system, uterus

SPECIALTIES AND RELATED FIELDS: Gastroenterology, gynecology, internal medicine, nephrology, urology

DEFINITION: The cavity in the central portion of the trunk that contains the vital organs most closely associated with the digestive process and the elimination of waste material.

KEY TERMS:

calculi: commonly called kidney stones; hardened concentrations of mineral salts that block the passage of urine from the kidneys through the ureters to the bladder

chyle: the product that results from the emulsification of fat by pancreatic juice during the digestive process

chyme: the semiliquid state of foods that have gone through the first stage of digestion in the stomach

Kupffer cells: specialized cells in the liver that perform the function of removing bacterial debris from the blood that has circulated throughout the body

urea: the major waste product produced in the kidneys that, when gathered in sufficient quantity and liquefied, flows into the bladder for elimination as urine

STRUCTURE AND FUNCTIONS

The abdomen is the portion of the body's trunk that begins immediately after the diaphragm, which is the main respiratory muscle in the chest cavity, and extends to the lower pelvic region. The abdominal area is defined by a muscular wall made up of fatty tissue and skin which determines the general shape of the body from chest to lower pelvis. The entire abdominal cavity is lined by a membrane called the peritoneum. This membrane encloses the essential organs of the abdomen: the stomach, small and large intestines, liver, gallbladder, bladder, pancreas, and kidneys. In females, the abdominal casing also contains the uterus, ovaries, and Fallopian tubes. At the front of the abdomen is the navel, essentially a scar which forms following the cutting of the umbilical cord after birth.

Any overview of the abdomen requires a composite view of the functions performed by each of the organs contained in it. With the exception of the female reproductive organs, all the organs contained in the abdominal cavity serve in one way or another in the process of food digestion, the transfer of diverse essential food by-products to the rest of the body, and the disposal of waste products via the urinary tract and the anal passage.

The esophagus is the tube through which all solid and liquid foods enter the stomach, which is the topmost organ in the abdominal cavity. Because it is essentially a bag, the stomach can assume different shapes and adjust in size to accommodate different volumes of food that reach it through the esophagus. In adult humans, the average capacity of the stomach is about one quart. The essential digestive function of the stomach is to convert foods from their original state to a general semiliquid state referred to as chyme.

This first stage of digestion is carried out by the chemical action of some thirty-five thousand gastric glands which make up the inner folds of the inner layer of the stomach, the gastric mucosa. As the gastric glands actively secrete gastric juice, the second layer of the stomach wall, which is muscle tissue, contracts and expands, providing the physical movement that is necessary for the gastric juice and food material to come into full contact.

Gastric juice actually begins to flow from the inner lining of the stomach even before food is present. This may occur when one smells food or even when one imagines the flavor of food. Among the component parts of gastric juice are the enzymes pepsin and rennin, hydrochloric acid, and mucus, which protects the lining of the stomach from the effects of high acidity. Pepsin and rennin begin to break down different types of proteins when an optimum acid environment (a pH between 1 and 3) exists.

Once the initial stage of digestion has occurred, food passes from the stomach into the upper portion of the small intestine, or duodenum, via the pyloric sphincter. This passageway will not allow food to enter the small intestine until it is suitably modified by the action of the stomach.

In the small and large intestines, partially broken-down food is reduced further by the action of gastric juices that are either secreted into the intestines from other abdominal organs (the pancreas and liver, most notably) or secreted by the mucous membranes of the intestines themselves. It is in the small intestine that most of the breaking-down digestive work of gastric juices takes place. Food particles reach a certain level of decomposition so that they may be absorbed into the bloodstream through the mucous membranes of the intestine. The bulk of what is left is allowed to pass, through a gatelike passageway called the cecum, from the small to the large intestine, or colon.

The function of the colon and the component juices that it contains is to separate out the three essential components that remain following the absorptive work of the small intestine: water, undigested foodstuff, and bacteria. Most of the water passes back into the body through the walls of the colon, while undigested food and bacteria are propelled further down the gastrointestinal tract for eventual elimination as feces.

The importance of other organs in the abdomen—the liver, kidneys, pancreas, gallbladder, and bladder—is as complex as that of the intestines and in several cases goes beyond the basic function of digestion. Closest to the stomach and the digestive process itself, perhaps, is the action of the pancreas. The pancreas is the glandular organ located directly beneath the stomach. It is connected to the duodenum, to which it provides pancreatic juice containing three digestive enzymes: trypsin, amylase, and lipase. These agents join the secretions of the small intestine, as well as bile flowing from the liver, to complete the digestive process that breaks down proteins, carbohydrates, and fats. They can then be absorbed through the walls of the intestine for the general nourishment of the body. In addition to its role in the digestive process, the pancreas possesses endocrine cells, called the islets of Langerhans, that secrete two hormones, insulin and glucagon, directly into the bloodstream. These two hormones work together to influence the level of sugar in the blood. When the insulin-secreting cells of the pancreas fail to function effectively, the disease diabetes mellitus may result.

Like the pancreas, the liver, which is the largest glandular organ of the body, shares in the digestive process by producing bile, a fluid essential for the emulsification of fats passing through the small intestine. Bile salts, as they are called, are stored in the gallbladder until they are released into the small intestine. This contribution to the digestive process, however, represents only a minimal part of the liver's functions, many of which have vital effects on body functions far beyond the abdominal cavity. Because blood filled with oxygen flows into the liver from the aorta through the hepatic artery on the one hand, and blood containing digested food enters the liver from the small intestine via the portal vein on the other, the relationship be-

tween "harmonizing" liver functions and the content of the blood is absolutely critical.

The metabolic cells that make up liver tissue, known as hepatic cells, are highly specialized. According to their specialized function, the hepatic cells in the four unequal-sized lobes of the liver may affect several processes: the amount of glycogen (converted and stored glucose) that should be reconverted to glucose and passed (for added energy) into the bloodstream; the conversion of excess carbohydrates and protein into fat; the counteraction of the harmful ammonia by-product of protein breakdown by the production of urea; the production of several essential components of blood, including plasma proteins and blood-clotting agents; the storing of key vitamins and minerals such as vitamins A, D, K, and B_{12}; and the removal of bacteria and other debris that collect in the blood itself—a function of the phagocytic, or Kupffer, cells in particular.

It is the next pair of vital abdominal organs, the kidneys, that separates many of the waste products associated with the liver's metabolic functions, including urea and mineral salts, out of the blood and removes them from the body in the form of urine. This separation is performed by millions of tiny filtering agents called nephrons. Blood penetrates the interior of the kidney by way of an incoming arteriole that branches off from the main renal artery. After the filtering process has been completed, cleansed blood flows

The Organs and Structures of the Abdomen

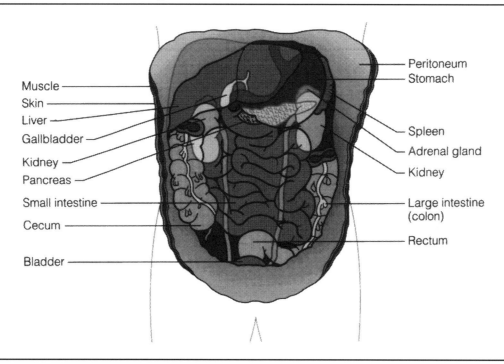

Abdominal organs and structures are those located between the rib cage and the pelvic bone.

back into the main bloodstream via an outgoing arteriole and a system of blood vessels leading to the main renal vein. Waste materials remain, after filtering, in a tubelike extension of each nephron until they can be concentrated, in the form of urine, in a chamber in the middle of the kidney, the kidney pelvis. From this chamber, urine is propelled by muscular compression through the ureter tubes leading to the bladder, the last organ (in males) contained within the lower abdominal cavity. In addition to removing waste products from the blood, the kidneys can adjust the level in the blood of other substances, such as sodium, potassium, and calcium, that are needed by the body but that may exist in excess at certain times. Because the two kidneys perform exactly the same functions, it is possible for the organism to survive as long as one of the two is healthy.

Although obviously essential for temporary storage of urine and final elimination of liquid waste through the process of urination, the bladder is the least complicated organ in the abdominal cavity. Essentially a sac with a liquid capacity of about one pint, the bladder's functions are governed by varied tension in, and loosening of, muscles in the walls of the sac and the external sphincter. When the pressure of collected urine reaches a certain point, nervous impulses cause the external sphincter to relax. Urine flow out of the bladder into the urethra tube can be controlled, up to a certain point, in humans and most mammals by conscious thought.

DISORDERS AND DISEASES

Given the concentration in the abdomen of vital regulatory organs, much medical research has focused on the pathology of this area of the body. Although there are a number of specific diseases that attack specific abdominal organs, the entire region is vulnerable to cancerous tumors. Medical science has tended to associate cancers in certain abdominal organs with dietary habits that are either of recent origin (consumption of highly processed foodstuffs in industrialized Western societies, for example) or geographically or ethnically distinctive—the East Asian, specifically Japanese, vulnerability to certain types of stomach cancer, for example. The latter vulnerability may, however, also be tied to dietary or other environmental considerations that vary in different populated areas of the globe.

Although cancers may strike any of the vital abdominal organs, chances of successful surgical intervention to remove tumors vary greatly according to the location of the cancer. Liver cancer, for example, is essentially untreatable through surgery, while the treatment of cancer of the colon has a significant success rate. This variation is partially attributable to the fact that the vital processes performed by the intestines may not be seriously threatened when a portion of the organ is removed in cancer surgery.

The most important specific diseases associated with the abdomen include peritonitis, hepatitis, and diabetes. Among these diseases, diabetes has received the most attention,

both for its widespread impact on all sectors of the population and for the amount of research that has gone into the task of finding a cure. Diabetes occurs when the pancreas fails to produce enough insulin to metabolize the sugar substance glucose. A breakdown in this function impairs proper cell nourishment and results in excessive sugar in the blood and urine. This state, referred to as hyperglycemia, can affect a number of body functions outside the abdominal cavity, leading, for example, to atherosclerosis and vascular degeneration in general. Because many diabetes patients must inject insulin into their bodies to counteract malfunctioning of the pancreas, an opposite, equally dangerous side effect, hyperinsulinism, may also occur. The most serious degenerative effect that menaces patients suffering from diabetes, however, occurs when the chemical and hormonal imbalance originating in the pancreas brings negative reactions to the kidneys, causing the latter to fail. Medical science has perfected various technical means for addressing this problem, most connected with the mechanical process called dialysis.

Hepatitis is an inflammation that attacks the liver. The two common forms are hepatitis A (formerly called infectious hepatitis) and hepatitis B (formerly called serum hepatitis). Both are transmitted as a result of unsanitary conditions, the first in food and water supplies and the second when unsterile hypodermic needles or infected blood come into contact with the victim's own bloodstream. Unlike most other diseases associated with the abdominal organs, hepatitis is extremely contagious. Hepatitis B can present dangers in using plasma supplied by donors, as there can be an incubation period from six weeks to six months before external signs of the disease occur.

Perhaps the most common abdominal disease, curable through the use of antibiotics if treated in time, is peritonitis. This is an acute inflammation of the peritoneum, the membrane that lines the entire abdominal cavity. It can occur as a result of direct bacterial invasion from outside the body or as a side effect of ruptures occurring in one of the organs contained in the abdomen. Peritonitis typically develops as a result of complications from appendicitis, bleeding ulcers, or a ruptured gallbladder.

PERSPECTIVE AND PROSPECTS

The history of medical analysis of disorders of the abdominal area goes back as far as written history itself, ranging from simple indigestion and painful (and possibly fatal) gallstones to very serious and only recently understood diseases such as diabetes.

Perhaps the most noteworthy advancement in medical knowledge affecting the organs of the abdominal region has been the development of more sophisticated means to counteract the effects of kidney disorders. While there were some striking advances (but not full levels of success) in organ transplant surgery beginning in the 1970's, a technique called dialysis made remarkable strides. First used shortly after World War II as an effective but costly and physically limiting treatment, dialysis involves the use of a machine that receives blood pumped directly from the patient's heart and processes this blood in place of the kidney. This involves filtering out excretory products, adding essential components that "refresh" blood needs (such as heparin, to combat clotting, and proper amounts of saline fluid), and then returning the blood to resume its vital function within the circulatory system.

Although the essential principles of dialysis did not change drastically in the last quarter of the twentieth century, levels of efficiency in a process that had to be repeated over a ten-hour period several times a week definitely did. Development of much smaller, portable dialysis devices made it possible for patients to follow their doctors' instructions in carrying out their own treatment between hospital or office visits, thus lessening the chances of very dangerous crises at the outset of kidney failure.

The most notable hope for patients afflicted with kidney disorders is successful transplant from a healthy or recently deceased donor. By the 1990's, transplants had also become foreseeable for those suffering from diseases that strike other organs in the abdominal cavity, especially the liver. Thus, healthy organ transplant technology can be said to represent one of the most important domains of future research, involving specialists of all the subsections of medicine relating to the abdominal cavity.

—*Byron D. Cannon, Ph.D.*

See also Abdomen; Abdominal disorders; Adrenalectomy; Amniocentesis; Anatomy; Appendectomy; Appendicitis; Bypass surgery; Cesarean section; Cholecystectomy; Colitis; Colon and rectal polyp removal; Colon and rectal surgery; Colon cancer; Colon therapy; Colonoscopy; Constipation; Crohn's disease; Cystectomy; Dialysis; Diarrhea and dysentery; Digestion; Diverticulitis and diverticulosis; Endoscopy; Enemas; Fistula repair; Gallbladder diseases; Gastrectomy; Gastroenterology; Gastroenterology, pediatric; Gastrointestinal disorders; Gastrointestinal system; Gastrostomy; Hernia; Hernia repair; Ileostomy and colostomy; Incontinence; Indigestion; Internal medicine; Intestinal disorders; Intestines; Kidney transplantation; Kidneys; Laparoscopy; Liposuction; Lithotripsy; Liver; Liver transplantation; Nephrectomy; Nephritis; Nephrology; Nephrology, pediatric; Obstruction; Pancreas; Pancreatitis; Peristalsis; Peritonitis; Pregnancy and gestation; Prostate cancer; Reproductive system; Roundworm; Splenectomy; Sterilization; Stomach, intestinal, and pancreatic cancers; Stone removal; Stones; Tubal ligation; Ultrasonography; Urethritis; Urinary disorders; Urinary system; Urology; Urology, pediatric; Worms.

FOR FURTHER INFORMATION:
Becker, Frederick F., ed. *The Liver: Normal and Abnormal Functions.* 2 vols. New York: Marcel Dekker, 1974-1975. Deals with most of the diseases that can affect the liver, ranging from alcohol-induced cirrhosis to various forms of cancer. Also valuable for its discussion of the early stages of experimentation with liver transplants.

Bernard, Claude. *Memoir on the Pancreas and on the Role of Pancreatic Juice in Digestive Processes.* Translated by John Henderon. New York: Academic Press, 1985. A new edition from the English translation of a classic mid-nineteenth century study, published by a physiologist concerned with the main organs of the abdominal cavity. Although the text may be somewhat dated, the detailed illustrations, not only of the pancreas but also of the interrelationship of several abdominal organs, are outstanding.

Deetjen, Peter, John W. Boylan, and Kurt Kramer. *Physiology of Kidney and of Water Balance.* New York: Springer-Verlag, 1975. Unlike H. E. de Wardener's general text on the kidney, this shorter monograph deals only with the normal functioning of the kidney, without examining kidney-related diseases. Concentrates mainly on the chemistry of absorptive processes occurring inside the organ, especially those involving calcium, sulfates, glucose, and amino acids.

De Wardener, H. E. *The Kidney: An Outline of Normal and Abnormal Function.* 5th ed. New York: Churchill Livingstone, 1985. Although this text on the functions and pathology of the kidney predates the impressive advances made in kidney transplant techniques in the 1980's and early 1990's, it is extremely comprehensive and comprehensible for the general, educated reader.

Stott, Robin. "Digestion and Absorption." In *Triumphs of Medicine,* edited by Harry Keen et al. London: Paul Elek, 1976. One of the few scientifically based essays that provides a comprehensive discussion of the technical functions of several of the key organs in the abdominal cavity, their pathology, and historical observations concerning discoveries of interrelations between the functioning of these organs, their secretions and hormones, and so on.

ABDOMINAL DISORDERS
DISEASE/DISORDER

ANATOMY OR SYSTEM AFFECTED: Abdomen, bladder, gastrointestinal system, intestines, kidneys, liver, stomach, urinary system

SPECIALTIES AND RELATED FIELDS: Emergency medicine, family practice, gastroenterology, internal medicine

DEFINITION: Disorders affecting the wide range of organs found in the torso of the body, including diseases of the stomach, intestines, liver, and pancreas.

KEY TERMS:

gastrointestinal: referring to the small and large intestines

pathogen: any microorganism that can cause infectious disease, such as bacteria, viruses, fungi, or other parasites

peritoneum: a membrane enclosing most of the organs in the abdomen

CAUSES AND SYMPTOMS

The main trunk, or torso, of the body includes three major structures: the chest cavity, contained within the ribs and housing the lungs and heart; the abdomen, containing the stomach, kidneys, liver, spleen, pancreas, and intestines; and the pelvic cavity, housing the sexual organs, organs of elimination, and related structures.

The abdomen is, for the most part, contained within a membrane called the peritoneum. The stomach lies immediately below the chest cavity and connects directly with the small intestine, a long tube. It fills the bulk of the abdominal cavity, winding around and down to the pelvic bones in the hips. The small intestine then connects to the large intestine, which extends upward and crosses the abdomen just below the stomach and then turns down to connect with the rectum. Other vital organs within the abdominal cavity include the liver, kidneys, spleen, pancreas, and adrenal glands. All these structures are subject to infection by viruses, bacteria, and other infective agents; to cancer; and to a wide range of conditions specific to individual organs and systems.

Diseases in the abdominal cavity are usually signaled by pain. Identifying the exact cause of abdominal pain is one of the most difficult and important tasks that the physician faces. The familiar stomachache may be simple indigestion, or it may be caused by spoiled, toxic foods, or by infection, inflammation, cancer, obstruction, and tissue erosion, among other causes. It may arise in the stomach, the intestines, or other organs contained within the abdominal cavity. In addition, pain felt in the abdomen may be referred from other sources outside the abdominal cavity. A good example would be a heart attack, which arises in the chest cavity but is often felt by the patient as indigestion. Another example is the abdominal cramping that is often associated with menstruation and premenstrual syndrome (PMS). Because abdominal pain could mean that the patient is in great danger, the physician must decide quickly what is causing the pain and what to do about it.

By far the most common cause of stomach pain is indigestion, but this term is so broad as to be almost meaningless. Indigestion can be brought on by eating too much, eating the wrong foods or tainted foods, alcohol, smoking, poisons, infection, certain medications such as aspirin, and a host of other causes. It may be merely an annoyance, or it may indicate a more serious condition, such as gastritis, gastroenteritis, ulcer, or cancer.

The stomach contains powerful chemicals to help digest foods. These include hydrochloric acid and chemicals called pepsins (digestive enzymes). In order to protect itself from being digested, the stomach mounts a defense system that allows the chemical modification of foods while keeping acid and pepsin away from the stomach walls. In certain people, however, the defense mechanisms break down and bring the corrosive stomach chemicals into direct contact with the stomach walls. The result can be irritation of the stomach lining, called gastritis. Gastritis may progress to a peptic ulcer, identified as a gastric ulcer if the inflammation occurs in the stomach wall or a duodenal ulcer if it occurs in the wall of the duodenum, the first section of the small intestine. In most cases, the ulcer is limited to the surface of the tissue. In severe cases, the ulcer can perforate the entire wall and can be life-threatening.

A common cause of stomach pain is the medication used to treat arthritis and rheumatism. These drugs include aspirin and a group of related drugs called nonsteroidal anti-inflammatory drugs (NSAIDs). As part of their activity in reducing bone and joint inflammation and pain, they interfere with part of the stomach's network of self-protective devices and allow acids to attack stomach and duodenal walls.

Bacterial and viral infections often result in abdominal distress. Foods that sit too long unrefrigerated can be infected by bacteria, or they can become infected by pathogens on the hands of people who prepare and serve them. The bacteria release toxins into the food. Once eaten, these poisons can cause pain and diarrhea. This can be a mere annoyance, a debilitating illness, or a deadly infection, depending upon the organism involved. Salmonella and staphylococcus are two of the many bacteria that can cause food poisoning. *Clostridium botulinum* is occasionally found in canned or preserved foods. It is probably the most serious infective agent in food; victims often do not recover.

Bacterial and viral infections of the gastrointestinal tract are also common causes of abdominal disease. Viral gastroenteritis is the second most common disease in the United States (after upper-respiratory tract infections) and a leading cause of death in infants and the elderly.

Appendicitis (inflammation of the appendix) is frequently seen. The appendix is a tiny organ at the end of the small intestine. It has no purpose in the physiology of modern humans, but occasionally it becomes infected. If the infection is not treated quickly, the appendix can burst and spread infection throughout the abdominal area, a condition that can be life-threatening.

Diarrhea, with or without accompanying abdominal pain, is a major symptom of gastrointestinal disease. It is commonly associated with bacterial or viral infection but may also be attributable to the antibiotics used to treat bacterial infections.

Other gastrointestinal diseases are peritonitis (inflammation of the membrane that covers the abdominal organs), diverticulitis, constipation, Crohn's disease, obstruction, colitis, and the various cancers that can afflict the gastrointestinal system, such as stomach and colon cancers.

The liver is the largest internal organ in the human body and perhaps the most complicated; it is subject to a wide range of disorders. It is the body's main chemical workshop and is responsible for a large number of activities that are vital to body function. The liver absorbs nutrients from the

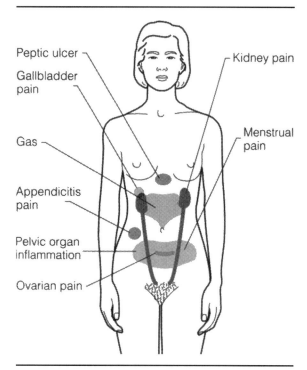

Peptic ulcer

Gallbladder pain

Gas

Appendicitis pain

Pelvic organ inflammation

Ovarian pain

Kidney pain

Menstrual pain

Abdominal disorders are many and varied; some common disorders and their sites are shown here.

intestinal tract and metabolizes them, that is, modifies them so that they can be used by the cells. The liver introduces nutrients into the bloodstream, supplying it with the glucose, protein, and other substances that the body needs. The liver detoxifies the blood and allows poisons, drugs, and other harmful agents to be eliminated. The liver also manufactures and stores many important substances, such as vitamin A and cholesterol.

Chief among liver disorders are the various forms of hepatitis and cirrhosis. Hepatitis can be caused by a viral infection, related to the use of alcohol or drugs, or the result of poisoning. There are many forms of viral hepatitis; the two most significant are hepatitis A and hepatitis B.

Hepatitis A is the most common form; it is caused by a virus that is transmitted through contaminated food or water. Hepatitis B is a blood-borne disease, that is, the virus is carried in the blood and other body fluids of the victim, such as semen and saliva. It can be transmitted only when infected body fluids are transferred from one person to another. The disease is commonly spread by sexual contact, bites, the use of contaminated needles, and during surgical and dental procedures. Nurses and other staff members in health care facilities are constantly exposed to hepatitis B when taking and handling infected blood samples. Pregnant women who are infected can pass the disease on to their children.

Cirrhosis develops when the liver is damaged by some substance such as alcohol. Liver cells are destroyed, and as the liver attempts to regenerate, scar tissue is formed. The steady flow of blood through the organ is impeded, as are vital functions such as the removal of waste materials from the blood.

The liver is also subject to a number of cancers. Cancer cells can spread to liver tissue from other parts of the body, or they can originate there as a result of hepatitis B or other chronic liver diseases such as cirrhosis.

The gallbladder is a small sac connected to the liver. The liver manufactures bile, a substance that aids in the digestion of fats. Bile is stored in the gallbladder and passes through the bile duct into the small intestine. A common disorder of the gallbladder is the formation of gallstones, crystalline growths that can be as fine as sand or as large as a golf ball. If the stones clog the passage to the bile duct, severe pain may result.

The pancreas, a vital gland situated near the liver, is subject to a number of disorders. The most prominent is diabetes mellitus, a condition in which the pancreas ceases to produce insulin or produces defective insulin. Pancreatitis is a disorder characterized by inflammation of the pancreas.

The other major organ system in the abdomen comprises the kidneys and the urinary tract. The system includes the two kidneys, which sit in the middle of the back on either side of the spine; the two ureters, which transport urine from the kidneys; the bladder, a pouchlike organ that collects the urine; and the urethra, which expels urine from the body. The kidneys and related organs are subject to several disorders, some inborn and some caused by infection, illnesses in other organs and systems, or cancer.

TREATMENT AND THERAPY

Many abdominal disorders are related to the overproduction of stomach acids, which damage the intestinal walls; the treatment of such conditions is often associated with changes in lifestyle. In treating gastrointestinal reflux disease, in which stomach acid backs up into the throat, physicians may suggest that the patient change habits that may be contributing to the condition, such as stopping smoking, reducing the intake of alcohol, losing weight, and avoiding certain foods and medications. Preparations to neutralize stomach acids are used, as well as drugs that reduce the amount of stomach acid produced. Surgery is rarely indicated.

Hiatal hernia, the protrusion of part of the stomach through the diaphragm, usually produces no symptoms. There may be reflux of stomach acids into the esophagus, which can be treated by the same methods used in treating gastrointestinal reflux disease. Surgery is sometimes indicated.

Gastritis is commonly treated with agents that neutralize stomach acid or others that reduce the production of stomach acid. When gastritis appears to be caused by drugs taken for arthritis or rheumatism (for example, aspirin or NSAIDs), the physician may change the drug or the dosage to reduce stomach irritation.

In treating gastric and duodenal ulcers, the physician seeks to heal the ulcer and prevent its recurrence. Acid-neutralizing agents are sometimes helpful, but more often agents that reduce the flow of stomach acids are used. It has been suggested that gastritis and ulcers are associated with certain bacteria. Consequently, some physicians add an antibiotic to the antacid regimen in order to destroy the pathogens. Surgery is sometimes required to heal ulcers.

Bacterial infections in the gastrointestinal tract are, as a rule, self-limiting. They run their course, and the patient recovers. Sometimes, however, appropriate antibiotics are needed. For viral infections, few medications are useful in eradicating the pathogens.

Appendicitis is usually treated surgically. Peritonitis, whether resulting from appendicitis or other gastrointestinal infection, is also treated surgically in order to remove infected tissue. In addition, antibiotic therapy is often used.

For two of the major liver diseases, hepatitis A and hepatitis B, there is no treatment once the person has become infected. For the most part, the diseases resolve without incident. Bed rest, dietary measures, and general support procedures are the only steps that can be taken. In a small percentage of patients, however, hepatitis B can progress to chronic active hepatitis, which may lead to liver failure, cirrhosis, liver cancer, and death. The main defense against hepatitis B is immunization. A vaccine is available and is recommended for all children and all adults who are at high risk. There is no treatment for cirrhosis, although physicians may be able to treat some of its complications.

PERSPECTIVE AND PROSPECTS

Medical science has made great progress in the treatment of disorders arising in the abdominal cavity, but there is much to be done. Most important is the identification of agents to treat or immunize against various viral diseases, particularly those that occur in the gastrointestinal tract and the liver.

A vaccine against hepatitis A is being sought. The vaccine against hepatitis B has been in use for years, but the incidence of the disease has remained relatively constant. In the United States, the practice now is to vaccinate all young children. If this immunization approach is successful, the rate of hepatitis B infection among American children should drop.

New treatment modalities are being developed for many of the diseases that occur in the abdominal cavity. One of the most significant successes has been in the treatment of peptic ulcers. The new drugs being used not only neutralize acid in the stomach but also cut off the secretion of acid into the stomach. One of these agents was the most-prescribed drug in the world for many years, indicating the importance of this therapeutic approach.

Innovations are also occurring in the treatment of diabetes mellitus, the disease caused by malfunction in the pancreas. Medications have been found that promise to treat and prevent some of the potentially fatal diseases that diabetes can cause.

Because the abdominal area contains so many vital organ systems, it is the seat of perhaps the widest range of diseases that afflict the human body—and hence, the target for the greatest amount of research and, potentially, the greatest advances in medicine. —*C. Richard Falcon*

See also Abdomen; Appendectomy; Appendicitis; Cholecystectomy; Colitis; Colon and rectal polyp removal; Colon and rectal surgery; Colon cancer; Colon therapy; Colonoscopy; Constipation; Crohn's disease; Cystectomy; Diabetes mellitus; Dialysis; Diarrhea and dysentery; Digestion; Diverticulitis and diverticulosis; Endoscopy; Gallbladder diseases; Gastroenterology; Gastroenterology, pediatric; Gastrointestinal disorders; Gastrointestinal system; Gastrostomy; Hernia; Hernia repair; Incontinence; Indigestion; Internal medicine; Intestinal disorders; Kidney transplantation; Kidneys; Laparoscopy; Lithotripsy; Liver; Liver transplantation; Nephrectomy; Nephritis; Nephrology; Nephrology, pediatric; Obstruction; Peristalsis; Peritonitis; Prostate cancer; Shunts; Splenectomy; Stomach, intestinal, and pancreatic cancers; Stone removal; Stones; Ultrasonography; Urethritis; Urinary disorders; Urinary system; Urology; Urology, pediatric.

FOR FURTHER INFORMATION:

Guillory, Gerard. *IBS: A Doctor's Plan for Chronic Digestive Disorders.* Point Roberts, Wash.: Hartley & Marks, 1991. Guillory includes both preventive and treatment recommendations for people suffering from chronic gastrointestinal problems, often referred to as irritable bowel syndrome (IBS).

Janowitz, Henry D. *Indigestion.* New York: Oxford University Press, 1992. This book covers upper-intestinal problems, such as heartburn, stomach disorders, ulcers, and gallstones. Designed for the lay reader.

Larson, David E., ed. *Mayo Clinic Family Health Book.* 2d ed. New York: William Morrow, 1996. Diseases of the abdominal cavity are discussed in chapters devoted to the individual organs or organ systems involved: "The Digestive System" (which includes liver disorders) and "The Kidneys and the Urinary Tract."

ABORTION

PROCEDURE

ANATOMY OR SYSTEM AFFECTED: Reproductive system, uterus

SPECIALTIES AND RELATED FIELDS: Ethics, gynecology

DEFINITION: The induced termination of pregnancy, which is usually legal only before the fetus is viable.

KEY TERMS:

dilation: making something wider or larger

embryo: the unborn young from conception to about eight
   weeks
fetus: the unborn young from about eight weeks to birth
quickening: the point at which a fetus first begins to move
   in the uterus
uterus: a hollow, muscular organ located in the pelvic cavity
   of females in which a fertilized egg develops
viability: the point at which a fetus is able to survive outside
   the uterus

THE CONTROVERSY SURROUNDING ABORTION

Abortion is the deliberate ending of a pregnancy before
the fetus is viable, or capable of surviving outside the
woman's body. It has been practiced in every culture since
the beginning of civilization. It has also been controversial.
The first law designating it as a crime dates to ancient
Assyria, where in the fourteenth century B.C. women who
were convicted of abortion were impaled on a stake and
left to die. Early Hebrew law also condemned abortion,
except when necessary to save the woman's life. The
Greeks allowed abortion, but the famous physician Hippocrates (460-370 B.C.) denounced the procedure and said
that it violated a doctor's responsibility to heal. Roman law
said that a fetus was part of a woman and that abortion
was her decision, although a husband could divorce his wife
if she had an abortion without his consent. Most abortions
in ancient times seemed to be related to unwanted pregnancies resulting from adultery or prostitution.

The Christian church called abortion a sin in the first
century. In the fifth century, however, Saint Augustine argued that the fetus did not have a soul before "quickening,"
that point in a pregnancy, usually between the fourth and
sixth months, when the woman first senses movement in
her womb. Until 1869, abortion until quickening was legal
in most areas of Europe. In that year, however, Pope Pius
IX declared abortion at any point outright murder. This position has been upheld by all subsequent popes.

In Protestant countries, the principal of legality until
quickening held true until around 1860. In that year, the
British parliament declared abortion a felony; that law remained on the books for more than a hundred years. In
1968, the Abortion Act passed by Parliament radically reduced the restrictions, allowing abortions in cases when
doctors determined that the pregnancy threatened the physical or mental health of the woman.

In the United States, abortion before quickening was legal until the 1840's. By 1841, ten states declared abortion
to be a criminal act, but punishments were weak and the
law frequently ignored. The movement against abortion was
led by the American Medical Association (AMA), founded
in 1847. Doctors were becoming increasingly aware that
the "first sign of life" took place well before the fetus actually moved. By this time, scientists had established that
fetal development actually began with the union of sperm
and egg. In 1859, the AMA passed a resolution condemning

abortion as a criminal act. Within a few years, every state
declared abortion a felony. Not until 1950 did the AMA
reverse its position, when it began a new campaign to lib-
eralize abortion laws. Many doctors were concerned about
the thousands of women suffering from complications and
even death from illegal abortions. In 1973, the Supreme
Court of the United States ruled in *Roe v. Wade* that abortions were generally legal. That ruling made abortions in
the United States available on the request of the pregnant
woman.

More than fifty countries, with about 25 percent of the
world's population, continue to make abortions illegal.
Most of the other 130 nations authorize abortions under
various conditions. The World Health Organization (WHO)
estimates that more than 50 million abortions occur per
year throughout the world and that about half of these are
illegal.

Before 1970, statistics on abortions in the United States
were generally not kept or reported, and they can only be
estimated. In the nineteenth century, it is believed that there
was one abortion for every four live births, a rate only a
bit lower than that in the latter part of the twentieth century.
The number of abortions in any year varied from 500,000
to 1 million, most of them illegal. In 1969, the Centers for
Disease Control (CDC), a branch of the U.S. Department
of Health and Human Services, began an annual abortion
count. Legal abortions in 1970 numbered about 200,000.
The number of illegal abortions is unknown. Ten years later,
legal abortions reached 1,200,000 and by 1990 had increased to 1,600,000; they have remained at that level fairly
consistently since then. The CDC estimated that there were
about 325 abortions for every 1,000 live births in the
1980's, a number consistent with findings for the 1990's.
The number of abortions in any year rarely fluctuated by
more of less than 3 percent from these figures.

Ireland, which has the most stringent abortion laws, performs 139 abortions per 1,000 live births. Czechoslovakia
and Hungary, on the other hand, perform more abortions
than births, with Czechs having 1,400 abortions for every
1,000 live births and Hungarians having 1,137. In China
and Japan, both of which use abortion as a method of official population control, the rate is not quite that high, but
it is estimated that in each country at least one out of two
pregnancies is ended with abortion. China alone performs
about 10,500,000 abortions per year.

In *Roe v. Wade*, the Supreme Court ruled that abortions
were legal under certain conditions. Those conditions included the welfare of the woman and the viability of the
fetus. During the first three months of pregnancy, according
to the Court, the government had no legitimate interest in
regulating abortions. The only exception was that states
could require that abortions had to be performed by a licensed physician in a "medical setting." Otherwise, the decision to abort was strictly that of the pregnant woman as

a constitutional right of privacy. During the second trimester, abortions were more restricted. They would be legal only if the woman's health needed to be protected and would require the consent of a doctor. The interest of the fetus would be protected during the third trimester, when it became able to survive on its own outside of the woman's body, with or without artificial life support. States, at this point, could grant abortions only to women for whom, according to medical opinion, the continued pregnancy would be life-threatening. The determination of viability would be made by doctors, not by legal authorities. This ruling effectively struck down all antiabortion laws across the United States.

In the aftermath of *Roe v. Wade*, abortion became an intensely emotional political issue in the United States. The Hyde Amendment of 1976 eliminated federal funding for abortions, and other legislation blocked foreign aid to programs such as family planning that members of Congress who were opposed to abortion saw as "pro-abortion." In *Webster v. Reproductive Health Services* (1989), the Supreme Court upheld its ruling in *Roe v. Wade*, but it also sustained a rule forbidding the use of public facilities or public employees for carrying out abortions. The Court also supported a requirement that a test for viability be done before any late abortion and said states could ban funding for abortion counseling. The issue continued to divide Americans, with opponents arguing that abortion at any point in the process of birth was murder.

A 1987 survey done by the Alan Guttmacher Institute of 1,900 women who had abortions revealed the most common reasons for making that decision. Ninety-three percent of the respondents gave more than one reason, but these reasons could usually be reduced to four basic notions. The most common was that having a baby would interfere with work or going to school. Next came not being able to afford a child. Third was a concern about relationship problems with the father. The last was that the potential mother did not want to be a single parent.

A study done by the CDC of what types of women wanted to have an abortion revealed that almost 60 percent were experiencing their first pregnancy. Women beneath the poverty level, regardless of race, religion, or ethnic background, were more likely to have an abortion than middle-class women. African American and Hispanic women had higher rates of abortion than did white women. The largest number of abortions were performed on white, single women, eighteen to twenty-five years of age. This same group, however, also had the highest number of live births.

Religion appeared to make little difference: The percent of Catholic women having abortions was actually a bit higher than the percent of Protestant women. The lowest percentage of abortions was found among Evangelical, "born-again" Christians. Teenagers under fifteen and women over forty had the highest rates of abortion of any age groups. The study showed that the reasons for late abortions, defined as those sixteen weeks or later after conception, differed somewhat from those given by women who had their abortions during the first trimester. Two key factors were involved in late abortions. Seventy-one percent of the women interviewed said that they had waited so long because they had not realized they were pregnant or did not know soon enough how long they had been pregnant. Fifty percent said that they had taken so long because they had problems raising enough money to pay for an abortion. Thus, poverty appears to be a leading cause of late abortions. Many in this latter group also reported that they had to leave their home states to obtain legal abortions because there were no facilities in these states. Almost 90 percent of counties in the United States do not have facilities or doctors who will perform abortions. Death rates for women who have abortions after sixteen weeks are thirty times higher than the rate at eight weeks.

TECHNIQUES AND PROCEDURES

A variety of techniques can be used to perform abortions. They vary according to the length of the pregnancy, which is usually measured by the number of weeks since the last menstrual period (LMP). Instrumental techniques are usually used very early in a pregnancy. They include a procedure called menstrual extraction, in which the entire contents of the uterine are removed. It can be done as early as fourteen days after the expected onset of a period. A major problem with this method is a high risk of error; the human

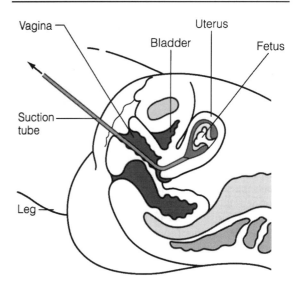

Elective or induced abortions can be performed in the first trimester using a simple suction technique; after the third month, much riskier and more complex methods are required.

embryo may still be so small at this age that it can be missed. It is also true that a high proportion of women undergoing this procedure turn out not to have been pregnant. Nevertheless, this method is easy to do and very safe. Death rates from this technique average less than 1 out of 100,000.

About 96 percent of all abortions in the United States are done by a procedure known as vacuum aspiration, or suction curettage. This technique can be used up to about fourteen weeks LMP. It can be performed with local anesthesia and follows these steps. First, the cervix is expanded with metal rods that are inserted into it one at a time, with each rod being slightly larger than the previous one. When the cervix is expanded to the right size, a transparent, hollow tube called the vacuum cannula is placed into the uterine cavity. This instrument is attached to a suction device, which looks something like a drinking straw. An electric or hand-operated vacuum pump then empties the uterus of its contents. Finally, a spoon-shaped device called a curette is used to check for any leftover tissue in the uterus. The entire procedure takes less than five minutes. This method, first used in China in 1958, is among the safest of procedures in medicine. There are about six times more maternal deaths during regular birth than during vacuum aspiration.

An older method, dilation and curettage (D & C), was common up to the 1970's, but it has largely been replaced by vacuum aspiration. In a D & C, the cervix was expanded or dilated and a curette was used to scrape out the contents of the uterus. The biggest difference was the use of general anesthesia during the process. Since most abortion-related deaths result from complications from anesthesia, a method that requires only local anesthesia, such as aspiration, greatly reduces the dangers of the procedure.

For the period from thirteen to twenty weeks, a method called dilation and evacuation (D & E) is usually preferred. The cervix is expanded with tubes of laminaria (a type of seaweed), and the fetus is removed with the placenta, the part of the uterus by which the fetus is nourished. Forceps, suction, or a sharp curette is sometimes used. The procedure is usually safe, but sometimes if the fetus is large, it must be crushed and dismembered in order to remove it through the cervix. This process can be upsetting for the doctor and the patient and is more dangerous than procedures done earlier in the pregnancy. Generally, the later abortions are performed, the more dangerous they are for the woman.

Along with the above methods of menstrual extraction, physicians can also use "medical induction" techniques when required. Amnioinfusion is an old example of this method that was used on fetuses from sixteen to twenty weeks old. This process has largely been replaced by D & E, which has proven far less dangerous.

Amnioinfusion usually required hospitalization, local an-

esthesia, and the insertion of a large needle into the uterus. Between 100 and 200 milliliters of fluid were withdrawn and a similar amount of hypertonic saline solution were infused into the uterine cavity. Within ninety minutes, the fetal heart would stop. The woman would go into labor and deliver a dead fetus within twenty-four to seventy-two hours. These kinds of abortions generally had much higher risks of complications than did D & E. On rare occasions, a fetus was born alive, but the main risk was infection, hemorrhage, and cervical injuries to the woman. The psychological difficulties associated with such long labor are very upsetting, especially with the knowledge that the fetus delivered will be dead.

Another method used prostaglandins, naturally occurring hormones that cause uterine contractions and expulsion of the fetus, rather than a saline solution. The hormones could be given to the patient in several different ways: intravenously, intramuscularly, through vaginal suppositories, or directly into the amniotic sac. Prostaglandins are used for inducing second trimester abortions and are as safe as saline solutions. Their major advantage is to reduce the time for the abortion, but they also have severe side effects. They cause intense stomach cramps and other gastrointestinal discomfort, and about 7 percent of the fetuses expelled show some sign of life.

Surgical techniques for abortion are very rare, although sometimes they prove necessary in special cases. Hysterotomy resembles a Cesarean section. An incision is made in the abdomen, and the fetus is removed. Hysterotomy is usually used in the second trimester, but only in cases where other methods have failed. The risk of death is much higher in this procedure than in most others. Even more rare is a hysterectomy, the removal of the uterus. This is done only in cases in which a malignant tumor threatens the life of the pregnant woman.

In the late 1980's, the French "abortion pill," RU-486, was approved for use in many parts of Europe. By the mid-1990's, it had been used in more than 50,000 abortions. Progesterone is a hormone that tells the uterus to develop a lining that can be used to house a fertilized egg. If the egg is not fertilized, the production of progesterone stops and the uterine lining is discarded during menstruation. RU-486 contains an antiprogesterone, which means that it prevents the production of progesterone. The pill has proven to be effective about 90 percent of the time if used in early pregnancy.

A few serious side effects sometimes occur with RU-486, the major one being sustained bleeding. About one out of a thousand users bleeds so much that a transfusion is required. Cramps and nausea are also reported in a number of cases. There is apparently no effect on subsequent pregnancies. The drug must be taken under medical supervision and requires, under French law, at least three visits to a doctor's office. The first visit is for testing and counseling.

On the second visit, the patient is given the drug. On the third, she receives an injection of prostaglandin. As of 1997, RU-486 was not legally available in the United States.

PERSPECTIVE AND PROSPECTS

Abortion is the most frequently performed surgical procedure in the United States. As long as women have unwanted pregnancies, that will continue to be true. Abortion is a very safe procedure, although there can be some complications. Generally, however, the earlier the procedure is performed, the less is the risk. The lowest chance of medical complications occurs during the first eight weeks of pregnancy. After eight weeks, the risk of complications increases by 30 percent for each week of delay. Nevertheless, the death rate per case is very low, about half that for tonsillectomy. These statistics apply only to those areas of the world where abortion is legal, since women in those places tend to have earlier abortions.

In parts of the world where it remains against the law, abortion remains a leading cause of death for women. WHO estimates that as many as 500,000 women a year die during abortions. About 200,000 of these deaths result from complications following abortions performed by unqualified medical personnel. About half of the total deaths take place in Southeast Asia and Africa. In the United States, deaths declined when abortions became legal in 1973. Before the *Roe v. Wade* decision, it was estimated that anywhere from a few hundred to several thousand American women died every year from the procedure. The best estimate was that in the 1960's, about 290 women died every year as a result of complications from abortions. In the 1980's, the average was twelve per year, mostly from anesthesia complications. More than 90 percent of abortions in the United States take place during the first twelve weeks of pregnancy.

—*Leslie V. Tischauser, Ph.D.*

See also Amniocentesis; Cervical, ovarian, and uterine cancers; Childbirth; Childbirth, complications of; Contraception; Embryology; Ethics; Fetal tissue transplantation; Genetic counseling; Genetics and inheritance; Gynecology; Hippocratic oath; Hysterectomy; Law and medicine; Pregnancy and gestation; Reproductive system; Sterilization.

FOR FURTHER INFORMATION:

Denney, Myron K. *A Matter of Choice: An Essential Guide to Every Aspect of Abortion.* New York: Simon & Schuster, 1983. A good overview of the subject that presents both pro-choice and antiabortion views. Discusses the medical and psychological problems involved and also presents alternatives to abortion.

Emmens, Carol A. *The Abortion Controversy.* New York: Julian Messner, 1987. Another useful and basic overview of the issues involved. Provides a history of abortion since earliest times. Provides help in understanding the statistics of abortion and compares the reactions of different ethnic and racial groups to the question of right to life.

Greer, Germaine. *Sex and Destiny: The Politics of Human Fertility.* New York: Harper & Row, 1984. Greer describes the attitudes of people in various cultures around the world on questions about children, birth control, abortion, infanticide, and the family.

McDonnell, Kathleen. *Not an Easy Choice: A Feminist Reexamines Abortion.* Toronto: Women's Press, 1984. This book discusses moral and philosophical questions. It examines men's roles as fathers and doctors. Describes new technologies such as genetic engineering and prenatal sex determination that may have an impact on the question of abortion.

Sachdev, Paul, ed. *International Handbook on Abortion.* Westport, Conn.: Greenwood Press, 1988. A extensive collection of data from thirty-three nations covering the legal status of abortion, abortion rates, and the availability of services.

Sciarra, John J., et al. *Gynecology and Obstetrics.* Vol. 6. Philadelphia: Harper & Row, 1991. A textbook that discusses methods, demographics, health concerns, and the psychological and medical consequences of abortions.

Sloan, Irving J. *The Law Governing Abortion, Contraception, and Sterilization.* Legal Almanac Series. London: Oceana, 1996. Covers historical and modern legislation relating to abortions, contraception, and the rights of minors to these services. Appendixes include selected state and federal laws.

ABSCESS DRAINAGE

PROCEDURE

ANATOMY OR SYSTEM AFFECTED: Brain, breasts, gallbladder, glands, gums, kidneys, liver, lungs, nervous system, pancreas, respiratory system, skin, spleen, stomach, urinary system

SPECIALTIES AND RELATED FIELDS: Dermatology, emergency medicine, family practice, general surgery

DEFINITION: The removal of a collection of pus in tissue through an opening in the skin.

INDICATIONS AND PROCEDURES

When bacteria infect a tissue, the body's defense systems attempt to isolate them and destroy the infective agent. An abscess develops when the bacteria become walled off from surrounding noninfected tissues and white blood cells enter the area to rid the body of the pathogen. The ensuing battle between the white blood cells and bacteria causes the death of these cells as well as of surrounding tissue. These dead cells form pus.

Staphylococci bacteria are the most common pathogens that cause abscesses to form, resulting in pain, swelling, and fever. If the abscess is near the skin, it is easily detected. The presence of abscesses in deeper tissues, however, may need to be confirmed using computed tomography (CT) scanning or magnetic resonance imaging (MRI).

The physician will usually prescribe antibiotics to help

destroy the bacteria. Unfortunately, the antibiotics may not have access to the site of infection since the abscess is usually encapsulated by tissue. If this is the case, the physician must drain the abscess cavity. He or she will make an incision into the cavity to allow the pus to drain. Occasionally, a tube will be inserted to maintain the opening for continued drainage of the cavity. The tube can be removed once the infection is gone.

The patient will be asked to watch for signs of recurrent infection after the abscess is removed, because some bacteria may remain. The abscess can reappear if these bacteria are not destroyed by the body's immune system or by antibiotics.

Uses and Complications

Abscesses can develop in any organ. Common sites, however, are under the skin, in the breasts, and around the teeth and gums. In rare cases, abscesses are found in the liver or brain. Fungi and protozoans are important pathogens in liver abscesses.

Most abscesses dissipate after they are drained and/or the patient is treated with antibiotics. Occasionally, antibiotic treatment alone will cause the abscess to subside. The rapid detection and treatment of abscesses in the liver and brain is a must because the damage to these vital organs is irreparable.

—Matthew Berria, Ph.D., and Douglas Reinhart, M.D.

See also Abscesses; Antibiotics; Bacterial infections; Biopsy; Breast biopsy; Breast disorders; Breasts, female; Culdocentesis; Cyst removal; Cysts and ganglions; Cytology; Cytopathology; Dermatology; Ganglion removal; Hydrocelectomy; Infection; Otorhinolaryngology; Periodontal surgery; Periodontitis; Root canal treatment; Skin; Skin disorders; Staphylococcal infections; Testicular surgery.

Abscesses

Disease/disorder

Anatomy or system affected: Brain, breasts, gallbladder, glands, gums, kidneys, liver, lungs, nervous system, pancreas, respiratory system, skin, spleen, stomach, urinary system

Specialties and related fields: Dermatology, family practice, microbiology

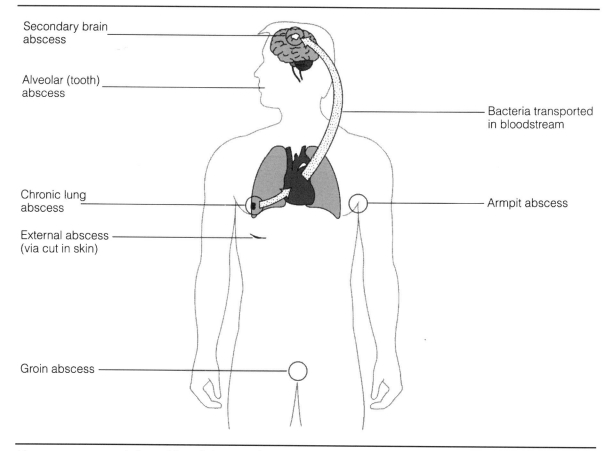

Abscesses are commonly located in soft tissues and near lymph nodes but may appear in internal organs and may cause other abscesses via bacterial migration.

DEFINITION: An abscess is a localized collection of pus resulting from infection, usually by bacteria such as staphylococci. The pus that fills an abscess contains leukocytes (white blood cells), microorganisms, and cells that have been destroyed by the infection. Abscesses generally form at sites where the immune system fights invading organisms, such as around lymph nodes, but they may develop anywhere in soft tissues or in any organ of the body. Common sites include the breasts, skin, lungs, and gums, but more serious sites can be the brain and liver. Abscesses in the skin may cause only localized swelling, tenderness, redness, and pain, while larger abscesses can cause fever, sweating, and general malaise. An abscess that does not subside on its own may be drained by a physician.

—*Jason Georges and Tracy Irons-Georges*

See also Abscess drainage; Acne; Brain disorders; Breast disorders; Cyst removal; Cysts and ganglions; Infection; Liver disorders; Lymphatic system; Skin; Skin disorders; Staphylococcal infections; Tumor removal; Tumors.

ACID-BASE CHEMISTRY
BIOLOGY
ANATOMY OR SYSTEM AFFECTED: Cells
SPECIALTIES AND RELATED FIELDS: Biochemistry, cytology, hematology, pharmacology
DEFINITION: The interaction between acids and bases in the cells of the body, the proper functioning of which is crucial in digestive metabolism, respiration, and the buffering capacity of body fluids.
KEY TERMS:
acidosis: condition of high blood carbon dioxide levels and low pH that results from such diseases as emphysema and pneumonia
alkalosis: a condition of abnormally low carbon dioxide levels that results from hyperventilation (rapid breathing)
Brønsted-Lowry definition (of an acid and a base): an acid is a substance that can donate protons, while a base is a proton acceptor
buffer: a solution which contains components that enable a solution to resist large changes in pH when small quantities of acids and bases are added
cellular respiration: the chemical utilization of oxygen and the production of carbon dioxide in the cell itself
extracellular respiration: the process of oxygen transport from the lungs to the cells and carbon dioxide transport from cells back to the lungs
general acid (or base) catalysis: the process in which a partial transfer of a proton from a Brønsted acid (or partial proton abstraction by a Brønsted base) lowers the free energy of a reaction's transition state
pH: a measure of acidity in a solution, which is equal to the negative logarithm of the hydrogen ion concentration; a neutral solution has a pH of 7, an acidic solution has a pH less than 7, and a basic solution has a pH greater than 7

STRUCTURE AND FUNCTIONS
The existence of acids and bases is critical to the functioning of the human body. An acid is a compound that contains hydrogen, can accept unshared electron pairs, has a pH that is less than 7, and is water-soluble. A base is a compound that contains a hydroxyl (OH) group, can give up unshared pairs of electrons, can accept protons, has a pH that is greater than 7, and is water-soluble. An acid and a base can react together to form a salt.

Both acids and bases can be classified further as either "hard" or "soft." Bases are classified as soft if they have high polarizability and low electronegativity, are easily oxidized, or have low-energy, empty orbitals. Opposite properties tend to classify them as hard bases. Hard acids are those that have low polarizability, small size, and a high oxidation state (valence) and that do not have easily removed outer electrons. Soft acids possess reversed properties. Generally, a hard acid always reacts with a hard base and a soft acid always reacts with a soft base. The reaction of a hard acid (or base) with a soft base (or acid) is always unfavorable. The hard-and-soft concept of acids and bases is only used as a way to classify and predict reactions. In the acid-base reactions of a living being, however, one must consider acids as proton donors and bases as proton acceptors.

A neutral solution is defined as one whose proton (hydrogen ion) and hydroxyl concentrations are equal. A solution that has more protons than hydroxyl groups is acidic, while a solution whose hydroxyl ions are more than its protons is basic. Expressing the hydrogen ion concentration in moles per liter is rather complex. Instead, the pH of a solution is used. The pH is the negative logarithm of the hydrogen ion concentration. Neutral solutions have a pH of 7, acidic solutions have a pH that is less than 7, and basic solutions have a pH that is higher than 7. Thus, a pH of zero is strongly acidic and a pH of 14 is strongly basic.

Buffers are solutions whose contents allow very small changes in pH upon the addition of small quantities of acids and bases. Usually, buffers are solutions of a weak acid and one of its salts, or solutions of a weak base and one of its salts. A buffer becomes ineffective when there are no more anions (if a weak acid is part of the buffer) or cations (if a weak base is involved). At this point, the buffer capacity of the solution is said to be exceeded.

General acid catalysis is a process in which partial proton transfer from an acid lowers the free energy of a reaction's transition state. A reaction can also be accomplished by a general base catalysis, in which a base enhances the rate by partially stealing a proton. Such reactions often have such a high activation energy that they cannot take place unless the specific catalysis is involved.

Many well-known substances encountered in everyday life are weak acids or bases. Aspirin (acetylsalicylic acid, a headache remedy), phenobarbital (a sedative), niacin (nicotinic acid, vitamin B), and saccharin (an artificial sweetener) are weak acids. The majority of drugs and narcotics (such as heroin, cocaine, and morphine) in their free-base state are weak bases. Among the components of deoxyribonucleic acid (DNA), which is a polymer of deoxyribonucleotide units, are nitrogenous bases, the purines and pyrimidines. Amino acids are either neutral, acidic, or basic, depending on the chemical group found in their side chain.

The normal metabolic processes of the body result in the continuous production of acids, such as carbonic acid (H_2CO_3), phosphoric acid (H_3PO_4), lactic acid, and pyruvic acid. In cellular oxidations, the main acid end product is carbonic acid, with 10 to 20 moles formed per day. In terms of acidity, this amount is equivalent to 1 to 2 liters of concentrated hydrochloric acid. Although some alkaline end products are also formed, the acid type predominates, and the body is faced with the necessity of continually removing the large quantities of acids that are formed within cells. The greatest restriction is that these products should be transported to the organs of excretion (via the extracellular fluids) with a minimal change in the hydrogen ion concentration.

Most biochemical processes are extremely sensitive to the level of hydrogen ions. The enzymes and other proteins involved in biological reactions, as well as many of the smaller molecules, are weak electrolytes whose state of ionization is a function of the hydrogen ion concentration. Most enzymes are active only within a narrow pH range, usually from 5 to 9. At a pH other than the optimum one, the binding of substrates to enzymes, the catalytic activity of enzymes, and changes in protein structure are seriously affected. Since the catalytic properties of enzymes are dependent on their state of ionization, it is not surprising that living cells cannot tolerate more than very minor changes in hydrogen ion levels. As a result, biological fluids are in general strongly buffered, so that their pH is maintained within narrow limits under physiological conditions.

Blood is buffered by plasma proteins and by hemoglobin, which can either accept or donate protons. The role of buffers can be understood by the following example. The addition of 0.01 mole hydrochloric acid in 1 liter of blood lowers the pH only from 7.4 to 7.2. When added to an isotonic saline (sodium chloride) solution, the same amount of hydrochloric acid lowers the pH from 7.0 to 2.0, since the saline solution has no buffering capacity. Another example of the effectiveness of the blood plasma indicates that 1.3 liters of concentrated hydrochloric acid are needed to drop the pH of the whole 5.5 liters of blood of an average human being from 7.4 to 7.0.

Metabolism in tissues leads to the production of carbon dioxide (CO_2), which when dissolved in water, forms carbonic acid and the following equilibrium:

$$CO_2 + H_2O \rightleftharpoons H_2CO_3 \rightleftharpoons H^+ + HCO_3^-$$

carbon dioxide — water — carbonic acid — bicarbonate anion

Carbon dioxide enters the bloodstream from tissues and is exchanged in the lungs for oxygen, which is then transported throughout the body by the hemoglobin in the blood. The fact that the ratio of bicarbonate to carbonic acid is relatively high (10:1) seems to make this buffer well outside its maximum capacity. Nevertheless, the system is appropriate, because the need to neutralize excess acid (such as lactic acid, which is produced during exercise) is much greater than the need to neutralize excess base. The excess bicarbonate serves this purpose. Strenuous exercise also leads to an increased formation of carbon dioxide by body tissues, which is accumulated in the air spaces of the lungs. Under normal circumstances, the bicarbonate in the blood buffer will lead to a shifting in the equilibrium toward the optimum 7.4 value. Should excess alkalinity take place, carbon dioxide from the lungs can be reabsorbed to form carbonic acid, which will help the neutralization process.

Many biochemically important reactions take place because of either acid or base catalysis, including the hydrolysis of peptides and esters, the reactions of phosphate groups, tautomerizations (ketoenol equilibria), and condensations of carbonyl groups. Sometimes, the side chains of several amino acid residues in aspartic acid, glutamic acid, histidine, cysteine, tyrosine, and lysine act in the enzymatic capacity of general acid and/or base catalysis.

The kidneys, which are usually seen as the organs of excretion, also act as regulators in water, electrolyte, and acid-base balance. Acid-base balance takes place in the tubules of the kidneys through the exchange of sodium ions and hydrogen ions. It is regulated by the pH of blood plasma and the ability of the tubular cells to acidify the urine through proton and ammonia formation. The glomerular filtrate contains the electrolytes, acids, and bases present in the blood plasma. The cations are mostly sodium ions, while the anions are either chloride, phosphate, or bicarbonate. At a pH of 7.4, 95 percent of the carbon dioxide is in the form of sodium bicarbonate, while 83 percent of the phosphate is disodium hydrogen phosphate. Normally, most of the sodium ions are taken up by the tubular cells in exchange for the protons formed in there. The sodium ions are then returned to the plasma after associating with the bicarbonate anions. The role of the kidneys is to stabilize the bicarbonate concentration and to neutralize the nonvolatile sulfuric and phosphoric acids. Base conservation by the kidneys takes place with the aid of ammonia formed by the decomposition of glutamine (via the enzyme glutaminase) and the amino acids (via amino acid oxidase).

DISORDERS AND DISEASES

Acids and bases are among the most important chemicals of the living being. Life depends on pH and acid-base reactions. The presence of buffers is also important for the optimum function of enzymes. Thus, in metabolic reactions enzymes have pH optima that allow the maximum catalysis of the substrate reactions. The means of accomplishing a steady pH of 7.4 in the blood involves a mechanism for the regulation of acid-base balance, which involves water and electrolyte balance, hemoglobin, and blood buffers, as well as the action of lungs and kidneys.

The pH of different body fluids in human beings varies greatly. For example, the pH range of gastric juices is 1 to 2, while that of intestinal juices is 8 to 9. If the blood plasma pH of 7.4 for a healthy individual varies by 0.2 or more units, then serious medical conditions arise; if not corrected, they may lead to death. Such reactions occur primarily because the functioning of enzymes is sharply pH-dependent.

Life can be described as a continuous fight against pH change. Nature has equipped the body with the buffers and the various mechanisms that keep organs functioning. The kidneys, lungs, and skin all share the common role of controlling the ionic balance of the organism, and thus controlling the bicarbonate concentration and pH. Cell pH regulation is complicated, however, because of the heterogeneous nature of the cell contents. For example, mitochondrial fluid is more alkaline than that of the cytoplasm, which allows the establishing of a hydrogen ion gradient between these two compartments of the cell. Basic functions such as oxidative phosphorylation, which is the transfer of metabolic energy to adenosinetriphosphate (ATP), are believed to depend on this hydrogen ion gradient.

When the blood pH is lower than 7.4, acidosis results. Most forms of acidosis are metabolic or respiratory in origin. Metabolic acidosis is caused by a decrease in bicarbonate and occurs with uncontrolled diabetes mellitus (as a result of ketosis, the excessive production of ketone bodies such as acetone), with certain kidney diseases, with poisoning by an acid salt, and in cases of vomiting when non-acid fluids are lost. Respiratory acidosis may occur with diseases that impair respiration, such as emphysema, asthma, and pneumonia. Under these conditions, carbon dioxide is not properly expired and, as a result, carbonic acid levels increase relative to those of bicarbonate.

Alkalosis results when bicarbonate becomes favored in the buffer ratio. Metabolic alkalosis is observed when excessive vomiting (loss of acid, in the form of hydrochloric acid) takes place, while respiratory alkalosis occurs with hyperventilation (such as that brought on by a high altitude). Mountain climbers reaching the summit of Mount Everest without supplemental oxygen were found to have their pH rise to 7.7 or 7.8.

The chief cause of dental decay is lactic acid, which is formed in the mouth by the action of specific bacteria, such as *Streptococcus mutans*, on the carbohydrates (and their by-products) that are attached to tooth surfaces in a sticky plaque. The normal pH of plaque is 6.8, but lactic acid lowers it to 5.5 or less, which speeds up the corrosion of enamel and leads to tooth decay. The application of fluoride-containing substances directly to the teeth or the drinking of fluoride-containing water changes the composition of teeth and forms a new substance called fluorapatite, which forms a new enamel that is much more resistant to acidity.

PERSPECTIVE AND PROSPECTS

Acids and bases have been known to human beings since ancient times. The word "acid" is derived from the Latin *acidus* (sour) and has been redefined several times over the centuries. Alchemists have considered an acid as a substance with a sour taste which dissolved many metals and reacted with alkalies to form salts. The French scientist Antoine-Laurent Lavoisier (1743-1794) insisted that an acid should involve the presence of oxygen. In 1810, the English chemist Sir Humphry Davy (1778-1829) showed that hydrogen is the element that all acids have in common. In 1840, German Justus von Liebig (1803-1873) redefined an acid as the compound that contains hydrogen and produces hydrogen gas upon reaction with metals. His definition coincided with the theories postulated separately by the Swedish chemist Svante A. Arrhenius (1859-1927) and the German chemist Carl W. Ostwald (1883-1943), who also pointed out that bases were substances that carried a hydroxyl group.

In 1909, the Danish chemist Søren Peter Lauritz Sørensen (1868-1939) proposed the pH system, which has become the standard measure of acidity. In separate works announced in 1923, Johannes N. Brønsted (1879-1947) and Thomas M. Lowry supported the Arrhenius-Ostwald theory and went further to postulate that the hydrogen ion is never found in the free state but instead exists in combination with another base (for example with water, when the hydrogen is in an aqueous solution). As a result, their work broadened the definition of a base, which according to them would include any compound that was a proton (hydrogen ion) acceptor. In 1938, American Gilbert N. Lewis (1875-1946) broadened even further the acid-base concept: An acid is an electron pair acceptor, while a base is an electron pair donor. In 1963, Ralph Gottfrid Pearson proposed the simple and effective way of classifying acids and bases as hard or soft.   —*Soraya Ghayourmanesh, Ph.D.*

See also Cells; Cytology; Enzymes; Fluids and electrolytes; Food biochemistry; Kidneys; Metabolism; Respiration.

FOR FURTHER INFORMATION:

Bishop, M. L., J. L. Duben-Von Laufen, and E. P. Fody, eds. *Clinical Chemistry: Principles, Procedures, Correlations*. Philadelphia: J. B. Lippincott, 1985. An advanced text on clinical chemistry. Chapter 11, "Blood Gases, pH, and Buffer Systems," discusses acid-base balance and ways of measuring the oxygen and carbon dioxide pressures. Also provides case studies.

Caret, R. L., K. J. Denniston, and J. J. Topping. *Principles and Applications of Organic and Biological Chemistry*. Dubuque, Iowa: Wm. C. Brown, 1993. A simple introductory text for the health sciences. Chapter 2, "Chemical Change," describes acid-base chemistry and its applications.

Kask, Uno, J. D. Rawn, and R. A. DeLorenzo. *General Chemistry*. Dubuque, Iowa: Wm. C. Brown, 1992. An undergraduate text that discusses acids and bases (chapter 14) and aqueous acid-base equilibria (chapter 15).

Matta, M. S., and A. C. Wilbraham. *General, Organic, and Biological Chemistry*. 2d ed. Menlo Park, Calif.: Benjamin Cummings, 1986. An excellent undergraduate text for health-related sciences. Discusses acids and bases (chapter 9), alkaloids (chapter 15), and acidosis and alkalosis (chapter 22).

Petrucci, R. H., and W. S. Harwood. *General Chemistry: Principles and Modern Applications*. 6th ed. New York: Macmillan, 1993. A general chemistry text for undergraduates. Chapters 17 and 18 discuss acids and bases and their equilibria. A section entitled "Focus On" (pages 556 and 557) describes buffers in the blood.

Routh, J. I. *Introduction to Biochemistry*. 2d ed. Philadelphia: W. B. Saunders, 1978. An excellent undergraduate text. The role of acid-base chemistry is well explained in chapter 14, "Body Fluids."

Stryer, Lubert. *Biochemistry*. 4th ed. New York: W. H. Freeman, 1995. An advanced text in biochemistry. Acids and bases are discussed in "Part I: Molecular Design of Life."

Voet, Donald, and Judith G. Voet. *Biochemistry*. New York: John Wiley & Sons, 1990. A text that approaches biochemistry via organic chemistry reactions. Chapter 2, section 2, discusses acids, bases, and buffers. Chapter 14, section 1A, covers acid-base catalysis.

ACNE

DISEASE/DISORDER

ANATOMY OR SYSTEM AFFECTED: Skin

SPECIALTIES AND RELATED FIELDS: Dermatology, family practice, pediatrics

DEFINITION: A group of skin disorders, the most common of which, acne vulgaris, usually affects teenagers; another form, acne rosacea, usually afflicts older people.

KEY TERMS:

acne rosacea: a skin eruption that usually appears between the ages of thirty and fifty; unlike acne vulgaris, it is not characterized by comedones

acne vulgaris: a skin eruption that usually occurs in puberty and is characterized by the development of comedones, which may be inflamed

comedo (pl. comedos, comedones): the major lesion in acne vulgaris; it occurs when a hair follicle fills with keratin, sebum, and other matter, and may become infected

pilosebaceous: referring to hair follicles and the sebaceous glands

sebaceous glands: glands in the skin that usually open into the hair follicles

sebum: a semifluid, fatty substance secreted by the sebaceous glands into the hair follicles

testosterone: the most potent male hormone, which exists in both sexes; it starts the chain of events that leads to acne vulgaris

CAUSES AND SYMPTOMS

Many skin disorders are grouped together as acne. The two most common are *acne vulgaris* and *acne rosacea*. Other acne diseases include *neonatal acne* and *infantile acne*, seen respectively in newborn babies and infants. *Drug acne* is a consequence of the administration of such medications as corticosteroids, iodides, bromides, anticonvulsants, lithium preparations, and oral contraceptives, to name some of the more common agents that are sometimes involved in acne outbreaks. *Pomade acne* and *acne cosmetica* are associated with the use of greasy or sensitizing substances on the skin, such as hair oil, suntan lotions, cosmetics, soap, and shampoo. They may be the sole cause of acne in some individuals or may aggravate existing outbreaks of acne vulgaris. *Occupational acne*, as the name implies, is associated with exposure to skin irritants in the workplace. Chemicals, waxes, greases, and other substances may be involved. *Acné excoriée des jeunes filles*, or acne in young girls, is thought to be associated with emotional distress. In spite of the name, it can occur in boys as well. Two forms of acne are seen in young women. One is *pyoderma faciale*, a skin eruption that always occurs on the face. The other is *perioral dermatitis (peri*, around; *ora*, the mouth), characterized by redness, pimples, and pustules. *Acne conglobata* is a rare but severe skin disorder that is seen in men between the ages of eighteen and thirty.

Acne vulgaris. In acne vulgaris, a disruption occurs in the normal activity of the pilosebaceous units of the dermis, the layer of the skin that contains the blood vessels, nerves and nerve endings, glands, and hair follicles. Ordinarily, the sebaceous glands secrete sebum into the hair follicle, where it travels up the hair shaft and onto the outer surface of the skin, to maintain proper hydration of the hair and skin and prevent loss of moisture. In acne vulgaris, the amount of sebum increases greatly and the hair shaft that allows it to escape becomes plugged, holding in the sebum.

Acne vulgaris usually occurs during puberty and is the result of some of the hormones released at that time to help the child become an adult. One of the major hormones is testosterone, an androgen (*andros*, man or manhood; *gen*, generating or causing), so called because it brings about bodily changes that convert a boy into a man. In boys, testosterone and other male hormones cause sexual organs to mature. Hair begins to grow on the chest and face, in pubic areas and armpits. Musculature is increased, and the larynx (voice box) is enlarged, so the voice deepens. In males, testosterone and other male hormones are produced primarily in the testicles. In girls, estrogens and other female hormones are released during puberty, directing the

Development of Acne

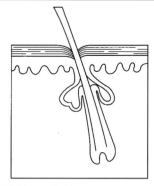

(1) Normal skin

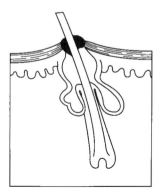

(2) Clogged sebaceous gland

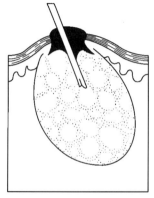

(3) Acne vulgaris

passage of the child from girlhood to womanhood. Testosterone is also produced, mostly in the ovaries and the adrenal glands.

In both sexes during puberty, testosterone is taken up by the pilosebaceous glands and converted to dihydrotestosterone, a substance that causes an increase in the size of the glands and increased secretion of the fatty substance sebum into hair follicles. At the same time, a process occurs that closes off the hair follicle, allowing sebum, keratin, and other matter to collect. This process is called intrafollicular hyperkeratosis (from *intra*, inside, *follicular*, referring to the follicle, *hyper*, excessive, and *keratosis*, production of keratin). Keratin buildup creates a plug that blocks the follicle opening and permits the accumulation of sebum, causing the formation of a closed comedo. As more and more material collects, the comedo becomes visible as a white-capped pimple, or whitehead. Closed comedones are the precursors of the papules, pustules, nodules, and cysts characteristic of acne vulgaris. *Papula* means "pimple," a pustule is a pimple containing pus, *nodus* means a small knot, and *kystis* means "bladder," or in this case a sac filled with semisolid material. Sometimes cysts are referred to generically as sebaceous cysts, but the material inside is usually keratin.

Another lesion in acne vulgaris, called an open comedo, occurs when a sac in the outer layer of the skin fills with keratin, sebum, and other matter. Unlike the closed comedo, it is open to the surface of the skin and the material inside appears black—hence the term "blackhead." Blackheads are unsightly, make the skin look dirty, and suggest that they are caused by bad hygienic habits. This is not true, but exactly why the material in the sac turns black is not fully understood. Some believe that the natural skin pigment melanin is involved.

Blackheads are usually easily managed and rarely become inflamed. It is the closed comedo, or whitehead, that causes the disfiguring lesions of acne vulgaris. As the closed comedo fills with keratin and sebum, colonies of bacteria, usually *Propionibacterium acnes*, develop at the site. The bacteria secrete enzymes that break down the sebum, forming free fatty acids that inflame and irritate the follicle wall. With inflammation, white blood cells are drawn to the area to fight off the bacteria.

The comedo enlarges with further accumulation of white blood cells, keratin, and sebum until the follicle wall ruptures, spreading inflammation. If the inflammation is close to the surface of the skin, the lesion will usually be a pustule. If the inflammation is deeper, a larger papule, nodule, or cyst may form.

Clothing, cosmetics, and other factors may exacerbate acne vulgaris. Headbands, chin straps, and other items can cause trauma that ruptures closed comedones and spreads infection. Ingredients in cosmetics, soaps, and other preparations used on the skin can contribute to the formation of comedones in acne vulgaris. Lanolin, petrolatum, laurel alcohol, and oleic acid are among the chemicals commonly found in skin creams, cosmetics, soaps, shampoos, and other preparations applied to the skin. They have been shown to aggravate existing acne in some people and to bring on acne eruptions in others.

It was long thought that fatty foods—such as chocolate, ice cream, desserts, and peanut butter—contributed to acne, perhaps because teenagers eat so much of them. This theory has been largely discarded. Except for specific allergic sensitivities, foods do not appear to cause or in any other way affect the eruptions of acne vulgaris.

Cases of acne vulgaris are classified as mild, moderate, or severe. In mild and moderate acne vulgaris, the number of lesions ranges from a few to many, appearing regularly or sporadically and occurring mostly in the top layer of the skin. Consequently, these cases are sometimes called "superficial acne." In severe cases, the acne lesions are deep, extending down into the skin, and characterized by inflamed papules and pustules.

Superficial acne, or mild-to-moderate acne vulgaris, is easily managed with the therapies available. The teenager goes through a year to two dealing with "zits." The problem may be irritating and may cause inconvenience and discomfort, but it is so common among teenagers that little lasting harm is done. With time and treatment, the skin clears and the problem is over.

With deep or severe acne, however, the condition can be devastating, physically and psychologically. In these cases, the lesions may come in massive eruptions that cover the face and extend to the neck, chest, and back. The lesions can be large and deep, frequently causing disfiguring pits and craters that become lifelong scars. The victims of severe acne can suffer profound psychological damage. The disease strikes at a time when most teenagers are especially concerned with being gregarious, popular, and well liked. The chronic, constant disfigurement effectively isolates the individual, however, often making him or her unwilling to risk social contact.

Acne rosacea. The other common form of acne is acne rosacea, so called because of the "rosy" color that appears on the face. Unlike acne vulgaris, it rarely strikes people under thirty years of age and is not characterized by comedones, although papules and pustules are common. It is predominantly seen in women, although its most serious manifestations are seen in men. The cause of acne rosacea is unknown, but it is more likely to strike people with fair complexions. It is usually limited to the center of the face, but eruptions may occur on other parts of the body.

Acne rosacea is progressive; that is, it gets worse as the patient grows older. It seems to occur most often in people who have a tendency to redden or blush easily. The blushing, whether it is caused by emotional distress, such as shame or embarrassment, or by heat, food, or drink, may be the precursor of acne rosacea. The individual finds that episodes of blushing last longer and longer until, eventually, the redness becomes permanent. Papules and pustules break out, and surface blood vessels become dilated, causing further redness. As the disease progresses, tissue overgrowth may cause the nose to swell and become red and bulbous. Inflammation may develop in and around the eyes and threaten vision. These severe symptoms occur more often in men than in women.

TREATMENT AND THERAPY

The majority of acne patients are treated at home with over-the-counter preparations applied topically (that is, on the skin). For years, many of the agents recommended for acne contained sulfur, and some still do. Sulfur is useful for reducing comedones, but it has been suggested that sulfur by itself may also cause comedones; however, sulfur compounds, such as zinc sulfate, are not suspected of causing comedones. Resorcinol and salicylic acid are commonly included in topical over-the-counter preparations to promote scaling and reduce comedones. Sometimes sulfur, resorcinol, and salicylic acid are used singly, sometimes together, and sometimes combined with topical antiseptics or other agents.

While most patients will be helped by the available over-the-counter agents, many will not respond adequately to such home therapy. These patients must be seen by a doctor, such as a family practitioner or dermatologist. The physician attempts to eliminate existing lesions, prevent the formation of new lesions, destroy microorganisms, relieve inflammation, and prevent the occurrence of cysts, papules, and pustules. If the patient's skin is oily, the physician may advise washing the face and other affected areas several times a day. This has little effect on the development of comedones, but it may improve the patient's appearance and self-esteem. The physician will also use medications that are similar to over-the-counter antiacne agents but more powerful. These include drying agents, topical antibiotic preparations, and agents to abrade the skin, such as exfoliants or desquamating (scale-removing) agents.

Various topical antibiotics have been developed for use in acne vulgaris, such as topical tetracycline, clindamycin, and erythromycin. One that is often used is benzoyl peroxide, a topical antibiotic that can penetrate the skin and reach the sites of infection in the hair follicle. It is also a powerful irritant that increases the growth rate of epithelial cells and promotes sloughing, which helps clear the surface of the skin. It is effective in resolving comedones and seems to suppress the release of sebum. Because it has a high potential for skin irritation, benzoyl peroxide must be used carefully. Physicians generally start with the weaker formulations of the drug and increase the strength as tolerance develops.

Vitamin A has been given orally to patients with acne vulgaris in the hope of preventing the formation of comedones. The effective oral dose of the vitamin for this purpose is so high, however, that it could be toxic. Therefore, a topical form of vitamin A was developed called vitamin A acid, retinoic acid, or tretinoin (marketed as Retin-A). Applied directly to the skin, it has proved highly beneficial in the treatment of acne vulgaris. It clears comedones from the hair follicles and suppresses the formation of new comedones. It reduces inflammation and facilitates the transdermal (through-the-skin) penetration of medications such as benzoyl peroxide and other topical antibiotics. Like benzoyl peroxide, vitamin A acid can be irritating to the skin, so it must be used carefully. When benzoyl peroxide and vitamin A acid are used in combination in the treatment of acne vulgaris, their therapeutic effectiveness is significantly increased. The physician generally prescribes a morning application of one and an evening application of the other.

When large comedones, pustules, or cysts form, the physician may elect to remove them surgically. The procedure is quite effective in improving appearance, but it does nothing to affect the course of the disease. Furthermore, it demands great skill on the part of the physician to avoid causing damage and irritating the surrounding skin, rupturing the comedo wall, and allowing inflammation to spread. The patient should be advised not to try to duplicate the process at home: Picking at pimples could create open lesions that may take weeks to heal and may produce deep scars. Sometimes, the physician will insert a needle into a deep lesion in order to drain the material from it. Sometimes, the physician tries to avoid surgery by injecting a minute quantity of corticosteroid, such as triamcinolone acetonide, into a deep lesion to reduce its size.

The physician may wish to add the benefits of sunlight to medical therapy. Sunlight helps dry the skin and promotes scaling and clearing of the skin, which is probably why acne improves in summer. The physician may suggest sunbathing, but an overzealous patient could become sunburned or chronically overexposed to the sun, thereby risking skin cancer. The beneficial effects of natural sunlight are not necessarily achievable with a sunlamp and, over a long period of exposure, the ultraviolet light produced by some lamps may actually increase sebum production and promote intrafollicular hyperkeratosis.

About 12 percent of patients with acne vulgaris develop severe or deep acne. In devising a treatment regime for these cases, the physician has many options to help clear the patient's skin, reduce the number and occurrence of lesions, and prevent the scarring that can disfigure the patient for life. Both the topical medications benzoyl peroxide and vitamin A acid are used, singly and in combination, as well as many other topical preparations. Nevertheless, these patients often also require oral antibiotics to fight their infection from within.

It may take weeks for oral antibiotic therapy to achieve results, and it may even be necessary for the patient to

continue the therapy for years. Therefore, the physician looks for an antibiotic that is effective and safe for long-term use. Oral tetracycline is often the physician's choice because it has been proven effective against *Propionibacterium acnes*, and it seems to suppress the formation of comedones. Oral tetracycline is usually safe for long-term therapy, and it is economical. Other oral antibiotics used to treat acne vulgaris are erythromycin, clindamycin, and minocycline.

Yet in long-term therapy with any broad-spectrum antibiotic, there is always the possibility that the agent being used will not only kill the offending organism but also destroy "friendly" bacteria that aid in bodily processes and help protect the body from other microorganisms. When this happens, disease-causing pathogens may be allowed to flourish and cause infection. For example, prolonged use of antibiotics in women may allow the growth of a yeastlike fungus, *Candida*, which can cause vaginitis. Prolonged use of clindamycin may allow the proliferation of *Clostridium difficile*, which could result in ulcerative colitis, a severe disorder of the lower gastrointestinal tract.

If, for any reason, the physician believes that oral antibiotics are not working or must be discontinued, there are other therapeutic agents and other procedures that may be helpful in treating severe, deep acne vulgaris. One medication that is highly effective, but also potentially very harmful, is isotretinoin. As the name implies, isotretinoin (meaning "similar to tretinoin") is derived from vitamin A, but it is both more effective and more difficult to use. Unlike the topical vitamin A acid preparations, isotretinoin is taken orally. It is highly effective in inhibiting the function of sebaceous glands and preventing the formation of closed comedones by reducing keratinization, but isotretinoin also produces a wide range of side effects. The majority of these are skin disorders, but the bones and joints, the eyes, and other organs can be affected. Perhaps the most serious adverse effect of isotretinoin is that it can cause severe abnormalities in the fetuses of pregnant women. Therefore, pregnancy is an absolute contraindication for isotretinoin. Before they take this drug, women of childbearing age are checked to ensure that they are not pregnant. They are advised to use strict contraceptive measures one month before therapy, during the entire course of therapy, and for at least one month after therapy has been discontinued.

Estrogens, female hormones, have been used to treat severe acne in women who are more than sixteen years of age. The aim of this therapy is to counteract the sebum-stimulating activity of circulating testosterone and to reduce the formation of comedones by reducing the amount of sebum produced. Estrogens cannot be used in males because the dose required to reduce sebum production could produce feminizing side effects.

Persistent lesions can be treated with cryotherapy. In this procedure, an extremely cold substance such as dry ice or liquid nitrogen is carefully applied to the lesion. This technique is effective in reducing both small pustules and deeper cysts. For patients whose skin has been deeply scarred by acne, a procedure called dermabrasion, in which the top layer of skin is removed, may help improve the appearance.

Although its cause is unknown, acne rosacea can be treated. The topical antiparasitic drug metronidazole, applied in a cream, and oral broad-spectrum antibiotics, such as tetracycline, have been found effective. It may be necessary to continue antibiotic therapy for a long period of time, but the treatment is usually effective. Surgery may be required to correct the bulbous nose that sometimes occurs with this condition.

PERSPECTIVE AND PROSPECTS

Most acne vulgaris (about 60 percent) is treated at home. There has been significant improvement in the treatment of mild-to-moderate acne vulgaris, so for most of these patients, the condition can be limited to an annoyance or an inconvenience of the teen years. Only recalcitrant cases of acne vulgaris are seen by physicians. Of those cases treated by doctors, the majority are seen by family physicians, general practitioners, and other primary care workers. Severe acne is usually referred to the dermatologist, who is skilled in the use of the more serious medications and the more exacting techniques that are required in treatment.

For at least 85 percent of those experiencing puberty, acne vulgaris is a fact of life. It is a natural consequence of the hormonal changes that occur at this time. It is not likely that any drugs or techniques will be found to avoid acne in the teenage years, as this would involve tampering with a fundamental growth process. It can be expected, however, that in this disease condition, as in so many others, progress will continue to be made, and newer, more effective, and safer agents will be developed.

—*C. Richard Falcon*

See also Abscesses; Cysts and ganglions; Dermatology; Keratoses; Pimples; Puberty and adolescence; Rosacea; Skin disorders.

FOR FURTHER INFORMATION:

Dvorine, William. *A Dermatologist's Guide to Home Skin Treatment*. New York: Charles Scribner's Sons, 1983. Offers descriptions of various skin diseases, including acne, and sensible instructions about how to deal with them at home.

Flandermeyer, Kenneth L. *Clear Skin*. Boston: Little, Brown, 1979. Billed as "a step-by-step program to stop pimples, blackheads, acne," a good general text for the layperson that details one dermatologist's views on acne and how to treat it.

Handbook of Nonprescription Drugs. 9th ed. Washington, D.C.: American Pharmaceutical Association, 1990.

Horton, Edward, Felicity Smart, and Trevor Weston, eds. *The Marshall Cavendish Illustrated Encyclopedia of*

Family Health. 24 vols. London: Marshall Cavendish, 1984. This multivolume set provides "doctor's answers" to common questions about various diseases. Acne is covered in volume 1.

Larson, David E., ed. *Mayo Clinic Health Book*. 2d ed. New York: William Morrow, 1996. One of the most thorough and accessible medical texts for the layperson.

ACQUIRED IMMUNODEFICIENCY SYNDROME (AIDS)

DISEASE/DISORDER

ANATOMY OR SYSTEM AFFECTED: Immune system, reproductive system

SPECIALTIES AND RELATED FIELDS: Epidemiology, family practice, immunology, internal medicine

DEFINITION: AIDS arises from chronic infection with the human immunodeficiency virus (HIV) and is characterized by progressive loss of immune function and susceptibility to secondary infections.

KEY TERMS:

CD4: an abbreviation for a protein found on the surface of certain human cells; CD4 is a specific receptor for HIV, and it determines the range of cells that HIV can infect

macrophages: cells involved in the presentation of antigen to the immune system, found in a number of tissues; macrophages, which have CD4 on their surfaces, may be a major reservoir of infection for HIV

opportunistic infections: infections caused by pathogens that take advantage of a dysfunctional immune system; much of the morbidity and mortality of AIDS results from opportunistic infections

retroviruses: the family of ribonucleic acid (RNA) viruses to which HIV belongs, characterized by a multiplication cycle that includes reverse transcription of the RNA into a deoxyribonucleic acid (DNA) copy

reverse transcriptase: an enzyme, encoded by an HIV gene, that causes a DNA copy of the HIV genes to be inserted into the chromosomes of the target cell; some drugs directed against HIV target reverse transcriptase

T helper cells: CD4-expressing cells involved in immune recognition and the coordination of immune responses; the destruction of T helpers by HIV multiplication contributes to AIDS immunodeficiency

zidovudine: a drug, also known as azidothymidine (or AZT), used to treat HIV infection; it interferes with the functioning of the virus' reverse transcriptase enzyme

CAUSES AND SYMPTOMS

Acquired immunodeficiency syndrome (AIDS) is a condition that occurs in persons infected with the human immunodeficiency virus (HIV). The morbidity and mortality attributed to AIDS result primarily from opportunistic viral and protozoal infections arising from a generalized failure in cell-mediated immunity caused by HIV infection, or from certain characteristic malignancies of uncertain etiology. There may also be tissue damage, especially in the central nervous system, that can be attributed directly to the destruction of HIV-infected cells. From a clinical standpoint, AIDS can be considered as a terminal manifestation of HIV infection, and there is no single diagnostic criterion to distinguish it from other disease states associated with HIV. AIDS is most widespread in central Africa and southern Asia, but it occurs with some degree of prevalence in most parts of the world.

HIV is a member of the Retroviridae, a family of enveloped viruses whose life cycles are characterized by the phenomenon of reverse transcription, by which the nucleotide sequence of the virus' ribonucleic acid (RNA) genome is used to synthesize deoxyribonucleic acid (DNA) that is subsequently incorporated into an infected cell's chromosomes; this is the reverse of the normal flow of genetic information in cells and is catalyzed by a unique viral enzyme, reverse transcriptase. There are two genetically distinct forms of HIV, HIV-1 and HIV-2, with HIV-1 being dominant worldwide.

HIV has evolved for transmission during sexual intercourse. HIV-susceptible cells are found in association with the epithelia of the vagina, rectum, and urethra. In HIV-infected persons, both HIV-infected cells and free virus particles (virions) may be found at these sites, as well as in seminal fluid and in vaginal secretions. There is evidence that the rate of HIV transmission (the proportion of sexual contacts between an infected and a susceptible individual that result in transmission of the virus), which is normally very low, may be increased by the presence of other sexually transmitted infections; presumably, the inflammation associated with these infections causes an increase in the number of HIV-infected and HIV-susceptible cell populations. Because HIV-infected cells and HIV virions are found in the blood of an infected person, HIV can be transmitted through accidental transfer of blood, as may occur in needle sharing by intravenous drug users, needle-stick injuries to health care workers, and the administration of blood products. Infection by vertical transmission to a developing fetus occurs in approximately one-third of children born to HIV-infected mothers. There is no evidence that HIV can be spread by airborne transmission, by indirect or direct nonsexual contact, or by arthropod vectors, such as mosquitoes.

The major cellular targets for the multiplication of HIV are macrophages and T-helper lymphocytes. Both of these cell populations display a surface protein designated as CD4, to which HIV can attach through interaction with proteins (gp120 and gp41) found on the surface of the virion. The presence of CD4 protein is necessary for infection but is not by itself sufficient for infection; additional coreceptors must also be present on the target cell. Interaction with the receptors leads to entry of the virus into the cell, probably involving fusion of the cell membrane and the viral envelope. After the nucleoprotein core (the HIV genome and associated proteins) migrates to the cell's nucleus, reverse transcriptase uses the viral RNA as a template for producing a DNA copy that is inserted into the chromosomal DNA of the cell.

At this point, the virus exists in the infected cell as a collection of genes. Conceivably, these genes could remain unexpressed, the virus persisting in this state without affecting the cell or giving evidence to the immune system of its presence; this condition of biological latency can be shown in cultured cells, though its significance in an infected person is unknown. For production of progeny virus particles (virions), HIV genes are expressed, leading to the synthesis of viral proteins and full-length RNA genomes. After assembly, the virions leave the cell by a process of budding through the cell membrane. The entire reproductive cycle is regulated by viral gene products and is influenced by the metabolic state of the cell. In culture, macrophages can continue releasing virions over a long period of time, while HIV infection of T helpers often leads to their rapid destruction. In an infected person, multiplication of HIV occurs primarily in lymphoid tissues, including lymph nodes and the spleen, where HIV-susceptible macrophages and lymphocytes are abundant.

HIV strains isolated from different persons, or even from the same person at different times in the course of an infection, may display genetic variability, especially in the genes encoding the virion surface proteins. Reproduction of HIV is associated with a high rate of spontaneous mutation, which may help the virus to evade an effective immune response. Such mutation places a significant restraint on development of an HIV vaccine.

The earliest stages of HIV infection may be unapparent or may be expressed in symptoms similar to those of many other viral infections, including mild fever, malaise, and swollen lymph nodes. Antibodies to HIV proteins are usually produced within twelve weeks of exposure, although they do not contain the infection.

Primary infection is followed by a period of clinical latency, during which signs and symptoms of HIV infection are absent or subtle. The length of this period varies and may exceed fifteen years. It is important to distinguish this state of clinical latency from biological latency of the virus. During clinical latency, HIV may continue to multiply, and the infected person continues to serve as a potential reservoir of infection, transmitting the virus to new hosts.

In virtually all HIV infections, continued multiplication of the virus eventually leads to a state of impaired cellular immunity. The mechanisms whereby this characteristic immunodeficiency of AIDS develops are complex. Both macrophages and T helpers are critical players in the immune response, and their destruction by HIV may be responsible in part for dysfunctional immunity. The immunodeficiency is not, however, entirely attributable to the

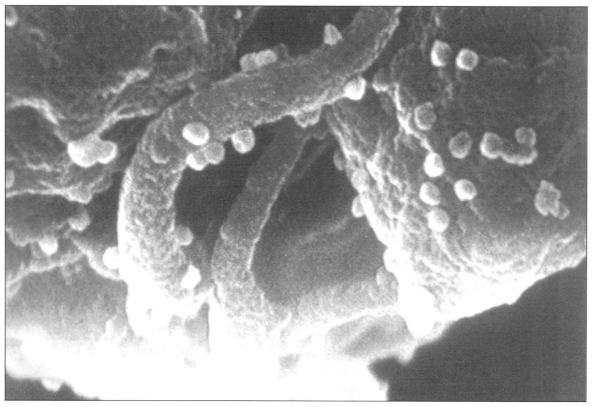

This electron micrograph shows human immunodeficiency viruses invading a lymphocyte. (Dan McCoy/Rainbow)

depletion of HIV-susceptible cells, since cells not infected by HIV also show aberrant behavior in infected persons; these include the cytolytic T lymphocytes that are essential to the defense against intracellular parasites and antibody-producing B lymphocytes. These indirect effects may arise from shifts in relative amounts of cytokines—small proteins produced by cells that influence the activity of surrounding cells—produced by HIV-infected cells.

Later stages of HIV infection, leading to AIDS, are distinguished by a measurable drop in absolute numbers of peripheral T helpers and weak delayed hypersensitivity responses. At this point the HIV-infected person becomes susceptible to a variety of opportunistic infections—infections caused by pathogens that are normally incapable of infecting humans but that can invade the tissues of a person whose immune response is impaired. Some of the opportunistic infections that afflict HIV-infected persons are also seen in other immunodeficiency states, such as those that occur in transplant patients receiving immunosuppressive drugs, while others are especially prominent in persons with AIDS.

The most common opportunistic infection accompanying advanced HIV infection, and one of the most commonly documented causes of death from AIDS, is pneumonia resulting from invasion by the eukaryotic parasite *Pneumocystis carinii*. *P. carinii* pneumonia can be treated with drugs, but unfortunately reinfection is common. Other fungal and parasitic infections common among persons with AIDS are oropharyngeal candidiasis, cryptococcal meningitis, and toxoplasmosis. Among bacterial pathogens, mycobacteria are especially important, including *Mycobacterium intracellulare* and *Mycobacterium tuberculosis*; persistence of *M. tuberculosis* in the United States is attributed in part to its association with AIDS. Herpesvirus infections, which are very common in the general population but are usually held in a state of biological latency by the immune system, may become reactivated in persons with AIDS, leading to systemic tissue damage.

Characteristic malignancies may also accompany advanced HIV infection, including Kaposi's sarcoma and non-Hodgkin's lymphomas. Kaposi's sarcoma is diagnosed primarily in the Western Hemisphere among homosexual and bisexual males; the significance of this unusual pattern of incidence is unclear but appears to be associated with a particular strain of herpesvirus.

Although opportunistic infections remain the major cause of death from AIDS, advanced HIV infections may also be accompanied by disease states more directly attributable to the viral infection. These include a wasting syndrome characterized by chronic or recurrent diarrhea and a pattern of neurological damage known as AIDS dementia.

The early stages of HIV infection are most commonly diagnosed by the identification of antibodies in patient serum that are specific for viral antigens, using an enzyme immunoassay (EIA). Test serum is incubated with a solid matrix coated with material containing HIV proteins; if the serum contains HIV-specific antibodies, these will bind to the matrix with high affinity. After the matrix is washed to remove nonspecific antibodies, it is incubated with a solution of secondary antibodies that are specific for human immunoglobulin; these will attach to any HIV-specific patient antibodies that are bound to the matrix. The secondary antibodies are covalently linked to an enzyme that catalyzes the formation of a detectable product, signaling the presence of the secondary antibodies and thus of HIV-specific antibodies in the test serum. While this test is very sensitive for the detection of HIV-specific antibodies, false-positive results may arise from the presence of antibodies in the test serum that bind to non-HIV proteins on the matrix.

Sera that test positive in the EIA test are therefore subjected to Western blot tests, which also detect antibodies in the serum but which allow greater discrimination of antibodies specific for HIV proteins. In terms of number of tests performed, the most significant application of the EIA and Western blot tests is in screening donor blood to prevent transfusion-associated HIV transmission. Immunoassays have also been developed to allow detection of HIV proteins in serum; these may have the advantage of allowing HIV infection to be diagnosed prior to the production of antibodies by the infected person. Methods for the detection of HIV that have been limited to the research setting include direct assay of viral activity in cell culture and amplification of the viral genome by polymerase chain reaction (PCR). PCR amplification of HIV nucleic acids was used to demonstrate the importance of lymphoid tissues as sites for HIV multiplication.

The course of HIV infection is commonly monitored by measuring the concentration, in cells per cubic millimeter, of peripheral blood lymphocytes displaying the CD4 protein, which is the major receptor for HIV. A drop in this CD4+ T-cell count below 500 may be an indicator of progression of HIV infection beyond the clinically latent phase, and CD4+ T-cell counts are one piece of information used to determine appropriate therapies, including the initiation of antiviral drug treatment and secondary infection prophylaxis. CD4+ T-cell counts can be obtained by a variation of flow cytometry known as fluorescence-activated cell sorting, or FACS. In FACS, leukocytes in a blood sample are incubated with antibodies specific for cell surface proteins such as CD4; the antibodies have fluorescent chemical groups attached to allow their detection by fluorometry. The antibody-labeled cells are subsequently channeled into a stream that carries them, one at a time, past a detector that measures the fluorescent intensity of each cell. FACS detectors can simultaneously distinguish fluorescent groups

attached to different antibodies, and consequently different cell surface proteins. This allows the counting of several cell populations in the same sample. For example, the ratio of lymphocytes displaying CD4 to those displaying CD8 (the cell surface protein found on cytotoxic T cells) may be significant in monitoring HIV infection.

TREATMENT AND THERAPY

By the early 1990's, the only available therapeutic agents for treating HIV infection directly were nucleoside analogues, the most widely used being zidovudine (formerly azidothymidine, or AZT). Nucleoside analogues such as zidovudine are phosphorylated in HIV-infected cells, where they interfere with the functioning of the virus' reverse transcriptase enzyme. This interference may block the production of a DNA copy of the virus' RNA genome, an essential step in HIV multiplication. Other nucleoside analogues used in HIV infection are deoxycytidine (ddC) and deoxyinosine (ddI).

Zidovudine produces measurable improvement in survival, immune reactivity, and quality of life in persons with AIDS; the benefit is significant enough that the earliest clinical trials were abandoned at six months so that placebo subjects could be offered the drug. Unfortunately, when given early in HIV infection, zidovudine has not been shown to lengthen the period of clinical latency significantly, and if given immediately after HIV exposure (as may be done in the case of needle stick injury to health care workers), may not block the establishment of HIV infection. Zidovudine therapy is usually initiated when CD4+ T-cell counts drop below 500.

Adverse reactions to zidovudine are common, the most important being suppression of blood cell formation in bone marrow, leading to leukopenia (a reduction in leukocytes) and anemia. Dosage adjustment may help, as may the co-administration of cytokines that promote granulocyte and erythrocyte formation. With severe anemia, administration of zidovudine may be temporarily withdrawn, or zidovudine may be replaced with another nucleoside analogue.

Continued administration of zidovudine can result in the selection of HIV strains that are resistant to the action of the drug, as a result of mutations in the gene for reverse transcriptase. The effect of this resistance on the clinical course of HIV infection is unknown. Concern with drug resistance and a desire to limit adverse reactions, however, has led to recommendations for multidrug therapies, in which different nucleoside analogues are administered either together or during alternate periods.

In addition to reverse transcription, potential targets for drug development include the process by which HIV attaches to host cells and the protein factors that regulate the expression of HIV genes.

Because opportunistic pathogens play such an important role in the pathology of AIDS, the control of opportunistic infections is central to the medical treatment of AIDS. Treatment of opportunistic infections is complicated by the fact that many of the relevant microorganisms are eukaryotic parasites, mycobacteria, or viruses, for which effective agents are often highly toxic and require long-term administration. Additionally, successful treatment with antimicrobials typically relies on immune responses that may not be effective in patients with AIDS. Nevertheless, early diagnosis and treatment of opportunistic infections can significantly improve the health and extend the life of persons infected with HIV. For example, treatment of *P. carinii* pneumonia with available antimicrobials, combined with the prophylactic administration of pentamidine, can dramatically limit episodes of this often-fatal opportunistic infection.

PERSPECTIVE AND PROSPECTS

There can be little doubt that the epidemiologic concentration of early Western AIDS patients among marginalized groups—homosexual men and intravenous drug users—contributed to a response that was tragically inadequate in terms of policy and resource allocation. Public concern became apparent only in the early 1980's, when the possibility of transmission by blood transfusion was revealed. This, in turn, led to a degree of irrational fear of casual transmission, contributing further to discrimination against persons infected with HIV. At one point, there was serious discussion of universal EIA testing of health care personnel, without regard to the tremendous cost of such an enterprise or the absence of evidence that health care workers could accidentally transmit HIV to their patients.

The HIV epidemic has dramatically influenced the health care system in the United States. In larger metropolitan areas, the presence of large numbers of young adults with a terminal infectious disease has contributed to a reassessment of health care objectives, with greater emphasis on patient care and health maintenance. Thanks in part to the efforts of patient advocacy groups, many HIV-infected persons are exceptionally well informed as to their medical options, leading physicians to recognize the importance of patient contribution to therapeutic decision making. One area of public health policy arising from the HIV epidemic that has affected large numbers of people is the implementation of workplace policies for preventing transmission of blood-borne pathogens. Along with minimizing exposure to HIV, such practices are likely to lead to reduced prevalence of infection with hepatitis B virus, which is far more readily transmitted.

The devastating manner in which AIDS progressively degrades the health of an HIV-infected person, along with its usually fatal outcome, tends to promote an aura of despair surrounding discussion of the disease. Certainly, AIDS has resisted many efforts at control, casting doubt on the traditional faith in biomedical solutions. It is important, however, to recognize that HIV is not a supernatural agent of evil. HIV is a virus and, from long experience, medical researchers know that viruses always possess points of vulnerability. One of these—the reverse transcriptase enzyme, which can be targeted by nucleoside analogues—has already been identified, as will others. With due recognition of predictable setbacks, there is every reason to expect continued progress in the effort to extend the lives and improve the health of persons infected with HIV.

—Kenneth A. Pidcock, Ph.D.
updated by Richard Adler, Ph.D.

See also Epidemiology; Human immunodeficiency virus (HIV); Immune system; Immunodeficiency disorders; Immunology; Kaposi's sarcoma; Sexually transmitted diseases; Terminally ill, extended care for the; Viral infections.

FOR FURTHER INFORMATION:

Biddle, Wayne. *Field Guide to Germs*. New York: Henry Holt, 1995. This comprehensive book is easily accessible to the nonspecialist and includes a discussion of nearly every virus, bacterium, and fungus known to cause human and nonhuman animal disease. The history of the microbe and the treatment of diseases are included.

Corey, Lawrence, ed. *AIDS: Problems and Prospects*. New York: W. W. Norton, 1993. A compiled collection of review articles first published in *Hospital Practice*. Some familiarity with medical terminology and concepts is helpful, though the authors have been careful to limit technical discussions. Outstanding illustrations and bibliographies are included.

Global AIDS Policy Coalition. *AIDS in the World*. Cambridge, Mass.: Harvard University Press, 1992. Considers the impact of AIDS as a global pandemic, looking at worldwide patterns of infection along with economic and political impacts. A useful source of information that is extensively documented with numerous graphs and tables.

Levy, Jay A. "Pathogenesis of Human Immunodeficiency Virus Infection." *Microbiological Reviews* 57 (March, 1993): 183-289. From a leader in AIDS research, a detailed overview of all aspects of HIV biology, including molecular events involved in its reproduction and its interaction with various host cells. Very difficult for the nonspecialist to read, but its depth makes it worth knowing about, and it should be available in almost all college libraries. Heavily referenced.

Miller, Roger, and Nava Sarver. "HIV Accesory Proteins as Therapeutic Targets." *Nature Medicine* 3, no. 4 (April, 1997): 389-394. A technical article, but one that updates the nature of HIV replication. The discussion of viral regulation illustrates potential targets for therapy.

Petrow, Steven, ed. *HIV Drug Book*. New York: Pocket Books, 1995. This book was produced by Project Information, the leading community-based AIDS treatment information and advocacy organization in the United States. Its user-friendly guide provides information on the most-used HIV/AIDS treatments.

Shilts, Randy. *And the Band Played On*. New York: St. Martin's Press, 1987. A thorough journalistic account of the United States' tragically limited response to AIDS through 1985 and the parts played by the biomedical community, politicians, journalists, and gay activists. Although the author is meticulous in placing blame, the book is admirably lacking in malice.

Sontag, Susan. *AIDS and Its Metaphors*. New York: Farrar,

New Research and Treatments

Not surprisingly, the second decade of research investigating AIDS and growth of HIV was characterized by both excitement and disappointment. Scientists developed a greater basis for understanding infection of cells by the virus, including the necessity for coreceptors working in cooperation with the CD4 protein. At the same time, a variety of therapeutic drugs were at best able to control only the progress of the disease. In 1997, it was estimated that by the end of the year, 30 million persons around the world would have contracted HIV. Through mid-1997, a total of 612,000 persons with AIDS was reported in the United States. The good news, at least in the United States, was that the rate of transmission had slowed.

Infection of cells by HIV requires the presence of the cell protein CD4, found primarily on macrophage and T helper cells. Several experiments suggested, however, that CD4 by itself was not sufficient for infection; chemokines, proteins secreted by the CD8 class of T cells, were found to modulate infection by HIV. In addition, some individuals who had been repeatedly exposed to HIV remained uninfected. Lymphocytes isolated from these persons had normal levels of CD4 protein expression.

The first coreceptor for HIV, named the fusin protein (also known as CXCR4), was discovered in 1996. Fusin was also found to bind several types of chemokines, providing an explanation for their ability to modulate HIV infection. Additional coreceptors were subsequently discovered and identified as members of the CC family of chemokine receptors: CC-CCR1-5. The CCR5 and CXCR4 coreceptors appeared to be the most crucial for HIV infection. The importance of the CCR5 coreceptor was noted with the discovery that persons resistant to HIV infection often lack a portion of the gene which encodes that protein.

Initially, the discovery of a new class of anti-AIDS drugs known as protease inhibitors provided hope for an additional means to control viral infection. Other drugs such as AZT (zidovudine) or ddI only targeted the viral reverse transcriptase, and resistant strains of the virus would shortly appear. Protease inhibitors targeted a second "weak point" of the virus: the cleavage and assembly of viral structural proteins. The first protease inhibitors, ritonavir and indinavir, were FDA-approved in 1996. Since treatment with single drugs at a time often resulted in selection of resistant strains of HIV, it was believed that combination therapy using several drugs at once might be more successful. The drug "cocktail" consisted of two inhibitors of reverse transcriptase, AZT and 3TC, plus the protease inhibitor indinavir.

Results were mixed. Although viral replication was suppressed during the course of the treatment, the virus itself remained associated with T cells in the body. The results showed no indication, however, of selection for drug-resistant strains of HIV. Nevertheless, the effectiveness of the new classes of drugs, and more aggressive treatments using existing therapies for both AIDS and AIDS-related diseases, was reflected in a decline of nearly 25 percent in the number of deaths among persons with AIDS between 1995 and 1997.

Researchers were also trying to find ways to limit mother-to-child transmission of the virus. In 1997, an estimated 850,000 children worldwide carried the virus, with an additional 300,000 infected babies born each year. Most were infected in utero by virus from the infected mother. It was found that treatment of the mother with zidovudine beginning at the fourteenth week of gestation significantly reduced transmission of the virus to the developing fetus.

Zidovudine was also found to be effective in limiting infection among health care workers accidently exposed to HIV. HIV transmission was associated with injuries among such workers when they were accidentally stuck with needles while working with HIV-positive patients. When these workers were treated prophylactically with zidovudine after exposure to the virus, the risk of transmission was significantly reduced. For this reason, the U.S. Public Health Service recommended such chemoprophylaxis after any type of occupational exposure to the virus. The eventual extension of such treatment to possible exposure related to sexual contact would seem logical.

With a greater understanding of the mechanisms by which HIV replicates, the potential grows for more effective means of treatments. Clearly, once the viral DNA has integrated into the host genetic material, elimination of the disease becomes progressively more difficult. New research is also aimed at targeting viral integrases, the enzymes utilized by HIV to insert itself into the host chromosome. Such drugs might serve to prevent the virus from "hiding," leaving it more vulnerable to existing therapies.

—*Richard Adler, Ph.D.*

Straus & Giroux, 1989. An extended essay on themes the author developed in her 1978 book *Illness as Metaphor*, applied to the AIDS epidemic. Sontag's dense writing style may not appeal to all readers, but her reflections on what AIDS is and is not contribute to rational discourse.

Stine, Gerald J. *AIDS Update: 1997*. Upper Saddle River, N.J.: Prentice Hall, 1997. An annual overview of research on AIDS. An excellent reference source on a disparate group of topics: viral replication, epidemiology, and anti-HIV therapy.

ACUPRESSURE

PROCEDURE

ANATOMY OR SYSTEM AFFECTED: Muscles, musculoskeletal system, nervous system, skin

SPECIALTIES AND RELATED FIELDS: Alternative medicine, preventive medicine, sports medicine

DEFINITION: A specialized form of massage used to stimulate the body's energy pathways.

INDICATIONS AND PROCEDURES

Acupressure is an ancient Chinese procedure which uses pressure from the fingertips, knuckles, or a blunt-tipped instrument called a *tei shin* to stimulate points on the body. (The Japanese version is known as shiatsu.) The rhythmic, moderately deep massage is used to treat muscular pain, migraines, insomnia, backaches, and gastrointestinal and gynecological problems. The procedure can be performed by the patient and is beneficial for relieving chronic pain and increasing the range of motion by loosening tight muscles. Practitioners claim that acupressure can alleviate fatigue because it opens blocked energy pathways.

USES AND COMPLICATIONS

Acupressure works on the body's organ, glandular, and muscular systems. Like acupuncture, acupressure targets designated points on the body along lines called "meridians." Meridians are not nerve pathways; rather, they correspond to energy pathways through which healthy Ch'i (pronounced "chee") energy flows. (Ch'i is comparable to the Western idea of vitality or life force.) These body points are believed to correspond to various organs and body functions. Practitioners believe that when these points are stimulated, the balance of energy in the body is restored and the patient finds relief from physical illness or disease.

Muscle tension causes the large muscle groups to contract and so restricts the flow of Ch'i. The body is then out of balance and the ability of the patient's body to deal with a physical problem is inhibited. Acupressure massage seeks to increase blood circulation, relieve muscle tension, and unblock energy pathways.

Practitioners of traditional Western medicine believe that acupressure stimulates the release of endorphins, the body's own chemicals that act as pain-blockers. Other benefits of acupressure have been recognized and accepted by tradi-

tional medicine. Acupressure is used in sports medicine to relieve muscle spasms and pain. The increased blood flow and muscle relaxation helps to minimize possible or further injury to the body. Acupressure is often used in connection with other traditional Western medical treatments because no known risks are associated with the procedure.

—*Virginia L. Salmon*

See also Acupuncture; Alternative medicine; Anxiety; Circulation; Holistic medicine; Motion sickness; Muscle sprains, spasms, and disorders; Muscles; Pain, types of; Pain management; Sports medicine; Stress; Stress reduction; Touch.

FOR FURTHER INFORMATION:

Bauer, Cathryn. *Acupressure for Everybody: Gentle, Effective Relief for More Than One Hundred Common Ailments*. New York: Henry Holt, 1991.

Gach, Michael R. *Acupressure's Potent Points: A Guide to Self-Care for Common Ailments*. New York: Bantam, 1990.

ACUPUNCTURE

PROCEDURE

ANATOMY OR SYSTEM AFFECTED: Skin

SPECIALTIES AND RELATED FIELDS: Alternative medicine, anesthesiology, preventive medicine

DEFINITION: An ancient therapy developed in China in which designated points on the skin are stimulated by the insertion of needles, the application of heat, massage, or a combination of these techniques in order to treat impaired body functions or induce anesthesia.

KEY TERMS:

Ch'i: Chinese concept of the vital essence; when Ch'i is unbalanced, disease results

meridians: designated points in the body that react to acupuncture stimulation

Yang: Chinese concept of the positive, male element of the universe

Yin: Chinese concept of the negative, female element of the universe

INDICATIONS AND PROCEDURES

The theory and practice of acupuncture is rooted in the Chinese concept of life—the Ch'i (pronounced "chee")—which, according to ancient writings, is the beginning and the end, life and death. The belief, which has been handed down for thousands of years, is that all things animate and inanimate have an internal source of energy. This energy stabilizes the chemical composition of matter, and when this matter is broken down, energy is released. The Chinese view differs from the Western view of life in its adherence to the belief that human beings are all one with the cosmos, obeying the rhythms of the natural order. This oneness with the entire universe is represented by two forces: Yin and Yang.

Yang, the positive force in human beings and nature, is

exemplified by powerful elements such as heat, energy, vitality, the lush growing period of summer, and the sun. Yin, on the other hand, is the passive, almost negative force that is most obvious during winter, when plant growth almost comes to a standstill and certain animals hibernate. The Yin force is believed to be at work nightly in humans when they sleep. People who suffer from rheumatic pains frequently claim that they can forecast a change in the weather by noting the onset of those pains, and many people respond emotionally to the flow of energy in their bodies. They can feel either full of life or deeply depressed for no apparent reason.

According to the ancient Chinese system of medicine, there are two categories of organs associated with the Ch'i: the Tsang and the Fou. The Fou is the group of organs that absorb food, digest it, and expel the waste products. They are all hollow organs such as the stomach, the large and small intestines, the bladder, and the gallbladder, and all are Yang by nature. Tsang organs are all associated with the blood—the heart, which circulates the blood around the body; the lungs, which oxygenate the blood; the spleen, which controls the red corpuscles; and the liver and the kidneys. These organs are Yin by nature. For the flow of energy to remain steady, it must pass unimpeded from one organ to another. If the organ is weak, the resultant energy that is passed on to the next organ is weakened. Acupuncture stimulates specifically designated points on the body (called "meridians") and corrects the problem.

According to the Chinese, the human "circuit" of energy is made up of twelve meridians, which stretch along the limbs from the toes and the fingers to the face and chest. There are six meridians in the upper limbs and six in the lower. Ten meridians are connected to a main organ by branches from the sympathetic nervous system, and each of these meridians contains the Ch'i, which varies in strength and is governed by the nerve impulses arising from the organs. The meridians and their attendant vessels contain the flow of energy that enables the body to function efficiently.

The meridian points that proved to be effective for certain ailments were organized, and specific names were given to each. Later, the meridian line concept was hypothesized in order to explain the effectiveness of the points. These meridian points were selected by observing the effects of stimulation on particular signs and symptoms.

According to modern medical concepts, some of these points are thought to be relating points at which the autonomic nervous system is stimulated by a specific visceral disorder. Anatomically, some of the meridian points appear to correspond to areas where a nerve appears to surface from a muscle or areas where vessels and nerves are relatively superficially located, such as areas between a muscle and a bone or between a bone and a joint. These areas are generally composed of connective tissue.

The meridians are stimulated by the insertion of needles. The needles that are commonly used range in size from the diameter of a hair to that of a sewing needle. In China, round and cutting needles are commonly used. The lengths of the needles range from approximately 0.14 millimeter to approximately 0.34 millimeter. In Europe, the needles are slightly shorter and slightly wider in diameter.

The needles are made of gold, silver, iron, platinum, or stainless steel. Stainless steel needles are most commonly used. Infection caused by needle puncture is said to be extremely rare. This may be the case because the minor injury created by the needle is controlled by biological reaction. It is routine to wipe the skin with alcohol before inserting the sterilized needle. The needle itself may be wiped with alcohol sponges before each insertion on the same patient. Needles are discarded after being used in patients with a history of jaundice or hepatitis.

Insertion of a needle requires great skill and much prac-

Meridians of the Body

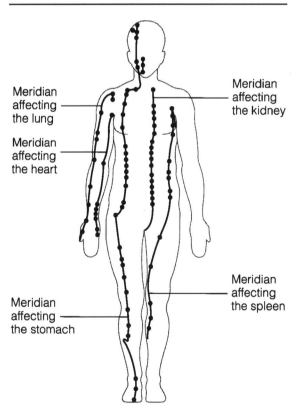

Acupuncture is an ancient Chinese medical practice based on the concept of meridians, channels in the body through which flows the life force called Ch'i; acupuncture involves the insertion and manipulation of tiny needles along these meridians.

tice. There are three different angles of penetration into the skin: perpendicular, oblique, and horizontal. These angles correspond to 90 degrees, 45 degrees, and a minimum angle, respectively. The angles may be chosen on the basis of the thickness of the skin and the proximity to muscle or bone at the desired puncture point. The depth of penetration will vary, with an average of 10, 30, and 40 millimeters in the head, shoulder, and back regions, respectively.

Tapping (the tube method) is one method of insertion: When the diameter of the needle is small, this method is extremely effective. The needle is placed into the tube from either direction, and the tube is shorter than the needle by 5 millimeters or more. Gentle tapping of the needle handle with the right index finger introduces the needle easily. The tapping finger must be removed from the needle head immediately; otherwise, it causes pain. The tube is removed gently with the right index finger and thumb.

In the twirling method (the freehand method), the left thumb and index finger make contact at the acupuncture point. The left hand is called the pushing hand. Next, the skin is cut with the needle tip, after which the needle is inserted by pushing and twirling it with the right hand.

The objective of the advancement of the needle and the needle motion is to create a needle feeling in the patient.

This is a dull, aching, paralyzing, or compressing feeling or a combination of these sensations that radiates to a distal or proximal portion of the body. When the patient notices the needle feeling, the operator increases the feeling by using various needle motions. Numerous motions are available, such as the single-stick, twirling, vibration, intermittent, and retention motions.

Light skin and muscle massage is recommended in order to prepare the body to accept needle stimulation. Prepuncture massage makes skin cutting easier and helps the patient relax. In addition to these advantages, massage may make it possible to detect pathologies such as nodules, spasms, pain, and depression. Postpuncture massage helps to confirm muscle hypersensitivity and the disappearance of pain or hard nodules that existed before the acupuncture was performed.

The amount of stimulation equals the strength of stimulation multiplied by the number of treatments; this is dependent on the sensitivity of the patient. Gradual increases of stimulation are essential. In general, for acute disease, treatment is usually given once a day for ten days and then terminated for three to seven days. For chronic ailments, treatment is administered once every two to three days for ten treatments and then terminated for seven days. The pa-

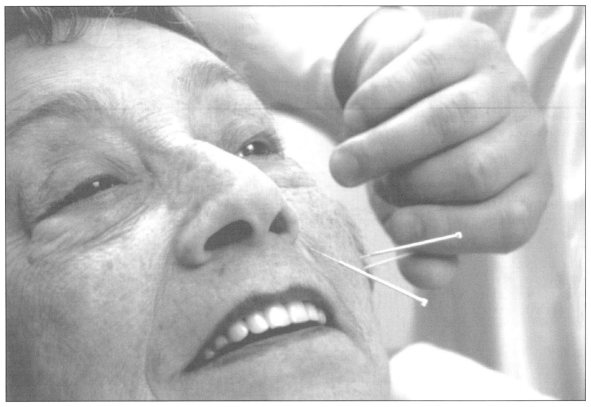

The use of acupuncture to supplement traditional medicine has been growing in acceptance. This woman is receiving acupuncture treatment to relieve pain. (Dan McCoy/Rainbow)

tient is placed in a supine, sitting, prone, or side position—the position that is most convenient for the patient and physician. A special position, however, may be needed in order to relax the painful area.

One of the most important factors to be considered in effective acupuncture is the accurate selection of acupuncture points. These points must be selected according to the specific ailment. The precise location of acupuncture points is crucial for obtaining the maximum therapeutic effect. This is difficult because of the different sizes and shapes of patients' bodies. Each acupuncture point is considered to be only about 3 millimeters in diameter.

USES AND COMPLICATIONS

Excluding pain caused by cerebral pathology, there are certain mechanisms of pain that are universally recognized. These are causal factors (stimuli), such as inflammation or trauma, the peripheral nervous system, and the brain. Acupuncture, which is one mode of stimulation therapy, works by changing the pattern of passage of stimulation from the peripheral nerves to the central nervous system. Stimulation treatments such as hot soaks and the management of certain pain problems with physical therapy have long been in existence. Chinese medicine has accumulated experiences, analyzed the quality of stimulation, and organized its findings into a medical system.

The basic approach of modern medicine involves removing the causal factor of disease. In this approach, the pain associated with disease or with a surgical procedure may not be eradicated instantaneously, however, and the management of pain becomes an issue until the disease is cured or until the surgery and recuperation are complete. Controlling chemical receptors and reducing the sensitivity of those receptors is one way of treating pain. Intensive studies of the stimulation that causes pain have indicated that intrinsic chemical substances (polypeptides) such as histamine and serotonin, which stimulate the receptors, are essential for pain. Therefore, an antagonistic drug for these chemicals is often effective in controlling pain.

Although acupuncture is used to treat conditions as diverse as allergies, circulatory disorders, dermatologic disorders, gastrointestinal disorders, genital disorders, musculoskeletal disorders, neurologic disorders, and psychiatric and emotional disorders, the use of acupuncture for pain control (analgesia) can be described as the most basic level of treatment.

The English words "anesthesia" and "analgesia" are misleading when used to describe the freedom from surgical or obstetrical pain that can be produced by acupuncture. If "analgesia" is described as insensibility to pain without loss of consciousness, it is a more appropriate word than "anesthesia," which is described as an insensibility, general or local, induced by anesthetic agents, and a loss of sensation of neurogenic or psychogenic origin.

Acupuncture does not alter the level of consciousness or produce numbness of any part of the body. The patient under acupuncture analgesia remains able to converse and cooperate with the surgical or obstetrical team. Obstetric patients are aware of uterine contractions and are able to use their muscles to bring forth the fetus. Surgical patients can tell when incisions are made but do not perceive them as painful. There is no loss of memory, as in hypnosis or general anesthesia, and no paresthesia (abnormal sensations) comparable to the sensations following local anesthesia.

Most operating room deaths and cardiac arrests in the United States are caused by chemical anesthesia rather than by surgery. Patients who are poor anesthetic risks because of heart, liver, or kidney disease tolerate acupuncture analgesia well. Infants and elderly individuals are also good candidates for acupuncture.

Although acupuncture does not alter the level of consciousness, it can be used to induce a feeling of well-being and calmness to allay the fear and apprehension most patients feel before surgery. It also appears to reduce both bleeding during surgical procedures and the incidence of shock. Postoperative acupuncture analgesia patients are spared from nausea and the difficulties with urinating and defecating that frequently follow chemical anesthesia. Acupuncture analgesia does not mask symptoms as chemical anesthetics and analgesics do. The patient remains aware of his or her symptoms, but acupuncture diminishes those symptoms to a tolerable level.

Postoperative pain does not usually occur for several hours after acupuncture analgesia has been terminated. When it does occur, acupuncture can be used again instead of narcotics, and the treatment seldom needs to be repeated more than once or twice. Some acupuncturists leave small needles superficially inserted for several days to give postoperative pain relief. Others give regular acupuncture treatments, leaving the needles in place for twenty minutes per day for as many days as are necessary.

The main disadvantage of acupuncture analgesia is that it is less reliable than chemical analgesia or anesthesia. In some cases, acupuncture analgesia cannot be induced or becomes inadequate during a surgical procedure. It may not produce the relaxation desirable for some abdominal surgery. For this reason, backup chemical anesthetics and analgesics are also available in most cases.

The actual induction of acupuncture analgesia takes about twenty minutes—slightly longer than chemical anesthesia. In most cases, electroacupuncture instruments must remain attached to all acupuncture needles during the entire procedure, but these can usually be kept away from the surgical field. The more skilled the acupuncturist, the fewer the needles required. In China, major surgical procedures have been performed with only one acupuncture needle as analgesia and without electric supplementation.

The same type of thin (usually 30-gauge) stainless steel needles that are used for acupuncture treatments are used for acupuncture analgesia. In general, the points that are used to relieve chronic pain in a specific area are the points of choice for analgesia. To obtain enough analgesia for surgery, it is usually necessary to heighten the effect of the acupuncture needles by twirling them continually or by attaching electronic instruments to them to deliver a current of about 200 microamperes, with a pulsating wave at a frequency of 200 per minute during the entire procedure. The use of electronic instruments will usually increase the depth of analgesia or prolong an analgesic effect that is beginning to wear off.

Besides the acupuncture points for analgesia of specific areas of the body, points are often used to relieve anxiety and promote a feeling of well-being. These are usually inserted for twenty minutes the evening before surgery as well as for at least twenty minutes before the actual surgery begins.

The theoretical principles of vital energy transmission are used in determining which acupuncture points should be effective for the anticipated surgery. Acupuncture points on meridians passing directly through, or in the vicinity of, the surgical area are usually selected. An attempt is made to use points on these meridians that are as far away from the surgical field as possible.

PERSPECTIVE AND PROSPECTS

According to most reports, acupuncture appears to have been developed in the northernmost area of the middle region of China around 300 B.C. People in this area were primarily nomads, moving from one area to another in an attempt to avoid cold weather. They were peace-loving people, but from time to time were forced to fight, either to repel invaders or to recover territory that had been occupied. The weapons they normally used were spears and bows and arrows, which inflicted grotesque wounds.

The high priests of China, like the high priests of biblical times in the Middle East, were also the society's physicians. These Chinese priests observed that men who were wounded in combat often reported the sudden disappearance of illnesses from which they had suffered for years. For example, a wound in a specific area of the foot would reduce blood pressure or relieve a headache or toothache, or an injury on the dorsal aspect of the knee joint would cure migraine. Over the years, the high priests recorded numerous observations of the phenomenon of a wound in one part of the body curing a long-standing complaint at another point. They discovered that it was the location of the wound that was significant. A pinprick in the correct location was enough to effect relief. It was noted that certain points of the body responded more noticeably to stimulation than other points and that frequently there was a direct correlation between the points that were responsive and a particular ailment. These points were subsequently named "meridian points."

At a later time, when metal was introduced to the culture,

needles were used as an irritant at meridian points, and it was thought that pain from a specific ailment was diverted in a linear fashion through the meridian points to the surface of the body. Thus the concept of the "meridian line" was developed. Thus acupuncture was discovered.

At first, the surgeon-priests used fish bones and sharpened splinters of bamboo to effect the pricks. Later came finely honed needles. The warlords and nobles were treated with needles forged from gold and silver. As the science of acupuncture developed, it was discovered that the needles needed only to be inserted in a point of skin measuring about one-tenth of an inch.

The earliest book describing acupuncture was written in 50 B.C. It described the clinical applications of acupuncture with anatomical physiological references that were based principally on the concept of the meridian lines of the body.

In 1911, Yüan Shih-K'ai, who had trained in a modern Western culture, formed the Republic of China. Under his rule, old Chinese medicine—including acupuncture—which had developed from tradition and experience, was unable to survive except in outlying areas of China. In 1949, however, when Mao Tse-tung formed the People's Republic of China, he tried to repopularize the old methods of Chinese medicine, which had been helpful to him. In the 1930's, when Mao and his followers were retreating to the north, he was forced to depend mainly on these traditional methods for medical treatment.

In 1955, Shyuken, a follower of Mao, stated his belief that acupuncture was effective in the management of illness. He wished to study the ancient Chinese way of medicine more systematically, comparing it to Western medicine, which he believed to be too analytical. Thus, a new medical movement began that united Western and Chinese medical practices.

Stimulation therapy using local heat, massage, and pressure has been known since ancient times. Long periods of observations and analysis by Chinese physicians of the effects on signs and symptoms of irritation of varying degrees at particular points on the body surface made it possible to relate specific points on the body (meridian points) to specific conditions.

According to ancient Chinese clinical concepts, the meridian points served as peeping holes into the body and passing holes for energy. The total number of meridian points was believed to be 365. Each was named according to its effect, anatomical location, appearance, and relation to the meridian line. These meridian points were selected initially according to measurements based on the patient's own unique anatomical standard (using the length between certain anatomical points; for example, between the shoulders). The exact location of a meridian point was then selected by the examiner, who felt with his or her fingertips the areas chosen by the initial measurement and observed the patient's response.

Acupuncture's popularity, like that of most techniques and discoveries, has waxed and waned throughout the years; for the most part, however, the Chinese have remained faithful to the five-thousand-year-old practice. The laws and method of acupuncture have endured, although these methods have been increasingly combined with Western medical techniques. Gradually, the practice of acupuncture has spread throughout the world, particularly in France, Russia, Japan, Switzerland, Germany, and the United States.
—*Genevieve Slomski, Ph.D.*

See also Acupressure; Addiction; Alternative medicine; Anesthesia; Anesthesiology; Anxiety; Circulation; Holistic medicine; Motion sickness; Muscle sprains, spasms, and disorders; Muscles; Pain, types of; Pain management; Sports medicine; Stress; Stress reduction.

FOR FURTHER INFORMATION:

Austin, Mary. *Acupuncture Therapy.* New York: ASI, 1972. As a physician and a student who has been trained in both Eastern and Western medicine, the author helps to dispel misconceptions about the philosophy, methods, and practice of acupuncture. The author stresses that all methods of acupuncture work with energy rather than disease—a concept that is foreign to orthodox Western medicine. Fully illustrated.

Duke, Marc. *Acupuncture.* New York: Pyramid House, 1972. An introductory account of the history, classical philosophy, and theory of medical acupuncture. The author argues that because of a combination of ignorance and prejudice in American physicians, the U.S. medical establishment lags behind every nation in the world in its knowledge of Chinese medicine. Bibliography and useful appendices.

Manaka, Yoshio, and Ian A. Urquhart. *The Layman's Guide to Acupuncture.* New York: Weatherhill, 1972. Two leading acupuncture authorities draw on their extensive clinical experience as well as current research findings to introduce the principles and practice of acupuncture. In addition, the authors discuss diagnosis, various treatment procedures, and empirical results. Numerous photographs, illustrations, and appendices.

Mann, Felix. *Scientific Aspects of Acupuncture.* London: William Heinemann, 1977. This scholarly work, written by a practicing acupuncture therapist, attempts to explain certain aspects of acupuncture in terms of science. It is not a scientific textbook of acupuncture; the book's purpose is to initiate the neurophysiological approach to acupuncture. Illustrated.

Stux, Gabriel, and Bruce Pomeranz. *Basics of Acupuncture.* 3d ed. New York: Springer-Verlag, 1995. An updated reference on acupuncture that provides details about the procedure. Also examines the history of acupuncture treatment.

Tan, Leong T., et al. *Acupuncture Therapy.* 2d rev. ed. Philadelphia: Temple University Press, 1976. A useful introduction to the theory and practice of acupuncture. The authors state that acupuncture, as a simple, efficient, and effective means of medical therapy, has successfully withstood the tests of time and scrutiny, earning acceptance in the United States. Numerous charts and illustrations. Bibliography.

ADDICTION
DISEASE/DISORDER
ANATOMY OR SYSTEM AFFECTED: Brain, nervous system, psychic-emotional system
SPECIALTIES AND RELATED FIELDS: Psychiatry, psychology
DEFINITION: A psychological and sometimes physiological process whereby an organism comes to depend on a substance; addiction is defined by a persistent need to use the substance and to increase the dosage used as a result of tolerance, as well as the experience of withdrawal symptoms when the substance is withheld or use is reduced.

KEY TERMS:
abstinence: complete, voluntary refrainment from the use of a substance of abuse
compulsion: a persistent, irresistible urge to perform a stereotyped behavior or irrational act, often accompanied by repetitious thoughts (obsessions) about the behavior
pharmacodynamics: changes in tissue sensitivity or physiologic systems in response to pharmacological substances
pharmacokinetics: the action of pharmacological substances within a biological system; pharmacologic substance absorption, distribution, metabolism, and elimination by an organism
physiological dependence: a state of tissue adaptation to a substance of abuse marked by tolerance and withdrawal
positive reinforcement: a process that increases the frequency or probability of a response and increases the strength of a learning process
psychological dependence: habitual substance use across various situations, or a persistent need for a substance for the sense of well-being provided by its reinforcing properties
substance abuse: the continued use of a psychoactive substance for at least one month despite impairment of psychological, social, occupational, or physical functioning
tolerance: a condition in which the same dose achieves a lesser effect, or in which successively greater doses of an abusable substance are required to achieve the same desired effect
withdrawal: a physical and mental condition following decreased intake of an abusable substance, with symptoms ranging from anxiety to convulsions

CAUSES AND SYMPTOMS
Addiction is a disorder that can affect any animal and may result from the use of a variety of psychoactive substances. Typically, it involves both psychological and physi-

ological dependence. Psychological dependence is marked by compulsions to use a substance of abuse because of its reinforcing qualities. Physiological dependence results when the body responds to the presence of the addictive substance. Tolerance, withdrawal, and significant decreases in psychological, social, and occupational dysfunction characterize physiological dependence.

Tolerance involves pharmacokinetics, pharmacodynamics, and environmental or behavioral conditioning. Pharmacokinetics refers to the way in which a biological system, such as a human body, processes a drug. Substances are subject to absorption into the bloodstream, distribution to different organs (such as the brain and liver), metabolization by these organs, and then elimination. Over time, the processes of distribution and metabolism may change, such that the body eliminates the substance more efficiently. Thus, the substance has less opportunity to affect the system than it did initially, reducing any desired effects. As a result, dose increases are needed to achieve the initial or desired effect.

Pharmacodynamics refers to changes in the body as a result of a pharmacologic agent being present. Tissue within the body responds differently to the substance at the primary sites of action. For example, changes in sensitivity may occur at specific sites within the brain, directly or indirectly impacting the primary action site. Direct changes at the primary sites of action denote tissue sensitivity. An example might be an increase in the number of receptors in the brain for that particular substance. Indirect changes in tissue remote from the primary action sites denote tissue tolerance, or functional tolerance. In functional tolerance, physiologic systems that oppose the action of the drug compensate by increasing their effect. Once either type of tolerance develops, the only way for the desired effect to be achieved is for the dose of the substance to be increased.

Finally, environmental or behavioral conditioning is involved in the development of tolerance. Organisms associate the reinforcing properties of substances with the contexts in which the drugs are experienced. Such contexts may be physical environments, such as places, or emotional contexts, such as when the individual is depressed or anxious. Over the course of repeated administrations in the same context, the tolerance that develops is associated with that specific context. Thus, an organism may experience tolerance to a drug in one situation, but not another. Greater doses of the reinforcing substance would be needed to achieve the same effect in the former situation, but not in the latter.

Tolerance develops differently depending on the type of substance taken, the dose ingested, and the routes of administration used. Larger doses may contribute to quicker development of tolerance. Similarly, routes of administration that produce more rapid and efficient absorption of a substance into the bloodstream tend to increase the likeli-

hood of an escalating pattern of substance abuse leading to dependence. For many drugs, injection and inhalation are two of the fastest routes of administration, while oral ingestion is one of the slowest. Other routes include intranasal, transdermal, rectal, sublingual, and intraocular administration.

For some substances, the development of tolerance also depends on the pattern of substance use. For example, even though two individuals might use the same amount of alcohol, it is possible for tolerance to develop more quickly in one person than in the other. Two individuals might each drink fourteen drinks per week, but they would develop tolerance at different rates if one consumes two drinks each of seven nights and the other consumes seven drinks each of two nights in a week. Because of their patterns of use, the first drinker would develop tolerance much more slowly than the second, all other things being equal.

Withdrawal occurs when use of the substance significantly decreases. Withdrawal varies by the substance of abuse and ranges from being minor or nonexistent with some drugs (such as hallucinogens) to quite pronounced with other drugs (such as alcohol). Mild symptoms include anxiety, tension, restlessness, insomnia, impaired attention, and irritability. Severe symptoms include convulsions, perceptual distortions, irregular tremors, high blood pressure, and rapid heartbeat. Typically, withdrawal symptoms can be alleviated or extinguished by readministration of the substance of abuse. Thus, a compounding problem is that the addicted individual often learns to resume drug use in order to avoid the withdrawal symptoms.

Addiction occurs with both legal and illegal drugs. Alcohol and nicotine are two of the most widely abused legal addictive drugs. Over-the-counter drugs, such as sleeping aids, and prescription drugs, such as tranquilizers (for example, sedative-hypnotics) and antianxiety agents, also have addiction potential. Common illegal addictive drugs include cocaine, marijuana, hallucinogens, heroin, and methamphetamine.

Not everyone who uses these substances will automatically become addicted. In the United States, for example, surveys have shown that approximately 65 percent of adults drink alcohol each year. In contrast, less than 13 percent of the population goes on to develop alcohol problems serious enough to warrant a medical diagnosis of alcohol abuse or dependence. Similarly, despite the fact that large numbers of individuals are prescribed opiates or sedative-hypnotics for pain while hospitalized, roughly 0.7 percent of the adult population is addicted to opiates and 1.1 percent is addicted to sedative-hypnotics or antianxiety drugs. Thus, the development of addiction often requires repeated substance administration, as well as other biological and environmental factors.

When addiction is present, the consequences are multiple and complex. While substance abuse involves deteriorated functioning in psychological, social, occupational, or physical functioning, substance dependence usually involves more severe problems in each of these areas for significantly longer amounts of time. Psychologically, problems with depression, anxiety, the ability to think clearly or remember information, motivation, judgment, and one's sense of self may result. Socially, one can become isolated from friends and family, or even unable to deal with the stresses and demands of normal, everyday relationships. Finally, occupational disruptions can result from the inability to plan, to manage one's feelings and thoughts, and to deal with social interactions.

In terms of health, there are many acute and chronic effects of addiction. With cocaine, for example, acute cardiac functioning may be affected, such that the risk of heart attacks is increased. Similarly, individuals addicted to opiates, alcohol, and sedative-hypnotics must contend with such risks as falling into a coma or experiencing depressed respiratory functioning. Finally, the acute effects of any of these drugs can impair judgments and contribute to careless behavior. As a result, accidents, severe trauma, and habitually dangerous behavior, such as risky sexual behavior, may be associated with addiction.

Chronic health consequences are common. Smoking is associated with cancers of the mouth, throat, and lungs, as well as premature deterioration of the skin. Alcohol is associated with cancers of the mouth, throat, and stomach, as well as ulcers and liver problems. General malnutrition is a risk for heroin and alcohol users, since they often fail to eat properly. Injected drugs such as heroin and cocaine are associated with problems such as hepatitis and acquired immunodeficiency syndrome (AIDS), since shared needles may transmit blood-borne diseases. Finally, addiction contributes to health problems in the unborn children of addicted individuals. Problems such as low birth weight in the children of smokers, fetal alcohol syndrome in the children of female drinkers, and withdrawal difficulties in the children born to other types of addicts are well documented.

TREATMENT AND THERAPY

Because of the combination of psychological and physiological dependence, addiction is a disorder that often demands both psychological and pharmacological treatments. Typically, interventions focus on decreasing or stopping the substance use and reestablishing normal psychological, social, occupational, and physical functioning in the addicted individual. Though the length and type of treatments may vary with the particular addictive drug and the duration of the addiction problem, similar principles are involved in the treatment of all addictions.

Psychological treatments focus primarily on extinguishing psychological dependence, as well as on facilitating more effective functioning by the addicted individual in other areas of life. Attempts to change the behavior and thinking of the addicted individual usually involve some combination of individual, group, and family therapy. Adjunctive training in new occupational skills and healthier lifestyle habits are also common.

In general, treatment focuses on understanding how the addictive behavior developed, how it was maintained, and how it can be removed from the person's daily life. Assessments of the situations in which the drug was used, the needs for which the drug was used, and alternative means of addressing those needs are primary to this understanding. Once these issues are identified, a therapist then works with the client to break habitual behavior patterns that were contributing to the addiction (for example, driving through neighborhoods where drugs might be sold, going to business meetings at restaurants that serve alcohol, or maintaining relationships with drug-using friends). Concurrently, the therapist helps the client design new behavior patterns that will decrease the odds of continued problems with addiction. Problems related to the drug use would then be addressed in some combination of individual, family, or group therapy.

The therapy or therapies selected depend on the problems related to drug use. For example, family therapy might be more appropriate in cases in which family conflicts are related to drug use. In contrast, individual therapy might be more appropriate for someone whose drug use is linked to thinking distortions or mood problems. Similarly, group therapy might be most appropriate for individuals lacking social support to deal with stress, or whose social interactions are contributing to their drug use. Regardless of the type of therapy, however, the basic goal remains: facilitating the client's solving of his or her specific problems. Additionally, the development of new ways of coping with intractable problems, rather than relying on drug use as a means of coping, would be critical.

Cognitive and behavioral therapies have been quite useful for breaking the conditioned effects of addiction. Some psychological dependence, for example, is based on placebo effects. A placebo effect occurs as a result of what people believe a drug is doing for them, rather than from anything that the drug actually has the power to accomplish. In addition, the practice of using addictive drugs within certain contexts is associated with drug tolerance, such that certain situations trigger compulsions leading to drug use. In this way, cognitive therapy can be used to challenge any faulty thinking associations that individuals have made about what the drugs do for them in different situations. This may involve increasing patients' awareness of the negative consequences of their drug use and challenging what they perceive to be its positive consequences. As a complement, such therapies correct distorted thinking that is related to coping with stressful situations or situations in which drug use might be especially tempting. In such situations, individuals might actually have the skill to handle the stress or temptation without using drugs. Without the confidence that they can successfully manage these situations, however, they may not even try, instead reverting to drug use. As such, therapy facilitating realistic thinking about stress and coping abilities can be quite beneficial.

Similarly, behavioral therapies are used to break down conditioned associations between situations and drug use. For example, smokers are sometimes made to smoke not in accordance with their desire to smoke, but according to a schedule over which they have no control. As a result, they are made to smoke at times or in situations where it is inconvenient, leading to an association between unpleasant feelings and smoking. While such assigned drug use would not be used with illegal drugs, the basic principles of increasing negative or unpleasant feelings with drug use in specific situations can be used. Rewarding abstinence has also been a successful approach to treatment. In this way, positive reinforcement is associated with abstinence and may contribute to behaviors related to abstinence being more common than behaviors related to drug use.

Pharmacological treatments concentrate on decreasing physical dependence on the substance of abuse. They rely on behavioral principles and on five primary strategies. The first strategy, based on positive reinforcement, is pharmacological replacement. Prescribed drugs with similar effects at the sites of action as the addictive drug are used. These prescribed drugs, however, usually fail to have reinforcing properties as powerful as the addictive drug and focus mainly on preventing the occurrence of withdrawal symptoms. Nicotine patches for smokers and methadone for heroin users are examples of replacement therapies.

A second strategy involves the use of both reinforcement and extinction, the behavioral process of decreasing and eventually extinguishing the drug-taking behavior. Partially reinforcing and partially antagonistic drugs are prescribed. The net effect is that the prescribed drug staves off withdrawal symptoms, but yields less reinforcement than drug replacement therapy, serving to facilitate the process of extinction for the drug taking.

Antagonists, or drugs that completely block the receptors responsible for the reinforcing effects of the drug action, are prescribed alone as a third strategy. With this strategy, extinction is the primary behavioral principle in effect. The prescribed drug blocks the primary receptor sites and does not yield positively reinforcing drug effects. Even if the addictive drug is taken in addition to the antagonist, no positively reinforcing effects are experienced. Thus, without reinforcement, drug-taking behavior should eventually cease. Naltrexone, typically used for opiate addiction, is a good example of this strategy.

Punishment is another behavioral principle used in pharmacological therapy. Metabolic inhibitors, or drugs that make the effects of the addictive substance more toxic, are often used to discourage drug use. Antabuse, a drug often given for problems with alcohol, is such a substance. When metabolic inhibitors are prescribed, individuals using these drugs in combination with their substance of abuse experience toxic and unpleasant effects. Thus, they begin to associate use of the addictive substance with very noxious results and are discouraged from continuing their drug use.

Symptomatic treatment of withdrawal effects is used as a fifth strategy. Based on reinforcement, this strategy simply encourages the use of drugs likely to reduce withdrawal effects. Unfortunately, these drugs may also have abuse potential. For example, when benzodiazepines are given to individuals with alcohol or opiate dependence, one dependency may be traded for another. As such, symptomatic treatment is helpful but is not a treatment of choice by itself. In fact, none of these pharmacological treatments is recommended for use in isolation; they are recommended for use with complementary psychological treatments.

PERSPECTIVE AND PROSPECTS

The use of substances to alter the mind or bodily experiences is a practice that has been a part of human cultures for centuries. Time and again, even through legislated acts such as Prohibition, drug and alcohol use have persisted. The continued use of drugs for recreational and medicinal practices seems virtually inevitable, and it is unlikely that substance abuse and dependence will disappear from the world's societies. Consequently, an understanding of substance use, how it leads to addiction, ways to minimize the development of addiction problems, and strategies for improving addiction treatments will be critical.

At different times in history, addiction has been viewed as strictly a moral, medical, spiritual, or behavioral problem. As the science of understanding and treating addiction has progressed, the variety of ways in which these aspects of addiction combine has been noted. Modern treatments and theories no longer view addiction from one strict point of view, but instead recognize the heterogeneity of paths leading to addiction. Such an approach has been helpful not only in treating addiction but also in preventing it. Efforts to curb the biological, social, and environmental forces contributing to addiction have become increasingly important.

Addiction remains a disorder with no completely effective treatment. Of individuals seeking treatment across all addictive disorders, fewer than 20 percent succeed the first time that they attempt to achieve long-term abstinence. As a result, individuals suffering from addiction often undergo multiple treatments over several occasions, with some individuals experiencing significant problems throughout their lives. Even though treatments for physiological and psychological dependence offer some improvement, much work remains to be done. In this context, the challenge ahead is not to prevent all substance use, but rather to decrease the odds that a person will become addicted. Improving the pharmacological and psychological treatments currently available will be important. Discoveries of new

New Research and Treatments

Recent advances in biological research on addiction have involved efforts to study the function of different areas of the brain. Nuclear magnetic resonance imaging (MRI) and positron emission tomography (PET) scans have both been used. The most recent research efforts in addiction are on the role of dopamine receptors in the reinforcing effects of different drugs. Studies in this area have focused primarily on alcohol and cocaine and have also examined the influence of comorbid disorders such as antisocial personality disorder.

Exciting developments in treatment have occurred. The first nationwide study examining the effects of matching treatments to clients with alcohol problems concluded its initial phase. This United States-based study, Project MATCH, was supported by the National Institute on Alcohol Abuse and Alcoholism. It was designed to examine the effect of matching clients to one of three individual treatment approaches—cognitive-behavioral, twelve-step facilitation, or motivational enhancement—based on psychosocial characteristics of the participants, such as severity of problems or the presence of other mental health problems. Results of this study suggested that all clients gain positive benefits from participating in assessment and treatment. Additionally, the data suggested that clients without other severe psychiatric symptoms do better in twelve-step facilitation treatment than clients with more severe problems, relative to the other two treatments.

Another exciting development has been the discovery of the utility of naltrexone, a drug commonly used in the treatment of opioid addiction, in the early phases of successful response to treatment for alcohol dependence when it is combined with psychosocial therapies. In ad-

dition, investigators have been studying how alternative medicine approaches might be of use for substance abuse treatment. Examples are the use of acupuncture and massage in the treatment of illicit substance use, such as stimulant use. While results in this area are promising, it is important to note that none of these treatments should be used alone, but rather as an adjunct to traditional treatment approaches.

Other areas where addiction research has developed includes study of a recent increase in heroin use in the United States among teenagers and young adults. Survey data suggest that these increases are being demonstrated in more individuals smoking heroin and other opioids, rather than through injection use. While this route of administration will prevent the transmission of HIV through needle-sharing, it remains dangerous, as overdose among inexperienced users is a likely possibility.

An emerging area of "new" addiction has been the phenomenon of Internet addiction, or compulsive use of on-line services such as e-mail and chat rooms. Such "addictions" (like gambling and workaholism) are not true addictions, but they share enough features with other addictive behaviors involving substance use to be studied together. Additionally, these behaviors may often coexist in persons who have dependence on substances of abuse, so there is a clear need to study them simultaneously.

Future investigation of such comorbities is likely to increase and expand into the study of such behavior in diverse populations, such as the elderly. Such work will be important as more elderly are in situations where they are required to use medicinal drugs that can interact with drugs of abuse. —*Nancy A. Piotrowski, Ph.D.*

ways of tailoring treatment for addiction to the needs and backgrounds of the different individuals affected will be one critical task for health professionals. Continued exploration of new pharmacological treatments to combat withdrawal and facilitate abstinence is necessary.

—*Nancy A. Piotrowski, Ph.D.*

See also Alcoholism; Eating disorders; Narcotics; Obsessive-compulsive disorder; Psychiatry; Psychology; Stress.

FOR FURTHER INFORMATION:

American Psychiatric Association. *Diagnostic and Statistical Manual of Mental Disorders*. 4th ed. Washington, D.C.: Author, 1994. This manual provides detailed descriptions of the behaviors and types of symptoms used to describe and diagnose different addictive disorders. It is written by mental health professionals from psychiatric, psychological, and social work backgrounds.

Brickman, Philip, et al. "Models of Helping and Coping." *American Psychologist* 37 (April, 1982): 368-384. This article describes a four-model perspective on helping and coping with problems related to addiction. A classic in the addiction field, providing a good review of historical factors influencing different treatment models.

Dupont, Robert L. *The Selfish Brain: Learning from Addiction*. Washington, D.C.: American Psychiatric Association, 1997. Discusses the commonalities across different types of addiction in an easy-to-understand manner.

Julien, Robert M. *A Primer of Drug Action*. 5th ed. New York: W. H. Freeman, 1988. A nontechnical guide to drugs written by a medical professional. Describes the different classes of drugs, their actions in the body, their uses, and their side effects. Basic pharmacologic principles, classifications, and terms are defined and discussed.

Miller, William R., and Nick Heather, eds. *Treating Addictive Behaviors: Processes of Change*. New York: Plenum Press, 1986. This book, written by medical and psychological scientists, is an overview of treatment strategies for problems ranging from nicotine to opiate addiction. Psychological, behavioral, interpersonal, familial, and medical approaches are outlined and discussed.

Schlaadt, Richard G., and Peter T. Shannon. *Drugs of Choice: Current Perspectives on Drug Use*. Englewood Cliffs, N.J.: Prentice Hall, 1982. A good introduction to the complex issues surrounding addiction and drug use. Describes different drugs of abuse, individual differences in drug use, legal and social issues, and continuing controversies. Also included is an overview of the differences between illegal and legal drugs, as well as drug myths and facts.

Weil, Andrew, and Winifred Rosen. *From Chocolate to Morphine: Everything You Need to Know About Mind-Altering Drugs*. Rev. ed. Boston: Houghton Mifflin, 1993. This book on psychoactive substances provides basic information to the general reader. Psychoactive substances are identified and defined. Also outlines the relationships between different types of drugs, the motivations to use drugs, and associated problems. As the title suggests, the discussion ranges from legal, caffeinated substances to illegal and prescription drugs.

ADDISON'S DISEASE
DISEASE/DISORDER

ANATOMY OR SYSTEM AFFECTED: Endocrine system, glands

SPECIALTIES AND RELATED FIELDS: Endocrinology

DEFINITION: Addison's disease, also known as adrenal insufficiency or adrenal hypofunction, is a chronic condition in which the adrenal glands do not produce adequate amounts of corticosteroid hormones. Symptoms include fatigue, dizziness, nausea, diarrhea, weight loss, a weak and irregular pulse, and a general darkening of the skin and mucous membranes. These symptoms are easily managed with corticosteroid drugs over the patient's lifetime, but with injury, surgery, or stress—when the body's immune system is compromised—acute episodes of the disease can occur. These Addisonian crises, or adrenal crises, require hospitalization. The disease was fatal before hormone replacement therapy was developed, but proper long-term care and prompt treatment when crises occur can allow patients to live with the disease.

—Jason Georges and Tracy Irons-Georges

See also Adrenalectomy; Endocrine disorders; Glands; Hormones.

ADENOID REMOVAL. *See* TONSILLECTOMY AND ADENOID REMOVAL.

ADOLESCENCE. *See* PUBERTY AND ADOLESCENCE.

ADRENAL DISORDERS. *See* ADDISON'S DISEASE; CUSHING'S SYNDROME.

ADRENALECTOMY
PROCEDURE

ANATOMY OR SYSTEM AFFECTED: Abdomen, endocrine system, glands, kidneys, urinary system

SPECIALTIES AND RELATED FIELDS: Endocrinology, general surgery

DEFINITION: Adrenalectomy is the surgical removal of the adrenal glands. The adrenal glands produce chemical substances which regulate the body's responses to stress, including the "fight or flight" response and less immediate physical changes. Occasionally, if the adrenal glands become diseased (for example, with cancer) or the hormones that they produce aggravate another condition (such as breast cancer), a physician may determine that they must be surgically removed. This major surgical procedure entails opening the abdomen with a transverse incision and exploring the organs of the abdominal cavity for disease. The colon and a portion of the small intestine are moved to expose the kidneys. After the adrenal veins and arteries are sealed, each gland is dissected from its position at the top of each kidney. Internal organs are replaced, drains are brought out through the incisions, and the incisions are closed. The procedure may also be performed by a posterior approach through the rib cage. Complications of abdominal surgery are possible, including infection and internal bleeding. The patient is closely monitored and given oral supplements for the hormones normally provided by the adrenal glands.

—Karen E. Kalumuck, Ph.D.

See also Abdomen; Abdominal disorders; Cancer; Endocrinology; Glands; Hormones; Kidneys; Nephrectomy.

AGING
BIOLOGY

ANATOMY OR SYSTEM AFFECTED: Psychic-emotional system, all bodily systems

SPECIALTIES AND RELATED FIELDS: Audiology, cardiology, emergency medicine, general surgery, genetics, geriatrics and gerontology, neurology, oncology, psychiatry, psychology

DEFINITION: The process of growing old, regardless of one's chronological age; with the number of old persons dramatically increasing, medical researchers are striving to understand the causes and effects of the aging process.

KEY TERMS:

Alzheimer's disease: a disorder characterized by progressive deterioration of intellectual capacity with memory loss, impaired judgment, and personality change

anitoxidant: a substance that neutralizes the damaging effects of free radicals in the body

arthritis: inflammation or degenerative joint change often marked by stiffness, swelling, and pain

atherosclerosis: a condition of an artery characterized by lipid deposits and a thickening of the inner wall

free radical theory: the idea that aging may be brought about by the production within the body of very reactive chemicals (free radicals) that damage chromosomes and other cell parts

geriatrics: the branch of medicine that treats the conditions and diseases associated with aging and old age

hypertension: a condition characterized by higher-than-normal blood pressure in the blood vessels

immunocompetence: the ability of the body to produce a proper immune response to infectious organisms

osteoporosis: a progressive loss of density in new bone as it replaces old bone

transient ischemic attack (TIA): a brief period of insufficient circulation to the brain

PROCESS AND EFFECTS

Aging is an ongoing process beginning at conception and eventually leading to death. The effects of aging, however, tend to be more observable after the age of forty. These age-related changes occur in every organ and system of the body.

Most changes that occur in the skin do not directly affect a person's physical health, but they may greatly affect one's self-concept and general attitude. Age spots form because pigment cells tend to clump together. Wrinkles become common when elastic fibers become less resilient and the fat layer below the skin is greatly reduced. The loss of many oil glands leaves skin dry and scaly. Hair gradually loses pigment and may become thin and fragile.

The chief age-related skeletal system change is a loss of calcium from bone. This loss begins at a younger age and progresses more rapidly in women than in men. Accompanied by a loss of protein fibers in the bone, calcium depletion leaves bones frail, brittle, and prone to break easily.

The cartilage in aging joints becomes thin and erodes away, causing discomfort and restricting movement. Cartilage between the ribs and breastbone hardens, becomes less flexible, and makes breathing more difficult. Progressive degeneration of cartilage discs between vertebrae leads to painful compression of the spine, especially in the neck and lower back.

A gradual reduction in strength, endurance, and coordination results from changes in aging muscle. As old muscle fibers are lost, new ones are not produced; instead, they are replaced by pockets of fat and of stringy connective tissue. In addition, the nerves that cause muscle contraction degenerate and lose their ability to bring about smooth, swift movement.

Because the nervous system directs and coordinates all other parts of the body, its age-related changes are of particular concern. Because nerve cells lose some ability to produce and receive neurotransmitters (chemicals that move

impulses from one nerve cell to another), impulses move more slowly in the elderly.

As nerve cells die, they are not replaced. This loss of neurons, especially in the brain, is believed to cause a decline in intelligence and in the capacity to learn new skills. It also triggers memory loss, especially of more recent memories. The loss of about 25 percent of the cells in the cerebellum of the brain adversely affects balance and the coordination of fine movements. Those exhibiting the most mental disabilities have a significant number of defects called neurofibrillary tangles within their nerve cells and neuritic plaques or debris between their nerve cells.

Age-related changes in the inner ear affect both hearing and balance. The spiral-organ cells in the cochlea, which enable sound to be perceived, die off as blood capillaries

Aging and the Body

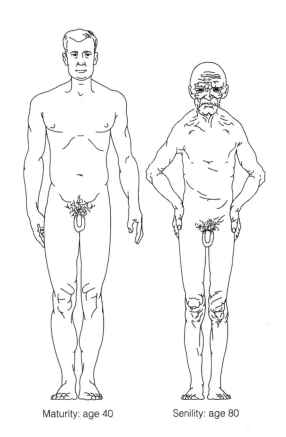

Maturity: age 40   Senility: age 80

Among the most obvious effects of aging are reduced body mass, a "shrinking" of height with loss of bone mass, sagging and wrinkling skin, and graying or loss of hair.

thicken and prevent nutrients from reaching the cochlea. The death of nerve cells in the semicircular canals greatly reduces the ability of the elderly to maintain equilibrium and to coordinate movements.

It is not unusual for an eighty-five-year-old to have lost 80 percent of his or her ability to see clearly. This dramatic difference in vision is caused by many cumulative changes. The cornea in front of the eye loses its ability to bend light correctly, while the lens becomes harder, thicker, less elastic, and unable to change shape as needed. The aqueous humor or fluid that cleanses and nourishes the lens and cornea becomes insufficient to do so in many older people, leaving the eye dry and irritated. In addition, the vitreous humor that gives shape to the eyeball may shrink and become opaque. This allows little light to reach the retina and images are, therefore, poorly received.

Elderly persons often fail to eat properly because food does not taste or smell appealing. A loss of taste stems from a decrease in the amount of saliva secreted, from changes in the taste-processing centers in the brain, and possibly from a decline in the number of taste buds. The loss of neurons involved in smell causes that sense to begin to decline in most people by middle age.

Structural changes occur in all parts of the digestive system with aging. There is a tendency to develop gum disease and to lose one's teeth. The degeneration of digestive glands leaves the mouth, stomach, and small intestine with less of their digestive juices. In spite of these changes, digestion and absorption are not appreciably diminished in otherwise healthy older persons.

Aging brings a major reduction in the elasticity of arteries and a narrowing of their diameter as a result of an accumulation of fats (lipids) in arterial walls. Blood pumped by the heart thus encounters more resistance to its easy movement through the vessels. The result is some degree of high blood pressure, or hypertension, in all the elderly. The heart of an older person is often enlarged and pumps less blood with less force than that of a young adult. Fat deposits gather on its surface, and valves may become less flexible. The heart, working much harder yet achieving increasingly less, is unable to supply adequate oxygen for all the body's needs.

The amount of red bone marrow also diminishes with age. Although sufficient marrow remains to form new blood cells under ordinary circumstances, it is not sufficient to form them rapidly should the elderly person bleed extensively for any reason.

Those who are aging experience a decreased ability of the respiratory organs to acquire and deliver the oxygen needed for normal physical activity. Hardening of the trachea and bronchi hampers the movement of air into the lungs, which themselves become inelastic. The walls of the alveoli, or lung air sacs, become increasingly unable to allow oxygen through them and into the blood.

Aging and the Brain

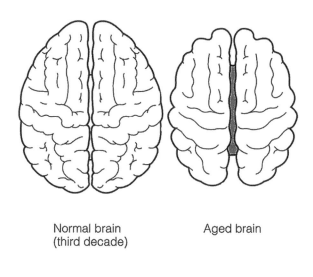

Normal brain
(third decade)

Aged brain

The human brain shrinks with age as nerve cells are lost and brain tissue atrophies.

In an aging woman, the degeneration of follicle cells in the ovary results in lowered secretion of estrogens and progesterone. These declining hormone levels cause changes in the uterus and the cessation of menstrual cycles known as the menopause. Some women experience hot flashes and irritability at this time. The diminished hormonal levels also cause fat to accumulate below the waist area, breast tissue to sag, and the vagina to become dry and thin.

Loss of estrogen during aging may explain the increased risk of heart disease among postmenopausal women. Estrogen has been shown to prevent or slow age-related complications such as heart disease, osteoporosis, mental deterioration, and colon cancer. Premenopausal women are believed to have a lower incidence of heart disease because of the protective role of estrogen.

In the older man, changes within the testes cause less testosterone to be produced, reducing muscle strength and resulting in a general wasting appearance. Sperm production is greatly decreased, although there may still be an adequate number to bring about fertilization at an advanced age. The penis tends to become smaller, and its erectile tissue becomes somewhat rigid; this inability to expand makes the attainment of an erection very difficult for many older men. Meanwhile, hard masses appear in the prostate, and the whole gland may double in weight. Its enlargement often constricts the urethra and makes urination difficult.

In both sexes, large numbers of glomeruli, the filters that make up the kidneys, are lost as one ages, as is an efficient blood supply to these vital organs. Consequently, the kidneys lose much ability to form urine and purify the blood correctly. By the age of seventy-five, the kidneys are usually only half as efficient as they are in a young adult.

COMPLICATIONS AND DISORDERS

The population is living longer than ever before because of advances in medicine. Degenerative diseases of aging—such as brain and bone disorders, cancer, and cardiovascular disease—are now the major complications of the aging population.

An accumulation of age-related changes can cause a serious dysfunction or disease to develop. Two major dysfunctions that medical science must treat in the skeletal system are arthritis and osteoporosis.

Arthritis is a general term used to describe the various kinds of degenerative changes or inflammation that occur in joints. These changes are seen in the membranes surrounding the joints, in the protective, cushioning cartilage at the ends of bones, and in the bones themselves. The most common form of arthritis, called osteoarthritis, is a chronic and debilitating degeneration of that protective, or articular, cartilage. The pain in stiff, swollen joints is caused by the wearing away of the smooth cartilage and the rubbing together of the rough, exposed bones. Bony growths or spurs may appear, causing the characteristic joint enlargement.

Osteoarthritis causes misshaped, painful fingers. More important, it affects the lower limbs and the vertebrae of the spine. It thus severely hampers posture and limits normal walking, while producing constant leg pain and backaches. No single cause of osteoarthritis has been discovered. It seems to result from a combination of the stress on joints and changes in the collagen and elastic fibers within the bones and cartilage. An additional cause may be the decreased blood supply to the joints found in most older people. It is thought that heredity also influences the degree to which cartilage thins, as well as the rate.

Osteoporosis ("porous bone") is a common dysfunction in elderly persons but especially in postmenopausal women. It is a progressive reduction in the density of the new bone that is replacing old bone. Osteoporosis can cause curvature of the spine, backache, diminished height, and brittle bones that are easily broken. From middle adulthood, everyone's bones begin a gradual decline in mass and strength. If bone volume reaches a level that is low enough, osteoporosis results. The cause of this disease is unclear, but contributing factors in both sexes include a deficiency of vitamin D and calcium in the diet over many years. Women may lose 50 percent of their bone mass by the age of seventy; their hormonal deficiencies after the menopause are believed to be the major factor in such extensive osteoporosis.

Two fairly common dysfunctions of the aging central nervous system are Parkinson's disease and Alzheimer's disease. The former is a chronic and slowly progressive condition which generally develops after the age of fifty.

More common in men than in women, Parkinson's disease involves useless contractions of skeletal muscles, a rhythmic tremor, and muscle rigidity. It becomes difficult for the patient to begin movement or to walk without a characteristic shuffling gait. Drooling from the mouth, slow and monotonous speech, and a loss of facial expression accompany this disease. Parkinson's disease is chacterized by deposits in the brain called Lewy bodies. Some degree of memory loss or decreased ability to comprehend new concepts afflicts patients with Parkinson's disease.

The disease results from loss of nerve cells in the part of the brain called the basal ganglia that controls movement. Loss of these cells leads to a deficiency of the neurotransmitter called dopamine. There is a direct relationship between the degree of dopamine deficiency and the severity of symptoms. Doctors usually prescribe levodopa (L-dopa) to replace the brain's supply of dopamine and to alleviate symptoms. Although once believed to be related to unknown factors in the environment, at least some cases of Parkinson's disease are linked to defects in a gene that codes for a nerve cell protein.

Alzheimer's disease is also progressive but has three recognizable stages. Impairment of recent memories, a lessening of spontaneous emotions, and confusion about one's surroundings are among the earliest symptoms seen. In the second stage, the ability to read, write, calculate, and think clearly are lost; the patient even becomes unable to recognize a spouse or other family members. Finally, the patient becomes unable to speak and begins to have seizures.

These symptoms may result from a deficiency of the neurotransmitter called acetylcholine. This lack is caused by the death of many neurons which had previously produced acetylcholine in the correct amount for normal brain functioning. The brains of Alzheimer's patients have a large number of neurofibrillary tangles and neuritic plaques. In addition, their brains tend to contain accumulations of metals such as aluminum. It has yet to be proven whether the tangles, the plaques, or the metal deposits are the causes or effects of this disease.

Alzheimer's disease is the leading cause of mental impairment in older people and appears to have a genetic basis, at least in part. An early form of the disease (early-onset) can afflict people in their thirties, forties, and fifties. A late-onset form occurs after the age of seventy. Genetic defects in a serum protein called apolipoprotein (Apo E) appear in half to two-thirds of all Alzheimer's patients. Defects in three other genes have been linked to the disease.

Dysfunctions of the circulatory system, all of which are potential causes of death, are more common in older people. Though patients who suffer from one often suffer from other, related conditions, the dysfunctions can be categorized by their primary symptoms as ischemic heart disease, myocardial infarction, cardiac arrhythmias, congestive heart failure, atherosclerosis and arteriosclerosis, and hypertension.

Coronary artery disease is an ischemic (anemic) condition in which the heart tissue does not receive an adequate supply of blood. The reduced blood flow is caused by a narrowing of the coronary arteries. Most sixty-year-olds are believed to have only one-third the blood flow through the heart's vessels when compared to a young adult. The most frequent cause of the constriction is a plaque which partially or completely blocks the vessel. If the plaque protrudes into the artery, its rough edges can cause a thrombus, or stationary blood clot, to block that vessel. If the thrombus detaches, it is called an embolus; it may then cause a blockage when it enters a smaller vessel.

A myocardial infarction, or heart attack, results when the muscle cells deprived of blood and oxygen are damaged and die. A heart thus damaged has much less, if any, ability to pump blood to the whole body.

When the heart does not contract in the regular manner with a predictable sequence of heartbeats, the condition is called cardiac arrhythmia. It may result from too few heartbeats or from many extra contractions per minute. The latter is more dangerous because it does not allow the heart chambers to fill properly and move the blood efficiently through the heart. An extremely rapid and irregular beat, known as fibrillation, puts great strain upon the heart.

Congestive heart failure may result from a heart attack, from valve damage, or from prolonged high blood pressure. It is also called cardiac insufficiency because the heart is not able to pump enough blood to meet the needs of the body. The insufficiency to the kidney causes less urine to be produced and blood volume to increase; the heart must work even harder to pump this greater blood volume and, in time, may fail.

Atherosclerosis and arteriosclerosis are very closely related conditions. Atherosclerosis is the presence in an artery wall of plaques composed of lipids, connective tissue, and abnormal smooth muscle cells. Plaques can cause ischemic heart disease directly by constricting a coronary artery or indirectly by causing a blood clot to form. Often, atherosclerotic plaques become hardened by the accumulation of calcium, producing arteriosclerosis, or "hardening of the arteries." These inelastic walls are one cause of hypertension, or high blood pressure. The excessive blood pressure creates kidney damage and thus more strain upon the heart.

Cardiovascular disease is the leading cause of death in the Western world. A major development in cardiovascular disease research is the finding that oxidation and immunology may play a central role in atherosclerosis. Cardiovascular disease is associated with low plasma concentrations of antioxidants such as ascorbate, tocopherol, and betacarotene. Oxidation of low-density lipoproteins (LDLs) in blood is believed to encourage the formation of foam cells and atherosclerotic plaques in arteries.

A malfunctioning cardiovascular system has great poten-

tial to damage the delicate nervous system. A transient ischemic attack (TIA) can result if the atherosclerosis prevents sufficient blood from reaching the brain for a very brief period. TIAs often serve as a prediction that a stroke will soon occur. A stroke or cardiovascular accident (CVA) involves either a blood clot or a rupture of a weakened blood vessel in the brain. A CVA is always accompanied by some destruction of fragile nervous tissue, and the severity of its effects depends on the size and location of the brain subdivision in which it occur.

PERSPECTIVE AND PROSPECTS

The understanding of the aging process holds a key position in modern medical science. Although people have observed and described many age-related changes for centuries, it was only in the twentieth century that scientists began to comprehend why the elderly suffer from so many diseases and dysfunctions. This understanding marked the birth of the science of geriatrics. In the 1980's, using the tools of biochemistry, microbiology, and genetics, gerontologists began to accumulate meaningful data to answer the ultimate question: What actually causes aging? If the underlying cause could be determined, it might be possible to interfere with the process and increase the human life span.

It seems most likely that there is no single cause of aging but rather a complex combination of causes. Many tentative theories have been advanced, including aging by program, gene-caused, gene mutation, cross-linkage, free radical, cellular garbage, and the wear-and-tear theories. The causes of aging seem closely interwoven with the role of the endocrine glands and the immune system.

There are strong arguments supporting the idea that aging is somehow programmed into all species. Some scientists believe the hypothalamus, located at the base of the brain, may be the timekeeper of life because of its key role in normal hormone production; others think the thymus gland might control life span because of its work in immunity. Still others assume that an individual organ is not responsible and that each cell has its own internal "life clock."

The gene-caused theory suggests that aging is programmed by harmful genes that only become active late in life or useful genes that are altered and become harmful over the years.

The gene mutation theory postulates that an accumulation of mistakes in deoxyribonucleic acid (DNA) production with the passage of time results in large numbers of altered, malfunctioning cells. This theory further assumes that the many methods of gene repair that are possessed by young cells become ineffective over the years.

The cross-linkage theory proposes that, with age, abnormal bonds form within numerous proteins, altering their structure and therefore the functioning of the organs in which they are found. These proteins include the thousands of enzymes responsible for body processes, and especially the collagen that makes up 30 percent of the protein found in organs.

The free radical theory postulates that highly reactive chemicals are formed in the course of normal living and combine with cell membranes and chromosomes, thus damaging and altering them. The number of free radicals can be suppressed by substances such as vitamins C and E, called antioxidants. If this theory is correct, there is hope that these vitamins could be used to increase life span and prevent age-related illnesses (see "Antioxidants" box).

The cellular garbage theory suggests that the accumulation over the years of large amounts of chemical waste products can interfere with normal cell activities and bring about the aging of all organs. The wear-and-tear theory includes the concept of cellular garbage and a possible accumulation of improperly produced proteins. It further focuses on the supposition that each animal has a specific amount of metabolic energy available to it; the length of life is determined by the rate at which that energy is used up.

Aging appears to be slowed by calorie or protein restriction. In rodents, calorie restriction greatly increases life span and lowers cancer rates. The beneficial effect may be attributable to reduced oxidative damage or enhanced immune responses in these animals.

The immune system seems to have a central role in aging for two reasons. First, autoimmune conditions, in which the person's immune system mistakenly attacks and destroys body parts, are very prevalent in the elderly. Second, the aging immune system's ability to recognize and destroy foreign invading organisms, its immunocompetence, becomes extremely reduced.

—Grace D. Matzen, updated by Linda Hart

The Use of Antioxidants

The role of antioxidants in preventing aging has received considerable interest in recent years. Antioxidants are substances that neutralize the harmful effects of free radicals in the body. Free radicals are highly reactive chemicals that form in normal metabolism or are produced by radiation and environmental stress. These volatile chemicals react with cell components, causing mutations in DNA and destroying cell proteins and lipids. The aging process and various degenerative diseases of aging are believed to be caused in part by the lifetime accumulation of cell damage caused by free radicals.

Antioxidant defenses occur naturally in the body to inactivate free radicals and repair damaged tissues. The body's natural supply of antioxidants is limited, however, and a small amount of destruction occurs to cells daily. Dietary antioxidants—in the form of fruits and vegetables or vitamin supplements—are believed to improve health and to slow aging by boosting the body's natural supply of antioxidants.

Extensive research, including many large-scale studies, have demonstrated the beneficial role of dietary antioxidants in preventing such age-related disorders as cardiovascular disease, cancer, immune dysfunction, brain and neurological disorders, and cataracts. Fruits and vegetables, long recognized for their protective and healthful effects, are particularly rich sources of antioxidants, which may be the basis for their antiaging and anticarcinogenic properties.

Vitamin E, vitamin C, and beta carotene are the main dietary antioxidants. Vitamin E (tocopherol) is a fat-soluble antioxidant found in oil, nuts, seeds, and whole grains. This antioxidant appears to protect arteries against damage. Two recent studies have shown that taking vitamin E supplements appears to reduce the risk of heart disease dramatically. In addition, studies in mice suggest that vitamin E supplements slow the decline of brain and immune system function caused by aging. Vitamin C (ascorbate) works in the water-soluble part of tissues. Citrus fruits, strawberries, sweet peppers, and broccoli are good sources of Vitamin C. This antioxidant boosts the immune system, strengthens blood vessel walls, and increases levels of a natural antioxidant, glutathione. Vitamin C also helps restore levels of active vitamin E in the body. Beta carotene, a precursor of vitamin A, is found in carrot juice, sweet potatoes, and apricots. Many studies have demonstrated the anticancer and antiaging effects of beta carotene.

Other antioxidants include coenzyme Q10, gingko, lipoic acid, grapeseed, and various substances found in green and black teas. The micronutrients zinc and selenium also have antioxidant properties; they aid the immune system and boost the levels of natural antioxidant enzymes in the body. Antioxidants appear to work together, as a combination of antioxidants is more potent than each substance alone.

Evidence for the beneficial role of antioxidants in human health is growing. Clinical studies have not definitively confirmed, however, whether consuming large amounts of antioxidants offers increased protection against aging. It is not clear what the optimal levels of antioxidants are to prevent the damaging effects of aging. Adequate levels of vitamins may vary greatly for each person, depending on levels of environmental stress, smoking, how well supplements are absorbed, and other factors. In addition, it is unclear whether vitamin supplements are superior to fruits and vegetables, since other factors in these foods (fiber, micronutrients) may be responsible for their healthful effects. —Linda Hart

See also Aging, extended care for the; Alzheimer's disease; Arteriosclerosis; Arthritis; Death and dying; Dementia; Depression; Diabetes mellitus; Estrogen replacement therapy; Geriatrics and gerontology; Hearing loss; Heart disease; Hormone replacement therapy; Memory loss; Menopause; Midlife crisis; Osteoarthritis; Osteoporosis; Parkinson's disease; Psychiatry, geriatric; Sense organs; Stress; Strokes and TIAs; Vitamins and minerals.

FOR FURTHER INFORMATION:

Bonner, Joseph, and William Harris. *Healthy Aging: New Directions in Health, Biology, and Medicine*. Claremont, Calif.: Hunter House, 1988. A brief but highly readable and informative book. Contains both theories of aging and practical applications. A useful glossary and an extensive bibliography are included.

Butler, Robert N., and Jacob A. Brody. *Delaying the Onset of Late-Life Dysfunction*. New York: Springer, 1995. A highly readible book on prevention of age-related diseases such as immune dysfunctions, heart disease, and Alzheimer's disease. Discusses research on evolutionary and molecular approaches to understanding the aging process.

Carper, Jean. *Stop Aging Now!* New York: HarperCollins, 1995. A consumer guide to the use of dietary antioxidants for boosting immunity and preventing aging. Includes suggested dietary levels of antioxidants, regimens, and a list of scientific references supporting the benefits of antioxidants.

Fries, James F. *Aging Well*. Reading, Mass.: Addison-Wesley, 1989. Offers precise explanations of all age-related changes and ways to prevent or cope with them. The format of the book makes information very easy to locate.

Kahn, Carol. *Beyond the Helix: DNA and the Quest for Longevity*. New York: Times Books, 1985. The story of the scientists working at laboratories throughout the United States to discover why organisms age and whether one can retard the aging process. Explains highly technical material in an exciting, comprehensible manner for the layperson.

Rossman, Isadore. *Looking Forward: The Complete Medical Guide to Successful Aging*. New York: E. P. Dutton, 1989. Offers sound medical advice on the prevention of most of the ills that can afflict the elderly. Contains reprints of innumerable, pertinent magazine and journal articles. Written in a warm, direct, personal style.

Rusting, Ricki L. "Why Do We Age?" *Scientific American* 267 (December, 1992): 130. An excellent summary of significant experiments in the 1980's and projected research in the 1990's on the genetic and biochemical causes of aging.

Schneider, Edward L., and John W. Rowe. *Handbook of the Biology of Aging*. 4th ed. San Diego: Academic Press, 1996. Part of a three-volume series that includes the biological, psychological, and social aspects of aging. Focuses on research approaches to understanding aging, including genetic studies, cellular and molecular biology, neurobiology, and nutrition.

Spence, Alexander P. *Biology of Human Aging*. Englewood Cliffs, N.J.: Prentice Hall, 1989. A general overview of the aging process. Spence makes a clear distinction between normal age-related changes and possible age-related dysfunctions. Contains a very thorough bibliography.

Weiss, Robert, and Genell J. Subak-Sharpe, eds. *Complete Guide to Health and Well-Being After Fifty*. New York: Times Books, 1988. An excellent volume sponsored by the Columbia University School of Public Health. Contains a clear, complete explanation of the aging process and what one can do to remain healthier to a more advanced age. Each chapter includes extensive lists of further resources.

AGING, EXTENDED CARE FOR THE

SPECIALTY

ANATOMY OR SYSTEM AFFECTED: All

SPECIALTIES AND RELATED FIELDS: Audiology, cardiology, critical care, dentistry, geriatrics and gerontology, neurology, nursing, nutrition, oncology, ophthalmology, optometry, pharmacology, physical therapy, psychiatry, psychology, public health, rheumatology

DEFINITION: The management of the health, personal care, and social needs of elderly people as they experience decreases in physical, mental, and/or emotional abilities.

KEY TERMS:

ageism: discrimination against individuals based on their age or the overlooking of individuals' abilities to make positive contributions to society because of their age

case management: an interdisciplinary approach to medical care characterized by the inclusion of physical, psychological, social, emotional, familial, financial, and historical data in patient treatment

cognitive functioning: a general term describing mental processes such as awareness, knowing, reasoning, problem-solving, judging, and imagining

malnutrition: a physical state characterized by an imbalance of dietary proteins, carbohydrates, fats, vitamins, and minerals, given an individual's physical activity and health needs

mental status exam: a comprehensive evaluation assessing general health, appearance, mood, speech, sociability, cooperativeness, motor activity, orientation to time and reality, memory, general intelligence, and other cognitive functioning

organic brain syndromes: clusters of behavioral and psychological symptoms involving impaired brain function, where etiology is unknown; includes delirium, delusions, amnesia, intoxication, and dementias

organic mental disorders: mental and emotional disturbances from transient or permanent brain dysfunction, with known organic etiology; includes drugs or alcohol ingestion, infection, trauma, and cardiovascular disease

psychosocial interventions: treatments that enhance individual psychological and social functioning by assisting with the development of the skills, attitudes, or behaviors necessary to function as independently as possible

THE PROBLEMS ASSOCIATED WITH AGING

The process of aging is inevitable. In the earlier stages of life, aging involves the acquisition and development of new skills and abilities, facilitated by the guidance and assistance of others. Later, the middle stages involve the challenges of maintaining and applying those skills and abilities in a manner that is primarily self-sufficient. Finally, in the end stages of life, aging involves the deterioration and loss of skills and abilities, with adequate functioning again being somewhat dependent on the assistance of others.

For many individuals, the final stages are brief, allowing them to live independently right up to their time of death. Thus, many experience little loss of their abilities to function independently. Others, however, endure more extended stages of later life and require greater care. For these individuals, losses in physical, emotional, and/or cognitive functioning frequently result in a need for specialized care. Such care involves whatever is necessary so that these individuals may live as comfortably, productively, and independently as possible.

The conditions leading to a need for long-term care are as varied as the elderly are themselves. Special needs for elders requiring extended care often include the management of physical, health, emotional, and cognitive problems. Physical problems dictating lifestyle adjustments include decreased speed, dexterity, and strength, as well as increased fragility. Changes to the five senses are also common. Visual changes include the development of hyperopia (farsightedness) and sometimes decreased visual acuity. Hearing loss is also common, such that softer sounds cannot be heard when background noise is present or sounds need to be louder in order to be perceived. Particularly noteworthy is that paranoia, depression, and social isolation often result as side effects of visual and hearing impairments in elders; they are not always signs of mental deterioration. Similarly, one's sense of touch may also be affected, such that the nerves are either more or less sensitive to changes in temperatures or textures. Consequently, injuries attributable to a lack of awareness of potential hazards or supersensitivities to temperature or texture may result. One example would be an elderly woman overdressing or underdressing for the weather because of an inability to judge the outside temperature properly. Another would be an elderly man cutting or wounding himself out of a lack of awareness of the sharpness of an object. Finally, both taste and smell may change, creating a situation in which subtle tastes and odors become imperceptible or in which tastes and smells that were once pleasant become either bland or unpleasant.

Health problems among the aged often demand increased management as well. Coordination of drug therapies and other medical interventions by a case manager is critical, as a result of increasing sensitivities in elders to physical interventions. Typical health conditions bringing elderly people into long-term care settings may include heart disease and strokes, hypertension, diabetes mellitus, arthritis, osteoporosis, chronic pain, prostate disease, and cancers of the digestive tract and other vital organs. Estimates are that approximately 86 percent of the aged are affected by chronic illnesses. Long-term care addresses both the medical management of these chronic illnesses and their impact on the individual.

An issue related to health and physical problems in the aged is malnutrition. For a variety of reasons, elders often fall victim to malnutrition, which can contribute to additional health problems. For example, calcium deficiency can increase the severity of heart disease and increase the likelihood of osteoporosis and tooth loss. Thus, a vicious cycle of medical problems can be put into motion. Factors contributing to malnutrition are multifaceted. Poverty, social isolation, decreased taste sensitivity, and tooth loss combine with lifelong dietary habits that can sometimes predispose certain elders to malnutrition. As such, attention toward the maintenance of healthy dietary habits in the elderly is critical to successful long-term care, regardless of the type of setting in which the care is being given.

Along with these physical aspects of aging come emotional and cognitive changes. Depression, anxiety, and paranoia over health concerns, for example, are not uncommon. Additionally, concerns about the threat of losing one's independence, friends, and former lifestyle may also contribute to acute or chronic mood disorders. Suicide is a particular danger with the elderly when mood disorders such as depression are present. Elderly people are one of the fastest growing groups among those who commit suicide. The stresses accompanying losing a spouse or enduring a chronic health problem can often be triggers to suicide for depressed elders. One should note, however, that elders are not particularly prone to depression or suicide because of their age but that they are more likely to experience significant stressors that lead to depression.

More common, less lethal problems associated with conditions such as depression, anxiety, and paranoia are weight change, insomnia, and other sleep problems. Distractibility, decreased ability to maintain attention and concentration, and rumination over distressing concerns are also common. Finally, some elders may be observed as socially isolated and prone to avoidance behavior. As a result, some become functionally incapacitated because of distressing emotions.

What is critical to remember, in addition to these signs, is that some elders may not describe their problems as emo-

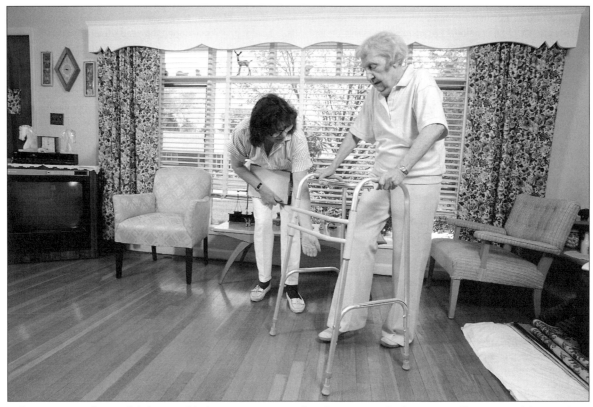

A home care professional helps an elderly woman use a walker for support. Such services allow many older people to have a more active and independent lifestyle. (Digital Stock)

tional at all, even though that is the primary cause of their discomfort. Individual differences in how people express themselves must be taken into account. Thus, while some elders may report being depressed or anxious, others may instead report feeling tired. Reports of low-level health problems that are vague in nature, such as aches and pains, are also common in elders who are depressed. It is not uncommon for emotional problems to be expressed or described indirectly as physical complaints.

Decreased cognitive functioning may result from more serious problems than depression, such as organic brain syndromes. These typically include problems such as dementias from Alzheimer's disease, Pick's disease, Huntington's chorea, alcohol-related deterioration, or stroke-related problems. Other causes may be brain tumors or thyroid dysfunction. With all dementias, however, the hallmark signs are a deterioration of intellectual function and emotional response. Memory, judgment, understanding, and the experience and control of emotional responses are affected. Functionally, these conditions reveal themselves as a combination of symptoms, including increased forgetfulness, decreased ability to plan and complete tasks, difficulties finding names or words, decreased abilities for abstract thinking, impaired judgment, inappropriate sexual behavior,

and sometimes severe personality changes. In some cases, affected individuals are aware of these difficulties, usually in the earlier stages of the disease processes. Later, however, even though their behavior and abilities may be quite disturbed, they may be completely unaware of the severity of their problems. In these cases, long-term care often begins as a result of outside intervention by concerned friends and family members.

OPTIONS FOR LONG-TERM CARE

Extended care for the aged requires an interdisciplinary effort that usually involves a team of physicians, psychologists, nurses, social workers, and other rehabilitative specialists. Depending on the nature of the problems requiring care and management, any of these professionals may take part in the care process. Additionally, the involvement of concerned individuals who are close to the elder needing care is critical. Family members (including the spouse, children, and extended family) and close friends are invaluable sources of information and of emotional and instrumental support. Their ability to assist an elder with instrumental tasks such as cooking, house cleaning, shopping, and money and medication management is crucial to the successful implementation of a long-term care plan.

In all cases, long-term care for the aged involves the

design of a comprehensive plan to address the multifaceted needs of the elder. Just as younger persons have psychological, social, intellectual, and physical needs, so do elders. As such, thorough assessment of an elder's abilities, goals, expectations, and functioning in each of these areas is required. A mental status exam and a thorough physical exam are usually the primary methods of evaluation. Once needs are identified, a plan can then be designed by the team of health care professionals, family and friends assisting with care, and, whenever possible, the elder. In general, the overarching goal is to design a case management plan that maximizes the independent functioning of the aged person, given certain physical, psychiatric, social, and other needs.

Specific management strategies are designed for the problems that need to be addressed. Physical, health, nutritional, emotional, and cognitive problems all demand different management settings and strategies. Additionally, care settings may vary depending on the severity of the problems that are identified. In general, the more severe the problems, the more structured the long-term care setting and the more intense the psychosocial interventions.

For less severe problems, adequate management settings may include the elder's own home, the home of a family member or friend, a shared housing setting, or a seniors' apartment complex. Shared housing is sometimes called group-shared, supportive, or matched housing. Typically, it refers to residences organized by agencies where up to twenty people share a house and its expenses, chores, and management. Ideal candidates for this type of setting include elders who want some daily assistance or companionship but who are still basically independent. Senior apartments, also called retirement housing, are usually "elderly-only" complexes that range from garden-style apartments to high-rises. Ideal candidates for this type of setting include nearly independent elders who want privacy, but who no longer desire or can manage a single-family home. In either of these types of settings, the use of periodic or regular at-home nursing assistance for medical problems, or "home-helpers" for more instrumental tasks, might be a successful adjunct to regular consultation with a case manager or physician.

Problems of moderate severity may demand a more structured setting or a setting in which help is more readily available. Such settings might include continuing care retirement communities or assisted living facilities. Continuing care retirement communities, also called life-care communities, are large complexes offering lifelong care. Residents are healthy, live independently in an apartment, and are able to use cafeteria services as necessary. Additionally, residents have the option of being moved to an assisted-living unit or an infirmary as health needs dictate. Assisted-living facilities—also called board-and-care, institutional living, adult foster care, and personal care settings—offer care that is less intense than that received in a medical setting or

nursing home. These facilities may be as small as a home where one person cares for a small group of elders or as large as a converted hotel with several caregivers, a nurse, and shared dining facilities. Such settings are ideal for persons needing instrumental care but not round-the-clock skilled medical or nursing care.

When more severe conditions such as incontinence, dementia, or an inability to move independently are present, nursing, convalescent, or extended care homes are more appropriate settings. Intense attention is delivered in a hospital-like setting where all medical and instrumental needs are addressed. Typical nursing homes serve a hundred clients at a time, utilizing semiprivate rooms for personal living space and providing community areas for social, community, and family activities. Often, the decision to place an elder in this type of facility is difficult to make. The decision, however, is frequently based on the knowledge that these types of facilities provide the best possible setting for the overall care of the elder's medical, health, and social needs. In fact, appropriate use of these facilities discourages the overtaxing of the elder's emotional and familial resources, allowing the elder to gain maximum benefit. An elder's placement into this type of facility does not mean that the family's job is over; rather, it simply changes shape. Incorporation of family resources into long-term care in a nursing home setting is critical to the adjustment of the elder and family members to the elder's increased need for care and attention. Visits and other family involvement in the elder's daily activities remain quite valuable.

Regardless of the management setting, some basic caveats exist with regard to determining management strategies. First and foremost is that the aged individuals should, whenever possible, be encouraged to maintain independent functioning. For example, even though physical deterioration such as decreased visual or hearing abilities may be present, there is no need to take decision-making authority away from the elder. Decreased abilities to hear or see do not necessarily mean a decreased ability to make decisions or think. Second, it is crucial to ask elders to identify their needs and how they might desire assistance. Some elders may wish for help with acquiring basic living supplies from outside the home, such as foods and toiletries, but desire privacy and no assistance within the home. In contrast, others may desire independence outside the home with regard to social matters but need more instrumental assistance within the home. Finally, it is important to recognize that even the smallest amount of assistance can make a significant difference in the lifestyle of the elder. A prime example is availability of transportation. The loss of a drivers' license or independent transportation signifies a major loss of independence for any elder. Similarly, the challenges posed by public transit may seem insurmountable because of a lack of familiarity or experience. As such, simple and small interventions such as a ride to a store or a doctor's office may provide great relief for elders by assisting their efforts to meet their own needs.

Special management strategies may be required for specific problem areas. For physical deterioration, adequate assessment of strengths and weaknesses is important, as are referrals to medical, rehabilitative, and home-help professionals. Hearing and visual or other devices to make lifting, mobility, and day-to-day tasks easier are helpful. Similarly, assisting the aged with developing alternative strategies for dealing with diminished sensory abilities can be valuable. Examples would be checking a thermometer for outdoor temperature to determine proper dress, rather than relying purely on sensory information, or having a phone that lights up when it rings. Health conditions also demand particular management strategies, varying greatly with the type of problem experienced. In all cases, however, medical intervention, drug therapies, and behavior modification therapies are commonly employed. Dietary problems (such as malnutrition or diabetes), cardiovascular problems (such as heart attacks), and emotional problems (such as depression) often require all three approaches. Finally, cognitive problems, particularly those related to depression, are sometimes alleviated with drug therapies. Others related to organic brain syndromes or organic mental disorders require both medical interventions and significant behavior modification therapies and/or psychosocial interventions for elders and their families.

PERSPECTIVE AND PROSPECTS

Advances in modern medicine are continually extending the human lifespan. Cures for dread diseases, improved management of chronic health problems, and new technologies to replace diseased organs are facilitating this evolution. For many, these advances translate into greater longevity, the maintenance of a high quality of life, and fewer obstacles related to ageism. For others, however, the trade-off for longevity is some loss of independence and a need for extended care and management. Thus, the medical field is also affected by the trade-off of extending life, while experiencing an increasing need to improve strategies for long-term care for those who are able to live longer and longer despite health conditions.

As a result of this evolution, long-term care for the aged presents special challenges to the medical field. Over time, medicine has been a field specializing in the understanding of particular organ systems and the treatment of related diseases. While an understanding of how each system impacts the functioning of the whole body is necessary, health care providers must struggle to understand the complexities in the case management required for high-quality long-term care for the aged. Care must be interdisciplinary, addressing the physical, mental, emotional, social, and family needs of the aged individual. Failure to address any of these areas may ultimately sabotage the successful long-term management of elderly individuals and of their problems. In this way, medical, psychiatric, social work, and rehabilitative specialists need to work together with elders and their families for the best possible results.

Integrated case management with a team leader is increasingly the trend so that a variety of services can be provided in an orchestrated manner. While specialty providers still play a role, managers, usually a primary care physician, ensure that complementary drug therapies, psychiatric, and other medical treatments are administered. Additionally, they are key in bringing forth family resources for emotional and instrumental support whenever possible, as well as community and social services when needed.

What was once viewed as helping a person to die with dignity is now viewed as helping a person to live as long and as productive a life as possible. Increasing awareness that old age is not simply a dying time has facilitated an integrated approach to long-term care. The news that elders can be as social, physical, sexual, intellectual, and productive as their younger counterparts has greatly stimulated improved long-term care strategies. No longer is old age seen as a time for casting elders aside or as a time when a nursing home is an inescapable solution in the face of health problems affecting the aged. Alternatives to care exist and are proliferating, with improved outcomes for both patients and care providers. —*Nancy A. Piotrowski, Ph.D.*

See also Aging; Alzheimer's disease; Arthritis; Audiology; Brain; Brain disorders; Critical care; Death and dying; Dementia; Depression; Endocrinology; Ethics; Euthanasia; Geriatrics and gerontology; Hearing loss; Hospitals; Incontinence; Malnutrition; Nursing; Nutrition; Ophthalmology; Optometry; Orthopedics; Osteoporosis; Pharmacology; Psychiatry, geriatric; Rheumatology; Sense organs; Terminally ill, extended care for the; Visual disorders.

FOR FURTHER INFORMATION:

American Psychiatric Association. *Diagnostic and Statistical Manual of Mental Disorders*. 4th ed. Washington, D.C.: Author, 1994. This manual provides detailed descriptions of the behavior symptoms used to diagnose psychiatric disorders, such as organic brain syndromes and affective disorders. Written by mental health professionals, this manual covers issues related to psychiatry, psychology, and social work.

Gerike, Ann E. *Old Is Not a Four-Letter Word: A Midlife Guide*. Watsonville, Calif.: Papier-Mache Press, 1997. This light-hearted book describes an alternative approach to aging that is focused on the positives.

Kane, Robert L., and Rosalie A. Kane. "Long-Term Care." In *Geriatric Medicine*, edited by Christine K. Cassel, Donald E. Riesenberg, Leif B. Sorensen, and John R. Walsh. 2d ed. New York: Springer-Verlag, 1990. This article describes trends in long-term care in the United States. Target populations, special risk factors, alternatives to long-term care, and case management issues are discussed.

Katz, Paul R., Robert L. Kane, and Mathy D. Mezey. *Advances in Long-Term Care*. Vol. 1. New York: Springer, 1991. One volume in an ongoing series covering issues related to the long-term care of elders by caregivers, both professional and nonprofessional. Written by medical, psychiatric, and nursing professionals, and discusses issues ranging from problem prevention to problem management.

Kübler-Ross, Elisabeth. *On Death and Dying*. New York: Collier Books, 1970. A classic in the study of grief. The nature of the grief process is outlined, and common emotional experiences related to grief and loss are described. Highly recommended for persons wanting to understand their own grief processes or the perspective of others who are experiencing loss.

Levin, Mora Jean. *How to Care for Your Parents: A Practical Guide to Eldercare*. New York: W. W. Norton, 1997. This book may be of practical use to individuals anticipating a need to care for disabled elders.

Mace, Nancy L., and Peter V. Rabins. *The Thirty-Six-Hour Day: A Family Guide to Caring for Persons with Alzheimer's Disease, Related Dementing Illnesses, and Memory Loss in Later Life*. Rev. ed. Baltimore: The Johns Hopkins University Press, 1991. An excellent reference for anyone dealing with dementia. It is appropriate both for individuals who are interested in learning about dementia because of personal concerns and for individuals who are concerned about managing a friend or relative. Symptoms, accompanying problems, management issues, and strategies for solutions are outlined.

Viorst, Judith. *Necessary Losses*. New York: Simon & Schuster, 1986. This book, written by a mental health specialist, focuses on clarifying losses that are common to all people at different times in the life cycle. An excellent and easy-to-read general resource for individuals experiencing losses caused by age and other factors or for those concerned about elders who are experiencing losses.

AIDS. *See* ACQUIRED IMMUNODEFICIENCY SYNDROME (AIDS).

ALBINISM
DISEASE/DISORDER
ANATOMY OR SYSTEM AFFECTED: Eyes, hair, skin
SPECIALTIES AND RELATED FIELDS: Dermatology, genetics, ophthalmology
DEFINITION: An inherited defect in the production of melanin, albinism is a rare condition characterized by a lack of pigmentation. Oculocutaneous albinism, the more common type, affects the skin and the eyes. Whites affected with albinism have extremely pale skin and white or yellow hair, and blacks with the defect have very light brown skin and hair that is white, slightly yellow, or yel-

lowish brown. Albinos with a less severe form of the disorder may experience some darkening of the skin and hair with age. Albinism causes such eye problems as myopia (nearsightedness), squinting, and photophobia (dislike of bright light), but its main danger is to the skin: Albinos have no melanin to protect them from the sun's harmful radiation and often develop skin cancers.

—Jason Georges and Tracy Irons-Georges
See also Myopia; Pigmentation; Skin; Skin cancer; Skin disorders; Visual disorders.

ALCOHOLISM
DISEASE/DISORDER
ANATOMY OR SYSTEM AFFECTED: Brain, liver, nervous system, psychic-emotional system
SPECIALTIES AND RELATED FIELDS: Family practice, internal medicine, psychiatry, psychology
DEFINITION: The compulsive drinking of and dependency on alcoholic beverages; viewed as psychological in origin, it can be arrested but not cured.

KEY TERMS:
cerebral cortex: the outer part of the cerebrum, responsible for higher nervous functions
cirrhosis: chronic liver disease; its symptoms include nonfunctional tissue, blocked blood circulation, liver failure, and death
delirium tremens: severe alcohol withdrawal syndrome, with symptoms including confusion, delirium, terrifying hallucinations, and severe tremors
distillation: the use of heat to separate mixtures of liquid chemicals that boil at different temperatures by vaporization and cooling back into the liquid state
Korsakoff's psychosis: brain damage that may require hospitalization because of disorientation and impaired or false memory
bipolar disorder: a disturbance of mood and behavior involving rapid alternations between extreme elation and depression
metabolism: the chemical and physical processes involved in the interconversion of foods and the maintenance of life
proof: a designation of beverage alcohol content; divided by two, it approximates the percentage of alcohol present
psychosis: a severe mental disorder characterized by loss of normal intellectual and social function and withdrawal from reality
substance abuse: the overuse of a controlled substance that causes physical dependence and psychological abnormality

CAUSES AND SYMPTOMS
The basis for alcoholism is physical dependence on alcoholic beverages and consequent problems in behavior and health. Problems related to alcohol probably developed soon after prehistoric humans discovered that fruit or grain,

Alcohol's Immediate Effects

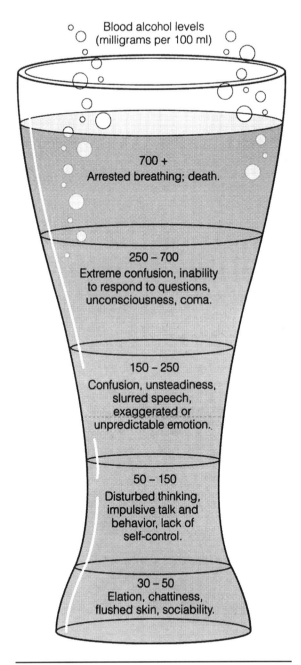

Blood alcohol levels
(milligrams per 100 ml)

700 +
Arrested breathing; death.

250 – 700
Extreme confusion, inability
to respond to questions,
unconsciousness, coma.

150 – 250
Confusion, unsteadiness,
slurred speech,
exaggerated or
unpredictable emotion.

50 – 150
Disturbed thinking,
impulsive talk and
behavior, lack of
self-control.

30 – 50
Elation, chattiness,
flushed skin, sociability.

The presence of 30-50 milligrams of alcohol per every 100 milliliters of blood, which represents the effects of an average drink (a glass of beer, wine, or an ounce of hard liquor), has immediate effects; as the amount increases, effects progress toward death.

mashed and suspended in water, fermented into beverages that produced euphoria in users. The first recorded production of fermented beverages was of beer and wine in ancient Babylon and Egypt, respectively.

The active ingredient in fermented beverages is ethyl alcohol (alcohol), a colorless, mild-smelling liquid that boils at 79 degrees Celsius. Alcohol content in such beverages is indicated as "proof." If divided by two, the proof number indicates the approximate percentage of alcohol present. For example, 20-proof wine contains about 10 percent alcohol. In contrast, 80-proof brandy and vodka—"hard liquors"—contain about 40 percent alcohol, because such hard liquors have been "fortified" by adding pure alcohol prepared via distillation.

Substance abuse of alcoholic beverages first became epidemic during the Middle Ages, when development of widespread alcohol distillation produced hard liquors and made it easy to attain alcoholic euphoria and stupor. In 1992, it was estimated that nearly 70 percent of Americans used alcoholic beverages, that more than ten million such people were involved in the severe substance abuse of alcohol, and that about 250,000 alcohol-related deaths occur each year.

Some deaths attributable to alcohol occur as a result of alcohol poisoning, from excessive consumption in a short time period. The drug primarily depresses the action of the central nervous system, creating the desired euphoric effects of alcohol consumption. Given a drink or two, a drinker may become relaxed and uninhibited. A few more drinks, however, may increase blood alcohol levels above .10 and further depress the central nervous system, causing lack of coordination, slurred speech, and stuporous sleep. If just a little more alcohol is imbibed before stupor occurs and blood alcohol levels rise much above .25, further depression of the central nervous system stops breathing and kills.

People engaged in substance abuse of alcohol, alcoholics, carry out repeated, compulsive abuse that may make them unable to retain their jobs, to obtain an education, or to engage in responsible societal roles. Eventually, alcoholics damage their brains and other body tissues irreversibly. Often, they die of these afflictions or by suicide triggered by depression or terrifying hallucinations. They also engage in behavior that is dangerous to themselves and others, such as driving under the influence or violence.

Chronic alcoholism damages many body organs. Best known is liver disease, or cirrhosis of the liver. Another common affliction is organic brain damage. Mental disorders caused by injury to the cerebral hemispheres may include delirium tremens (the D.T.'s) and Korsakoff's psychosis. Both the D.T.'s, characterized by hallucination and other psychotic symptoms, and Korsakoff's psychosis, which is characterized by short-term memory loss and confabulation, or stories to cover this loss, may be accompanied by severe physical debility requiring hospitalization.

In addition, alcoholism damages the kidneys, the heart,

and the pancreas. In fact, a large number of instances of diseases of other organs are thought to arise from alcohol abuse. Also, much evidence suggests that alcoholism greatly enhances the incidence of mouth and throat cancer resulting from smoking tobacco.

Severe effects in the liver occur because most ingested alcohol is metabolized there. In the presence of alcohol, most other substances normally metabolized by the liver—the factory bloc of the body—are not changed into useful and essential forms. One example has to do with fat, a major dietary source of energy. Decreased fat metabolism in the livers of alcoholics results in the fat accumulation—a fatty liver—that precedes cirrhosis of the liver. Cirrhosis results in the replacement of liver cells with nonfunctional fibrous tissue.

Another problem that results from excessive alcohol metabolism is that the liver no longer destroys the many other toxic chemicals that are eaten. This defect adds to problems seen in cirrhosis and leads to dissemination of such chemicals through the body, where they can damage other body parts. In addition, resistance to the flow of blood through the alcoholic liver develops, which can burst blood vessels and cause dangerous internal bleeding. As a consequence of these problems, alcoholic liver disease, or cirrhosis, has become a major, worldwide cause of death from disease.

There is no one clear physical explanation for the devel-opment of alcoholism. Most often, it is viewed as the result of a biological predisposition to addiction and/or social problems and psychological stresses, especially in those socio-economic groups in which consumption of alcoholic beverages is equated with manliness or sophistication. Other proposed causes of behaviors that lead to alcoholism include habitual drinking, other mental health problems, domineering parents, adolescent peer pressure, personal feelings of inadequacy, loneliness, job pressures, and marital discord.

The fact that 20 percent of children of alcoholics tend to develop the disease, compared to 4 percent of the children of nonalcoholics, has led to investigations of the genetic proclivity for alcoholism. The fact that 80 percent of the progeny of alcoholic parents escape alcoholism, however, diminishes support for such theories. On the other hand, there are clearer indications that genetic factors are important to distaste for alcohol, precluding the development of alcoholism in some ethnic and national groups.

Another disease attributable to alcoholism is fetal alcohol syndrome, which occurs in many children of mothers who drank heavily during pregnancy. Such children may be hyperactive, mentally retarded, and facially disfigured, and they may exhibit marked growth retardation. Fetal alcohol syndrome is becoming more frequent as alcohol consumption increases worldwide.

Commonly observed symptoms of alcoholism are physi-

Alcohol's Long-Term Effects

Brain/nervous system: depressed; permanently impaired following prolonged alcohol abuse.

Skin: flushed; typically pink or red in habitual drinkers.

Heart and circulatory system: hypertensive, leading to heart disease, heart failure, stroke.

Gastrointestinal system: greater incidence of disorders such as ulcers.

Liver: fatty hepatitis, cirrhosis, cancer in advanced stages of abuse.

Urinary system: diuretic effects of alcohol lead to excessive urination, renal failure.

Genital system: increased sexual confidence, reduced performance leading to impotence.

The abuse of alcohol has extensive and serious effects on the body; unarrested, alcohol abuse will lead inevitably to death.

cal dependence on alcohol consumption shown by tremor, shakes, other physical discomfort, and excitability reversed only by alcohol intake; blackout and accompanying memory loss; diminished cognitive ability, exhibited as an inability to understand verbal instructions or to memorize simple series of numbers; and relaxed social inhibitions. These symptoms are attributable to the destruction of tissues of the central nervous system. Diminished sexual activity and sexual desire may also result from excessive alcohol consumption. A high level of alcohol appears to cause diminished libido and impotence. In addition, alcohol may even increase the rate of destruction of existing testosterone in the body.

TREATMENT AND THERAPY

In the mid-1930's, alcoholism, previously viewed as criminal and immoral behavior, was first conceived to be a disease.

There is no known immediate, miracle cure for alcoholism. Treatments for alcohol problems with demonstrated effectiveness, however, do exist. Treatments involving a combined biological, psychological, and social approach, complete with follow-up, often appear most helpful. For most individuals, however, an important phase—or possibly even a permanent feature—of treatment involves total abstinence from alcoholic beverages, all medications that contain alcohol, and any other potential sources of alcohol in the diet.

The recognition of alcoholism as a medical problem has led to the establishment of alcoholic rehabilitation centers, where psychiatric treatment, medication, and other therapies are used in widely different combinations. The supportive programs of the organization Alcoholics Anonymous are also viewed as effective deterrents to a return to alcohol problems.

Two well-known medical treatments for enforcing sobriety are the drugs disulfiram (Antabuse) and citrated calcium carbonate (Abstem). These drugs are given to alcoholics who wish to avoid all use of alcoholic beverages and who require a deterrent to drinking to achieve this goal. Neither drug should ever be given secretly by well-meaning family or friends because of the serious dangers that Antabuse and Abstem pose if an alcoholic backslides and drinks alcohol.

These dangers are the result of the biochemistry of alcohol utilization via the two enzymes (biological protein catalysts) alcohol dehydrogenase and aldehyde dehydrogenase. Normally, alcohol dehydrogenase converts alcohol to the toxic chemical acetaldehyde, and aldehyde dehydrogenase quickly converts the acetaldehyde to acetic acid, the main biological fuel on which the body runs. Either Abstem or Antabuse will turn off aldehyde dehydrogenase and cause acetaldehyde levels to build up in the body when alcohol is consumed. The presence of acetaldehyde in the body then quickly leads to violent headache, great dizziness, heart palpitation, nausea, and vertigo. When the amount of alcohol

found in a drink or two (or even the amount taken in cough medicine) is consumed in the presence of either drug, these symptoms can escalate to the extent that they become fatal.

An interesting sidelight is the view of many researchers that abstinence from alcohol may be genetically related to the presence of too much alcohol dehydrogenase and/or too little aldehyde dehydrogenase in the body. Either of these unbalanced conditions is thought to produce enough acetaldehyde from a small amount of any alcohol source to cause aversion to all alcohol consumption. This is viewed as particularly relevant in Japan, where about 50 percent of the population lacks aldehyde dehydrogenase, and this lack correlates well with the low predisposition of many Japanese to become alcoholics.

As a result of the symptoms of alcohol withdrawal common during detoxification and the presence of other mental health disorders in nearly half of all individuals diagnosed with alcohol dependence, other therapeutic drugs are often used in treatment. Examples include lithium (more often given when bipolar disorder is present), tranquilizers, and sedative hypnotics. The function of these psychoactive drugs is to diminish the discomfort of alcohol withdrawal. Lithium treatment, which must be done with great care because it can become very toxic, appears to be effective only in the alcoholics who drink because of depression or bipolar disorder.

The use of tranquilizers and the related sedative hypnotics must also be done with great care, under close supervision of a physician. Many such drugs are addictive. In addition, some of these drugs have strong synergistic (additive) effects when mixed with alcohol, and such synergism can be fatal. Detailed information on the uses and dangers of these therapeutic drugs in the treatment of alcoholism can be found in *The Merck Manual of Diagnosis and Therapy* (1987), edited by Robert Berkow and Andrew J. Fletcher.

It is believed that the advent of Alcoholics Anonymous in the 1930's has been crucial to the perception of alcoholism as a disease to be treated, rather than as immoral behavior to be condemned. This organization operates on the premise that abstinence is the best course of treatment for alcoholism—an incurable disease that can, however, be arrested by the cessation of all alcohol intake. The methodology of the organization is psychosocial. First, alcoholics are brought to the realization that they can never use alcoholic beverages without succumbing to alcoholism. Then, the need for help from a "higher power" is identified as crucial to abstinence. In addition, the organization develops a support group of people in the same situation. As stated by Andrew M. Mecca in *Alcoholism in America* (1980), "Alcoholics Anonymous never pronounces the disease as cured. . . . [I]t is arrested." More detailed information on Alcoholics Anonymous is found in most of the bibliography citations for this article.

Estimates of the membership of Alcoholics Anonymous in 1992 ranged between 1.5 and 4 million, meaning up to one-third of American alcoholics were affected by its tenets. These people, ranging widely in age, achieve results varying from periods of sobriety (lasting longer and longer as membership in the organization continues) to lifelong sobriety. A deficit of the sole utilization of Alcoholics Anonymous for alcoholism treatment—in the opinion of some experts—is lack of medical, psychiatric, and trained sociological counseling. The results of the operation, however, are viewed by most as beneficial to all parties who seek help from the organization.

Alcohol rehabilitation centers apply varied combinations of drug therapy, psychiatric counseling, and social counseling, depending on the treatment approach for the individual center. Group therapy, however, is the dominant mode of treatment in the United States. The great value of the psychotherapist in alcoholism therapy can be identified from various sources, including David H. Knott's *Alcohol Problems: Diagnosis and Treatment* (1986). Knott points out that, while psychotherapists cannot perform miracles, psychotherapy can be very valuable in helping the alcoholic patient. It can identify the factors leading to "destructive use of alcohol," explore and help to rectify the problems associated with inability to abstain from alcohol abuse, provide emotional support that helps patients to rebuild their lives, and refer patients to Alcoholics Anonymous and other long-term support efforts. The psychotherapist also has experience with managing clients who use or have used psychoactive drugs, understands behavioral modification techniques, and can determine whether an individual requires institutionalization.

Knott and others also point out the importance of behavior modification as a cornerstone of alcoholism psychotherapy and make it clear that many choices are available to all alcoholics desiring psychosocial help. An interesting point made by several sources is that autopsy and a variety of other sophisticated medical techniques, including CT (computed tomography) and PET (positron emission tomography) scans, identify the atrophy of the cerebral cortex of the brain in many alcoholics. This damage—and cortical damage that is not extensive enough to see with existing technology—is viewed as participating in the inability of alcoholics to stop drinking, their loss of both cognitive and motor skills, and the eventual development of serious conditions such as Korsakoff's psychosis and the D.T.'s.

PERSPECTIVE AND PROSPECTS

Modern efforts to deal with alcoholism are often considered to have begun in the early twentieth century, with the activities of the American temperance movement and the Anti-Saloon League. These activities culminated in the period called Prohibition after Congress passed the 1919 Volstead Act, proposed by Minnesota congressman Andrew J. Volstead. The idea behind the act was that making intoxi-

cating beverages impossible to obtain would force sobriety on Americans. Prohibition turned out to be self-defeating, however, and several sources point out that it increased the incidence of alcoholism. Subsequently, the act was repealed in 1933, ending Prohibition.

The next, and much more useful, effort to combat alcoholism was the psychosocial Alcoholics Anonymous organization, started in 1935 by William Griffith Wilson and Robert Holbrook Smith. Because that organization does not reach the majority of alcoholics, other efforts have evolved as treatment methodologies. Among these have been psychiatric counseling, alcohol rehabilitation centers, family counseling, and alcohol management programs in the workplace. These endeavors, funded by the federal government and private industry, reached workable levels in the last quarter of the twentieth century.

Alcoholics Anonymous and all the other options for treating alcoholism, alone or in various combinations, have had considerable success in reaching alcoholics, and combined alcoholism therapy seems to work best. It has not yet been possible to cure the disease, however, partly because there is no clear understanding of the cause of alcoholism. It is obvious that solving the riddle of alcoholism is essential because of its epidemic proportions. Frightening observations of the late twentieth century were estimates that up to 25 percent of American teenagers got drunk weekly and that 50 percent of alcoholics were children of alcoholic parents. The main hope for curing alcoholism is ongoing basic research in the areas of behavioral science, biochemistry, pharmacology, physiology, and psychiatry.

—Sanford S. Singer, Ph.D.
updated by Nancy A. Piotrowski, Ph.D.

See also Addiction; Cirrhosis; Dementia; Fetal alcohol syndrome; Intoxication; Jaundice; Liver disorders; Manic-depressive disorder; Psychosis.

FOR FURTHER INFORMATION:

Becker, Charles E. "Pharmacotherapy in the Treatment of Alcoholism." In *The Diagnosis and Treatment of Alcoholism*, edited by J. H. Mendelson and N. K. Mello. New York: McGraw-Hill, 1979. This article describes the uses and pitfalls of therapeutic drugs. Topical coverage includes managing intoxication, alcohol withdrawal syndrome, and related problems; chronic assistance; and handling depression in patients.

Bennett, Abram E. *Alcoholism and the Brain*. New York: Stratton International Medical Book, 1977. The relationships between brain function and alcoholism as a brain disease are considered. Coverage includes alcohol action in the brain; tests for alcoholism-related brain disease; constructive relationships between psychiatry and other alcoholism treatments; and rehabilitation methodology.

Berkow, Robert, and Andrew J. Fletcher, eds. *The Merck Manual of Diagnosis and Therapy*. 13th ed. Rahway, N.J.: Merck Sharp & Dohme Research Labs, 1977. This book contains a compendium of data on the etiology, diagnosis, and treatment of alcoholism. Contains good cross-references to the psychopathology related to the disease, drug rehabilitation, and Alcoholics Anonymous. Designed for physicians, it is also valuable to less specialized readers.

Collins, R. Lorraine, Kenneth E. Leonard, and John R. Searles, eds. *Alcohol and the Family*. New York: Guilford Press, 1990. This book is divided into genetics, family processes, and family-oriented treatment. Genetic testing and markers are well covered, and adolescent drinking, children of alcoholics, and alcoholism's effect on a marriage are also discussed. Evaluates the ability of the family to cope with stresses of alcoholism and its treatment.

Cox, W. Miles, ed. *The Treatment and Prevention of Alcohol Problems: A Resource Manual*. Orlando, Fla.: Academic Press, 1987. This work contains much information on the psychiatric and behavioral aspects of alcoholism. It is also widely useful in many other related issues, including Alcoholics Anonymous, marital and family therapy, and alcoholism prevention.

Eskelson, Cleamond D. "Hereditary Predisposition for Alcoholism." In *Diagnosis of Alcohol Abuse*, edited by Ronald R. Watson. Boca Raton, Fla.: CRC Press, 1989. This article provides useful data on the genetic aspects of alcoholism, concentrating on metabolism, animal and human studies, teetotalism, familial alcoholism, and genetic markers. Sixty-five references are included.

Knott, David H. *Alcohol Problems: Diagnosis and Treatment*. New York: Pergamon Press, 1986. This book provides physicians with useful information. Topics include alcohol use and abuse; biochemical factors; epidemiology, diagnosis, and treatment; information on special populations affected by the disease; and perspectives on control and prevention.

Mecca, Andrew M. *Alcoholism in America: A Modern Perspective*. Belvedere, Calif.: California Health Research Foundation, 1980. Entertaining reading about the history of alcoholic beverages, the nature of alcoholism, its effects on the body, its treatment, community alcoholism prevention, and future perspectives. Includes a useful glossary.

Rix, Keith J. B., and Elizabeth Lumsden Rix. *Alcohol Problems: A Guide for Nurses and Other Health Professionals*. Bristol, England: John Wright and Sons, 1983. This book, with more than two hundred references, provides nurses with "information that will contribute to . . . improved education." Contains information on the causes of alcoholism, its epidemiology, characteristics of alcohol intoxication and withdrawal, medical treatment, psychosocial aspects, and intervention models.

Watson, Ronald R., ed. *Diagnosis of Alcohol Abuse*. Boca Raton, Fla.: CRC Press, 1989. This work contains chapters on various aspects of alcoholism research. They in-
clude basic science issues in biochemistry, genetics, enzymology, and nutrition. Other topics covered are the diagnosis of alcoholic liver disease, the identification of problem drinkers, and alcohol testing and screening.

ALLERGIES

DISEASE/DISORDER

ANATOMY OR SYSTEM AFFECTED: Gastrointestinal system, immune system, lungs, nose, skin, stomach

SPECIALTIES AND RELATED FIELDS: Dermatology, family practice, immunology, internal medicine, otorhinolaryngology, pediatrics, pharmacology

DEFINITION: Exaggerated immune reactions to materials that are intrinsically harmless; the body's release of pharmacologically active chemicals during allergic reactions may result in discomfort, tissue damage, or, in severe responses, death.

KEY TERMS:

allergen: any substance that induces an allergic reaction

anaphylaxis: an immediate immune reaction, triggered by mediators that cause vasodilation and the contraction of smooth muscle

basophil: a type of white blood cell which contains mediators associated with allergic reactions; represents 1 percent or less of total white cells

histamine: a compound released during allergic reactions which causes many of the symptoms of allergies

IgE: a type of antibody associated with the release of granules from basophils and mast cells

mast cell: a tissue cell with granules containing vasoactive mediators such as histamine, serotonin, and bradykinin; the tissue equivalent of basophil

CAUSES AND SYMPTOMS

Allergies represent inappropriate immune responses to intrinsically harmless materials, or antigens. Most allergens are common environmental antigens. Approximately one in every six Americans is allergic to material such as dust, molds, dust mites, animal dander, or pollen. The effects range from a mere nuisance, such as the rhinitis associated with hay fever allergies or the itching of poison ivy, to the life-threatening anaphylactic shock that may follow a bee sting. Allergies are most often found in children, but they may affect any age group.

Allergy is one of the hypersensitivity reactions generally classified according to the types of effector molecules that mediate their symptoms and according to the time delay that follows exposure to the allergen. P. G. H. Gell and Robin Coombs defined four types of hypersensitivities. Three of these, Types I through III, follow minutes to hours after the exposure to an allergen. Type IV, or delayed-type hypersensitivity (DTH), may occur anywhere from twenty-four to seventy-two hours after exposure. People are most familiar with two of these forms of allergies: Type I, or immediate hypersensitivity, commonly seen as hay fever or asthma; and Type IV, most often following an encounter with poison ivy or poison oak.

Type I hypersensitivities have much in common with any normal immune response. A foreign material, an allergen, comes in contact with the host's immune system, and an antibody response is the result. The response differs according to the type of molecule produced. A special class of antibody, IgE, is secreted by the B lymphocytes. IgE, when complexed with the specific allergen, is capable of binding to any of several types of mediator cells, mainly basophils and mast cells.

Mast cells are found throughout skin and tissue. The mucous membranes of the respiratory and gastrointestinal tract in particular have high concentrations of these cells, as many as ten thousand cells per cubic millimeter. Basophils, the blood cell equivalents of the mast cells, represent 1 percent or less of the total white-cell count. Though the cells are not identical, they do possess features related to the role that they play in an allergic response. Both basophils and mast cells contain large numbers of granules composed of pharmacologically active chemicals. Both also contain surface receptors for IgE molecules. The binding of IgE/allergen complexes to these cells triggers the release of the granules.

A large number of common antigens can be associated with allergies. These include plant pollens (as are found in rye grass or ragweed), foods such as nuts or eggs, bee or wasp venom, mold, or animal dander. A square mile of ragweed may produce as much as 16 tons of pollen in a single season. In fact, almost any food or environmental substance could serve as an allergen. The most important defining factor as to whether an individual is allergic to any particular substance is the extent and type of IgE production against that substance.

Type I allergic reactions begin as soon as the sensitized person is exposed to the allergen. In the case of hay fever, this results when the person inhales the pollen particle. The shell of the particle is enzymatically dissolved, and the specific allergens are released in the vicinity of the mucous membranes in the respiratory system. If the person has had prior sensitization to the materials, IgE molecules secreted by localized lymphocytes bind to the allergens, forming an antibody/antigen complex.

Events commonly associated with allergies to pollen—a runny nose and itchy, watery eyes—result from the formation of such complexes. A sequence of events is set in place when the immune complexes bind to the surface of the mast cell or basophil. The reactions begin with a cross-linking of the IgE receptors on the cell. Such cross-linking is necessary because, in its absence, no release of granules occurs. On the other hand, artificial cross-linking of the receptors in laboratory experiments, even in the absence of IgE, results in the release of vasoactive granules.

Following the activation of the cell surface, a series of biochemical events occurs, the key being an influx of calcium into the cell. Two events rapidly follow: The cell begins production of prostaglandins and leukotrienes, two mediators that play key roles in allergic reactions, and preexisting granules begin moving toward the cell surface. When they reach the cell surface, the granules fuse with the cell membrane, releasing their contents into the tissue.

The contents of the granules mediate the clinical mani-

The Body's Response to Allergens

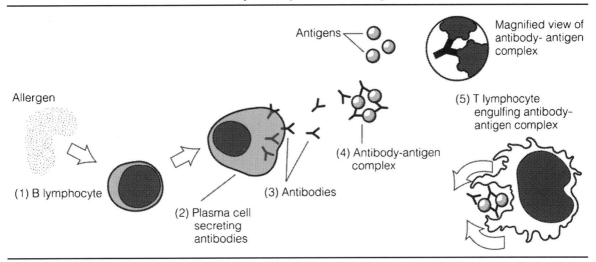

An allergic reaction is caused when foreign material, or antigens, enter the immune system, which produces B lymphocytes (1) that cause blood plasma cells to secrete antibodies (2). The antibodies (3) link with antigens to form antigen-antibody complexes (4), which then are engulfed and destroyed by a T lymphocyte (5).

festations of allergies. These mediators can be classified as either primary or secondary. Thus, clinical responses are divided into immediate and late-phase reactions. Primary mediators are those found in preexisting granules and that are released initially following the activities at the cell surface. They include substances such as histamine and serotonin, associated with increased vascular permeability and smooth muscle contraction. Histamine itself may constitute 10 percent of the weight of the granules in these cells. The result is the runny nose, irritated eyes, and bronchial congestion with which so many are familiar. Secondary mediators, which are released in the late phase, are synthesized following the binding of the immune complexes to the cell surface. These substances include the leukotrienes (also called slow reactive substances of anaphylaxis, or SRS-A) and prostaglandins. Pharmacological effects from these chemicals include vasodilation, increased capillary permeability, contraction of smooth muscles in the bronchioles, and, more important, a group of chemotactic activities that attract many different white cells in the site to magnify the inflammatory reaction. This is why an allergic reaction is divided into two phases and the late reaction may last for days.

Foods to which one is allergic may trigger similar reactions in the gut. Mast cells in the gastrointestinal tract also contain receptors for IgE, and contact with food allergens results in the release of mediators similar to those in the respiratory passages. The result may be vomiting or diarrhea. The allergen may also pass from the gut into the circulation or other tissues, triggering asthmatic attacks or urticaria (hives).

In severe allergic reactions, the response may be swift and deadly. The venom released during a bee sting may trigger a systemic response from circulating basophils or mast cells, resulting in the contraction of pulmonary muscles and rapid suffocation, a condition known as anaphylactic shock. The leukotrienes, platelet-activating factor, and prostaglandins play key roles in these reactions.

Delayed-type hypersensitivities, also known as contact dermatitis reactions, are most commonly manifested following the presentation of a topical allergen. These may include the catechol-containing oils of poison oak, the constituents of hair dyes or cosmetics, environmental contaminants such as nickel or turpentine, or any of a wide variety of environmental agents. Rather than being mediated by antibodies, as are the other types of hypersensitivities, DTH is mediated through a specific cellular response. These cells appear to be a special class of T (for thymus-derived) lymphocytes.

DTH reactions are initiated following the exposure to the appropriate antigen. Antigen-presenting cells in the skin bind and "present" the allergen to the specific T lymphocytes. This results in the secretion by these T cells of a variety of chemicals mediating inflammation. These media-

tors, or cytokines, include gamma interferon, interleukin-2, and tumor necrosis factor. The result, developing over a period of twenty-four to seventy-two hours, is a significant inflammatory response with subsequent localized damage to tissue.

The other classes of hypersensitivity reactions, Types II and III, are less commonly associated with what most people consider to be allergies. Yet they do have much in common with Type I, immediate hypersensitivity. Type II reactions are mediated by a type of antibody called IgG. Clinical manifestations result from the antibody-mediated destruction of target cells, rather than through the release of mediators. One of the most common forms of reaction is blood transfusion reactions, either against the A or B blood group antigen or as a result of an Rh incompatibility. For example, if a person with type O blood is accidentally transfused with type A, an immune reaction will occur. The eventual result is destruction of the incompatible blood cells. Rh incompatibilities are most commonly associated with a pregnant woman who is lacking the Rh protein in her blood (that is, Rh negative) carrying a child who is Rh positive (a blood type obtained from the father's genes). The production of IgG directed against the Rh protein in the child's blood can set in motion events that result in the destruction of the baby's red blood cells, a condition known as erythroblastosis fetalis.

Type III reactions are known as immune complex diseases. In this case, sensitivity to antigens results in formation of IgG/antigen complexes, which can lodge in the kidney or other sites in the body. The complexes activate what is known as the complement system, a series of proteins which include vasoactive chemicals and lipolytic compounds. The result can be a significant inflammation that can lead to kidney damage. Type III reactions can include autoimmune diseases such as arthritis or lupus, or drug reactions such as penicillin allergies.

It should be kept in mind, however, that none of these reactions is inherently abnormal. Under normal circumstances, these same reactions mediate an inflammatory defense against foreign pathogens. For example, the normal role of IgE appears to be associated with the destruction of parasites such as are found in helminthic infections (such as parasitic worms). The release of mediators under these conditions is important as a defensive reaction leading to the expulsion or destruction of worms. It is only when these same mediators are released inappropriately that one observes the symptoms of allergies.

Most individuals are familiar with immediate hypersensitivities as reactions involving a localized area. The most common form of allergy is rhinitis, known as hay fever, which affects approximately 10 percent of the population. When a person inhales an environmental allergen such as ragweed pollen, the result is a release of pharmacologically active mediators from mast cells located in the upper respiratory tract. If the release occurs in the lower respiratory tract, the condition is known as asthma. In both instances, the eyes and nose are subject to inflammation and the release of secretions. In mild cases, the person suffers from watery discharges, coughing, and sneezing. In more severe asthma attacks, the bronchioles may become constricted and obstruct the air passages.

TREATMENT AND THERAPY

There exist three methods for dealing with allergies: avoidance of the allergen, palliative treatments, and desensitization. Ideally, one can attempt to avoid the allergen. For example, cow's milk, a common allergen, should not be given to a child at too young an age, and one can stay away from patches of poison ivy or avoid eating strawberries if one is allergic to them.

Yet avoidance is not always possible or desirable, as the problem may be the fur from the family cat. In any event, it is sometimes difficult to identify the specific substance causing the symptoms. This is particularly true when dealing with foods. Various procedures exist to identify the irritating substance, skin testing being the most common. In this procedure, the patient's skin is exposed to small amounts of suspected allergens. A positive test is indicated by formation of hives or reddening within about twenty to thirty minutes. If the person is hypersensitive to a suspected allergen and finds a skin test too risky, then a blood test (RAST) may be substituted. In addition to running a battery of tests, a patient's allergy history (including family history, since allergies are in part genetic) or environment may give clues as to the identity of the culprit.

The most commonly used method of dealing with allergies is a palliative treatment—that is, treatment of the symptoms. Antihistamines act by binding to histamine receptors on target cells, interfering with the binding of histamine. There exist two types of histamine receptors: H-1 and H-2. Histamine binding to H-1 receptors results in contractions of smooth muscles and increased mucous secretion. Binding to H-2 receptors results in increased vasopermeability and swelling. Antihistamines that act at the level of the H-1 receptor include alkylamines and ethanolamines and are effective in treating symptoms of acute allergies such as hay fever. H-2 blockers such as cimetidine are effective in the symptomatic treatment of duodenal ulcers through the control of gastric secretions.

Many antihistamines can be obtained without a prescription. If they are not used properly, however, the side effects can be serious. Overuse may result in toxicity, particularly in children; overdoses in children can be fatal. Because antihistamines can depress the central nervous system, side effects include drowsiness, nausea, constipation, and drying of the throat or respiratory passage. This is particularly true of H-1 blockers. There is a new generation of H-1 antihistamines available on the market. They are long-acting and are free of the sedative effect of other antihistamines.

Other symptomatic treatments include the use of cromolyn sodium, which blocks the influx of calcium into the mast cell, and thus is called a mast cell stabilizer. It acts to block steps leading to degranulation and the release of mediators. In more severe cases, the administration of steroids (cortisone) may prove useful in limiting symptoms of allergies.

Anaphylaxis is the most severe form of immediate hypersensitivity, and unless treated promptly, it may be fatal. It is often triggered in susceptible persons by common environmental substances: bee or wasp venom, drugs such as penicillin, foods such as peanuts and seafood, or latex protein in rubber. Symptoms include labored breathing, rapid loss of blood pressure, itching, hives, and/or loss of bladder control. The symptoms are triggered by a sudden and massive release of mast cell or basophil mediators such as histamine, leukotrienes, or prostaglandin derivatives. Treatment consists of an immediate injection of epinephrine and the maintenance of an open air passage into the lungs. If cardiac arrest occurs, cardiopulmonary resuscitation must be undertaken. Persons in known danger of encountering such a triggering allergen often carry with them an emergency kit containing epinephrine and antihistamines.

Contact dermatitis is a form of delayed-type hypersensitivity, developing several days after exposure to the sensitizing allergen. Rather than resulting from the presence of IgE antibody, the symptoms of contact dermatitis result from a series of chemicals released by sensitized T lymphocytes in the area of the skin on which the allergen (often poison ivy or poison oak) is found. Treatments generally involve the application of topical corticosteroids and soothing or drying agents. In more severe cases, systemic use of corticosteroids may be necessary.

In some persons, the relief of allergy symptoms may be achieved through desensitization. This form of immunotherapy involves the repeated subcutaneous injection of increasing doses of the allergen. In a significant number of persons, such therapy leads to an improvement in symptoms. The idea behind such therapy is that repeated injections of the allergen may lead to production of another class of antibody, the more systemic IgG. These molecules can serve as blocking antibodies, competing with IgE in binding to the allergen. Because IgG/allergen complexes can be phagocytosed (destroyed by phagocytes) and do not bind receptors on mast cells or basophils, they should not trigger the symptoms of allergies. Unfortunately, for reasons that remain unclear, not all persons or all allergies respond to such therapy.

The type I immediate hypersensitivity reactions commonly run in families. This is not so surprising if one realizes that the regulation of IgE production is genetically determined. Thus, if both parents have allergies, there is little chance that their offspring will escape the problem. On the other hand, if one or both parents are allergy-free, the odds are at least even that the offspring will also be free from such reactions.

PERSPECTIVE AND PROSPECTS

Though allergies in humans have probably existed since humans first evolved from ancestral primates, it was only in the nineteenth century that an understanding of the process began to develop. Type I hypersensitivity reaction was first described in 1839 through experiments in which dogs were repeatedly injected with egg albumin and developed an immediate fatal shock. The term "anaphylaxis" was coined for this phenomenon in 1902, when Paul Portier and Charles Richet observed that dogs repeatedly immunized with extracts of sea anemone tentacles suffered a similar fate. Richet was awarded the 1913 Nobel Prize in Physiology or Medicine for his work on anaphylaxis.

In the 1920's, Sir Henry Dale established that at least some of the phenomena associated with immediate hypersensitivity were caused by the chemical histamine. Dale sensitized guinea pigs against various antigens. He then observed that, when the muscles from the uterus were removed and exposed to the same antigen, histamine was released and the muscles underwent contraction (known as the Schultz-Dale reaction).

The existence of a component in human serum which

Multiple Chemical Sensitivity Syndrome

Multiple chemical sensitivity syndrome (MCS), reactive airway dysfunctions, and the "sick building" syndromes are overlapping disorders caused by intolerance of environmental chemicals. Exactly how many people are affected by MCS is unknown. The onset is often associated with initial acute chemical exposure; patients may report the onset of MCS after moving into a new home, after exposure to chemicals in the workplace, or following the use of pesticides in the home. Patients often describe an increasing intolerance to commonly encountered chemicals at concentrations well tolerated by other people.

Symptoms usually wax and wane with exposure and are more likely to occur in patients with preexisting histories of migraine or classical allergies. Idiosyncratic medication reactions (especially to preservative chemicals) are common in MCS patients, as are dysautonomic symptoms (such as vascular instability), poor temperature regulation, and food intolerance. It is thought that patients with MCS have organ abnormalities involving the liver, the nervous system (including the brain and the limbic, peripheral, and autonomic systems), the immune system, and perhaps porphyrin metabolism, probably reflecting chemical injury to these systems. There is often a substantial overlap of MCS symptoms with fibromyalgia and chronic fatigue syndrome.

The common clinical symptoms may include headaches (often migraine), chronic fatigue, musculoskeletal aching, chronic respiratory inflammation (rhinitis, sinusitis, laryngitis, asthma), attention-deficit disorder, and hyperactivity (affecting younger children). Less common complaints include tremor, seizure, and mitral valve prolapse. Agents associated with the onset of MCS include gasoline, kerosene, natural gas, pesticides (especially chlordane and chlorpyrifos), organic solvents, new carpet and other renovation materials, adhesives and glues, fiberglass, carbonless copy paper, fabric softener, formaldehyde and glutaraldehyde, carpet shampoo (lauryl sulfate) and other cleaning agents, isocyanates, combustion products (poorly vented gas heaters, overheated batteries), and medications (dinitrochlorobenzene for warts, intranasally packed neosynephrine, prolonged antibiotics, and general anesthesia with petrochemicals).

It is believed that the mechanisms that lead to MCS may be multifactorial and include neurogenic inflammation (respiratory, gastrointestinal, and genitourinary symptoms), kindling and time-dependent sensitization (neurologic symptoms), and immune activation or impaired porphyrin metabolism (multiple-organ symptoms). Pathological findings of MCS have rarely been examined. A preliminary study of nasal pathology of these patients indicate that they are characterized by defects in the junctions between cells, desquamation of the respiratory epithelium, glandular hyperplasia, lymphocytic infiltrates, and peripheral nerve fiber proliferation. A consistent physiologic abnormality in these patients has not been established.

Psychiatric, personality, cognitive/neurologic, immunologic, and olfactory studies have been conducted comparing MCS subjects with various control groups. Thus far, the most consistent finding is that patients with MCS have a higher rate of psychiatric disorders across studies and relative to diverse comparison groups. Since these studies are cross-sectional, however, causality cannot be implied. Various working groups have proposed several research questions addressing the relationship between neurogenic inflammation and toxicant-induced loss of tolerance with the development of MCS.

The management of patients with MCS at present is symptomatic and supportive therapy. There is a general consensus among researchers and clinicians that in order to treat patients with MCS effectively, a double-blind, placebo-controlled study performed in an environmentally controlled facility, with rigorous documentation of both objective and subjective responses, is needed to help elucidate the nature and origin of MCS.

—Shih-Wen Huang, M.D.

mediates hypersensitive reactions was demonstrated by Otto Prausnitz, a Polish bacteriologist, and Heinz Kustner, a Polish gynecologist, in 1921. Kustner had a strong allergy to fish. Prausnitz removed a sample of serum from his colleague and injected it under his own skin. The next day, Prausnitz injected fish extract in that same region. Hives immediately appeared, indicating that the serum contained components that mediated the allergy. For some time, the Prausnitz-Kustner test, or P-K test, remained a means of testing for allergens under circumstances in which a person could be tested for sensitivity. (It is no longer in use because of safety concerns.) In this test, a serum sample from the test subject was injected under the skin of a surrogate (usually a relative) and later followed with test allergens. The presence of a wheal and flare reaction (hives) indicated sensitivity to the allergen. The serum component responsible for this sensitivity was later identified as the antibody IgE by K. and T. Ishizaka and S. G. O. Johansson in 1967. The target cells to which the IgE bound were later identified as mast cells and basophils.

The discovery of IgE allowed scientists to develop a blood test called a radioallergosorbent test (RAST) that could measure a specific IgE antibody to an allergic substance. RAST is equally sensitive as a skin test and thus can be a substitute in some clinical circumstances. Furthermore, discoveries of numerous mediators form mast cells and other white cells such as cytokines, chemokines, interleukins, growth factors, and interferon have helped scientists understand the pathology of allergy at the molecular level. It helps clinically to divide the allergic reaction into immediate reaction (onset within a few minutes after exposure to allergens) and delayed or late-phase reaction (onset hours after exposure to antigens and a reaction that may last for days). The definition of allergy now expands from the traditional, immediate allergic reaction to the inclusion of chronic inflammatory process in the tissues. With a better understanding of how allergies develop, better treatments can be offered to patients who suffer from this disorder.

The eventual goal of the research was to understand the molecular defects that result in allergies and ultimately to find a means to eliminate the problem, rather than simply offer palliative measures. For example, it is now known that interleukin-4 (one of the mediators of T cells) raises IgE production, while interferon (another mediator of T cells) lowers IgE production. By understanding the regulation of IgE production, it may become possible to inhibit IgE production in allergic persons selectively, without affecting the desired functions of the immune response.

—Richard Adler, Ph.D.
updated by Shih-Wen Huang, M.D.

See also Asthma; Autoimmune disorders; Bites and stings; Dermatitis; Dermatology; Food poisoning; Gastroenterology; Gastroenterology, pediatric; Gastrointestinal disorders; Gastrointestinal system; Host-defense mechanisms;

Immune system; Immunization and vaccination; Immunology; Lungs; Poisonous plants; Pulmonary medicine; Pulmonary medicine, pediatric; Rashes; Shock; Skin; Skin disorders.

FOR FURTHER INFORMATION:

Cutler, Ellen W. *Winning the War Against Asthma and Allergies.* Albany, N.Y.: Delmar, 1998. This clearly written book provides practical information on all aspects of allergies—what they are, their causes, testing, diagnosis, and treatment, including nontraditional therapies. Preventive measures are covered, as are scenarios for various allergy elimination therapies.

Joneja, Janice M. V., and Leonard Bielory. *Understanding Allergy, Sensitivity, and Immunity.* New Brunswick, N.J.: Rutgers University Press, 1990. The authors provide extensive discussion on allergies and the roles played by the immune system. They describe the means by which one can learn to cope with allergies and discuss various testing methods for the identification of allergens. Written for the nonscientist.

Kuby, Janis. *Immunology.* New York: W. H. Freeman, 1992. The section on hypersensitivity in this immunology textbook is well written and includes a mixture of detail and overview of the subject. Particularly useful are discussions of the various types of hypersensitivity reactions. Some knowledge of biology is useful.

Life, Death, and the Immune System. New York: W. H. Freeman, 1994. This comprehensive collection of articles from *Scientific American* provide basic information and research directions on AIDS, autoimmune disorders, allergies, and an excellent discussion of the immune system in general.

Norback, Craig T., ed. *The Allergy Encyclopedia.* New York: Penguin Books, 1981. A concise discussion of allergies and their causes. Much of the book is in the form of questions or terms related to the subject. Describes the symptoms associated with various types of allergies, as well as the role of psychosomatic disorders. Written for the nonscientist.

Roitt, Ivan. *Essential Immunology.* 7th ed. Boston: Blackwell Scientific Publications, 1991. Written by a leading author in the field, the text provides a fine description of immunology. The section on hypersensitivity is clearly presented and profusely illustrated. Though too detailed in places, most of the material can be understood by individuals who have taken high school-level biology. The first choice as a reference for the subject.

Shaw, Michael, ed. *Everything You Need to Know About Diseases.* Springhouse, Pa.: Springhouse Press, 1996. This well-illustrated consumer reference, compiled by more than one hundred doctors and medical experts, describes five hundred illnesses and conditions, their causes, symptoms, diagnosis, treatment, and prevention. A valuable reference book for everyone interested in health and disease.

Walsh, William. *The Food Allergy Book*. St. Paul, Minn.: ACA, 1995. In this excellent guide to one highly prevalent form of allergy, the author presents useful background information on food allergies and a pragmatic guide to identifying and eliminating food allergens from your diet.

Young, Stuart, Bruce Dobozin, and Margaret Miner. *Allergies*. Yonkers, N.Y.: Consumer Reports Books, 1991. An excellent review of the subject from Consumer Reports. In addition to discussing the diagnosis and treatment of allergies, the authors evaluate the various remedies on the market at the time of publication. Also useful are lists of organizations to contact for further information and various clinics that specialize in the treatment of allergies.

ALLIED HEALTH
HEALTH CARE SYSTEM
DEFINITION: A designation used to describe the services and personnel that support the providers of direct patient care within the larger health care system.

KEY TERMS:

anesthetist: a health care specialist who administers an agent (anesthetic) that makes the patient insensitive to sensation or pain

audiologist: a hearing impairment specialist involved in evaluation, measurement, and rehabilitation

chiropractic: a health care strategy which teaches that disease can be caused by the pinching of spinal nerves, the treatment of which involves spinal adjustment

kinesiotherapist: a health care specialist who provides therapy to a patient's muscles through muscular movement and exercise

nuclear medicine: an area of medicine that uses radioactive nucleotides in diagnostic and treatment procedures

optometry: a specialty that deals with problems in the refractive power of the eyes and with the making of corrective lenses

paramedical: related to the science or practice of medicine

perfusionist: a health care specialist who operates extracorporal circulation equipment when it is necessary to support or replace a patient's circulatory or respiratory function

podiatry: the specialty that deals with the diagnosis and treatment of foot problems, including minor surgery

sonographer: a health care specialist who records and displays the results of an ultrasonic scan which produces a sonogram of a specific anatomical area

THE BOUNDARIES OF ALLIED HEALTH WITHIN MEDICINE

Allied health refers to a field of health care workers who participate with physicians and/or nurses in a team effort to promote health and prevent disease in the patient. Allied health occupations may be either professional or technical, depending on the extent and caliber of didactic learning and clinical study as well as on the duties associated with the occupation.

Throughout the evolution of the American health care system, the role of the physician has remained relatively stable and of primary importance. The American Medical Association (AMA) successfully developed specialty categories to solidify the role of physician and to protect the doctorate in medicine.

The designation "allied health" appears to be a creation of the AMA to describe those paramedical occupations that developed within the evolving health care system in response to the advancing technology and expanding health care facilities, such as hospitals, clinics, medical centers, and laboratories. The AMA, through its various societies and committees, guided the formation of a variety of occupations to perform tasks that would not or could not be performed by the medical doctor or nurse. These occupations were carefully husbanded by strict job descriptions, educational guidelines, and evaluation criteria. For the most part, allied health professionals are those fields that the Committee on Allied Health Education and Accreditation (CAHEA) of the AMA has scrutinized according to essential criteria that have been adopted by the particular profession. These criteria are primarily the standards that are established by a profession as a means to establish education programs that instruct new professionals, to perform a self-study by each program, and to be evaluated by an outside visiting team. A profession is also characterized by the establishment of a society or association by those practitioners of the occupation for the purpose of supporting the research, teaching, and learning of its members. The society sets standards of job performance and evaluation and also establishes a code of ethics to which its members adhere.

Those professions not accredited by the CAHEA are dentistry, optometry, podiatry, chiropractic, veterinary medicine, physical therapy, and nursing. Whether a profession finds the designation "allied health" complimentary or acceptable appears to depend on the status of the profession with respect to its age, the amount of education and responsibility required, and whether autonomy from the AMA is desired. The more autonomous a profession, the more impressive the identity and social status of its practitioners with respect to salary, power, and influence. For example, although a physical therapist can have a private practice rather than be employed in a hospital or another setting that guarantees a certain number of patients, a therapist is not legally allowed to treat a patient without an order from a physician. In 1987, the average salary for a hospital physical therapy (PT) supervisor was $38,000, while those in private practice earned $40,000 or more. In order to have a private practice, a physical therapist must cultivate a list of local physicians for referrals.

The nursing profession is a good example of a health profession that, to a greater or lesser extent, is not under the allied health umbrella. It is not listed by either the CAHEA or the Association of Schools of Allied Health Professions (ASAHP). Although the U.S. government provided scholarships for nurses in the Allied Health Personnel Training Act of 1966, nursing is excluded from the definition in the Health Professions Education Amendment of 1991. Nursing has been continuously able to maintain its integrity as a profession for a number of reasons: It has always had solidarity provided by the National League of Nursing (NLN), it has continued to develop its education requirements and responsibilities, it requires government licensure, and it has a very visible role in health care delivery—to some extent more than that of the physician.

The nursing profession continues to develop and is reaching into areas that were traditionally considered to be the domain of the physician. Nurse practitioners are able to take medical histories, read X rays, order and read tests, and diagnose conditions. They are able to prescribe medications in thirty-five states and can be reimbursed for some services by Medicare and Medicaid. Nurse anesthetists can work independently of a doctor in a variety of health care delivery settings.

According to the 1991 federal legislation cited above, the term "allied health profession" excludes both the nurse and the physician assistant. It includes all those who have had educational training in a science program relating to health services, earning anything from a certificate to a doctorate. It further defines allied health care personnel as individuals who share in the responsibility of the delivery of health care services or those related to health care. Such services include the identification, evaluation, and prevention of disease and disorders, as well as those related to diet and nutrition, health promotion, rehabilitation, and health systems management.

Those professionals who are excluded from the label of allied health care personnel by the government are doctors of medicine, osteopathy, dentistry, veterinary medicine, optometry, podiatry, pharmacy, chiropractic, and clinical psychology. Also excluded are pharmacists with bachelor's degrees, social workers, and those with graduate degrees in public health and health administration. It is confusing, however, to have physician assistant excluded from allied health by the government and the CAHEA but included in the designation by the ASAHP. Physical therapy is included by the government and the ASAHP but excluded by the CAHEA. The reason for such apparent confusion rests with the various points of view. The government is interested in the service provided by the particular occupation. The ASAHP is interested in promoting allied health education, professional growth, and collaboration between the professions and in influencing public policy as it relates to the above. The CAHEA has the responsibility of overseeing the allied health education programs that are under the AMA umbrella.

According to the ASAHP, allied health professionals serve in a variety of autonomous and service positions. Therapists and counselors function in private practice and are directly involved with their patients. The medical technologist practices in a laboratory profession at least once removed from patient contact. Allied health care professionals work in every aspect of the health delivery system in a variety of disciplines with a variety of educational experiences. They work throughout the country in a number of physical settings, including hospitals, physicians' office laboratories, clinics, hospices, community programs, schools, and extended care facilities.

Because of the dynamic state of health care, many allied health care occupations eventually become professions. The expansion of knowledge and evolving technology require increased learning and understanding. The aspiring practitioner of a particular occupation is confronted with a body of information that must be mastered. Those involved with the occupation must organize the information, find new applications, and teach what they know to students interested in the occupation. Essentials or standards are adopted, and a new allied health profession is born. The evolution of the medical technologist or clinical laboratory scientist from the help hired by the pathologist provides a good example of how a profession begins and then sustains itself. The first allied health professions to establish essential criteria and have their education programs evaluated by the AMA were occupational therapy, medical technology, and physical therapy.

SCIENCE AND PROFESSION

Allied health is a designation that can only be understood in the context of direct health care providers and patients. Direct health care providers are those who are licensed to interact directly with the patient in diagnosis and/or treatment. Examples are medical doctors of various specialties, nurses, dentists, optometrists, chiropractors, and podiatrists. Ancillary activities that support direct care would be described as allied health. Those careers that are involved with these activities are allied health careers or professions.

The ancillary activities to primary care have come about for many reasons. Among them are the advances in technology that have resulted in more sophisticated diagnostic testing. Only the direct caregiver such as a medical doctor (and in some cases, a nurse practitioner) can make a diagnosis. This activity may require data, however, that are provided by the medical technologist, audiologist, diagnostic medical sonographer, or radiologic technologist; some data are provided only after time-consuming and specialized laboratory activity provided by the cytotechnologist or the blood bank technology specialist. Health care often involves specialized equipment and someone specifically trained in running it, such as the perfusionist, the radiation therapy technologist, and the cardiovascular technologist; the more mundane but very important task of medical record keeping is performed by an administrator and technicians; highly specialized areas of therapy have resulted in careers that require a very narrow area of medical understanding or a specialized area that complements the medical activity of the doctor, such as art therapist, music therapist, occupational therapist, physical therapist, and respiratory therapist.

Allied health has become an important aspect of the American health care system. Sophisticated technology and equipment, new therapeutic techniques, routine record keeping, complex laboratory tests, and specialized therapies have resulted in careers that complement the duties of the direct caregiver. Clinical care can only be as good as the primary care professionals supported by allied health care professionals. An adequate allied health system depends on the support of allied health educational institutions, professional organizations, and clinical settings that support service delivery, research, and education.

If the designation "allied health" is to be related to those professions whose essential criteria for their education programs are adopted by the CAHEA, then three things must be considered when describing each of the allied health professions: first, the educational background in terms of degree requirements and of didactic and clinical experience; second, the occupational duties to be performed; and third, the association or organization that takes on the responsibility of sponsoring the profession with regard to organizing, developing, teaching, and evaluating.

For a number of allied health occupations, either a bachelor's degree is not required or this requirement varies among programs. Examples of such occupations often use the designation "technician" as in emergency medical technician, histologic technician, medical laboratory technician, medical record technician, and respiratory therapist technician. Others receive very specialized training, such as the diagnostic medical sonographer and the perfusionist. Examples of those allied health professionals in fields whose essential criteria are evaluated and accredited by the CAHEA that have maintained the bachelor's degree are anesthesiology assistants, athletic trainers, specialists in blood bank technology, cytotechnologists, medical illustrators, medical records administrators, nuclear medicine technologists, occupational therapists, radiation therapy technologists, radiographers, and respiratory therapists.

Even under the aegis of the AMA, however, CAHEA evaluation and accreditation are not enough to be used to define allied health personnel. The ASAHP lists the twenty-eight careers regulated by the AMA (except physician assistant) and thirty-nine others that fall under the definition of allied health professions as outlined by the federal government. Among those careers found are art therapist, audiologist, dance therapist, dental assistant, dietitian, educational therapist, genetic counselor, health care administrator,

histotechnologist, kinesiotherapist, music therapist, nutritionist, ophthalmic medical technologist, optician, optometric technician, physical therapist, psychiatric technician, recreational therapist, speech/language pathologist, veterinary technician, and vocational rehabilitation counselor. The ASAHP listing of allied health careers demonstrates an allied health view that extends beyond the medical profession into autonomous professional areas such as dentistry, optometry, dietetics, nutrition, physical therapy, and veterinary medicine.

Credentials such as certification, registry, or licensure of occupation/profession is the final aspect that has an impact on the allied health professions. Certification implies that an individual has met certain ethical criteria and has achieved the minimal standards required to practice a particular occupation. Certification is usually provided by a nongovernment agency. Registry, which is usually provided by a government agency, involves being placed on a government listing. It is usually used with occupations that involve a minimal threat to public safety.

Licensure is an important part of the health care system because it attempts to protect both the public (which must rely on competent care) and the health care personnel (who must protect the profession to which they belong). Public safety is achieved when a government agency is given the responsibility to oversee the credentials of a person who attempts to practice a particular occupation or use a particular title. The health care worker is protected because licensure prevents unqualified practitioners from entering the occupation or profession. It also appears to increase salary benefits and prestige, as well as to provide the profession with greater visibility with respect to legislative government and the public in general.

Probably one of the most important aspects of licensure is that it legally defines the extent of the activities that are performed in the profession or occupation. For example, medical technologists and respiratory therapists can monitor arterial blood gases and electrolytes. If licensure to perform the tests were given to only one of the occupations, however, it would be illegal for individuals in the unlicensed profession to perform the tests. Licensure is particularly significant to the allied health professions because duties may overlap, especially in the variety of health care settings that are being developed.

The negative aspects to licensure should also be considered for their impact on allied health and most health care professions. There is a decrease in mobility when each state has its own licensing commission or agency. Some studies indicate that many rural areas do not have adequate care, and it is believed the licensure of professions not already licensed in some states, such as medical technology, could add to this problem by discouraging the movement of health care workers to these areas.

Finally, licensure affects not only individuals but also the facilities in which health care is practiced. Laboratories and direct care facilities such as hospitals are usually regulated by government licensure. The movement of health care treatment from hospitals to the many alternative facilities that now exist may also require that standards be established and evaluated.

Because of the uniformity of the health care system, there is ease of mobility horizontally (from location to location) for those in allied health occupations. There is consistency of facilities, equipment, job opportunity, job description, operating procedures, and regulations. Yet the very reason for the creation of most allied health occupations or professions—the requirement for specialized knowledge, procedures, or technology—makes them narrow in focus. Consequently, many people agree that there is less vertical mobility within some allied health positions.

Nevertheless, the educational requirements for some allied health occupations, particularly a bachelor's degree in liberal arts, provide greater opportunity for advancement. Job advancement opportunities can also increase with advanced degrees. For example, a bachelor's degree in medical technology or a master's degree in business administration provides an individual with professional opportunities in many of the ancillary industries that support the American health care system.

PERSPECTIVE AND PROSPECTS

The health care system in the United States is the product of three major forces: private enterprise, government, and charity. Although each of these forces may have had different objectives, their united goal has been the improved health of the American population. The primary location for the delivery of health care has been the hospital. The health care professions that evolved within this system and that have, in large part, given direction to its evolution are the medical profession and the nursing profession.

With the establishment of hospitals as the site of health care delivery, the nursing profession made itself fundamental to the continued evolution of health care. The hospital became the keystone of the entire health care system, as well as the focal point where each of the three forces would exert its influence.

As a result of health care moving from the private home to the public setting of the hospital, the health care of the patient became better, but at the same time it became more technology-oriented and more costly. Since the 1950's, technological advances have had a direct effect on patient care and therefore on the ever-evolving professions of medicine and nursing. During this same time of technological growth and specialized care, new areas of health care have begun to develop that are outside the accepted areas of medicine and nursing but allied to them because their common goal is the health of the patient.

As many as sixty-seven professions can be described as allied health. They complement the activities of not only the physician and nurse but also a variety of direct caregivers such as dentists, optometrists, and clinical psychologists. Allied health activities take place in hospitals, physicians' office laboratories, private laboratories, clinics, schools, extended care facilities, and the variety of other facilities utilized by direct care providers.

Advanced technology, the professions that constitute the health care team, and the administrative bureaucracy form the 500 billion-dollar health care industry in the United States. In 1988, it was estimated that health care spending would grow to 15 percent of the gross national product (GNP) of the United States by the year 2000, up from 12 percent. The health care system provides one of the most rapidly expanding areas for job opportunities in the American economy. In the 1980's, allied health—and in fact the entire health care system—was projected by the United States Department of Labor to be an area of growth through the remainder of the twentieth century.

Allied health occupations and professions are an integral part of the American health care system. Their role is indispensable to those professions responsible for patient diagnosis and treatment. Allied health provides a vast market for scientific products and instrumentation. It is composed of and supported by an array of professional organizations and educational institutions that will provide the impetus for its continued growth and evolution.

—*Patrick J. DeLuca, Ph.D.*

See also American Medical Association; Anesthesiology; Audiology; Blood bank; Cardiac rehabilitation; Cytopathology; Environmental health; Health maintenance organizations (HMOs); Hospitals; Imaging and radiology; Laboratory tests; Nuclear radiology; Occupational health; Paramedics; Physical rehabilitation; Physician assistants; Preventive medicine; Pulmonary medicine; Sports medicine; Surgical technologists.

FOR FURTHER INFORMATION:
Allied Health Education Directory. 23d ed. Chicago: American Medical Association, 1995. This directory is an excellent catalog of those allied health professions that have been developed and regulated by the AMA through the CAHEA. Professions are listed and described with regard to their duties and educational requirements. This text is useful for both students and educators because it identifies changes within the guidelines for educational programs of allied health professions.

Clerc, Jeanne M. *An Introduction to Clinical Laboratory Science*. St. Louis: Mosby Year Book, 1992. This introductory text provides an excellent treatment of the development of the clinical laboratory and the clinical laboratory scientist as they relate to the health care system. Describes the evolution of an allied health occupation to a profession and differentiates between the two.

Corder, Brice W., ed. *Strategy for Success: A Handbook for Prehealth Students*. Champaign, Ill.: National Association of Advisors for the Health Professions, 1990. An excellent resource for students, health profession advisers, and anyone who is interested in learning about health professions. Careers are described in the context of the health care settings in which they are practiced. Their educational and licensing requirements, as well as average compensation, are discussed.

ALTERNATIVE MEDICINE

SPECIALTY

ANATOMY OR SYSTEM AFFECTED: All

SPECIALITES AND RELATED FIELDS: Osteopathic medicine, preventive medicine, public health

DEFINITION: A wide variety of medical practices and therapies which falls outside traditional, Western medical practice. The approaches emphasize the individual as a biopsychosocial whole, or, in some cases, as a biopsychosocial-spiritual whole. They deemphasize focusing treatment on specific diseases or symptoms.

KEY TERMS:

physiological: characteristic of or appropriate to an organism's healthy or normal functioning

therapeutic: relating to the treatment of disease or disorders

toxin: a poisonous substance that is a product of the chemical processes of a living organism

SCIENCE AND PROFESSION

Alternative medicine—known also as natural healing, complementary medicine, or holistic medicine—focuses on the relationship among the mind, body, and spirit. The underlying philosophy is that people can maintain health by preventing disease in the first place by keeping the body in "balance" and by utilizing the body's "natural" healing processes when people succumb to disease. Alternative medicine approaches contrast with Western medicine's traditional focus on treating symptoms and curing disease and its underemphasis of preventive medicine. Thought "way-out" at one time, complementary medicines and therapies are gaining wide appeal as their anecdotal efficacy and reputation grows.

Alternative medicine practitioners treat everything from diseases such as cancer and acquired immunodeficiency syndrome (AIDS) to chronic pain and fatigue, stress, insomnia, depression, high blood pressure, circulatory and digestive disorders, allergies, arthritis, diabetes mellitus, and drug and alcohol addictions.

The major risks associated with alternative medicine include costly delays in seeking appropriate treatment, misinformation, side effects from self-administered remedies, and psychological distress if patients believe that they are responsible for their own illness or lack of recovery. In addition, many alternative medicine practitioners have little or no formal health training and may discourage traditional medical treatment or oppose proved health measures such as immunization and pasteurization.

DIAGNOSTIC AND TREATMENT TECHNIQUES

Numerous alternative medicine treatments exist, and they vary widely in the nature of their claims, their acceptability to conventional doctors, and the manner in which they can and cannot be tested. The treatments can be divided into three main types.

The first type consists of those treatments that deal with the mind/body connection or that have recognized benefits and accepted applications and so are often used together with conventional medicine. These approaches include acupuncture and acupressure, biofeedback, chiropractic, hydrotherapy, light therapy, meditation, oxygen therapy, qi gong, sound therapy, Tai Chi Chuan, and yoga. The second type comprises treatments that can be tested by conventional methods and have some accepted applications. These treatments include aromatherapy, cell therapy, colon therapy, detoxification, energy medicine, enzyme therapy, homeopathy, kinesiology, magnetic field therapy, and neural therapy. The third type of treatments are very difficult to study because they seem to be at odds with Western medicine and cannot readily be tested through standard methods. An example of this type of treatment is herbal medicine.

Acupressure and acupuncture. These treatments are both based on the belief that the body has a vital energy that must be balanced in order to maintain good health. Acupressure uses pressure from the fingertips or knuckles to stimulate specific points on the body, while acupuncture uses needles inserted into the skin to restore the balance of energy. Both acupressure and acupuncture have been shown to stimulate the release of endorphins, the body's natural painkillers. Acupressure is useful for relieving chronic pain and fatigue and increasing blood circulation. Acupuncture is used successfully for relieving chronic pain and treating drug and alcohol withdrawal symptoms. Although hepatitis, transmission of infectious disease, and internal injuries have been reported in connection with acupuncture, such risks are uncommon.

Biofeedback. This technique involves learning to control automatic physiological responses such as blood pressure, heart rate, circulation, digestion, and perspiration in order to reduce anxiety, pain, and tension. The patient concentrates on consciously controlling the body's automatic responses while a machine monitors the results and displays them for the patient. Biofeedback can be useful in treating asthma, chronic pain, epilepsy, drug addiction, circulatory problems, and stress.

Chiropractic. Chiropractic treatment uses traditional medicine techniques such as X rays, physical examinations, and various tests in order to diagnose a disorder. Muscle spasms or ligament strains are treated by manipulation or adjustment to the spine and joints, thus reducing pressure on the spinal nerves and providing relief from pain. Recent research suggests chiropractic should be considered in treating certain types of lower back pain, as it is often superior to conventional interventions. Practitioners should be state licensed, and caution should be taken with practitioners who often repeat full-spine X rays or who ask patients to sign contracts at any time during treatment. Chiropractic is practiced either "straight," involving only spinal manipulation, or "mixed," involving other biomedical technologies such as electrical stimulation. Chiropractic treatment can be harmful if it is practiced in patients with fractures or undetected tumors or if it is practiced incorrectly.

Hydrotherapy. The use of water for healing or therapeutic purposes is termed hydrotherapy. It is used to treat chronic pain; to relieve stress; to improve circulation, mobility, strength, and flexibility; to reduce swelling; and to treat injuries to the skin. Because the buoyancy of water offsets gravity, more intense exercise can be done when standing in water, while a lower heart rate is maintained and pain is decreased. The risks associated with hydrotherapy are minimal, such as overdoing exercise, or rare, such as slipping or drowning.

Light therapy. Phototherapy, or light therapy, is used to treat health disorders that are related to problems with the body's inner clock, or circadian rhythms. These rhythms govern the timing of sleep, hormone production, body temperature, and other biological functions. People need the full wavelength spectrum of light found in sunlight in order to maintain health. If the full wavelength is not received, the body may not be able to absorb some nutrients fully, resulting in fatigue, tooth decay, depression, hostility, hair loss, skin conditions, sleep disorders, or suppressed immune functions. Treatment involves spending more time outdoors, exercising, and using light boxes that mimic natural sunlight. It is commonly used to treat seasonal affective disorder, a recognized subtype of depressive illness.

Meditation. Meditation is used to relax the mind and body, to reduce stress, and to develop a more positive attitude. By focusing on a single thought or repeating a word or phrase, a person can release conscious thoughts and feelings and enter deep relaxation. Meditation can affect the pulse rate and muscle tension and so is effective in treating high blood pressure, migraines, insomnia, and some digestive disorders.

Oxygen therapy. Hyperbaric oxygenation therapy, or oxygen therapy, is used to treat disorders in which the oxygen supply to the body is deficient. This therapy can help with heart disease, circulatory problems, multiple sclerosis, gangrene, and strokes. Oxygen therapy is also used for traumas such as crash injuries, wounds, burns, bedsores, and carbon monoxide poisoning. Treatment consists of exposing the patient to 100 percent pure oxygen under greater-than-normal atmospheric pressure. The body tissues receive more than the usual supply of oxygen and so can compensate for conditions of reduced circulation. The increased oxygen helps keep the tissues alive and promotes healing.

Qi gong. Qi gong (pronounced "chee-kung") translates from the Chinese as "breathing exercise." The Chinese believe that exercise balances and amplifies the vital energy force—Ch'i or qi—within the body. Qi gong is used to increase circulation; to reduce stress; to promote health, fitness, and longevity; and to cure illness. The most common exercises involve relaxation, strengthening, and inward training. Because the exercise involves movement done with gentle circular and stretching movements, people with decreased flexibility or disabilities can participate.

Sound therapy. The use of certain sounds can reduce stress, lower blood pressure, relieve pain, improve movement and balance, promote endurance and strength, and overcome learning disabilities. The body has its own rhythm, and illness can arise when the rhythm is disturbed. Tests have shown that particular sounds can slow breathing and a racing heart, create a feeling of well-being, alter skin temperature, influence brain-wave frequencies, and reduce blood pressure and muscle tension.

Tai Chi Chuan. Originally designed as a form of self-defense, Tai Chi Chuan is now practiced as physical exercises based on rhythmic movement, equilibrium of body weight, and effortless breathing. The exercises involve slow and continuous movement without strain. Tai Chi Chuan is beneficial because it demands no physical strength initially. The exercises increase circulation, stimulate the nervous system and glandular activity, and help joint movement and concentration.

Yoga. The ancient art of yoga seeks to achieve the balance of mind, body, and spirit. Practitioners believe that good health is created through proper breathing, relaxation, meditation, proper diet and nutrition, and exercise. The deep breathing and stretching exercises bring relaxation, release of tension and stress, improved concentration, and oxygenation of the blood. The exercises can also provide muscle toning and aerobics, which is beneficial to the heart.

Aromatherapy. Used extensively in Europe and Japan, aromatherapy involves the use of the essential oils or essence from the flowers, stems, leaves, or roots of plants or trees. These essences can be absorbed through the skin, eaten, or inhaled in vapor form. There is evidence that inhaling some scents may help prevent secondary respiratory infections and reduce stress. Practitioners believe that aromatherapy can benefit people suffering from muscle aches, arthritis, digestive and circulatory problems, and emotional or stress-related problems. Absorption through the skin and inhalation are considered safe, but eating any essence could result in poisoning.

Cell therapy. Although not approved in the United States, cell therapy is widely used worldwide. It involves the injection of cells from the organs, fetuses, or embryos of animals and humans. These cells are used for revitalization purposes; that is, they promote the body's own healing process for damaged or weak organs. Cell therapy seems to stimulate the immune system and is used to treat cancer, immunological problems, diseased or underdeveloped organs, arthritis, and circulatory problems.

Colon therapy. This technique involves the cleaning and detoxification of the colon by flushing with water, using enemas, or ingesting herbs or other substances. A healthy colon will absorb water and nutrients and eliminate wastes and toxins. Most modern diets, however, are low in fiber, a substance which helps clean out the colon. If not completely eliminated, layers of wastes can build up in the colon and toxins can leak into the bloodstream, causing many health problems. Although not a specific cure for any disease, colon therapy removes the source of toxins and allows the body's natural healing processes to function properly. Practitioners claim that symptoms related to colon dysfunction, such as backaches, headaches, bad breath, gas, indigestion and constipation, sinus or lung congestion, skin problems, and fatigue can be relieved when the toxins are removed from the colon.

Detoxification. This therapy focuses on ridding the body of the chemicals and pollutants present in water, food, air, and soil. The body naturally eliminates or neutralizes toxins through the liver, kidneys, urine, and feces and through the processes of exhalation and perspiration. Detoxification therapy accelerates the body's own natural cleansing process through diet, fasting, colon therapy, and heat therapy. Symptoms of an overtaxed body system include respiratory problems, headaches, joint pain, allergy symptoms, mood changes, insomnia, arthritis, constipation, psoriasis, acne, and ulcers.

Energy medicine. Bioenergetic medicine, or energy medicine, uses an energy field to detect and treat health problems. A screening process to measure electromagnetic frequencies emitted by the body can detect imbalances that may cause illness or warn of possible chemical imbalances. One of several machines is then used to correct energy-level imbalances. Energy medicine claims to relieve conditions such as skin diseases, headaches, migraines, muscle pain, circulation problems, and chronic fatigue.

Enzyme therapy. This treatment uses plant and pancreatic enzymes to improve digestion and the absorption of nutrients. Since enzymes provide the stimulus for all chemical reactions in the body, improper eating habits may cause a lack of certain enzymes, resulting in general health problems.

Homeopathy. Based on the belief that "like cures like," homeopathy is thought to provide relief from most illnesses. During therapy, the patient receives small doses of prepared plants and minerals in order to stimulate the body's own healing processes and defense mechanisms. These substances mimic the symptoms of the illness. While studies on this approach remain inconclusive, homeopathic medicine has wide appeal, possibly because most (but not all) homeopathic practitioners are traditionally trained medical physicians.

Kinesiology. This therapy employs muscle testing and standard diagnosis to evaluate and treat the chemical, structural, and mental aspects of the patient. The principle behind kinesiology is that certain foods can cause biochemical reactions that weaken the muscles. Diet and exercise, as well as muscle and joint manipulation, are part of the treatment. There are risks of injury caused by an unqualified practitioner.

Magnetic field therapy. Also called biomagnetic therapy, magnetic field therapy uses specially designed magnets or magnetic fields applied to the body. Electrically charged particles are naturally present in the bloodstream, and when magnets are placed on the body, the charged particles are attracted to the magnets. As a result, currents and patterns are created that dilate the blood vessels, allowing more blood to reach the affected area. Magnetic field therapy is used to speed healing after surgery, to improve circulation, and to strengthen and mend bones. It is also used to improve the quality of healing in sprains, strains, cuts, and burns, as well as to reduce or reverse chronic conditions such as degenerative joint disease, some forms of arthritis, and diabetic ulcers.

Neural therapy. This therapy is used to treat chronic illness or trauma (injury) caused by changes in the natural electrical conductivity of the nerves and cells. Every cell has its own frequency range of electricity, and tissue remains healthy as long as the energy flow through the body is normal. Neural therapy uses anesthetics injected into the body to deliver energy to cells blocked by disease or injury. Conditions that respond to neural therapy are allergies, arthritis, asthma, kidney, liver and heart disease, depression, head and back pain, and muscle injuries.

Herbal medicine. This field uses plants and flowers to treat most known symptoms of physical and emotional illnesses. Almost 75 percent of the world's population relies on herbal remedies as their primary source of health care, and much of traditional medicine is derived from plants. Herbal medicine mixtures can be complicated, however, and some, like any medications, are toxic if taken incorrectly.

PERSPECTIVE AND PROSPECTS

Many alternative or complementary therapies, while new to Western society and medicine, are ancient and derive from nontechnologically based understandings of how the human body and the world work. What specifically works for whom, when, and for what conditions remains a complex problem. Anecdote and hearsay, and the limits and failures of Western medicine, guide and motivate interest in these approaches.

Renewed interest in alternative therapies occurred in the 1970's and has grown since. By 1998, an estimated one-third of all Americans had used some form of complementary therapy. In 1992, with Americans spending more than 14 billion dollars annually on alternative medicine, the U.S.

government established the Office of Alternative Medicine as a part of the National Institutes of Health (NIH). This office evaluates complementary treatments on a scientific basis and provides public information. Health insurers maintain a key interest in alternative medicine, and an increasing number are paying for it. Many traditionally trained physicians are prescribing or recommending some form of alternative medicine as a complement to their own.

—*Virginia L. Salmon, updated by Paul Moglia, Ph.D.*

See also Acupressure; Acupuncture; Allied health; Aromatherapy; Cell therapy; Chiropractic; Colon therapy; Enzyme therapy; Herbal medicine; Holistic medicine; Homeopathy; Hydrotherapy; Hypnosis; Kinesiology; Light therapy; Magnetic field therapy; Meditation; Oxygen therapy; Pain management; Qi gong; Stress reduction; Tai Chi Chuan; Yoga.

FOR FURTHER INFORMATION:

The CQ Researcher 2, no. 4 (January 31, 1992). This entire issue discusses the topic of alternative medicine. Offers a balanced viewpoint and contains a valuable bibliography for further reading.

Goldberg, Burton, comp. *Alternative Medicine: The Definitive Guide*. Puyallup, Wash.: Future Medicine, 1993. A well-written reference work which includes long, illustrated entries on various treatments. Provides sources of further information and recommended readings.

Guernsey, Diane. "Alternative Medicine: A T&C Report." *Town and Country*, January, 1977, pp. 97-104. A well-written, solid, and responsible overview of complementary medicines with much practical advice on how to get started.

Jacobs, Jennifer, ed. *The Encyclopedia of Alternative Medicine: A Complete Family Guide to Complementary Therapies*. Boston: Journey Edition, 1996. Discusses current alternative medicine approaches.

Kastner, Mark, and Hugh Burroughs. *Alternative Healing: The Complete A-Z Guide to over 160 Different Alternative Therapies*. La Mesa, Calif.: Halcyon, 1993. The encyclopedic, one-page to four-page entries are brief but include sources of additional information. Also offers a useful resource section and bibliography.

Mauskop, Alexander, and Brill Marietta Abrams. *The Headache Alternative: A Neurologist's Guide to Drug-Free Relief*. New York: Dell Paperbacks, 1997. A practical review of how to apply complementary and alternative approaches to treating migraine, sinus, and tension headaches. Contains excellent resources and a bibliography section.

Mills, Simon, and Steven J. Finando. *Alternatives in Healing*. New York: New American Library, 1988. Provides detailed introductory chapters discussing the principles, philosophy, and techniques of diagnosis and treatment with alternative medicine. Includes case studies comparing various treatment methods.

ALTITUDE SICKNESS
DISEASE/DISORDER

ANATOMY OR SYSTEM AFFECTED: Brain, ears, head, lungs, nervous system, respiratory system

SPECIALTIES AND RELATED FIELDS: Emergency medicine, neurology, occupational health

DEFINITION: A condition resulting from altitude-related hypoxia (low oxygen levels).

CAUSES AND SYMPTOMS

There are four types of altitude sickness: acute mountain sickness, high-altitude pulmonary edema (HAPE), high-altitude cerebral edema (HACE), and high-altitude retinopathy (HAR). Though most patients have mild symptoms, death is not uncommon in severe cases. Illness is associated with rapid ascent to mountain areas by tourists, skiers, and mountaineers. Residents of mountainous regions are less susceptible because their bodies have adapted to lower oxygen levels. It is estimated that up to one-quarter of tourists skiing in the mountains of the western United States have experienced some manifestations, although mild ones, of altitude sickness.

Acute mountain sickness is characterized by headache, decreased appetite, insomnia, fatigue, nausea, and onset at altitudes above 1,980 meters (6,500 feet). The risk of becoming affected increases with young age, quick ascent, and a past history of acute mountain sickness. Symptoms usually last for a few days. Between 5 and 10 percent of patients with acute mountain sickness progress to HAPE, which occurs when the small pulmonary blood vessels leak, allowing fluid accumulation in the lungs. Mortality from HAPE ranges from 11 to 44 percent. The related condition HACE occurs when fluid accumulation in the brain causes increased pressure within the skull. Neurologic signs such as confusion and coma may be noted.

TREATMENT AND THERAPY

Prevention is crucial to the reduction of morbidity and mortality from altitude sickness. Ascents should be slow, especially when involving physical exertion. Sedatives and salt should be avoided. Most people adapt to altitude changes within three days. Returning to lower altitudes at night is advised. Premedication with acetazolamide, a prescription drug, will hasten adaptation and reduce symptoms. In serious cases, descent to lower altitudes is vital. Corticosteroids, oxygen, and hyperbaric treatments may be used. Chronically ill persons should check with their doctors before attempting strenuous activity at high altitudes.

—*Louis B. Jacques, M.D.*

See also Asphyxiation; Brain; Brain disorders; Coma; Edema; Lungs; Nervous system; Neurology; Neurology, pediatric; Pulmonary diseases; Pulmonary medicine; Pulmonary medicine, pediatric; Respiration.

FOR FURTHER INFORMATION:

Auerbach, Paul S. *Medicine for the Outdoors*. Rev. and updated ed. Boston: Little, Brown, 1991.

Rennie, D. "The Great Breathlessness Mountains." *JAMA* 256 (July 4, 1986): 81-82.

Wilkerson, James A., ed. *Medicine for Mountaineering and Other Wilderness Activities.* 4th ed. Seattle: Mountaineers, 1992.

ALZHEIMER'S DISEASE

DISEASE/DISORDER

ANATOMY OR SYSTEM AFFECTED: Brain, nervous system, psychic-emotional system

SPECIALTIES AND RELATED FIELDS: Family practice, genetics, geriatrics and gerontology, neurology, psychiatry

DEFINITION: The most common cause of dementia in old age, affecting between 3 and 11 percent of those over sixty-five.

KEY TERMS:

agnosia: an inability to recognize persons or various objects even though the patient sees them clearly

anomia: an inability to remember the names of persons or objects even though the patient sees and recognizes the persons or objects

aphasia: difficulty in understanding and talking to other people in the absence of hearing impairment

apraxia: difficulty in carrying out coordinated voluntary activities (such as dressing, undressing, or brushing one's teeth) in the absence of any muscular weakness

benign senescent forgetfulness: a common source of frustration in old age, associated with memory impairment; unlike dementia, it does not interfere with the individual's social and professional activities

brain imaging techniques: tests performed to examine brain anatomy and functioning; these include computed tomography (CT) scans, magnetic resonance imaging (MRI), and single photon emission computed tomography (SPECT)

cognitive deficit: an impairment in mental functions, including anomia, agnosia, aphasia, and apraxia; it is usually associated with an impairment in the ability to make rational decisions

dementia: also called dementing illness; a disease characterized by memory impairment of sufficient severity to interfere with the individual's daily social and professional activities

neuropsychological testing: a series of tests administered by a neuropsychologist to examine the efficiency of various parts of the brain

neurotransmitters: chemical substances inside the brain that allow the flow of electrical impulses from one part of the brain to another; at least five neurotransmitters are absent with Alzheimer's disease

CAUSES AND SYMPTOMS

Alzheimer's disease is the most common dementing illness in old age. In the United States, it is estimated that its prevalence increases from 3 percent in those aged sixty-five to seventy-four years, to 18.7 percent in those seventy-five to eighty-four years of age, to as much as 47.2 percent of those over the age of eighty-five. While both sexes are about equally affected, there are more women than men with Alzheimer's disease because women tend to live longer. As with other dementing illnesses, the characteristic memory impairment initially affects the recent, rather than the remote, memory and interferes with the patient's daily social and professional activities; the patient's attention span is also significantly reduced.

The disease typically has a slow, insidious onset, and a very slow, gradual progress. Caregivers observing this decline are often unable to agree about when the symptoms began to manifest themselves. The memory deficit is usually accompanied by an impaired ability to make good, rational decisions. One of the most common and earliest problems is an inability to take care of one's financial affairs. In addition to being unable to balance a checkbook, the patient may attempt to pay the same bill several times, while disregarding other financial obligations. Similarly, the patient may be overly generous at times and extremely mean on other occasions.

In Alzheimer's disease, the dementing process is also associated with other evidence of cognitive deficit. When anomia is present, patients often use paraphrases to describe various objects because they have difficulty finding the correct words. For example, they may say "milk pourer" instead of "milk jug." This condition is usually present very early in the disease process, but it is often so slight that it may only be detected by neuropsychological testing. Agnosia develops later and can be quite hazardous. For example, a patient may confuse a knife with a comb. As the disease progresses, a patient may develop aphasia and find it difficult to communicate with other people. Finally, the patient develops apraxia, experiencing difficulty carrying out coordinated activities such as dressing or undressing, even though there is no loss of muscular power. The apraxia may also be responsible for unsteadiness, and the patient may fall repeatedly and may become chairbound or bedfast. Anomia, agnosia, aphasia, and apraxia are sometimes referred to as the "four A's" that accompany the memory deficit seen in Alzheimer's disease.

Alzheimer's disease is progressive, and there is much individual variability in the rate of progress. A number of staging classifications, most of them arbitrary, are available. One of the most practical is the three-stage classification. In stage 1, the memory impairment and degree of cognitive deficit are so slight that patients may still be able to function socially and even professionally, although family members and close associates may have observed strange behavioral patterns. Superficially, the patients may appear "normal," although somewhat eccentric. Although the memory deficit and impaired mental functions are present, patients may use various tricks to mask this deficit. They may ask a partner

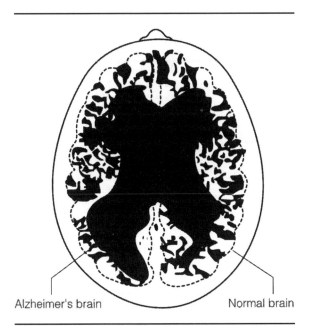

Alzheimer's brain   Normal brain

Alzheimer's disease causes the volume of the brain to shrink substantially.

to keep score of a game they are playing because they have "left their reading glasses at home" or may decline invitations to play card games or socialize altogether. Patients with this disease may also stop engaging in their favorite hobbies and activities. Patients at this stage usually have difficulties balancing their checkbooks. Errors of judgment are not infrequent, although they are initially often attributed by family and friends to age, to eccentricity, or to the patient's having too many things on his or her mind. Patients may buy large quantities of the same item and start hoarding various articles. As time progresses, they may lose their way, and their errors in judgment while driving may result in traffic accidents. One of the main problems in this stage is the inability to learn and retain new information. This mental deficit becomes particularly problematic if the patient's work is being reorganized or if the patient relocates. Agitation, irritability, and anxiety are not uncommon in this stage and probably represent the patient's inability to cope with a loss of control over the environment and a declining mental ability.

In stage 2, the memory impairment, cognitive deficit, and degree of impaired judgment are so great that even a stranger who has never met the patient cannot help but conclude that there is something wrong with the patient's mental functions. In this stage, patients frequently become lost, even in very familiar surroundings, such as in their own houses. They may no longer be able to find their way to the toilet, they may no longer recognize people they know well, and they are unable to take care of their own hygienic needs. They tend to walk aimlessly and wander constantly

and are likely to become agitated, irritable, and even aggressive. These symptoms are often pronounced late in the afternoon or early evening and are often referred to as "sundowning syndrome."

In stage 3, in addition to their mental impairment, patients become unsteady on their feet and may sustain repeated falls. Because they have become physically frail, they tend to wander much less and to spend most of their time confined to a chair or bed. They are completely dependent on their caregivers for most activities. Swallowing is often difficult, and feeding through a small tube inserted in the nose (a nasogastric tube) may be required. Patients are at risk of becoming dehydrated and malnourished, and urinary and even fecal incontinence are not uncommon. Mutism gradually sets in, and communication with the patient becomes difficult. Flexion (bending) contractures gradually develop, and the patient slowly adopts the fetal position, with the arms and knees bent. The development of pressure ulcers, or bedsores, is likely. The common cause of death is septicemia (blood poisoning) resulting from a respiratory tract infection, a urinary tract infection, or an infected pressure ulcer.

Alzheimer's disease is characterized by a loss of brain cells, affecting in particular the cerebral cortex. The brain appears smaller in size and atrophic, with the gyri (grooves) much less prominent and the ventricles (cavities inside the brain) enlarged. Multiple deficiencies in the neurotransmitters, chemical substances inside the brain that carry impulses from one cell to another, have been identified with this disease.

Diagnosis. At present, there are no positive tests available to make a definitive diagnosis of Alzheimer's disease without examining brain tissue under the microscope. Before such a diagnosis can be considered, several factors should be present. First, the memory impairment should be of sufficient magnitude and consistency to interfere with one's social and professional activities, and it should be accompanied by evidence of cognitive deficit and impaired judgment. These are the main differentiating features between Alzheimer's disease and benign senescent forgetfulness, which is also very common in old age. Although the latter can be quite irritating, it does not significantly interfere with the person's professional and social activities and tends to be selective, with one's forgetting only unimportant and relatively trivial matters. The forgetfulness seen in Alzheimer's disease, on the other hand, is global and does not distinguish between trivial and important matters.

Second, in Alzheimer's disease, the onset of memory impairment is insidious, and the progress is slow. This differentiates it from multiple infarct dementia, which is caused by multiple strokes and which has an abrupt onset and progress marked by bouts of deterioration. Whenever a stroke develops, the patient's condition deteriorates and then stabilizes until the next stroke occurs.

Third, the patient must be alert, not drowsy—one of the main distinctions between Alzheimer's disease and delirium. The latter, in addition to having a sudden onset, is associated with clouding of consciousness, a rambling and incoherent speech, disorganized thinking, hallucinations, and sensory misperceptions.

Finally, as the diagnosis of Alzheimer's disease is still based on a process of exclusion, all other possible causes of impaired mental functions must be ruled out. These causes are numerous and can be conveniently remembered by the mnemonic device DEMENTIA.

The D stands for drugs. Older patients are particularly susceptible to the effects of many medications that may impair mental functions. These indications include not only those acting specifically on the brain, such as the sedatives and hypnotics, but also other medications such as those that lower blood pressure. Finally, alcohol is often abused by older people and may significantly interfere with the older person's mental abilities.

The E stands for emotional disorders. Depression is very common in old age and may manifest itself with cognitive impairment. Unlike patients with Alzheimer's disease, who except in the very early stages of the disease are not aware of their deficit, those with depression are acutely aware of their problem and often exaggerate it. Often, patients with depression also have a long list of complaints. They lack animation, their appetite is reduced, and they take a diminished interest in their environment and pleasure in their daily activities. Sleep disturbances, in the form of insomnia or increased sleepiness, are common. Although most cases of depression are easily recognized, some may be difficult to diagnose and therefore may require neuropsychological testing to differentiate them from Alzheimer's disease. This differentiation is important, because unlike Alzheimer's disease, depression can be treated, and the outlook is good. Additionally, it is important to emphasize that about 20 percent of patients with Alzheimer's disease have a coexistent depression that often responds to appropriate therapy.

The M stands for metabolic disorders. In old age, both overactivity and underactivity of the thyroid gland may be responsible for mental impairment without a patient's exhibiting any of the characteristic clinical features. Dehydration is a common cause of confusion in older patients because their sense of thirst is often reduced. Liver and kidney diseases also may be responsible for impaired mental functions. Similarly, patients with diabetes mellitus are susceptible to a number of metabolic disorders, including an increased or decreased blood sugar level, both of which may cause cognitive impairment. Serum electrolyte disorders also may result in confusional states and can be precipitated by severe vomiting, diarrhea, or the intake of medication. Finally, vitamin B_{12} deficiency may be responsible for impaired mental functions, occasionally without there being any other clinical evidence of this deficiency. Patients who

have had a gastrectomy (surgical removal of their stomach) and no vitamin B_{12} replacement are likely to develop B_{12} deficiency a few years after surgery. By this time, however, the patient may have relocated, changed physicians, and probably "forgotten" about the surgery.

The E stands for both eyes and ears. For individuals to interact appropriately with others and the environment, they must be aware of the various circumstances surrounding them. If an individual cannot hear properly and guesses at the questions asked, he or she often will not give an appropriate answer and may give the impression of being confused. Hearing impairment is very common among the older population, and often older people choose not to wear a hearing aid because of difficulties manipulating the controls or because of embarrassment. Visual impairment may also interfere with an individual's appropriate interaction with the environment and give the impression of dementia. There are many causes of visual impairment in old age, including glaucoma, cataracts, and macular degeneration (a progressive disorder of the retina).

The N stands for neurological disorders; these include other dementias such as multi-infarct dementia and hydrocephalus (increased fluid in the brain).

The T stands for both tumors and trauma. A subdural hematoma (a collection of blood inside the skull) may be precipitated by trauma that is usually trivial. The symptoms do not become apparent until a few days or even weeks after the trauma, by which time the patient and caregivers may have forgotten about the physical trauma. Brain tumors may also manifest themselves with impaired mental functions. The computed tomography (CT) scan and magnetic resonance imaging (MRI) are useful tools in diagnosing these conditions.

The I stands for infections. Infections, regardless of their location but especially those of the respiratory and urinary tracts, may be associated with confusional states in older people. Unlike younger people, they often do not exhibit a rise in body temperature, thus making the diagnosis of infection difficult. Acquired immunodeficiency syndrome (AIDS) is another cause of dementia that is related to infection; this condition must be suspected when mental functions deteriorate rapidly, especially if the patient has risk factors for AIDS.

The A stands for atherosclerosis and includes arteriosclerotic cardiovascular diseases. Older patients who experience myocardial infarction (a "heart attack" caused by a sudden reduction of blood flow to the heart muscle) may not experience any chest pain but may nevertheless develop an acute confusional state. Generalized arteriosclerosis also might be responsible for multiple, small, repeated strokes that can eventually interfere with the patient's cognitive functions.

The accuracy of the clinical diagnosis of Alzheimer's disease can be increased to about 90 percent if a few investigations are conducted. These include a complete blood count, Chem-18 (a series of blood tests to check on the blood levels of many substances and the functioning of the kidneys and liver), thyroid function tests, serum B_{12} measurement, electrocardiogram, and brain imaging tests. Single photon emission computed tomography (SPECT) seems to be a promising test in the diagnosis of Alzheimer's disease and may represent the first step toward being able to make a diagnosis without examining brain tissue microscopically.

TREATMENT AND THERAPY

Although the understanding of the pathophysiology of Alzheimer's disease has increased tremendously since it was first described by Alois Alzheimer in the early years of the twentieth century, this understanding has not been translated into effective therapeutic opportunities. A large number of compounds have been and are being tried for the treatment of Alzheimer's disease but, unfortunately, without any significant degree of success. At present, therefore, it is essentially a disease without a cure.

Nevertheless, many things can be done to aid a patient with Alzheimer's disease. It is important to detect the presence of any other disease that may worsen the patient's condition, and unnecessary medications must be avoided for the same reason. Medication may nevertheless be required to control agitation and the sundowning syndrome. Physicians will generally start with the smallest possible dose of medication and then gradually increase it according to the patient's symptoms.

The patient's environment and daily routine should be left as constant as possible, as any change may precipitate or worsen the symptoms and degree of confusion. The patient should be spared the task of having to choose an option among several ones (such as which dress to wear) and to make decisions (such as which activity in which to become involved). Instead, the daily routine should be as structured as possible and yet retain enough flexibility for the patient to withdraw from any activity that is disliked and to join any that is enjoyed.

The patient with Alzheimer's disease should be treated not in isolation but by caregivers and family members, who will also need support and help if they are to cope effectively with their loved one's illness. Social workers and various community agencies can help develop a management program tailored to the individual patient's needs and

New Research

By the mid-1990's, two drugs were developed that showed promise in improving function in patients with Alzheimer's disease: tacrine, marketed under the name Cognex, and donepezil, marketed under the name Aricept. The reasoning that underlies the development of these medications was as follows: The biological basis of many cognitive disorders involves low levels of the neurotransmitter acetylcholine. One reason for these low levels is the presence of a recently discovered brain enzyme, acetylcholinesterase, that breaks down or destroys acetylcholine. Without sufficient levels of acetylcholine, major intellectual functions such as recall and recognition, reasoning, and judgment become compromised. Tacrine and donepezil are cholinesterase inhibitors that reduce the breakdown of acetycholine, although they do not replace it.

In mild and moderate Alzheimer's disease, when there are higher amounts of the neurotransitter to preserve, the medications have provided some benefit, at least for the short term. Memory improves, as does reasoning ability. Tacrine has come into disuse, however, largely because of both irritating side effects such as nausea, vomiting, diarrhea, and tremulousness and potentially serious side effects such as liver toxicity. Although donepezil is chemically quite similar to tacrine, the associated side effects are far fewer, and the medication remains in wide use.

Other promising medications, developed using the same underlying rationale as tacrine and donepezil, include metrifonate, long-acting physostigmine, and ENA 713. Unfortunately, while this class of medicine, the cholinesterase inhibitors, has proved beneficial to Alzheimer's patients, the improvement is relatively short term. Even with their use, the disease continues to progress, but the rate of cognitive deterioration is slowed. There is no cure and no current way to arrest the disease. Extract from the gingko tree and estrogen supplements, to date inadequately studied, also are showing promise in improving patients' memories.

In addition to memory loss and confusion, Alzheimer's patients suffer numerous behavioral and attitudinal changes. This class of medications usually does little to improve behavior directly. Changes in personality, depression, loss of interest and ability to enjoy oneself, aggression, anxiety, and sleep disturbances are often the most difficult symptoms to manage and the most difficult for loved ones and caregivers to witness. It is now the standard that those taking care of Alzheimer's patients themselves need support and must utilize available resources in order to sustain their own well-being. Practical, hands-on planning ideas such as keeping a daily schedule for the patient, ensuring that one's own personal time includes time off and away from caregiving demands, getting individual counseling or participating in a support group are often the best long-term interventions. The treatment of Alzheimer's patients now involves the treatment of Alzheimer's caregivers, family members, and professional staff. —*Paul Moglia, Ph.D.*

those of his or her caregivers. A number of community programs are available, and the Alzheimer's Association and support groups are very useful resources. Caregivers and family members should also be given advice concerning financial, legal, and ethical issues, such as obtaining a durable power of attorney and finding out the patient's wishes concerning advance directives prior to incapacitation.

PERSPECTIVE AND PROSPECTS

Alzheimer's disease has been compared to other brain diseases that reduce neurotransmission, how the brain communicates with itself, and the actual number of brain cells. Clinical and experimental drugs have become available that attempt to treat age-related cognitive decline, Alzheimer's disease, and other dementias. By the late 1990's, no panacea had been developed, but research in this area continued to be vigorous and well funded, and expectations were high.

—Ronald C. Hamdy, M.D., Louis A. Cancellaro, M.D., and Larry Hudgins, M.D.; updated by Paul Moglia, Ph.D.

See also Aging; Aging, extended care for the; Amnesia; Brain; Brain disorders; Dementia; Geriatrics and gerontology; Memory loss; Neurology.

FOR FURTHER INFORMATION:

American Psychiatric Association. *Practice Guideline for the Treatment of Patients with Alzheimer's Disease and Other Dementias of Late Life.* Washington, D.C.: Author, 1997. May be helpful for individuals seeking information on what to expect in future treatment and assessment for family members.

Coons, Dorothy H., ed. *Specialized Dementia Care Units.* Baltimore: The Johns Hopkins University Press, 1991. Contains articles that assess the treatment of dementia patients in care units designed to address their special needs. The advantages of such specialized care are weighed against the problems that these units encounter.

Cummings, Jeffrey L., and Bruce L. Miller, eds. *Alzheimer's Disease.* New York: Marcel Dekker, 1990. Explores the available therapies for Alzheimer's disease patients, including the management of behavioral symptoms and the need to provide long-term care. The various authors of this edited text also speculate on future treatments for this disease.

Hamdy, Ronald C., J. M. Turnbull, L. D. Norman, and M. M. Lancaster, eds. *Alzheimer's Disease: A Handbook for Caregivers.* St. Louis: C. V. Mosby, 1994. Offers practical advice for researchers and caregivers about how to deal with the patient with Alzheimer's disease or another type of dementia. Presents a thorough discussion of the symptoms of these disorders, as compared to normal brain structure and function and the natural effects of aging.

Howe, M. L., M. J. Stones, and C. J. Brainerd, eds. *Cognitive and Behavioral Performance Factors in Atypical Aging.* New York: Springer-Verlag, 1990. Using younger

patients as a point of reference, this work addresses the factors that control brain function and behavior in older individuals.

Mace, Nancy L., and Peter V. Rabins. *The Thirty-Six-Hour Day: A Family Guide for Caring for Persons with Alzheimer's Disease, Related Dementing Illnesses, and Memory Loss in Later Life.* Rev. ed. Baltimore: The Johns Hopkins University Press, 1991. Possibly the best practical and informational guide to the myriad difficulties that caregivers and family members face. Highly regarded within the field.

Terry, Robert D., ed. *Aging and the Brain.* New York: Raven Press, 1988. The structure and function of the brains of both normal elderly people and those with various types of dementias (including Alzheimer's disease) are compared. Reviews the neurobiological and technological concepts developed in the 1980's in this field of study.

U.S. Congress. Office of Technology Assessment. *Confused Minds, Burdened Families: Finding Help for People with Alzheimer's and Other Dementias.* Washington, D.C.: Government Printing Office, 1990. This official government report describes the current system of services in the United States set up to care for those with Alzheimer's disease and other dementias. Details its many inadequacies and presents an alternative vision of a more efficient system, including recommendations for congressional policy options to make it a reality.

U.S. Congress. Office of Technology Assessment. *Losing a Million Minds: Confronting the Tragedy of Alzheimer's Disease and Other Dementias.* Washington, D.C.: Government Printing Office, 1987. Offers a comprehensive assessment of the impact of Alzheimer's disease on the United States, including the psychoeconomic effects of this disease on patients and caregivers, personnel training and quality assurance in public and private programs that serve patients with dementia, and future governmental policies regarding these issues.

West, Robin L., and Jan D. Sinnott, eds. *Everyday Memory and Aging.* New York: Springer-Verlag, 1992. This work discusses the methodology of research into the human memory. Focuses on the changes in memory that occur naturally with age, as well as those that are brought about by various forms of dementia in the older individual.

AMENORRHEA

DISEASE/DISORDER

ANATOMY OR SYSTEM AFFECTED: Reproductive system, uterus

SPECIALTIES AND RELATED FIELDS: Gynecology

DEFINITION: In girls or women suffering from amenorrhea, menstruation has not occurred or is abnormally suppressed. Primary amenorrhea is diagnosed if a young woman has not experienced menarche (the first menstruation) by the age of eighteen; it may be caused by a hormone imbalance, a tumor in the pituitary or adrenal glands, or an underactive thyroid. Secondary amenorrhea is defined as the cessation of menstruation for at least three months in a woman who has menstruated previously; in addition to the above causes, it may be attributable to rapid weight loss or gain, overly strenuous exercise, prolonged use of oral contraceptives, or emotional trauma. Treatment depends on the cause of the amenorrhea, such as hormone therapy for imbalances, surgery for tumors, or psychiatric counseling for self-destructive behaviors.

—*Jason Georges and Tracy Irons-Georges*
See also Eating disorders; Gynecology; Hormones; Menstruation; Weight loss and gain.

AMERICAN MEDICAL ASSOCIATION
ORGANIZATION
DEFINITION: The largest voluntary association of physicians in the United States, with most of its members engaging directly in the practice of medicine.

KEY TERMS:

Accreditation Council for Continuing Medical Education (ACCME): the organization that promotes and accredits continuing education for physicians, which the AMA sponsors

Accreditation Council for Graduate Medical Education (ACGME): the council that accredits physician residency programs in 1,500 U.S. medical schools; it is sponsored by the AMA and four other organizations

House of Delegates: the representative body that decides official policy and action on the behalf of the AMA membership; state medical societies are allocated most of the delegate positions in the house, since 90 percent of all physicians affiliate with them, while medical specialty societies, military and other federal service groups, and five special sections also are given representation

Liaison Committee on Medical Education (LCME): an organization formed by the AMA and the Association of American Medical Colleges to set standards and accredit all U.S. and Canadian medical schools offering M.D. degrees

THE ROLE OF THE AMA IN THE UNITED STATES

Since its inception, the American Medical Association (AMA) has worked to improve the credibility of medicine as a profession in the United States. The AMA helped to shape and develop the physician licensing system used now in every state. Through the auspices of various accreditation bodies that it sponsors, such as the LCME, ACGME, and ACCME, the AMA monitors medical education programs to ensure that they continue to meet high standards. The AMA established a professional code of ethics for physicians and revises it periodically to guide physicians through the ever-changing health care environment. The AMA Council on Ethical and Judicial Affairs regularly issues in-

terpretations of the principles of medical ethics; the council can censure, suspend, or expel a physician who violates the code of ethics. The *Journal of the American Medical Association* (or *JAMA*) was first published in July, 1883, and is now the world's most widely circulated medical journal. The AMA also publishes ten medical specialty journals and the weekly *American Medical News*. In addition, the AMA produces and distributes press releases, video news releases, and radio and television news programs.

The AMA advocates a "patient's bill of rights," which supports patient autonomy, dignity, confidentiality, and ongoing access to needed medical care. The AMA believes that the practice of medicine should be based on sound scientific principles, which are promulgated in *JAMA* and in the many specialty journals that it sponsors and publishes. The AMA also houses one of the nation's largest medical libraries, subscribes to more than 150 computer databases, and maintains comprehensive computer files on all physicians and medical students in the United States.

GUIDELINES FOR HEALTH

The AMA acknowledged early in its development the role that it should play in promoting the improvement of public health. Among the public health initiatives that the AMA has sponsored are the clear labeling of poison containers, early childhood screening for hearing and vision problems, the inspection of milk to ensure its quality, the installation of seat belts in automobiles, low tolerance in state laws regarding drunk driving, and the banning of tobacco product advertisement. More recently, the AMA was among the first professional associations to advocate significant reform of the American health care delivery system, especially to respond to the needs of uninsured and underinsured people. The communications arm of the AMA produces services and products designed to increase public knowledge regarding significant health care issues and medical care advances.

PERSPECTIVE AND PROSPECTS

Nathan Smith Davis, a medical doctor and a delegate of the New York State Medical Society, introduced resolutions that led to the holding of the first national medical convention in May, 1846. Davis' tireless leadership during the first convention enabled the establishment of the American Medical Association in May, 1847. Davis also served as an AMA president and the first editor-in-chief of the *Journal of the American Medical Association*.

The original AMA constitution set out several enduring principles for the organization. The AMA would be governed by representatives elected from the membership, and officers would serve only one year. The purposes of the AMA would be to advance medical knowledge, to work to improve medical education, to establish high ethical and practice standards, to encourage the formation and maintenance of state and local medical societies, and to work against medical quackery.

In order to ensure that the association speaks with a unified voice, the AMA has used, since its founding, the principle of representative democracy. State medical societies are entitled to a voting delegate and an alternate for each one thousand members; this represents the overwhelming majority of voting delegates. Other organizations, such as the Veterans Administration and medical schools sections, are also given one delegate and one alternate. The delegates form the AMA House of Delegates, which meets twice a year to evaluate and decide on policy issues. In order to prepare properly for a meeting of the House of Delegates, reference committees consider and hold open hearings on important medical issues, such as testing for acquired immunodeficiency syndrome (AIDS). The reference committees then make recommendations to the House of Delegates, which often decides hundreds of policies during each session.

The American Medical Association is a powerful lobbyist in Washington, D.C., where it seeks to influence national legislation affecting the delivery of medical care. The AMA also represents the interests of its members in important cases brought before various courts.

—*Russell Williams, M.S.W.*

See also Animal rights vs. research; Education, medical; Ethics; Hippocratic oath; Law and medicine.

FOR FURTHER INFORMATION:

Campion, Frank. *The AMA and U.S. Health Policy Since 1940.* Chicago: Chicago Review Press, 1984.

Caring for the Country: A History and Celebration of the First 150 Years of the American Medical Association. Chicago: American Medical Association, 1997.

Fishbein, Morris. *A History of the American Medical Association, 1847 to 1947.* Philadelphia: W. B. Saunders, 1947.

AMNESIA

DISEASE/DISORDER

ANATOMY OR SYSTEM AFFECTED: Brain, nervous system, psychic-emotional system

SPECIALTIES AND RELATED FIELDS: Neurology, psychiatry, psychology

DEFINITION: The loss of memory due to physical and/or psychological conditions.

KEY TERMS:

anterograde: referring to amnesia in which events following a biological or psychological trauma are forgotten; new learning is impaired

episodic memory: the remembrance of personal information in one's life, such as the events of the previous day

procedural memory: the ability to reproduce learned skills, particularly perceptual-motor activities such as riding a bike

retrograde: referring to amnesia in which events preceding a biological or psychological trauma are forgotten; retrieving previously formed memories is impaired

semantic memory: the storage of factual information, such as the meaning of words

CAUSES AND SYMPTOMS

The primary attribute of amnesia is a loss of memory for a specific time period. The extent, duration, and type of that memory loss can vary greatly. The most common amnesia forms are anterograde, in which the formation of new memories is impaired. In rare cases, anterograde amnesia is continuous, in which there is great impairment of memory formation for the remainder of a person's life. Retrograde amnesia in rare cases may be generalized, in which the totality of an individual's personal memory preceding the onset of amnesia is lost. More commonly, both anterograde and retrograde amnesias are localized, in which the memory of a period of time ranging from seconds to minutes (although occasionally days or longer) is lost. The memory loss may be selective, with only some aspects of a particular time period being absent. In all these forms of amnesia, the most common type of information lost is episodic; rarely are procedural memories destroyed.

Amnesia is typically caused by either psychological circumstances, in which case it is termed psychogenic, or by biological processes, where it is referred to as biogenic or organic. Sometimes, however, the cause involves both psychological and biological factors. Psychogenic amnesias are usually caused by some sort of emotional trauma. Emotional trauma is the common thread that runs through the amnesia associated with the following disorders: dissociative amnesia (the inability to recall significant personal information); fugue (memory loss accompanied by sudden, unexpected travel from home); dissociative identity disorder (the presence of two or more distinct personalities, with inability to recall extensive time periods); and post-traumatic stress disorder (significant distress and memory disturbances following an extreme traumatic event). Emotional trauma is typically absent in posthypnotic amnesia, which is induced by hypnotic suggestion, and childhood amnesia, in which adult memories of early childhood experiences before the age of five are typically vague and fragmentary. Psychogenic memories, while principally involving episodic information, may extend to semantic information, which is rarely seen in biogenic amnesia.

Biogenic amnesia is usually the result of trauma to the brain or disease processes. Anterograde and retrograde amnesia are common following a concussion or brain surgery, particularly involving the temporal lobe. Electroconvulsive treatments induced by a current passed through electrodes on the forehead (sometimes used to treat depression) tends to have a more anterograde effect. A diversity of toxic and infectious brain illnesses can lead to Korsakoff's syndrome, first described in chronic alcoholics. The primary feature is anterograde disturbance with the ability to store new information limited to a few seconds. Dementia typically begins with the loss of recent memories and gradually spreads retrograde into the person's more distant past as the condition progresses. Hardening of the brain arteries, Alzheimer's disease, and numerous infectious agents can lead to dementia. Transient global amnesia is an abrupt anterograde and retrograde loss leaving some degree of permanent memory loss; it is thought to be caused by temporary reductions in the blood supply to specific brain regions.

TREATMENT AND THERAPY

As time passes from the emotional and physiological traumas that precipitate amnesia, there is usually some degree of memory recovery. The less severe the trauma, the better the prognosis. Psychological interventions involving the use of careful interrogation, the use of emotionally significant stimuli, or hypnosis can help the amnesic fill in the gaps of memory deficits. Drugs that affect levels of neurotransmitters such as acetylcholine, aspartate, glutamate, norepinephrine, and serotonin can also have an impact on memory recovery. For example, John Krystal reported in 1993 that Vietnam War veterans given yohimbine, a drug that activates norepinephrine, experienced vivid flashbacks of combat trauma.

Some amnesias can be either prevented—using electrodes on only one side of the head in electroconvulsive treatment lessens the likelihood of amnesia—or significantly improved by psychological and/or biological intervention. Severe amnesias, however, such as in dementia, have no effective treatment. Major memory loss in the elderly has a particularly poor prognosis for recovery and is often indicative of imminent death. Where memory recovery is poor, optimizing the use of the remaining mental abilities and available environmental resources can help those with amnesia better adapt to their living environments.

PERSPECTIVE AND PROSPECTS

The first scientific explanations of amnesia came in the late nineteenth century. Théodule-Armand Ribot (1839-1916) proposed a "law of regression," in which memory loss was thought to progress from the least stable to the most stable memories. Sergey Korsakoff (1853-1900) was one of the first to demonstrate that amnesia need not be associated with the loss of reasoning abilities found in dementia. While Ribot and Korsakoff focused on organic causes of amnesia, Pierre Janet (1859-1947) described amnesics who apparently had no underlying biological disease. He explained these cases in terms of mental fragmentation that he called dissociation.

Prevention, rather than treatment, of amnesia became the focus of attention as the twentieth century drew to a close. Two examples of promising research areas include drugs to limit the effects of brain damage and the beneficial impact of a stimulating environment in staving off the effects of aging on the brain.

—*Paul J. Chara, Jr., Ph.D., and Kathleen A. Chara, M.S.*
See also Aging; Aging, extended care for the; Alcohol-

ism; Alzheimer's disease; Brain; Brain disorders; Dementia; Electroconvulsive therapy; Geriatrics and gerontology; Hypnosis; Memory loss; Psychiatric disorders; Psychiatry; Psychiatry, child and adolescent; Psychiatry, geriatric; Stress.

FOR FURTHER INFORMATION:

Damasio, Antonio, R. *Descartes' Error: Emotion, Reason, and the Human Brain*. New York: G. P. Putnam's Sons, 1994.

Herman, Judith L. *Trauma and Recovery*. New York: Basic Books, 1992.

Schacter, Daniel L. *Searching for Memory: The Brain, the Mind, and the Past*. New York: Basic Books, 1996.

AMNIOCENTESIS

PROCEDURE

ANATOMY OR SYSTEM AFFECTED: Abdomen, reproductive system, uterus

SPECIALTIES AND RELATED FIELDS: Embryology, genetics, obstetrics, perinatology

DEFINITION: The removal of amniotic fluid from a pregnant woman for analysis; this fluid provides biochemical and genetic information about the fetus, enabling physicians to identify hereditary problems in the baby well before it is born.

KEY TERMS:

amniotic sac: a thin, very tough membranous sac that contains amniotic fluid and the embryo or fetus of a mammal, bird, or reptile

chorionic villi: the fingerlike projections of the placenta that function in oxygen, nutrient, and waste transportation between a fetus and its mother

Down syndrome: an inherited disease that produces moderate to severe mental retardation

embryo: an organism in the early stages of development, before it has reached a recognizable form

Fallopian tube: one of the two tubes through which egg cells travel from the ovaries, in which they originate, to the uterus

fetus: the recognizable unborn young of humans and other viviparous organisms; in humans, the unborn child from the eighth week after its conception to birth

respiratory distress syndrome: a disease of lung immaturity which can be fatal and is likely to be found in children who will be born prematurely

Rh factor: a blood substance of Rh-positive people, absent in Rh-negative individuals; an Rh-negative woman and an Rh-positive man can produce an Rh-positive fetus at risk for a dangerous form of anemia

trimester: any of the three consecutive three-month periods during pregnancy

ultrasonography: the use of sound waves, directed at the body, to create visual images of the tissues being examined

INDICATIONS AND PROCEDURES

Human pregnancy begins after an egg cell and a sperm cell unite to become a fertilized egg. This process, called conception, occurs in a Fallopian tube, and about a week later the fertilized egg enters the uterus. Cell division during the time period between fertilization and its entry into the uterus converts the fertilized egg into an organized cell cluster that attaches to the endometrial lining of the uterus. Following this attachment, the cluster penetrates the lining and becomes intimately commingled with uterine tissues, developing three parts: the placenta, the embryo, and an amniotic sac filled with the fluid in which the embryo is suspended within the uterus. Two months after conception, the embryo—then an inch-long fetus—possesses all the anatomic features that will be present when it is born. During the remainder of the pregnancy, the fetus will grow much larger and all its internal and external anatomic details will be perfected.

When a woman visits her physician and learns that she is pregnant, she may begin to worry about possible birth defects. Such fears lead the expecting mother to seek assurance that her baby will be normal and healthy. Many factors, inferred from the medical history of a pregnant woman, can tell physicians whether a baby is likely to be healthy or whether birth defects are probable. For example, pregnant women who are over age thirty-five and those suffering from diabetes mellitus have higher-than-usual chances of giving birth to babies with defects.

In a small percentage of cases, the birth defects in a fetus will be so severe that the termination of a pregnancy may be considered as a necessary personal choice. Such situations include the occurrence of very severe mental damage or of a fatal genetic disease that will cause tremendous havoc in the affected family. In such cases, great tragedy can sometimes be averted by election of therapeutic abortion.

In a much larger number of cases, the knowledge of existing physical or biochemical problems in a fetus may allow treatment while the fetus is still in the uterus. Such treatment, promptly applied, may save the newborn baby from problems that could persist throughout life or prove lethal at a young age. Such information is often obtained by examination of the amniotic fluid in which the fetus is maintained throughout pregnancy. In order to carry out such an examination, a sample of the amniotic fluid must be procured. The procedure that is most often utilized for obtaining such samples is called amniocentesis.

Amniocentesis is used to provide diagnostic information before a fetus is born. It is carried out most often on fourteen- to sixteen-week-old fetuses because, at that stage of development, the procedure can be carried out very safely, amniotic fluid samples large enough for detailed genetic and biochemical analysis may be obtained without harming a fetus, and adequate time is available both to obtain data

and to use them to solve any problems that are encountered.

Modern amniocentesis is usually carried out in six consecutive steps. First, the position of the placenta in the uterus is located using ultrasonography. Then, the physician who will carry out the procedure locates the fetus by gentle, careful palpation of the mother's abdomen. Next, the mother is usually, but not always, given a dose of a local anesthetic. This is followed by the careful insertion of a long hypodermic needle through the abdominal wall and into the amniotic sac. As soon as amniotic fluid is seen in an attached sterile hypodermic syringe, a 20-milliliter sample (about four teaspoons) of fluid is carefully drawn up into the syringe. Finally, the needle and syringe are removed from the mother's abdomen.

Amniocentesis is reported to be almost painless: Even when patients are subjected to the procedure without being given an anesthetic, most report only an initial needle prick and a feeling of pressure during the process. Amniocentesis is also deemed to be very safe for both mother and fetus: Even if repeated several times, it has been reported to produce a risk factor of well under 1 percent.

The amniotic fluid of early pregnancy is very like the blood serum from which it arises. As pregnancy continues, the content in the fluid of substances derived from fetal urine and other fetal secretions increases greatly. Amniotic fluid also contains fetal cells arising from the skin, the stomach and other parts of the gastrointestinal organs, the reproductive organs, and the respiratory organs. Conse-

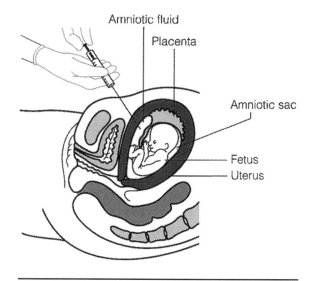

Amniocentesis

Amniotic fluid

Placenta

Amniotic sac

Fetus

Uterus

Removal and analysis of fluid from the amniotic sac that surrounds a fetus during gestation can be used to rule out or confirm the presence of serious birth defects or genetic diseases.

quently, this fluid is a very valuable diagnostic tool. Immediately after the amniotic fluid is collected, these fetal cells are separated out to be used for genetic analysis. The remaining, cell-free amniotic fluid is examined using a wide variety of biochemical techniques.

Important tests of the amniotic fluid and the cells that it contains include the determination of lecithin and sphingomyelin content, sex determination, and the identification of chromosomal diseases. Lecithins and sphingomyelins are two kinds of fatlike molecules known as lipids. Lecithins are the essential components of the pulmonary surfactant that acts, at lung surfaces, to prevent the collapse and dysfunction of tiny lung air sacs (alveoli) when a person exhales. Subnormal production of the pulmonary surfactant in a fetus may indicate the presence of the potentially fatal respiratory distress syndrome or hyaline membrane disease. Thus an important measurement made after amniocentesis is the ratio of lecithin and sphingomyelin content in the amniotic fluid. Lecithin-sphingomyelin ratio values of about 2.0 are deemed to be healthy, and those of 1.5 or less indicate a likelihood of risk to the fetus. Many other biochemical problems can be identified by similar analysis of other components of the amniotic fluid.

Both the sex of the fetus and the presence of chromosomal diseases can be diagnosed by examining the hereditary material, the deoxyribonucleic acid (DNA), from fetal cells grown in tissue cultures derived from the cells that were obtained by amniocentesis. Both sex determination and the presence of some diseases caused by abnormal chromosomes are identified by examination of the number and shape of the chromosomes in the fetal cells, a process known as karyotyping. Human beings usually possess twenty-three pairs of chromosomes, each of which has a characteristic size, shape, and overall appearance. A number of chromosomal diseases are associated with the presence of too many or too few chromosomes. A classical example is Down syndrome, which is always caused by the presence of an extra copy of chromosome number 21 (that is, there are three such chromosomes instead of the usual pair).

Some chromosomal abnormalities are caused by much more subtle DNA changes that do not alter human chromosome numbers. Rather, they are attributable to changed DNA in a chromosome that alters a small part of that chromosome. These diseases are discovered using DNA sequence analysis, which identifies existing abnormalities in the organization of parts of DNA molecules. A gene—a piece of DNA in a chromosome that carries genetic information—can be likened to the bar code used in supermarkets to identify a product at the cash register. Changes in that gene are like the changes in the bar code that indicate another, similar product. The bar code in a gene is a sequence of chemical units, and its alteration may signal the presence of a severe disease.

USES AND COMPLICATIONS

Amniocentesis may be utilized either to identify the sex of a human fetus or to explore its normalcy, its well-being, and its developmental maturity. Any of this information can be obtained both safely and successfully from this procedure at any time after the fourteenth week of pregnancy. The use of amniocentesis to explore the well-being and developmental maturity of a given fetus is carried out at intervals during the pregnancy. When a serious health or developmental aberration is identified, medical efforts can be made to correct this condition, if possible. If diseases such as Down syndrome (a cause of moderate to severe mental retardation) or fetal respiratory distress syndrome (a potentially lethal metabolic defect) are expected from a family medical history or from an actual occurrence in prior children, it is essential to carry out amniocentesis as soon as it becomes possible to do so.

Where amniocentesis identifies an exceptionally severe chromosomal disease in a fetus, the parents are informed concerning what to expect. In some cases, the decision to terminate the pregnancy may be made, and in others the pregnancy is continued with knowledge regarding the child's likely physical and mental status. A second amniocentesis procedure is often carried out to confirm the existence of the problem before any kind of action is taken by the parents.

It is important to note that, in many cases, amniocentesis will identify a treatable disease that can be handled while the fetus is still in the uterus. One such example is respiratory distress syndrome. When this disease is diagnosed early in the third trimester of a pregnancy, it can be treated successfully with hormones. In such cases, the amniocentesis procedure is then repeated at appropriate intervals after treatment, to assure both the parents and the physician that the problem has been solved.

The use of amniocentesis has replaced and has come to supplement the uncertainty of indirect genetic counseling, which had been used exclusively. The decision to choose or to exclude a particular course of action in family planning had been based entirely on a calculation of the mathematical odds of an inheritable disease being passed on to the children of those who were counseled. For example, when a family history indicated that both of the prospective parents carried a harmful gene—that is, when there was a history of the frequent occurrence of a disease in past generations—some risk was identifiable. On the other hand, if one or both of the parents actually suffered from a genetic disease, the odds of its being passed on increased to a point at which it was assumed that a child would develop that disease.

The use of amniocentesis is most valuable when, because of parental genetics, such a disease is likely but not assured. Genetic and/or biochemical information obtained by testing can either confirm the existence of the problem and suggest a corrective course of action or put the prospective parents' minds at rest. In such testing, it is important to identify the appropriate maternal group to test for each of the many diseases that are detectable by amniocentesis. Testing only the appropriate cases will ensure that the accompanying small but existent risks of amniocentesis to mothers and their fetuses can be minimized.

Amniocentesis is usually indicated when an Rh-negative woman and an Rh-positive man conceive a child because of the chance of hemolytic anemia in Rh-positive offspring. In fact, this use of amniocentesis was the basis of the pioneering effort, by Douglas Bevis in the 1950's, that first demonstrated the great predictive value of this procedure.

Additional group selection of subjects appropriate for amniocentesis is possible in many other cases. For example, the use of the procedure to identify Down syndrome is most important in mothers over the age of thirty-five, for whom the risk to a fetus is much higher than that seen in younger women. Likewise, the exploration of the possibility of respiratory distress syndrome is very valuable when there is family history of previous premature children because premature infants are always at high risk for developing the disease.

A test, via amniocentesis, of the lecithin-sphingomyelin ratio is also quite important in pregnant women who suffer from diabetes mellitus. The babies of such mothers are very likely to have subnormal lecithin levels and thus be at risk for various lung disorders. When amniocentesis identifies an at-risk lecithin-sphingomyelin ratio value, the potentially endangered fetus is injected with hormones that help it to produce mature lungs by raising the lecithin-sphingomyelin ratio value. The success or failure of such efforts is confirmed by the repetition of the amniocentesis. Numerous other biochemical problems that may be present in fetuses can be identified through a similar analysis of other components of the amniotic fluid.

Pregnancy in women who are more than thirty-five years old is currently viewed as the best reason for carrying out amniocentesis. The main fear, in this circumstance, is the presence of severe chromosomal diseases, the incidence of which is far greater for older women than for younger women. For example, the severe mental retardation caused by Down syndrome occurs in 3 percent of all live births of children to mothers over forty-five, an incidence about one thousand times greater than that in the offspring of a twenty-year-old woman.

Some other chromosomal diseases that can be identified by amniocentesis and DNA analysis are spina bifida, anencephaly, sickle-cell anemia, cystic fibrosis, muscular dystrophy, Huntington's chorea, and Klinefelter's syndrome. A number of these potentially devastating diseases can be corrected while a fetus is in the uterus, if they are diagnosed quickly enough. Where such treatment is not possible, an early diagnosis will usually make it possible to choose whether to undergo a therapeutic abortion or have the baby within a time window that ensures the safety of the former option.

PERSPECTIVE AND PROSPECTS

Until 1952, with the appearance of the article that Bevis wrote about the value of amniocentesis, neither parents nor physicians were able to see, touch, or otherwise examine any human fetus inside the uterus. This limitation had produced significant problems in obstetric care and in the diagnosis of the mental and physical characteristics of human offspring. With Bevis' observation that amniocentesis could be utilized to assess the risk factors in Rh incompatibility, this block disappeared. The development of modern technology soon led to all the uses of amniocentesis that have been cited for diagnosis of maturity, sex, health, and genetic defects in the fetus.

Numerous consequences of improvements in the methodologies associated with amniocentesis have produced still more effective avenues of exploration of the state of the fetus in the uterus. One example is the use of telescope-like fetoscopes to examine fetuses directly. In a procedure similar to that used to enter the uterus for amniocentesis, a fetoscope is utilized to examine the fetus for physical defects. In some cases, these defects are repaired via surgery, hormone administration, or chemotherapy. Such avenues of fetal monitoring and care are components of the medical specialty called fetology.

Another technique of obtaining fetal cells is chorionic villus sampling. It arose from the demonstration of the clear value of the information derived from fetal cells obtained from amniotic fluid. This useful procedure was devised to shorten the several-week-long time period, after amniocentesis, that is needed to grow enough fetal cells in tissue culture to provide the amount of tissue required for successful karyotyping or DNA sequencing work. Another advantage of the chorionic villius sampling procedure is that it can be carried out with younger fetuses, as young as twelve weeks old, although the risk to such a fetus is somewhat higher than that which is seen after amniocentesis. When an abortion or another type of corrective action is indicated by the results of chorionic villius sampling, however, it is often safer to carry out such actions because the testing procedure was performed much earlier in the pregnancy.

In chorionic villus sampling, a catheter is usually inserted into the uterus through the vaginal opening. This catheter is then guided by ultrasonography until its tip reaches the many chorionic villi that edge the placenta at its connection to the uterus. Gentle suction is applied, and a few of the villi are sucked out, first into the catheter and then into a sampling device. The cells that are obtained are tested in the same manner as with cells obtained after amniocentesis.

According to Aubrey Milunsky, the author of *The Prenatal Diagnosis of Hereditary Disorders* (1973), positive consequences of the use of amniocentesis, chorionic villus testing, and related prenatal diagnostic methods include better lives for children born in at-risk situations, reduced parental anguish, and huge monetary savings to society. The advantages to the children whose physical and/or mental state is improved are the most obvious. Similarly, the short-term mental anguish of parents decreases if it becomes clear that their baby will not be born impaired or can be treated medically. Long-term parental anguish can be diminished by such treatment or, where deemed necessary, via an abortion. Moreover, society spends considerable money on the institutionalization of hopelessly impaired children; such costs are unnecessary when the damage to such children can be repaired or prevented.   —*Sanford S. Singer, Ph.D.*

See also Abortion; Biopsy; Birth defects; Chorionic villus sampling; Cystic fibrosis; Down syndrome; Embryology; Genetic counseling; Genetic diseases; Genetics and inheritance; Gynecology; Laboratory tests; Mental retardation; Multiple births; Muscular dystrophy; Obstetrics; Pregnancy and gestation; Rh factor; Screening; Sickle-cell anemia; Spina bifida; Ultrasonography.

FOR FURTHER INFORMATION:

Bevis, Douglas. "The Antenatal Prediction of Haemolytic Disease of Newborn." *Lancet* 1 (February 23, 1952): 395-398. This article describes pioneering work on amniocentesis and its value in identifying the risk of hemolytic anemia in a fetus produced by an Rh-negative mother and an Rh-positive father. The methodology of diagnosis and the implications of the work are discussed.

Filkins, Karen, and Joseph Russo, eds. *Human Prenatal Diagnosis.* 2d ed. New York: Marcel Dekker, 1990. This book attempts to "clarify and rationalize aspects of diagnosis, genetic counseling, and intervention." It is meant as a guide for health professionals and is useful to general readers. The fourteen chapters cover a wide range of useful topics, including DNA analysis.

Holtzman, Neil A. *Proceed with Caution: Predicting Genetic Risks in the Recombinant DNA Era.* Baltimore: The Johns Hopkins University Press, 1989. This quite technical text describes the use of karyotyping and numerous other forms of hereditary material testing for identifying genetic problems. Included among these topics are applications associated with amniocentesis.

Milunsky, Aubrey. *The Prenatal Diagnosis of Hereditary Disorders.* Springfield, Ill.: Charles C Thomas, 1973. Covers the practice and use of amniocentesis; chromosomal, sex-linked, and biochemical hereditary disorders and congenital malformations; and genetic counseling. A detailed description of many hereditary diseases is included, as are hundreds of references.

Sherwood, Lauralee. *Human Physiology: From Cells to Systems.* 3d ed. Belmont, Calif.: Wadsworth, 1997. This college textbook contains useful biological information about pregnancy and genetic defects, as well as facts useful to understanding amniocentesis and its advantages and disadvantages. Provides many valuable definitions and diagrams. Clearly written, the book is a mine of information for interested readers.

Siggers, D. C. *Prenatal Diagnosis of Genetic Disease.* Oxford, England: Blackwell Scientific Publications, 1978. This brief but useful book discusses chromosomal disorders, neural tube defects, and biochemical problems in fetuses and newborns. Also contains a comprehensive description of amniocentesis. Useful tables, figures, and references are included.

Verp, Marion S., and Albert B. Gerbie. "Amniocentesis for Prenatal Diagnosis." *Clinical Obstetrics and Gynecology* 24 (1981): 1007-1021. This concise, technical review of amniocentesis covers much material, including genetic counseling, the composition of amniotic fluid, the risks associated with amniocentesis, and Rh sensitization. Seventy-five references are made available to interested readers.

AMPUTATION

PROCEDURE

ANATOMY OR SYSTEM AFFECTED: Arms, bones, hands, joints, knees, legs, muscles, musculoskeletal system, nervous system, skin

SPECIALTIES AND RELATED FIELDS: Critical care; emergency medicine; general surgery; oncology; orthopedics; physical therapy; plastic, cosmetic, and reconstructive surgery; vascular medicine

DEFINITION: The removal of a limb or other body part in order to prevent more serious harm to the patient.

KEY TERMS:

disarticulation: the amputation of a limb through a joint, without cutting the bone

edema: the accumulation of an excessive amount of fluid in cells or tissues

fascia: a sheet of fibrous tissue which envelops the body beneath the skin and also encloses the muscles or groups of muscles, separating their many layers or groups

gangrene: necrosis (tissue death) caused by obstruction of the blood supply; it may be localized to a small area or involve an entire extremity

ischemia: a local anemia or area of diminished or insufficient blood supply caused by mechanical obstruction (commonly narrowing of an artery) of the blood supply

periosteum: the thick, fibrous membrane that covers the entire surface of a bone except for the cartilage within a joint

peripheral: referring to a part of the body away from the center

prosthesis: a fabricated, artificial substitute for a missing part of the body, such as a limb

prosthetist: an individual skilled in constructing and fitting prostheses

vascular: relating to or containing blood vessels

INDICATIONS AND PROCEDURES

Amputations are performed in order to preserve life or to avoid more extensive damage or destruction to an individual or a portion of the body. They are performed in response to pathological processes (bacterial or viral infections, ischemia, or cancer, for example) that do not respond to treatment or to address the aftereffects of violent trauma (accidents, crushing injuries, or bullet wounds) in which tissues have been injured so extensively that they cannot be repaired, restored, or otherwise salvaged or saved.

Extremities are the most common sites for amputations, and there are four reasons for removing all or part of an extremity. The first is trauma which is so severe that surgical or other repair is not possible. The second reason is the presence of a tumor in the bones, soft tissues, muscles, blood vessels, or nerves of the extremity. A third cause is extensive infection that does not respond to usual or conservative treatment or that may lead to septicemia, a generalized infection which spreads throughout the entire body. The final indication for performing an amputation is the presence of peripheral vascular disease, a group of conditions that compromise or reduce the blood supply in an extremity.

Most amputations of the leg are performed because of impaired circulation, or ischemia. Several conditions may lead to ischemia, the most common of which is inadequately controlled diabetes mellitus. Others include atherosclerosis (a buildup of plaque in a blood vessel which restricts circulation), cellulitis, and vascular diseases. Bacterial infection can also lead to impaired circulation. When circulation continues to be inadequate, gangrene develops; infection can also contribute to or accelerate existing gangrene.

There are three general classes of amputation: provisional or open, conventional or standard, and osteomyoplastic. The techniques for each are briefly described.

The technique for a provisional amputation is often referred to as guillotine. In the past, this approach was commonly used in battle situations where speed was important to minimize both blood loss and subsequent infection. Currently, the technique is used mainly to remove a victim from a dangerous situation, typically one causing a crushing injury in which the alternative to amputation is death. All tissues are cut circularly. Skin is retained to the greatest degree possible, muscle and fascia are cut shorter, and the bone is cut shorter still. The hope is that the soft tissues (skin and muscles) will ultimately cover the bone, but the results are generally unsatisfactory. Large scars are common, and muscle frequently adheres to the bone. Long periods are required for healing, infections are common, and prostheses do not fit well. Another, more definitive amputation is usually required at a later date.

In a conventional amputation, skin, underlying tissues, muscle, and fascia are all cut in curved flaps that originate at the end of the remaining, unamputated bone. The muscles, fascia, bone, and major blood vessels are divided at the base of the remaining bone; nerves are cut at a slightly higher level, approximately 2.5 centimeters (1 inch) above the end of the bone. The nerves will retract somewhat into the muscle, minimizing postoperative pain. Muscles are tapered so that large masses of tissue are not present over the end of the stump; this will enhance the fit of a later prosthesis. At the cut end of the bone, the outer layer of bone is removed in order to reduce the possibility of bone spurs forming at some time in the future. The skin over the amputation site is closed loosely to avoid stretching as it heals.

The purpose of an osteomyoplastic amputation is to improve function after a prosthesis is fitted. The preparation of skin and fascia is the same as for a conventional amputation. Nerves and blood vessels are also divided. Muscles are separated for about 5 centimeters (2 inches) past the point where the bone will be cut. A portion of the outer surface (periosteum) from the bone to be amputated is sutured to the divided muscle. The bone is then cut. The prepared flap of periosteum and muscle is sutured to the periosteum of the stump. This procedure covers the marrow cavity of the stump, helps to preserve the remaining bone, and reduces postoperative infections. The remaining muscles are then sutured across the end of the stump. The skin is closed as in a conventional amputation. In an alternative procedure, holes are drilled in the bone of the stump. Muscles are inserted in the holes and sutured in place. The net effect of these osteomyoplastic procedures is to strengthen the musculature of the stump and to improve mobility for a prosthesis.

There are several common sites of levels for amputations of the leg. Syme's amputation is performed when most of the foot has been destroyed by trauma or compromised by poor circulation. In this type of amputation, the bones of the foot are removed, and the end of the tibia becomes the weight-bearing surface for the prosthesis.

A below-the-knee (BK) amputation is used to provide additional mobility for a prosthesis. It also leads to more complete rehabilitation because the knee is still available for movement. It is also associated with a reduction in phantom limb pain.

An above-the-knee (AK) amputation is frequently selected when gangrene extends into the muscles or skin of the calf. When the muscles of the leg are contracted, a prosthesis is not likely to be fitted or used; thus there is no advantage to a BK amputation in this situation. The AK amputation is associated with the highest healing rate for amputations among patients with peripheral vascular disease. The rate of a repeat amputation performed at a higher level on the leg is also low. Prostheses that permit walking, however, are less efficient with amputations at this level.

Both amputations have about the same rate of healing,

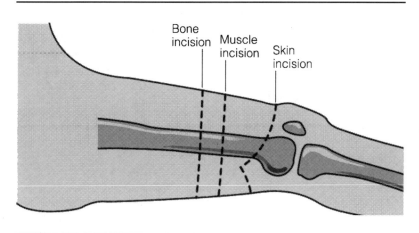

In above-the-knee amputation, incisions in the bone, muscles, and skin are made in such a way that the muscles and skin can be folded over the remaining bone, thus creating a stump to which a prosthesis may later be molded and attached.

cipal concern is a wide excision of any apparent tumor. When amputation is performed after the patient has sustained significant trauma or to treat peripheral vascular disease, the major factor determining the best site is usually the extent of healthy tissue. Other important factors include preserving sufficient length in the remaining bone or stump so that a prosthesis may be used. Furthermore, the prosthesis must be functional, must have adequate space for attachment, and must be cosmetically acceptable. The scar must be placed so that it will not break down from mechanical traction or interfere with the fit of the prosthesis.

In general, the more bone that can be left in place, the more functional a prosthetic limb will be; patients will

but a higher percentage of individuals with BK amputations walk on prostheses than do those with AK amputations. The choice between BK and AK amputation is determined by the general health of the patient and the potential for rehabilitation. The most important determinant of level of amputation, however, is the vascular status of the patient.

The leg can also be amputated at either the knee or the hip; such a procedure is a disarticulation, an amputation through a joint. A knee disarticulation is most commonly used with children to preserve the growing portion (epiphysis) of the remaining thigh bone. A hip disarticulation is used with tumors or extensive soft tissue injuries in the thigh. Special prostheses that permit walking after such procedures are available, but they are relatively uncommon.

Portions of the upper extremity are usually amputated after extensive trauma. Malignant disease of the bone or muscle is a less common reason for amputation at these sites. The considerations described for the lower extremity are applicable for the upper extremity, namely preserving as much tissue as possible for later rehabilitation and recovery of function. The sites for amputation are also analogous. Individual fingers can be amputated, or the entire hand can be amputated at the wrist (a location similar to the Syme's amputation of the foot). Similarly, the forearm can be amputated either below the elbow or above the elbow. Portions of the arm can be disarticulated at the elbow or at the shoulder. Restoration of function is far more difficult, however, in an upper extremity amputation than for a lower extremity amputation. It is easier to restore the ability to walk than it is to restore hand function.

USES AND COMPLICATIONS

The level or site of an amputation is critical to recovery and rehabilitation. When an amputation is performed because of cancer or some other malignant disease, the prin-

also have better control of their prostheses. Frequently, special procedures will have to be used to save skin or to graft skin to the site of an amputation so as to preserve the length of the bone. The issue of bone length is especially critical in amputations of the upper extremities, as arms, hands, and fingers are so important in daily functions. The prospects for rehabilitation are also considered when an amputation is contemplated. For example, there is less need to preserve bone for a prosthesis if an individual is not inclined—because of temperament, age, or physical condition—to rehabilitate a lost body part.

There are different regional considerations for patients requiring an amputation for peripheral vascular disease. The ability of the skin and other tissues to heal is directly dependent on an adequate supply of blood. Injections of dye into local small arteries, a procedure called arteriography, are used to determine if the vessels can deliver sufficient blood to a proposed amputation site or around joints such as the knee.

Amputations for extensive trauma should be performed soon after the injury is sustained in order to reduce the chances for contamination or infection. This practice will also assist in subsequent psychological adjustment to the loss of the body part.

Bedridden patients frequently suffer from ulcers of the skin, or bedsores, lesions that do not heal well if at all. In combination with impaired circulation (ischemia), these ulcers can lead to the need for amputations. This group of patients must be carefully prepared for surgery by conditioning muscles that will remain after the amputation. Before an amputation is attempted, extensive efforts must be made to heal all skin ulcers. Physical therapy is frequently used before the surgery to strengthen and improve the tone of muscles. Antibiotics, moist heat, and frequently changed dressings are employed to fight infection. Patients should be moved frequently to avoid the formation of new skin ulcers. Special beds are often used to avoid concentrating pressure on body parts; this can be accomplished with pillows and lambskin mats. In some cases, ice packs are used in the days immediately prior to amputation to limit the spread of infection and to reduce pain.

Conventional postoperative care for amputation focuses on providing optimal tissue care: movement and specific exercises to prevent contractures (the loss of use for muscles), the compression of tissue to prevent edema, and the initiation of physical therapy to regain or retain the optimum use of the remaining body part. The ultimate goal is to provide a prosthesis wherever possible and appropriate in order to improve the patient's quality of life and vocational opportunities.

Edema is minimized by applying tight dressings to the amputation site. After sutures are removed, elastic bandages are used for the next several weeks. Exercises and movement of the stump will prevent contractures. These exercises should be started as soon as possible after the amputation. When a portion of an arm or leg has been removed, it is important to move and stretch the entire limb.

One problem associated with amputations is called phantom limb pain: the perception of pain in a body part that is no longer attached to the body. Typically, a patient who has lost a limb will experience pain or other sensation as if the limb were still intact. This phenomenon occurs because of stimulation in the nerve endings of the remaining stump. Such sensations are amplified in the posterior horn, a portion of the spinal cord. The nervous impulses are processed by the brain and interpreted as pain; it is this subjective feeling that the patient experiences. Phantom limb pain can usually be prevented by surgical techniques employed at the time of amputation.

Traumatically amputated body parts can sometimes be reattached. Portions of fingers, hands, and entire upper extremities have been successfully reattached; lower extremity reattachments are less common. The regeneration of nerves, however, is not uniformly accomplished. The myelin sheaths of nerves—the cells that surround many nerves to provide insulation and to increase the velocity of nerve impulse conduction—must be approximated for successful regeneration. The lack of nerve regeneration can affect either motor or sensory aspects of the body part. Lack of motor nerve regeneration leads to disuse atrophy and loss of functional use of the body part. Cosmetically, the body usually appears normal. Loss of sensory innervation requires adaptation, but the ability to move the body part is not affected. If the sensory loss is from skin only, the deficit is usually not significant. Sensory loss in fingers and toes is more serious; other senses such as sight and position receptors in joints must be relied upon to compensate for the lack of direct input from fingers or toes. These deficits can be overcome with rehabilitation.

Amputations performed by surgeons skilled in techniques appropriate for ischemic or necrotic tissue have the lowest incidence of postoperative complications and the highest degree of success for subsequent rehabilitation. The death rate for amputations required for isolated trauma, infection, or tumors is less than 3 percent. In contrast, amputations related to vascular diseases result in death for approximately one patient in four. Mortality rates rise with the removal of increasing amounts of a body part: The removal of a toe or foot is less likely to end in death than the removal of an entire leg.

PERSPECTIVE AND PROSPECTS

Historically, techniques for amputation evolved on the battlefield. Amputation was the only treatment available for battle casualties; the alternative was death. Military surgeons were known for speed. In the early part of the twentieth century, antibiotics were discovered. Improved instrumentation and operative techniques were first developed in the 1950's. Microscopic procedures have been perfected more recently. The net effect of these developments has been to reduce the need for amputation following trauma. These same techniques have enabled the reattachment or reimplantation of fingers or other extremities.

When amputation is necessary, however, the surgeon must weigh the desires of the patient against his or her best interests. It is natural for patients to want to retain as much original tissue as possible, but surgeons prefer to perform an amputation only once. Impaired circulation compromises tissues. When individuals with conditions such as diabetes require amputation and insufficient tissue is removed, the result is frequently another amputation. Individuals with poorly controlled diabetes may lose their entire legs in a series of amputations.

After an amputation, physical therapy begins the rehabilitation process. As soon as the patient can tolerate movement, exercises are undertaken. The goal of these activities is to return the person to as normal a level of function as possible. The services of an occupational therapist are used to regain old motor skills or to learn new ones. An artificial body part is fitted by a prosthetist. The sooner a prosthesis is fitted, the greater is the probability that the patient will adapt successfully to it. Temporary prostheses initially fitted within the first twenty-four hours following surgery have had high degrees of acceptance.

Prostheses typically are of two varieties: functional and cosmetically appealing. Prostheses with wires attached to movable hooks allow limited motor function of hands. Muscles of the forearm are retrained to provide movement of the hook. Lower limb prostheses are usually more anatomically correct and cosmetically appealing. They allow walking and other movements but do not usually allow fine motor control of toes. This does not preclude the adaptation and eventual recovery of fairly complex motor skills, including those required for participation in sports activities.

One predictor of eventual success with the prosthesis is the age at which it is fitted. Young children adapt rapidly, but the older the patient is, the more difficult adaptation to a prosthesis becomes. Older persons often merely tolerate an artificial limb while younger persons accept the prosthesis and continue with the activities of their lives. Much of the rehabilitation after an amputation is psychological. With appropriate support and therapy, the potential for a nearly normal life exists for most persons experiencing an amputation. —*L. Fleming Fallon, Jr., M.D., M.P.H.*

See also Arteriosclerosis; Bacterial infections; Bone cancer; Bone disorders; Bone grafting; Bones and the skeleton; Cancer; Circulation; Critical care; Critical care, pediatric; Diabetes mellitus; Emergency medicine; Fracture and dislocation; Fracture repair; Frostbite; Gangrene; Grafts and grafting; Ischemia; Lower extremities; Muscles; Oncology; Orthopedic surgery; Orthopedics; Orthopedics, pediatric; Physical rehabilitation; Plastic, cosmetic, and reconstructive surgery; Skin; Tumor removal; Tumors; Upper extremities; Vascular medicine; Vascular system; Wounds.

FOR FURTHER INFORMATION:

Burgess, C. M. "General Principles of Amputation Surgery." In *Atlas of Limb Prostheses: Surgical and Prosthetic Principles.* St. Louis: C. V. Mosby, 1981. A fairly technical account of surgical techniques of amputation. General readers are advised to approach this work with a medical dictionary for assistance.

Friedmann, Lawrence W. *The Psychological Rehabilitation of the Amputee.* Springfield, Ill.: Charles C Thomas, 1978. Discusses problems related to rehabilitation after amputation, providing greater depth than is possible in this entry. Well written and useful for the general reader.

Sabiston, David C., Jr., ed. *Textbook of Surgery.* 15th ed. Philadelphia: W. B. Saunders, 1997. A standard textbook of surgery that contains an extensive discussion of different types of fractures and dislocations and how they are treated. Intended for practicing professionals but can be generally understood by the layperson.

Schwartz, Seymour I., G. Tom Shires, and Frank C. Spencer, eds. *Principles of Surgery.* 6th ed. New York: McGraw Hill, 1994. A standard textbook of surgery that contains sections on fractures and dislocations. Its intended audience is practicing surgeons, and thus technical language is used. The serious reader can find greater detail in this work.

ANATOMY

ANATOMY OR SYSTEM AFFECTED: All
SPECIALTIES AND RELATED FIELDS: All
DEFINITION: The structure of the human body—its parts, systems, and organs.
KEY TERMS:
abdomen: the rib-free part of the trunk, below the diaphragm

head: the part of the body containing the major sense organs (such as the eyes and ears) and the brain
lower extremities: the thigh, lower leg, and foot
thorax: the part of the trunk above the diaphragm, containing the ribs; the chest
trunk: the central part of the body, to which the extremities are attached
upper extremities: the arm, forearm, and hand

STRUCTURE AND FUNCTIONS

The body's parts can be categorized either regionally or functionally. Regionally, the body consists of a trunk to which are attached two upper extremities, two lower extremities, and a head, attached by means of a neck. Functionally, the body consists of a digestive system, a circulatory system, an excretory system, a respiratory system, a reproductive system, a nervous system, an endocrine system, an integument (skin), a skeleton, and a series of muscles.

Regionally, the body consists of a central portion called the trunk, to which other parts are attached. The trunk itself may be divided into an upper portion called the chest (or thorax), containing ribs, and a lower, rib-free portion called the abdomen. Internally, the thorax and abdomen are separated by a muscular sheet called the diaphragm. Attached to the trunk are two upper extremities, two lower extremities, and a head. The upper extremities include the arms, forearms, and hands; the lower extremities include the thighs, lower legs, and feet. The head includes the brain and the major sense organs such as the eyes and ears; the neck is the narrower, flexible part that connects the head to the trunk. The ventral (front) surface of the abdomen is often divided around the umbilicus into upper-left, upper-right, lower-left, and lower-right quadrants.

Functionally, the body consists of a number of organ systems: a digestive system, a circulatory system, an excretory system, a respiratory system, a reproductive system, a nervous system, an endocrine system, an integument (skin), a skeleton, and a series of muscles. The digestive system breaks down foods into simpler substances and absorbs them. The circulatory system transports oxygen and other materials around the body. The excretory system rids the body of many waste products, while the respiratory system rids the body of carbon dioxide and adds oxygen to the blood. The reproductive system produces sex cells and, in females, provides an environment for the development of an embryo. The nervous system sends signals in the form of nerve impulses from one part of the body to another, and the endocrine organs send chemical messengers (hormones) through the bloodstream. The integument, or skin, protects the outer surface of the body from infection, from injury, and from drying out (desiccation); it also maintains the body's internal temperature by providing insulation and preventing the body from overheating during exercise through sweating. The skeleton serves as the body's framework and consists of 206 separate bones; these bones support the body's other organs and also protect the heart, lungs, and especially the central nervous system (including the brain and the spinal cord). The muscles produce movements by their contractions.

Each major organ system is constructed of several major organs. The major organs contained within the thorax are the heart, lungs, and thymus body. The major organs contained within the abdomen include the stomach, spleen, liver, pancreas, small intestine (consisting of the duodenum, ileum, and jejunum), large intestine (consisting of the caecum, colon, and rectum, with the colon further divided into an ascending colon, transverse colon, descending colon, and sigmoid colon), and bladder. The kidneys and urinary ducts lie along the dorsal body wall of the abdomen. Also contained within the lower abdomen are the uterus, ovaries, and Fallopian tubes in the female and the vas deferens and prostate gland in the male. In males, two downward extensions of the abdominal cavity form the scrotal sacs that surround the testes.

The thoracic and abdominal cavities (and the scrotal cavities in males) are all considered part of the general body cavity, or coelom. Each part of the coelom is lined on all sides with a thin, single layer of flat (squamous) cells known as the peritoneum. The peritoneum forming the outer wall of these cavities is called the parietal peritoneum; the peritoneum on the outer surface of the internal organs, or viscera, is called the visceral peritoneum.

Each type of organ is made of a number of different tissues. The four major types of tissues are epithelium, connective tissue, muscle tissue, and nervous tissue. Epithelial tissues (or epithelium) include those tissues that originate in broad, flat surfaces; their functions include protection, absorption, and secretion. Epithelia can be one-layered (simple) or many-layered (stratified). Their cells can be flat (squamous), tall and skinny (columnar), or equal in height and width (cuboidal). Some simple epithelia have nuclei at two different levels, giving the false appearance of different layers; these tissues are called pseudostratified. Some simple squamous epithelia have special names: The inner lining of most blood vessels is called the endothelium, while the lining of the body cavities (including all parts of the coelom) is called the mesothelium. Kidney tubules and most small ducts are also lined with simple squamous epithelia. The pigmented layer of the retina and the front surface of the lens are examples of simple cuboidal epithelia. Simple columnar epithelia form the inner lining of most digestive organs and the linings of the small bronchi and the gallbladder. The epithelia lining the Fallopian tubes, nasal cavities, and bronchi are ciliated, meaning that the cells have small, hairlike extensions called cilia.

The outer layer of skin is a stratified squamous epithelium; other stratified squamous epithelia line the inside of the mouth, esophagus, and vagina. Sweat glands and other glands in the skin are lined with stratified cuboidal epithelia. Most of the urinary tract is lined with a special kind of stratified cuboidal epithelium, called a transitional epithelium, that allows a large amount of stretching. Parts of the pharynx, larynx, urethra, and the ducts of the mammary glands are lined with stratified columnar epithelium.

Glands are composed of epithelial tissues that are highly modified for secretion. They may be either exocrine glands (in which the secretions exit by ducts to targets nearby) or endocrine glands (in which the secretions are carried by the bloodstream to targets some distance away). The salivary glands in the mouth, the glandular lining of the stomach, and the sebaceous glands of the skin are examples of exocrine glands. The thyroid gland, adrenal gland, and pituitary gland are examples of endocrine glands. The pancreas has both exocrine and endocrine portions: The exocrine parts secrete digestive enzymes, while the endocrine parts, called the islets of Langerhans, secrete the hormones insulin and glucagon.

Connective tissues are tissues containing large amounts of material called extracellular matrix, located outside the cells. The matrix may be a liquid (such as blood plasma), a solid containing fibers of collagen and related proteins, or an inorganic solid containing calcium salts (as in bone). Blood and lymph are connective tissues with a liquid matrix (plasma) that can solidify when the blood clots. In addition to plasma, blood contains red cells (erythrocytes), white cells (leucocytes), and the tiny platelets that help form clots. The many kinds of leucocytes include granular types (basophils, neutrophils, and eosinophils, all named according to the staining properties of their granules), the monocytes, and the several types of lymphocytes. Lymph contains lymphocytes and plasma only.

Most connective tissues have a solid matrix which includes fibrous proteins such as collagen and elastic fibers in some cases. If all the fibers are arranged in the same direction, as in ligaments and tendons, the tissue is called regular connective tissue. The dermis of the skin is an example of an irregular connective tissue in which the fibers are arranged in all directions. Loose connective tissue and adipose (fat) tissue both have very few fibers. The simplest type of loose connective tissue, with the fewest fibers, is sometimes called areolar connective tissue. Adipose tissue is a connective tissue in which the cells are filled with fat deposits.

Hemopoietic (blood-forming) tissue occurs in bone marrow and in the thymus, and it contains the immature cell types that develop into most connective tissue cells, including blood cells. Cartilage tissue matrix contains a shock-resistant complex of protein and sugarlike (polysaccharide) molecules. Cartilage cells usually become trapped in this matrix and eventually die, except for those closest to the surface. Bone tissue gains its supporting ability and strength from a matrix containing calcium salts. Its typical cells, called osteocytes, contain many long strands by which these cells exchange nutrients and waste products with other osteocytes, and ultimately with the bloodstream. Bone also contains osteoclasts, large cells responsible for bone resorption and the release of calcium into the bloodstream.

Mesenchyme is an embryonic connective tissue made of wandering, amoeba-like cells. During embryological development, the mesenchyme cells develop into many different cell types, including hemocytoblasts, which give rise to most blood cells, and fibroblasts, which secrete protein fibers and then usually differentiate into other cell types.

Muscle tissue are tissues specially modified for contraction. When a nerve impulse is received, overlapping fibers of the proteins actin and myosin slide against one another to produce the contraction. The three types of muscle tissue are smooth muscle, cardiac muscle, and skeletal muscle. The term "striated muscle" is sometimes used to refer to cardiac and skeletal muscle, both of which have cylindrical fibers marked by cross-bands, also called cross-striations. The striations are caused by the lining up of the contractile proteins actin and myosin. Smooth muscle contains cells with tapering ends and centrally located nuclei. Muscular contractions are smooth, rhythmic, and involuntary, usually not subject to fatigue. The cells are not cross-banded. Smooth muscle occurs in many digestive organs, reproductive organs, and skin, as well as in many other organs. Cardiac muscle occurs only in the heart. Its cross-striated fibers branch and come together repeatedly. Contractions of these fibers are involuntary, rhythmic, and without fatigue. Nuclei are located in the center of each cell; cell boundaries are marked by dark-staining structures called intercalated disks. Skeletal muscle occurs in the voluntary muscles of the body. Their cylindrical, cross-striated fibers contain many nuclei but no internal cell boundaries; a multinucleated fiber of this type is called a syncytium. Skeletal muscle is capable of rapid, forceful contractions, but it fatigues easily. Skeletal muscle tissue always attaches to connective tissue structures.

Nervous tissues contain specialized nerve cells (neurons) that respond rapidly to stimulation by conducting nerve impulses. All neurons contain RNA-rich granules, called Nissl granules, in the cytoplasm. Neurons with a single long extension of the cell body are called unipolar, those with two long extensions are called bipolar, and neurons with more than two long extensions are called multipolar. There are two types of extensions: Dendrites conduct impulses toward the cell body, while axons generally conduct impulses away from the cell body. Many axons are surrounded by a multilayered fatty substance called the myelin sheath, which is composed of many layers of cell membrane wrapped around the axon.

Nervous tissues also contain several types of neuroglia, cells that hold nervous tissue together. Many neuroglia cells have processes that wrap around the neurons and help nourish them. The many types of neuroglia include the tiny microglia and the larger protoplasmic astrocytes, fibrous astrocytes, and oligodendroglia.

Two major tissue types make up most of the brain and spinal cord, or central nervous system. The first type, gray matter, contains the cell bodies of many neurons, along with smaller amounts of axons, dendrites, and neuroglia cells. The second type, white matter, contains mostly the axons, and sometimes also the dendrites, of neurons whose cell bodies lie elsewhere, along with the myelin sheaths that surround many of the axons. Clumps of cell bodies are called nuclei when they are found within the brain and ganglia when they occur elsewhere. Bundles of axons are called tracts within the central nervous system and nerves when they appear peripherally.

The body can be described by the use of directional terms, which are defined in a relative manner according to the location of a given body part or segment. Some important directional terms are "superior," "inferior," "cranial," "caudal," "dorsal," "ventral," "medial," "lateral," "radial," "ulnar," "anterior," and "posterior."

Directional Terms for the Body

Superior: upward; toward the top of the head
Inferior: downward; toward the ground or the feet
Cranial: toward the head; the same as superior in humans
Caudal: toward the tail
Dorsal: toward the back
Ventral: toward the belly surface
Medial: toward the midline
Lateral: away from the midline
Radial: on the medial side (or thumb side) of the arm, forearm, and hand
Ulnar: on the lateral side (or little finger side) of the arm, forearm, and hand; the same side that contains the ulna
Anterior: forward, in the customary direction of motion; equivalent to ventral in humans, but the same as cranial in other animals
Posterior: toward the rear, opposite to the customary direction of motion; equivalent to dorsal in humans, but the same as caudal in other animals

DISORDERS AND DISEASES

Diseases or disorders that affect the entire body are called systemic or multisystem diseases. For example, fevers or febrile diseases raise the body's temperature. Many fevers are caused by infectious diseases such as influenza (actually a series of different viral infections). Influenzas cause fever, sore throat, muscle aches, coughs, headache, fatigue, and a general feeling of malaise.

Edema, or tissue swelling, is marked by an increase in the amount of extracellular fluid in several parts of the body at once. In the case of pulmonary edema, the fluid stains pink and fills the usually empty lung spaces (alveoli).

Most cancers are recognized by abnormalities of the cells in which they occur. The most dangerous cancers are marked by large tumors with ill-defined, irregular margins. If the cancer tumor is well-defined, small, and has a smooth, circular margin, then it is much less of a threat. Cancers are especially dangerous when they undergo metastasis, a process by which they produce wandering cells that spread throughout the body.

Juvenile diabetes mellitus (also called diabetes mellitus, Type I, and insulin-dependent diabetes mellitus, or IDDM), like most endocrine disorders, has systemic consequences throughout the body, including damage to nearly all the blood vessels. The primary defect in this disorder is a lack of insulin, which impairs the body's ability to use glucose. Another endocrine disorder with systemic consequences is Addison's disease, which is caused by a deficiency of the hormone adrenal corticotrophic hormone (ACTH) normally produced by the cortex of the adrenal gland. Symptoms include weakness, loss of appetite, fatigue, weight loss, and reduced tolerance to cold. These symptoms result from imbalances in the levels of glucose and mineral salts throughout the body.

Lupus erythematosus, a connective tissue disease, often produces red skin lesions marked by degeneration and flattening of the lower layers of the epidermis, drying and flaking of the outermost layer, dilation of the blood vessels under the skin, and the leakage of red blood cells out of these vessels, adding to the red color. (The word "erythematosus" means "red.")

Muscular dystrophy has several forms; the most common form is marked in its advanced stages by enlarged muscles in which the muscle tissue is replaced by fatty substance. Another muscular disease, myasthenia gravis, is often marked by overall enlargement of the thymus and an increase in the number of thymus cells. Myocardial infarction, a form of heart disease marked by damage to the heart muscle, is noticed in histological section by dead, fibrous scar tissue replacing the muscle tissue in the heart wall. In patients with arteriosclerosis, the usually elastic walls of the arteries become thicker and more fibrous and rigid; many of the same patients also suffer from atherosclerosis, a buildup of deposits on the inside of the blood vessel, partially or completely blocking blood flow.

In nervous tissue, damage to peripheral nerves often results in a process called chromatolysis in the cell bodies of the neurons from which these axons arise. The nuclei of these cells enlarge and become displaced to one side, while the Nissl granules disperse and the cell body as a whole undergoes swelling. Increased deposits of fibrous tissue characterize multiple sclerosis and certain other disorders of the nervous system. Some of these diseases are also marked by a degeneration of the myelin sheath around nerve fibers. In the case of a cerebrovascular stroke, impaired blood supply to the brain causes degeneration of the neuroglia, followed by general tissue death and the replacement of the neuroglia by fibrous tissue. Cranial hematoma (abnormal bleeding) results in the presence of blood clots (complete with blood cells and connective tissue fibers) in abnormal locations. Alzheimer's disease is marked by granules of a proteinlike substance called amyloid, often containing aluminum, surrounded by additional concentric layers of similar composition.

PERSPECTIVE AND PROSPECTS

The Latin names that are used today for most body parts are derived in large measure from the writings of Galen, or Caius Galenus, the physician to the Roman army in the second century. The study of anatomy was furthered in the Renaissance by artists such as Leonardo da Vinci (1452-1519) and Michelangelo (1475-1564), both of whom dissected human corpses illegally in order to gain further knowledge of the anatomical structures visible on the body's surface. Such studies were followed by the well-illustrated anatomical texts of Andreas Vesalius (1514-1564), who corrected many of Galen's errors regarding the structure of the human body.

A medical understanding of the circulatory system began with the studies of the Renaissance physician William Harvey (1578-1657), who examined the veins in the arms of many patients. It was Harvey who first described the presence of valves in the veins and who proved that the blood circulates outward from the heart, throughout the body, and then back again to the heart.

Microscopes were first developed around 1700 by Antoni van Leeuwenhoek (1632-1723) and others. Electron microscopes first became commercially available in the 1950's. These two types of microscopy were widely used for distinguishing between healthy and diseased tissue, in tissue taken either from bodies at autopsy or from biopsies of living patients. Modern diagnostic radiology began with the discovery of X rays by Wilhelm Conrad Röntgen (1845-1923). Computed tomography (CT) scanning, which was developed in the 1960's and 1970's, allows for the creation of a three-dimensional X-ray picture.

—Eli C. Minkoff, Ph.D.

See also Physiology; Systems and organs; *specific parts or systems.*

FOR FURTHER INFORMATION:

Agur, Anne M. R., and Ming J. Lee. *Grant's Atlas of Anatomy.* 9th ed. Baltimore: Williams & Wilkins, 1991. Offers many excellent, detailed illustrations of the human body.

Anson, Barry J. *An Atlas of Human Anatomy.* 2d ed. Philadelphia: W. B. Saunders, 1963. Anson provides excellent color-coded illustrations but little explanatory text.

Crouch, James E. *Functional Human Anatomy.* 4th ed. Philadelphia: Lea & Febiger, 1985. An easy-to-read book which offers helpful explanations. A good reference source for the beginning anatomy student or nonscientists.

Gray, Henry. *Gray's Anatomy*. Edited by Peter L. Williams et al. 38th ed. New York: Churchill Livingstone, 1995. The classic anatomy text. Thorough descriptions and excellent, detailed color illustrations are provided.

King, Barry G., and Mary Jane Showers. *Human Anatomy and Physiology*. 6th ed. Philadelphia: W. B. Saunders, 1969. Contains excellent functional explanations of the workings of most organs, but muscle actions are not as thoroughly explained as in the other works cited in this bibliography.

McMinn, R. M. H., and R. T. Hutchings. *Color Atlas of Human Anatomy*. 3d ed. St. Louis: Mosby Year Book, 1993. A useful set of color illustrations covering all parts of the body.

Netter, F. H. *The CIBA Collection of Medical Illustrations*. 8 vols. West Caldwell, N.J.: CIBA Pharmaceutical, 1983. A large-format set of excellent medical illustrations for college students.

Rohen, J. W., and Chihiro Yokochi. *Color Atlas of Anatomy: A Photographic Study of the Human Body*. 3d ed. New York: Igaku-Shoin, 1993. An excellent compendium of color photographs of various anatomical structures.

Rosse, Cornelius, and Penelope Gaddum-Rosse. *Hollinshead's Textbook of Anatomy*. 5th ed. Philadelphia: Lippincott-Raven, 1997. Good descriptions and illustrations are highlights of this thorough, modern, and detailed reference work.

Sobotta, Johannes. *Sobotta Atlas of Human Anatomy*. Edited by Helmut Ferner and Jochen Staubesand. Translated and edited by Walther J. Hild. 10th ed. 2 vols. Baltimore: Urban & Schwarzenberg, 1982. This reference work contains excellent illustrations of the human body.

ANEMIA

DISEASE/DISORDER

ANATOMY OR SYSTEM AFFECTED: Blood

SPECIALTIES AND RELATED FIELDS: Family practice, hematology, internal medicine, serology

DEFINITION: A pathological deficiency in the oxygen-carrying material of the blood. Not a disease but a sign of the presence of a variety of diseases, anemia is a frequent and significant worldwide health problem.

KEY TERMS:

aplastic anemia: anemia caused by lack of a functioning bone marrow; also known as bone marrow aplasia

erythrocytes: red blood cells

hemoglobin: the protein whose major function is to transport oxygen throughout the body

hemolytic anemia: anemia resulting from hemolysis, the excessive destruction of red blood cells

hypoxia: a deficiency in the amount of oxygen reaching the body tissues

iron-deficiency anemia: anemia characterized by low serum iron concentration

megaloblastic anemia: anemia caused by the failure of red blood cells to mature; also known as pernicious anemia, Addisonian anemia, or maturation failure anemia

microcytic or hypochromic anemia: anemia that ensues after blood loss

CAUSES AND SYMPTOMS

Hemoglobin, the red blood pigment, is a protein whose major function is to transport oxygen throughout the body. It is contained in the erythrocytes (red blood cells), which are flexible, biconcave disks that can squeeze through capillary blood vessels that are smaller in diameter than they are and ensure the rapid diffusion of oxygen. Anemia is defined as a reduction in either the volume of red blood cells or the concentration of hemoglobin in a sample of venous blood when compared with similar values obtained from a reference population. The anemic condition is considered to exist if hemoglobin levels are below 13 grams per 100 milliliters of blood in males and below 12 grams per 100 milliliters in adult, nonpregnant females.

The initial symptoms of patients with anemia are related to efforts by the body to compensate for the diminished oxygen supply. Later symptoms reflect the failure of these compensatory mechanisms. The viscosity of the blood is dependent almost entirely on the concentration of red blood cells. In severe anemia the blood viscosity may fall to as low as one and a half times that of water, rather than the normal value of around three times the viscosity of water. The greatly decreased viscosity decreases the resistance to blood flow in the blood vessels so that far greater than normal quantities of blood return to the heart. Also, hypoxia caused by the diminished transport of oxygen by the blood causes the tissue vessels to dilate, increasing the return of blood to the heart. As a result, the cardiac output can increase to as much as two to three times its normal value.

The increased cardiac output in anemia offsets many of its symptoms: Even though each unit quantity of blood carries only small quantities of oxygen, the rate of blood flow may be increased so much that normal quantities of oxygen are delivered to the tissues. As long as an anemic person's rate of activity is low, he or she can live without fatal hypoxia of the tissues, even when his or her concentration of red blood cells may be reduced to a quarter of the normal quantity. When the patient begins to exercise, the heart is not capable of pumping much greater quantities of blood than it is already pumping. Therefore, during exercise, which increases tissue demand for oxygen, extreme tissue hypoxia results and acute cardiac failure can ensue.

Anemia is a process that evolves within a clinical context produced by any condition that causes the quantity of oxygen transported to the tissues to decrease. Some of the most important types of anemia are microcytic or hypochromic anemia, iron-deficiency anemia, aplastic anemia, mega-loblastic anemia, and hemolytic anemia.

Microcytic or hypochromic anemia is the type of anemia that ensues after blood loss. In the case of rapid hemorrhage, the body normally replaces plasma within one to two days, but this leaves a low concentration of red blood cells, creating the anemia condition. If another hemorrhage does not occur, the red blood cell count goes back to normal within three to four weeks. In the case of chronic blood loss, the person cannot absorb enough iron through the intestines to form hemoglobin as fast as it is lost. Therefore, red blood cells are produced in too few numbers and with too little hemoglobin in them, again creating the anemic condition. The symptoms of microcytic anemia depend on whether the anemia is sudden in onset, as in severe hemorrhage, or gradual. In all cases, it is frequently manifested by pallor of the skin and mucous membranes, shortness of breath, palpitations of the heart, soft systolic murmurs in the heartbeat, lethargy and fatigability, and low blood pressure.

Iron-deficiency anemia is characterized by low serum iron concentration. There are two possible causes of this type of anemia. One is a condition in which the storage sites in macrophages are depleted of iron and cannot supply it to the plasma. The other possibility is a chronic disorder, in which the macrophage iron level is normal or increased but iron flow to the plasma appears to be partially blocked.

Both abnormalities are among the most common causes of anemia. Iron deficiency in macrophages predominates in children and young women, while chronic disorders are the most common cause of this type of anemia among elderly individuals.

Aplastic anemia is serious and usually lethal. It is caused by an inability of the bone marrow to function properly, a condition also known as bone marrow aplasia. Red blood cell numbers are greatly reduced, and the bone marrow does not regenerate them. Examples of patients with this type of anemia are persons exposed to gamma radiation, excessive X-ray treatments, certain industrial chemicals, and even drugs. Symptoms include paleness and a tendency to suffer hemorrhages under the skin and mucous membranes.

Megaloblastic anemia—also known as pernicious anemia, maturation failure anemia, or Addisonian anemia— occurs when red blood cells fail to mature. In pernicious anemia, there is atrophy of the stomach mucosa, or loss of the stomach lining. Patients with intestinal sprue, in which folic acid and other vitamin B compounds are poorly absorbed, also experience maturation failure. The bone marrow cannot proliferate rapidly enough to form normal numbers of red blood cells, and the cells that are formed are oversized and have bizarre shapes and fragile membranes. These cells rupture easily, leaving the patient in dire need of an adequate number of red blood cells. This is commonly a disease of

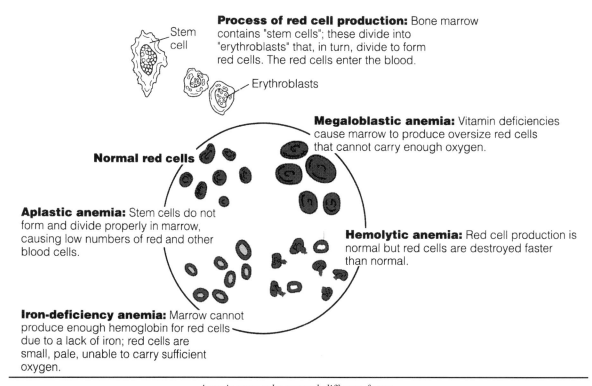

Anemia may take several different forms.

the middle aged, rarely occurring before the age of forty. It affects both men and women, and because its onset is insidious, it is usually well developed before medical help is sought. Patients have a lemon yellow complexion, and their tongue is sore and appears thinner and redder than normal. Other symptoms include soreness of and cracks in the skin at the corners of the mouth, slight enlargement of the spleen, and a complete absence of free hydrochloric acid in the stomach. One of the most serious complications of this anemia is a degenerative condition of the spinal cord (subacute combined degeneration) that can be cured by treating the anemia. The adult form of pernicious anemia is particularly common among individuals of Scandinavian, English, and Irish ancestry and is most common in late adult life.

Vitamin B_{12} is required for nuclear maturation and division. Since tissues that produce red blood cells are among the most rapidly growing and proliferating of all the body's tissues, lack of vitamin B_{12} especially inhibits the rate of red blood cell production. Therefore, it is said that deficiency of vitamin B_{12} causes maturation failure. In the mucus secreted by the stomach is a mucopolysaccharide or mucopolypeptide called intrinsic factor which combines with the vitamin B_{12} of the food and makes it available for absorption by the gut. The intrinsic factor binds tightly with the vitamin, and in this bound state the vitamin is protected from digestion by the gastrointestinal enzymes. Still in the bound state, the B_{12} and intrinsic factor attach to the membranes of the small intestine. The combination is then transported into the cells and, about four hours later, free vitamin B_{12} is released into the blood. Lack of intrinsic factor causes loss of much of the vitamin and also results in failure of absorption. Therefore, either a lack of the intrinsic factor in gastric secretions or a lack of the vitamin will produce this type of anemia. Once the vitamin has been absorbed from the gastrointestinal tract, it is stored in large quantities in the liver and then released slowly as needed. Consequently, there is normally a long period of defective B_{12} absorption before anemia results.

Hemolytic anemia results from hemolysis, the excessive destruction of red blood cells. Different abnormalities of the red blood cells, most of which are hereditary, make the cells very fragile so that they rupture easily as they go through the capillaries, especially through the spleen. Therefore, even when the number of red blood cells produced is normal, the cell life span is so short that serious anemia results. Acquired hemolytic anemia can also result from transfusion reactions, malaria, reactions to certain drugs such as penicillin, sulfonamides, and burns or as an autoimmune process. Some of these types of anemia are hereditary spherocytosis, sickle-cell anemia, thalassemia, and erythroblastosis fetalis.

In hereditary spherocytosis, the red cells are very small in size and spherical in shape rather than biconcave disks. They cannot be compressed because they do not have the normal loose, baglike cell membrane structure of the disks. Therefore, they are easily ruptured by even slight compression when they pass through capillaries.

With sickle-cell anemia, the red cells contain an abnormal type of hemoglobin called hemoglobin S, caused by abnormal composition of the globin portion of the hemoglobin. When this type of hemoglobin is exposed to small amounts of oxygen, it precipitates into long crystals inside the red blood cell. The crystals elongate the cell and give it the appearance of a sickle instead of a biconcave disk. The precipitated hemoglobin also damages the cell membranes so that the cells are highly fragile, leading to anemia. Patients sometimes enter a cycle in which low oxygen tension in tissues causes sickling, impeding the blood flow through the tissue and causing a further decrease in oxygen tension. Once this process starts, it progresses rapidly, leading to a serious decrease in red blood cell mass in a few hours. These episodes or crises are characterized by severe pain because of microvascular occlusions. The sickle-cell trait and disease occur mainly in persons of equatorial African descent.

Thalassemia is also called Cooley's anemia or Mediterranean anemia. In this type of hemolytic anemia, the red cells are small and have fragile membranes and are therefore easily ruptured. This type of anemia is common in people from Mediterranean regions and areas of Asia where malaria is prevalent. The disease is characterized by a reduction in the rate of synthesis of the beta chain of hemoglobin, and severely affected individuals do not survive childhood.

In erythroblastosis fetalis, Rh-positive red blood cells in the fetus are attacked by antibodies from an Rh-negative mother. The antibodies make the red cells fragile, and the child is born with serious anemia.

TREATMENT AND THERAPY

Fundamentally, anemia is attributable to loss of blood, excessive destruction of red blood cells, or impaired red cell production. The optimal treatment of anemia requires eradication of its cause or, if that is not possible, at least modification of the underlying disorder.

Anemia is usually insidious in its onset and in some cases has no specific symptoms to alert the physician to its presence. Unusual fatigue is the earliest and most common complaint, but other, more subtle changes such as loss of libido or alterations in mood or sleep patterns may be elicited. The level of anemia at which symptoms occur is highly variable among individuals. Since oxygen transport is much more compromised by impaired circulation than by diminished oxygen-carrying capacity per se, patients with vascular or cardiac disease may show stronger symptoms with milder degrees of anemia.

The first step in the treatment of the anemic patient is evaluation. First, the physician should make sure that the symptoms are not caused by other diseases. If the condition is proven to be anemia, it must be determined whether it is inherited or acquired. Evidence of blood loss is sought, such as pregnancy, ulcers, cancers, anomalous vessels, or parasites. Hemolytic anemias are considerably less common than the anemias of iron deficiency or chronic disease and may be more difficult to recognize, since inherited disorders show a wide spectrum of severity. Therefore, the practitioner would ask the patient about jaundice, dark urine, gallbladder disease, or other conditions. It should also be determined if there has been exposure to medication or toxins that can result in anemia; drug-induced anemias may be associated with marrow aplasia, maturational effects, and hemolysis by both direct or immune-mediated mechanisms. Lastly, the physician should determine if there is a systematic illness or nonhematologic organ dysfunction. The anemia of chronic disease is present in most patients with active inflammatory disease or advanced malignant disease. Chronic infections such as subacute bacterial endocarditis and active inflammatory processes such as rheumatoid arthritis and inflammatory bowel syndrome are almost always associated with it. Patients with diminished renal, hepatic, or endocrine function are often anemic. In each case, a significant degree of organ failure must be present to result in anemia, so these conditions are easily excluded by measuring renal, hepatic, thyroid, or pituitary function. Red blood cell production and destruction are intimately modulated by the immune system, so immune dysfunction is commonly complicated by anemia.

Therapy for anemia may be specific, as in the replacement of deficient iron, vitamin B_{12}, or folate; diagnostic, as in the therapeutic trial; or symptomatic, as in the administration of blood transfusions. Specific therapy requires a definitive diagnosis. The duration of treatment must be correlated with response and based on a thorough understanding of the requirements and body stores to avoid harm to patients. For megaloblastic anemia, administration of vitamin B_{12} by injection for the rest of the patient's life is the normal treatment. For microcytic or hypochromic anemia, treatment consists primarily of giving sufficient iron by mouth to restore and then maintain a normal blood picture. The main iron preparation is ferrous sulfate. Iron can also be given intravenously, but only when rapid results are needed. If there is hemorrhage, however, this process must be arrested, and if the loss of blood is severe, a blood transfusion may be necessary. In the case of aplastic anemia, the treatment consists primarily of regular blood transfusion. The disease is often fatal, but 25 percent of the patients recover when adequately treated and others survive several years. Promising results are reported with the use of bone marrow transplantation.

PERSPECTIVE AND PROSPECTS

The study of the blood has a long history, since it is likely that even primitive humans realized that loss of blood, if sufficiently great, is associated with death. The therapeutic use of iron was mentioned in Greek mythology in the story of Iphiclus, who was cured of impotence by drinking iron rust dissolved in wine. Iron was used to treat a variety of ailments in ancient Egypt and the Roman Empire, but the specific use of iron salts was not reported until the 1700's. In the 1830's, anemia, hypochromia, and lack of iron in the blood were detected.

Credit for reporting the first case of pernicious (megaloblastic) anemia is generally given to George Combe in 1822, while Thomas Addison is given credit for recognizing the condition as a clinical entity in 1855. As early as 1860, Austin Flint expressed the view that the anemia resulted from deficient gastric secretions and consequent inadequate assimilation of food. The relation of the gastric defect to the cause of pernicious anemia was demonstrated by William Castle and coworkers in 1929. In 1926, two Americans, G. R. Minot and W. P. Murphy, reported that pernicious anemia responded to treatment with liver. Vitamin B_{12} is needed for the formation of normal red blood cells. The efficient absorption of this vitamin into the body is dependent on the presence of the intrinsic factor that is produced normally by the mucous lining of the stomach. It is the inability of the patient to produce the intrinsic factor that leads to the onset of pernicious anemia. The use of whole liver by mouth led to the development of liver extracts of increasing potency that could be administered parenterally. The search for the active principle of liver extract culminated in the discovery of vitamin B_{12} in 1948.

In 1945, Linus Pauling correctly hypothesized that sickle-cell anemia is the result of the presence of a mutant hemoglobin. He and his coworkers demonstrated an ionic difference between normal human hemoglobin (HbA) and sickle-cell hemoglobin (HbS). In 1956, Vernon Ingram developed the technique of peptide mapping in order to pinpoint the difference between HbA and HbS—one peptide in the beta subunits. This discovery marked the first time that an inherited disease was shown to arise from a specific amino acid change in a protein. Some individuals are homozygous (cells have two copies of the gene for sickle-cell anemia) or heterozygous (one copy of the gene). Heterozygous individuals, who are said to have sickle-cell trait, can live normally even though their erythrocytes have a shortened life span.   —*Maria Pacheco, Ph.D.*

See also Blood and blood components; Blood testing; Hematology; Hematology, pediatric; Serology; Sickle-cell anemia; Thalassemia; Vitamins and minerals.

FOR FURTHER INFORMATION:

Guyton, Arthur C., and John E. Hall. *Textbook of Medical Physiology.* 9th ed. Philadelphia: W. B. Saunders, 1996. An in-depth presentation of various medical subjects. Several chapters deal with the different types of anemias, their diagnosis and treatment.

Landau, Sidney I., ed. *International Dictionary of Medicine and Biology.* Vol. 1. New York: John Wiley & Sons, 1986. Offers an accessible and concise presentation of various medical terms and subjects.

Leavell, Byrd S., and Oscar A. Thorup, Jr. *Fundamentals of Clinical Hematology.* 4th ed. Philadelphia: W. B. Saunders, 1976. A comprehensive presentation of the fundamentals of hematology. Relatively easy to read, although it uses a large number of medical terms. A good science background is recommended for those who use this reference.

Lee, G. Richard, et al. *Wintrobe's Clinical Hematology.* 9th ed. Vol. 1. Philadelphia: Lea & Febiger, 1993. An extensive treatise on blood and its diseases. Includes excellent, very detailed coverage of the different types of anemia, their discovery, symptoms, and treatment. A good background in chemistry and biology is recommended for use of this reference.

ANESTHESIA

PROCEDURE

ANATOMY OR SYSTEM AFFECTED: Brain, muscles, musculoskeletal system, nerves, nervous system, psychic-emotional system, skin, spine

SPECIALTIES AND RELATED FIELDS: Anesthesiology, critical care, dentistry, emergency medicine, general surgery, neurology, ophthalmology

DEFINITION: The administration of drugs to block the transmission of nerve impulses and thus to prevent pain, especially during surgery or childbirth; anesthesia may be general (causing total unconsciousness) or regional and local (deadening sensation and decreasing awareness, without causing loss of consciousness).

KEY TERMS:

epidural anesthesia: anesthesia produced by injecting a local anesthetic between the vertebral spines and beneath the ligamentum flavum into the extradural space; also known as extradural anesthesia

local anesthesia: anesthesia produced by injecting a local anesthetic solution directly into the tissues; also known as local block

local anesthetics: drugs that produce a reversible blockade of nerve impulse conduction

regional anesthesia: insensibility caused by the interruption of nerve conduction in a region of the body

spinal anesthesia: anesthesia produced by injecting a local anesthetic around the spinal cord; also known as subarachnoid block

INDICATIONS AND PROCEDURES

Anesthetics are given primarily to prevent the pain of surgery during operations. They also are given to reduce fear, relax tissues, and prevent a sympathetic nervous system response to surgery. Some believe, erroneously, that being "put to sleep" with a general anesthetic is the only way an operation can be performed pain-free.

General anesthesia is a type of anesthesia that produces total unconsciousness and affects the entire body. Regional anesthesia, another type of anesthesia, does not produce unconsciousness but allows surgery to be performed without pain by producing loss of sensation in a region of the body—by interrupting the transmission of nerve impulses from the area to be incised.

With general anesthesia, patients receive drugs that are delivered both intravenously and by inhalation. With regional anesthesia, the anesthetic agents are deposited either on the surface of the area to be anesthetized or near a particular nerve or pathway that lies between the area and receptors for painful stimuli that are part of the central nervous system. As a result, transmission of noxious stimuli to the brain is effectively "blocked," allowing a surgical procedure to be performed without the patient's feeling pain. Regional anesthesia is frequently referred to as regional nerve blockade.

Local anesthetics operate in several ways. Those injected near the nerves diffuse into the nerves and bind to receptors on their membranes. Once in the nerve sheath, local anesthetic agents prevent sodium from moving into the nerve interior by physically occluding sodium channels. Impulses traveling from the surgical area to the central nervous system are blocked such that nerves transmitting touch, temperature, and pain sensation are temporarily interrupted. Nerve impulses traveling from the central nervous system to the surgical area are also blocked, leading to an interruption of motor power to the surgical area.

The number of nerves blocked depends on where the local anesthetic is deposited—that is, on the type of regional anesthetic technique utilized. The duration of the nerve blockade depends on the type and dosage of local anesthetic injected as well as on the technique utilized. Diffusion of the local anesthetic out of the nerve and its absorption into the vascular bed causes the effect of the local anesthetic to be terminated. The blood flowing around the nerve removes the drug from the area. Decreasing the flow of blood to the area by adding vasoconstricting agents, such as epinephrine, to the local anesthetic to be injected is a method commonly utilized to prolong the duration of the nerve block.

Local anesthetics are weak bases whose structure consists of an aromatic moiety connected to a substituted amine through an ester or amide linkage. The two major families of local anesthetics are the amino amides and the amino esters. The clinical differences between the ester and amide local anesthetics involve their potential for producing adverse side effects and the mechanisms by which they are metabolized.

Local anesthetics are also classified on the basis of their potency and duration of action: a short duration of action (thirty to forty-five minutes), an intermediate duration of action (one to two hours), or a long duration of action (four to eight hours). The range in duration of nerve blockade is attributable primarily to two factors: the concentration of the drug used and the addition of vasoconstricting agents, such as epinephrine.

Local and regional anesthesia are excellent ways of supplying surgical anesthesia and postoperative analgesia (pain control). Local anesthetics are now being given in combination with narcotic analgesics (painkillers). Narcotics injected in combination with local anesthetics work through a different mechanism of action; they bind to narcotic receptors in the area and provide analgesia without interrupting nerve transmission. The combination of local anesthetic agents with narcotics is gaining popularity in postoperative and labor pain control; longer durations of pain relief can be obtained while avoiding the systemic side effects of intravenously administered narcotics.

There are six categories of regional anesthesia: topical anesthesia, local block and field block, nerve block, intravenous (IV) neural blockade, subarachnoid block (spinal anesthesia), and epidural anesthesia, including caudal block. The major differences are the size of the region that is anesthetized and the duration of the neural blockade.

Topical anesthesia. In this technique, also known as surface anesthesia, an anesthetic drug is sprayed or dropped onto an area to be desensitized. This short-acting form of anesthesia blocks nerve endings in the skin as well as mucous membranes, such as those of the nasopharynx (nose and throat), mouth, rectum, and vagina. Topical anesthesia is employed in minor procedures such as eye or rectal examinations. The advantages of topical anesthesia include quick onset of action, ease of administration, and general nontoxicity. Disadvantages include lack of deeper-tissue anesthesia and lack of tissue relaxation. A frequently used topical anesthetic is the drug benzocaine, often utilized for traumatic tissue pain secondary to sunburn.

Local blocks and field blocks. In local blocks, the local anesthetic is injected with a needle and syringe into the skin and tissues of an area to be incised. As a result, the nerves in the area of the incision are blocked. Local blocks are used in short minor operations and prior to the insertion of intravenous or spinal needles. A field block is another type of local block. In a field block, the area surrounding the incision is also injected with local anesthetics, preventing impulses transmitted from a larger area from reaching the central nervous system.

Nerve blocks. Nerve blocks interrupt the transmission of nerve impulses by nerves or by bundles of nerves that are further removed from the surgical site. Nerve blocks may be used to anesthetize a single finger or toe (digital nerve block), a foot (ankle block) or hand, or an entire arm (axillary, supraclavicular, and interscalene blocks) or leg (leg block). In each type of neural blockade, the physician or nurse anesthetist injects local anesthetic agents around the major nerves that supply the area to be incised. The number of injections depends on the location of the nerves to be blocked. For example, in performing a leg block, four nerves—the femoral, sciatic, lateral femoral cutaneous, and obturator nerves—because of their separate locations, may be blocked individually. An arm block can be accomplished by a single injection of a larger volume of local anesthetic into the axillary sheath or between the middle and anterior scalene muscles in the neck. Upper extremity blocks can be performed with a single injection because the brachial plexus (the nerves innervating the arm) is collectively encased in a sheath. Distal to the axillary area, the nerves innervating the arm are no longer encased in a sheath. Consequently, separate injections of the radial, median, and ulnar nerves are required to block the arm at the elbow or wrist.

Intercostal nerve blocks. Intercostal nerves innervate the outer and inner surfaces of the abdominal wall. Intercostal nerve blockade is utilized for postoperative pain control following thoracic or upper abdominal surgeries. A sterile needle is inserted into the skin over the lower margin of the rib along the posterior axillary line. The needle is then directed toward the intercostal groove located inferior to the rib. A local anesthetic is injected into the intercostal space containing the intercostal nerve, vein, and artery. The anesthetic lasts from six to twelve hours and may be prolonged by the addition of epinephrine to the solution.

Intravenous neural blockade. Intravenous (IV) neural blockade was discovered by August Bier in 1908; he was also the first to utilize spinal anesthesia routinely. Today, IV regional neural blockade is also referred to as Beir blockade. With Beir blockade, the local anesthetic agent is injected into a vein, lying distal to a tourniquet, in an upper or lower extremity (instead of around a nerve). Inflation of the tourniquet prevents the local anesthetic from being released into the general circulation. The local anesthetic, thus contained in the extremity, travels to the major nerves in the limb and blocks neural transmission. The duration of the neural blockade is governed by the length of time that the tourniquet is inflated. Once the tourniquet is deflated, the local anesthetic enters the systemic circulation, the neural blockade recedes, and normal sensation and power to the extremity are rapidly returned. Intravenous regional blockade of the extremities has many advantages: ease of performance, rapid onset, controllable duration of action, and rapid recovery. The disadvantages include possible tourniquet discomfort, possible reaction to the local anesthetic when it is released into the general circulation, and rapid return of sensation, including pain.

Spinal anesthesia. Spinal anesthesia, also called subarachnoid block, is a commonly utilized form of anesthesia. Spinal anesthesia can be used for almost any type of surgical procedure below the umbilicus, such as surgical procedures performed on the legs and hips, hysterectomies, appendectomies, and cesarean sections.

A lumbar puncture (spinal tap) is performed in the lower

back, usually between the second and third lumbar verte-brae, the third and fourth lumbar vertebrae, or the fifth lumbar and first sacral vertebrae. The patient is placed on his or her side in a flexed position (or sometimes in a sitting position). The physician or nurse anesthetist, wearing sterile gloves, prepares the skin in the area to be punctured with a skin antiseptic, such as betadine, and then drapes the area with a sterile towel. The anesthetist then infiltrates the area of the puncture with lidocaine, producing a local block. Once the skin is anesthetized, the lumbar puncture is performed; a needle is inserted through the intraspinous space into the subarachnoid space. The needle passes through the supraspinous ligament, intraspinous ligament, and ligamentum flavum. Proper placement of the needle is identified through an observation of freely flowing spinal fluid. A local anesthetic agent is then injected into the spinal fluid. Cerebrospinal fluid (CSF) is a clear, colorless ultrafiltrate of the blood that fills the subarachnoid space. The total volume of CSF is 100 to 150 milliliters; the volume contained in the subarachnoid space is 25 to 35 milliliters.

Once injected into the subarachnoid CSF, the local anesthetic agent spreads in both a cephalad (toward the head and anterior) and a caudad (toward the feet and posterior) direction. Factors influencing this spread include the dose and volume of the agent used, patient position, and the specific gravity (weight) of the anesthetic solution relative to the CSF. One of three types of solutions—isobaric, hypobaric, or hyperbaric—can be used. Hyperbaric solutions are heavier than CSF; thus placing the patient in Trendelenburg's position (with the head tilted downward) will increase the cephalad spread of the anesthetic. With the patient in Trendelenburg's position, hypobaric solutions (with a specific gravity less than that of CSF) of local anesthetic agents spread caudally. Spread of the local anesthetic in the subarachnoid space usually stops (fixation) within five to thirty-five minutes after injection. After fixation has occurred, patient position changes will not influence the spread of local anesthetic or the subsequent level of anesthesia.

Within minutes after a subarachnoid injection of a local anesthetic, patients experience a warm sensation in their lower extremities, followed by a loss of sensation and inability to move the legs. The duration of the neural blockade is dependent on the type of local anesthetic utilized, as well as the addition of any vasoconstrictor.

Epidural anesthesia and caudal block. Like spinal anesthesia, epidural blockade can be used for the prevention of pain during surgery. It can also be used to relieve pain after surgery, chronic pain, and the pain in labor; to supplement a light general anesthetic; and to diagnose and treat autonomic nervous system dysfunction. The technique is excellent for the operations performed on the lower abdomen, pelvis, and perineum; for laminectomies; and in obstetrics for the relief of labor pains and the facilitation of delivery.

As with spinal anesthesia, the patient is placed on his or her side in a flexed position (or sometimes in a sitting position). The physician or nurse anesthetist, wearing sterile gloves, prepares the skin in the area of the puncture with an antiseptic such as betadine and drapes the area with a sterile towel. The anesthetist infiltrates the area of the puncture with lidocaine, producing a local block. Once the skin is anesthetized, an epidural needle is inserted between the appropriate lumbar vertebrae (occasionally between thoracic vertebrae). With epidural blockade, however, the needle is not advanced into the subarachnoid space; needle advancement is terminated when the needle tip is in the epidural space. Thus, the dura is not penetrated as in spinal anesthesia. (As a result, postdural puncture headache does not occur with a properly placed epidural needle.) Once the epidural space has been identified, local anesthetic agents (in larger volumes than utilized with subarachnoid anesthesia) are injected through the needle or through a small catheter threaded through the needle. Placement of a catheter through the needle allows reinjection to take place without subsequent needle punctures; this is particularly desirable for long surgeries, postoperative pain control, and the control of labor pains. Local anesthetic agents injected through a catheter for postoperative or labor pain control are usually given at lesser concentrations so that nerve motor fibers are not interrupted.

Caudal block is another type of epidural anesthesia. In this case, the needle (with or without a catheter) is placed through the sacrococcygeal ligament just superior to the coccyx. The technique is gaining popularity as an adjunct to general anesthesia in children, for the purpose of postoperative pain control.

USES AND COMPLICATIONS

Regional anesthesia has several advantages over general anesthesia. The first is ease of administration: The agents used are injectable, the equipment required is minimal, and the costs are reasonable. Second is relative safety: A localized area of the body can be operated upon while avoiding most of the undesirable and potentially harmful side effects of general anesthesia, such as loss of consciousness and the depression of the cardiovascular and respiratory systems. In addition, advantages include excellent muscle relaxation, which is often required in order to facilitate surgical procedures; improved peripheral blood flow; an antithrombitic effect; a decreased loss of blood in some cases; and postoperative pain relief, a benefit most patients find highly desirable. Regional anesthesia is also utilized in combination with general anesthesia in an effort to increase the benefits of both while decreasing the adverse side effects of each.

Yet regional anesthesia has some disadvantages. First, some operations cannot be performed under regional anesthesia (for example, major surgical procedures involving the brain, heart, and lungs). Second, some patients may be allergic to the local anesthetics. Local anesthetics of the amino ester type may result in allergic reactions because of the metabolite p-aminobenzoic acid. Local anesthetics of the amino amide class are essentially devoid of allergic potential. Many anesthetic solutions, however, contain methylparaben as a preservative, and this compound can produce an allergic reaction in persons sensitive to p-aminobenzoic acid. Third, some patients desire to be unaware of the operation and may be anxious at the thought of being "awake." They erroneously believe that the total unconsciousness produced by general anesthesia is the only method to produce unawareness. In the majority of cases, patients who receive a regional anesthetic also receive intravenous sedation to decrease their level of awareness. Subsequently, many patients report having no recollection whatsoever of the surgical procedure.

In addition, the advantages of spinal anesthesia, one of the most popular types of regional anesthesia, far outweigh the disadvantages, which include hypotension, a high level of anesthesia, and postdural puncture headache. Hypotension is treated with intravenous fluids and, if necessary, the administration of vasoconstricting drugs. Postdural puncture headache (spinal headache) is thought to be caused from a loss of spinal fluid (which cushions the brain) through the dural hole produced by the spinal needle. Recent advances in the technique of spinal anesthesia administration, including the use of very small needles introduced in a manner that separates the dural fibers, have significantly decreased the incidence of postdural puncture headache. Should this complication arise, however, it is treated with analgesics, intravenous fluids, and, if necessary, an injection of saline (or a sample of the patient's own blood) around the site of the dural puncture, effectively "patching" the dural hole created by the spinal needle.

The first successful demonstration of anesthesia (diethyl ether) by William T. G. Morton occurred in 1846 at the Massachusetts General Hospital. The discovery of anesthesia occurred prior to the discovery of germ theory and aseptic techniques: Although anesthesia made surgery painless in the early nineteenth century, there was still a high rate of surgical morbidity and mortality as a result of infection. In the late 1860's, germ theory had evolved from the work of Robert Koch and Louis Pasteur, and Joseph Lister's subsequent work on principles of asepsis contributed significantly to a decline in surgical mortality from infection by the late 1880's. There remained, however, a high surgical mortality rate caused by anesthesia. At that time, general anesthetic agents were commonly utilized, and few, if any, practitioners specialized in the administration of anesthesia.

Regional anesthesia was first utilized in 1884 when a German physician named Carl Koller performed an operation to correct glaucoma using a local anesthetic. In this case, cocaine, an alkaloid obtained from the coca plant, was instilled into the eye. This successful operation brought significant acceptance to the principle of local anesthesia. The great advantage of local anesthesia was that it anesthetized only the part of the body on which the operation was to be performed: Patients could be spared the depressive effects of general anesthesia, especially those on the cardiovascular and respiratory systems.

By the 1930's, various regional anesthesia techniques had been developed, including subarachnoid block (spinal anesthesia), lumbar epidural, caudal epidural, intravenous, and brachial plexus anesthesia. The occurrence of these regional anesthetic techniques, along with the evolution of local anesthetic agents, allowed anesthetists to tailor the type and duration of regional anesthesia to the requirements of each patient. As a result, regional anesthesia has become a popular choice among surgeons, anesthetists, and patients.

—Maura S. McAuliffe

See also Acupuncture; Anesthesiology; Catheterization; Hypnosis; Lumbar puncture; Narcotics; Nervous system; Neurology; Neurology, pediatric; Pain, types of; Pain management; Pharmacology; Surgery, general; Surgical procedures.

FOR FURTHER INFORMATION:

Cousins, Michael J., and P. O. Bridenbaugh, eds. *Neural Blockade in Clinical Anesthesia and Management of Pain.* 2d ed. Philadelphia: J. B. Lippincott, 1988. This bible of regional anesthesia principles and techniques contains chapters written by experts in the field. Offers historical information about the subject, as well as reports of contemporary research pertaining to all types of regional anesthesia.

Katz, Jordan. *Atlas of Regional Anesthesia.* 2d ed. Norwalk, Conn.: Appleton and Lange, 1994. An atlas of nerve block techniques explained in a simple and straightforward manner. The exquisite drawings and meticulous details of the illustrations make this an exceptional text.

Lee, J. A., R. S. Atkinson, and M. J. Watt. *Sir Robert Macintosh's Lumbar Puncture and Spinal Analgesia: Intradural and Extradural.* 5th ed. New York: Churchill Livingstone, 1985. A classic text on spinal and epidural anesthesia, updated periodically to reflect advances in the field. Contains chapters devoted to the anatomy, physiology, pharmacology, techniques, and management of, and the complications associated with, spinal and epidural anesthesia.

Stoelting, R. K. *Pharmacology and Physiology in Anesthetic Practice.* Philadelphia: J. B. Lippincott, 1987. Chapter 6, "Local Anesthetics," provides a comprehensive discussion of local anesthetics, including structure and activity relationships, mechanisms and durations of action, absorption, elimination, clearance, and side effects. Tables and graphs make comparisons among the various drugs used for regional anesthesia easy to understand.

Winnie, A. P. *Plexus Anesthesia: Perivascular Techniques of Brachial Plexus Block.* Philadelphia: W. B. Saunders,

1983. This book, written by the leading expert in regional anesthesia for the upper extremities, is the best of its kind. A well-organized, comprehensive text that also contains a wealth of practical information related to normal anatomy and regional anesthetic techniques for upper extremities. Contains excellent illustrations.

ANESTHESIOLOGY

SPECIALTY

ANATOMY OR SYSTEM AFFECTED: Brain, muscles, musculoskeletal system, nerves, nervous system, psychic-emotional system, skin, spine

SPECIALTIES AND RELATED FIELDS: Anesthesiology, critical care, dentistry, emergency medicine, general surgery, neurology, ophthalmology

DEFINITION: The science of administering anesthesia during a surgical procedure.

KEY TERMS:

anesthesia: a new word coined in the 1840's, derived from a Greek word meaning "not feeling"

electric anesthesia: the use of pulses of electricity to deaden nerve cells or cause unconsciousness

endotracheal tube: a flexible tube inserted through the mouth or nose into the trachea (windpipe) to carry anesthetic gas and oxygen directly to the lungs

ether: a volatile liquid that causes unconsciousness when inhaled; first demonstrated during surgery in 1846

nitrous oxide: called "laughing gas" because people appeared to become intoxicated from inhaling it; first used in 1844 to pull a tooth painlessly

novocaine: a local anesthetic, commonly used in dentistry, whose chemical structure is similar to that of cocaine

sodium pentothal: a fast-acting anesthetic that is injected into the vein; first developed for military hospitals during World War II

spinal anesthesia: the injection of an anesthetic at the base of the spine to produce loss of feeling in the lower part of the body and legs

THE HISTORY OF ANESTHESIOLOGY

In a modern hospital, the surgical operating room normally is a very quiet place. The anesthesiologist, surgeon, assisting doctors, and nurses perform their duties with little conversation while the patient sleeps. Family members sit quietly in a nearby waiting room until the operation is over. Before the advent of anesthesiology in the 1840's, however, surgery had been a thoroughly gruesome experience. Patients might drink some whiskey to numb their senses, and several strong men were recruited to hold them down. Surgeons cut the flesh with a sharp knife and sawed quickly through the bone while patients screamed in agony. The operating room in the hospital was located as far as possible from other patients awaiting surgery so that they would not hear the cries so plainly.

Many kinds of operations were performed before anes-

thetics were discovered. Among these were the removal of tumors, the opening of abscesses, amputations, the treatment of head wounds, the removal of kidney stones, and cesarean sections and other surgeries during childbirth. The frightful ordeal of "going under the knife," however, often caused patients to delay surgery until it was almost too late. Also, for the surgeon it was nerve-racking to work without anesthetics, trying to operate while the patient screamed and struggled.

Sir Humphry Davy (1778-1829) was a distinguished British chemist who studied the intoxicating effect of a gas called nitrous oxide. While suffering from the pain of an erupting wisdom tooth, he sought relief by inhaling some of the gas. In 1800, he published a paper suggesting the use of nitrous oxide to relieve pain during surgery. There was no follow-up on his idea, however, and it was forgotten until after anesthesia had been discovered independently in America.

The next episode in the history of anesthesiology was the work of Crawford W. Long (1815-1878), a small-town doctor in Georgia. In the early 1800's, "ether frolics" had become popular, in which young people at a party would inhale ether vapor to give them a "high" such as from drinking alcohol. One young man was to have surgery on his neck for a tumor. Long was the town druggist as well as the doctor, so he knew that this fellow had purchased ether and enjoyed its effects. Long suggested that he inhale some ether to ready himself for surgery. On March 30, 1842, the tumor was removed with little pain for the patient. It was the first successful surgery under anesthesia.

Unfortunately, Long did not recognize the great significance of what he had done. He did not report the etherization experiment to his colleagues, and it remained relatively unknown. He used ether a few more times in his own surgical practice, one time while amputating the toe of a young slave. Long finally wrote an article for a medical journal in 1849 telling about his pioneering work, three years after anesthesia had been publicly demonstrated and widely adopted by others.

The story of anesthesiology then moved to Hartford, Connecticut, where a young dentist named Horace Wells (1815-1848) played a major role. P. T. Barnum, of show business and circus fame, was advertising an entertaining "GRAND EXHIBITION of the effects produced by inhaling NITROUS OXIDE or LAUGHING GAS!" Wells decided to attend. He was one of the volunteers from the audience and "made a spectacle of himself," according to his wife.

Another volunteer who had inhaled the gas began to shout and stagger around; finally he ran into a bench, banging his shins against it. The audience laughed, but the observant Wells noticed that the man showed no pain, even though his leg was bleeding. This demonstration gave Wells a sudden insight that a person might have a tooth pulled or even a leg amputated and feel no pain while under the influence of the gas.

Wells became so excited by the idea of eliminating pain that he arranged to have some nitrous oxide gas brought to his office on the next day. Then he had a long talk with a young dentist colleague, John Riggs, about the potential risks of trying it out on a patient. Finally, Wells decided to make himself the first test case, if Riggs would be willing to extract one of his wisdom teeth.

On the morning of December 11, 1844, a bag of nitrous oxide gas was delivered by the man who had been in charge of the previous evening's exhibition. Wells sat in the dental chair and breathed deeply from the gas bag until he seemed to be asleep. Riggs went to work with his long-handled forceps to loosen and finally pull out the tooth, with no outcry from the patient. After a short time, Wells regained consciousness, spit out some blood, and said that he had felt "no more pain than the prick of a pin."

After this success, Wells immediately set to work on further experiments. He acquired the apparatus and chemicals to make his own nitrous oxide. Within the next month, he used the gas on more than a dozen patients. Other dentists in Hartford heard about the procedure and started using it. By the middle of January, 1845, Wells was confident enough to propose a demonstration to a wider audience.

Wells was able to arrange for a demonstration at Massachusetts General Hospital in Boston. While the audience watched, he anesthetized a volunteer patient with gas and extracted his tooth. Unfortunately, the patient groaned at that moment, causing laughter and scornful comments from the onlookers. Wells was viewed as another quack making grandiose claims without evidence. His demonstration had failed, and he returned to Hartford in discouragement. He later commented that he had probably removed the gas bag too soon, before the patient was fully asleep.

It was another dentist, William T. G. Morton (1819-1868), who finally provided a convincing demonstration of anesthesia. Morton tried to obtain some nitrous oxide from a druggist, who did not have any on hand and suggested that ether fumes could be substituted. Morton then used ether on several dental patients, with excellent results. In 1846, he obtained permission for a demonstration at the same hospital where Wells had failed two years earlier. Famous Boston surgeon John Warren and a skeptical audience watched as Morton instructed a patient to breathe the ether. When the patient was fully asleep, Warren removed a tumor from his neck. To everyone's amazement, there was no outcry of pain during the surgery. After the patient awoke, he said that he felt only a slight scratch on his neck. Warren's words have been recorded for posterity: "Gentlemen, this is no humbug!" Another doctor said, "What we have seen here today will go around the world."

The result of this dramatic demonstration of October 16, 1846, spread quickly to other hospitals in America and Europe. Several hundred surgeries under anesthesia were done in the next year. In England, John Snow experimented with a different anesthetic, chloroform, and began to use it for women in childbirth. In 1853, Queen Victoria took chloroform from Snow during the delivery of her eighth child. Acceptance of anesthesia, and the science of anesthesiology, by the medical profession and the general public grew rapidly.

SCIENCE AND PROFESSION

Nitrous oxide, ether, and chloroform were the big three anesthetics for general surgery and dentistry for nearly a hundred years after their discovery. All three were administered by inhalation, but there were differences in safety, reliability, and side effects for the patient.

Wells, the dentist who had unsuccessfully tried to demonstrate nitrous oxide anesthesia in 1844, came to a tragic end in 1848 because of chloroform. He was testing the gas on himself to find out what an appropriate dosage should be. Unfortunately, he became addicted to the feeling of intoxication that it gave him. While under the influence of a chloroform binge, he accosted a woman on the street and was arrested. He committed suicide while in prison.

Nitrous oxide is a nearly odorless gas that must be mixed with oxygen to prevent asphyxiation. Storing the gases in large, leakproof bags was awkward. By comparison, ether and chloroform were much more convenient to use because they are liquids that can be stored in small bottles. The liquid was dripped onto a cloth and held over the patient's nose. Ether is hazardous, however, because it is flammable, and it also has a disagreeable odor. Chloroform is not flammable but is more difficult to administer because of the danger of heart stoppage.

Anesthesiology was practiced primarily by dentists, eye doctors, chemists, and all types of surgeons for many years. The Mayo Clinic in Rochester, Minnesota, was one of the first hospitals to recognize the need for specialists to administer anesthesia. In 1904, a nurse from Mayo named Miss Magaw gave a talk on what she had learned from eleven thousand procedures performed under anesthesia. Her concluding comment was that "ether kills slowly, giving plenty of warning, but with chloroform there is not even time to say good-by." Ether takes more time to induce anesthesia, but Miss Magaw asserted that the patient's life was in less danger than from chloroform.

A Scottish physician, James Y. Simpson, was one of the early advocates of using chloroform for partial anesthesia during childbirth. The woman could breathe the vapor intermittently for several hours as needed without the disagreeable odor of ether. She would remain conscious, but the anesthetic apparently produced a kind of amnesia so that the pain was not fully remembered. Simpson received much public acclaim for his help to women in labor, including a title of nobility. (One humorist of the day suggested a coat-of-arms for Sir Simpson, showing a newborn baby with the inscription, "Does your mother know you're out?")

In the 1920's, several new anesthetic gases were created by chemists working closely with medical doctors. The advantages and drawbacks of each new synthesized compound were tested first on animals, then on human volunteers, and finally during surgery. One of the most successful ones was cyclopropane: It was quick-acting and nontoxic and could be mixed with oxygen for prolonged operations. Like other organic gases, however, it was explosive under certain conditions and had to be used with appropriate caution.

A major development in 1928 was the invention of the endotracheal tube by Arthur Guedel. A rubber tube was inserted into the mouth and down the trachea (windpipe) to carry the anesthetic gas and oxygen mixture directly to the lungs. The space around the rubber tube had to be sealed in some way in order to prevent blood or other fluid from going down the windpipe. Guedel's ingenious idea was to surround the tube with a small balloon. When inflated, it effectively closed off the gap between the tube and the trachea wall. He gave a memorable demonstration at a medical meeting using an anesthetized dog with a breathing tube in its throat. After inflating the seal, the dog was submerged under water for several hours and then revived, showing that no water had entered its lungs.

The first local anesthetic was discovered in 1884 by Carl Koller, a young eye doctor in Vienna. He was a colleague of the famous psychoanalyst Sigmund Freud, and together they had investigated the psychic effects of cocaine. Koller noticed that his tongue became numb from the drug. He had the sudden insight that a drop of cocaine solution might be usable as an anesthetic for eye surgery. He tried it on a frog's eye, with much success. Following the tradition of other medical pioneers, he then tried it on himself. The cocaine made his eye numb. Koller published a short article, and the news spread quickly. Within three months, other doctors reported successful local anesthesia, using cocaine for dentistry, obstetrics, and many kinds of general surgery.

Chemists investigated the molecular structure of cocaine and were able to develop synthetic substitutes such as novocaine, which was faster-acting and

less toxic. Another improvement was to inject local anesthetic under the skin with a hypodermic needle. With this technique, it was possible to block off pain from a whole region of the body by deadening the nerve fibers. A spinal or epidural block is often used to relieve the pain of childbirth or for various abdominal surgeries.

There is another class of anesthetic drugs called barbiturates which were originally developed for sleeping pills. Any medication that induces sleep automatically becomes a candidate for use as an anesthetic. The most successful barbiturate anesthetic has been sodium pentothal. It is normally administered by injection into a vein in the arm and puts the patient to sleep in a matter of seconds. When the surgery is over, the needle is withdrawn and consciousness returns, with few aftereffects for most people. The anesthesiologist may use sodium pentothal in combination with an inhaled anesthetic if the surgery is expected to be lengthy.

DIAGNOSTIC AND TREATMENT TECHNIQUES

Suppose that a man is scheduled to have some kind of abdominal surgery, such as the repair of a hernia or hemorrhoids or the removal of the appendix, an intestinal blockage, or a cancerous growth. The anesthesiologist would select a sequence of anesthetics that depends primarily on the expected length of the operation and the physical condition of the patient.

About an hour before surgery, the patient receives a shot of morphine to produce relaxation and drowsiness. After

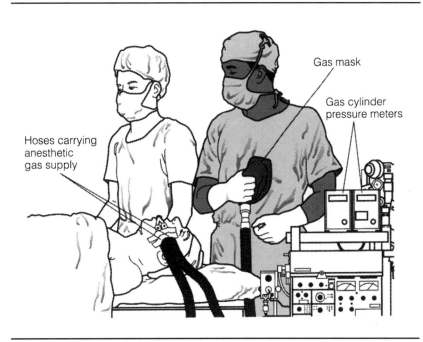

The anesthesiologist, as a crucial team member in every major surgery, must constantly monitor the vital signs and level of consciousness of the anesthetized patient.

he is wheeled into the operating room, the anesthesiologist inserts a needle into a vein in the patient's arm and injects a barbiturate such as sodium pentothal. This drug puts him to sleep very quickly because it is rapidly distributed through the body, but it is not suitable for maintaining anesthesia.

A muscle-paralyzing agent such as curare is now injected, which allows the anesthesiologist to insert an endotracheal tube into the lungs. The tube delivers a mixture of nitrous oxide and oxygen, supplemented with a small amount of other organic additives or of a more potent gas such as ether. The seal around the tube must be inflated to prevent fluids from entering the windpipe. The patient is now in a state of surgical anesthesia.

For a difficult surgery, additional curare may be injected to paralyze the abdominal muscles completely. In this case, the breathing muscles would also become paralyzed, which means that a mechanical respirator would be needed to inflate and deflate the lungs.

The anesthesiologist monitors the patient's condition with various instruments, such as a stethoscope, blood pressure and temperature sensors, and an electrocardiograph (EKG or ECG) with a continuous display. A catheter may be inserted into a vein to inject drugs or to give a blood transfusion if necessary. When the surgery is completed, the anesthesiologist is responsible for overseeing procedures undertaken in the recovery room as the patient slowly regains consciousness.

Perspective and Prospects

Many modern surgeries would be impossible without anesthesia. Kidney or other organ transplants, skin grafts for a burn victim or microsurgery for a severed finger all require that the patient remain still for an extended period of time. Anesthesiologists choose from a variety of local and general anesthetics as the individual situations require.

In the emergency room of a hospital, patients are brought in with injuries from industrial, farm, or car accidents. Gunshot and knife wounds, the ingestion of toxic chemicals, or sports injuries often require immediate action to reduce pain and preserve life. Soldiers who are wounded or burned in battle can be given relief from pain because of the available anesthetics. Beyond operating room patients, another category of people who benefit greatly from anesthesia are those who suffer from chronic pain, including arthritis, back pain, asthma, brain damage, cancer, and other serious ailments.

A more recent innovation is electric anesthesia, which employs an electric current. It is widely used for animals and is gaining acceptance for humans. A marine biologist can submerge two electrodes into water and cause nearby fish to become rigid and unable to swim. After being netted and tagged, the fish are released with no harmful aftereffects. Veterinarians can use a commercially available device with two electrodes that attach to the nose and tail of a farm animal. Pulses of electricity are applied, causing the

animal to remain immobilized until surgery is completed.

The most common human application of electric anesthesia is in dentistry. The metal drill itself can act as an electrode, sending pulses of electric current into the nerve to deaden the sensation of pain. The discomfort of novocaine injections and the possible aftereffects of the drug are avoided. Another application is to provide relief for people with chronic back pain, using a small, battery-powered unit attached to the person's waist.

Experiments have been done using electricity for total anesthesia, both on animals and on human volunteers. Electrodes are strapped to the front and back of the head. When an appropriate voltage is applied, the subject falls into deep sleep in a short time. When the electricity is turned off, consciousness is regained almost immediately. In one experiment, two dogs underwent "electrosleep" for thirty days with no apparent ill effects. Long-term studies with more subjects are needed to establish this new technology.

People who have misgivings about becoming a subject for electric anesthesia today perhaps can appreciate the feelings of anxiety that the early volunteers for inhalation anesthesia experienced in the 1840's. Moreover, the contribution of anesthesiology to modern medicine, in all of its forms, has been spectacular when one recalls the suffering of preanesthesia patients.   —*Hans G. Graetzer, Ph.D.*

See also Acupuncture; Anesthesia; Hypnosis; Narcotics; Neurology; Neurology, pediatric; Nursing; Pain management; Pharmacology; Physician assistants; Surgery, general; Surgical procedures.

For Further Information:

Goldman, Brian. "Electric Anesthesia," *Omni* 6 (July, 1984): 22. Describes the electric anesthesia device developed by Aime Limoge, a professor of physiology in Paris. By the mid-1980's, more than two hundred of his machines had been sold for human use, mostly at European hospitals. In electric anesthesia, small currents through the brain, produced by electrodes on the head, cause unconsciousness.

Gross, Amy, and Dee Ito. "All About Anesthesia: What Are the Choices When It Comes to Childbirth and Surgery?" *Parents Magazine* 65 (April, 1990): 213-221. A question-and-answer format is used to clarify the differences between spinal, epidural, and general anesthesia during childbirth. Several questions deal with potential recovery problems for mother and baby, especially when emergency cesarean surgery is necessary.

Kreig, Margaret B. *Green Medicine: The Search for Plants That Heal*. Chicago: Rand McNally, 1964. Drugs such as quinine and digitalis were successful folk medicines long before being adopted by the medical profession. One chapter in this book tells the story of curare, which was used as a poison by South American tribes to hunt game with a blowgun. Its applications in modern surgery for muscle relaxation are described.

Modell, Walter, and Alfred Lansing. *Drugs*. New York: LIFE Science Library, Time-Life Books, 1967. One chapter deals with anesthetic drugs, including a sixteen-page photographic essay on the vanquishing of pain. Contains informative, clear explanations. Highly recommended.

Postotnik, Pauline. "Anesthesia: A Long Way from Biting Bullets." *FDA Consumer*, June, 1984, p. 24-27. A brief history of the development of anesthesia. Provides a good overview of sedatives, barbiturates, narcotics, muscle relaxants, and gaseous anesthetics. The monitoring equipment used during surgery is also described.

Raper, Howard Riley. *Man Against Pain: The Epic of Anesthesia*. New York: Prentice Hall, 1945. A well-written account of the discovery of anesthetics in the 1840's that offers many historical details and twenty-four pages of photographs. Further developments in anesthesiology during the next hundred years are described. Highly recommended as a classic in the history of medicine. Available through university or medical school libraries.

Rushman, G. B., N. J. H. Davies, and R. S. Atkinson. *A Short History of Anaesthesia*. Oxford, England: Butterworth-Heinemann, 1996. A historical text that examines the first one hundred fifty years of the practice of anesthesia. Includes a bibliography and an index.

Senz, Laurie S. "Doing Away with Dental Pain." *Saturday Evening Post* 260 (October, 1988): 20. Describes how a small, pulsed electric current inside the patient's mouth blocks the perception of pain by the brain. The discomfort of a novocaine injection is avoided, and afterward there are no problems of numbness or slurred speech.

Winter, Peter M., and John N. Miller. "Anesthesiology." *Scientific American* 252 (April, 1985): 124-131. Explains the sequence of anesthetics used for a typical operation at a modern American hospital. The important role of the anesthesiologist in adjusting dosages and monitoring the functions of vital organs during and after surgery is described. Well written.

ANEURYSMECTOMY

PROCEDURE

ANATOMY OR SYSTEM AFFECTED: Bones, blood vessels, brain, circulatory system, head, heart, nervous system

SPECIALTIES AND RELATED FIELDS: Cardiology, emergency medicine, general surgery, neurology, vascular medicine

DEFINITION: The removal and/or repair of a weak area in the wall of a blood vessel. Aneurysms are balloonlike enlargements of weak areas of blood vessels that may rupture, leading to sudden death. They usually occur in areas of high blood flow and pressure, such as in the brain and the vessels leading from the heart. To locate

cerebral aneurysms, angiography and computed tomography (CT) scans of the brain are performed. Surgeons access the affected area through a craniotomy flap made in the skull. Once located, the aneurysm may be clipped out and the edges of the vessel stitched together; if this is not feasible, it may be coated with a plastic to prevent rupture. Aneurysms in the aorta, a major artery, are located through ultrasound. The chest is opened and internal organs moved to reveal the aneurysm. Clamps are applied to the margins of the aneurysm while it is surgically removed. Often, a graft made of Dacron is inserted, with the healthy portions of the aorta sutured to it. Complications associated with these major surgeries include hemorrhage and damage to internal organs.

—*Karen E. Kalumuck, Ph.D.*

See also Aneurysms; Angiography; Brain; Brain disorders; Cardiology; Circulation; Computed tomography (CT) scanning; Craniotomy; Heart; Neurosurgery; Vascular medicine; Vascular system.

ANEURYSMS

DISEASE/DISORDER

ANATOMY OR SYSTEM AFFECTED: Blood vessels, brain, circulatory system, head, heart, nervous system

SPECIALTIES AND RELATED FIELDS: Cardiology, emergency medicine, general surgery, neurology, vascular medicine

DEFINITION: A localized dilatation of a blood vessel, particularly an artery, that results from a focal weakness and distension of the arterial wall.

CAUSES AND SYMPTOMS

The arterial distension associated with aneurysms will take one of several forms. For example, fusiform aneurysms create a uniform bulge around an artery, while those of the saccular variety distend on one side of the blood vessel. Some saccular aneurysms found in the brain are called berry aneurysms for their protruding shapes.

Hypertension and arteriosclerosis commonly produce dilatation of the thoracic aorta. Very large aneurysms of the abdominal aorta (possibly the most common type) are usually caused by advanced atherosclerosis. The pathologic processes associated with the production of aortic aneurysms are varied, but certain factors are common to all. The media (middle arterial layer) of the normal aorta must remain intact in order for the aorta to withstand the systolic blood pressure. When the media is damaged, there is progressive dilation of the weakened area and an aneurysm develops. An aortic aneurysm is a serious disease with poor prognosis. Many such aneurysms rupture and cause death before surgical intervention can take place.

There are several types of aneurysms. Dissecting aneurysms are actually hematomas. Blood enters the wall of the aorta and splits the media of the vessel. The dissection of the media usually begins as a transverse tear in the re-

Types of Aneurysm

Saccular   Fusiform   Dissecting   Berry

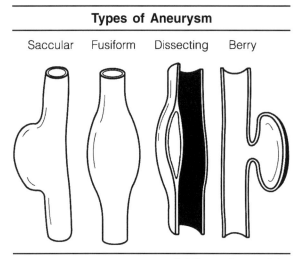

Aneurysms may cause a variety of different shapes of distension of the affected blood vessel.

gion above the aortic valve. Some believe that hypertension promotes the tear by increasing the tension on the aorta. Traumatic aneurysm is usually caused by penetrating wounds or by blunt trauma; the most common cause of such injuries is automobile accidents. Mycotic aneurysms of the aorta may be associated with bacterial endocarditis and sometimes with organisms such as salmonella. Aneurysms of the sinuses of Valsalva may be attributable to syphilitic aortitis, bacterial endocarditis, or congenital defect.

TREATMENT AND THERAPY

Surgical therapy for thoracic aortic aneurysms varies with the type and location of the lesion. Aneurysms involving the aortic arch are often surgically corrected by employing a bypass technique. One method sutures a large prosthetic graft between the ascending and descending aortas, thus bypassing the diseased area. Surgical techniques sometimes offer the only hope for the survival of a patient with aneurysm.   —*Jane A. Slezak, Ph.D.*

See also Aneurysmectomy; Arteriosclerosis; Brain; Brain disorders; Bypass surgery; Cardiology; Cardiology, pediatric; Circulation; Heart; Hypertension; Neurology; Neurology, pediatric; Neurosurgery.

FOR FURTHER INFORMATION:

Bennett, J. Claude, et al., eds. *Cecil Textbook of Medicine*. 20th ed. Philadelphia: W. B. Saunders, 1996. A comprehensive text which provides a valuable reference for all diseases, disorders of the nervous and neuromuscular systems, and environmental and physical factors in disease.

Burch, George E. *A Primer of Cardiology*. 3d ed. Philadelphia: Lea & Febiger, 1963. A text covering fundamental clinical cardiology and basic hemodynamic phenomena in healthy individuals and those with cardiac disease.

Kernicki, Jeanette, Barbara Bullock, and Joan Matthews. *Cardiovascular Nursing*. New York: G. P. Putnam's Sons, 1970. A book covering the clinical aspects of dealing with cardiac patients. Includes chapters on the anatomy and physiology of the cardiovascular system, problems of fluid and electrolyte disturbances, congestive heart failure, and cardiac arrhythmias.

Yao, James S. T., and William H. Pearce, eds. *Aneurysms: New Findings and Treatments*. Norwalk, Conn.: Appleton & Lange, 1994. Discusses the diagnosis of aneurysms and therapies to treat them. Includes bibliographic references and an index.

ANGINA

DISEASE/DISORDER

ANATOMY OR SYSTEM AFFECTED: Circulatory system, heart

SPECIALTIES AND RELATED FIELDS: Cardiology, family practice, internal medicine

DEFINITION: Chest pain ranging from mild indigestion to a severe crushing, squeezing, or choking sensation.

CAUSES AND SYMPTOMS

Usually located below the sternum, angina may radiate down the left arm and/or left jaw, or down both arms and jaws. It is ischemic in nature, meaning that the pain is produced by a variety of conditions that result in insufficient supply of oxygen-rich blood to the heart. Some examples include arteriosclerosis (hardening of the arteries), atherosclerosis (arteries clogged with deposits of fat, cholesterol, and other substances), coronary artery spasms, low blood pressure, low blood volume, vasoconstriction (a narrowing of the arteries), anemia, and chronic lung disease.

Precipitating factors for angina include physical exertion, strong emotions, consumption of a heavy meal, temperature extremes, cigarette smoking, and sexual activity. These factors can cause angina because they may increase heart rate, cause vasoconstriction, or divert blood from the heart to other areas, such as the gastrointestinal system. Angina usually lasts from three to five minutes and commonly subsides when the precipitating factors are relieved. Typically, it should not last more than twenty minutes after rest or treatment.

Diagnosis consists of a physical examination which includes a chest X ray to determine any cardiac abnormalities; blood tests to screen risk factors such as lipids or to detect enzymes that can indicate if a heart attack has occurred; electrocardiography (ECG, or EKG); nuclear studies such as Thallium stress tests, which measure myocardial perfusion; coronary angiography to evaluate the anatomy of the coronary arteries and to note the location and nature of artery narrowing or constriction; cardiac catheterization to measure cardiac output; and Holter monitor studies to evaluate chest pain during the performance of daily activities for a twenty-four-hour period.

Treatment depends on the specific cause of the angina. Three types of drugs are the most common form of treatment: nitrates, to increase the supply of oxygen to the heart by dilating the coronary arteries; beta blockers, to lower oxygen demand during exercise and improve oxygen supply and demand; and calcium blockers, to decrease the work of the heart by decreasing cardiac contractility.

—*John A. Bavaro, Ed.D., R.N.*

See also Arteriosclerosis; Cardiology; Cardiology, pediatric; Chest; Heart; Heart attack; Heart disease; Hyperlipidemia; Hypertension; Ischemia; Pain, types of; Thrombosis and thrombus.

ANGIOGRAPHY
PROCEDURE

ANATOMY OR SYSTEM AFFECTED: Blood, blood vessels, brain, circulatory system, head, heart

SPECIALTIES AND RELATED FIELDS: Cardiology, emergency medicine, radiology, vascular medicine

DEFINITION: The X-ray analysis of the cardiovascular system following the injection of a radiopaque contrast dye into an artery.

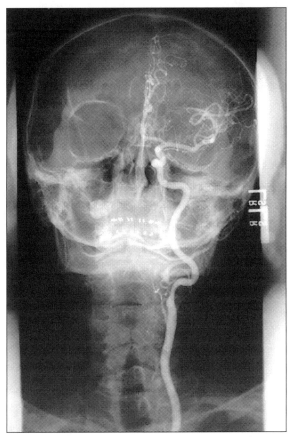

This angiogram shows the path of the carotid artery through the head and neck. (Digital Stock)

INDICATIONS AND PROCEDURES

Angiography (also called arteriography) is a procedure utilized for the detection of abnormalities in arteries of the heart, brain, or other organs. The procedure is carried out when symptoms suggest the narrowing or blockage of an artery, most frequently in the heart or brain. Such symptoms include chest pain or similarly associated discomfort in the region of the stomach or left side of the body. Even if pain is absent, shortness of breath may indicate a cardiac or pulmonary problem. Slurred speech or vision may likewise suggest narrowing of an artery in the brain. Angiography can therefore indicate the likelihood of a heart attack or stroke, as well as other problems which may produce similar symptoms, such as blood clots or cancer.

The patient must avoid food or drink for approximately eight hours prior to the procedure. A catheter is inserted through the skin, usually in the groin area, and placed into the artery to be examined. A sedative is not necessary, although it may be given to the patient to aid in relaxation.

Once the catheter is in place, a radiopaque dye is injected, and X-ray photographs of the area in question are taken. The procedure generally takes about three hours.

USES AND COMPLICATIONS

Since any blockage or narrowing of an artery will result in accumulation of the radiopaque dye, the radiologist can pinpoint the site of the block. Based on the symptoms, the physician can discuss the diagnosis and recommend further procedures.

The most common complication associated with angiography is the mild discomfort resulting from insertion of the catheter. The dye itself may cause a slight burning sensation, and on rare occasions it may trigger an allergic response. In 1 to 2 percent of cases, more serious complications develop. If the blockage results from an atherosclerotic plaque or from a blood clot, in rare circumstances a piece of this material may break off and lodge elsewhere in the arterial system. The result can be a stroke or heart attack.

—*Richard Adler, Ph.D.*

See also Angioplasty; Arteriosclerosis; Bypass surgery; Cardiology; Catheterization; Circulation; Heart; Heart attack; Imaging and radiology; Radiopharmaceuticals, use of; Strokes and TIAs; Vascular medicine; Vascular system.

ANGIOPLASTY
PROCEDURE

ANATOMY OR SYSTEM AFFECTED: Blood vessels, circulatory system, heart

SPECIALTIES AND RELATED FIELDS: Cardiology, vascular medicine

DEFINITION: The insertion of a long, flexible tube into a narrowed or blocked blood vessel in order to repair it; in balloon angioplasty, a small balloon at the end of the tube is inflated to compress a fatty blockage in the blood vessel and thus increase blood flow.

INDICATIONS AND PROCEDURES

Angioplasty, particularly balloon angioplasty, may be performed on any blocked or narrowed blood vessel, such as in the legs, but it is most commonly used to open heart valves blocked by coronary artery disease.

More than six million people in the United States have a history of heart disease, a condition often signaled by chest pain known as angina pectoris. Other symptoms include shortness of breath, heart palpitations, or an actual heart attack. Probable causes of heart disease can be diagnosed by stress tests and angiography. If the cause results from blockage of the coronary arteries, the cardiologist may order angioplasty to open the blocked vessels and restore a better blood flow to the heart muscle.

The patient cannot eat or drink anything after midnight the day before the procedure is to be performed. A mild sedative may be given. The site for insertion of the catheter, often the inside of the elbow or the groin, is shaved and is cleaned with an antiseptic solution. A local anesthetic is injected at the insertion site, but the patient remains awake during the procedure. The surgeon makes a small opening in the skin at the insertion site, inserts the catheter into an artery, watches the progress of the catheter on an X-ray monitor, and guides the tip into the blocked arteries.

In balloon angioplasty, the most common type, the tube is equipped with a balloon. Once the tip is in place in the blocked area, the balloon is inflated and deflated several times in order to compress the fatty material (plaque) and increase blood flow through the artery. The catheter then is slowly withdrawn.

If the arm site was used, the small incision is stitched closed. If the groin site was used, the puncture opening is closed with pressure. A dressing is applied to the insertion site. Barring any complications, the usual hospital stay is four to seven days.

Angioplasty

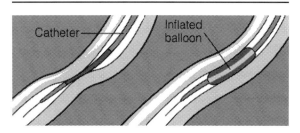

Balloon angioplasty involves the insertion of a catheter into an artery that has narrowed and the inflation of a small balloon in order to expand the vessel; this procedure is usually performed to counteract the effects of atherosclerotic disease, in which plaque deposits accumulate in the arteries.

USES AND COMPLICATIONS

The cardiac catheters used in angioplasty can also remove plaque with special cutting or laser tips. The balloon tip may be used to place a stent, a metal device, permanently in the coronary artery to keep it open.

About 80 percent of the angioplasty treatments are successful, with the patient being able to resume a reasonably normal lifestyle and enjoy a good quality of life. Complications of coronary artery angioplasty seldom occur, but they may include bleeding or clotting, an abnormal heartbeat, perforation of the heart muscle or artery, and, rarely, a heart attack, stroke, or even death. *—Albert C. Jensen*

See also Angina; Angiography; Arteriosclerosis; Bypass surgery; Cardiology; Catheterization; Heart; Heart attack; Heart disease; Heart valve replacement; Palpitations; Thrombolytic therapy and TPA; Vascular medicine; Vascular system.

ANIMAL RIGHTS VS. RESEARCH
ETHICS

DEFINITION: The debate concerning medical research techniques using animals as test specimens in order to obtain information regarding procedures, drugs, or products to be used on human beings.

KEY TERMS:

amyloidosis: a condition characterized by the deposit of waxy substances in animal organs

biomedical research: investigation or experimentation relating to biological, medical, and physical science

biomedicine: the branch of medical science concerned with the capacity of human beings to survive and function in abnormally stressful environments and with the protective modification of such environments

cardiomyopathy: a typically chronic disorder of heart muscle that may involve obstructive damage to the heart

commissurectomy: the removal of a connecting band of tissue in the brain or spinal cord

endocarditis: inflammation of the lining of the heart and its valves

hemophilia: a hereditary blood defect (occurring almost exclusively in males) characterized by delayed clotting of the blood and consequent difficulty in controlling hemorrhage after even minor injuries

neuritis: an inflammatory or degenerative lesion of a nerve, marked by pain and the loss of normal reflexes

toxoplasmosis: an infection caused by parasitic microorganisms that invade tissues and that may cause damage to the central nervous system, especially in infants

uveitis: inflammation of the uvea of the eye

THE CONTROVERSY SURROUNDING ANIMAL EXPERIMENTATION

The practice of utilizing animals as test subjects in research has resulted in the informal formation of two basic factions: those who support its role as providing information regarding the contagion and transmission of diseases, their treatment, and their potential cure; and those who deplore the use of animals, citing miserable living conditions for captive animals, which are subjected to painful and debilitating experiments that sometimes result in disfigurement, permanent injury, or death. Those in the first party include doctors, medical researchers, and the patients and their families who have benefited from the information gained. They believe that the performance of experiments on animals has been invaluable, leading to the discovery of many medical treatments and cures for humans afflicted with disease, as well as information related to the risks and benefits of other drugs or products. The second party, often referred to as animal rights activists, is made up of people dedicated to halting the testing and killing of animals in experiments. Groups such as People for the Ethical Treatment of Animals (PETA) and the Animal Liberation Front (ALF) have picketed laboratories, incensed the media, and, in extreme cases, destroyed testing facilities and released the animals kept in them in order to prevent or impede further testing. These groups believe that animals have a right to live in their normal habitats without human intervention.

Since second century Rome, doctors and scientists have conducted experiments on animals, including dissections. The discoveries have yielded untold amounts of information which can be assimilated to human medical conditions. Animal experiments have become so commonplace, however, that animals are sometimes regarded as mere tools in the laboratory. "To me, a monkey was as expendable as a screwdriver or a pair of pliers," indicates Donald Barnes, a former experimental psychologist who has become an animal activist.

Animal rights activists seek an end to animal experimentation, claiming that much of it is unnecessary. According to PETA, the major infectious diseases, such as poliomyelitis, tuberculosis, cholera, and typhoid fever, are dying out in developing countries mostly because of improved living conditions and sanitation, rather than because of vaccines. Furthermore, the ALF reminds scientists that insulin, a treatment for diabetes mellitus that was created using animal research, is not a cure for the disease. Some test procedures, such as scalding or electrocution, are pointless, as the outcome of the experiment is already known. Barnes explains why he was fired from a research position: "One day I refused to carry out a particular military experiment on four perfectly healthy primates, but only because we already knew the answer to the question. It was an invalid experiment, and as the principal investigator I knew that its only purpose was to ensure further funding for the lab."

Animal rights activists can take two different approaches to the issue. The more conventional and more peaceful method is the pursuit of stricter regulations for animal research. In announcements and letters to researchers, activists may state that they are seeking the enactment of laws and regulations that ban all research using animals. Bills to prevent or limit animal research have been introduced in several American states. Other efforts include an attempt to win legal standing to act on behalf of animals and endeavors to divert federal funds earmarked for biomedical research into the development of alternatives for experimentation.

Other activists have taken extreme measures to display their disgust through demonstrations, break-ins, and vandalism to research laboratories across the United States. Such acts cost research firms more than $17 million annually. Damage to the laboratories and equipment and the releasing or stealing of animals impede the research process and call attention to the activists' concerns. The efforts of some of these activists have become increasingly violent, including the use of bombs and other explosives at or near testing facilities. PETA, an organization of more than 325,000 members, says that it disavows violence, but the ALF has actually claimed credit for some of the attacks.

In direct contrast to the activists' perceptions of animal research are doctors, scientists, beneficiaries, and others who argue in favor of animal biomedical testing. According to David Chernof, the president of the Los Angeles County Medical Association, "Animal research has been the basis for every medical advance which has benefited humanity in the past 100 years—from insulin to heart surgery to polio and a cure for childhood leukemia." The American Medical Association (AMA) and other medical organizations support the use of animal testing for its importance in advancing the treatment and cure of human diseases. Animals are considered indispensable in biomedical research because of structural similarities between animals and humans, who often react to illnesses in the same way and suffer from many of the same diseases. The AMA actively opposes all laws, regulations, and social protesting that seek to limit such research. The medical field believes that it is only through continued support of the research process, including funding and experimentation, that the United States can continue to be a leader in medical discoveries.

Consumers of a variety of health, hygiene, and beauty products also benefit from animal testing. Such testing has protected consumers from pain, discomfort, and allergic reactions to such products as shampoo, lipstick, and dyes. While testing that does not involve the use of animals often can achieve these goals, sometimes animal testing is the only way to establish the safety of a product for use by humans.

Scientists point out that the information gained from the research often benefits the animals as well. For example, research has shown that feeding monkeys a low-cholesterol diet helps to relieve arteriosclerosis in that particular animal. Other experiments have resulted in the discovery of vaccines to treat infected cattle, poultry, horses, cats, and dogs. In addition, the researchers indicate that the federal government's rules and regulations regarding the housing conditions and care of test animals are so strict that the medical centers probably provide better care for these animals than that received by human patients.

Another group that supports animal biomedical research are the patients who have survived an illness or catastrophe because research had allowed the development of proper treatments, or patients currently receiving treatment. The Incurably Ill for Animal Research (IIFAR), a U.S. organization made up of people suffering from chronic diseases (and their families), supports the humane use of animals for research. In 1990, the group presented the U.S. Congress with a petition signed by 70,000 members requesting that such research be allowed to continue. While the members of IIFAR express regret that animals have been sacrificed, they argue that the technology and information gained have helped many of them cope with illness and receive treatment and have sometimes cured diseases that otherwise would have proven fatal to humans.

Caught in the middle of the controversy are veterinarians, who by trade seek to alleviate pain and illness of animals. Veterinarians are the caretakers of research animals and at the same time are the targets of the campaigns of animal rights activists. The American Veterinary Medical Association basically agrees with the AMA on this issue, but it has not taken such a high-profile role in proclaiming this position. Some veterinarians believe that they are fighting a war of facts-versus-emotions and that education is the only answer, that the public should be informed that animal welfare is not necessarily equated with animal rights.

A go-between group needs to be established, one that could assuage the fears of animal rights activists while still promoting humane methods of experimentation with animals. One organization, the Physicians for Responsible Medicine, could perhaps lead the way for more answerable research practices.

THE BENEFITS OF ANIMAL RESEARCH

Whether the use of animals in experiments is ethical is a matter of debate. Not all animal experimentation is equal. The goals of animal experimentaation for product safety, such as for cosmetics versus a drug for heart disease, may need to be weighed separately. The merit and the pros and cons may differ substantially in the eyes of both animal testing advocates and animal rights advocates.

Nevertheless, such research has had many successes. Breakthroughs using animal research have resulted in the development of a vaccine for polio, treatments for cancer, safer heart surgery, and even the artificial heart. Some other medical discoveries made through animal research, listed in the *Journal of the American Medical Association*, are in aging, anesthesia, behavioral studies, cardiovascular medicine, the study of hearing (audiology), ophthalmology, organ transplantation, pulmonary medicine, radiology, repro-

ductive biology, virology, and the treatment and study of AIDS, cancer, hemophilia, hepatitis, malaria, rabies, and toxoplasmosis.

Aging. Direct relationships between infections and immunologic disease have made dogs an excellent example to study in cases of amyloidosis. Dogs also serve as models for the study of Alzheimer's disease because of similar pathological changes—an increase in neuritic plaques— seen with Alzheimer's disease in humans. Primates also exhibit this abundance of neuritic plaques. Mice have been used in aging studies because their functional ability declines with age in a fashion similar to that of humans. Rats have been studied extensively for their age-related characteristics and behavior.

Anesthesia. The development of equipment and use of positive-pressure ventilation in performing chest surgery on dogs led to an adapted use for humans. A classic success story in the development of anesthetic techniques was when the first lung cancer patient to have a lung removed survived another forty years.

Behavioral studies. Research involving dogs, rats, and mice provides feedback on environmental adaptation, hereditary characteristics, and learned behaviors. Relationships between behaviors such as fear and stress and between physiological changes such as cardiac rate changes and anorexia nervosa can provide assimilations for humans. Research on depression in primates provides information about sleep disturbances, which can resemble depression and disordered physiology in humans. The study of the communicative abilities of primates helps in the development of teaching practices for mentally retarded children. Animals who suffered from intractable epilepsy have undergone commissurectomy, which has led to the understanding of left-right brain hemisphere cognitive differences in humans. Experiments with rats have shown that obesity shortens the life span. Finally, mice have been utilized as principal research subjects because of the availability of inbred strains and mutants with differing neuroanatomy and biochemistry. Furthermore, the generally short life span of a mouse allows researchers to observe the animal and its changes in its normal lifetime, yielding information within a short time frame.

Cardiovascular medicine. Endocarditis develops naturally in dogs—no inducement or intervention is necessary—and provides scientists with information on bacterial endocarditis in humans. Many inherited cardiovascular problems occur in dogs, and the surgical techniques to correct such defects have also proven effective in humans. Rats develop hypertension spontaneously, increasing with age and occurring more frequently in male rats. Tests of blood pressure controls and the use of antihypertensive agents work on both rats and humans. Cats are used as models to evaluate therapeutic approaches to cardiomyopathy, as well as the role of the liver and how the gastrointestinal tract functions.

Audiology. Hearing loss patterns in mice closely resemble those in humans. The mouse has become an excellent source of information about age-induced hearing loss as well as about the effects of noise exposure.

Ophthalmology. Common retinal diseases such as glaucoma, cataracts, and uveitis occur in dogs; these animals have been used to find effective strategies for alleviating these eye conditions in humans. Cat research involving cataracts has provided information on postsurgical corneal healing. Primates have also been used in the study of visual disorders and visual maturation in children.

Organ transplantation. The first successful kidney transplants were performed on dogs in the late 1950's, which led to correct procedures for human organ transplantation. Studies of tissue rejection in rats can be assimilated to the same affliction in humans.

Pulmonary medicine. Rats have proven valuable in the study of decompression sickness as well as of the effects of air emboli in the lungs. Dogs have been used to study emphysema, pulmonary edema, and thermal burns of the lung associated with fire or the ingestion of chemicals. Lung surgery on dogs led to the development of the pulmonary pump oxygenator.

Radiology. Research in radiology shows that some animals are more sensitive to radiation than others and that survival is dependent on the age when the first dosages of radiation were received.

Reproductive biology. Primates, rats, and mice are excellent subjects for reproductive research, including studies on endocrinology and menstruation. This research has led to advances in fertility control methods for humans. Pregnancy, fetal development, and birth are studied in primates because of their similarities to the human condition of pregnancy. The identification of the Rh factor was an immunological breakthrough resulting from tests on primates.

Virology. Understanding of viral transmissions and diseases has been furnished by research done on mice; these findings have led to the formulation of vaccines for influenza, polio, encephalomyelitis, and rabies.

Acquired immunodeficiency syndrome (AIDS). Simians provide an excellent study for AIDS because their immunodeficiency symptoms, syndromes, and viruses are almost identical to those of humans. In addition, the AIDS virus itself was isolated in captive Rhesus monkeys.

Cancer. One of the first studies of chemotherapy was performed on dogs, which resulted in the knowledge that some cancers may be caused by infectious agents. Cats are used as subjects in breast cancer studies because of similarities in structure to humans. In addition, rats and mice are used extensively in cancer research, especially in the study of tumors and in the screening of carcinogenic (cancer-causing) compounds.

Hemophilia. Hemophilia in dogs is nearly identical to that in humans, so the dog has served as a model for this research. The first successful bone marrow transplant occurred in laboratory mice and served as the example for such transplants in humans.

Hepatitis. The dog is used as a research subject because viral hepatitis occurs naturally in dogs. The dog also is used for comparative studies of cirrhosis of the liver. Research involving chimpanzees led to the discovery of the hepatitis B vaccine.

Malaria. Potential therapies for malaria, which affects 200 million people worldwide, can be discovered through tests on primates.

Rabies. The original vaccine produced for the treatment of rabies resulted from experimentation on rabbits.

Toxoplasmosis. The study of cats infected with toxoplasmosis has led to treatments for the 4,500 human babies born annually in the United States with this infection.

PERSPECTIVE AND PROSPECTS

Through the use of animals as test subjects, benefits have been gained for both humans and animals. Many therapies and cures have been discovered through careful experimentation with animals in which a particular animal is found to be suited to a particular test. Animal research has been performed for centuries, and the information gleaned from the procedures has provided modern medicine with many vaccines and treatments that probably would not have been possible without such research.

Animal rights activists have struck a nerve in the field of research and have increased awareness among animal researchers about ensuring the use of humane methods of experimentation. Continued dialogue between these groups will be necessary to avoid the halting of important medical research and to discourage the unnecessary use of animals when other methods are available.   *—Carol A. Holloway*
updated by Nancy A. Piotrowski, Ph.D.

See also American Medical Association; Ethics; Laboratory tests; Veterinary medicine.

FOR FURTHER INFORMATION:

"Animals in Research." *JAMA: The Journal of the American Medical Association* 261 (June 23, 1989): 3602. A well-written article containing an extensive listing of many research topics. Discusses how the use of animals has contributed to the study of each topic.

Breo, Dennis L. "Animal Rights vs. Research? A Question of the Nation's Scientific Literacy." *JAMA: The Journal of the American Medical Association* 264 (November 21, 1990): 2564. An excellent source of information regarding all aspects of animal biomedical research.

Cooke, Patrick. "A Rat Is a Pig Is a Dog Is a Boy: The Debate over Animal Rights Is Full of Equations That Don't Add Up." *Health* 5 (July/August, 1991): 58-64. An excellent article examining the highly emotional issue of animal experimentation in medical research.

Groves, Julian McAllister. *Heart and Minds: The Controversy over Laboratory Animals*. Philadelphia: Temple

University Press, 1997. This book describes the contro-versies involved in the use of laboratory animals for different types of testing.

Jackson, Christine. "Dissection: Science or Violence?" *Mothering*, no. 9 (Spring, 1991): 91. A list of sources for further information is provided at the end of the article, as well as a directory of sources offering alternatives to the dissection of animals.

Lynch, Berkley A., Peter Singer, and Susan Sperling. "Unkind to Animals." *The New York Review of Books* 36 (April 13, 1989): 52-53. A letter to the editor on the subject of animal experimentation.

ANOREXIA NERVOSA
DISEASE/DISORDER

ANATOMY OR SYSTEM AFFECTED: Psychic-emotional system, reproductive system, many other systems

SPECIALTIES AND RELATED FIELDS: Endocrinology, gynecology, internal medicine, nutrition, psychiatry, psychology

DEFINITION: Anorexia nervosa is an eating disorder characterized by a compulsive aversion to food. The anorectic (usually a young woman) fears obesity and creates a false body image; as a result, she intentionally starves herself. The extreme weight loss that often results can cause such medical problems as skeletal muscle atrophy, dental car-

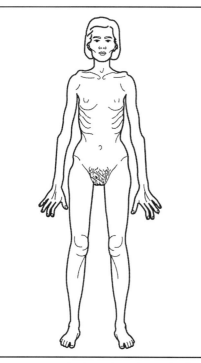

Anorexia nervosa results in undereating and other behaviors that lead to emaciation and, if unchecked, death; although this condition is most often seen in women, its incidence among men is on the rise.

ies, constipation, hypotension, hair loss, amenorrhea (cessation of menstruation), electrolyte imbalance, and osteoporosis. Cardiac arrest or circulatory collapse can occur and may prove fatal. Intensive psychiatric counseling and perhaps hospitalization to correct the symptoms of severe malnutrition are required.

—*Jason Georges and Tracy Irons-Georges*

See also Addiction; Amenorrhea; Anxiety; Depression; Eating disorders; Malnutrition; Nutrition; Obsessive-compulsive disorder; Psychiatric disorders; Psychiatry; Psychiatry, child and adolescent; Puberty and adolescence; Sports medicine; Stress; Vitamins and minerals; Weight loss and gain.

ANTIBIOTICS
PROCEDURE

ANATOMY OR SYSTEM AFFECTED: All

SPECIALTIES AND RELATED FIELDS: Bacteriology, immunology, microbiology, pharmacology

DEFINITION: The use of drugs that are selectively toxic to microorganisms.

KEY TERMS:

chemotherapeutic index: for antibiotics, the ratio of the maximum dose that can be administered without causing serious damage to a person to the minimum dose that will cause serious damage to the infecting microorganism; a measure of selective toxicity

minimal inhibitory concentration: the amount of an antibiotic needed to inhibit the growth of a microorganism in the laboratory; may be correlated to the dose of the antibiotic needed to control an infection

normal microbiota: the collection of microorganisms that inhabit tissues of healthy persons and that to some degree establish environments hostile to pathogens (the causative agents of disease)

resistance determinants: genes found in some bacteria that permit them to resist the action of particular antibiotics; these genes can be transferred between cells, allowing rapid spread of antibiotic resistance among bacteria

semisynthetic: used to refer to natural products, such as antibiotics, that have been chemically modified to be more useful for a particular application

spectrum of activity: the range of microbial species that can be inhibited by an antibiotic; broad-spectrum antibiotics can control more than one kind of infection, but narrow-spectrum antibiotics avoid unintentional damage to the normal microbiota

superinfection: an infection caused by destruction of the normal microbiota by antibiotic therapy, which allows for proliferation of a pathogen other than the one targeted by the antibiotic

INDICATIONS AND PROCEDURES

Humans live in the midst of a microbial world of bacteria, fungi, and protozoa. Microorganisms were the first inhabitants of the earth, and when multicellular animals arose, some microbes adapted to use them as a source of nutrients. Most of these microorganisms did no harm to their hosts—humans carry around bacteria numbering in the trillions—but some possessed the means to penetrate tissues and invade internal organs. In animals, in turn, a variety of defensive strategies evolved, referred to as immune responses, to resist such invasion. Infections develop when these responses fail to repel the invaders. At this point, humans can turn to antibiotics.

Antibiotics are drugs that kill, or inhibit the reproduction of, microorganisms. In the strict use of the term as defined by Selman Waksman, the discoverer of streptomycin, an antibiotic is "a chemical substance produced by microorganisms which has the capacity to inhibit the growth of bacteria and even destroy bacteria and other microorganisms in dilute solution." In everyday communication, however, use of the term has been expanded to include a variety of synthetic and semisynthetic chemicals exhibiting antimicrobial activity.

The effectiveness of antibiotics arises from their selective toxicity, which relies on differences between the fundamental biology of pathogenic microorganisms and that of an infected person. The sulfonamides, or sulfa drugs, the first class of antimicrobial compounds to achieve widespread use, are chemically similar to molecules used by bacteria for the synthesis of folic acid, an essential vitamin. When sulfonamides are present, they interfere with folic acid synthesis, preventing growth of the bacteria. Because humans lack the ability to synthesize folic acid (which is obtained from food), their cells are unaffected by sulfonamides. The beta-lactams, a class of antimicrobial chemicals that includes the penicillins and cephalosporins, interfere with the synthesis of peptidoglycan, an essential component of bacterial cell walls that is totally lacking in human cells. Other antibiotics target unique aspects of microbial protein synthesis and nucleic acid metabolism. Antibiotics are sometimes used in combination; for example, beta-lactams may be used to weaken bacterial cell walls, promoting access of a second antibiotic directed against an internal target.

The clinical microbiology laboratory can assist physicians in determining appropriate antibiotic therapy by identifying infectious agents and determining the susceptibility or resistance of the agent to a range of potential antibiotics. An increased need for such services has accompanied the evolution of pathogenic microorganisms in response to the use of antibiotics. In the early days of antimicrobial chemotherapy, it was often sufficient to diagnose an infection from its symptoms, from which one could infer the type of microorganism causing the infection (for example, gram-positive or gram-negative bacteria) and prescribe one of a limited number of broad-spectrum agents with confidence that it would be effective. Today, while immediate application of broad-spectrum antibiotics may be called for to con-

tain a serious infection, concern over creating resistant pathogens leads more physicians to request the identification and testing of microorganisms. Furthermore, the extensive resistance encountered among pathogens suggests that a broad-spectrum agent may be ineffective.

Advances in clinical microbiology are directed toward increasing the speed and accuracy of the identification of infectious agents, with a primary goal of providing information useful in prescribing antimicrobial chemotherapy. Clinical samples (infected fluids, biopsy samples, or tissue swabs) are used to inoculate selective and differential media that favor the growth of a suspected pathogen. Material from isolated colonies is then subjected to a variety of tests designed to characterize aspects of the microorganism's physiology and metabolic biochemistry, which provide criteria for the taxonomic identification of the organism. While some smaller laboratories rely on the manual inoculation of test media and reference to printed diagnostic tables for identification, the trend is toward greater automation to allow more rapid processing of multiple samples. Panels of test media prepared in multiwell plates can be simultaneously inoculated, and because many of the tests are evaluated by color changes, test results can be read with spectrophotometers designed to scan the individual tests. Test data are entered into computer programs that match the test results with probability matrices to provide a probable identification of the organism used to inoculate the tests. In the largest laboratories, efficiency can be enhanced by using robotics to conduct many of the steps, from inoculation to the reporting of test results and probable identification.

While automation can help to speed up the rate at which test information is obtained, classic identification tests are limited by the need for the incubation and growth of the test organism; this limitation can be particularly burdensome in the case of microorganisms that are especially slow-growing, among which are the mycobacteria that cause tuberculosis. In response, laboratories increasingly rely on identification methods that allow direct examination of the microorganism. Serological tests, which use antibodies directed against antigens specific to a particular microbe, and DNA probes, targeted to species-specific genes, are being applied to an increasing range of pathogenic microorganisms. Some of these tests have advanced to the point that infectious agents can be identified directly in clinical samples, circumventing the need for isolation in the laboratory.

In evaluating the susceptibility of a microorganism to an antibiotic, microbiologists seek to determine the minimal inhibitory concentration (MIC) at which an antibiotic will inhibit the growth of the microbe in a standard growth medium; the MIC can be correlated with an effective dose of the antibiotic. In broth dilution tests, a defined number of microbial cells is inoculated into a series of broth tubes containing different concentrations of an antibiotic; the

MIC is reported as the lowest concentration of the antibiotic that prevents growth of the organism in the broth. The same technologies used to automate identification can be used to allow a large number of broth dilution tests to be carried out in multiwell plates, so that susceptibility to a range of antibiotics can be determined simultaneously.

Where automation is unavailable, broth dilution testing is impractical because of the labor involved, and laboratories may rely on an indirect method called a disk diffusion test, or Kirby-Bauer assay. In this method, disks of filter paper impregnated with a defined amount of antibiotic are placed on a plate of solid growth medium that has been seeded with cells of the microorganism being tested. During incubation, the antibiotic diffuses from the disk, leading to a gradient of antibiotic concentration extending in all directions from the disk. If the microbe is susceptible to the antibiotic, its growth will be inhibited in a circular zone surrounding the disk; the diameter of the zone of inhibition varies directly with the MIC for that antibiotic. As with traditional identification methods, tests for antibiotic susceptibility are limited by the requirement that the test organism be allowed time to grow in the laboratory. It is likely that commercial DNA probes will be developed to allow the direct detection of genes that encode resistance to individual antibiotics.

USES AND COMPLICATIONS

Given the importance of differences between the biology of infectious microorganisms and the biology of the infected host to the effectiveness of antibiotics, it is not surprising that antibiotics have been used most successfully to control infections caused by bacteria, whose molecular and cellular biology differs vastly from that of humans. Consequently, most antibiotics directed against bacteria show a favorable chemotherapeutic index, which is the ratio of the maximum dose that can be administered without causing serious harm to the recipient of the drug to the minimum dose that will be effective in controlling the infection.

Infections caused by eukaryotic fungi and protozoa are particularly difficult to treat because of the similarities between the cell structure and function of these organisms and those of human cells. While the topical application of antifungal agents such as miconazole is very effective in the treatment of fungal skin infections and vaginal candidiasis, the treatment of systemic fungal infections (usually with amphotericin B) is much more difficult to perform and is more likely to cause serious side effects. Similar complications accompany efforts to treat protozoal infections with antimicrobial agents; this situation is especially frustrating, since parasitic infections such as malaria and schistosomiasis pose a major worldwide health problem. The number of methods available for the chemical treatment of viral infections is extremely limited, in view of the fact that viruses rely on the molecular machinery of the infected host for their reproduction. One antiviral strategy that has met with limited success is to design nucleotide analogues that interfere with viral nucleic acid synthesis; both acyclovir, used for infections caused by the herpes simplex virus, and azidothymidine, the first agent shown to affect the course of human immunodeficiency virus (HIV) infection, belong to this class of drugs.

In addition to potential toxicity, other factors need to be considered when choosing an antibiotic for treatment of a particular infection. Attention must be given to the fate of an antibiotic once it is administered, so that a sufficient concentration is maintained at the site of infection. If an antibiotic is administered orally, then it must be able to survive the environment of the gastrointestinal tract in order to reach the targeted tissues. Only certain antibiotics are able to cross the blood-brain barrier for effective treatment of infections of the central nervous system. Although the rapid clearance of an antibiotic may be detrimental in the treatment of many infections, it can be advantageous in the treatment of urinary tract infections, in which effectiveness requires the accumulation of the antibiotic in the bladder.

Antibiotics can be classified according to their spectrum of activity (the range of pathogenic organisms that they effectively kill or inhibit); broad-spectrum antibiotics are effective against many species, while narrow-spectrum antibiotics target a specific group. A broad-spectrum antibiotic can be prescribed upon diagnosis of an infection, without identification of the particular pathogen responsible; this trait can be important when immediate containment of the infection is essential to the health of the patient. Yet the indiscriminate use of broad-spectrum antibiotics can harm microorganisms other than those causing an infection. One's external surfaces, including the skin, gastrointestinal tract, upper-respiratory tract, and vagina, are inhabited by large numbers of microorganisms, collectively referred to as the normal microbiota. While this relationship is hardly a symbiotic one, such organisms do help to maintain environments that inhibit the growth of pathogenic microbes. Administration of broad-spectrum antibiotics can cause the depletion of normal microbiota organisms, leading to conditions favoring superinfection by a pathogen other than the one targeted by the antibiotic. For example, vaginal candidiasis (often called a yeast infection) can develop with the administration of antibacterial drugs. The bacteria that normally inhabit the vagina maintain an acidic environment that inhibits the growth of the pathogenic fungus *Candida albicans*, which may nevertheless persist in low numbers. If these bacteria are adversely affected by antibiotic treatment, then the vagina may become less acidic, allowing *C. albicans* to grow and cause tissue damage. Other superinfections can lead to serious damage to the gastrointestinal tract. There is also concern that the use of broad-spectrum antibiotics may encourage the growth of antibiotic-resistant strains among the microorganisms that constitute the normal microbiota. Because antibiotic resistance can be transferred from one bacterial species to another, conditions that favor the growth of any antibiotic-resistant microbes can contribute to the development of antibiotic-resistant pathogens.

Specific resistance to the action of antibiotics is a matter of great concern to medical personnel who deal with infectious diseases. In the early 1940's, when the first antibiotics came into widespread use, virtually all strains of *Staphylococcus aureus* (a bacterium that causes a variety of infections) were susceptible to penicillin G, a beta-lactam that can be administered orally. By the 1990's, it was rare to isolate a strain of *S. aureus* from an infection that was not resistant to multiple beta-lactams. Similar situations prevail with other pathogenic microorganisms, seriously impairing the ability to control many infections. Antibiotic resistance usually develops when a pathogen possesses specific genes encoding proteins that allow the organism to avoid the action of the antibiotic. Such proteins may inactivate the antibiotic molecule, interfere with the uptake of the antibiotic, or modify the target of the antibiotic so that it is no longer affected by the antibiotic. In bacteria, the genes encoding antibiotic resistance (called resistance determinants, or R-factors) are usually found on plasmids, small circular deoxyribonucleic acid (DNA) molecules that are separate from the bacterial chromosome. A single plasmid may contain genes for resistance to several antibiotics. Many plasmids also contain genes that allow them to be transferred from one cell to another, even if the cells are of different species. These genes can cause antibiotic resistance to spread rapidly among microorganisms.

Because the presence of an antibiotic in an animal's tissues favors the survival of bacteria carrying resistance determinants for that antibiotic, continued application of an antibiotic tends to increase the incidence of resistance to that antibiotic. Overcoming this dilemma is difficult. Narrow-spectrum antibiotics should be used whenever practical, since they limit the range of species subject to selection for antibiotic resistance. Some microbiologists have urged that the nontherapeutic application of antibiotics, such as the use of tetracycline as a growth-promoting factor in animal feeds, be discontinued because it can contribute to the spread of resistance determinants. The identification of new natural and synthetic compounds for which resistance has not yet been encountered can help to defeat pathogens that have developed resistance to the current repertoire of antibiotics, but experience teaches one to expect that such victories will be temporary; the implementation of each new antibiotic will lead to the discovery of new resistance determinants. Humans must accumulate knowledge of the biology of their adversaries in order to design narrow-spectrum drugs that are precisely targeted to the metabolism of a pathogen.

PERSPECTIVE AND PROSPECTS

The latter decades of the nineteenth century are often referred to as the golden age of microbiology, because it was during this time that microbiologists identified many of the pathogenic microorganisms responsible for infectious diseases. Although such knowledge was very useful in helping to control the transmission of infectious diseases in populations through public health measures and vaccination programs, it did little to alleviate the suffering of the individual already infected with the now-identifiable pathogen. Actual treatment of infections required the identification of chemical compounds that would be selectively toxic to the

The Action of Antibiotics

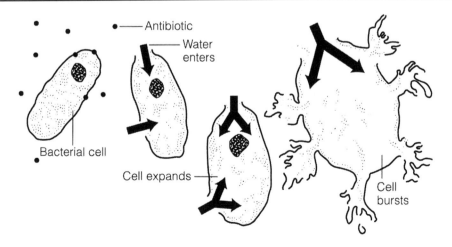

An antibiotic destroys a bacterium by causing its cell walls to deteriorate; water will then enter the bacterium unchecked until it bursts.

microorganisms, and such compounds were unknown at that time. Nevertheless, the potential value of such compounds motivated many scientists to devote their research to the search for chemicals that would destroy microorganisms without damaging an infected person.

The few compounds used at this time (mostly heavy metal salts) tended to exhibit a very low chemotherapeutic index, and some scientists despaired of finding poisons that were poisonous for only some forms of life. Then, in 1910, Paul Ehrlich demonstrated that Salvarsan (arsphenamine), an arsenical compound, was selectively toxic to the bacterial agent of syphilis. Although Salvarsan was useless for other infections, it provided evidence that selective toxicity was possible and encouraged the medical community to find other selective toxins. Extensive chemical screening programs led, in 1935, to the commercial production of the sulfanilamides, which are active against multiple species of bacteria.

The greatest conceptual advance in the development of antimicrobial drugs was made by those bacteriologists who concentrated on the phenomenon of antagonism, whereby certain microorganisms produce compounds that inhibit others. Study of these compounds eventually led to the practical application of gramicidin (described by René Dubos in 1939), penicillin (described by Alexander Fleming in 1928), and streptomycin (described by Selman Waksman in 1943). Penicillin receives special attention in the history of antibiotics because the industrial processes developed to allow production of massive quantities of the drug proved valuable in the commercial exploitation of other antibiotics. With the goal of increasing the yield of penicillin—motivated in part by a desire to have an alternative to the sulfonamides for the treatment of infections attending World War II—industrial microbiologists optimized the composition and aeration of the growth media and selected mutant strains of the penicillin-producing fungus that secreted the drug in amounts far greater than those seen by Fleming. In doing so, they established some of the engineering principles that allowed for the growth of biotechnology.

Eventually, major pharmaceutical companies committed themselves to extensive screening programs to identify additional natural antibiotics. Microorganisms isolated from soil were tested for their ability to inhibit the growth of pathogens. Eventually it was realized that, although a diverse range of organic molecules possess antibiotic properties, such compounds are produced by a limited range of microorganisms. More than half of the natural antibiotics currently in use are produced by mycelial bacteria called actinomycetes. One approach that has complemented the identification of new natural antibiotics is the chemical modification of such drugs through the addition or removal of groups of atoms. Compared to natural antibiotics, such semisynthetic derivatives may have properties that promote accumulation at high levels in the target tissue or prevent recognition of the antibiotic molecule by products of resistance determinants. All the beta-lactams in common use today are semisynthetic molecules.

While microbiologists have been discovering further natural antibiotics and synthesizing others, they have also been learning more about the molecular biology of infectious pathogens. This knowledge will allow antibiotic development to become increasingly focused as humans attempt to stay ahead of the evolution of their ancient adversaries.   —*Kenneth A. Pidcock, Ph.D.*

See also Bacterial infections; Bacteriology; Candidiasis; Chemotherapy; Cytology; Cytopathology; Drug resistance; Fungal infections; Genetic engineering; Gram staining; Laboratory tests; Immune system; Immunology; Immunopathology; Infection; Microbiology; Parasitic diseases; Pharmacology; Pharmacy; Protozoan diseases; Viral infections.

FOR FURTHER INFORMATION:

Black, Jacquelyn G. *Microbiology: Principles and Practices.* 3d ed. Upper Saddle River, N.J.: Prentice Hall, 1996. Numerous microbiology textbooks are in print, each of them having strengths and weaknesses in the presentation of different topics. Black's book has an especially good chapter on antimicrobial therapy that uses excellent illustrations to outline both the agents themselves and issues attending their use.

Brock, Thomas, ed. *Milestones in Microbiology.* Englewood Cliffs, N.J.: Prentice Hall, 1961. A collection of classical papers in microbiology published before World War II. Includes papers by Paul Ehrlich, Alexander Fleming, and Gerhard Domagk describing the first classes of antimicrobial compounds.

Gale, E. F., et al. *The Molecular Basis of Antibiotic Action.* London: John Wiley & Sons, 1981. The definitive scientific reference work on antibiotics. The text is organized by target of antimicrobial effect, with extensive citation of original papers that provide the current models of antibiotic action.

Moberg, Carol L., and Zanvil A. Cohn, eds. *Launching the Antibiotic Era.* New York: Rockefeller Press, 1990. A collection of papers from a 1989 symposium at Rockefeller University honoring René Dubos, whose discovery of gramicidin provided evidence that microbial antagonism could be exploited for chemotherapy. The testimony of leading scientists gives some indication of the challenges faced by researchers in the early "antibiotic era."

Neu, H. C. "The Crisis in Antibiotic Resistance." *Science* 249 (August 21, 1992): 1064-1073. One of a series of articles in this issue of *Science* that deal with "emerging pathogens," microorganisms that have been found to be unexpectedly difficult. Contains somewhat technical but clear descriptions of the molecular mechanisms used by bacteria to defeat antibiotic action.

ANXIETY

DISEASE/DISORDER

ANATOMY OR SYSTEM AFFECTED: Heart, nervous system, psychic-emotional system, skin

SPECIALTIES AND RELATED FIELDS: Cardiology, internal medicine, psychiatry, psychology

DEFINITION: Heightened fear or tension that causes psychological and physical distress; the American Psychiatric Association recognizes six types of anxiety disorders, which can be treated with medications or through counseling.

KEY TERMS:

anxiety: abnormal fear or tension, which may occur without any obvious trigger

brain imaging: any of several techniques used to visualize anatomic regions of the brain, including X rays, magnetic resonance imaging, and positron emission tomography

compulsion: a repetitive, stereotyped behavior performed to ward off anxious feelings

GABA/benzodiazepine receptor: an area on a nerve cell to which gamma aminobutyric acid (GABA) attaches and that causes inhibition (quieting) of the nerve; benzodiazepine drugs enhance the attachment of GABA to the receptor

obsession: a recurrent, unwelcome, and intrusive thought

panic: a sudden episode of intense fearfulness

CAUSES AND SYMPTOMS

Anxiety is a subjective state of fear, apprehension, or tension. In the face of a naturally fearful situation, anxiety is a normal and understandable condition. When anxiety occurs without obvious provocation or is excessive, however, anxiety may be said to be abnormal or pathological (existing in a disease state). Normal anxiety is useful because it provides an alerting signal and improves physical and mental performance. Excessive anxiety results in a deterioration in performance and in emotional and physical discomfort.

There are several forms of pathological anxiety, known collectively as the anxiety disorders. As a group, they constitute the fifth most common medical or psychiatric disorder. In the United States, 14.6 percent of the population will experience anxiety at some point in their lives. More women suffer from anxiety disorders than do men, by a 2:1 ratio.

The anxiety disorders are distinguished from one another by characteristic clusters of symptoms. These disorders include generalized anxiety disorder, panic disorder, obsessive-compulsive disorder, phobias, adjustment disorder with anxious mood, and post-traumatic stress disorder. The first three disorders are characterized by anxious feelings that may occur without any obvious precipitant, while the latter three are closely associated with anxiety-producing events in a person's life.

Generalized anxiety disorder is thought to be a biological form of anxiety disorder in which the individual inherits a habitually high level of tension or anxiety that may occur even when no threatening circumstances are present. Generally, these periods of anxiety occur in cycles which may last weeks to years. The prevalence is unknown, but this disorder is not uncommon. The male-to-female ratio is nearly equal.

Evidence suggests that generalized anxiety disorder is related to an abnormality in a common neurotransmitter receptor complex found in many brain neurons. These complexes, the GABA/benzodiazepine receptors, decrease the likelihood that a neuron will transmit an electrochemical signal, resulting in a calming effect on the portion of the brain in which they are found. These receptors exist in large numbers in the cerebral cortex (the outer layer of the brain), the hippocampus (the sea horse-shaped structure inside the temporal lobe), and the amygdala (the almond-shaped gray matter inside the temporal lobe). The hippocampus and amygdala are important parts of the limbic system, which is significantly involved in emotions. Benzodiazepine drugs enhance the efficiency of these receptors and have a calming effect. In contrast, if these receptors are inhibited, feelings of impending doom result.

Panic disorder is found in 1.5 percent of the United States population, and the female-to-male ratio is 2:1. This disorder usually begins during the young adult years. Panic disorder is characterized by recurrent and unexpected attacks of intense fear or panic. Each discrete episode lasts about five to twenty minutes. These episodes are intensely frightening to the individual, who is usually convinced he or she is dying. Because people who suffer from panic attacks are often anxious about having another one (so-called secondary anxiety), they may avoid situations in which they fear an attack may occur, in which help would be unavailable, or in which they would be embarrassed if an attack occurred. This avoidance behavior may cause restricted activity and can lead to agoraphobia, the fear of leaving a safe zone in or around the home. Thus, agoraphobia (literally, "fear of the marketplace") is often secondary to panic disorder.

Panic disorder appears to have a biological basis. In those people with panic disorder, panic attacks can often be induced by sodium lactate infusions, hyperventilation, exercise, or hypocalcemia (low blood calcium). Normal people do not experience panic attacks when these triggers are present. Highly sophisticated scans show abnormal metabolic activity in the right parahippocampal region of the brain of individuals with panic disorder. The parahippocampal region, the area surrounding the hippocampus, is involved in emotions and is connected by fiber tracts to the locus ceruleus, a blue spot in the pons portion of the brain stem that is involved in arousal.

In addition to known biological triggers for panic attacks, emotional or psychological events may also cause an attack.

To be diagnosed as having panic disorder, however, a person must experience attacks that arise without any apparent cause. The secondary anxiety and avoidance behavior often seen in these individuals result in difficulties in normal functioning. There is an increased incidence of suicide attempts in people with panic disorder; up to one in five have reported a suicide attempt at some time. The childhoods of people with panic disorder are characterized by an increased incidence of pathological separation anxiety and/or school phobia.

Obsessive-compulsive disorder (OCD) is an uncommon anxiety disorder with an equal male-to-female ratio. It is characterized by obsessions (intrusive, unwelcome thoughts) and compulsions (repetitive, often stereotyped behaviors that are performed to ward off anxiety). The obsessions in OCD are often horrifying to the afflicted person. Common themes concern sex, food, aggression, suicide, bathroom functions, and religion. Compulsive behavior may include checking (such as repeatedly checking to see if the stove is off or the door is locked), cleaning (such as repetitive handwashing or the wearing of gloves to turn a doorknob), or stereotyped behavior (such as dressing by using an exact series of steps that cannot be altered). Frequently, the compulsive behaviors must be repeated many times. Sometimes, there is an exact, almost magical number of times the behavior must be done in order to ward off anxiety. Although people with OCD have some conscious control over their compulsions, they are driven to perform them because intense anxiety results if they fail to do so.

The most common psychological theory for OCD was proposed by Sigmund Freud, who believed that OCD symptoms were a defense against unacceptable unconscious wishes. Genetic and brain imaging studies, however, suggest a biological basis for this disorder. Special brain scans have shown increased metabolism in the front portion of the brain in these patients, and it has been theorized that OCD results from an abnormality in a circuit within the brain (the cortical-striatal-thalamic-cortical circuit). Moreover, OCD is associated with a variety of known neurological diseases, including epilepsy, brain trauma, and certain movement disorders.

Phobias are the most common anxiety disorders. A phobia is an abnormal fear of a particular object or situation. Simple phobias are fears of specific, identifiable triggers such as heights, snakes, flying in an airplane, elevators, or the number thirteen. Social phobia is an exaggerated fear of being in social settings where the phobic person fears he or she will be open to scrutiny by others. This fear may result in phobic avoidance of eating in public, attending church, joining a social club, or participating in other social events. Phobias are more common in men than in women, and they often begin in late childhood or early adolescence.

In classic psychoanalytic theory, phobias were thought to be fears displaced from one object or situation to another. For example, fear of snakes may be a displaced fear of sex because the snake is a phallic symbol. It was thought that this process of displacement took place unconsciously. Many psychologists now believe that phobias are either exaggerations of normal fears or that they develop accidentally, without any symbolic meaning. For example, fear of elephants may arise if a young boy at a zoo is accidentally separated from his parents. At the same time that he realizes he is alone, he notices the elephants. He may then associate elephants with separation from his parents and fear elephants thereafter.

Adjustment disorder with anxious mood is an excessive or maladaptive response to a life event in which the individual experiences anxiety. For example, an individual may become so anxious after losing a job that he or she is unable to eat, sleep, or function and begins to entertain the prospect of suicide. While anxiety is to be expected, this person has excessive anxiety (the inability to eat, sleep, or function) and a maladaptive response (the thought of suicide). The exaggerated response may be attributable to the personality traits of the individual. In this example, a dependent person will be more likely to experience an adjustment disorder than a less dependent person.

Adjustment disorders are very common. In addition to adjustment disorders with anxious mood, people may experience adjustment disorders with depressed mood, mixed emotional features, disturbance of conduct, physical complaints, withdrawal, or inhibition in school or at work. These disorders are considered to be primarily psychological.

Post-traumatic stress disorder (PTSD) is similar to adjustment disorder because it represents a psychological reaction to a significant life event. PTSD only occurs, however, when the precipitating event would be seriously emotionally traumatic to a normal person, such as war, rape, natural disasters such as major earthquakes, or airplane crashes. In PTSD, the individual suffers from flashbacks to the precipitating event and "relives" the experience. These episodes are not simply vivid remembrances of what happened but a transient sensation of actually being in that circumstance. For example, a Vietnam War veteran may literally jump behind bushes when a car backfires.

People who suffer from PTSD usually are anxious and startle easily. They may be depressed and have disturbed sleep and eating patterns. They often lose normal interest in sex, and nightmares are common. These individuals usually try to avoid situations that remind them of their trauma. Relationships with others are often strained, and the patient is generally pessimistic about the future.

In addition to the anxiety disorders described, abnormal anxiety may be caused by a variety of drugs and medical illnesses. Common drug offenders include caffeine, alcohol, stimulants in cold preparations, nicotine, and many illicit drugs, including cocaine and amphetamines. Medical illnesses that may cause anxiety include thyroid disease, heart failure, cardiac arrhythmias, and schizophrenia.

Treatment and Therapy

When an individual has difficulty with anxiety and seeks professional help, the cause of the anxiety must be determined. Before the etiology can be determined, however, the professional must first realize that the patient has an anxiety disorder. People with anxiety disorders often complain primarily of physical symptoms that result from the anxiety. These symptoms may include motor tension (muscle tension, trembling, and fatigue) and autonomic hyperactivity (shortness of breath, palpitations, cold hands, dizziness, gastrointestinal upset, chills, and frequent urination).

When an anxiety disorder is suspected, effective treatment often depends on an accurate diagnosis of the type of anxiety disorder present. A variety of medications can be prescribed for the anxiety disorder. In addition, several types of psychotherapy can be used. For example, patients with panic disorder can be educated about the nature of their illness, reassured that they will not die from it, and taught to ride out a panic attack. This process avoids the development of secondary anxiety, which complicates the panic attack. Phobic patients can be treated with systematic desensitization, in which they are taught relaxation techniques and are given graded exposure to the feared situation so that their fear lessens or disappears.

The origin, diagnosis, and treatment of anxiety disorders can best be portrayed through case examples. Three fictional cases are described below to illustrate typical anxiety disorder patients.

Hypothetical case examples. Ms. Smith is a twenty-four-year-old married mother of two young children. She works part-time as a bookkeeper for a construction company. Her health had been good until a month ago, when she began to experience spells of intense fearfulness, a racing heart, tremors of her hands, a dry mouth, and dizziness. The spells would come on suddenly and would last between ten and fifteen minutes. She was convinced that heart disease was causing these episodes and was worried about having a heart attack. As a result, she consulted her family physician.

Physical examination, electrocardiogram, and laboratory studies were all normal. Her physician had initially considered cardiac arrhythmia (abnormal rhythm of the heartbeat) as a cause but diagnosed panic disorder on the basis of Ms. Smith's history and the outcome of the tests. Treatment consisted of medication and comforting explanations of the nonfatal nature of the disorder. Within three weeks, the panic attacks stopped altogether.

This case illustrates many common features of panic disorder. The patient is a young adult female with classic panic attacks striking "out of the blue." Most patients fear that they are having a heart attack or a stroke or that they are going insane. Typically, they present their symptoms to gen-

eral medical physicians rather than to psychiatrists. Treatment with medication and simple counseling techniques are usually successful.

Mr. Jones is a thirty-five-year-old single man who works as an accountant. He has always been shy and has adopted leisure activities that he can do alone, such as reading, gardening, and coin collecting. As a child, he was bright but withdrawn. His mother described him as "highstrung," "a worrier," and "easily moved to tears." Recently, he has been bothered by muscle achiness, frequent urination, and diarrhea alternating with constipation. He thinks constantly about his health and worries that he has cancer.

Mr. Jones makes frequent visits to his doctor, but no illness is found. His doctor tells him that he worries too much. The patient admits to himself that he is a worrier and has been his whole life. He ruminates about the details of his job, his health, his lack of friends, the state of the economy, and a host of other concerns. His worries make it hard for him to fall asleep at night. Once asleep, however, he sleeps soundly. Finally, Mr. Jones is given a tranquilizer by his physician. He finds that he feels calm, no longer broods over everything, falls asleep easily, and has relief from his physical symptoms. To improve his social functioning, he sees a psychiatrist, who diagnoses a generalized anxiety disorder and an avoidant (shy) personality disorder.

This case illustrates many features of patients with generalized anxiety disorder. These individuals have near-continuous anxiety for weeks or months that is not clearly related to a single life event. In this case, some of the physical manifestations of anxiety are prominent (muscle tension, frequent urination, and diarrhea). Difficulty falling asleep is also common with anxiety. In contrast, patients who are depressed will often have early morning wakening. In this case example, the patient also has a concomitant shy personality that aggravates his condition. Such a patient usually benefits from treatment. Medication may be required for many years, although it may be needed only during active cycles of anxiety. Because some patients attempt to medicate themselves with alcohol, secondary alcoholism is a potential complication.

Ms. Johnson is a forty-two-year-old married homemaker and mother of four children. She works part-time in a fabric store as a salesclerk. She is friendly and outgoing. She has also been very close with her family, especially her mother. Ms. Johnson comes to her family physician because her mother has just had a stroke. Because her mother lives on the other side of the country, Ms. Johnson needs to take an airplane if she is to get to her mother's bedside quickly. Unfortunately, Ms. Johnson has a long-standing fear of flying; even the thought of getting into an airplane terrifies her. She has not personally had a bad experience with flying but remembers reading about a plane crash when she was a teenager. She denies any other unusual fears and otherwise functions well.

Her family physician refers her to a psychologist for systematic desensitization to relieve her phobia for future situations. As a stop-gap measure for the present, however, she is taught a deep-muscle relaxation technique, is shown videotapes designed to reduce fear of flying, and is prescribed a tranquilizer and another drug to reduce the physical manifestations of anxiety (a beta-blocker). This combination of treatments allows her to visit her mother immediately and, eventually, to be able to fly without needing medication.

This case illustrates a typical patient with an isolated phobia. Phobias are probably the most common anxiety disorders. Treatments such as those described above are usually quite helpful.

PERSPECTIVE AND PROSPECTS

Anxiety has been recognized since antiquity and was often attributed to magical or spiritual causes, such as demonic possession. Ancient myths provided explanations for fearful events in people's lives. Pan, a mythological god of mischief, was thought to cause frightening noises in forests, especially at night; the term "panic" is derived from his name. An understanding of the causes of panic and other anxiety disorders has evolved over the years.

Sigmund Freud (1856-1939) distinguished anxiety from fear. He considered fear to be an expected response to a specific, identifiable trigger, whereas anxiety was a similar emotional state without an identifiable trigger. He postulated that anxiety resulted from unconscious, forbidden wishes that conflicted with what the person believed was acceptable. The anxiety that resulted from this mental conflict was called an "anxiety neurosis" and was thought to result in a variety of psychological and physical symptoms. Psychoanalysis was developed to uncover these hidden conflicts and to allow the anxiety to be released.

Freud's theories about anxiety are no longer universally accepted. Many psychiatrists now believe that several anxiety disorders have a biological cause and that they are more neurological diseases than psychological ones. This is primarily true of generalized anxiety disorder, panic disorder, and obsessive-compulsive disorder. It is recognized that anxiety can also be triggered by drugs (legal and illicit) and a variety of medical illnesses.

Psychological causes of anxiety are also recognized. Adjustment disorder with anxious mood, phobias, and posttraumatic stress disorder are all thought to be primarily psychological disorders. Unlike with Freud's conflict theory of anxiety, most modern psychiatrists consider personality factors, life experiences, and views of the world to be the relevant psychological factors in such anxiety disorders. Nonpharmacological therapies are no longer designed to uncover hidden mental conflicts; they provide instead support. Specific therapies include flooding (massive exposure to the feared situation), systematic desensitization (graded exposure), and relaxation techniques.

—*Peter M. Hartmann, M.D.*

See also Arrhythmias; Death and dying; Depression; Emotions, biomedical causes and effects of; Grief and guilt; Hypochondriasis; Manic-depressive disorder; Midlife crisis; Neurosis; Obsessive-compulsive disorder; Palpitations; Panic attacks; Paranoia; Phobias; Postpartum depression; Psychiatric disorders; Psychiatry; Psychiatry, child and adolescent; Psychiatry, geriatric; Psychoanalysis; Psychosomatic disorders; Sexual dysfunction; Stress; Stress reduction; Suicide.

FOR FURTHER INFORMATION:

American Psychiatric Association. *Diagnostic and Statistical Manual of Mental Disorders: DSM-IV*. 4th ed. Washington, D.C.: Author, 1994. This textbook contains the official diagnostic criteria and classification for all the anxiety disorders. Provides useful descriptions, definitions, and prevalence data.

Bourne, Edmond J. *The Anxiety and Phobia Workbook*. Oakland, Calif.: New Harbinger, 1995. This is an excellent self-help book for problems related to anxiety. It may also be helpful for family members seeking to understand anxiety better or to support those affected by anxiety.

Greist, John H., James W. Jefferson, and Isaac M. Marks. *Anxiety and Its Treatment*. Washington, D.C.: American Psychiatric Press, 1986. A short book written by three psychiatrists with a special interest in the anxiety disorders. Intended for a lay audience, it describes the nature of the anxiety disorders and their treatment.

Kleinknecht, Ronald A. *Mastering Anxiety: The Nature and Treatment of Anxious Conditions*. New York: Plenum Press, 1991. This book provides a good overview, with statistics and good explanations of the different types of anxiety disorder.

Leaman, Thomas L. *Healing the Anxiety Diseases*. New York: Plenum Press, 1992. A helpful text written by a family physician with an interest in anxiety disorders. Provides a good overview to the subject in nontechnical terms, and contains practical advice on dealing with anxiety.

Sheehan, David V. *The Anxiety Disease*. New York: Bantam Books, 1983. A classic book written for the layperson that explains the nature of anxiety, the different types of anxiety disorder, and treatment approaches.

Weekes, Claire. *Hope and Help for Your Nerves*. New York: Hawthorne Books, 1969. A classic text describing the nature of panic disorder. Weekes describes her pioneering approach to the nonpharmacological management of this disorder.

APHASIA AND DYSPHASIA
DISEASE/DISORDER

ANATOMY OR SYSTEM AFFECTED: Brain, nervous system, psychic-emotional system

SPECIALTIES AND RELATED FIELDS: Neurology, speech pathology

DEFINITION: Dysphasia is a disturbance of such language skills as speaking, reading, writing, and comprehension, while aphasia is the total absence of these skills. Both conditions occur with damage to areas of the brain that are important to language, usually as a result of a head injury or stroke. Damage to Broca's area causes slow, labored speech. When there is damage to Wernicke's area, comprehension of speech becomes difficult (that of others as well as of the patient's own speech), resulting in grammar and word selection errors. Nominal aphasia refers to a difficulty in naming objects, while widespread brain damage can cause global aphasia, the complete inability to speak, write, or understand words.

—*Jason Georges and Tracy Irons-Georges*
See also Brain; Brain disorders; Neurology; Neurology, pediatric; Speech disorders; Strokes and TIAs.

APNEA

DISEASE/DISORDER

ANATOMY OR SYSTEM AFFECTED: Lungs, nervous system, respiratory system

SPECIALTIES AND RELATED FIELDS: Neurology

DEFINITION: Apnea is the temporary cessation of breathing; sleep apnea, the most common type, occurs during the night and causes frequent waking. This condition can be physical, caused by obstruction of the upper airway, or neurological, caused by a failure of the respiratory center to stimulate adequate breathing. The occurrence of sleep apnea is linked to stress, strokes, senility, obesity, smoking, excess alcohol consumption, and the use of mind-altering drugs. As an extreme, chronic condition, sleep apnea can result in sleep deprivation, permanent brain damage, and cardiac arrhythmias leading to heart failure. In babies, it is sometimes associated with sudden infant death syndrome (SIDS). Sleep apnea can usually be avoided by sleeping on one's side, rather than on the back. —*Jason Georges and Tracy Irons-Georges*
See also Asphyxiation; Lungs; Respiration; Sleep disorders; Sudden infant death syndrome (SIDS).

APPENDECTOMY

PROCEDURE

ANATOMY OR SYSTEM AFFECTED: Abdomen, gastrointestinal system, intestines

SPECIALTIES AND RELATED FIELDS: Emergency medicine, general surgery

DEFINITION: Corrective surgery to remove the appendix, which is required when acute appendicitis produces severe abdominal pain and the probability of peritonitis or health complications, which may be fatal if untreated.

KEY TERMS:
cecum: a pouchlike portion of the large intestine
fecalith: a hardened piece of fecal matter which often begins events leading to appendectomy by blocking the appendix

peritonitis: infection of the abdominal (peritoneal) cavity in which the visceral organs are found
septic pyelophlebitis: inflammation of the veins which carry blood away from the kidneys, it results from neglecting symptoms of acute appendicitis and can be fatal

INDICATIONS AND PROCEDURES

The appendix, more correctly named the veriform appendix, is a hollow tube of muscle attached to the pouchlike beginning of the large intestine (the cecum) and closed at the end farthest from this point of attachment. It does not serve a known purpose and is thought to be a disappearing vestige of an organ that once had a purpose. Hence the appendix is called a vestigial organ.

A veriform appendix exists only in humans and other primates. In humans, it is approximately 7.6 to 10.2 centimeters (3 to 4 inches) long and 1.3 centimeters (0.5 inch) in diameter. The cavity of the appendix (its lumen) is narrowest at the point of attachment to the cecum, and the muscular walls of the organ normally contract periodically to expel into the cecum both mucus made by the appendix and intestinal contents which may have accidentally entered the lumen.

When the narrow opening of the appendix into the cecum is blocked so as to prevent expulsion of mucus or fecal material, the organ becomes infected, a condition called appendicitis. The most frequent obstructions found in appendix openings are fecaliths. These objects are hardened pieces of fecal matter that entered the appendix from the large intestine. Swelling of the inner walls of the appendix as a result of other causes, (such as bacterial infection) can also begin such a blockage.

Following blockage, the events leading to appendicitis usually occur in the following order. First, fluids and mucus secreted by the cells lining the walls of the appendix collect in the blocked organ. This makes the appendix swell, causing the blood vessels that feed the organ's tissues gradually to close off. In the absence of an adequate blood supply, the tissue begins to die. At the same time, bacteria originating in the cecum grow vigorously in the affected appendix, increasing the inflammation and swelling of the dying organ.

Quick and appropriate treatment by surgical removal of the infected appendix—appendectomy—is often required at this time. Otherwise, the walls of such an appendix, one weakened by tissue death and subjected to increasing pressure by both bacterial growth and the buildup of mucus, may burst. When this happens, the contents spill into the abdominal cavity and infect the membranes which line it. Such infection, peritonitis, can be very painful. In most cases, however, the use of antibiotics will keep peritonitis from becoming fatal.

Where appendectomy is required, the patient is usually given a general anesthetic. A 5- to 7.6-centimeter (2- to 3-inch) incision is made directly over the site of the appen-

The Removal of the Appendix

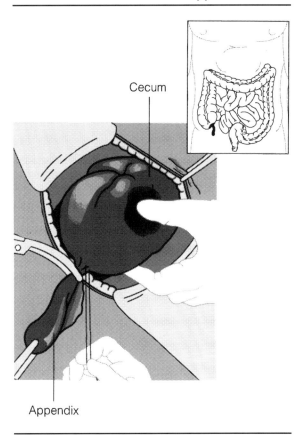

Cecum

Appendix

Inflammation of the appendix, a vestigial organ attached to the colon, usually requires an emergency appendectomy to avoid rupture and more extensive, life-threatening infection; the inset shows the location of the appendix.

dix, and the surgeon ties off and cuts the blood vessels that feed the organ. The appendix is then tied off near its connection to the cecum and carefully cut free without allowing its contents to enter the abdominal cavity. The operation usually takes under an hour and produces minor postoperative discomfort for a few days. The surgical risks of this procedure are very slight.

USES AND COMPLICATIONS

Acute infection of the appendix, requiring its surgical removal, is the most frequent cause for abdominal surgery. It is most likely to occur between the ages of eight and thirty, but no age group is exempt. Acute appendicitis is often symptomized by initial generalized abdominal pain which rapidly becomes localized. The pain, which can be quite severe and which is felt whenever the patient moves or coughs, frequently occurs in the lower-right quadrant of the abdomen (an area between the navel and the front edge of the right hipbone). This location is common because

many appendixes are located in the underlying abdominal cavity. The appendix may be found, however, in any of several other positions. Hence, the pain can occur elsewhere in the abdomen, and acute appendicitis may be mistaken for other abdominal disorders.

Other symptoms useful in diagnosing acute appendicitis are nausea and vomiting, increased pulse rate, and mild fever. In addition, the patient's white blood count will often increase from the normal range of 7,000 to 10,000 per cubic millimeter to 25,000. When symptoms of acute appendicitis occur, medications should not be given unless quick access to surgical facilities is available. For example, cathartics are a poor treatment choice because they stimulate intestinal contractions that may accelerate intestinal rupture. Similarly, the use of hot water bottles to relieve pain is inappropriate because it may also speed rupture. In cases of acute pain, the patient should be taken to a hospital emergency room as quickly as possible.

The dangers associated with appendicitis arise from its neglect. Peritonitis is rarely fatal because of the use of antibiotics. Much more serious are localized abscesses of the abdominal wall and the inflammation of the veins that carry blood away from the kidneys (septic pyelophlebitis). Both of these problems can be fatal, even when extensive and aggressive antibiotic therapy is carried out.

If a clear diagnosis of acute appendicitis cannot be made, it has become customary, in recent years, to wait and observe the patient's symptoms for up to twenty-four hours before surgery. This waiting period allows the physician an exact diagnosis without unduly subjecting the patient to the risk of peritonitis. In some cases, abdominal X rays are useful diagnostic tools. During such waiting periods, patients are under careful surveillance, and a surgical facility is kept ready for quick use, if needed. —*Sanford S. Singer, Ph.D.*

See also Abdomen; Abdominal disorders; Appendicitis; Emergency medicine; Gastroenterology; Gastroenterology, pediatric; Gastrointestinal system; Infection; Inflammation; Intestinal disorders; Intestines; Laparoscopy; Pediatrics; Peritonitis.

FOR FURTHER INFORMATION:

Berkow, Robert, and Andrew J. Fletcher, eds. *The Merck Manual of Diagnosis and Therapy.* 16th ed. Rahway, N.J.: Merck Sharp & Dohme Research Laboratories, 1992.

Maingot, Rodney. *Maingot's Abdominal Operations.* 10th ed. Edited by Michael J. Zinner et al. Stamford, Conn.: Appleton and Lange, 1997.

Tierney, Lawrence M., Jr., et al., eds. *Current Medical Diagnosis and Treatment.* 37th ed. Norwalk, Conn.: Appleton and Lange, 1998.

APPENDICITIS

DISEASE/DISORDER

ANATOMY OR SYSTEM AFFECTED: Abdomen, gastrointestinal system, intestines

SPECIALTIES AND RELATED FIELDS: Emergency medicine, gastroenterology, pediatrics

DEFINITION: Inflammation of the human vermiform appendix.

CAUSES AND SYMPTOMS

Appendicitis may be acute or chronic. The inflammation characteristic of the condition may be associated with infection or the causes may be various or even unknown.

In the human digestive system, the small intestine empties into the large intestine, or colon, in the lower right abdomen. Movement of waste from that point is generally upward through the ascending colon, but the colon begins with a downward-projecting blind end called the cecum, to which is attached the vermiform ("wormlike") appendix. The appendix is 7.5 to 15 centimeters long and less than 2.5 centimeters in diameter, and it has no known function. Occasionally, its opening into the cecum becomes obstructed, and inflammation, swelling, and pain follow. Sometimes the cause of the obstruction is identifiable, such as pinworms or other parasites, or hardened fecal material;

more often, it is not. Symptoms, including pain that is general at the outset but localizes in the lower right abdomen, can include nausea, fever, and an elevated white blood cell count. If the swollen appendix bursts, peritonitis—infection and poisoning of the abdominal cavity—can result. Peritonitis is usually signaled to the patient by an abrupt cessation of pain, when the swelling is relieved, but is followed by serious and life-threatening complications.

TREATMENT AND THERAPY

The treatment of choice is almost invariably surgical removal of the inflamed appendix, an operation that is no longer considered major surgery. The patient is usually out of bed in a day or two and fully recovered in a few weeks. Peritonitis, however, calls for emergency surgery to remove the toxic material released by the ruptured appendix, as well as the appendix itself. Because a greater or lesser portion of the abdominal cavity must be cleansed with saline solution and treated with antibiotics, this surgery can become a major procedure.

—Robert M. Hawthorne, Jr., Ph.D.

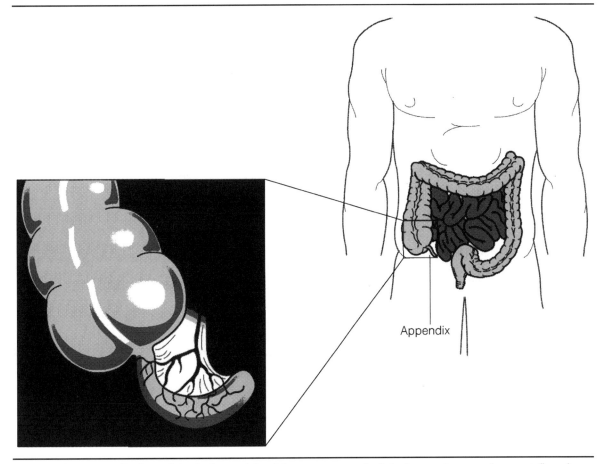

Appendix

The vermiform appendix, located in the lower-right abdomen at one end of the large colon, may become inflamed as a result of obstruction; surgery is nearly always required to avoid bursting and the release of deadly toxins into the body.

See also Abdomen; Abdominal disorders; Appendectomy; Gastroenterology; Gastroenterology, pediatric; Gastrointestinal disorders; Gastrointestinal system; Infection; Intestinal disorders; Intestines; Obstruction; Pediatrics; Peritonitis.

FOR FURTHER INFORMATION:

Clayman, Charles B., ed. *The American Medical Association Encyclopedia of Medicine.* New York: Random House, 1989.

Larson, David E., ed. *Mayo Clinic Family Health Book.* 2d ed. New York: William Morrow, 1996.

Wagman, Richard J., ed. *New Complete Medical and Health Encyclopedia.* 4 vols. Chicago: J. C. Ferguson, 1992-1993.

AROMATHERAPY
PROCEDURE

ANATOMY OR SYSTEM AFFECTED: Brain, nervous system, nose, psychic-emotional system

SPECIALTIES AND RELATED FIELDS: Alternative medicine, otorhinolaryngology, preventive medicine, psychology

DEFINITION: The use of scents to facilitate physical, mental, and emotional well-being.

INDICATIONS AND PROCEDURES

Aromatherapy is best thought of as a complement to other procedures or treatments. Essential oils and aromatic plants are used to stimulate memories, bring about feelings of calm, aid meditation, and enhance visualization exercises. Aromatherapy benefits conditions requiring the enhanced ability to concentrate, mental or physical relaxation, or the discussion of personal information or memories. As such, aromatherapy may be an appropriate adjunctive treatment for stress-related disorders or disorders treated with psychotherapies. Some practitioners suggest that specific scents have extraordinary properties (such as memory enhancers or aphrodisiacs), but little scientific evidence exists for such claims.

Methods of aromatherapy are varied but chiefly involve scent inhalation alone or in combination with massage. With massage, essential oils (oils from aromatic plants) are applied directly to the body and massaged into the skin. Otherwise, essential oils are inhaled briefly, as one might use "smelling salts," or in a more diffuse manner, as with incense or perfume. Oils may be dabbed on pulse points, disbursed by fragrance diffusers, simmered in potpourri vessels, added to boiling water to be diffused by steam, or added to baths.

USES AND COMPLICATIONS

Allergic reactions to the aromatic oils are the greatest complication of aromatherapy. The substances typically used are highly concentrated and not safe for internal use. In the hands of an unskilled user, the oils may create unpleasant odors or medically dangerous allergic reactions. Aromatherapy is probably not advisable for adults or children without the consultation of an allergist. In addition, the long-term effects of such inhalants on lung functioning are not well documented; caution must be advised.

PERSPECTIVE AND PROSPECTS

Historically, perfumes were sacrificed to the gods among Greeks, were essential for burial rites among Egyptians, and attracted good spirits among American Indians. Today, scents are used widely by therapists and individuals alike to facilitate well-being. Future work will likely include greater research on aromatherapy's safety and the role of olfaction on memory functioning.

—*Nancy A. Piotrowski, Ph.D.*

See also Allergies; Alternative medicine; Anxiety; Stress; Stress reduction.

FOR FURTHER INFORMATION:

Ryman, Daniele. *Aromatherapy: The Complete Guide to Plant and Flower Essences for Health and Beauty.* New York: Bantam, 1993.

ARRHYTHMIAS
DISEASE/DISORDER

ANATOMY OR SYSTEM AFFECTED: Circulatory system, heart

SPECIALTIES AND RELATED FIELDS: Cardiology, internal medicine

DEFINITION: An arrhythmia is an irregularity in the heartbeat, in rhythm or rate. The heartbeat is an electrical impulse that normally originates in the sinoatrial node (S-A node) and then travels to the atrioventricular node (A-V node). A disturbance in either node can cause such cardiac abnormalities as sinus tachycardia (a regular, rapid beat), ventricular tachycardia (an irregular, rapid beat originating in the ventricles), supraventricular tachycardia (a regular, very rapid beat originating in the tissue above the ventricles), sinus bradycardia (a regular, slow beat), atrial fibrillation (a very irregular, rapid beat), and heart block (alternating tachycardia and bradycardia). Arrhythmias are usually caused by coronary heart disease, especially after a myocardial infarction (heart attack) occurs. In the case of heart block, the implantation of an artificial pacemaker may be required.

—*Jason Georges and Tracy Irons-Georges*

See also Arteriosclerosis; Cardiology; Cardiology, pediatric; Heart; Heart attack; Heart disease; Hypertension; Ischemia; Mitral insufficiency; Pacemaker implantation; Palpitations; Panic attacks.

ARTERIOSCLEROSIS
DISEASE/DISORDER

ANATOMY OR SYSTEM AFFECTED: Blood vessels, circulatory system, heart

SPECIALTIES AND RELATED FIELDS: Cardiology, internal medicine, vascular medicine

DEFINITION: Also called atherosclerotic disease or "hardening of the arteries," a generalized disease that causes narrowing of the arteries because of deposits on the arterial walls and leading to a multitude of serious medical conditions, notably stroke and heart attack.

KEY TERMS:

angina: chest, jaw, or shoulder pain with exercise or stress—a symptom of atherosclerotic heart disease

embolus: a small piece of atherosclerotic plaque, thrombus, or other debris that breaks off and lodges in a blood vessel

infarct: tissue death resulting from lack of blood flow

intermittent claudication: a symptom of lower-extremity arteriosclerosis manifested by pain or cramping in the leg while walking, relieved by rest; from the Latin word *claudicatio,* "to limp"

ischemia: lack of blood in a particular tissue

rest pain: pain noted in the most distal portion of the extremity at rest, relieved by analgesics

revascularization: procedures to reestablish the circulation to a diseased portion of the body

thrombosis: aggregation of platelets and other blood cells to form a clot

CAUSES AND SYMPTOMS

The human body's arterial system is designed to carry oxygen, hormones, various types of blood cells (such as red and white blood cells), and other nutrients in the blood from the heart to the periphery and all organ structures of the body. The arteries are composed of three separate layers: adventia (the outer layer), media (the middle layer), and intima (the inner layer). Atherosclerosis or arteriosclerosis, derived from the Greek words that mean "hardening of the arteries," refers to the different diseases that compromise one or more of the layers of the large-or medium-sized arteries or smaller arterioles. Most commonly, fat, cholesterol, and calcium deposits are laid down along the intima and inner portion of the media. These components build up, forming plaques, which then may produce stenosis (narrowing) or occlusion (closure) of the arterial lumen. Accumulation of platelets and other blood cells can form a thrombus along with plaque buildup, which also obstructs the arteries. Pieces of plaque or thrombotic material can break off, causing emboli to lodge in the vessels acutely. Atherosclerosis begins with some form of damage to the delicate lining of the intima (the endothelium), by infections, inflammation, hypertension, or even natural toxins. That damage induces platelet adherence and other repair mechanisms, creating an opportunity for the accumulation of fat and calcium deposits in plaques.

Depending on the arterial segment in the body that is affected, various diseases and symptoms may occur. As the blood vessels become diseased with plaque buildup, the body will try to compensate by the development of collaterals, small vessels that bypass the diseased artery. Collateral vessels are smaller than the native arteries and cannot accommodate the same amount of blood. Normally, during

exercise, there is an increased demand for additional blood flow to the muscles; flow will increase and the arteries will dilate. With atherosclerosis, since the arteries are blocked and collaterals cannot accommodate the additional blood volume, waste products in the muscles build up, causing pain. In the heart, this process affects the flow in the coronary arteries, and angina (chest pain) may occur. In lower-extremity arteriosclerosis, stenosis or occlusions of the aorta, iliac, femoral, popliteal, or tibial arteries may occur, producing intermittent claudication.

As the disease progresses, more blood vessels become stenosed or occluded and collateral formation will maximize, but the circulation is severely limited and ischemia may result. In atherosclerotic heart disease, significant ischemia may then result in a myocardial infarct, or heart attack. In the lower extremities, patients may develop rest pain. The most severe symptoms of lower-extremity arteriosclerosis are the development of nonhealing ulcers and gangrene (tissue death) in the lower portion of the foot, similar to a heart attack. When the disease process has become this severe, there are multisegmental areas of arterial occlusions and no further compensatory mechanisms.

Acute arterial ischemia is a sudden onset of ischemia as opposed to the more common chronic processes described above. The usual cause of acute arterial ischemia is an embolus (portion of a clot) that lodges in the arteries. The most common source of embolization is the heart; embolization from the heart occurs in patients who have recently

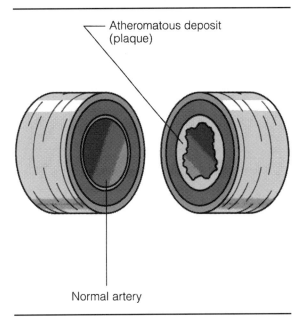

Atheromatous deposit (plaque)

Normal artery

Arteriosclerosis leads to the buildup of fatty plaques on the walls of arteries, which inhibits blood flow and may lead to obstructions resulting in stroke, heart attack, and other life-threatening events.

had a heart attack, who have mitral valvular disease, or who have atrial fibrillation (irregular heartbeats). Another cause of acute arterial ischemia is thrombosis of, or embolization from, an aneurysm. In such cases, since no significant collaterals have developed in the area of the acute blockage, immediate revascularization is mandatory to prevent significant tissue death.

Aneurysms—another disease entity that may be associated with the atherosclerotic disease process—produce a weakening of the adventia and a "ballooning" of the arteries with a thrombus (clot). Rupture or thrombosis (clotting off) may be a consequence of aneurysmal disease.

In cerebrovascular disease, atherosclerosis affects the arteries supplying the circulation to the brain (the carotid and vertebral-basilar system). The most common symptoms noted are transient ischemic attacks (TIAs), also referred to as ministrokes. TIAs usually last less than twenty-four hours. Most TIAs are produced by embolization, in which pieces of plaque in the major arteries break off and temporarily block the blood flow to certain areas of the brain. Once the symptoms last more than twenty-four hours, a cerebrovascular accident (CVA), cerebral infarct, or stroke has occurred. Atherosclerosis in the cerebrovascular system will behave in a manner similar to that previously described, with increasing stenosis and eventual occlusion. Collateral development seems to be especially prominent in the cerebrovascular system, since the brain is a greedy organ needing blood at all times. The majority of CVAs are caused by occlusion or thrombosis of a major vessel, producing significant ischemia in a portion of the brain.

Other sources of CVAs are hemorrhaging (bleeding) from ruptured cerebral aneurysms or from uncontrolled hypertension. This significant bleeding can cause spasm of the arteries in the brain and eventual ischemia. Monckeberg's sclerosis, not usually thought of as a true form of atherosclerosis, refers to the disease in which calcification of the tibial arteries is noted, often in diabetic patients.

Contributing or significant risk factors in the development of atherosclerosis include hypertension (high blood pressure), hyperlipidemia (high amounts of fats or lipids in the blood), smoking, diabetes mellitus, and family history. The role of inflammation, especially from infections, is a newly discovered and significant risk factor as well. Also, depending on the significance and the location of atherosclerosis, a variety of symptoms and conditions can result. In atherosclerotic heart disease, the first symptom is angina. As in intermittent claudication, chest, shoulder, or upper back pain may occur during exercise or stress as a result of the decreased blood supply to the tissues of the end-organ, the myocardium (heart muscle). As the disease progresses, the angina will become more unstable and patients will become progressively limited in minor activities. Symptoms of a heart attack may include severe, crushing chest pain, shortness of breath, pain in the left arm, and

tingling of the fingers. Cessation of breathing and cardiac arrest indicate a significant heart attack. Immediate medical attention during the severe symptomatic phase or with cardiac arrest will aid in reducing further damage to the heart muscle and may prevent death. Many heart attacks are "silent" in that, although portions of the cardiac muscle are "dead," symptoms will have been negligible or minor, because of sufficient collateralization.

In lower-extremity atherosclerosis, patients with intermittent claudication will complain of pain or cramping in their calves, thighs, or buttocks while walking or exercising; symptoms will be relieved by rest. Claudication is usually described by distances, such as "one block" claudication or "half a mile" claudication. Rest pain occurs mostly at night at the most distal portion of the extremity, usually the toes and forefoot. Often patients will sleep in chairs or with their legs hanging off the bed to relieve the pain. On physical examination, the foot is usually cool to the touch, with a slightly bluish discoloration. There is hardening of the nails, dryness of the skin, and loss of hair in the lower portion of the leg. Pulses are absent or diminished. Often, when the leg is in a dependent position, *dependent rubor*, a purplish discoloration of the leg is seen, produced by dilation of the small blood vessels in the skin to provide the maximum amount of blood. Elevating the leg will produce a cadaverous white pallor. Because of the limited blood supply, ulcers will not heal and gangrene can develop. Patients with symptoms of severe claudication, rest pain, or neuropathic diabetes should be evaluated prior to undergoing any podiatry procedures because their compromised circulation will result in poor healing. Patients with acute arterial ischemia of the lower extremity will complain of the "five P's": pain, pallor, pulselessness, parathesias (loss of feeling), and paralysis. As previously described, emergent revascularization of the acutely ischemic limb is necessary to prevent limb loss or amputation.

Although aneurysmal disease is a separate entity, it may be associated with atherosclerotic disease in certain cases. Most aneurysms produce no symptoms. Detection of aneurysms is usually incidental; during a physical examination, for example, a physician may note a pulsatile mass in the abdomen (aorta, iliac), in the groin (femoral), or behind the knee (popliteal). Incidental diagnosis of aneurysms may also occur during routine chest X rays; the X ray may reveal a calcium rim around the body of the aneurysm. As aneurysms increase in size, the probability of rupture increases; therefore, elective surgery is usually recommended once certain sizes are achieved: more than 6 centimeters for an abdominal aneurysm and more than 2 centimeters for femoral and popliteal aneurysms. Symptoms of a rupturing abdominal aneurysm include severe lower back pain and a decrease in blood pressure, whereas thrombosis of a popliteal or femoral aneurysm will cause an acutely ischemic leg. Symptomatic aneurysms are considered medical emergencies, since ruptures may result in death and thrombosis in limb loss.

Symptoms of TIAs in the carotid arteries, which supply the front of the brain, include hemiparesis (numbness) or hemiplegia (weakness) of an arm and/or leg, affecting the carotid artery on the side opposite the symptom; aphasia (speech disorder), usually affecting the left carotid artery; or amaurosis fugax (blindness in one eye, similar to the sensation of a shade over the eye), which is from the carotid artery on the same side as the blindness. Other symptoms include dizziness, vertigo, imbalance, and other visual disturbances. These more generalized symptoms are referable to the vertebral-basilar circulation, which supplies the back portions of the brain, or are a result of multisegmental cerebrovascular disease in which a low-flow state can affect multiple areas of the brain and produce diverse symptoms. A stroke is an event whose symptoms will last more than twenty-four hours. Often these are permanent deficits, affecting the patient for the rest of his or her life.

Many patients will be asymptomatic (have no symptoms) and not develop TIAs but will have a stroke, which may result from eventual occlusion or thrombosis of the cerebral vessels and infarcts in a particular section of the brain. Asymptomatic cerebrovascular disease is often detected by the presence of a bruit (French for "noise"). Stenosis in arteries resembles rapids in a river: Flow will go very fast through the blockage and then be turbulent. The turbulence will produce a bruit which can be detected with a stethoscope. Turbulence from stenoses ranging from 20 to 80 percent can cause a bruit. The absence of a bruit does not mean that the arteries are disease-free. Once the stenosis reaches critical proportions, the flow is diminished and turbulence may be negligible. An occluded artery will also have no bruit, since there is no flow. Once the narrowing has reached 60 to 80 percent, many doctors will recommend elective surgery to reestablish flow and prevent eventual occlusion and possible stroke. About 75 percent of strokes are ischemic, resulting from this process. Bruits may be appreciable in other parts of the body and can also indicate the presence of atherosclerosis in those areas.

Atherosclerosis of the renal arteries, which supply the kidneys, may cause a condition known as renovascular hypertension. This type of high blood pressure is often difficult to control with medication, and continued high blood pressure will contribute to progression of the atherosclerotic process elsewhere in the body.

Another condition that results from atherosclerosis is chronic mesenteric ischemia. Here the blood vessels supplying the intestines, stomach, and many of the organs associated with the digestive process are affected. Patients may experience pain with eating and significant weight loss. This condition is often missed until an extensive workup for cancer or other chronic diseases yields negative results. In acute mesenteric ischemia, by contrast, thrombosis of the superior mesenteric artery occurs. As with other acute arterial conditions, emergent revascularization is necessary to prevent gangrene of the intestines.

TREATMENT AND THERAPY

A complete history and physical examination are usually the first methods of diagnosing atherosclerosis. Eliciting symptoms, noting significant risk factors and physical findings, will aid the physician in determining areas at risk.

In lower-extremity atherosclerosis, a common noninvasive method utilizes Doppler ultrasound. A series of blood pressure cuffs are attached to the extremity, and segmental blood pressure and plethysmographic (a technique which measures a change in volume) waveforms are measured. A drop of more than 20 millimeters of mercury (mm Hg) of pressure between segments or extremities is indicative of a significant stenosis at that level. Exercise testing will demonstrate whether there are significant drops in pressure, confirming the diagnosis and severity of claudication. A similar method, ocular pneumoplethysmography (OPG), developed by William Gee, utilizes eye cups placed in the eye to measure the ocular pressure. A vacuum is applied to the eyes, effectively occluding the ophthalmic arteries, the first major branch of the internal carotid artery. As the vacuum is released, the blood flow is reestablished and the appearance of arterial pulsations is noted on a strip chart, denoting the systolic ophthalmic pressures. A difference of 5 mm Hg is consistent with significant (greater than 50 to 70 percent) carotid disease.

Duplex ultrasound machines utilize B-mode (brightness-mode) ultrasound to visualize the vessels and type of plaque, while Doppler ultrasound can audibly evaluate the blood flow in the vessels. Using real-time spectrum analyzers, the Doppler signals are then analyzed in terms of velocities and waveform characteristics. The greater the velocities, the greater the amount of stenosis. Absence of blood flow will denote occlusions. The use of color duplex ultrasound, in which the Doppler signals are color-coded in terms of flow direction and speed to denote the various flow patterns in normal and diseased vessels, has enhanced the diagnostic accuracies in the examinations. The use of color Doppler in many of the ultrasound machines is aiding in more rapid detection of arterial lesions in the heart, cerebrovascular, and lower-extremity arterial circulation.

Arteriography or angiography is an invasive procedure. The delineation of the blockages and collateral pathways detected through this method—in which the patient is hospitalized and a catheter is used to inject dye containing iodine into the arteries—is then used to plan a revascularization procedure.

Ultrasound is the primary diagnostic tool for detecting and measuring the size of aneurysms. Computed tomography (CT) scanning is an alternative radiological modality to visualize aneurysms.

The majority of patients with mild to moderate intermittent claudication can be treated conservatively. Cessation of smoking, alterations to diet, and a carefully controlled exercise plan will alleviate or decrease the progression of symptoms. Less than 5 percent of patients with intermittent claudication will develop gangrene sufficient to warrant a major amputation within a five-year period.

Some medications available work by decreasing the stickiness of the platelets in the blood; these are often prescribed for patients with claudication. Aspirin is often prescribed to alleviate symptoms of TIAs and to protect patients from strokes or heart attacks. Although it is a powerful drug in decreasing the incidence of embolization, a national study has demonstrated that patients with TIAs and severe stenosis of the carotid arteries should undergo surgical revascularization to protect against major strokes. It has become clear that aspirin may also be helpful because of its anti-inflammatory properties, particularly now that the role of damage to the endothelium from inflammation and infections is understood.

Severe disabling claudication, rest pain, ulceration or gangrene of the lower extremity, and unstable angina and heart attacks require some sort of surgical intervention. Usually bypass surgery is planned to revascularize the ischemic portion of the extremity or myocardial tissue to prevent limb loss or further cardiac events. The arteriogram will illustrate the areas of blockage, and, depending on the results of this test, various types of bypasses can be performed. Inflow procedures refer to bypasses performed above the groin: Aorto-iliac or aorto-femoral are the most common types performed, usually utilizing a prosthetic (plastic) material. Outflow procedures are those performed below the groin: femoral-popliteal or femoral-tibial bypasses. Prosthetics are sometimes used, but the best bypass material in terms of durability is the patient's own vein, either removed and reversed, or in situ (in place). Depending on the type of bypass procedure performed, the five-year patency rates (number of bypasses open at five years) exceeds 85 percent for aorto-iliac/aorto-femoral bypasses and 75 percent for lower-extremity reconstructions. Coronary artery bypass grafts (CABGs) typically employ the saphenous veins of the legs or the mammary artery of the chest wall to bypass the diseased segments in the heart vessels.

Endarterectomy, a surgical technique in which the intima and part of the media are excised, effectively "scrapes out" atherosclerotic plaques. Although used in other arterial segments, endarterectomy is the most common surgical procedure used to revascularize the carotid arteries.

Other interventional modalities have been developed. Percutaneous balloon angioplasty involves placing a balloon catheter in the diseased segment during an angiogram and opening up the area of stenosis or small segmental occlusion. This method has been employed in the coronary arteries as well as in the vessels of the aorta, iliacs, and lower extremities.

New lytic drugs, which "dissolve" clots, are sometimes employed alone, or in combination with balloon angioplasties or surgery, especially in the more acute cases of lower-extremity arterial ischemia and myocardial infarctions.

PERSPECTIVE AND PROSPECTS

Atherosclerosis of the coronary and cerebrovascular system is a major cause of death. Heart attacks are the primary cause of death in the United States, with approximately 650,000 people dying annually. Half of those deaths are sudden, with no prior significant symptoms. Stroke is the third leading cause of death in the United States, with approximately 155,000 deaths annually. There are 400,000 strokes annually, and about one-fourth of all nursing home patients are permanently impaired from strokes. These statistics have a great impact on the amounts of health care monies spent annually to care for victims of heart disease and strokes.

Since the 1960's, the rates of death from both heart attacks and strokes in the United States have decreased significantly. Control of blood pressure and diet, the development of new drugs and diagnostic techniques, and the advent of cardiovascular surgery in the early 1950's have aided in this decrement. Unfortunately, atherosclerotic diseases are still prevalent. Autopsies of Korean and Vietnam War American soldiers demonstrated that atherosclerotic plaque was evident even at an early age. This was attributed to the high-fat diet of most Americans. It is recognized that this disease is more prevalent in young males and that females are more protected until the onset of menopause; then the death rates tend to equalize. High-salt diets, which may increase the incidence of hypertension, also contribute to the development and progression of atherosclerosis. Since the 1960's, extensive education of the American public regarding dietary control has had a favorable impact. More recently, the benefits of exercise have helped to stem the atherosclerotic process.

The 1950's saw the development of cardiovascular surgery. The first bypass (arterial autograft) probably occurred during the Korean War. Coronary artery bypass surgery and carotid endarterectomies are the most common surgical procedures performed today. Recognition of and prompt treatment of symptomatic cardiac and cerebrovascular symptoms remain the key to better survival rates. With development of newer bypass materials for lower-extremity bypass surgery in the 1970's, as well as better surgical techniques for utilization of the saphenous veins, the amputation rate has significantly decreased. Research into graft materials that better mimic the native arteries and veins continues. The use of lasers to obliterate atherosclerotic plaque, popular in the 1980's and early 1990's, is being discontinued, since the results are not as favorable. Atheroscopy devices, which suction out the diseased segments, are being investigated in some centers.

Since the 1950's, a number of noninvasive and invasive procedures have been developed to diagnose atherosclerotic disease. The development of ultrasound devices in the 1950's initiated the research into using these noninvasive devices to diagnose atherosclerotic disease. The duplex devices, introduced commercially in the late 1970's and early 1980's, opened a new diagnostic field for detection of atherosclerotic disease. These devices allow for visualization of plaque morphology (composition of the plaque such as thrombus, calcium, and hemorrhage) and the blood-flow characteristics for a better understanding of the atherosclerotic process. Future developments in the field of ultrasound include holographic imaging for three-dimensional visualization of plaques. These noninvasive technologies will also allow physicians to monitor the effects of new drugs and techniques in the treatment of atherosclerosis. Advances in digital subtraction and computer enhancement of angiographic techniques, along with new contrast media, are making arteriograms safer and more accurate.

Technologies being developed for future diagnostic use include magnetic resonance imaging (MRI), a nonradiological modality for visualizing structures in the brain and other portions of the body. MRI is being expanded with the aid of computerization to do MR angiography. Magnetic resonance is also being utilized to measure, noninvasively, actual flow in individual arterial segments of the body in terms of cubic centimeters per minute. Positron emission tomography (PET) scans, the newest non-X-ray method, gives brilliant, color-enhanced visualization of blood flow to tissues. —*Silvia M. Berry, M.Sc., R.V.T.*
updated by Connie Rizzo, M.D.

See also Angina; Angiography; Angioplasty; Bypass surgery; Cardiology; Cholesterol; Circulation; Claudication; Edema; Embolism; Endarterectomy; Heart attack; Heart disease; Heart failure; Hypercholesterolemia; Hyperlipidemia; Hypertension; Ischemia; Phlebitis; Strokes and TIAs; Thrombolytic therapy and TPA; Thrombosis and thrombus; Vascular medicine; Vascular system; Venous insufficiency.

FOR FURTHER INFORMATION:

American Heart Association. *AHA Focus Series: Arteriosclerosis.* Washington, D.C.: Author, 1988. This pamphlet helps educate patients on the causes and symptoms of arteriosclerosis.

Bennett, J. Claude, ed. *Cecil Textbook of Medicine.* 20th ed. Philadelphia: W. B. Saunders, 1996. This is the standard textbook of medicine. Although it is somewhat difficult, it is complete, beginning with normal conditions and progressing through disease process, diagnosis, and treatment.

The New Good Housekeeping Family Health and Medical Guide. New York: Hearst Books, 1989. A general reference guide on medical problems and the subspecialties associated with medical care.

Rutherford, Robert B., ed. *Vascular Surgery.* 4th ed. Philadelphia: W. B. Saunders, 1995. The definitive textbook for the understanding, diagnosis, and treatment of vascular disorders.

Tierney, Lawrence M., Jr., et al., eds. *Current Medical Diagnosis and Treatment.* 37th ed. Norwalk, Conn.: Appleton and Lange, 1998. This text, updated yearly, is the point of reference for physicians and other health care practitioners. It incorporates each year's biomedical research discoveries that have immediate, relevant, and applicable use for the patient.

ARTHRITIS

DISEASE/DISORDER

ANATOMY OR SYSTEM AFFECTED: Bones, hands, hips, immune system, joints, knees, legs, musculoskeletal system

SPECIALTIES AND RELATED FIELDS: Internal medicine, orthopedics, physical therapy, rheumatology

DEFINITION: A group of more than one hundred inflammatory diseases that damage joints and their surrounding structures, resulting in symptomatic pain, disability, and systemwide inflammation.

KEY TERMS:

anti-inflammatory drugs: drugs to counter the effects of inflammation locally or throughout the body; these drugs can be applied locally or introduced by electric currents (in a process called ionthophoresis), by injections into the joint or into the muscles, or by mouth; the three classes of these drugs are steroidal, immunosuppressant, and nonsteroidal

cartilage: material covering the ends of bones; it does not have a blood supply or nerve supply but may swell or break down

inflammation: the body's defensive and protective responses to trauma or foreign substances by dilution, cellular efforts at destruction, and the walling-off of irritants; characterized by pain, heat, redness, swelling, and loss of function mediated through a chemical breakdown

physical modalities: the physical means of addressing a disease, which include heat, cold, electricity, exercises, braces, assistive devices, and biofeedback

rehabilitation: a physician-led program to evaluate, treat, and educate patients and their families about the sequelae of birth defects, trauma, disease, and degenerative conditions, with the goals of alleviating pain, preventing complications, correcting deformities, improving function, and reintegrating individuals into the family and society

synovium: the cellular lining of a joint, having a blood supply and a nerve supply; the synovium secretes fluid for lubrication and protects against injury and injurious agents

CAUSES AND SYMPTOMS

Approximately one in six people (more than 15 percent) suffers from one of approximately one hundred varieties of arthritis, and 2.6 percent of the population suffer from ar-

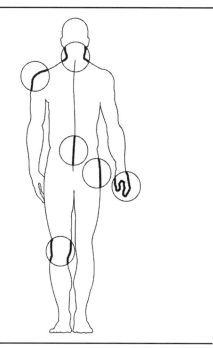

Arthritis most commonly affects the joints of the neck, shoulders, hands, lower back, hips, and knees.

thritis that limits their activities. Although many people over seventy-five years of age experience arthritis, the disease can occur in the young as a result of infections, rheumatic conditions, or birth defects. Young and middle-aged adults experience the disease as a result of trauma, infections, and rheumatic or immune reactions. Arthritis may be located in joints, joint capsules, the surrounding muscles, or diffusely throughout the body. Inflammation of the joint lining (synovium) can similarly afflict the linings of other organs: the skin, colon, eyes, heart, and urinary passage. Those suffering from the disease may therefore suffer from psoriasis and rashes, spastic colitis and diarrhea, dryness of the eyes, inflammations of the conjunctiva or iris, frequent urination, discharge and burning upon urination, and other symptoms.

The collagen-type arthritic diseases involve the binding materials in the body or connective tissues and may be rheumatologic, generally more diffuse and in the distal joints (as in juvenile rheumatoid arthritis and rheumatic fever), or located in the skin and muscles (dermatomyositis). Psoriatic arthritis causes severe punched-out defects in the joints. Reiter's and Sjögren's syndromes involve the eyes and the joints. Genetic conditions, such as Gaucher's disease, frequently run in families. Metabolic disturbances, such as gout, can leave uric acid deposits in the skin and in the joints. Gout sufferers experience very painful, hot, tender, and swollen joints—often in the large toe. Immunologically mediated arthritides may be associated with in-

fections, liver diseases, bowel disturbances, and immune deficiencies. Localized infections may be bacterial, viral, or fungal. "Miscellaneous disorders," a basket category, include conditions that do not fit into any of the aforementioned categories: Psychogenic disorders and arthritis associated with cystic disorders are examples. Arthritis may also be associated with tumors that grow from cartilage cells, blood vessels, synovial tissue, and nerve tissue. Blood abnormalities may give rise to hemorrhages into joints (a side effect of sickle-cell anemia and hemophilia) and can be disabling and very painful, sometimes requiring surgery. Traumatic and mechanical derangements—sports and occupational injuries, leg-length disparity, and obesity—may elicit acute synovial inflammation with subsequent degenerative arthritis. Finally, wear-and-tear degeneration can occur in joints after years of trauma, repetitive use, and (especially in the obese) weight-bearing. The most common arthritic entities are rheumatoid arthritis (also called atrophic or proliferative arthritis), osteoarthritis, hypertrophic arthritis, and degenerative arthritis.

The inflammatory reactions in response to injury or disease consist of fluid changes—the dilation of blood vessels accompanied by an increase in the permeability of the blood vessel walls and consequent outflow of fluids and proteins. Injurious substances are immobilized with immune reactions and removed by the cellular responses of phagocytosis and digestion of foreign materials, resulting in the proliferation of fibrous cells to wall off the injurious substances and in turn leading to scar formation and deformities. The chemical reactions to injury commence with a degradation of phospholipids when enzymes are released by injured tissue. Phospholipids—fatty material that is normally present—break down into arachidonic acid, which is further broken down by other enzymes, lipoxygenase and cycloxygenase, resulting in prostaglandins and eicosanoid acids. Most anti-inflammatory medications attempt to interfere with the enzymatic degradation process of phospholipids and could be damaging to the liver and kidneys and to the body's blood-clotting ability.

The physician bases the diagnosis of arthritic disease on the patient's medical history and a physical examination. Specific procedures such as joint aspiration, laboratory studies, and X-ray or magnetic resonance imaging may help to establish the diagnosis and the treatment. The history will elicit the onset of pain and its relation to time of day and difficulties performing the activities of daily living. A functional classification has evolved that is similar to the cardiac functional classification: Class 1 patients perform all usual activities without a handicap; class 2 patients perform normal activities adequately with occasional symptoms and signs in one or more joints but still do not need to limit their activities; class 3 patients find that they must limit some activities and may require assistive devices; and class 4 patients are unable to perform activities, are largely or wholly incapacitated, and are bedridden or confined to a wheelchair, requiring assistance in self-care.

A person's medical history or surgical conditions and the medications that he or she is taking can influence the physician's diagnosis and prescription for treatment. Patients may present a gross picture of the body to the physician showing the joints involved in their symmetry (whether distal or proximal, and whether weight-bearing or post-traumatic in distribution). Physicians may ask (verbally or by questionnaire) for a history of other system complaints, which can then be checked more thoroughly. During a physical examination, the physician will check the joints, skin, eyes, abdomen, heart, and urinary tract. The neuro-muscular evaluation may reveal localized tenderness of the joints or muscles, swelling, wasting, weakness, and abnormal motions. Joints may have weakened ligamentous, muscle, and tendon supports that could give rise to instability or grinding of joints, with subsequent roughening of cartilage surfaces. The arthritides are frequently associated with muscular pains, called fibrositis and myofascial pain syndromes.

Fibrositis is a diffuse muscular pain syndrome with tenderness in the muscles, no muscle spasm, and no limitations in motion; all laboratory tests are within normal limits. It is frequent in postmenopausal women who have a history of migraines, cold extremities, spastic colitis, softening of the bone matrix accompanied by loss of minerals, and irritability. Myofascial trigger points can be found in both men and women, at all ages, with acutely tender nodules or cords felt in muscles. The pain of these trigger points is referred to more distal areas of the muscles that may not be tender to touch. Physicians may frequently miss the acutely tender trigger points. Tests will show whether pain

Osteoarthritis

Bone forms from cartilage at edge of joint.

Outgrowth forms irregular bone (osteophyte).

Osteoarthritis results when irregular bone growth occurs at the edge of a joint, causing impaired movement of the joint and pressure on nerves in the area.

is elicited when muscles are contracted with motion, when muscles are contracted without motion, or when motion is carried out passively by the examiner without muscular effort by the patient.

Joint pathology is generally associated with some limitation in the range of motion. Sensation testing, muscle strength, and reflex changes may also indicate nerve tissue damage. Nerves occasionally pass close to joints and may be pinched when the joint swelling encroaches upon the passage opening. This condition may result in carpal tunnel syndrome, in which the median nerve at the wrist becomes pinched, causing pain, numbness, and weakness in the hand. Pinched nerves may also be associated with tarsal tunnel syndrome, in which the nerve at the inner side of the ankle joint may be compressed and cause similar complaints in the feet. Other nerves may be constricted in exiting from the spine and when passing through muscles in spasm.

The medications used to treat arthritis can involve the nervous system. An evaluation and estimation of the severity of the disease can be obtained by electrical testing, as in electroneuromyography. The nerves are stimulated and their rate of transmitting the stimulus is measured. The normal transmission rate for nerves is 45 meters per second. Delays at areas of impingement can be determined by measuring the transmission rate of a stimulus from different points along the nerve paths. Abnormal or damaged muscles will cause muscle fibers to contract spontaneously, or "fibrillate." Chest expansion during inspiration and after expiration may be limited because of arthritis at the spine or because of lung pathology. Involvement of the spine can also be measured by the posture, the ability to move the neck, and the ability to move the lower back.

Arthritis of the spine leads to progressive loss in motion. The amount lost can be measured by comparing the normal motion with the restricted motion of the patient. The neck may be limited in all directions, rotation of the head to the sides can restrict the driving view, and the head may gradually tilt forward. The lower back may also exhibit restriction in all directions; for example, it may be limited in forward bending because of spasms in the muscles in the back. Tilting backward of the trunk may be limited and painful when the vertebral body overgrowth of osteoarthritis or degenerative arthritis restricts the space for the spinal cord. The nerves pinched in their passage from the vertebrae may thus cause radiculitis, irritation of the nerves as they exit from the spine that leads to pain and muscle involvement. Circumferential measurements of the involved joints and the structures above and below can confirm swelling, atrophy from disuse or inaction, or atrophy from a damaged nerve supply. When measurements are repeated, they can indicate improvement or deterioration.

Testing of blood for cells, chemicals, or enzymes is helpful. The simplest test—the sedimentation (or "sed") test—

measures the rate at which blood cells settle out of the plasma. Normally, women have a more rapid rate of sedimentation than men. When this rate exceeds the normal range, active inflammation in the body is indicated. Comparisons of sed tests performed at different stages can reveal the disease's rate of progression or improvement. The chemicals tested may include uric acid for gout and sugar for diabetes. Blood tests for immune substances and antibodies are also possible. The joint fluid can be aspirated and analyzed, particularly for appearance, density, number of blood cells, and levels of sugar. Cloudy fluid, the tendency to form clots, a high cell count, and lower-than-normal levels of sugar in the joint fluid (compared to the overall blood sugar level) indicate abnormalities. With inflammatory arthritides, the X rays will show the results of synovial fluid and cellular overabundance. Clumps of pannus break off and may destroy the cartilage and bone. Bones about these joints, because of increased vascularity and blood flow, have less minerals and will appear less dense, a condition known as osteoporosis.

Deformities in inflammatory arthritis may be the result of unequal muscle pulls or the destruction or scarring of tissues; such deformities can occasionally be prevented by the use of resting splints, which is most important for the hands.

Degenerative and post-traumatic arthritis show joint narrowing, thinning of the cartilage layer, hardening of the underlying bone (called eburnation), and marginal overgrowth of the underlying bone (called osteophytes), result-

ing in osteoarthritis. Osteophytes, or marginal lipping in the back, may enhance symptoms of lower back pain. The cushions between the vertebrae, called discs, are more than 80 percent water, a figure which diminishes with aging, bringing the joints in the back (the facets) closer together and compressing the facet joints between the vertebrae. Irritation and arthritis of these joints are the result. Other organ structures may be involved as well.

A diagnosis of rheumatoid arthritis should include two to four of the following criteria: morning stiffness, three or more joints involved symmetrically (especially the hands), six weeks or longer in duration, rheumatoid nodules that can be felt under the skin, blood tests showing a serum rheumatoid factor, and the radiographic evidence described above.

TREATMENT AND THERAPY

Treatment of arthritis may vary from home treatment to outpatient treatment to hospitalization for acute, surgical, and/or rehabilitative care. Educating patients as to their condition, the prognosis, the treatment goals, and the methods of treatment is necessary. Patients must be made aware of warning signs of progression, drug effects, local and systemic side effects of drug therapy, and diet associated with relieving pain, stiffness, and inflammation. If surgery is contemplated for joint replacement or other reasons, patients should be fully informed as to expectations and rate of functional activities. Postoperative restrictions in the range of motion must be given; in hip replacement, for example, hip bending should not exceed 90 degrees. The ro-

Rheumatoid Arthritis

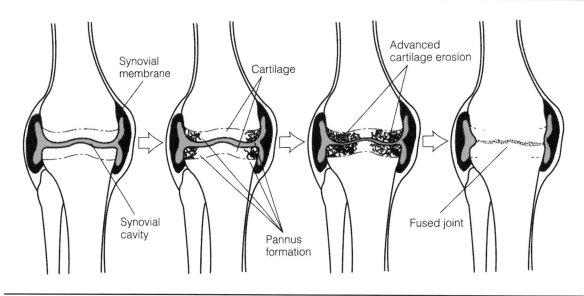

Rheumatoid arthritis begins with the inflammation of the synovial membrane and progresses to pannus formation and erosion of cartilage; eventually, the joint cavity is destroyed and the bones (here, the knee bones) become fused.

tation and overlapping of legs must be limited initially after surgery.

Some physicians provide a questionnaire that outlines the activities of daily living and recommends how a patient should perform such activities and how much time should be spent at rest. The goals generally are to maintain function, to alleviate pain, to limit the progression of deformities, to prevent complications, and to treat associated and secondary disease states. In patients with degenerative arthritis—most often the elderly, who are at risk for other organ failures—arthritides associated with systemic diseases and other organ involvements may require care. Patients with rheumatoid arthritis, for example, frequently are anemic. Anti-inflammatory drugs, normally used to treat the arthritis, may cause blood loss through the gastrointestinal tract and even ulcerations. The physician may therefore prescribe alternative therapies.

Other therapies can include assistive devices, counseling patients and their families regarding home management, medicinal regimen and compliance, behavior modification, sexual advice, and biofeedback. The aim is to reduce the need for and frequency of medical care, through a balance between rest and activity and between effective drug dose, toxicity, and physical modalities. To protect joints and allow function, various braces and assistive devices may be needed. Scarring of a wrist joint can be alleviated by avoiding positions that inhibit function. Shoulders should not be left with arms close to the body, since frozen shoulders aggravate neck and arm problems.

Physicians may offer physical therapy, occupational therapy, assistive devices for self-care, ambulation, or home and automobile modifications. Assistive devices may include reachers, an elongated shoehorn handle, thickened handles for utensils, walkers, canes, crutches, and wheelchairs. Homes may require ramps for easier access, widened doors to allow wheelchair passage, grab bars in bathtubs, or raised toilet seats for easier transference from a wheelchair.

Heat therapy may reduce the pain, loosening and liquefying tightened tissues. Somewhat like gelatin, tissue liquifies when heated and solidifies when cooled. Patients frequently will be stiffer after protracted rest periods (for example, on waking) and feel better after some activity and exercise. Heated pools offer an excellent heating and exercise modality. The type of heat modality used will depend upon the depth of heating desired. Hot packs and infrared lamps will heat predominantly the skin surface areas and some underlying muscles. Diathermy units heat the muscular layers, and ultrasound treatments heat the deepest bony layers. Ultrasound (but no diathermy) can even be used in patients who have metallic implants such as joint replacements.

Transcutaneous electrical nerve stimulation can be used to alleviate pain. The units can regulate the frequency of electrical impulses. The usual starting rate is 100 cycles, which can alleviate pain in a few minutes; this rate is later changed to 4 cycles, which will give hours of relief even when discontinued. The intensity can also be varied. The sensation desired is a slight tingle. The effect described induces an increase in the release of beta endorphin, a substance naturally produced by the body with effects similar to those of morphine. Endorphin is produced by other physical therapy procedures as well: hypnosis, acupuncture, suggestion, and stress, among others.

Patients in chronic pain may show a reduced level of the beta endorphin and an increase in a substance P, and they may find no relief of pain with physical therapy. The P chemical increases the nerves' sensitivity to stimuli, producing greater pain. Patients with chronic pain may show depression, hysteria, and hypochondriasis on the Minnesota Multiphasic Personality Inventory test and may require antidepressants. Exercise programs can help to increase endorphin levels. These exercises may range from simple movements performed by a therapist (the patient remaining passive) to active exertion against loads for strength. Stretching or gentle, intermittent traction may gradually decrease contractures, but neck traction should not be used in patients with rheumatoid arthritis of the neck.

Surgery may occasionally be necessary to alleviate pain, to replace joints, or to alleviate contactures. Isometric or static exercises can mobilize muscles without joint movement and maintain muscle viability during joint pain. Individuals can, however, be trained to perform activities more efficiently and effectively, thus saving energy. Posture training may alleviate postural muscle fatigue. In acute stages of inflammation, the treatment choices are rest, ice, compression, and proper positioning and medicinals for pain and inflammation. The stepped-up medicinal approach utilizes nonsteroidal anti-inflammatory drugs (NSAIDS), adding other drugs as necessary, including antimalarials and gold, immune suppressants, and systemic corticosteroids. Irradiation of lymphoid tissues may also be used at the acute stages. Heat modalities should not be used in acute cases, since the speed of chemical reactions increases on heating; the chemical enzyme activity of collagenase that destroys cartilage could increase the rate and extent of damage. The simplest way to prepare cold applications is to fill a plastic container with water and refrigerate it. Physicians may also use fluoromethane or other refrigerant sprays. The hot packs sold in pharmacies can similarly be soaked in water and placed in the refrigerator to create an ice pack.

PERSPECTIVE AND PROSPECTS

Historically, arthritis was treated with electric eels (as the source of electric shocks) and warm baths or sands. Some experimental treatments presently being tried include electric current to joints to bring about reductions in intra-articular pressures and in the fluid and cellular content in joints. Acupuncture has been shown to bring an increase in the beta endorphin levels and consequent relief of pain. Topical use of capsaicin, an extract from peppers, is reported to counteract substance P. One group is attempting the experimental procedure of washing out inflamed joints with a saline-type solution. Exercises continue to maintain and improve strength, dexterity, the range of motion, and endurance. Good health habits—including adequate rest, good nutrition, and nutritional supplements—can be beneficial.

—*Eugene J. Rogers, M.D.*

See also Bone disorders; Bones and the skeleton; Bursitis; Fracture and dislocation; Gout; Hip fracture repair; Inflammation; Muscle sprains, spasms, and disorders; Orthopedic surgery; Orthopedics; Orthopedics, pediatric; Osteoarthritis; Pain management; Physical rehabilitation; Rheumatoid arthritis; Rheumatology; Spinal disorders; Spine, vertebrae, and disks; Tendon disorders; Tendon repair.

FOR FURTHER INFORMATION:

Dachman, Ken, and John Lyons. *You Can Relieve Pain.* New York: HarperCollins, 1990. This book approaches pain from a psychological point of view. Discusses methods for behavior modification, relaxation techniques, and mental imagery. Lists the names and addresses of various support groups and offers a suggested reading list for pain management.

Dong, Collin, and Jane Banks. *New Hope for the Arthritic.* New York: Ballantine Books, 1990. The emphasis in this book is predominantly on nutrition. The authors believe that food allergies and chemical additives in foods contribute to arthritis. They outline exercise programs to benefit arthritic patients.

Fries, James F. *Arthritis: A Take-Care-of-Yourself Guide to Understanding Your Arthritis.* 4th ed. Reading, Mass.: Addison-Wesley, 1995. This book is recommended by the Arthritis Foundation. Discusses the major categories of arthritis, as well as pathology, quackery, surgery, employment, prevention, home treatment, and the effects of medications.

Gach, Michael R. *Acupressure's Potent Points: A Guide to Self-Care for Common Ailments.* New York: Bantam Books, 1990. Outlines the various acupressure points for treatment of various pain sites. The instructions for self-administration of acupressure techniques are specific and outlined in a steplike manner. The author also includes tips on proper eating and lifestyles.

Gordon, Neil F. *Arthritis: Your Complete Exercise Guide.* Champaign, Ill.: Human Kinetics, 1993. The author is eminently qualified to discuss and illustrate the various types of exercise modalities; he suggests a schedule of frequencies and durations for each. The illustrations are easily understood and followed.

Lorig, Kate, and James F. Fries, eds. *The Arthritis Handbook: A Tested Self-Management Program for Coping with Your Arthritis.* 3d ed. Reading, Mass.: Addison-Wesley, 1990. This book states that it is recommended by the Arthritis Foundation. The contributors, who include allied health professionals from the fields of physical therapy, occupational therapy, and public health, address pain management principles, body mechanics, and exercises.

MacLean, Helene. *Relief from Chronic Arthritis Pain.* New York: Dell Medical Library, 1990. This small book describes how to make a diagnosis of arthritis, stresses the importance of making the right diagnosis, and discusses treatments from aspirin to gold. Also includes chapters on alternative treatments, exercises, and vitamins and minerals. The glossary and index are helpful.

Pisetsky, David S., and Susan Trien Flamholtz. *The Duke University Medical Center Book of Arthritis.* New York: Fawcett Columbine Press, 1992. Discusses some of the major types of arthritis in three sections. The first discusses the major facts about arthritis, including its effects and some of the tests for the disease. The second portion delves into the major forms of arthritis. The third section goes into detail about the Duke University Basic Treatments, including physical therapy, diet, rest, exercises, and early medical interventions.

Yates, George, and Michael Shermer. *Meeting the Challenges of Arthritis: Motivational Program to Help You Live a Better Life.* Los Angeles: Lowell House, 1990. The book describes the personal struggle in overcoming marked disability from arthritis. Discusses the mental and physical effort expended and the techniques used to overcome the hardship of arthritic disabilities experienced by a young adult.

ARTHROPLASTY

PROCEDURE

ANATOMY OR SYSTEM AFFECTED: Hips, joints, knees, legs
SPECIALTIES AND RELATED FIELDS: Orthopedics, rheumatology
DEFINITION: The science of treating damaged and diseased joints.

KEY TERMS:

pathology: a disease condition; also, the science that studies diseases

prosthesis: a device, made of metal or plastic, that is implanted to replace damaged bone tissue

INDICATIONS AND PROCEDURES

Arthroplasty, a term which comes from *arthro,* meaning "joint," and *plasty,* meaning "to form or shape," covers many surgical procedures that are used to treat faulty or damaged joints.

Rheumatoid arthritis is the most common condition requiring arthroplasty, although other diseases, traumatic events (such as accidents), or congenital malformations may cause joints to become diseased. In an arthroplastic procedure, the surgeon attempts to alter damaged joint structures to relieve pain, restore mobility, and/or correct deformity.

This may involve reshaping or replacing bones, or it may be restricted entirely or largely to soft tissues surrounding the joint.

For example, when rheumatoid arthritis attacks the fingers, the result may be a drastic, painful deformity that twists the hands out of shape. The surgeon may operate to alter bony structures and may realign and reattach surrounding ligaments, tendons, and other soft tissues. Sometimes the results achieved are cosmetic, improving the appearance of the hand, and sometimes the surgeon can achieve significant relief of pain and restore some mobility.

One class of arthroplastic procedures has been quite successful in some patients and holds great promise for many others: total or partial replacement of the bones of a joint by a prosthesis fabricated in metal, plastic, or other material. The most successful of these procedures is total hip replacement. Total knee and total elbow replacements are also performed, but they have not achieved the same success rate.

The practice of replacing bones with prostheses dates from about 1939, although as a theory it had been hypothesized for years. Orthopedic surgeons knew that replacement of massively damaged joints or individual bones would be ideal therapy in many situations. There were significant problems, however, paramount among them the lack of a suitable material for the prosthetic device. All metals and alloys available at the time were unstable inside the body, subject to interaction with body substances and to rejection by the immune system. No cements were available for fixing the prostheses, and other procedures for fixation, such as screwing or bolting the prosthesis into place, could not guarantee long-term stability.

The problem of an appropriate metallic alloy was solved by two German metallurgists working in the United States. They developed an alloy named Vitallium which had remarkable resistance to interaction with substances found in the body. It was virtually inert and was not rejected by the body. It was extremely hard and durable, difficult to machine, but it could be cast. The metallurgists were able to mold Vitallium into virtually any configuration required by the orthopedic surgeon. The components of a joint were sculpted in wax. The wax model was encased in a hard, heat-proof medium and heated. The wax melted out, leaving a hollow mold into which molten Vitallium was poured. When the mold was removed, the result was a perfect replica of the required bone formation, with appropriate modifications to allow it to be affixed to living bone.

One of the first surgeons to use Vitallium was M. N. Smith-Petersen of Harvard Medical School. He developed the first successful total hip replacement. His procedure, which is quite similar to procedures practiced today, involved replacing both the top of the femur (the thighbone) and the cup in which it rotates with prosthetic devices exactly duplicating the configuration of a healthy hip joint. Since then, many newer and better total hip configurations

Arthroplasty

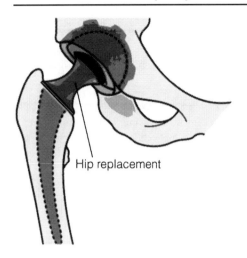

Hip replacement

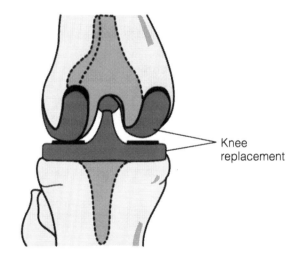

Knee replacement

The hip and knee joints can be replaced by metal or plastic ball-and-socket prostheses when disease or injury is too extensive to repair the existing joints.

have been fashioned. In addition, other joints and individual bone structures have been developed in metal, plastic, and silicone.

USES AND COMPLICATIONS

Arthroplastic surgery as it is known today has been practiced only since the 1930's. Its uses span a wide range of joint problems, and it is successful in relieving pain and deformity in many conditions. Total hip replacements are quite successful, total knee replacements are successful in some patients, and total elbow replacements have been attempted with varying success. Finger bones can be replicated; shoulder and ankle replacements are projected for the future.

Among the major problems and complications of arthroplasty is the progressive nature of rheumatoid arthritis, the chief cause of joint disease. Many arthroplastic procedures are temporary and may have to be repeated, or new procedures may have to be performed to ameliorate the patient's pain, discomfort, and disfigurement as the disease progresses.

As the populations of Western countries continue to live longer, the number of candidates for total joint replacement grows. More patients are receiving total hip replacements, and the incidence of complications is relatively rare. Complications and failures are common, however, with other total joint replacement procedures at this time.

PERSPECTIVE AND PROSPECTS

The success of an arthroplastic surgical procedure is often limited both by the extent of joint damage and by the limitations of current surgical techniques. In the case of massively deformed fingers, for example, there is often little that a surgeon can do.

With damaged knees, many procedures can give the patient relief, such as synovectomy (removal of all or part of the synovial membrane that surrounds the joint). For patients with significant destruction of bone tissue, total knee replacement would be ideal, but this procedure is successful in only about a third of patients.

With total joint replacement, the criteria for success can be severe. For example, in a total hip replacement, the surgeon hopes to promise the patient at least five or six years, or much more, of trouble-free service. For an elderly patient, this may be satisfactory. As total hip surgery is performed on younger patients, however, such a short life span

for the prosthesis is a major concern. Nevertheless, practitioners are optimistic that new techniques and materials will solve the problem.

Arthroplastic surgery has come a long way in a short time. It brings relief and restores mobility in millions of patients. The future holds the promise that many patients who cannot be successfully treated today can be helped tomorrow. —*C. Richard Falcon*

See also Arthritis; Arthroscopy; Bones and the skeleton; Fracture and dislocation; Fracture repair; Hip fracture repair; Kneecap removal; Orthopedic surgery; Orthopedics; Osteoarthritis; Rheumatoid arthritis; Rheumatology; Sports medicine.

FOR FURTHER INFORMATION:

Larson, David E., ed. *Mayo Clinic Family Health Book*. 2d ed. New York: William Morrow, 1996.

Yates, George, and Michael Shermer. *Meeting the Challenge of Arthritis*. Los Angeles: Lowell House, 1990.

ARTHROPOD-BORNE DISEASES

DISEASE/DISORDER

ANATOMY OR SYSTEM AFFECTED: Blood, nervous system, skin

SPECIALTIES AND RELATED FIELDS: Environmental health, epidemiology, public health

DEFINITION: Diseases that employ arthropods as vectors to animal or human hosts.

KEY TERMS:

arbovirus: an abbreviation for "arthropod-borne virus"

enzootic: referring to a disease that maintains itself in an animal reservoir

Arthropod-Borne Viral Diseases

Disease	Principal Vectors
Colorado tick fever	Tick: *Dermacentor andersoni*
Encephalitis, California	Mosquitoes: *Culex tarsalis, Aedes* species
Encephalitis, Eastern equine	Mosquitoes: *Aedes sollicitans, Culiseta melanura*
Encephalitis, Far East Russian	Tick: *Ixodes persulcatus*
Encephalitis, St. Louis	Mosquitoes: *Culex pipiens pipiens, C. p. quinquefasciatus, C. tarsalis*
Encephalitis, Venezuelan	Mosquitoes: *Aedes serratus, Ae. scapularis, Ae. taeniorhynchus, Anopheles aquasalis, Culex vomifer, C. taeniopus, Haemogogus* species, *Mansonia titillans, Psorophora confinnis, P. ferox*
Encephalitis, Western equine	Mosquitoes: *Culex tarsalis* and others
Louping ill	Tick: *Isodes ricinus*
Pappataci or sandfly fever	Sandfly: *Phlebotomus papatasii*
Rift Valley fever	Mosquitoes: *Eretmapodites chrysogaster, Aedes caballus, Ae. deboeri, Ae. circumluteolus, Ae. tarsalis, Culex theileri*
Yellow fever	Mosquitoes: *Aedes aegypti* (urban and jungle strains), *Ae. africanus, Ae. simpsoni, Ae. leucocelaenus, Sabethes chloroterus,* and others

filariasis: infection with filaria, very slender parasitic worms mostly found in the tropics

helminthic: worm-related

host: the organism that harbors a disease agent, usually providing habitat and nourishment and often suffering harm from the infection or infestation

pathogen: a disease-causing agent (usually a virus, bacterium, protozoan, or parasitic worm)

vector: the agent that transfers a disease organism from host to host; may also be an intermediate site of propagation of the disease agent

zoonosis: a disease continuously transmitted in an animal population and for which humans are a side infection

CAUSES AND SYMPTOMS

From the perspective of a disease agent (virus, bacteria, protozoan, or parasitic worm) there are two major problems: adjusting to live in the host organism and avoid its defenses, and moving to new victims when the host eventually dies. Arthropods—the very successful group of small animals that includes mites, ticks, insects, and related organisms—are major vectors that shuttle many diseases to new hosts.

Size is a major factor in the success of arthropods. To both the massive blue whale and the microscopic bacterium, food items and natural media appear fairly uniform. It is at the size of insects and other arthropods that the world is most varied, and their more than one million known species outnumber all other animals and plants together. Because different arthropods live on roots and stems or infest the specific parts of all animals, disease agents that evolved an ability to live in ticks, fleas, or mosquitoes have shared the success of the arthropods. The control of these diseases requires a knowledge of the biology of insects and their relatives in order to interrupt this route of transmission.

Yet disease agents are not simply ingested and expelled by roving mosquitoes. Disease organisms must be finely adapted to survive the harsh gut environment of an insect or be able to migrate across insect membranes, migrate to salivary ducts, or proliferate wildly in the arthropod's own body fluids. Many disease agents simply cannot cross these barriers and are therefore not arthropod-borne. The range of disease agents includes viruses, protozoa, bacteria, and parasitic worms. That such a wide range of organisms have succeeded in using this route of transmission indicates that the strategy of using arthropod vectors has evolved many times.

In a strict sense, viruses are not living entities that can metabolize or move on their own. Merely elegant chunks

Arthropod-Borne Bacterial and Rickettsial Diseases

Disease	Disease Agent	Principal Vectors
Anthrax	*Bacillus anthracis*	Various horse flies by mechanical transmission
Boutonneuse fever	*Rickettsia conori*	Ticks: *Rhipicephalus sanguineus, R. secundus*, and species of *Haemaphysalis, Hyalomma, Amblyomma, Boophilis, Dermacentor*, and *Ixodes*
Carrion's disease	*Bartonella bacilliformis*	*Phlebotomus* sandflies
Food poisoning	*Shigella* and *Salmonella*	Various flies by mechanical transmission
Plague	*Yersinia pestis*	*Xenopsylla cheopis* and some other fleas
Q fever	*Coxiella burneti*	Ixodid ticks
Relapsing fever	*Borrelia*	*Ornithodoros* ticks
Rickettsialpox	*Rickettsia akari*	Mite: *Liponyssoides sanguineus*
Rocky Mountain spotted fever	*Rickettsia rickettsi*	Ticks: *Dermacentor andersoni, D. variabilis, Amblyomma americanus, Haemaphysalis leporispalustris* (rabbit-to-rabbit transmission)
Trench fever	*Rickettsia quintana*	Human body louse *Pediculus humanus humanus*
Tularemia	*Francisella tularensis*	Deer flies and ticks
Typhus, louse-borne	*Rickettsia prowazekii*	Human body louse *Pediculus humanus humanus*
Typhus, murine	*Rickettsia mooseri*	Rat flea *Xenopsylla cheopis*; the rat louse *Polyplax spinulosa* and the tropical rat mite *Ornthonssus bacoti* are zoonotic vectors
Typhus, scrub	*Rickettsia tsutsugamushi*	Mites: *Leptotrombidium akamushi* and *L. deliensis*
Yaws	*Treponema pertenue*	*Hippelates* gnats

of hereditary material protected by protein, viruses resemble living agents and are infectious only when they are taken in and reproduced by host cells. Plant bugs transmit many serious plant virus diseases; likewise a limited number of human viruses are transmitted by arthropods.

Some species of bacteria have adapted to transmission through arthropods. In some cases, they serve as simple mechanical carriers; other insects and ticks serve as true vectors by providing the pathogen with a medium in which to propagate and then actively injecting the bacteria into a new host. Rickettsias are smaller relatives of the bacteria that are particularly adapted for arthropod transmission. Rickettsias develop only inside the cells of susceptible hosts and vectors.

Protozoa are cellular organisms that are more complex than bacteria. Amebic dysentery caused by *Entamoeba histolytica* may occasionally be transmitted mechanically by cockroaches and flies. Yet some of the most serious tropical human afflictions—malaria, sleeping sickness, and leishmaniasis (kala-azar)—are also caused by protozoans. The trypanosomes and *Leishmania* are flagellates that belong to the subphylum Mastigophora; the malaria organisms are part of the Apicomplexa, a group of protozoa specialized for parasitism.

The last group of organisms that are transmitted with the help of arthropods is the parasitic worms. "Worms" is a nonscientific term that includes the flatworms (Trematoda), spiny-headed worms (Acanthocephalans), tapeworms (Cestoda), and roundworms (Nematoda). Many are quite large in size, but those that utilize arthropod vectors have microscopic stages. While most of the nematode parasites need to enter the bloodstream and are vectored by various blood-sucking flies, the other worms—those that mostly target the digestive system—are contracted when people ingest the arthropod host.

The involvement of arthropods in carrying diseases varies greatly. House flies and horseflies may merely pick up bacteria and mechanically transmit it to food or a wound. In such cases, it is difficult to determine accurately the extent to which such casual transmission is involved in diseases. Other arthropods are actually required by the disease agent for the completion of their developmental stages; without some time in the insect's gut, for example, a pathogen may be unable to infect another host. Finally, some arthropods are critical because they seek out and target the host with accuracy.

TREATMENT AND THERAPY

Unlike some viral and bacterial infections that have been thoroughly controlled or even eliminated, most arthropod-borne diseases remain serious health threats, especially in tropical areas. For example, smallpox (which is not insect-borne) was easier to control and eliminate because it only

Arthropod-Borne Protozoan Diseases

Disease	Disease Agent	Principal Vectors
Chagas disease	*Trypanosoma cruzi*	Assassin bugs: *Panstrongylus megistus* and many species of *Triatoma*
Kala-azar	*Leishmania donovani*	Sandflies: *Phlebotomus chinensis, P. major, P. argentipes, P. perniciosus*
Leishmaniasis, American mucocutaneous	*Leishmania braziliensis*	Sandflies: *Phlebotomus intermedius, P. longipalpus, P. pessoai*
Leishmaniasis, Mexican	*Leishmania mexicana*	Sandfly: *Phlebotomus flaviscutellatus*
Malaria, benign tertian	*Plasmodium vivax*	Mosquitoes: species of *Anopheles*
Malaria, malignant tertian	*Plasmodium falciparum*	Mosquitoes: *Anopheles stephensi, A. labranchiae*
Malaria, ovale tertian	*Plasmodium ovale*	Mosquitoes: *Anopheles gambiae, A. funestus*
Malaria, quartan	*Plasmodium malariae*	Mosquitoes: many species of *Anopheles*
Nagana (cattle, etc.)	*Trypanosoma brucei*	Tsetse fly: *Glossina morsitans*
Oriental sore	*Leishmania tropica*	Sandflies: *Phlebotomus papatasii* and *P. sergenti*
Sleeping sickness, East African	*Trypanosoma rhodesiense*	Tsetse flies: *Glossina morsitans* and *G. swynnertoni*
Sleeping sickness, West African	*Trypanosoma gambiense*	Tsetse flies: *Glossina tachinoides* and *G. palpalis*
Surra (camels, etc.)	*Trypanosoma evansi*	Horse flies in the family Tabanidae
Texas cattle fever	*Babesia bigemina*	Ticks: *Boophilus annulatus, B. microplus, B. decoloratus, Haemaphysalus punctata,* and species of *Rhipicephalus*

occurred in humans; it was transferred directly from human to human; a survivor or inoculated person had lifetime immunity from further infection; inoculation was cheap and provided long-term protection; and smallpox was easy to diagnose (few other diseases could be mistaken for it).

In contrast, arthropod-borne diseases generally reside in an animal reservoir. This animal reservoir may provide the natural cycle for the parasite or disease agent; this is known from cases in which the disease agent is mild in its natural animal host, indicating that the organism and the disease have evolved together over a long time. For both parasites and disease agents, mild strains that preserve the host are selected over time, and virulent strains that rapidly kill the host have less chance of surviving themselves. Therefore, when a new arthropod-borne disease appears that is extremely virulent, it is an indication that humans are a new host with little adaptation to the parasite.

Arthropod-borne diseases may be unusually resistant to the human immune system, which usually eliminates invaders in a short time. Some organisms such as malaria *Plas-modium* are constantly changing the stage that they present to the immune system. Parasitic worms, on the other hand, may seal themselves up in cysts or inside protective cuticles and live protected lives. Because one often cannot reach the infective agent in the human body, attempts to control arthropod-borne diseases have centered heavily on interrupting the transmission by the vectors.

Because humans do not form immunity to worms and some other disease agents, an individual can be infected repeatedly. Moreover, the symptoms of many of these diseases are fevers easily confused with other ailments. Thus, in many tropical regions it is the norm for people to have a parasite load. Since the disease agents are generally protected inside the relatively uniform environment of the body of host animals and humans, the fact that many of these diseases do not extend to the temperate areas of the world indicates that harsh winters are important in controlling the range of insect vectors. This fact also explains why tropical diseases do not spread in a temperate country when immigrants bring them: The arthropod vector is absent.

Arthropod-Borne Worm (Helminthic) Diseases

Contracted Through Ingesting Arthropod Host

Disease	Parasite	Arthropod Host
Broad tapeworm	*Dibothriocephalus latus*	Crustaceans eaten by fish that in turn are eaten by humans
Dog tapeworm	*Dipylidium caninum*	Dog flea *Pulex irritans* and lice
Dracunculosus or guinea worm	*Dracunculus medinensis*	Copepod crustaceans: *Cyclops* species
Oriental lung fluke	*Paragonimus westermani*	Snails via crabs and crayfish
Rodent tapeworm	*Hymenolepis diminuta*	Fleas including *Xenopsylla cheopis*; also roaches, moth and beetle larvae
Spiney-headed worm	*Macracanthorhynchus hirudinaceus*	Beetle larvae

Contracted from Blood-Sucking Flies

Disease	Parasite	Principal Vectors
Acanthocheilonemasis	*Acanthocheilonema perstans*	Biting midges: *Culicoides austeni* and *C. grahami*
Bancroft's filariasis	*Wuchereria bancrofti*	Mosquitoes: *Culex pipiens quinquefasciatus* and other *Culex*, *Aedes*, *Anopheles*, and *Mansonia* species
Brug's filariasis	*Brugia malayi*	Mosquitoes: *Mansonia*, *Anopheles*, *Aedes*, and *Armigeres* species
Dog heartworm	*Dirofilaria immitis*	Mosquitoes: *Culex pipiens*, *Aedes aegypti*, and others
Loiasis or African eyeworm	*Loa loa*	Mango flies: *Chrysops dimidiatus* and *C. silaceus*
Onchocerciasis	*Onchocerca volvulus*	Black flies: *Simulium damnosum*, *S. neavei*, *S. ochraceum*, and others
Ozzard's filariasis	*Mansonella ozzardi*	Biting midge *Culicoides furens*

Mosquito-Borne Diseases

Mosquito	Habits	Features	Diseases
Aedes	Day biter, urban or rural	Head bent, body parallel to surface, black and white in color	Dengue, yellow fever, viral encephalitis
Anopheles	Night biter, mainly rural	Head and body in line, at angle to surface	Malaria, filariasis
Culex	Day biter, urban or rural	Shaped like *Aedes* but brown; whines in flight	Viral encephalitis, filariasis

Perspective and Prospects

Following the work of Louis Pasteur and Robert Koch and their students, the late 1800's saw a shift away from a belief in night air miasmas ("malaria" means "bad air") toward germ theory—that disease agents are at the cause of all ailments. Indeed, nutritional deficiencies such as pellagra were even suspected to be caused by some disease agent. Therefore, in 1878 when Patrick Manson observed the development of *Wuchereria bancrofti* in the bodies of *Culex* mosquitoes, it did not take long for him and other workers to prove that this insect was the intermediate host and vector for this medically important worm infection. The discovery of vector-borne diseases gave birth to the field of medical entomology, and a sequence of important discoveries followed: malaria parasites in the blood of humans; tsetse fly transmission of nagana, cattle sleeping sickness, and human sleeping sickness; malaria parasites in mosquitoes; mosquito transmission of yellow fever; transmission of the plague organism through sick rats by fleas; and the role of the body louse in carrying typhus fever (1909).

Whenever science becomes aware of a new infectious disease—as in the cases of Lyme disease, Legionnaires' disease, AIDS, or Hantavirus—the possibility that the disease is arthropod-borne is an early concern. (Of these new diseases, only Lyme disease involves an arthropod vector.) In addition to working out the etiology—the mechanisms by which the disease agent actually causes the illness—it is important to confirm if an insect or mite is spreading the disease in order to put effective control measures into place.

Clues that a new disease may be arthropod-borne could include epidemiological evidence, such as a pattern of disease occurrence that matches the range of a mosquito or the common report of insect bites by all patients. Eventually, confirmation of the role of an arthropod as a vector for the disease will come after extensive clinical work proves the identity of the disease agent and additional laboratory work shows this disease agent to be present in natural populations of the vector. This knowledge proves beneficial when control of arthropod populations results in dramatic improvements in the health of human populations.

—John Richard Schrock, Ph.D.

See also Bites and stings; Elephantiasis; Encephalitis; Epidemiology; Leishmaniasis; Lice, mites, and ticks; Lyme disease; Malaria; Parasitic diseases; Plague; Sleeping sickness; Tropical medicine; Yellow fever; Zoonoses.

For Further Information:

Busvine, James R. *Disease Transmission by Insects: Its Discovery and Ninety Years of Effort to Prevent It*. New York: Springer-Verlag, 1993. Discusses insects as carriers of disease and methods of controlling them.

_____. *Insects, Hygiene, and History*. London: Athlone Press, 1976. An accurate summary of human relationships with ectoparasites, primarily insects and mites. With abundant illustrations and further references to classics in parasite biology.

Desowitz, Robert S. *The Malaria Capers: More Tales of Parasites and People, Research, and Reality*. New York: W. W. Norton, 1991. The best modern overview of how social and political factors are involved in the science of public health medicine is this set of two stories on kala-azar and malaria. Honest false leads in early research contrast with modern research fraud impeding the effort to hold the line against these two major world diseases.

James, Maurice T., and Robert F. Harwood. *Herm's Medical Entomology*. 6th ed. New York: Macmillan, 1969. Entomologists, scientists who study insects, are also called upon to identify noninsect arthropods involved in bites, stings, and vector-transmitted diseases. An authoritative text for training medical entomologists and a standard reference.

Learmonth, Andrew. *Disease Ecology: An Introduction to Ecological Medical Geography*. Oxford, England: Basil Blackwell, 1988. Important chapters on the history of diseases, tropical diseases, mosquito-borne diseases, and onchocerciasis place arthropod-borne diseases in a wider perspective.

McKelvey, John J., Jr., Bruce F. Eldridge, and Karl Maramorosch. *Vectors of Disease Agents: Interactions with Plants, Animals and Man.* New York: Praeger, 1981. Authorities in the biology of vectored diseases explain the problems encountered by disease agents and by humans trying to control their transmission.

Shaw, Michael, ed. *Everything You Need to Know About Diseases.* Springhouse, Pa.: Springhouse Press, 1996. This well-illustrated consumer reference, compiled by more than one hundred doctors and medical experts, describes five hundred illnesses and conditions, their causes, symptoms, diagnosis, treatment, and prevention. A valuable reference book for everyone interested in health and disease.

Snow, Keith R. *Insects and Disease.* New York: John Wiley & Sons, 1974. A clear and simple explanation of the biology of both insects and pathogens.

ARTHROSCOPY

PROCEDURE

ANATOMY OR SYSTEM AFFECTED: Hips, joints, knees, legs

SPECIALTIES AND RELATED FIELDS: Orthopedics, rheumatology

DEFINITION: A technique for examining joints through a thin scope inserted into the joint; it may be used to visualize and perform surgical procedures.

INDICATIONS AND PROCEDURES

The arthroscope is a rigid tube enclosing a series of lenses around which are wrapped glass fibers for transmitting light. The arthroscope is placed inside a larger metal sheath which allows fluid to flow between the components. After disinfecting the skin, the surgeon inserts a cannula (tube) into the desired cavity using an obturator, a prosthetic device which is removed and replaced by the arthroscope.

Instruments passed through the cannula include probes, forceps, knives, scissors, and a variety of clamps. Cutting may be done manually or with a motor-driven tool. The eyepiece of an arthroscope may be replaced by a video camera to allow viewing on a television monitor.

After the skin is prepared and the instruments are inserted, diagnostic or operative procedures are begun. The joint or tissue is thoroughly explored before any further steps are taken. An assistant positions the body part, freeing the surgeon to operate. The most common site for an arthroscopic procedure is the knee; other sites include the elbow, shoulder, and ankle.

After the procedure is completed, the joint is flushed to remove all debris. The instruments are withdrawn, and the skin punctures are closed with a single suture or bandage closure. The patient returns in a week for a postarthroscopic examination and removal of sutures. Rehabilitation is important; it should begin on the day following arthroscopy and can require up to several months, depending on the site and procedure.

USES AND COMPLICATIONS

Arthroscopy is a technique originally developed for diagnosis in joints; it is now used for surgical procedures as well. A thin, tubular arthroscope is inserted into a joint cavity. The surgeon uses a small light and lens on the instrument to see the operative field. Modified instruments can be passed through the tube. In this way, operative procedures can be performed using the arthroscope.

Many simple procedures can be done using local anesthesia, although regional or general anesthesia is preferred. Arthroscopy can be carried out in either a fluid or a gas environment within the joint. A saline solution is often used; it disperses light more evenly but requires a system to pump the fluid in and out. A gas environment is more useful for visualizing surface irregularities of cartilage.

Such techniques have significantly changed orthopedic surgery. The use of arthroscopy for diagnosis and treatment reduces postoperative infections, the time needed for rehabilitation, and costs. Most arthroscopic procedures are now done on an outpatient basis.

—*L. Fleming Fallon, Jr., M.D., M.P.H.*

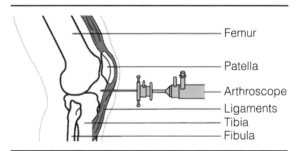

Arthroscopy is a diagnostic procedure in which a fiberoptic instrument is inserted into a joint for direct examination without the complications that accompany a larger incision; sometimes surgical instruments are also passed through the arthroscope.

See also Arthritis; Arthroplasty; Bones and the skeleton; Endoscopy; Fracture and dislocation; Fracture repair; Hip fracture repair; Kneecap removal; Laparoscopy; Orthopedic surgery; Orthopedics; Osteoarthritis; Rheumatoid arthritis; Rheumatology; Sports medicine.

ASPHYXIATION

DISEASE/DISORDER

ANATOMY OR SYSTEM AFFECTED: Lungs, respiratory system

SPECIALTIES AND RELATED FIELDS: Emergency medicine, occupational health

DEFINITION: The state of unconsciousness or death resulting from oxygen deprivation.

The phenomenon whereby the body experiences a decrease in oxygen below normal levels is called hypoxia; extreme cases of hypoxia lead to anoxia, a complete lack of oxygen. The difference between anoxia and asphyxia is that in asphyxia an accumulation of excess carbon dioxide (hypercapnia) takes place, as the normal exchange of oxygen and carbon dioxide in the lungs is obstructed.

Respiration is regulated in the medulla, while chemoreceptors present in the aortic arch and the carotid sinus respond to levels of oxygen, carbon dioxide, and the pH in blood and the cerebrospinal fluid. The concentration of carbon dioxide pressure in the plasma is proportional to the oxygen pressure. Generally, oxygen deprivation may be the consequence of one or more of several conditions. In all cases, damage results that leads first to hypoxia and eventually to death.

Types of oxygen deprivation. In the first condition, respiration may be slowed or stopped by injury or foreign material blocking the air passage. The most common example of this case is asphyxia that results from the inhalation of water by exhausted swimmers or persons who cannot swim. Large quantities of water fill the lung and cut off the oxygen supply. Other examples include the entrapment of food or liquid in the respiratory tract, strangulation, and residence in high altitude. In these cases, the carbon dioxide pressure is drastically increased. Artificial respiration may save the victim's life; it should be performed as soon as possible and after the removal of the inhaled foreign substance via vomiting. Strangulation provides the more serious problem of capillary rupturing and internal bleeding.

A second condition, hypoxic anoxia, is caused by an inadequate concentration of oxygen in the atmosphere, which occurs in poorly ventilated enclosed spaces such as in mine tunnels, sewers, or industrial areas. Odorless gases such as methane (which is produced in decomposing sewage) or nitrogen may be dangerous because they generally go undetected. A former way of detecting such gases involved taking along a bird in a cage and monitoring its well-being during the exploration of unknown caves or ancient tombs.

In anemic anoxia, respiration may not be effective because of the reduced capacity of the blood to become oxygenated; as a result, less oxygen is transferred to the tissues. Carbon monoxide behaves differently than methane or nitrogen, since it binds much more strongly to hemoglobin than oxygen does. Thus the hemoglobin, which is the oxygen-carrying component of blood, does not transfer oxygen to the tissues, which are starved of it. The passage of oxygen from the lung alveoli to the adjacent blood capillaries may also be affected, such as with chronic lung disease, infections, or developmental effects.

A fourth category is stagnant anoxia, whereby a reduced flow of blood through the blood tissues takes place. This may be a generalized condition, attributable to heart disease, or localized, which may take place in a pilot during aerial maneuvers. The blackout of the aviator is a result of the heart's inability to pump enough blood to these regions against the high centrifugal force. In some cases, the carbon dioxide pressure cannot be removed in the usual manner by the lung. Any lung disease will decrease the effective removal of carbon dioxide and therefore result in elevated levels of it in the blood. Thus in emphysema, a disease in which the alveoli increase in size and which leads to a reduction of the surface area available for gas exchange, carbon dioxide will be retained in the blood. In bronchopneumonia, the alveoli contain secretions, white cells, bacteria, and fibrin, which prevent an efficient gas exchange.

In histotoxic anoxia, the failure of cellular respiration is observed. The body's cells are unable to utilize oxygen as a result of poisoning, as from cyanide. The supply of oxygen is normal, but the cells are unable to metabolize the oxygen that is delivered to them.

Symptoms. All cases of anoxia may lead to oxygen deprivation in the brain, which may be fatal if it lasts more than a few minutes. Nerve cell degeneration may start and continue, despite the fact that the original cause of anoxia is removed and normal breathing is resumed. Many health conditions may interfere with the blood transport of oxygen, which is accomplished via the red blood cells. Such diseases include cases of anemia, trauma, hemorrhage, and circulatory disease.

The body responds toward oxygen deprivation with an increase in the rate of depth of breathing. The normal, sea-level oxygen pressure of the air is approximately 160 millimeters (6.2 inches) of mercury. When the oxygen pressure is reduced to 110 millimeters (4.2 inches) of mercury at an altitude of about 3,000 meters (10,000 feet), the pulse rate increases and the volume of blood pumped from the heart also increases. Although prolonged exposure to low oxygen pressure may bring the pulse rate back to normal, the output of the heart remains elevated. Despite the lack of oxygen, both the heart and the brain function because of the dilation of their blood cells and the increased oxygen extraction from the blood. Anoxia leads to vision problems first, while hearing is generally the last sense to go. It is not unusual for a person who is suffering from anoxia to be incapable of moving but able to hear.

—Soraya Ghayourmanesh, Ph.D.

See also Altitude sickness; Apnea; Asthma; Choking; Emphysema; Lungs; Pulmonary medicine; Pulmonary medicine, pediatric; Respiration; Resuscitation; Unconsciousness.

ASTHMA
DISEASE/DISORDER
ANATOMY OR SYSTEM AFFECTED: Chest, immune system, lungs, respiratory system
SPECIALTIES AND RELATED FIELDS: Environmental health, immunology, pulmonary medicine

DEFINITION: A chronic inflammatory obstructive pulmonary disease that obstructs the airways to the lungs and makes it difficult or, in severe attacks, nearly impossible to breathe.

KEY TERMS:

allergen: any substance that causes an overreaction of the immune system; also called an antigen

allergic reaction: the presence of adverse symptoms that are part of the body's overreaction to an antigen

allergy: an overreaction of the immune system to a substance that does not affect the general population; the tendency to be allergic is inherited

beta-agonists: chemicals that attach to the beta-receptors on cells; often used in inhalers, they cause the bronchioles to dilate, or open

bronchioles: small air tubes leading to the air sacs of the lungs; the functional units of the airway that are involved in asthma

mast cells: cells in connective tissue capable of releasing chemicals that cause allergic reactions

trigger: the substance or event that sets off an asthma attack; triggers may be allergens or some other type of stimulus

CAUSES AND SYMPTOMS

Asthma is a Greek word meaning "grasping" or "panting." It is a chronic obstructive pulmonary (lung) disease that involves repeated attacks in which the airways in the lungs are suddenly blocked. The disease is not completely understood, but asthma attacks cause the person to experience tightening of the chest, sudden breathlessness, wheez-

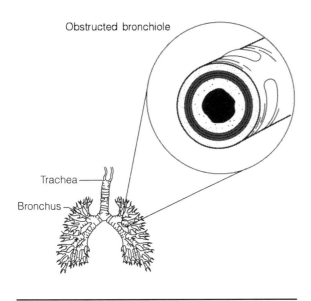

During an asthma attack, obstructed bronchioles limit or halt airflow, resulting in severely restricted breathing.

ing, and coughing. Death by asphyxiation is rare but possible. Fortunately, the effects can be reversed with proper medication. The severity of symptoms and attacks varies greatly among individuals, and sufferers can be located on a continuum running from mild to severe. Mild asthmatics have fewer than six minimal attacks per year, with no symptoms between attacks, and they require no hospitalizations and little or no medication between attacks. Severe asthmatics have more than six serious attacks each year, have symptoms between attacks, lose more than ten school days or workdays, and require two or more hospitalizations per year. Attacks are typically spaced with symptom-free intervals but may also occur continuously. Rather than focusing only on the specific attacks, one should view and treat asthma as a chronic disease, a nagging, continuing condition that persists over a long period of time.

A review of the path of air into the body during normal breathing helps in understanding asthma. During inhalation, air travels into the nose and mouth and then into the trachea (windpipe); it then divides into the two tubes called bronchi and enters the lungs. Inside each lung, the tubes become smaller and continue to divide. The air finally moves into the smallest tubes, called bronchioles, and then flows into the millions of small, thin-walled sacs called alveoli. Vital gas exchange occurs in the alveoli.

This gas exchange involves two gases in particular, oxygen and carbon dioxide. Oxygen must cross the membrane of the alveoli into the blood and then travel to all the cells of the body. Within the cells, it is used in chemical reactions that produce energy. These same reactions produce carbon dioxide as a by-product, which is returned by the blood to the alveoli. This gas is removed from the body through the same pathway that brought oxygen into the lungs.

The parts of this airway that are involved in asthma are the bronchioles. These tubes are wrapped with smooth, involuntary muscles that adjust the amount of air that enters. The lining of the bronchioles also contains many cells that secrete a substance called mucus. Mucus is a thick, clear, slimy fluid produced in many parts of the body. Normal production of mucus in the lungs catches foreign material and lubricates the pathway to allow smooth airflow. People suffering from asthma have very sensitive bronchioles.

Three pathological processes in the bronchioles contribute to an asthma attack. One is an abnormal sensitivity and constriction of the involuntary muscles surrounding the airways, which narrows the diameter of the airway. Another is an inflammation and swelling of the tissues that make up the bronchioles themselves. The third is an increased production of mucus, which then blocks the airways. These three mechanisms may work in combination and are largely caused by the activation of mast cells in the airways. The result can be extreme difficulty in taking air into the lungs until the attack subsides. The characteristic "wheeze" of asthma is caused by efforts to exhale, which is more difficult than inhaling. In the most serious attacks, the airways may close down to the point of suffocating the patient if medical help is not given.

Attacks can vary in severity at different times because of variations in tension within the bronchiole muscles. Although there is still debate about the general function of these muscles, they probably help to distribute the air entering the alveoli evenly. Control of the tension in these smooth muscles is involuntary and follows a circadian (twenty-four-hour) rhythm influenced by neurohormonal control. Accordingly, for most people this cycle causes maximum constriction to occur at about 6:00 A.M. and maximum relaxation to occur at about 6:00 P.M. Hence, asthma attacks tend to be more severe in the late night and early morning.

Following a given asthma attack, patients are sometimes susceptible to additional, more severe attacks. This period of high risk, called a late-phase response, occurs five or six hours after the initial symptoms pass and may last as long as several days. Some researchers believe that the increase in deaths from asthma in the United States may be tied to this danger, which often goes unrecognized.

The initial cause and mechanism of an asthma attack can vary from person to person. Accordingly, asthma is usually divided into two types. One type is extrinsic, that is, caused by external triggers that bring about an allergic response. Allergic reactions involve the immune system. Normal functioning of the immune system guards the body against harmful substances. With an allergy, the body incorrectly identifies a harmless substance as harmful and reacts against it. This substance is then called an allergen. If the symptoms of this reaction occur in the lungs, the person has extrinsic or allergic asthma. Pollens, dust, dust mites, animal dander, molds, cockroaches, and feathers are common allergens.

When allergens enter the body, the white blood cells make specific IgE antibodies that can bond with the invaders. Next, the IgE antibodies attach to the surfaces of mast cells; these cells are found all over the body and are numerous in the lungs. The allergens attach to the IgE antibodies located on the mast cells, and the mast cells are stimulated to produce and release chemicals called mediators, such as histamine, prostaglandin D_2, and leukotrienes. These mediators cause sneezing, tighten the muscles in the bronchioles, swell the surrounding tissues, and increase mucus production.

The second type of asthma is intrinsic and does not involve allergies. People who suffer from intrinsic asthma have hyperactive or twitchy airways that overreact to irritating factors. The mechanism for this form is not always understood, but no IgE antibodies for the irritant are placed on the mast cells. Examples of such nonallergic stimuli are cigarette smoke, house dust, artificial coloring, aspirin, ozone, or cold air. Odors from insecticides, cleaning fluids,

cooking foods, and perfume can also trigger attacks. Also included in this category are attacks that are caused by viral infections (including colds and flu), stress, and exercise. Asthma can be triggered by many different substances and events in different people. While the symptoms are the same whether the asthma is intrinsic or extrinsic, asthmatics need to identify what substances or events trigger their attacks in order to gain control of the disease.

Why people develop asthma is not well understood. Asthma can begin at any age, but it is more likely to arise in childhood. While it is known that heredity predisposes an individual to asthma, the pattern of inheritance is not a simple one. Most geneticists now regard allergies as polygenic, which means that more than one pair of genes is involved. Height, skin color, and intelligence are other examples of polygenic traits. Exposure to particular external conditions may also be important. The children who develop asthma are more likely to be boys, while girls are more likely to show signs of the disease at puberty (about age twelve). Childhood asthma is also most likely to disappear or to be "outgrown" at puberty; about half of the cases of childhood asthma eventually disappear.

Early exposures to some triggers may be a key in the development of asthma. Smoking by mothers can cause children with a genetic disposition to develop asthma. Apparently, the early exposure to secondhand smoke develops an allergy. Early studies in this area were confusing until the data were sorted by level of education. Lung specialist Fernando Martinez of the University of Arizona believes that less-educated women who smoke are more likely to cause this effect because their homes are likely to be smaller and therefore expose the children to more smoke. Another study, this one in Great Britain, indicated that more frequent and thorough housecleaning might keep children from developing asthma. Early exposure by genetically susceptible children to dust and the mites that thrive in dust may also cause some to develop asthma.

Asthma is a major health problem in the United States. As many as 20 million Americans may have the disease, and the number has been mysteriously increasing since 1970. While attacks can cause complications, there is no permanent damage to the lungs themselves, as there is in emphysema. Complications include possible lung collapse, infections, chronic dilation, rib fracture, a permanently enlarged chest cavity, and respiratory failure. Furthermore, millions of days of work and school are lost as victims recuperate; asthma is the leading cause of missed school days. Even though attacks can be controlled by medication, occasionally fatalities do occur. The total number of deaths from asthma in the United States reached 4,600 in 1987.

TREATMENT AND THERAPY

The key to gaining control of asthma is discovering the particular factors that act as triggers for an attack in a given individual. These factors vary and at times can be surprising; for example, one person found that a mint flavoring in a particular toothpaste was a trigger for his asthma. Nevertheless, most common triggers fall in the following groups: allergies; irritants, including dust, fumes, odors, and vapors; air pollution, temperature, and dryness; colds and flu; and stress. Even types of food may be important. Diets low in vitamin C, fish, or a zinc-to-copper ratio, as well as diets with a high sodium-to-potassium ratio, seem to increase the risk of asthma attacks and bronchitis. There have also been correlations between low niacin levels in the diet and tight airways and wheezing.

Various medications are available to keep the airways open and to lower their sensitivity. In an emergency, drugs may be injected, but medications are usually either inhaled or taken orally as pills. Because inhaling transports the medication directly to the lungs, lower doses can be used. Many asthmatics carry inhalers, which allow them to breathe in the medication during an attack. Because this action requires a person to coordinate inhaling with the release of the spray, young children are sometimes better off with a device that requires them to wear a mask. The choice and dosage of medicine vary with the patient, and physicians need to determine what is safest and most effective for each individual. Self-treatment with nonprescription drugs should be avoided.

Some of the most commonly prescribed drugs are bronchodilators, inflammation reducers, and trigger-sensitivity reducers. The bronchodilators include albuterol, metaproterenol, and terbutaline. They are beta-agonists that mimic the way in which the body's nervous system relaxes or dilates the airways. (Any drug that functions as a beta-blocker should be avoided by asthmatics because of its opposite effects.) Another bronchodilator is adrenaline (or epinephrine), but it is a less specific drug that also affects the heart and pulse rate. Theophylline, a stimulant chemically related to caffeine, relaxes the airways and also helps clear mucus. The use of corticosteroids (or steroids) for asthma has been increasing because they reduce inflammation and relax airways. Initially, corticosteroids were used if other drugs were ineffective, but in 1991 they were strongly recommended for long-term preventive use. As another way of addressing asthma as a long-term problem, cromolyn sodium is sometimes inhaled on a daily basis to prevent attacks by decreasing sensitivity to triggers.

The concern for safety with these medications increases when asthmatics use high doses (more than two hundred inhalations monthly) of beta-agonist inhalers. A higher risk of fatal or near-fatal attacks has been found with a high usage of fenoterol, a beta-agonist that is not used in the United States. Paul Scanlon, a chest physician at the Mayo Clinic, warns that individuals should not exceed their prescribed dosage when using an inhaler. An individual who feels the need to use an inhaler more often to obtain adequate relief should see a doctor. The increased need is a

sign of worsening asthma, and a doctor needs to investigate and perhaps change the treatment.

Some doctors have improved their diagnosis of asthma with a tool called the peak flow meter. The meter can also be used by patients at home to predict impending attacks. This inexpensive device measures how fast air can be moved out of the lungs. Therefore, it can be discovered that airways are beginning to tighten before other symptoms occur. The early warning allows time to adjust medications to head off attacks. This tool can help asthmatics take charge of their disease.

Research is continuing with a new family of drugs that interfere with the chemical moderators, such as leukotriene, released by mast cells. Two drugs, zileuton and MK-571, have shown promise. Zileuton interferes with leukotriene production in the mast cells. MK-571 does not affect production but blocks the receptor sites for leukotriene on the smooth muscle. Zileuton reduced the feeling of congestion in volunteers in one experiment and allowed another group to withstand much more cold air before having an attack. MK-571 reduced airway constriction by about 70 percent during a stationary bicycle test. This line of research represents a hopeful new direction for asthma sufferers.

Over-the-counter drugs are often used by asthmatics to treat their symptoms. These drugs often use ephedrine, metaraminol, phenylephrine, methoxamine, or similar chemicals. All these drugs are structurally related to amphetamine or adrenaline. Unfortunately, some people may be getting relief without discovering the cause of their asthma. The National Asthma Education Panel (NAEP) maintains that self-treatment without a doctor's guidance is risky.

That asthmatics should generally avoid exercise is a myth. With a doctor's approval, regular sports and exercise may be pursued. Furthermore, exercise may be helpful in reducing the frequency and severity of attacks. Many athletes compete at high levels in spite of their asthma. An outstanding example is Olympic gold medalist Jackie Joyner-Kersee, who is asthmatic and who was named the best all-around female athlete in the world in 1988. Another is Jeanette Bolden, who had been especially affected as a child but sprinted to an Olympic gold medal in 1984. Sports that do not require continuous activity or exposure to cold, dry air are preferred. Swimming is considered ideal. Doctors can help the athlete with a pre-exercise medication plan and a backup plan if symptoms occur during or after the exercise.

Another damaging belief about asthma needs comment. Early Freudian psychology held that asthma could be caused by a mother who failed to answer her baby's crying. Accordingly, the onset of asthma, with its gasping for air, was seen as a continuation of that crying. This sad hypothesis is false: Asthma is not connected to any abnormal relationships between mother and child, and it is not caused by early or deep psychological problems.

Researchers continue to search for new ways to reduce the frequency and the effects of asthmatic attacks. The National Heart, Lung, and Blood Institute in Bethesda, Maryland, found that caffeine in coffee seems to help. The study showed that asthmatics who are regular coffee drinkers suffer one-third fewer symptoms (particularly, less wheezing) than those who do not drink coffee. The most promise, however, seems to be in developing a new line of drugs that will prevent the mast cells from releasing their chemicals. Such a medication could stop inflammation before it takes hold, either by curbing the production of leukotrienes or by preventing these chemicals from acting on the airways.

PERSPECTIVE AND PROSPECTS

Asthma was recognized in ancient times in both the East and the West. The Chinese people have a rich collection of traditional remedies going back more than two thousand years that includes the use of *ma huang*, an Asiatic species of the genus *Ephedra*, for asthma and other lung conditions. *Ma huang* is a vinelike, shrubby, almost leafless gymnosperm. In 1887, the alkaloid ephedrine was isolated from *Ephedra* as the active ingredient in the plant; the drug is similar in effect to adrenaline. Alkaloids are bitter in taste and often affect the nervous system. Scientists used the ending *-ine* to identify alkaloids, many of which have strong physiological effects on humans (such as caffeine, morphine, nicotine, and cocaine). *Ma huang* was used in both ancient China and India.

Pliny the Elder (A.D. 23-79) believed that everything had been created for the sake of humans and therefore that nature was a complete storehouse of natural remedies. His encyclopedia *Historia Naturalis* recommended ephedron, a source of ephedrine, for asthma, coughing, and hemorrhages. Some believe that Pliny may have suffered from asthma. He died from the fumes of Mount Vesuvius while investigating the volcano and trying to help refugees.

In the eighteenth century, the discovery of oxygen, nitrous oxide, and other gases led to serious efforts to determine medical uses for these gases. Inhalation allowed a gaseous medication to be removed as soon as the effect was achieved; precise dosage did not have to be calculated. There were legitimate efforts to find painkillers for surgery and dentistry. Soon charlatans falsely claimed, however, to be able to use the new gases to cure asthma and other diseases. Anesthetics such as ether, nitrous oxide, and chloroform were used by doctors in the 1850's to treat asthma and other conditions.

As early as 1190, Maimonides, the physician to the court of Sladin, the sultan of Egypt, noted that asthma tended to run in families. Unfortunately, Maimonides' thoughts about heredity were forgotten until much later. Early in the twentieth century, researchers did find that 48 percent of the asthmatics surveyed had an immediate family history of allergies.

In 1991, the NAEP, a federal panel of experts brought together by the National Heart, Lung, and Blood Institute, issued the first national guidelines for the diagnosis and treatment of asthma. These guidelines recommended that doctors should not approach asthma as treatment for the attacks alone. Rather, NAEP experts urged a focus on long-term prevention, increasing the use of inhaled steroids especially with severe and moderate asthmatics. The report also urged increased use of the peak flow meter to predict attacks.
—*Paul R. Boehlke, Ph.D.*
updated by Shih-Wen Huang, M.D.

See also Allergies; Asphyxiation; Environmental diseases; Lungs; Pulmonary diseases; Pulmonary medicine; Pulmonary medicine, pediatric; Respiration.

FOR FURTHER INFORMATION:

Haas, François, and Sheila Sperber Haas. "Living with Asthma." In *The World Book Medical Encyclopedia*. Chicago: World Book, 1988. This special report carefully explains the disease and encourages asthmatics to take control of their lives. A chart details how a house can be asthma-proofed. Side effects and drawbacks of various drugs are charted.

Krementz, Jill. *How It Feels to Fight for Your Life*. Boston: Little, Brown, 1989. A collection of fourteen case studies of children who have serious chronic diseases. In one chapter, Anton Broekman, a ten-year-old, describes what living with asthma is like.

Ostrow, Williams, and Vivian Ostrow. *All About Asthma*. Morton Grove, Ill.: Albert Whitmany, 1989. A children's book written to inform and encourage. The writers, a boy and his mother, tell about his experience with asthma. He explains causes, symptoms, and ways to lead a normal life. A must for children with asthma.

Paul, Glennon H., and Barbara A. Fafoglia. *All About Asthma and How to Live with It*. New York: Sterling, 1988. A valuable book with tips for coping with asthma at home, in school, and in the workplace. The chapter on drugs is very helpful, pointing out both benefits and risks.

Weinstein, Allan M. *Asthma: The Complete Guide to Self-Management of Asthma and Allergies for Patients and Their Families*. New York: Fawcett Crest, 1987. An excellent guide to asthma which contains an extensive section on the identification of triggers that may be causing an individual's attacks.

ASTIGMATISM

DISEASE/DISORDER

ANATOMY OR SYSTEM AFFECTED: Eyes

SPECIALTIES AND RELATED FIELDS: Ophthalmology, optometry

DEFINITION: An astigmatism is a relatively common condition in which either the cornea of the eye or the lens is not symmetrical, being flatter or more curved in some places. The vision is blurred because the image that reaches the retina is distorted or out of focus. Astigmatism may occur in combination with myopia (nearsight-edness) or hyperopia (farsightedness). The condition can be corrected by placing a cylindrical lens (such as an eyeglass or contact lens) in front of the eye in order to focus the image on the retina.

—*Jason Georges and Tracy Irons-Georges*

Astigmatism results when either the cornea or the lens is irregular, distorting the image that reaches the retina.

See also Eye surgery; Eyes; Myopia; Ophthalmology; Optometry; Sense organs; Visual disorders.

ATAXIA
DISEASE/DISORDER
ANATOMY OR SYSTEM AFFECTED: Muscles, musculoskeletal system, nervous system

SPECIALTIES AND RELATED FIELDS: Neurologists

DEFINITION: Ataxia is characterized by an inability to coordinate the muscles in voluntary movement. The sufferer may have an awkward, unsteady gait with little balance, jerky movement of the limbs, and slurred speech. It may have many causes, ranging from brain damage from a stroke or tumor to a disorder of the inner ear to excessive alcohol consumption. The symptoms are much more severe and longer lasting, if not permanent, when the cause is neurological, as with brain disorders or multiple sclerosis.
—*Jason Georges and Tracy Irons-Georges*

See also Alcoholism; Brain; Brain disorders; Ears; Multiple sclerosis; Muscle sprains, spasms, and disorders; Muscles; Strokes and TIAs.

ATHLETE'S FOOT
DISEASE/DISORDER
ANATOMY OR SYSTEM AFFECTED: Feet, skin

SPECIALTIES AND RELATED FIELDS: Dermatology, family practice, podiatry, sports medicine

DEFINITION: Athlete's foot is a contagious fungal infection of the skin on the feet. It usually affects the soles of the feet and can be identified by moist, grayish or red scales,

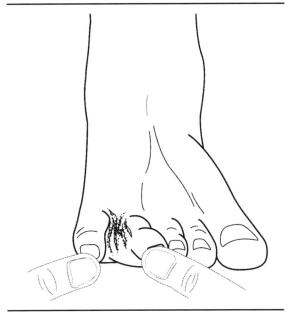

Athlete's foot can be identified by the itchy scaling that appears between the toes.

especially between the toes. Sometimes, small blisters may form. It is common for itching to occur in inflamed areas. Athlete's foot is caused by infection by a trichophyton fungus, which can occur with poor hygiene and/or hot or humid weather. Symptoms can be treated by keeping the affected areas cool and dry. Additionally, nonprescription medication may be applied after cleansing.   —*Jason Georges and Tracy Irons-Georges*
See also Foot disorders; Fungal infections; Lower extremities; Skin; Skin disorders.

ATTENTION-DEFICIT DISORDER (ADD)
DISEASE/DISORDER
ANATOMY OR SYSTEM AFFECTED: Brain, nervous system, psychic-emotional system
SPECIALTIES AND RELATED FIELDS: Family practice, genetics, neurology, pediatrics, psychiatry, psychology
DEFINITION: A condition characterized by an inability to focus attention or to inhibit impulsive, hyperactive behavior; it is associated with poor academic performance and behavioral problems in children.
KEY TERMS:
antianxiety medication: a medication that acts in the brain to decrease a negative reaction to stress and anxiety
antidepressant: a medication that acts in the brain to decrease a sad or depressed mood
nervous system: the system in the body, including the brain, that receives and interprets stimuli and transmits impulses to other organs; the brain is the center of thinking and behavior
neurotransmitter: a chemical in the brain that sends a signal from one brain cell to another
nontraditional therapy: a form of treatment that has not been generally accepted by the scientific professional community as a result of lack of scientifically proved usefulness

CAUSES AND SYMPTOMS
Most experts think that 2 to 5 percent of children may have attention-deficit disorder (ADD), which is also known as attention-deficit hyperactivity disorder (ADHD). The cause of ADD is unknown, although the fact that it often occurs in families suggests some degree of genetic inheritance. The condition is more common in boys, but it does occur in girls. ADD is usually diagnosed when a child enters school, but it may be discovered earlier. Adolescents and even adults who escaped earlier detection may be diagnosed when their symptoms cause particularly severe problems. Some causes of ADD that have been suggested, but never proved, include low blood sugar, food additives, the sweetener aspartame, allergies, and vitamin deficiencies.

Children who do not have ADD may, at times, have some of the symptoms of this disorder, but children who can be diagnosed with ADD must have most of the symptoms most of the time—in school, at home, or during other activities.

The symptoms are usually grouped into three main categories: inattention, hyperactivity, and impulsiveness.

Children who have symptoms of inattention often make careless mistakes at school or do not pay close attention to details in play or work. They may have problems sustaining attention over time and frequently do not seem to listen when spoken to, especially in groups. Children with ADD have difficulty following instructions and often fail to finish chores or schoolwork. They do not organize well and may have messy rooms and desks at school. They also frequently lose things necessary for play or school. Because they have trouble sustaining attention, children with ADD dislike tasks that require this skill and will try to avoid them. One of the key symptoms is distractibility, which means that children with ADD are often paying attention to extraneous sights, sounds, smells, and thoughts rather than focusing on the task that they should be doing. Particularly frustrating to parents is the symptom of forgetfulness in daily activities, in spite of numerous reminders from parents about such common, everyday activities as dressing, hygiene, manners, and other behaviors. Children with ADD have a poor sense of time; they are frequently late or think that they have more time to do a task than they really do.

Not all children with ADD have symptoms of hyperactivity, but many have problems with fidgeting, or squirming. It is common for these children to be constant talkers, often interrupting others. Other symptoms of hyperactivity include leaving their seat in school, church, or similar settings and running around excessively in situations where they should be still. Children with ADD have difficulty playing quietly, although they may watch television or play video games for long periods of time. Some of these children seem to be driven by a motor, or are continuously on the go.

All children with ADD will have some symptoms of impulsiveness, such as blurting out answers before questions are completed or intruding on others by "butting in." They often have difficulty standing in lines or waiting for their turn in games.

Russell A. Barkley reports in his book *Taking Charge of ADHD* (1995) that ADD "is a developmental disorder of self-control. It consists of problems with attention span, impulse control, and activity level." He also states that ADD is "reflected in impairment in a child's will or capacity to control his or her own behavior relative to the passage of time—to keep future goals and consequences in mind." Children with ADD often make the same mistakes repeatedly because they lack hindsight and forethought. Their primary problem is not that they cannot pay attention but that they pay attention to everything. Consequently, they cannot focus on the most important sensory input, such as a parent's order or a teacher's assignment.

It is important to recognize that children with ADD are not bad children who are hyperactive, impulsive, and inattentive on purpose. Rather, they are usually bright children who would like to behave better and to be more successful in school, in social life with peers, and in family affairs, but they simply cannot. One way to think about ADD is to consider it a disorder of the ability to inhibit impulsive, off-task, or undesirable attention. Consequently, the child with ADD cannot separate important from unimportant stimuli and cannot sort appropriate from inappropriate responses to those stimuli. It is easy to understand how someone whose brain is trying to respond to a multitude of stimuli, rather than sorting stimuli into priorities for response, will have difficulty focusing and maintaining attention to the main task.

It is also important to remember that it is not only the presence of symptoms that categorizes a child as having ADD but also the intensity and prevalence of the symptoms in more than one setting. For example, a child may not seem to pay attention in school and often be disruptive in class but be a normal child at home, playing Little League baseball, and in church school. This child may have a learning disability without ADD or a specific conflict with the teacher.

Children most likely to be diagnosed correctly with ADD will have many of the following characteristics. They will have a short attention span, particularly for activities that are not fun or entertaining. They will be unable to concentrate because they will be distracted by peripheral stimuli. They will have poor impulse control so that they seem to act on the spur of the moment. They will be hyperactive and usually rather clumsy, resulting in their being labeled "accident-prone." They will certainly have school problems, especially when classwork requires more thinking and planning—often seen about third grade and beyond. They may display attention-demanding behavior and/or show resistant or overpowering social behaviors. Last, children with ADD often act as if they were younger, and "immaturity" is a frequent label. Along with this trait, they have wide mood swings and are seen as very emotional.

Many experts think that ADD is a developmental problem, caused by the failure of the brain and nervous system to grow and mature normally. Most people would agree that an average, normal two-year-old child is a perfect definition for ADD: short attention span, impulsive, distracted by almost anything new, highly emotional, demanding, often clumsy and reckless, unable to plan well, and sometimes aggressive. All these characteristics are acceptable for the toddler. When those symptoms persist into and beyond kindergarten, however, an unusually slow brain and nervous system development seems likely. This slow development may improve during childhood or may persist into adolescence.

Adolescents who have ADD are usually not hyperactive, although they may have problems with impulsive talking and behavior. They have considerable difficulty complying with rules and following directions. They may be poorly organized, causing problems both with starting projects and with completing them. Their inability to monitor their own behavior leads to problems making and keeping friends and causes them to have conflicts with parents and teachers beyond those normally seen in teenagers. Adolescents with ADD usually have problems in school in spite of average or above-average potential. They may have poor self-esteem and a low frustration tolerance.

Several other neurologic or psychiatric disorders have symptoms that can overlap with ADD, so diagnosis is often difficult. When a child is suspected of having ADD, he or she should have a thorough medical interview with, and physical examination by, a physician familiar with child development, ADD, and related conditions. A psychological evaluation to determine intelligence quotient (IQ) and areas of learning and performance strengths and weaknesses should be obtained. School records need to be reviewed, and teachers may be asked to submit rating forms or similar instruments to document school performance. A thorough family history and a discussion of family problems such as divorce, violence, alcoholism, or drug abuse should be part of the evaluation. Other conditions that might be found to exist along with ADD, or to be the underlying cause of symptoms thought to be ADD, include oppositional defiant disorder, conduct disorder (usually seen in older children), depression, or anxiety disorder. Some physicians, teachers, psychologists, and parents do not believe that ADD is a "real" condition, but this disorder is usually widely accepted in the United States as a credible diagnosis for a child who demonstrates many of the above symptoms at home, at play, and at school.

TREATMENT AND THERAPY

The medical treatment of ADD is one of the most controversial issues in education and in medicine. Although scientific studies clearly show the value of certain medications, and scores of parents and teachers have noticed remarkable improvement with treatment, some people take issue with using medications to change a child's behavior. Clearly, medications alone are not the answer for ADD. Families and children need guidance and support in the form of counseling, as well as considerable information about the condition. Special accommodations can be arranged with most schools and are mandated by federal law. Once educational adjustments have been made and counseling is in place, however, medications can play an important role.

The most frequently prescribed medications are stimulants; they include dexedrine, methylphenidate (Ritalin), and a combination of dexedrine salts (Adderall). A similar medication, pemoline (Cylert), has been related to side effects, which may limit its usefulness. The stimulant medications may function by influencing chemicals in the brain called neurotransmitters, which help transmit messages among brain and nerve cells. In ADD, it is thought that the medications improve the function of cells that direct the brain to focus attention, resist distraction, control behavior, and perceive time correctly. These medications are generally thought to be safe and effective, although they can have such adverse effects as headache, stomachache, mood changes, heart rate changes, appetite suppression, and interference with going to sleep. All children receiving medication must be monitored at regular intervals by a physician.

Other medications that may be used for ADD include antidepressants and antianxiety medications. Some children are treated with combinations of two medications; in unusual circumstances, there may be even more than two. Some of these medications are Imipramine and Desipramine, antidepressants that act mainly to control impulsiveness and hyperactivity; Bupropion, an antidepressant, and Buspar, an antianxiety medicine, both of which have been used largely in older children and adolescents; and clonidine and guanfacine, which work on brain nerve message transmitters and are sometimes helpful in calming aggressive behavior.

Several nontraditional therapies can be used for ADD, but no scientific proof exists that any of them are useful. Some of the nontraditional therapies are sensory integration therapy, vision therapy (using tinted lenses to help with reading), and taking extra vitamins or using "natural" products, usually sold in health food stores, by local, independent distributors, or over the Internet. Parents of children with ADD may read untrue statements in the media about the dangers of medication, and they may receive numerous suggestions from friends and relatives about the benefits of one or another of the nontraditional therapies. Costs and risks for adverse effects should be discussed with the physician who has made the diagnosis of ADD before implementing any treatment, to ensure safety and a reasonable expectation of efficacy.

PERSPECTIVE AND PROSPECTS

Attention-deficit disorder remains controversial, largely because of the subjective nature of its symptoms. For about 5 percent of all children and adolescents, however, ADD is a real issue that can cause great harm if not recognized and managed correctly. Diagnosis should be based on documentation of the child's and family's history, careful examination, and educational and psychological assessment. Treatment should always include educational accommodations and counseling for the child and the family. When symptoms create problems at home and at school, properly prescribed and managed medications have been shown to offer great relief in most cases.

Children and parents in the United States can share experiences and resources through organizations that aim to assist families who are dealing with attention-deficit disorder. The national organization Children and Adults with Attention Deficit Disorder (CHADD) has state and local chapters helping families cope with the condition. CHADD chapters often have libraries and provide resources on ADD. Learning Disabilities Association of America (LDA) has state and local chapters helping schools and families cope with a wide range of learning disabilities, including ADD. —*Robert W. Block, M.D.*

See also Anxiety; Brain; Brain disorders; Emotions, biomedical causes and effects of; Learning disabilities; Pediatrics; Psychiatry, child and adolescent; Puberty and adolescence; Stress.

FOR FURTHER INFORMATION:

Barkley, Russell A. *Taking Charge of ADHD.* New York: Guilford Press, 1995. A comprehensive guide for parents that discusses how to understand ADD, how to be a successful parent, how to cope with the child at home and at school, and how to evaluate medications.

Block, Robert W., and Elaine King Miller. "The Maladroit Adolescent: Learning Disorders and Attentional Deficits." In *Advances in Pediatrics.* Vol. 33. Chicago: Year Book Medical Publishers, 1986. This article was written for parents as well as for medical and educational professionals. It describes ADD and several learning disabilities and recommends appropriate interventions.

Wender, Paul H. *The Hyperactive Child, Adolescent, and Adult.* New York: Oxford University Press, 1987. This book offers concise information about ADD in children, adolescents, and adults. Clearly defines the characteristics of individuals with symptoms of ADD and discusses the reasons for using medications.

Zeigler Dendy, Chris A. *Teenagers with ADD: A Parents' Guide.* Bethesda, Md.: Woodbine House, 1995. This resource is a workbook for parents and teachers of adolescents who have ADD. Includes useful lists of problem behaviors at home and at school, with practical solutions to these problems.

AUDIOLOGY

SPECIALTY

ANATOMY OR SYSTEM AFFECTED: Ears

SPECIALTIES AND RELATED FIELDS: Neurology, otorhinolaryngology, speech pathology

DEFINITION: The study of the auditory system and its measurement, including the assessment of the medical, surgical, or rehabilitation implications arising from a number of disorders affecting hearing.

KEY TERMS:

audiologist: one who is specifically trained at an approved institution of learning to provide diagnostic testing and rehabilitative training to those with hearing disorders

audiometer: a calibrated electronic device for the purpose of measuring human hearing to determine the magnitude of loss and the probable rehabilitative course

auditory system: the human hearing mechanism, including the pinna, the external ear canal, the middle ear structures, the cochlea, and the ascending neural pathway that terminates in the auditory cortex of the brain *auditory system disorder:* any condition or state that interferes with or alters the normal function of acoustic information transfer from the outer ear to the brain

aural rehabilitation: a program for hearing-impaired individuals which may include auditory prostheses, auditory training, and speech-reading training

communicative skills: those skills required to express thoughts, desires, and feelings effectively through verbal communication

habilitative: referring to the process of creating or teaching a function involving human behavior, thought, and reason

mixed hearing loss: the combined effects of the loss of sensory or neural integrity and the presence of a barrier to the normal transmission of sound (such as wax in the ear, a hole in the eardrum, or some congenital anomaly affecting the transmission pathway of the auditory system)

rehabilitative: referring to the process of re-creating or teaching a function that has been impaired as a result of injury, disease, or aging

retrocochlear hearing loss: any disruption of neural information processing beyond the cochlea

sensorineural hearing loss: the loss of sensory or neural tissue of the auditory system as a result of disease, age, and acquired or congenital factors

SCIENCE AND PROFESSION

The field of audiology has become an indispensable adjunct in the objective diagnosis of hearing loss and auditory disorders. The scope of audiology practice is rather extensive and includes broad categorical services. According to the U.S. Department of Labor, the audiologist "specializes in diagnostic evaluation of hearing, prevention, habilitative and rehabilitative services for auditory problems and research related to hearing and attendant disorders." Among other functions, the audiologist

> determines range, nature, and degree of hearing function . . . using electroacoustic instrumentation; . . . coordinates audiometric results with other diagnostic data, such as educational, medical, social, and behavioral information; . . . differentiates between organic and nonorganic hearing disabilities through evaluation of total response pattern and use of acoustic tests; . . . [and] plans, directs, conducts, or participates in conservation, habilitative and rehabilitative programs, including hearing aid selection and orientation, counseling guidance, auditory training, speech reading, language rehabilitation, and speech conservation.

Audiologists may have primary affiliations in private practice, clinics and hospitals, military installations, universities and colleges, or in public and private school systems.

Because of the significant advances that have been made in providing differential diagnosis of impaired auditory behavior, the number of institutions providing audiology programs increased dramatically in the latter half of the twentieth century. Although the highest degree offered in audiology is the Ph.D., there is a strong movement supporting the introduction of a professional doctorate of audiology, which would stress clinical diagnosis, auditory prosthetic evaluation, and rehabilitative practice.

The membership of the American Speech-Language-Hearing Association (ASHA) consists of speech pathologists and audiologists, with the former having significantly greater numbers. ASHA provides two major, bimonthly sources of information: the *Journal of Speech and Hearing Research* and the *Journal of Speech and Hearing Disorders*. In 1988, James Jerger and other prominent audiologists in the United States formed the American Academy of Audiology. Its members consist exclusively of audiologists holding a masters or Ph.D. degree in that field. A quarterly publication of the Academy is the *Journal of the American Academy of Audiology*. Its content reflects the increase in knowledge of the human auditory system, its measurement and rehabilitative care.

DIAGNOSTIC AND TREATMENT TECHNIQUES

One of the most common services associated with the practice of audiology is the basic assessment of the auditory system relative to pure-tone air conduction thresholds. This is a procedure in which the patient's ability to just detect the presence of a tone delivered through earphones or speaker is determined. Additionally, speech threshold detection is determined by assessing the patient's ability to identify correctly 50 percent of a list of two-syllable words. Measurements of the acoustic reflex provide information about hearing loss, as do reflex-eliciting auditory tests. The acoustic reflex is the contraction of the stapedial muscle produced by a strong acoustic signal. The strength of the response and the level at which it is elicited are important diagnostic indicators of system malfunction, as is the absence of a reflex response. The degree to which the reflex response deviates in morphology and amplitude from normal is diagnostically significant. Communication handicap inventories also are an essential part of the basic assessment procedure. Such inventories provide useful information as to the degree of social handicap as a concomitant part of hearing impairment. Serial communication inventories serve as indicators of the effectiveness of habilitative or rehabilitative programs designed to enhance communicative skills. The term "basic" is applied to indicate a routine assessment of auditory function. Basic assessment does not provide the preponderance of clinical evidence needed to determine the site of injury or disease or to suggest its medical or surgical management.

Another service associated with audiology is an extended evaluation of the auditory system, which is composed of all anatomical structures that contribute to human hearing. Such an evaluation may include the determination of air conduction, bone conduction, and speech thresholds, as well as the administration of word and sentence recognition tests. Air conduction tests are performed by placing calibrated headphones over the patient's ears and presenting a broad range of discrete frequencies. In practice, that frequency range extends from 250 to 8,000 hertz. Even though the normal human ear is capable of perceiving a much broader frequency range (from 20 hertz to 20,000 hertz), the range between 250 hertz and 8,000 hertz contains all the essential frequencies needed to understand speech. Bone conduction thresholds are determined by placing a vibrator, or bone oscillator, at the mastoid bone and presenting the same frequency range. Often, differences in the patient's response to air-conducted and bone-conducted signals provide essential diagnostic information and suggest the site of injury or disease.

Speech threshold and word or sentence evaluations provide the clinician with performance scores that indicate the degree to which speech understanding has been compromised by the hearing disorder. Such measurements also indicate the probability of understanding connected discourse in communicative situations. There are a number of speech tests that provide information about the status of the auditory system. The most commonly used speech stimuli are two-syllable words to determine an individual's speech reception threshold and one-syllable words to assess the auditory system's discrimination function.

Another standard audiological practice is a comprehensive behavioral evaluation to determine the sensorineural site of lesion, that is, the place in the auditory system from which the hearing disorder originates. For most hearing disorders affecting auditory performance, it is critical that this site be located. It may be found in the peripheral system (the cochlea), which contains specialized sensory tissue that responds to sound pressure changes. The problem could also lie in the ascending auditory pathway, including its terminal projection in the auditory cortex of the brain. To arrive at an accurate diagnosis, the audiologist employs a number of advanced tests, such as sophisticated acoustic reflex tests, tests of frequency discrimination (the ability to detect differences between two or more signals), tests of intensity discrimination, and tests of auditory adaptation. The latter is a clinical procedure in which one determines whether a continuous sound decays over time to the point of inaudibility; such abnormal decay of the test signal indicates possible malfunction of the neural pathway of the auditory system. The results of these several tests increase significantly the probability that the site of lesion can be found.

One of the most promising clinical advances in audiology has been the development of evoked response audiometry (ERA). ERA is best defined as the measurement of neuroelectrical activity generated in the brain stem or of higher orders of brain function elicited by an acoustic signal. Acoustic signals, clicks, and tone pips are submitted to the external auditory ear. If the signals are detected by the auditory system, there is a change in neuroelectrical activity for each signal presented. A computer stores these minute changes in activity. When a sufficient number of acoustic signals have been processed, the computer prints out a response pattern consistent with the transmission of the electrical response from cochlear and subsequent responses as the signal travels to the brain. Response patterns have been classified as first (from the cochlea, 0 to 2 milliseconds), fast (from the acoustic nerve and auditory brain stem, 2 to 10 milliseconds), slow (from the primary and secondary areas of the cerebral cortex, 50 to 300 milliseconds), and late (from the primary and associated areas of the cerebral cortex, more than 300 milliseconds). More recent terminology of these time-related events refers to them as early, middle, and late responses.

Evoked potential measurement is significant because it offers a method of auditory assessment for those patients unwilling or unable to give reliable voluntary responses to acoustic stimuli. For example, evoked response audiometry provides a means of detecting hearing impairment in the neonate and very young. It also provides a clinical method of determining normal or abnormal hearing function for those who are mentally retarded. Evoked responses to acoustic stimuli aid in the diagnosis of various types of tumors or neuromas that affect the transmission of auditory signals to the brain. If such lesion sites are detected early, it may be possible to remove them surgically and save the patient's hearing. Certainly, early detection of retrocochlear pathology increases the probability that surgical intervention will preserve auditory system performance.

In 1978, D. T. Kemp published a germinal paper identifying the presence of otoacoustic emissions. Spontaneous emissions are generated within the cochlea and can be measured by a probe microphone assembly inserted into the external ear canal. Not all individuals have spontaneous otoacoustic emissions that can be measured by current probe microphone systems. Evoked otoacoustic emissions can be measured, however, in individuals having normal hearing or hearing loss of no more than 40 to 45 decibels. Such emissions are evoked by presenting a series of clicks or other compatible acoustic stimuli to the patient's auditory system. The cochleomechanical activity induced by these acoustic signals is "picked up" by a probe microphone and processed by a computer. The graphic information obtained has proven to be of significant benefit in the screening of neonates and the very young. The literature would seem to suggest that otacoustic emission measurement is fast, reliable, and repeatable. Research is under way to assess the range of losses that can be measured and the most appropriate stimuli to be employed in order to gain specific bits of information about cochlear behavior.

Auditory prosthetic evaluations have become common practice in audiology. When tests for hearing function de-

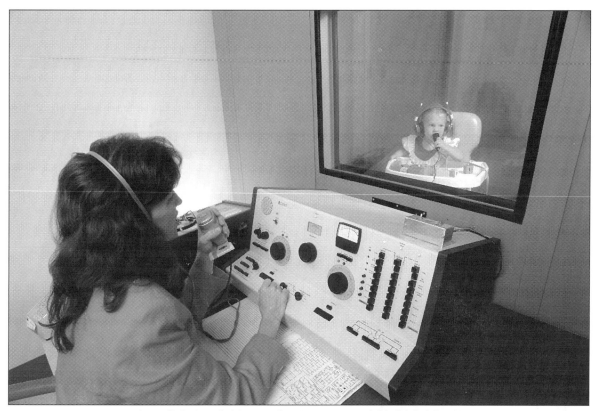

An audiologist administers a hearing test to a child. (Digital Stock)

termine that a hearing impairment exists, medical referral is mandatory for appropriate clinical management. For a sizable number of hearing-impaired individuals, however, medical or surgical intervention will not alter the hearing loss. For cases in which hearing impairment is a permanent sensorineural condition, a hearing aid or assistive listening device (or both) is often the preferred treatment modality in the rehabilitative process. To determine the appropriate electroacoustic characteristics of the hearing aid device to compensate best for the hearing deficit, special tests are conducted. Such tests may measure differences in word and speech understanding with and without the hearing aid. Another important test measures the degree of comfort or discomfort resulting from the sound level that is produced by the hearing aid device; if such a test is not performed, the patient may reject the hearing aid because it is too loud and unpleasant. Other tests designed to help determine the appropriate level of amplified sound involve narrow-band noise thresholds and various environmental sounds to which the patient may be periodically exposed during the activities of daily living. The use of environmental sound recordings provides the audiologist with objective indications of the electroacoustic responses that will yield maximum speech discrimination in the presence of specific background noises.

Audiology has helped many children and adults with hearing impairment through the use of hearing aids and the practice of aural rehabilitation. The selection and fitting of hearing aid devices have become important parts of the professional responsibilities of the clinical audiologist. With the many advances in hearing aid technology that have occurred, the audiologist has been given a much broader array of electroacoustic devices from which to select the one that offers the best correspondence with a patient's needs. For example, some commercial hearing aid systems can be digitally programmed to meet the specific acoustic requirements of the hearing-impaired individual. In some cases, programmable hearing aids provide more than one acoustic response at the immediate command of the user. Should the device fail to meet the acoustic requirements of the patient, it can be reprogrammed in a short period of time to achieve a better correlation with the patient's need for amplification.

Auditory (aural) rehabilitation is also of clinical concern to the audiologist, and a major branch of audiological practice is in this field. In this context, rehabilitation refers to the development and conduct of special programs to assist the hearing impaired in utilizing and understanding more efficiently verbal language (speech). For example, for those children born with a severe auditory deficit, the early introduction of aural rehabilitation programs is paramount to the development of verbal language. Consistent with the development of rehabilitation programs in the early detection of hearing impairment that cannot be ameliorated by surgical or medical intervention. From a rehabilitative point of view, early introduction of hearing aid amplification and supportive auditory and speech-reading training programs have been of inestimable value in speech and language development for the hearing-impaired child. In some of the major school systems throughout the United States, there is an "educational audiologist" whose task it is to develop and maintain special programs intended to assist hearing-impaired children.

Equally as important are auditory rehabilitation programs for the hearing-impaired adult. Hearing impairment is a rather insidious phenomenon, gradually worsening over time. Consequently, adult patients are somewhat unaware of hearing loss until they fail to recognize enough of speech sounds to understand intended messages. When speech understanding has been degraded by hearing impairment, rehabilitative programs stress the use of hearing aid amplification and the value of speech reading. Training programs may assist the adult in learning speech-reading skills or in adapting to a hearing aid device. It is important that the audiologist be aware of attitudes or behaviors that may restrict or limit a patient's acceptance of and participation in programs designed to assist the hearing impaired.

Perspective and Prospects

Audiology, as a recognized academic discipline, originated during World War II. At that time, thousands of military personnel needed diagnostic and rehabilitative services for ear injuries incurred during active service. It was essential that an organized program be developed to meet the demand. Several military hospitals and selected universities and colleges undertook the task of developing programs to accomplish these diagnostic and rehabilitative tasks. One of the first textbooks dealing exclusively with audiological practice was authored by Dr. Hayes Newby in 1958 while he was teaching at Stanford University. Since that memorable introduction, hundreds of special texts have been published relative to various aspects of audiological practice.

Since the early pioneering days during the World War II, the field of audiology and the clinical skills of audiologists have expanded appreciably. Significant advances in auditory disorder diagnosis and in prosthetic and rehabilitative care have been made. Although audiology is a relatively new academic and professional discipline, its contributions to the understanding and treatment of auditory system disorders have greatly advanced the understanding of its role in human communication. —*Robert Sandlin, Ph.D.*

See also Aging; Aging, extended care for the; Biophysics; Dyslexia; Ear infections and disorders; Ear surgery; Ears; Hearing loss; Ménière's disease; Motion sickness;

Neurology; Neurology, pediatric; Otorhinolaryngology; Sense organs; Speech disorders.

For Further Information:

Davis, Hallowell, and S. Richard Silverman. *Hearing and Deafness*. 4th ed. New York: Holt, Rinehart & Winston, 1978. Considered to be one of the classical texts in audiology. Reviews the development and growth of audiology as an academic discipline, and covers many of the processes of hearing function that lend themselves to measurement and interpretation. While this is a rather basic text, it does require that the reader have some knowledge relative to physics and sound production. Yet even these concepts are explained in simple terms that should be clear to most readers interested in the practice of audiology.

Jerger, James, ed. *Pediatric Audiology*. San Diego: College Hill Press, 1984. This text is devoted exclusively to explaining the various clinical tests conducted to determine the extent of hearing disorders in children. Brings together a number of distinguished authors dealing with specific aspects of pediatric audiology.

Katz, Jack, ed. *Handbook of Clinical Audiology*. 4th ed. Baltimore: Williams & Wilkins, 1994. This text is really not intended for the beginner. It reviews in considerable detail the various diagnostic tests currently employed in the audiological sciences. The work's main contribution is to give a much more detailed picture relative to the wide range of clinical activities inherent in audiology.

Newby, Hayes, and Gerald Popelka. *Audiology*. 5th ed. Englewood Cliffs, N.J.: Prentice Hall, 1985. A well-organized introductory text on the practice of audiology. Each chapter reviews in reasonable depth a specific aspect of audiological practice from the bases of hearing to the various audiological tests designed to yield clinical information about the normal and abnormal behavior of the human auditory system.

Rose, Darrell E., ed. *Audiological Assessment*. 2d ed. Englewood Cliffs, N.J.: Prentice Hall, 1978. Although this well-written text is not as current as some presented in this bibliography, the general scope of knowledge offered is sufficient for those wanting more extensive background in audiological practice. Unfortunately, very few texts about clinical audiology are intended primarily for the layperson.

Autism

Disease/disorder

Anatomy or system affected: Nervous system, psychic-emotional system

Specialties and related fields: Psychiatry, speech pathology

Definition: An emotional disturbance found in children in which communication, social interactions, and language skills are severely impaired.

CAUSES AND SYMPTOMS

Autism was first delineated in 1943 by Dr. Leo Kanner, who observed that some children seemed unable to relate properly to people. Later, those who worked with autistic children became convinced that the disorder was caused by cold, distant parents. Intensive treatment designed to break through this problem was unsuccessful, and parents were no longer seen as causing the disorder. Investigators now believe autism is the result of brain damage caused by any of several factors, including genetic errors, infectious diseases, metabolic disturbances, and neurological disorders. Autism does not progress, but it has no cure and is a lifelong disability. While some people with autism have normal or better intelligence, most are mentally retarded.

Autistic children demonstrate delays in speech, deficits in interpersonal skills, hearing or sight impairment, severe problems in eating and sleeping, attachments to unusual objects, persistent attention to spinning objects, and endlessly repeated behaviors such as hand flapping. Autism is a relatively rare disorder, occurring in fewer than 15 of every 10,000 children. People with autism may also suffer from other sensory deficits, hyperactivity, obsessive-compulsive disorder, depression, or Tourette's syndrome.

TREATMENT AND THERAPY

Children diagnosed with autism need psychological testing so that the child's deficits and strengths are well understood. A few autistic children are gifted in a specialized area, such as puzzle-solving. Proper plans of treatment draw upon the person's strengths to compensate for deficits and are individualized, community-based, family-focused, and well structured. Treatment should emphasize developing the person's social and communication skills. Family members need special training and support to cope with the needs of the autistic person. Psychoactive medication is used increasingly when treating the autistic person. People with autism can have normal life spans, and, with treatment, can live successfully in a community. —*Russell Williams, M.S.W.*

See also Learning disabilities; Mental retardation; Psychiatric disorders; Psychiatry; Psychiatry, child and adolescent.

FOR FURTHER INFORMATION:

Baron-Cohen, Simon, and Patrick Bolton. *Autism.* Oxford, England: Oxford University Press, 1993.

Batshaw, Mark L., ed. *The Child with Developmental Disabilities.* Philadelphia: W. B. Saunders, 1993.

Dulcan, Mina K., and Charles W. Popper. *Concise Guide to Child and Adolescent Psychiatry.* Washington, D.C.: American Psychiatric Press, 1991.

Gillberg, Christopher, ed. *Diagnosis and Treatment of Autism.* New York: Plenum Press, 1989.

AUTOIMMUNE DISORDERS
DISEASE/DISORDER

ANATOMY OR SYSTEM AFFECTED: Immune system, all physical systems

SPECIALTIES AND RELATED FIELDS: Genetics, immunology, internal medicine, rheumatology

DEFINITION: Disorders in which the immune system attacks an individual's own body.

KEY TERMS:

antibodies: proteins of the immune system formed by lymphocytes in response to a specific antigen

antigen: a molecule, usually a foreign invader to the body, which induces the production of antibodies which will bind to it in a highly specific manner

inflammation: a by-product of the attack upon an antigen by antibodies and other cells of the immune system; the aggregation of these cells causes swelling and pain, and increased blood flow to the area results in redness and a sensation of heat

lymphocyte: the major cells of the immune system; one type of lymphocyte produces antibodies

CAUSES AND SYMPTOMS

The body's immune system is a complex, highly coordinated defense system against foreign invaders. Phagocytes digest microorganisms, dust particles, allergens, pollutants, and other cellular debris that does not belong in the body. Macrophages, a type of phagocyte, act in concert with other cell types such as T lymphocytes to destroy invading viruses. B lymphocytes are responsible for the production of antibodies, which in turn are designed to react with and destroy an invader which displays a particular antigen on its surface. Suppressor T cells call off the immune response once the foreign bodies have been eradicated. A low level of antibodies will remain circulating in the bloodstream, poised to eliminate a recurring invasion swiftly.

During fetal development, the cells of the immune system learn to recognize the markers on the cells and tissues of the body as "self" and are programmed to ignore all such components. Occasionally, the immune system is somehow disrupted and components of the body are mistakenly identified as foreign invaders. In this case, antibodies against body components are formed and attack these self cells and tissues. The attack of the body by its own immune system is the basis of autoimmune diseases.

Systemic lupus erythematosus, often simply called lupus, is a chronic disease characterized by inflammation that can affect the skin, blood, kidneys, and joints. Symptoms include a butterfly-shaped rash across the face, fatigue, shortness of breath and/or chest pains caused by inflamed lung or heart lining, sensitivity to light, arthritis, anemia, and oral or nasal lesions. Normally, the immune system will eliminate the body cells that die naturally. In lupus, antibodies are made against these dead self cells. They attach to the debris and form large complexes that cannot be eliminated from the body. These complexes may lodge in the small blood vessels of any body tissue, causing an inflammatory response. Other damage is caused by the direct attack of body cells by these misguided antibodies, as in the destruction of red blood cells. The cause of lupus is unknown.

Multiple sclerosis and diabetes mellitus are two relatively common disorders of an autoimmune nature. In multiple sclerosis, the immune system attacks the insulation along the outside of nerve fibers, called myelin. The holes are replaced with scar tissue that cannot conduct nerve impulses, resulting in symptoms such as blurred vision, muscular weakness, and loss of coordination. In diabetes, the cells of the pancreas that produce insulin are targeted and gradually destroyed by the immune system. Lack of insulin prevents the proper regulation of the uptake of glucose by the brain and other body cells, resulting in severe complications and possible death. The cause of these disorders is unknown, but evidence suggests that an infection of viruses harboring antigens similar in structure to myelin or pancreatic cells may be involved in their onset.

In rheumatoid arthritis, the body manufactures antibodies which attack the membranes that cover the joints. Pain, fatigue, and inflammation in the fingers, knees, hips, and back are common symptoms. In severe cases, the heart, lungs, and kidneys can be affected, as well as the cartilage and tendons, leading to joint degeneration. Myasthenia gravis is a serious disorder in which the immune system attacks and destroys the muscle cell receptors for the neurotransmitter acetylcholine. Thus the muscles are prevented from responding to signals from the brain, and the result is severe muscle weakness.

Pernicious anemia is a potentially fatal disorder in which immune cells attack the intestinal cells that absorb vitamin B_{12}, thus denying the body this vitamin. B_{12} is necessary for the production of red blood cells and for a healthy nervous system; therefore, lack of it produces severe consequences. In a disorder called Hashimoto's thyroiditis, a protein called thyroglobulin which is normally sequestered inside the thyroid cells accidentally leaks into the bloodstream, forming antibodies that destroy the thyroid gland.

Fibromyalgia is characterized by pain and stiffness of the muscles and is often accompanied by sleep disturbances, fatigue, headaches, numbness, and tingling. No cause is known, but it may be associated with damage to the muscle cell membranes. In Sjögren's syndrome, the immune cells attack the body's salivary and tear glands, resulting in a host of mouth and eye disorders as well as fatigue and central nervous system disturbances. Sjögren's syndrome can mimic and coexist with other autoimmune disorders. Scleroderma is an autoimmune disorder which damages the blood vessels and causes thickening and scarring of the skin and malfunction of internal organs. The symptoms can be limited to a small area or can spread throughout the body.

Chronic fatigue syndrome, formerly known as chronic Epstein-Barr virus, is a debilitating disorder characterized by extremely severe fatigue that may last months or years.

While the cause is unknown, it is believed that the overproduction of some of the chemicals involved in the immune response are the causative agents. Abnormalities in the levels of specific immune cells are also implicated.

Rheumatic fever is the result of cross-reaction of antibodies produced in response to the bacterium that causes strep throat. These antibodies also recognize the heart valves, attacking them and causing inflammation and damage. Other autoimmune diseases include those targeted against a man's sperm, resulting in severe inflammation of the reproductive tract (orchitis, epididymitis); destruction of the eye (sympathetic ophthalmia); destruction of platelets within the blood (thrombocytopenia); and inflammation of the arteries (periarteritis). Leakage of the silicone from breast implants has been associated with the development of scleroderma and lupus.

TREATMENT AND THERAPY

While for many types of autoimmune disorders there are theories as to the cause—for example, the involvement of a virus or hereditary factors—the actual cause of any of these diseases is unknown. Because of this lack of fundamental information, no cures for autoimmune diseases are available and treatment is based on alleviating the symptoms of the disorders and strengthening the body when appropriate.

Treatment for systemic lupus erythematosus varies from individual to individual. Rest, proper nutrition, and avoiding the sun, which seems to trigger symptomatic episodes, can help to limit symptoms. Other treatments which are used include anti-inflammatory drugs such as aspirin; antimalarial drugs, which can cause eye problems; and steroids, which have a variety of negative side effects. While not normally fatal, this disease can be extremely debilitating. Kidney involvement can lead to serious consequences, perhaps necessitating the use of kidney dialysis to remove wastes from the body. Because symptoms are so broad and tend to come and go, physicians frequently misdiagnose lupus as a psychological disorder. Choosing a knowledgeable physician and participating in a support group, such as those provided through the National Lupus Foundation, can be extremely helpful in coping with this disorder.

Multiple sclerosis is generally a manageable disease, treated with a variety of drugs and a therapeutic lifestyle. Steroid hormones are prescribed to alleviate symptoms of a severe attack. These drugs function by suppressing the immune system and reducing inflammation, but prolonged use can have serious side effects. The drug baclofen (Lioresal) is used to help reduce jerkiness and spasticity. Physical therapy is also successful in limiting spasticity, as well as in improving flexibility and range of motion. Mild exercise, rest, proper nutrition, health maintenance, and occupational therapy all contribute to maintaining a high level of daily functioning for multiple sclerosis patients.

Individuals affected by diabetes must monitor the sugar

levels in their bodies closely, and in the insulin-dependent form of the disease must administer daily injections of insulin. Failure to do so can result in repeated episodes of coma that may lead to death. All forms of diabetes can be controlled by proper diet, exercise, and weight control. If appropriate, drug therapy may be prescribed. Proper monitoring of this disease is critical since it can lead to such complications as blindness, kidney disease, and neurological disorders.

Exercise, relaxation, and nutrition are all useful in the prevention and treatment of rheumatoid arthritis. Walking, yoga, and swimming are examples of exercise that helps to preserve the joints. A diet low in fat has been shown to reduce pain, swelling, and stiffness. Eliminating foods that trigger attacks is important; some of these foods are alcohol, sugar, chocolate, beef, pork, monosodium glutamate (MSG), and artificial preservatives. Drug therapies include the use of aspirin or ibuprofin for mild arthritis. Severe arthritis can be treated with immunosuppressant drugs, steroids, and anti-inflammatory drugs. Unfortunately, all these medications have dangerous side effects. Surgery to repair damaged joints is sometimes performed on individuals with a crippling form of the disease.

Fibromyalgia is treated with muscle exercises and low-impact aerobic exercise, massage, heat, and stress-reduction techniques. Small doses of antidepressants may be used to improve sleep and reduce pain. No therapy has been shown to be totally effective for long periods of time, so the best approach is for individuals to become familiar with the treatments to which their own disorders respond best and to locate and participate in a support group.

So little is known about scleroderma that no generalized treatment exists; however, therapy is aimed at body organs such as the lungs, heart, and kidneys that may become severely affected by the disorder, frequently to the point of fatality. The treatment for Sjögren's syndrome is based on the severity of the symptoms and is aimed at preventing progression of the disease to a debilitating stage.

Once chronic fatigue syndrome has been diagnosed properly, a variety of therapeutic approaches may be tried. Regular periods of uninterrupted rest are essential, especially during the most acute phase of the disorder. A healthy diet including many vegetables and complex carbohydrates, as well as vitamin supplements, can be helpful. Meditation, acupuncture, and avoidance of stress are some techniques that provide relief in some patients. Low dosages of antidepressants can be helpful in combating insomnia and pain, and certain medications to reinforce the immune system are sometimes prescribed. Emotional support for those suffering from chronic fatigue syndrome is comforting to most people, and in the United States there is an active national organization for sufferers of this disorder which can guide individuals to appropriate resources within their communities.

PERSPECTIVE AND PROSPECTS

Autoimmune disorders are, in general, a group of "modern" diseases. Recorded incidents of few, if any, of these disorders are nonexistent prior to the late nineteenth century. According to historical accounts, multiple sclerosis was unheard of prior to the mid-1800's. Some scientists believe that the disease existed at that time but was not properly diagnosed; however, there are no earlier records of any symptoms resembling those of multiple sclerosis. Other disorders seem to have arisen in the latter half of the twentieth century, such as chronic fatigue syndrome. Some speculate that industrial pollutants and toxins, which are unfortunate by-products of contemporary life, may trigger autoimmune diseases in individuals with susceptible immune systems. No specific chemicals or toxins have yet been shown to be the cause of any of these diseases.

The number of new cases of autoimmune disorders is steadily increasing, in part because of improved diagnostic tests. For years, disorders such as fibromyalgia and chronic fatigue syndrome were misdiagnosed or attributed to a psychological disorder. Many of these disorders seem to have a genetic component, in that individuals directly related to an affected individual may have a slightly higher risk of developing the same autoimmune disorder. This knowledge has permitted closer monitoring of at-risk individuals in an effort to begin treatment at the earliest signs of distress.

Before cures can be developed for autoimmune disorders, the causes must be determined. Therapies targeted against the causative agent may completely alleviate the disease. Improved means of enhancing the immune system through greater knowledge of its mechanics will be a huge step in improved maintenance of affected individuals. While treatment that focuses on symptoms does not cure a disease, improvement in the management of symptoms of autoimmune diseases will allow individuals a greater degree of comfort and an improved ability to conduct a normal life.

—*Karen E. Kalumuck, Ph.D.*

See also Anemia; Arthritis; Asthma; Chronic fatigue syndrome; Diabetes mellitus; Immune system; Immunodeficiency disorders; Immunology; Lupus erythematosus; Multiple sclerosis; Rheumatic fever; Rheumatoid arthritis; Thyroid disorders.

FOR FURTHER INFORMATION:

Boston Women's Health Book Collective. *The New Our Bodies, Ourselves.* New York: Simon & Schuster, 1992. This comprehensive book on women's health issues provides detailed discussions of the most common autoimmune diseases. Includes a useful list of national support organizations and other resources in the United States.

Carroll, David L., and Jon D. Dorman. *Living Well with MS.* New York: HarperPerennial, 1993. This informative book covers all aspects of multiple sclerosis, including its history and diagnosis, a detailed description of the disease, therapies, and research.

Desowitz, Robert S. *The Thorn in the Starfish*. New York: W. W. Norton, 1987. This very accessible book is written in a narrative style and wonderfully simplifies the story of the immune system and how it works. An excellent source for anyone interested in the history or mechanics of immunity, immune health maintenance, and the future of immune research.

Dwyer, John M. *The Body at War: The Story of Our Immune System*. 2d ed. London: J. M. Dent, 1993. This easy-to-read text is an excellent introduction to the functions of the immune system and such related topics as pregnancy, allergies, immune disorders, and research.

Feiden, Karyn. *Hope and Help for Chronic Fatigue Syndrome*. New York: Prentice Hall, 1990. An invaluable resource for those suffering from chronic fatigue syndrome or for anyone with an interest in the topic. Symptoms, treatments, and support resources are thoroughly covered.

Life, Death, and the Immune System. New York: W. H. Freeman, 1994. This comprehensive collection of articles from *Scientific American* provides basic information and research directions on AIDS, autoimmune disorders, allergies, and an excellent discussion of the immune system in general.

Nilsson, Lennart. *The Body Victorious*. New York: Delacorte Press, 1987. This clearly and concisely written description of the human immune system is fabulously illustrated with photographs of the immune processes in action.

Shaw, Michael, ed. *Everything You Need to Know About Diseases*. Springhouse, Pa.: Springhouse Press, 1996. This well-illustrated consumer reference, compiled by more than one hundred doctors and medical experts, describes five hundred illnesses and conditions, their causes, symptoms, diagnosis, treatment, and prevention. A valuable reference book for everyone interested in health and disease. Of particular interest is chapter 18, "Immune Disorders."

AUTOPSY

PROCEDURE

ANATOMY OR SYSTEM AFFECTED: All

SPECIALTIES AND RELATED FIELDS: Biochemistry, forensic medicine, histology, microbiology, pathology

DEFINITION: The postmortem (after-death) examination of a body in order to determine the cause of death; it involves both a systematic, orderly inspection of the external and internal structures of the body systems and a chemical and microbiological analysis of visceral contents.

KEY TERMS:

anatomic pathologist: a doctor who is especially concerned with the study of the structural and functional changes in tissues and organs that cause or are caused by disease; this doctor performs autopsies

coroner: an officer, often a layperson, who holds inquests in regard to violent, sudden, or unexplained deaths

diener: a person who assists the pathologist in the morgue and at the autopsy; a morguetrician

forensic autopsy: a systematic investigation to determine the cause of death, providing the pathologist with information to state an informed opinion about the manner and mechanism of death in cases that are of public interest

gross pathology: that which is visible to the naked eye, or "macroscopic," during inspection

histopathology: the histologic or microscopic description of abnormal pathologic tissue changes; these changes can be seen under the microscope

morgue: a place, usually cooled, where dead bodies are temporarily kept, pending proper identification, autopsy, or burial

THE FUNDAMENTALS OF PATHOLOGY

Translated literally, pathology is the study (*logos*) of suffering (*pathos*). As a science, pathology focuses on the study of the structural and functional consequences of injury on cells, tissues, and organs and ultimately the consequences on the entire organism (that is, the patient). Oftentimes, cells and fragments of tissues are obtained surgically from living patients; this procedure, called biopsy, is for the purpose of evaluating the nature and extent of injury. The results of a biopsy help direct the treatment. Autopsy, by contrast, is performed to examine the dead body and the internal organs systematically, in order to determine why the patient died.

Four aspects of a disease process form the core of pathology and are searched for diligently during autopsy studies. These are etiology, or cause; pathogenesis, the mechanism of development of disease; morphologic changes, the structural alterations induced in cells, tissues, and organs of the body; and clinical significance, the functional consequences of these morphologic changes.

There are two major classes of etiologic causation factors: genetic and acquired. Examples of acquired factors are infections, physical trauma, chemical injury and poisoning, nutritional factors, and radiation and solar injury (sunburn). When an autopsy is performed, this etiology is sought, but it has been acknowledged that the classic concept of one cause leading to one disease—developed largely from the discovery of specific infectious agents as the causes of specific diseases—is no longer sufficient. More often than not, multiple factors are acting at once. Genetic factors also affect environmentally induced diseases: For example, not all alcoholic patients develop significant liver disease (cirrhosis). Conversely, environment may have a profound influence on genetically induced disease: For example, not all individuals with the chemical and genetic markers for gout will develop that disease. During autopsies, systematic samplings of blood, body fluids, and tissues are taken in order to test for microbial causes and often chemical causes.

Pathogenesis refers to the sequence of events in the cells and organs that results from injury, from the initial responses to the ultimate expression of disease. It has become clear, for example, that many events at the subcellular and molecular levels are interacting and taking shape long before a disease becomes clinically observable. For example, the acquired immunodeficiency syndrome (AIDS) virus destroys lymphocytes (special white blood cells) and causes a gradual loss of immunity in the body long before AIDS becomes clinically observable as a disease.

Morphologic changes are the structural and associated functional alterations in cells, tissues, and organs that are characteristic of a disease process. They are directly observed at the autopsy table by "gross" or "macroscopic" inspection of the body and organs and later by "microscopic" or histologic study of tissue samples removed from these organs. These morphologic studies can be carried out in extreme detail using the electron microscope (ultrastructural studies) and immunologic or even genetic and molecular analysis. In forensic medicine, deoxyribonucleic acid (DNA) evidence is at times used as a definitive "thumbprint" of specific genetic makeup and can be obtained from even a few hairs.

The nature of these morphologic changes and their distribution in different organs influence normal function and determine the observed clinical features—the signs and symptoms of disease, such as fever and pain—and the disease's course and outcome. Thus, the clinical significance of these alterations can be used to assess the cause of death.

PROCEDURES AND TECHNIQUES

Autopsies are performed for several generally recognized purposes, which are closely related. Medical autopsies are performed to improve the diagnosis of disease and to help the practicing or treating physician avoid repeating errors in diagnosis and therapy; it has been repeatedly shown that autopsies contribute to improvements in medical care. The College of American Pathologists (CAP) has stressed the importance and necessity of the autopsy as a service to both the medical community and the public, recognizing it as a useful medical procedure performed by a qualified physician to assess the quality of patient care and evaluate clinical diagnostic accuracy. The autopsy is also a valuable tool for determining the effectiveness and impact of treatment modalities, discovering and defining new and/or changing diseases (as in AIDS), increasing the understanding of biological processes of disease (pathogenesis), and augmenting clinical and basic research. Information gathered from autopsies is used to provide accurate public health and vital statistical information and education as it relates to disease. Finally, the autopsy is used for obtaining legal, factual information.

In the United States, permission to perform an autopsy must be granted. A legal action can arise when the autopsy consent has not been obtained or when it has not been obtained from the proper person. The statutes of individual states usually establish who can consent to the autopsy. In general, a surviving spouse has first priority for authorizing an autopsy, and in the absence of the spouse, the next of kin has legal custody of the body and the right to authorize an autopsy. Some statutes indicate that whoever assumes custody of the body for burial may give permission for autopsy.

At large medical centers, there usually is an autopsy service, the director of which is a qualified anatomic pathologist. At times, there is also a perinatal pathologist, an anatomic pathologist specializing in the pathology of newly born babies. House officers who are medical doctors-in-training often assist in performing the autopsies. The autopsy suite is a well-equipped theater usually in close proximity to the morgue and is served by a diener.

Thus the usual autopsy is performed by professional pathologists. After carefully examining the body as a whole and recording its various attributes, the pathologist makes a surgical incision to allow for the detailed inspection of the body cavities and the organ systems, looking for gross abnormalities. Every organ is thus examined, measured, and weighed and its description recorded. Sampled sections of the organs are then taken for histologic studies, and samples of blood and other body contents may be taken for microbiologic and chemical studies.

The objectives of the autopsy will vary among institutions and even among cases within an institution. For example, an academic institution with a training program in pathology, a private hospital without a training program, and a medical examiner's office might be expected to approach a specific autopsy with very different objectives. Nevertheless, a minimum basic and standard level of examination, description, and tissue sampling is usually done. Photography is also used to document the gross findings.

Histologic study of the tissue samples is completed, and the results of microbiologic and chemical analysis are obtained. After the patient's record is carefully reviewed and all the findings are correlated, often in consultation with the decedent's treating physician, a final document, the autopsy report, is produced.

In many autopsies, the basic gross, histologic, chemical, and microscopic examination will be inadequate to resolve fully all questions raised by the circumstances of the patient's clinical course and death. The ability to carry out additional studies may then become critical to resolving these questions. Ancillary studies to which pathologists may resort include injections of substances into blood vessels to observe blockages (angiography), chromosomal studies, toxicology, X-ray defractions, and histochemical procedures. The results of these studies are also recorded in the final autopsy report.

Two standard techniques are generally used to perform autopsies. They differ from each other in the order in which the organs are removed and in whether single organs or intact organ systems are removed from the body. In Virchow's technique, organs are removed one by one. Originally, the first step was to expose the cranial cavity, the spinal cord, and the thoracic, cervical, and abdominal organs, in that order. This technique, with some modifications, is still widely used. In Rokitansky's technique, the dissection is initially carried out in situ (before the removal) and then combined with en bloc removal. This technique is often modified when used in medical centers, where the en bloc removal of the cervical, thoracic, and abdominal organs is done. Dissection of the various organ systems is performed after removal.

Another technique, Potter's technique, is often used in pediatric autopsies. The external examination, particularly of fetuses and newborns, concentrates on the search for congenital malformations; the face, ears, or hands may reveal characteristic symptoms of a disorder, such as with Down syndrome. The placenta and umbilical cord must be studied in all autopsies for fetuses and newborns.

Few autopsies offer more difficulties than postoperative cases, in which death has occurred during or shortly after a surgical operation. The pathologist must evaluate his or her findings in the light of their medicolegal implications, such as complications from surgical intervention, anesthesia, or drug administration. At times, obtaining permission to conduct an autopsy may require certain restrictions in its performance. In such restricted autopsies, access can be confined to only the chest or abdomen, or to the reopening of surgical wounds.

Medicolegal autopsies are best carried out by forensic pathologists, who must first ascertain that death has, in fact, occurred. (Failure to do so has, on occasion, led to embarrassment and serious repercussions.) Not all medicolegal autopsies deal with violent or unnatural deaths. Generally, more than half of all cases investigated by the office of the chief medical examiner in New York are deaths from natural causes that occur suddenly, unexpectedly, or in an unusual manner. Coronary heart disease (heart attacks) and respiratory infections (pneumonias) are the most common causes of death in such cases, and the greatest incidence is in persons forty-five to fifty-five years of age. Strenuous physical or emotional activity may bring about a heart attack in a patient with undetected but severe narrowing of the coronary vessels.

When a crime is suspected, evaluation of the circumstances of death and investigation of the scene where the body was found may be crucial. The position of the body, the distribution of the blood lost by the victim or the assailant, or objects found in the vicinity may offer important clues. Identification of the body can be a complex issue, especially with mutilated or decomposed bodies, and may involve X-ray and dental studies, as well as detailed studies of body contents and hair samples.

Estimation of the time of death is another concern of the forensic pathologist; at times, this can be determined very simply by the circumstantial evidence. For example, when, after a rainy night, the ground under the body is found to be dry, death probably occurred before the onset of rain. More often, however, the time of death is estimated from physical or chemical measurements of values whose rate of postmortem change has been found to be rather constant, such as body temperature or the chemical analysis of certain body and blood constituents. These methods can be useful for short postmortem intervals. For longer intervals, a determination of the level of potassium in the vitreous humor (a gelatinous fluid in the eyeball) is fairly reliable.

Special procedures are used by the forensic pathologist to investigate questions related to criminal abortion, vehicular and aircraft accidents, air embolism, decompression sickness, drowning, exposure to elements, gunshot wounds, rape, and infanticide (in which the main objective is to decide whether the infant was born alive or was a stillbirth).

Toxicologic autopsies, in which poisoning is suspected, are also the responsibility of the forensic pathologist. The sampling of tissues, especially from the brain, liver, lung, kidneys, fat, hair, fingernails, and stomach contents, is done, and samples are also collected from urine, blood, bile, and the vitreous humor of the eyeball. The list of possible poisons and drugs that can be abused is endless, and the investigation of which poison may be the cause of death is both an art and a science.

Perspective and Prospects

The field of pathology is, next to therapeutics (the study of medicinal substances), the oldest division of the healing arts because it is the study of disease itself. Its historical development can be broadly sketched in five different periods, each one highlighted by a fundamental change in the concept of the "seat of disease." An examination of the steps by which pathology has reached its present state provides a useful perspective on the subject.

At the dawn of history, primitive humans believed that there was only a single disease, one that could produce disturbances as varied as headaches, blood vomit, epilepsy, or the death of mother and child during labor. While, in some of those cases, there were apparent causes of death, the real causes were thought to be hidden and supernatural. Thus, the concept of disease was not localized to any specific organ or even to a war wound or broken bone.

The idea of "humors" soon took over. It began in ancient Egypt, was well articulated by the Greeks, and came to dominate the medical thought in the Western world up to the Renaissance. The humoral theory of disease proposes that illness is the result of disturbance in the equilibrium between four qualities (hot, cold, wet, and dry) and four elements (air, water, fire, and earth) to affect four body constituents (blood, yellow bile, black bile, and phlegm). This theory was championed by such intellectual giants as Aristotle, Pythagoras, and even Hippocrates and was fine-tuned by Galen in the second century.

The theory of the "equilibrium of humors" implies that disease affects not the entire organism but only such fluids, or humors, indicated by the specific disease. Thus a man has jaundice because of an imbalance of his humors caused by an excess of yellow bile, an excess resulting from the winds blowing in the wrong direction. One disease had become many diseases, with specific seats within the body, but these seats were not subject to anatomic evaluation.

The study of anatomy and gross pathology (that is, autopsy) became generalized in the sixteenth century, and it sounded the death knell for humoral pathology. Antonio Benivieni (1443-1502) is rightfully considered the founder of gross pathology. He is the first physician who performed autopsies, and his medical text appears to be the first to deal with anatomic and gross changes in different organs in relation to clinical symptoms. He worked in the same hospital in Florence, Italy, where the great anatomist Leonardo da Vinci conducted his anatomic dissections. His book contains the protocols for fifteen autopsies performed to ascertain the cause of death, or the seat of disease. Also of great significance in this period is the work of Jean-François Fernel (1497-1558), from Paris, whose book *Medicina* (1554) was divided into three parts: physiology, pathology, and therapeutics. The section on pathology contains 120 chapters and separates diseases into special groups, with brief autopsy presentations for clinical correlation.

The seventeenth century saw the emergence of a small group of physicians who collected the accounts of all available experiences and published them in enormous volumes. Théophile Bonet (1620-1689) is the most important of these reviewers, and his book, *Corps de medecine et de chirurgie* (1679), appearing about two hundred years after Benivieni's, contains summaries of more than three thousand autopsy protocols, including those of Benivieni himself and other masters such as Andreas Vesalius. This book was the stimulus for the monumental contribution of Giovanni Battista Morgagni (1682-1771), whose work marks the official inauguration of anatomic pathology and autopsy as a science. His classic text, *De sedibus et causis morborum per anatomen indagatis* (1761), contains the clinical histories and autopsy protocols of more than seven hundred cases, correlating the morphologic and clinical findings. More important, he committed his autopsy studies to the revelation of the cause of disease, thus establishing the general principle that "seats of disease" are internal body organs, not humors, and that localization in different organs explains different symptoms. This concept served as the basis for the fundamental work of anatomic pathologists-clinicians

such as René-Théophile-Hyacinthe Laënnec and Richard Bright.

The next great step in the development of pathology, and establishing the premiership of autopsy as its medium of study, is the French pathologist Marie-François-Xavier Bichat (1771-1802), who established in *Recherches physiologiques sur la vie et la mort* (1800) that organs are formed of elements called tissues. The work of Rudolf Virchow (1821-1902) raised pathology to the premier medical science; he placed the concept of the microscopic cell as the unit of life at the center of medicine and his theory of cellular pathology, thus making cells the unit and "seat" of disease.

Impressive strides in subcellular and molecular pathology have established many morphologic lesions within subcellular structures, even within genes. Such studies can be performed on minute samples of tissues obtained through fine probes. These biopsy techniques and the great technological advances in nuclear and radiologic investigative techniques have allowed the physician to study the cause and extent of disease during the patient's lifetime and with a high level of sophistication. Thus, the role of the autopsy has declined somewhat as an educational tool, but the practice continues to be used in clinical research, medical statistics, public health, and population genetics and to procure organs for tissue transplantation. In fact, many of the functions of autopsy will be extended and improved. For example, the demand for transplantable tissues and organs, procured from cadavers, is likely to increase. Also, recognition of new diseases will occur, aided by postmortem exams and the application of new technologies and ancillary studies. The autopsy still has much to contribute to education and research, as it constitutes a priceless, continuing, and intimate contact with the natural history of disease.

—*Victor H. Nassar, M.D.*

See also Anatomy; Biopsy; Blood testing; Death and dying; Disease; Forensic pathology; Law and medicine; Malpractice; Pathology; Wounds.

FOR FURTHER INFORMATION:

Compton, Carolyn C., et al. *Pathologic Basis of Disease.* 4th ed. Philadelphia: W. B. Saunders, 1995. The standard textbook of pathology for medical students.

Hutchins, Grover M., ed. *Autopsy: Performance and Reporting.* Northfield, Ill.: College of American Pathologists, 1990. A multiauthored, detailed manual which is concisely written and illustrated. The chapters examine techniques, various medicolegal and ethical questions, contemporary issues related to the decline in autopsy rates in the 1980's, autopsy utilization, quality assurance, and reimbursement.

Ludwig, Jurgen. *Current Methods of Autopsy Practice.* Philadelphia: W. B. Saunders, 1972. A standard manual which contains detailed descriptions of autopsy techniques for all purposes. The chapters are written by specialists and aimed at the practicing pathologist-in-training.

Perez-Tamayo, Ruy. *Mechanisms of Disease: An Introduction to Pathology*. 2d ed. Chicago: Year Book Medical Publishers, 1985. A fascinating review of the study of disease as life under abnormal conditions. Considers the history and future of pathology, with up-to-date information on new technologies. A textbook for medical students.

BACK DISORDERS. *See* SPINAL DISORDERS.

BACTERIAL INFECTIONS
DISEASE/DISORDER

ANATOMY OR SYSTEM AFFECTED: Gastrointestinal system, immune system, intestines, lungs, lymphatic system, respiratory system

SPECIALTIES AND RELATED FIELDS: Bacteriology, epidemiology, immunology, internal medicine, microbiology

DEFINITION: Infectious diseases caused by bacteria, of which hundreds exist.

KEY TERMS:

antibiotic: a substance that kills microorganisms, including bacteria; antibiotics are used as a primary therapy in combating bacterial diseases

bacteria: small, single-celled organisms with a very simple structure; they live virtually everywhere and most varieties are harmless, although some types are capable of causing disease

cell: the smallest unit of a living thing; a bacterium consists of one cell, whereas humans are made of billions

immune system: the natural defenses of the body, which kill invading organisms such as harmful bacteria

immunity: resistance to infection by a particular disease-causing microorganism, often acquired by vaccination

infectious disease: diseases that can be passed from person to person through direct or indirect contact; many bacterial diseases are infectious

inflammation: signs and symptoms of the body's immune response to some bacterial infections; may include redness, swelling, heat, pain, and the production of pus

metabolism: the chemical reactions in an organism that sustain life and lead to growth and reproduction

microorganism: any small organism, including bacteria, protozoans, mold, fungi, and viruses; in this context, refers to those which cause disease

vaccination: the process of injecting into an individual a substance that provides immunity to a particular disease

CAUSES AND SYMPTOMS

Bacteria are very small, one-celled organisms (the cell being the smallest unit of a living organism) with an average size of thousandths of a millimeter. Based on their relatively simple structure, they are classified as prokaryotic cells. Prokaryotic cells have a rigid outer cell wall, very simply organized hereditary material (deoxyribonucleic acid, or DNA) floating free within the cell, and only a few other structures necessary for their survival, growth, and reproduction. Eukaryotic cells, such as those found in humans, plants, and other animals, have highly organized DNA and many more internal structures. Despite the fact that bacteria are relatively "simple," they are still very complex living organisms.

The many types of bacteria can be divided into three categories based on their shape: coccus (round), bacillus (rod-shaped), or spirillum (spiral). Another major distinction between types of bacteria is based on the sugar and lipid (fat) composition of their cell walls. This difference can be identified by Gram-staining bacteria, the result of the stain determining whether the organism is gram-positive or gram-negative. Various types of bacteria may have additional structures that are useful in their identification. Capsules and slime layers are water-rich sugary materials secreted by the bacteria which cling to their surfaces and form halolike structures. Flagella are long, thin, whiplike structures found in one location on the bacterium or occasionally covering its entire surface. These structures are used to enhance the motility, or movement, of the bacteria.

Some bacteria are normal, harmless inhabitants of human bodies, such as those on the surface of the skin. Others, such as those which live in the human intestinal tract, aid in digestion and are essential for good health. Yet the warm, moist, nutrient-rich human body also provides an excellent breeding ground for numerous harmful bacterial invaders. For bacteria to cause infectious disease, several stages must occur. The bacteria must enter the person; they must survive and multiply on or in the person; they must resist the natural defenses of the human body; and they must damage the infected person. Most bacterial diseases are infectious because of the ease with which they can be transmitted from individual to individual by physical contact with the person, a contaminated object, or bacteria expelled into the air, such as by coughing or sneezing. A few bacterial diseases, such as food poisoning, are not classified as infectious.

Bacterial infections cause disease by a variety of mechanisms. Many of them produce chemical compounds that are toxic to human beings. For example, *Salmonella* and *Staphylococcus aureus* are two types of bacteria that are capable of causing food poisoning. *Clostridium botulinum* produces the deadly botulism toxin. In each case, ingestion of the toxin in contaminated food can lead to serious illness. *Clostridium tetanii* can enter the body through puncture wounds and will multiply rapidly deep in tissue where there is little exposure to the air. The toxin that it produces acts on the central nervous system and causes severe muscle spasms, which can lead to death from respiratory failure. Water that has been contaminated with raw sewage is a potent source of disease-causing bacteria. *Vibrio cholera* produces a potent toxin which causes severe diarrhea leading to death if it is not vigorously treated. Certain varieties of *Escherichia coli* and *Shigella* found in contaminated water can also cause severe intestinal disorders. Toxic shock syndrome is associated with the production of toxins by *Staphylococcus aureus*.

Another common cause of disease from bacterial infections is the result of the physical destruction of tissue by the invading organisms. Leprosy (also called Hansen's disease), caused by *Mycobacterium leprae*, if left untreated can lead to severe deterioration and disfiguration of large areas of a person's body. If a wound interrupts the blood supply to an area of the body such as a hand or foot, the tissues begin to decay, thereby providing nutrients for many bacteria, especially *Clostridium perfringens*. These bacteria can greatly accelerate the destruction of the tissue, which causes the condition known as gas gangrene.

In many cases, disease results when the infecting bacteria are recognized by the body's natural defense system (the immune system) as "nonself," that is, as invaders. Certain cells within the body are designed to attack intruders and eliminate them. During this process, disease symptoms that

The Body's Response to Bacterial Infection

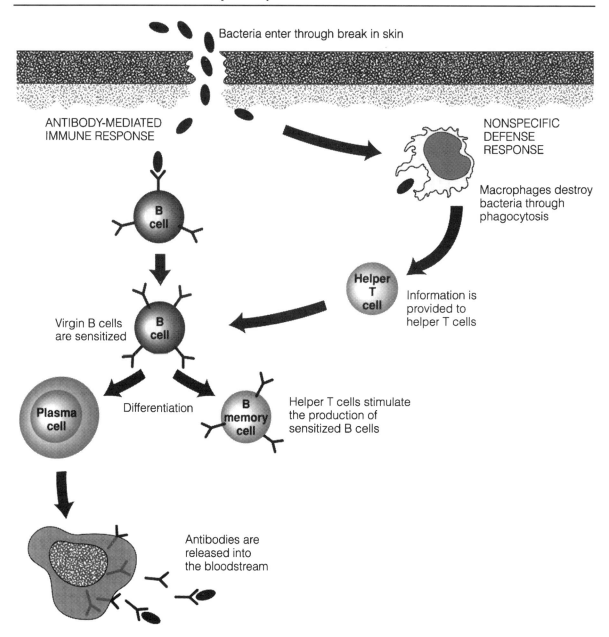

Bacterial infections cause the body to respond with either antibody production or phagocytosis leading to antibody production.

are consequences of the immune system's response may be evident: inflammation (redness and swelling), the production of pus, and fever, among other symptoms. In some cases, certain components of the bacteria, such as capsules and slime layers, may protect them from being eliminated by the immune system. The bacteria may also multiply exceedingly rapidly, producing increasing amounts of toxins that overwhelm the capacity of the immune system to eliminate them. In these cases, continued and increasingly elevated disease symptoms such as fever can cause severe, even fatal, damage unless an alternate method for eliminating the infection is found. Failure to eliminate the bacterial invaders can also lead to a long-term, chronic infection that damages body tissues.

Many respiratory diseases are associated with the body's immune response to bacterial invasion. *Streptococcus pyogenes* is the causative agent of strep throat, whose features include severe redness, inflammation, pain, and the production of pus in throat tissue. In a small percentage of cases, strep throat can also lead to an infection of and potential permanent damage to the heart valves in a disease called rheumatic fever. In tuberculosis, *Mycobacterium tuberculosis* enters the lungs through inhalation. The body's defense system walls off the intruders and forms a nodule called a tubercle deep in the lung tissue. Nevertheless, the bacteria continue to multiply in the nodule and can travel to new sites in the lung. Tubercle formation occurs at these new sites. Eventually, this repeated cycle of infection and nodule formation becomes a chronic disease and leads to the destruction of lung tissue. Bacterial pneumonia can be caused by several different organisms, including *Klebsiella pneumoniae* and *Mycobacterium pneumoniae*. A pneumonia-like disease, Legionnaires' disease, was first identified in 1976 after twenty-nine delegates to an American Legion convention died from a mysterious respiratory disorder. The lengthy process of identifying a causative agent led to the discovery of a type of bacteria not previously known, *Legionella pneumophila*.

The human urinary and genital tracts are also potential havens for invading bacteria. Cystitis (bladder infections) are caused by many different types of bacteria. Kidney infections can be acquired as corollaries of urinary tract infections. Sexually transmitted diseases (STDs) are contracted through sexual contact with an infected partner, and two common STDs have a bacterial origin. Gonorrhea is caused by *Neisseria gonorrhoeae* and leads to a severe inflammatory response and rapid spread of the organisms throughout the body. If not treated, it can lead to sterility as well as to diseases of the joints, heart, nerve coverings, eyes, and throat. Syphilis, caused by *Treponema pallidum*, can also have serious consequences if left untreated, including dementia and death. In addition, it can be passed to a fetus developing inside an infected mother in a condition known as congenital syphilis.

TREATMENT AND THERAPY

The medical management of the many bacterial infections and the diseases they cause begins with diagnosis. Diagnosis relies on a variety of biochemical tests that are analyzed in conjunction with the signs and symptoms exhibited by the infected individual. Treatment is then designed so that it not only eliminates the disease symptoms but also eradicates all invading bacterial organisms, thereby minimizing the chance of a recurrence of the disease. Prevention involves steps that the individual takes to avoid potential contact with infectious diseases, as well as the use of medical procedures that protect against specific bacterial diseases.

In order to treat a bacterial disease properly, the invading organism must be identified correctly. In some cases, symptomology can be specific enough to identify the offending bacterium, but since there are literally thousands of different types of disease-causing organisms, a systematic approach using a variety of tests is undertaken to make a definitive diagnosis. First, a specimen from the infected person is collected. This may be a blood or urine sample; a swab of the infected area, such as the throat or another skin surface; or a secretion, such as sputum, mucus, or pus. Since human bodies are normally inhabited by a variety of harmless bacteria, the individual types of bacteria are isolated in pure cultures, in which each bacterium present is of the same type. The pure cultures are then tested to determine the identity of the organisms. Staining procedures, such as Gram's stain, and microscopic examination of the stained bacteria to determine the Gram reaction and the shape of the bacteria can narrow down the identity of the organisms considerably.

Based on these results, a standard series of tests is performed, continually narrowing down the possible identities until only one remains. One test measures the organisms' growth requirements. Many identifications are aided by analyzing the types of sugars and proteins that the organisms can use as food sources. The by-products of their metabolism (chemical reactions occurring inside the bacteria), such as acids and gas, are identified. Oxygen requirements, motility, and the presence of a capsule are three other common characteristics that are examined. For cases in which the identification of a particular variety of one type of bacteria is necessary, more complex tests may be undertaken, such as an analysis of the particular sugars and proteins on the surface of the organism or tests for the production of specific toxins. Once the bacterium's identity is confirmed, treatment may begin.

The most common type of treatment for bacterial infection is antibiotic therapy. Antibiotics are chemical compounds that kill bacteria. Originally discovered as antibacterial compounds produced by bacteria, molds, and fungi (such as penicillin from bread mold), many more are synthetically produced. Antibiotics work in a variety of fashions. Some, such as penicillin and the cephalosporins, interfere with the synthesis of cell walls by bacteria, thus preventing the organisms from multiplying. Other commonly used antibiotics prevent the bacteria from synthesizing the proteins that they need to survive and multiply. These includes the tetracyclines (a class of antibiotics which act against a large range of bacteria), erythromycin, and streptomycin. A host of other antibiotics target a variety of bacterial functions, including specific chemical reactions and the propagation of genetic material, and the structural components of the bacteria. Each class of antibiotics works best on certain types of bacteria. For example, penicillin is most efficient in killing cocci (such as *Streptococcus* and *Staphylococcus*) and gram-positive bacilli.

Frequently, the symptoms of a bacterial disease may disappear rapidly after the beginning of antibiotic therapy. This reaction is attributable to the inhibition of bacterial multiplication and the destruction of most of the microorganisms. A small number of the bacteria may not be killed during this initial exposure to antibiotics, however, and if antibiotic therapy is ended before all are killed, a recurrence of the disease is likely. A full prescription of antibiotics should be taken to avoid this situation. For example, effective treatment and eradication of all bacteria in tuberculosis may take six months to a year or more of antibiotic treatment, despite the fact that the symptoms are alleviated in a few weeks.

Upon repeated exposure to a type of antibiotic, some bacteria develop the capacity to degrade or inactivate the antibiotic, thus rendering that drug ineffective against the resistant microorganism. In these cases, other antibiotics and newly developed ones are tested for their effectiveness against the bacteria. Such situations have arisen in the bacteria that cause gonorrhea and tuberculosis.

While antibiotics exist to combat infections of most types of bacteria, in some cases the human immune system is capable of clearing the infection without additional intervention. In these instances, the symptoms of the infection are treated until the body heals itself. This is the common treatment path in mild cases of food poisoning, such as those caused by some *Salmonella* and *Staphylococcus* varieties. Diarrhea and vomiting are treated by replacing water and salts, by drinking large volumes of fluids, and perhaps

"Flesh-Eating Bacteria"

Necrotizing fasciitis is an invasive bacterial infection of the connective tissue between the skin and muscle known as the fascia. It must be urgently treated surgically and, even in the best circumstances, has a high mortality rate.

Although it had been identified in the past, in 1994 there were numerous headline newspaper reports describing a new "flesh-eating bacteria." These articles detailed the devastating effect of seemingly minor wounds infected with streptococcal bacteria. Patients quickly become very sick, with a rapidly progressive downward course, even from trauma resulting in a deep muscle bruise or muscle strain or in "minor" cuts and scrapes.

In the former nonpenetrating injuries, it is likely that the bacteria were already present in the blood and then seeded the site of damage. Most of these patients, however, did not recall any prior recent infection that may have made them susceptible. Penetrating injuries, where the normally protective barrier of the skin has been broken, were often minor and not originally treated as contaminated or infected. Other cases of necrotizing fasciitis are caused by surgical infections and bowel contamination. These cases are more rare and often found to have a mixture of bacteria, such as staphylococci or *Escherichia coli* (*E. coli*).

Patients with necrotizing fasciitis have fever, inflammation, severe pain, and blistering at the site of infection. If this cellulitis is not recognized and urgently treated, the infection will quickly spread in the layers of connective tissue just under the skin known as the fascia. As the bacteria multiply, they cause blood vessels supplying the skin to form clots and thus cut off blood flow to the skin. Without nutrients, oxygen, and the ability to remove waste products, the skin dies. Once this occurs, the nerves are destroyed and the patient no longer has the excruciating pain. The skin at this point appears to be "eaten away." The possibility exists that the underlying muscle adjacent to the fascia will become infected. Thus, the potential for muscle death as well as skin death is of great concern, particularly if the infection begins in the arms, legs, abdomen, or back, as these areas have large muscle groups directly underlying the skin. In necrotizing fasciitis, the extremities and the area around the genitals and anus (perineum) are most commonly and extensively involved.

Multiplication and movement of these streptococcal bacteria and their toxins into the bloodstream produces a shocklike state. The patient must quickly be stabilized in an intensive care unit, where fluids can be administered and heart and lung condition can be closely monitored. The only lifesaving treatment available is extensive surgical debridement to remove the necrotic (dead) tissue and slow the spread of the bacteria. Antibiotics including penicillins, clindamycin, and gentamicin are given to help eradicate the pathogen. Because the infection spreads so rapidly, death often results even with heroic surgical and drug therapy unless the condition is diagnosed and treated early. Fortunately, these infections remain relatively rare. —*Matthew Berria, Ph.D.*

by using over-the-counter remedies to ease some of the symptoms.

Many bacterial diseases can be easily prevented through good hygiene. Foods that are not thoroughly cooked, such as eggs and meats, may become quickly contaminated by the rapid growth of food-poisoning organisms present on their surfaces. Proper cooking kills these organisms. Similarly, foods that are not properly stored but left out in warm places can also provide a potent breeding ground for toxin-producing bacteria. Picnic food not properly refrigerated is a common source of food poisoning. Similarly, questionable water sources should never be used for drinking or cooking water without proper treatment. Filtering with an ultrafine filter specifically designed to remove bacteria is one safeguard, as is boiling for the required time period based on altitude. Food that may have been washed with contaminated water sources should always be cooked or peeled before consumption.

Many diseases can be prevented with vaccinations. A bacterial vaccine is a mixture of a particular bacterium, its parts, or its inactivated toxins. When this solution is injected into an individual, it provides immunity (resistance to infection) to the particular organism contained in the vaccine. Some vaccines provide lifetime immunity when enhanced with an occasional booster shot, while some are relatively short-acting. Many types of vaccines that are directed against specific diseases are part of standard preventive care given to children. For example, the DPT vaccine confers immunity to diphtheria, pertussis (whooping cough), and tetanus. Some vaccines are useful for individuals who are living, working, or traveling in areas where certain diseases are endemic, or for those who regularly come into contact with infected individuals. Examples of these sorts of vaccines include those for plague (*Yersinia pestis*), typhoid fever (*Salmonella typhi*), cholera, and tuberculosis.

PERSPECTIVE AND PROSPECTS

Bacteria were first described as "animalcules" by the Dutch scientist Antoni van Leeuwenhoek in 1673 after he observed them in water-based mixtures with a crudely designed microscope. In 1860, Louis Pasteur recognized that bacteria could cause the spoiling of wine and beer because of the by-products of their metabolism. Pasteur's solution to this problem was heating the beverages enough to kill the bacteria, but not change the taste of the drink—a process known as pasteurization, which is used today on milk and alcoholic beverages. In addition, Pasteur settled a long-standing debate on the origin of living things that seemed to arise spontaneously in fluids exposed to the air. He demonstrated that these life-forms were seeded by contaminating bacteria and other microorganisms found in the air, in fluids, and on solid surfaces. Pasteur's work led to standard practices in laboratories and food processing plants to prevent unwanted bacterial contamination; these practices are referred to as aseptic techniques.

Prior to the late 1800's, deaths from wounds and simple surgeries were quite common, but the reason for these high mortality rates was unknown. In the 1860's, Joseph Lister, an English surgeon, began soaking surgical dressings in solutions that killed bacteria, and the rate of survival in surgical and wound patients was greatly improved. In 1876, Robert Koch, a German physician, discovered rod-shaped bacteria in the blood of cattle that died from anthrax, a disease which was devastating the sheep and cattle population of Europe. When he injected healthy animals with these bacteria, they contracted anthrax, and samples of their blood showed large numbers of the same bacteria. By these and other experiments, Koch, Lister, and others proved the "germ theory of disease"—that microorganisms cause disease—and appropriate measures were instituted to protect against the transmission of bacteria to humans through medical procedures and food.

A milestone in the prevention of infectious diseases was the development of vaccinations. The first vaccine was developed in 1798, long before the germ theory of disease was proven. The British physician Edward Jenner first used vaccination as a preventive step against the contraction of deadly smallpox, a viral disease. How vaccinations work and their use as a protection against bacterial diseases were discovered around 1880 by Pasteur.

The first antibiotic, penicillin, was discovered by Alexander Fleming in 1928. Since then, scores of others, produced both naturally and synthetically, have been analyzed and used in the treatment of bacterial diseases. All these discoveries have made bacterial disease a much less deadly category of illness than it was in the late 1800's. Yet bacterial diseases are by no means conquered. Overuse of antibiotics in medical practice and in cattle feed results in the appearance of new varieties of bacteria that are resistant to standard antibiotic therapy. Research will continue to develop new means of controlling and destroying such infective organisms. Bacteria also play an important role in synthesizing new antibiotics and other pharmaceuticals in the laboratory through recombinant DNA technology. These organisms will continue to provide challenges and opportunities for human health in the years to come.

—*Karen E. Kalumuck, Ph.D.*
updated by Matthew Berria, Ph.D.

See also Antibiotics; Botulism; Childhood infectious diseases; Cholecystitis; Cholera; Cystitis; Diphtheria; Drug resistance; *E. coli* infection; Endocarditis; Gangrene; Glomerulonephritis; Gonorrhea; Gram staining; Infection; Laboratory tests; Legionnaires' disease; Leprosy; Lyme disease; Mastitis; Microbiology; Microscopy; Pelvic inflammatory disease (PID); Pertussis; Plague; Pneumonia; Salmonella; Scarlet fever; Serology; Shigellosis; Staphylococcal infections; Strep throat; Streptococcal infections; Syphilis; Tetanus; Tonsillitis; Toxemia; Tropical medicine; Tuberculosis; Typhoid fever and typhus.

FOR FURTHER INFORMATION:

Biddle, Wayne. *Field Guide to Germs*. New York: Henry Holt, 1995. This comprehensive book is easily accessible to the nonspecialist and includes a discussion of nearly every virus, bacterium, and fungus known to cause human and nonhuman animal disease. The history of the microbe and the treatment of diseases are included.

Dixon, Bernard. *Magnificent Microbes*. New York: Atheneum, 1976. This well-written book, written in a narrative style, imparts classic information to those curious about the world of microbes from the perspective of their importance in maintaining health and life. The reader will come away with a true appreciation for the virtues and helpfulness of microbes, including bacteria, to humans—indeed of their necessity for maintaining life.

Finegold, Sydney M., and William J. Martin. *Bailey and Scott's Diagnostic Microbiology*. 6th ed. St. Louis: C. V. Mosby, 1982. A well-organized text that is accessible to the general reader. Describes in detail methods for the isolation and identification of microorganisms, in particular diagnostic procedures for the identification of bacterial infectious diseases. Includes many illuminating color plates illustrating diagnostic tests.

Gest, Howard. *The World of Microbes*. Menlo Park, Calif.: Benjamin/Cummings, 1987. A very readable, jargon-free book written in an engaging narrative style. Includes a discussion of the history of microbiology, the basic biology and chemistry of microorganisms with an emphasis on bacteria, the roles microorganisms play in the environment and their impact on humans, disease pathology, prevention and cure, and the use of bacteria in biotechnology.

Joklik, Wolfgang K., and Hilda P. Willett, eds. *Zinsser: Microbiology*. 20th ed. East Norwalk, Conn.: Appleton and Lange, 1992. This is the bible of microbiology, with a heavy emphasis on medical microbiology. Features a detailed analysis of the biochemistry of bacteria and other microorganisms. Recommended for its extensive discussions of the many types of diseases and their causative agents.

Pelczar, Michael J., Jr., E. C. S. Chan, and Noel R. Krieg. *Microbiology*. 5th ed. New York: McGraw-Hill, 1986. This general textbook is accessible to the general reader and is a good source of information on bacterial physiology and genetics, diagnostic testing, the prevention and cure of bacterial diseases, and environmental microbiology. Includes many informative photographs and illustrations, as well as an excellent glossary of terms.

Rossmoore, Harold W. *The Microbes, Our Unseen Friends*. Detroit: Wayne State University Press, 1976. An excellent, narrative-style book intended to be read for knowledge and pleasure. In addition to a discussion of bacteria and disease, it includes excellent material on the benefits to human health of microorganisms and their ubiquity and importance in everyday life.

Schlegel, Hans G. *General Microbiology*. 6th ed. Cambridge, England: Cambridge University Press, 1986. This compact version of a classic German textbook provides a concise yet broad account of bacteriology and microbiology for readers with all levels of interest. Topics include cell structure, biochemistry, microbes in the environment, the practical applications of microbes, and the cause, prevention, and cure of diseases.

Shaw, Michael, ed. *Everything You Need to Know About Diseases*. Springhouse, Pa.: Springhouse Press, 1996. This well-illustrated consumer reference, compiled by more than one hundred doctors and medical experts, describes five hundred illnesses and conditions, their causes, symptoms, diagnosis, treatment, and prevention. A valuable reference book for everyone interested in health and disease. Of particular interest is chapter 19, "Infection."

BACTERIOLOGY

SPECIALTY

ANATOMY OR SYSTEM AFFECTED: Cells, immune system

SPECIALTIES AND RELATED FIELDS: Biochemistry, epidemiology, microbiology, pathology, pharmacology, public health

DEFINITION: The study of bacteria.

KEY TERMS:

anaerobic: free of oxygen

fermentation: a chemical reaction that splits complex organic compounds into relatively simple substances

infection: the invasion of healthy tissue by a pathogenic microorganism, resulting in the production of toxins and subsequent injury of tissue

SCIENCE AND PROFESSION

Bacteriology is the study of bacteria, unique life-forms that maintain the basic physiological and genetic processes of all other types of cellular life but that have the unusual characteristic of chemicophysiological diversity. Many bacteria live in totally anaerobic environments, converting carbohydrates to acids and alcohol by fermentation, nitrate to nitrogen gas, sulfate to hydrogen sulfide, and hydrogen and carbon dioxide to methane gas. Some bacteria live by photosynthetic processes similar to plants, while others survive by using energy obtained through the oxidation of sulfur, hydrogen, ammonia, or ferric minerals.

The history of life on Earth is closely linked to the presence of bacteria. Geologic evidence suggests the early increase in the earth's atmospheric oxygen more than two billion years ago was the direct result of bacteriological activity. Throughout time, bacteria have continued to play a crucial role in recycling materials necessary for the survival of plants and animals. In the biosphere, bacteria are responsible for degrading and converting complex substances into useful products. Bacteria break down carbohydrates, proteins, and lipids to form carbon dioxide, and they convert ammonia to nitrate and nitrogen gas to amino acids, all of which are essential to the life cycle of plants. Bacteria are the basis of many industrial processes. Bacteria colonies are involved in producing cheeses and fermented foods such as pickles, sausage, and sauerkraut. Bacteria thriving in sewage and landfills produce methane gas, which is used as an alternative energy source by humans. The exploitation of bacteria as a detoxifying agent of environmental pollutants is becoming widespread. Almost all medically important antibiotics are produced by bacteria cultures.

Many types of bacteria live in association with animals. Most bacteria associated with humans live on the surface of the skin, in the mouth, or in the intestinal tract; the majority are harmless, many are quite beneficial. Some bac-

The Culturing of Bacteria

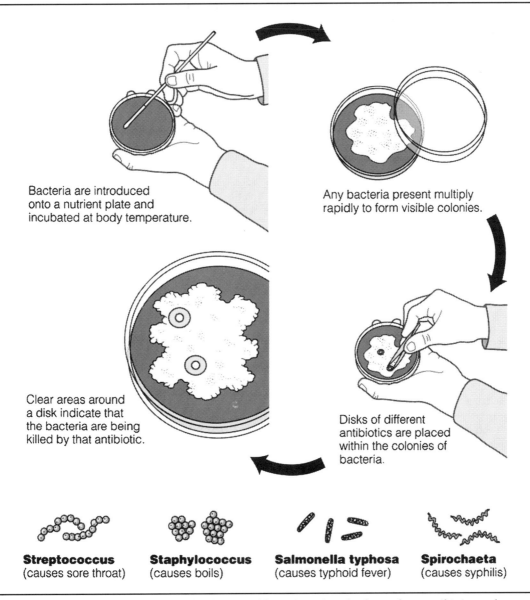

Bacteria are introduced onto a nutrient plate and incubated at body temperature.

Any bacteria present multiply rapidly to form visible colonies.

Disks of different antibiotics are placed within the colonies of bacteria.

Clear areas around a disk indicate that the bacteria are being killed by that antibiotic.

Streptococcus
(causes sore throat)

Staphylococcus
(causes boils)

Salmonella typhosa
(causes typhoid fever)

Spirochaeta
(causes syphilis)

Bacteriologists use culturing techniques to identify types of bacteria and to develop and test antibiotics to destroy them; some bacteria are either harmless or helpful to humans, but harmful bacteria can cause a number of diseases, such as syphilis, typhoid fever, streptococcal infections, and staphylococcal infections.

teria, known as pathogens, are opportunistic and able to establish themselves in the body of a host, multiply, and produce local or systemic infections. Many pathogens are the causes of severe diseases in humans; most notable are anthrax, tuberculosis, bubonic plague, typhoid fever, pneumonia, gonorrhea, syphilis, gangrene, meningitis, botulism, diphtheria, scarlet fever, tetanus, streptococcal infections, and pertussis (whooping cough).

Medical bacteriology involves the study of infectious diseases produced by bacteria. Medical bacteriologists isolate bacteria suspected of being infectious, relate their role to the disease in question, study the life cycle of the bacteria colony, and seek means to provide therapy to infected victims and prevent further spread of the infectious pathogen.

Bacteriologists are highly skilled scientists having undergone advanced studies in the fields of biology, microbiology, and chemistry; many have additional training in medical specialties such as pathology, epidemiology, and serology.

DIAGNOSTIC AND TREATMENT TECHNIQUES

The way in which bacterial infections develop usually follows a consistent pattern. Transmission may occur by one of four pathways: direct contact, such as sneezing or sexual intimacy; inhalation; common source contacts, such as food, water, or blood; and vector-borne spreading by insects or parasites. Bacteria first invade the body through some opening, such as a wound or the skin, nose, throat, lung, intestine, urethra, or bloodstream. The bacteria then target specific cells and begin to reproduce, establishing a primary infection. If the infection remains unchecked, it may spread to the lymphatic system or bloodstream, and multiple sites of infection may develop. The resulting infection destroys local tissue by producing toxins that damage cells or by producing compounds that interfere with body metabolism.

The control of bacterial infections is accomplished by breaking the links in the chain of transmission. This can be done by altering the behavior of potential hosts through education programs, quarantine, health inspections of common source contacts, and pest eradication programs. Other efforts to control infections involve altering the defensive capability of the host. The most effective means has been through vaccination. Vaccination immunizes individuals so that they are no longer susceptible to the targeted infection. Additionally, many bacterial infections can be treated with injections or topical and oral applications of antibiotics.

PERSPECTIVE AND PROSPECTS

During the mid-nineteenth century, studies by Louis Pasteur into undesirable fermentation of beers and wines led him to the conclusion that infections in animals might be the result of some type of fermentation process. Pasteur experimented with the microbiological cause of infections by studying the characteristics of anthrax and cholera bacilli. Pasteur noted that the introduction of dead bacterial

pathogens into a healthy host did not result in disease. Furthermore, if the host was injected with a virulent supply of the subject bacteria, the host did not contract the disease. The result of this work was the discovery of a method for acquired immunity to disease.

Working during the same period, German physician Robert Koch provided proof that anthrax and tuberculosis are caused by bacteria. Earlier in his career, Koch developed methods for isolating pure cultures of bacteria, then identifying, staining, and cataloging bacilli. The result of this work was that Koch and other investigators were able to view infected blood samples, then quickly isolate and cross-reference noted bacilli with previously identified pathogens.

The work of these two pioneering bacteriologists quickly led to the development of bacterial toxins for diphtheria and tetanus. The groundwork that they provided helped to establish the role that microorganisms play in the development of infectious disease and ushered in a golden age of discovery into the cause of infectious diseases and their control by immunization. —*Randall L. Milstein, Ph.D.*

See also Antibiotics; Bacterial infections; Cells; Cholecystitis; Cystitis; Cytology; Cytopathology; Drug resistance; *E. coli* infection; Endocarditis; Gangrene; Glomerulonephritis; Gram staining; Immunology; Immunopathology; Infection; Laboratory tests; Mastitis; Microbiology; Microscopy; Pathology; Pharmacology; Staphylococcal infections; Strep throat; Streptococcal infections; Tonsillitis; Toxemia; Tropical medicine.

FOR FURTHER INFORMATION:

Braude, Abraham I. *Medical Microbiology and Infectious Diseases.* Philadelphia: W. B. Saunders, 1981.

Parker, M. T., and L. H. Collier, eds. *Topley and Wilson's Principles of Bacteriology, Virology, and Immunity.* 8th ed. 5 vols. St. Louis: B. C. Decker, 1990.

Salle, A. J. *Fundamental Principles of Bacteriology.* 7th ed. New York: McGraw-Hill, 1973.

Volk, Wesley A. *Essentials of Medical Microbiology.* 5th ed. Philadelphia: Lippincott-Raven, 1996.

BALDNESS. *See* HAIR LOSS AND BALDNESS.

BASAL CELL CARCINOMA. *See* SKIN CANCER.

BED-WETTING
DISEASE/DISORDER

ANATOMY OR SYSTEM AFFECTED: Bladder, muscles, musculoskeletal system, urinary system

SPECIALTIES AND RELATED FIELDS: Family practice, geriatrics and gerontology, pediatrics, psychology, urology

DEFINITION: A condition characterized by an inability of the bladder to contain the urine during sleep, often a developmental condition in children.

KEY TERMS:

alarm therapy: the practice of utilizing mechanical or electronic devices to detect bed-wetting as it occurs

bed-wetting: the passage of urine during sleep

bladder: a membranous sac in the body that serves as the temporary retention site of urine

diaphragm: a body partition of muscle and connective tissue separating the chest and abdominal cavities

enuresis: an involuntary discharge of urine; incontinence of urine

nervous system: the bodily system that receives and interprets stimuli and transmits impulses to the organs

neurophysiological: pertaining to the nervous system in the human body

phrenic: of or relating to the diaphragm

sphincter: a muscle surrounding and able to contract or close a bodily opening (such as the opening to the bladder)

CAUSES AND SYMPTOMS

Primary enuresis is defined medically as the inability to hold one's urine during sleep. The condition is quite common and occurs most often in children; approximately 20 percent of children under the age of six suffer from the condition. These percentages decrease to about 5 percent at age ten, 2 percent at age fifteen and only about 1 percent of adults. Secondary enuresis is bed-wetting in a child who had previously achieved bladder control. (These terms do not apply, however, to urination problems caused by physical illness, disease, or anatomical defect.) The condition is more common in boys than in girls. Bed-wetting usually occurs during the first third of sleep, although it can occur during all sleep stages and without relation to awakening periods.

It is important to realize that enuresis is considered to be a developmental concern rather than an emotional, behavioral, or physical one. Donald S. Kornfeld and Philip R. Muskin report in *The Columbia University College of Physicians and Surgeons Complete Home Medical Guide* (Rev. ed., 1989) that "enuresis is due to a lag in development of the nervous system's controls on elimination." Many parents fail to understand this neuropsychological element and thus punish the child for a wet bed. Punishing, ridiculing, or shaming the child does not correct the situation; in fact, in many cases, it may prolong the problem as well as cause other unnecessary and undesirable psychological problems. Emotional problems have resulted from enuresis, as the child may be too embarrassed to partake in normal childhood activities such as camping or sleepovers.

TREATMENT AND THERAPY

Techniques for helping the enuretic child achieve dryness range from withholding liquids near bedtime to alarm systems to medical intervention. Generally, restriction of liquid intake after dinner is the first course of action. This treatment method, however, does not have a very high success rate. Should this treatment fail after a trial period of a few weeks, other methods may be employed.

Alarm therapy can help a child achieve control within four months, sometimes in only a few weeks. A beeper- or buzzer-type alarm sounds when moisture touches the bedding or underwear; the desired result is that the child, while sleeping, will eventually recognize the need to urinate and awaken in time to get to the bathroom. Electronic alarms are generally of two types. The first is a wired pad, consisting of two screens, which is placed under the sheets to detect wetness; when the child wets, the moisture activates the battery-operated alarm. The second is a device worn on the body, either in the underpants and connected by a wire to an alarm or a wristwatch-type alarm; the underwear serves as a separating cloth for the contact points. In either case, as wetness occurs, the alarm sounds, thus wakening the child; the child can then be directed to the bathroom to complete urination.

Barry G. Powell and Lynda Muransky cite several case histories in which alarm therapy proved to be effective in stopping enuresis. For example, a six-year-old who never had a dry bed achieved dryness within a week through the use of an alarm. In another case, a fifteen-year-old had been trying to overcome his bed-wetting problem for ten years. Several trips to the doctor showed that he had no physical cause for enuresis. His parents labeled him "lazy, inconsiderate, and difficult." His desire to join his hockey team in overnight travel gave him the impetus to seek help. Powell and Muransky found his problem to be primary enuresis aggravated by family ridiculing. Through the use of his alarm, he achieved dryness within two weeks.

A case involving secondary enuresis is described as well. A child who had suffered through primary enuresis, then achieved dryness, was found to be wetting again. This second bout of bed-wetting seems to have been the result of his parents' marital separation. After a medical examination revealed no physical problems, it appeared the problem was psychological, caused by emotional upset. He resumed dryness in three weeks (although an alarm system on his bed for six months gave him more confidence). It is important to note, however, that alarms can take up to several months' time before a child feels comfortable in stopping its use. Also, parental supervision is imperative in order for this type of therapy to work properly.

Chiropractic spinal manipulation has been found to be effective in the treatment of some cases of enuresis. Some believe that a spinal reflex is involved in bed-wetting. As nighttime breathing slows down (a normal reaction), carbon dioxide builds up in the body. When the carbon dioxide buildup reaches a certain level, a breathing mechanism called the phrenic reflex is triggered. This mechanism normally causes the diaphragm to return breathing to its normal pattern. If the mechanism does not work properly, however, the carbon dioxide continues to increase, resulting in an involuntary relaxation of the sphincter muscle at the opening to the bladder. Fluid (urine) is released and leaks out of the bladder. A child in a deep state of sleep does not recognize that the bed has been wet. Generally, chiropractors believe that the bed-wetting child sleeps in a state of high carbon dioxide intoxication.

While immature development of the phrenic reflex is the most common cause of bed-wetting, in some children a misalignment of the bones in the neck and spine (referred to as "subluxation" by chiropractors) is thought to cause pressure on the nerves that are related to the phrenic reflex. Through chiropractic adjustments, it is argued, the subluxation can be corrected, thus relieving pressure on the nerves. With the spine realigned and bodily functions working normally, enuresis can be eliminated. One child had never had a dry bed in his first ten years of life; after only two spinal adjustments by a licensed chiropractor, the child stopped wetting immediately. Chiropractors usually recommend a series of adjustments in order to realign the spine and nerves and keep them in the proper position.

Drug therapy solely for the treatment of enuresis is controversial. However, when an illness such as diabetes mellitus is the underlying cause of the bed-wetting, the use of drugs may be indicated. The drug imipramine hydrochloride (an antidepressant agent) has been studied to assist in contraction of the sphincter; however, because of the high toxicity and limited effectiveness of such antidepressants, its use is not widespread. Relapse rates are high, and a cure rate of only 25 percent is seen. More success has been achieved with desmopressin acetate, an antidiuretic drug. There is an immediate improvement in 70 percent of treated children. Relapse rates are lower than those associated with imipramine but higher than with the use of bed-wetting alarms, probably because the sphincter muscle is not fully developed in the enuretic child. In general, drug therapy yields a final success rate of 25 percent.

PERSPECTIVE AND PROSPECTS

The history of bed-wetting is probably a lengthy one. The term "enuresis" was first coined around 1800 and has plagued children from every ethnic background and socioeconomic level around the world. It continues to be a problem for many children today and probably will be so in the future as well.

Most enuretics are deep sleepers who are usually quite active during their waking hours. This sleeping pattern, combined with urinary systems that are not yet fully developed, is generally the main cause of bed-wetting. There are some indications that enuresis is hereditary; many children who suffer from the condition have a parent who was enuretic as a child. It is reassuring to know that almost all affected children outgrow the problem by adulthood. While no immediate cure is available, continued experiments with alarm systems and drugs will certainly alleviate the discomfort and embarrassment until the body's lag in development corrects itself.

—*Carol A. Holloway*

See also Anxiety; Geriatrics and gerontology; Incontinence; Psychology; Sleep disorders; Stress; Urinary disorders; Urinary system; Urology; Urology, pediatric.

FOR FURTHER INFORMATION:

"Alarm Bells for Enuresis." *The Lancet* 337 (March 2, 1991): 523. Alarm therapy is discussed as a treatment for enuresis (nocturnal bed-wetting) in children. Attention is given to the importance of parental supervision, family stress, environmental obstacles, and behavioral problems that can contribute to bed-wetting.

Clayman, Charles B., ed. *American Medical Association Family Medical Guide.* Rev. and updated 3d ed. New York: Random House, 1994. An informative article detailing the subject. Medical myths concerning the problem are discussed. Related articles covering such topics as urinary infections in children and nephritis are conveniently located in the same chapter of the book.

"Defining Enuresis." *FDA Consumer* 23 (May, 1989): 10. This article, written for the layperson, is easy to understand and even offers a helpful pronunciation guide for difficult terms. The links between enuresis and sleep patterns, sleepwalking, and nightmares are examined.

Kornfeld, Donald S., and Philip R. Muskin. "Enuresis, or Bed-wetting." In *The Columbia University College of Physicians and Surgeons Complete Home Medical Guide,* edited by Donald Tapley et al. 3d rev. ed. New York: Crown, 1995. A well-written article explaining the causes, effects, and treatments of bed-wetting in children. Offers the encouraging suggestion that even if all treatments fail, the problem is usually outgrown by adulthood.

Powell, Barry G., and Lynda Muransky. *Bedwetting: Questions and Answers for Parents.* Missasauga, Ontario: Helpful Publications, 1984. This booklet is dedicated to assisting parents in understanding bed-wetting. A strong emphasis on alarm systems is evident, as the writers have also established their own bed-wetting alarm company.

BELL'S PALSY

DISEASE/DISORDER

ANATOMY OR SYSTEM AFFECTED: Muscles, musculoskeletal system, nerves, nervous system

SPECIALTIES AND RELATED FIELDS: Family practice, neurology, physical therapy

DEFINITION: Bell's palsy is a sudden paralysis of one side of the face, including muscles of the eyelid. Pain behind the ear on the affected side, distorted facial expressions, and changes in salivation are common symptoms. The cause is unknown, although reduced blood supply to the facial nerves is believed to trigger most cases. The symptoms of Bell's palsy can be treated by applying heat to painful areas twice a day and by wearing goggles or an eye patch to keep the eye moist and protected. As muscle strength returns, facial massage and exercise may be

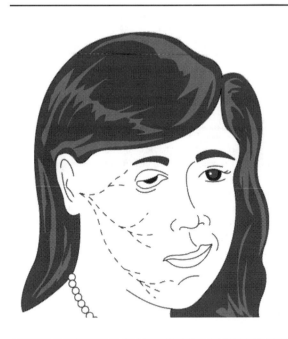

Bell's palsy results in a temporary sagging and paralysis of one side of the face; dashed lines show the main neural pathways affected.

helpful. The mouth should be kept clean with increased brushing and flossing.

—*Jason Georges and Tracy Irons-Georges*

See also Muscle sprains, spasms, and disorders; Muscles; Nervous system; Neuralgia, neuritis, and neuropathy; Neurology; Neurology, pediatric; Palsy; Paralysis.

BERIBERI
DISEASE/DISORDER

ANATOMY OR SYSTEM AFFECTED: Muscles, musculoskeletal system, nervous system

SPECIALTIES AND RELATED FIELDS: Family practice, internal medicine, nutrition, public health

DEFINITION: Beriberi is a serious vitamin deficiency caused by an inadequate dietary intake of thiamine (B_1). Thiamine, which can be found in green vegetables, whole grains, meat, nuts, and potatoes, is required in order to digest carbohydrates. Its absence in the diet can result in neurological and muscular problems such as numbness and muscle wasting ("dry" beriberi) or heart failure ("wet" beriberi). Except for chronic alcoholics, elderly people who are undernourished, or those in extreme poverty, the disease is rare in developed countries. It is more common, however, in poor countries and is a possibly fatal complication of severe malnutrition. Treatment with thiamine brings about a complete recovery.

—*Jason Georges and Tracy Irons-Georges*

See also Alcoholism; Malnutrition; Nutrition; Vitamins and minerals.

BIOFEEDBACK
PROCEDURE

ANATOMY OR SYSTEM AFFECTED: Brain, circulatory system, endocrine system, glands, heart, muscles, musculoskeletal system, nerves, nervous system, psychicemotional system

SPECIALTIES AND RELATED FIELDS: Alternative medicine, cardiology, exercise physiology, family practice, internal medicine, neurology, occupational health, physical therapy, preventive medicine, psychology, sports medicine, vascular medicine

DEFINITION: The learned self-regulation of the autonomic nervous system through monitoring of the physiological activity occurring within an individual.

KEY TERMS:

biodisplay: audio or visual information about the physiological activity within an organism displayed by various instruments and processes

biofeedback: the provision of information about the biological or physiological processes of an individual to him or her, with the objective of empowering the individual to make conscious changes in the processes being monitored; it can be instrumental (using devices that monitor physiological or biological processes) or noninstrumental (using bodily sensations)

biofeedback instrument: a device (usually electronic) that is capable of measuring and displaying information about a physiologic process in a way that allows an individual to monitor the physiologic activity through his or her own senses

electrodermal response (EDR) biofeedback: the monitoring and displaying of information about the conductivity of the skin; used for anxiety reduction, asthma treatment, and the treatment of sleep disorders

electroencephalographic (EEG) biofeedback: the monitoring and displaying of brain wave activity; used for the treatment of substance abuse disorders, epilepsy, attention deficient disorders, and insomnia

electromyograph (EMG): an instrument that is capable of monitoring and displaying information about electrochemical activity in a group of muscle fibers

neuromuscular rehabilitation: the process of employing electromyographic biofeedback to correct physiological disorders that have both muscular and neurological components, such as the effects of strokes and fibromyalgia; also called myoneural rehabilitation

physiological autoregulation: the process by which an individual utilizes information about a physiological activity to effect changes in that activity in a direction which contributes to normal (or desirable) functioning

INDICATIONS AND PROCEDURES

Biofeedback has been utilized in both research and clinical applications. The term itself denotes the provision of information (feedback) about a biological process. It has been found that individuals (laboratory animals included), when given feedback that is reinforcing, are able to change physiological processes in a desired direction; homeostatic processes being what they are, these changes are in a positive direction. In the case of humans, the feedback is provided about a physiological function of which the individual would not otherwise be aware if it were not for the provision—via a biodisplay—of information about that process.

It has been observed that for persons employing biofeedback, the equipment used serves as a kind of a sixth sense. Quoting from the publication *Biofeedback*, by the National Institute of Mental Health,

> This sixth sense allows the person to "see" or "hear" activity inside of their bodies—activity that they would otherwise be unaware of. For the individual who now knows what the physiological activity actually is (and knowing in what direction the physiological process should be heading) the biofeedback equipment now serves as a "mirror." The "mirror" provides the feedback which the individual uses in order to make corrections (physiological autoregulation) in the given physiological process in the desired direction.

Human maladies range from the purely structural to the purely functional, with various gradations. An example of a structural disorder is a broken bone, while an example of a functional disorder might be a person who manifests symptoms of blindness for which there is no known or identifiable organic cause. Looking at the spectrum of human maladies, one can consider the continuum as "structural," "psychophysiological," "mental-emotional," "hysterical," and "feigned." The category of psychophysiological lies midway between structural and mental-emotional. A psychophysiological disorder has elements of both mind and body interactions; it is a physiological disorder brought about by thoughts, feelings, and emotions. There are those who take the position that all human maladies and disorders have a mental-emotional component to them, that there can be no change in the mental-emotional state without a corresponding change in the physiological state and no change in the physiological state without a corresponding change in the mental-emotional state.

It is currently the preference of many scientifically and technologically oriented practitioners to deal with the more structural disorders (or to treat the disorder as if it were mostly structural). It is also the case that many mental health practitioners prefer to deal with disorders that fall more into the mental-emotional category. There is, however, a growing number of practitioners who have an interest in and training for dealing with psychophysiological disorders. This emerging field is referred to as behavioral medicine,

and a large percentage of the practitioners in this field employ biofeedback as a modality.

A classic example of biofeedback being used to correct a physiological problem would be the employing of electromyograph (EMG) biofeedback for the correction of a simple tension (or psychophysiologic) headache. The headache is caused by inappropriately high muscle tension in the neck, head, or shoulders. In surface electromyographic biofeedback, the biofeedback practitioner attaches electronic sensors to the muscles of the forehead, neck, or shoulders of the patient. The electronic sensors pick up signals from electrochemical activity at the surface of the skin in the area of the involved muscle groups. The behavior of the muscles being monitored is such that minute changes in the electrochemical activity in the muscles—tension and relaxation—occur naturally.

The sensitivity of the biofeedback instrument (the magnification of the signal may be as high as one thousand times) and the display of the signal make the individual aware of these changes via sound or visual signals (biodisplays). When the biofeedback signal indicates that the muscle activity is in the direction of relaxation, the individual makes an association between that muscle behavior and the corresponding change in the strength of the signal. The individual can then increase the duration, strength, and frequency of the relaxation process. Having learned to relax the involved muscles, the individual is able to prevent or abort headache activity.

It is axiomatic that any physiological process (behavior) that is capable of being quantified, measured, and displayed is appropriate for biofeedback applications. The following are some of the more commonly used biofeedback instruments.

An electromyograph is an instrument that is capable of monitoring and displaying information about electrochemical activity in a group of muscle fibers. Common applications of surface electromyography (in which sensors are placed on the surface of the skin, as opposed to the insertion of needles into the muscle itself) would be stroke rehabilitation. Surface electromyography is also used in the treatment of tension headaches and fibromyalgia.

An electrodermal response (EDR) biofeedback instrument is capable of monitoring and displaying information about the conductivity of the skin. An increase in the conductivity of the skin is a function of moisture accumulating in the space recently occupied by blood. The rate of blood flow depends on the amount of autonomic nervous system arousal present within the organism at the time of measurement. The higher the level of autonomic nervous system arousal, the greater the amount of skin conductivity. Common applications of EDR biofeedback are the reduction of anxiety caused by phobic reactions, the control of asthma (especially in young children), and the treatment of sleep disorders. For example, many insomniacs are unable to drop off to sleep because of higher-than-appropriate autonomic nervous system activity.

An instrument that is capable of monitoring and displaying the surface temperature of the skin, as correlated with an increase in vascular (blood flow) activity in the area of the skin in question, can also be used for biofeedback. Such an instrument is helpful in the treatment for high blood pressure and migraine headaches.

Electroencephalographic (EEG) biofeedback involves the monitoring and displaying of brain wave activity as a correlate of autonomic nervous system activity. Different brain waves are associated with different levels of autonomic nervous system arousal. Common applications of EEG biofeedback are in the treatment of substance abuse disorders, epilepsy, attention-deficit disorders, and insomnia.

USES AND COMPLICATIONS

Biofeedback is gaining in popularity because of a number of factors. One of the principal reasons is a growing interest in alternatives to the lifetime use of medications to manage a disorder.

To understand the rationale for biofeedback in a clinical setting, it is essential to discuss the types of disorders for which it is commonly employed. As pointed out in the publication *Biofeedback*, the more common usages of biofeedback treatment techniques include "migraine headaches, tension headaches, and many other types of pain; disorders of the digestive system; high blood pressure and its opposite, low blood pressure; cardiac arrhythmias (abnormalities, sometimes dangerous, in the rhythm of the heartbeat); Raynaud's disease (a circulatory disorder that causes uncomfortably cold hands); epilepsy; paralysis and other movement disorders."

Thus, biofeedback can be safely and effectively employed in the alleviation of numerous disorders. One example worth noting—in terms of the magnitude of the problem—

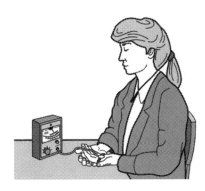

In biofeedback therapy, patients monitor their own autonomic physiological responses, such as blood pressure or pulse rate, in order to gain some control over these responses or to reduce stress.

is the treatment of cardiovascular disorders. Myocardial infarctions, commonly known as heart attacks, are one of the major health problems in the industrialized world and an area of special concern to those practitioners with a psychophysiological orientation. In the United States alone, approximately 700,000 persons die of heart attacks each year.

One of the principal causes of heart attacks is hypertension (high blood pressure). Emotions have much to do with the manifestation of high blood pressure (hypertension), which places this condition in the category of a psychophysiological disorder. Researchers have demonstrated that biofeedback is an effective methodology to correct the problem of high blood pressure. The data reveal that many individuals employing biofeedback have been able to decrease (or eliminate entirely) the use of medication to manage their hypertension. Studies also show that these individuals maintain normal blood pressure levels for as much as two years following the completion of biofeedback training.

Because of its noninvasive properties and its broad applicability in the clinical setting, biofeedback is also increasingly becoming one of the more commonly utilized modalities in many fields, such as behavioral medicine. Researchers have provided documented evidence showing that biofeedback is effective in the treatment of so-called stress-related disorders. It is recognized that the four major causes of death and disability in the United States fall into the "stress-related" category. Research has also shown that biofeedback has beneficial applications in the areas of neuromuscular rehabilitation (working with stroke victims to help them develop greater control and use of afflicted muscle groups) and myoneural rehabilitation (working with victims of fibromyalgia and chronic pain to help them obtain relief from debilitating pain).

Research in the 1960's pointed to the applicability of EEG biofeedback for seizure disorders (such as epilepsy). Advanced technology and later research findings, however, have demonstrated EEG biofeedback to be effective in the treatment of attention-deficit disorder, hyperactivity, and alcoholism as well.

Biofeedback appears to have particular applicability for children. Apparently, there is an innate ability on the part of the young to learn self-regulation skills much more quickly than older persons, such as the lowering of autonomic nervous system activity. Since this activity is highly correlated with respiratory distress, biofeedback is often used in the treatment of asthma in prepubescent children. Biofeedback is also being successfully used as an alternative to prescription medications (such as Ritalin) for youngsters with attention-deficit disorder.

The use of biofeedback is also found in the field of athletics and human performance. Sports psychologists and athletic coaches have long recognized that there is an inverted "U" pattern of performance where autonomic nervous system activity and performance are concerned. In the field of sports psychology, this is known as the Yerkes-Dobson law. The tenets of this law state that as the level of autonomic nervous system arousal rises, performance will improve—but only to a point. When autonomic nervous system arousal becomes too high, a corresponding deterioration in performance occurs. At some point prior to an athletic competition, it may be desirable for an athlete to experience an increase (or a decrease) in the level of autonomic nervous system activity (the production of adrenaline, for example). Should adrenaline levels become too high, however, the athlete may "choke" or become tense.

To achieve physiological autoregulation (often referred to in this athletic context as self-regulation), athletes have used biofeedback to assist them with establishing better control of a variety of physiologic processes. Biofeedback applications have ranged from hand-warming techniques for cross-country skiers and mountain climbers to the regulation of heartbeat for sharpshooters (such as biathletes and archers) to the lowering of adrenaline levels for ice-skaters, gymnasts, and divers.

Biofeedback, apart from empirical studies or research on both animal and human subjects, is seldom used in isolation. In most treatment protocols, it is employed in combination with such interventions as behavioral management, lifestyle counseling, exercise, posture awareness, and nutritional considerations. In most biofeedback applications, the individual is also taught a number of procedures that he or she is encouraged to use between therapy sessions. The conscientious and effective practice of these recommended procedures has been proven to be a determining factor in the success rate of biofeedback. The end aim of biofeedback is self-regulation, and self-regulation must extend to situations outside the clinical setting.

Biofeedback (when employed as a part of a behavioral medicine program) is usually offered as a component of a treatment team approach. The biofeedback practitioner commonly interfaces with members of other disciplines to design and implement a treatment protocol implemented to correct the presenting problem (for example, fibromyalgia) for which the referral was made.

One commonly found model of biofeedback is for the patient, the biofeedback practitioner, and the primary medical care provider to constitute a team. The team concept applies even to the extent that the biofeedback practitioner (in many ways acting as a coach) will give the patient a number of procedures to follow between treatment sessions and will then evaluate, with the patient and the medical practitioner, the effectiveness of the procedure. Modifications in the modalities and in the interventions follow from these evaluations. Biofeedback interventions are dynamic and measurable so that the effectiveness of the protocol can be adjusted to meet the needs of the patient.

PERSPECTIVE AND PROSPECTS

Biofeedback, as a treatment modality, is relatively new.

The history of biofeedback as a research tool, however, dates back to early attempts to quantify physiological processes. From the time of Ivan Pavlov and his research on the salivary processes in canines, both psychologists and physiologists have long been interested in the measurement of human behavior (including physiological processes).

Early in the twentieth century, the work of Walter B. Cannon, with his book *The Wisdom of the Body* (1932), helped to set the stage for the field of self-regulation. Another landmark publication was that of Edmund Jacobson's *Progressive Relaxation*, published in 1929. More recently, the work of such pioneers as John V. Basmajian, Neal Miller, Elmer Green, Joseph Kamiya, and many others spawned research and development efforts that by 1975 produced more than twenty-five hundred literature references utilizing biofeedback as a part of a study.

The evolution of biofeedback as a treatment modality has its historical roots in early research in the areas of learning theory, psychophysiology, behavior modification, stress reactivity, electronics technology, and biomedical engineering. The emerging awareness—and acceptance by the general public—that individuals do in fact have the potential to promote their own wellness and to facilitate the healing process gave additional impetus to the development of both the theory and the technology of biofeedback treatment. Several other factors have combined to produce the climate within which biofeedback has gained recognition and acceptance. One of these was widespread recognition that many of the disorders that afflict humankind today have, as a common basis, some disruption of the natural feedback processes. Part of this recognition is attributable to the seminal work of Hans Selye on stress reactivity.

Developments in the fields of electronics, physiology, psychology, endocrinology, and learning theory produced a body of knowledge which spawned the evolution and growth of biofeedback. Further refinement and an explosion of technology have resulted in procedures and techniques that have set the stage for the use of biofeedback as an effective intervention with wide applications in the treatment of numerous disorders.

The practice of biofeedback has extended to a number of disciplines. Included in the membership of the Association of Applied Psychophysiology and Biofeedback (formerly the Biofeedback Society of America) are representatives from the fields of medicine, psychology, physical therapy, social work, occupational therapy, and chiropractic. The professional journal of the association is *Biofeedback and Self-Regulation*, published by Plenum Press. The accrediting arm of the Association of Applied Psychophysiology and Biofeedback is the Biofeedback Certification Institute of America.   —*Ronald B. France, Ph.D.*

See also Alternative medicine; Anxiety; Arrhythmias; Asthma; Attention-deficit disorder; Brain; Cardiac rehabilitation; Cardiology; Electrocardiography (ECG or EKG);

Electroencephalography (EEG); Epilepsy; Exercise physiology; Headaches; Heart attack; Hypertension; Hypnosis; Meditation; Nervous system; Neurology; Pain management; Paralysis; Phobias; Physical rehabilitation; Physiology; Preventive medicine; Respiration; Sleep disorders; Sports medicine; Stress; Stress reduction.

FOR FURTHER INFORMATION:

Basmajian, John V., ed. *Biofeedback: Principles and Practice for Clinicians.* 3d ed. Baltimore: Williams & Wilkins, 1989. A collection of writings dealing with the uses of biofeedback for various disorders. This work contains chapters on instrumentation and theory as well.

Brown, Barbara Banter. *Stress and the Art of Biofeedback.* New York: Harper & Row, 1977. This work, by a pioneer researcher and clinician, is one of the earliest references on the use of biofeedback. Brown developed much of her material while working for the Veterans Administration medical system.

Green, Elmer, and Alyce Green. *Beyond Biofeedback.* New York: Delta, 1977. Observations about the future of not only biofeedback but behavioral medicine as well. Written by two of the key researchers and clinicians in the field. Their work at the Menninger Foundation in Topeka, Kansas, served as one of the wellsprings of biofeedback theory and practice.

Olton, David S., and Aaron R. Noonberg. *Biofeedback: Clinical Applications in Behavioral Medicine.* Englewood Cliffs, N.J.: Prentice Hall, 1980. A practical overview of the applicability of biofeedback in the practice of behavioral medicine. This reference contains a basic overview of the development of biofeedback, as well as fundamental clinical applications in the treatment of various disorders.

Schultz, J. H., and Wolfgang Luthe. *Autogenic Methods.* Vol. 1 in *Autogenic Therapy.* New York: Grune & Stratton, 1969. One of the early formalized statements concerning the innate ability to regulate and control physiologic processes by virtue of self-monitoring. One of two volumes of therapeutic formulations and methods for treating various disorders through the influence of the mind on the functions of the body.

Schwartz, Mark S. *Biofeedback: A Practitioner's Guide.* 2d ed. New York: Guilford Press, 1995. One of the more recent references in the field of biofeedback. The chapters contain updated information concerning the fundamentals of and (as of 1987) state-of-the-art methodologies concerning biofeedback.

Schwartz, Mark S., and Les Fehmi. *Applications Standards and Guidelines for Providers of Biofeedback Services.* Wheatridge, Colo.: Biofeedback Society of America, 1982. A statement of the professional and ethical foundations for the practice of biofeedback. An important reference for anyone considering the employment of biofeedback in a clinical setting.

BIONICS AND BIOTECHNOLOGY

PROCEDURES

ANATOMY OR SYSTEM AFFECTED: All

SPECIALTIES AND RELATED FIELDS: Biotechnology, cytology, genetics, immunology, microbiology

DEFINITION: The integration and application of biological and engineering knowledge to the medical sciences; bionics applies this knowledge to the design of artificial systems that act in the place of natural systems, while biotechnology applies this knowledge at the molecular and genetic levels of these natural systems in order to diagnose, treat, cure, or learn more about diseases.

KEY TERMS:

bioengineering: the combination of biological principles and engineering concepts and/or methodology to improve knowledge in both areas

biological principles: knowledge concerned with living organisms and their natural systems, particularly at the cellular, molecular, and genetic levels

biological systems: any of several levels of life, from that of the individual organism to the functional level (for example, the circulatory system, respiratory system, or limbs), the organ level (such as the heart or liver), the cellular level, and the molecular level; also called natural systems

cybernetics: a field of study closely associated with bionics which is concerned with communication and control in living systems and their application to artificial systems

engineering concepts and methodology: an analysis of how systems work (in particular, the step-by-step processes involved) and how these systems can be duplicated

monoclonal antibodies: antibodies (proteins that protect the body against disease-causing foreign bodies such as bacteria and viruses) produced in large quantities from cloned cells

recombinant DNA technology: manipulation of the genetic material DNA whereby pieces are separated and interchanged in order to obtain a desired result

INDICATIONS AND PROCEDURES

Bionics and biotechnology are part of the larger arena of bioengineering. This broad interdisciplinary field integrates the many disciplines of biology and engineering for use in the medical sciences, as well as in other areas such as agriculture, chemical manufacturing, environmental studies, and mining. Because of the interdisciplinary nature of these studies, an often-confusing array of terms may be used, such as biochemical engineering, bioelectronics, biofeedback, biological modeling, biomaterials, biomechanics, environmental health engineering, genetic engineering, human engineering, and medical engineering. When applied to the medical sciences, these various areas of knowledge can be pulled together under the headings of bionics and biotechnology when considering the diagnosis, investigation, prevention, or treatment of diseases and damaged biological systems.

Within the medical sciences, bionics is concerned with applying engineering concepts and methodology to constructing artificial systems, such as organs or limbs, in order to replace damaged or diseased natural systems. In order to duplicate biological systems and replace them successfully, knowledge of how these systems function biologically, chemically, and mechanically is required. Creating artificial systems has evolved from the making of crude imitations, such as an artificial kidney machine, to the making of sophisticated replicas of the natural system, with the replacement being made in the living organism. While it is necessary to apply engineering knowledge to duplicate these natural systems, the fact that these are natural systems requires the application of biological knowledge to the engineering effort. Some animals have the ability to regenerate lost or destroyed limbs; humans, however, must rely on their ingenuity. Biotechnology is an interdisciplinary field that seeks to replace, if not re-create, nature.

Within the medical sciences, biotechnology is concerned with the manipulation and study of biological systems at the molecular and genetic level. In addition to a basic understanding of how these systems function at these levels, biotechnology is used for practical purposes as well. A significant application is the synthesis of biological products, such as antibiotics, biochemicals used in diagnostic tests, drugs, enzymes, vaccines, and vitamins. This field is also concerned with the manipulation of genetic material to improve this synthetic process, as well as the study of genetic diseases and the manipulation of the associated genes to prevent or cure these diseases. These kinds of syntheses and studies involve the use of molecules, cells, or genes as raw materials in biological processes that are duplicated under artificial conditions in order to improve or increase the quantities of needed biological products. The techniques and methodologies used to achieve these results are the basis of the technology. So, once again, a thorough knowledge of biology and engineering are needed to understand the natural system and to improve the process by which the natural system works in order to accomplish an imposed artificial result.

Much of this work has been carried out through the use of recombinant DNA technology. Since genes provide the instructions controlling those processes by which biological products are made, it is possible to change the processes, or the rate of the processes, by changing the genes. Through genetic engineering, cell cloning, and other techniques, it is possible to make naturally produced antibiotics, vaccines, vitamins, and other needed biological products rather than duplicating these products with artificial materials using artificial means. Also, the rate at which these products are naturally produced can be increased so that large quantities can be obtained (under natural conditions, these products are produced in extremely small amounts). Another aspect of recombinant DNA technology has to do with diseases that result from biological processes that are improperly controlled by genes at critical points. Genetic engineering is used to replace or correct the genetic structure in order to replace or correct the instructions used to guide the biological process.

There is still much to be learned about biological processes and about the genetic material. It is estimated that there are about 100,000 genes constructed from some 3 billion base pairs. Discovering how these genes interact and about the biological processes that each controls is a formidable task. A comprehensive effort known as the Human Genome Project seeks to map the entire human genetic structure from which all biological processes are controlled, including the flawed ones that cause diseases. Eventually, studies of other genomes, such as those of bacteria and viruses, will treat or prevent diseases and illnesses caused by them as well. This study of genetic material, along with the ongoing study of genetic diseases and of other diseases at the molecular level, will have an increasingly important impact on the overall study of diseases.

Biotechnology has contributed much to the medical sciences in a relatively short time. It has provided a better understanding of human physiology and an improved fundamental knowledge of disease itself. Knowledge has been gained about the physiological control networks (in part resulting from related studies in cybernetics), the key regulatory agents and processes, the target molecules needed for therapeutic intervention, and the molecular and genetic causes of disease.

With rapid advances in biotechnology, however, the scientific and medical professions are entering sensitive and controversial areas that have raised legal and regulatory concerns. The alteration of genes, the creation of modified organisms, the development of new drugs, the safety and side effects of new biochemicals, the detection of genetic diseases in the fetus, experimental therapies, the ability to clone, the ability to enhance brain functions, and the national and international competition to produce pharmaceuticals are some of the concerns facing medical practitioners, the biomedical industry, government, society, and the individual. These concerns will continue as biotechnological advances delve even deeper into the molecular and genetic basis of life in order to achieve improved health benefits.

USES AND COMPLICATIONS

While there are many applications of biotechnology, some of the more significant ones include the production of pharmaceuticals and biochemicals, the production of monoclonal antibodies, the improved understanding and control of complex diseases such as cancer and acquired immunodeficiency syndrome (AIDS), and the improved understanding of genetic diseases. Many of the biotechnology techniques and methodologies are still experimental, as are the resulting products (for example, antibodies, drugs, enzymes, vaccines, vitamins, cloned cells, and recombinant

DNA). Some are considered useful and practical, but are not yet approved for use.

The production of pharmaceuticals and biochemicals has been one of the most practical outgrowths of biotechnology research. It has produced both the knowledge of what needs to be done to correct a certain disease process and the ability to make the needed corrections. Some diseases result from deficiencies in particular proteins, as is the case with diabetes, hemophilia, and dwarfism. Others result from deficiencies in enzymes that would normally break down other chemicals, thus resulting in an accumulation of these chemicals, such as in Fabry's, Gaucher's, and Tay-Sachs disease. Still others result from a lack of cellular control, such as cancers.

It has been possible to produce deficient proteins (insulin for diabetes, factor VIII for hemophilia, and growth hormone for dwarfism), deficient enzymes, and missing bioregulatory proteins (interferon for cancer). This is done by learning how these proteins are produced naturally and then engineering the cells or biochemical processes that can produce these proteins in quantity. In addition to these various kinds of proteins, other biochemical products can be made, including antibiotics, vaccines, and vitamins. Scientists may produce natural, unaltered biochemicals; altered biochemicals (for improved results); or synthetic versions of the biochemicals.

Monoclonal antibodies are a significant group of naturally produced, unaltered biochemicals. They are highly specific biochemicals used for the diagnosis of infectious diseases, for monitoring cancer therapy, for determining the blood concentrations of therapeutic drugs and hormones, for use in some pregnancy tests, for suppressing immune responses, and, to some extent, for disease therapy (for example, to kill cancer cells). While much of this work is still experimental, there is a great potential for the development of highly specific vaccines and for reagents used in diagnostic tests. In addition to being highly specific, these vaccines and reagents would be free of any biological contamination and tend to be reliably stable at room temperature. The vaccines would also be safer since their production would not require the handling of large quantities of the pathogenic agent (which is how vaccines have traditionally been obtained). Possible use could involve immunological protection against hepatitis B, herpes simplex, polio myelitis, rabies, and malaria.

Molecular pharmacologists also develop biochemicals from nonhuman sources. In fact, the diversity of animal and plant life in the world is a natural pharmacy of potentially useful biochemicals. Many medicinal plants are already known, and systematic studies of other species are under way. Animals also contribute useful biochemicals. For example, excretions from the skin of tropical frogs have been used to treat skin diseases, diabetic ulcers, eye infections, and cancers. Through the study of fifty species of poison arrow frogs, scientists have discovered more than three hundred chemicals. Only about 5 percent of the world's frog species have been studied, and this is only one group in the world's great biodiversity. Biotechnology has made it possible to study natural biochemicals in small amounts and at the molecular level and has provided the necessary techniques and methodologies for using these biochemicals in the study of diseases.

Cancers form a complex group of diseases that continue to defy the best attempts to understand them. A cancer is composed of normal cells that have proliferated uncontrollably. This response may be caused by a mutated gene, by carcinogenic agents (for example, chemicals or ultraviolet light), or by viruses. Cancers develop in multiple stages that involve different physiological mechanisms. Understanding these mechanisms and the genes and biochemicals that are involved has been possible in large part because of the techniques and methodologies of biotechnology research.

The same can be said of the efforts to study AIDS. This syndrome is caused by a virus that infects and kills certain kinds of T lymphocytes that are needed to initiate and maintain normal immune system responses; therefore, AIDS is characterized by the occurrence of unusual infections or by Kaposi's sarcoma (a rare cancer). The nucleotide sequence of the viral genome has been determined through recombinant DNA technology, and the functions of the genes are being characterized. Diagnostic tests to determine if blood is contaminated by the virus have been developed, and efforts are under way to develop a vaccine. The proteins used in these immunological investigations are made in large quantities by genetically engineered microorganisms. Other vaccine studies are concerned with using recombinant DNA technology to disable the AIDS virus genetically (by removing or altering its genes) so that it will infect and generate protective immunity without actually causing the disease.

Genetic diseases are also beginning to be understood as a result of biotechnology. Many of these diseases are caused by gene mutations that cause the absence of a protein or the production of a defective protein, affecting biochemical processes. Recombinant DNA technology is providing methods of detecting these defects, as well as providing therapies for correcting or replacing them. Many of these defects can even be diagnosed in the fetus and in previously undetectable carriers. Some of the commonly known genetic diseases include Alzheimer's disease, cystic fibrosis, hemophilia, Huntington's disease, muscular dystrophy, sickle-cell anemia, and thalassemia. There are approximately three thousand genetic diseases resulting from single-gene mutations. In addition to studying these numerous mutations, efforts are being made to study diseases associated with specific normal genes (such as the susceptibility for heart attacks by individuals with genes producing specific cholesterol-carrying proteins) and to cure genetic disorders by replacing the mutated gene with a cloned normal gene.

One advantage of learning more about common genetic diseases is that more can be learned about normal genomes by comparing them to mutated genomes. These diseases are few in number, however, and much remains to be done. In the process of studying the human genome (as well as the genome of other animals, plants, bacteria, and viruses), biotechnology, and its usefulness to the medical sciences, will advance significantly. The Human Genome Project is an effort to learn about the entire human genetic structure, mapping every gene in the twenty-four chromosomes. It is estimated that there are about 100,000 genes with about 3 billion base pairs. In addition, there are about 3 million differences per genome from one individual to another. These differences are responsible for such things as personality differences and inherited diseases. In order to find and understand some of the rarest disease-causing genes, it is estimated that the differences between the genomes of some 4 billion individuals will need to be studied. This would create a database that would strain even state-of-the-art computers, not to mention the researchers who will compile the database.

PERSPECTIVE AND PROSPECTS

Artificial limbs have been in use for centuries, but no attempt was made to duplicate natural limbs except in the crudest sense. The use of microorganisms for the production of fermented beverages (such as beer, wine, and vinegar) and food (such as bread) goes back many centuries. Likewise, folk medicine made use of natural biochemicals to treat diseases for as many centuries. These traditional processes, however, did not involve an understanding of what was occurring and may only be considered biotechnology by default. The knowledge needed for biotechnology required the development of several scientific disciplines, all of which only occurred after the 1950's, when scientifically understood and controlled processes were developed to produce biological products. It was not until the 1970's that recombinant DNA technology allowed significant advances in the understanding of many molecular and genetic processes.

The advancement of bionics and biotechnology after the 1950's was the result of advances made in related scientific fields during earlier decades, primarily after 1900. These developments included the discovery that enzymes were proteins and the theory of enzyme action; the discovery of the structure and function of vitamins; the discovery of the composition of nucleic acids; the discovery of the structure of carbohydrates; the development of a better understanding of the cellular infrastructure; work on natural and experimentally induced mutation; the study of hereditary metabolic errors; a better understanding of immunology, viral and bacterial diseases, tumors, and cell pathology; the realization that genes were found in the chromosomes; early studies concerning chromosome recombinations and the

mechanisms of genetic expression; the ultraviolet analysis of DNA and RNA; the increased use of electron microscopy; the development of the technology involved in the large-scale production of penicillin; and the further development and integration of studies in genetics, biochemistry, and physiology.

The 1950's and 1960's saw important advances in the discovery of the structure of DNA, the breaking of the genetic code, the discovery of how gene actions were regulated, the structure of the gene and of numerous proteins, the discovery and study of numerous hereditary diseases, the development of medical procedures for organ transplants, the evolution of the branch of science known as molecular biology, and the continuing synthesis of discoveries and theories from a variety of scientific disciplines. The 1970's saw the development of technologies that further developed these areas of study, in particular recombinant DNA technology and monoclonal antibody technology. The future will see an increased refinement of these technologies and further developments resulting from the Human Genome Project. —*Vernon N. Kisling, Jr., Ph.D.*

See also Amputation; Biofeedback; Biophysics; Cloning; Computed tomography (CT) scanning; Dialysis; DNA and RNA; Electrocardiography (ECG or EKG); Electroencephalography (EEG); Gene therapy; Genetic engineering; Genetics and inheritance; Heart transplantation; Heart valve replacement; Magnetic resonance imaging (MRI); Mutation; Pacemaker implantation; Pharmacology; Physical rehabilitation; Plastic, cosmetic, or reconstructive surgery; Positron emission tomography (PET) scanning.

FOR FURTHER INFORMATION:

Abelson, Philip H., ed. *Biotechnology and Biological Frontiers*. Washington, D.C.: American Association for the Advancement of Science, 1984. A technical overview of specific applications of biotechnology. These are updated and corrected articles that have appeared in the journal *Science*.

Albertini, Alberto, Claude Lenfant, and Rodolfo Paoletti, eds. *Biotechnology in Clinical Medicine*. New York: Raven Press, 1987. A technical review of specific applications of biotechnology in various areas of medicine.

Blank, Robert H., and Miriam K. Mills, eds. *Biomedical Technology and Public Policy*. New York: Greenwood Press, 1989. Contains reviews of the ethical implications of rapidly advancing medical technologies and examinations of government activities dealing with these issues.

Marx, Jean L., ed. *A Revolution in Biotechnology*. New York: Cambridge University Press, 1989. An excellent general review of the various areas of study encompassed by biotechnology. Begins with an explanation of heredity, genes, and DNA and then goes on to describe the study and practical applications of biotechnology. Well illustrated and contains lists of additional reading in each chapter.

Rehm, Hans-Jürgen, and Gerald Reed, eds. *Biotechnology.* 8 vols. Deerfield Beach, Fla.: Verlag Chemie, 1981-1988. An eight-volume set covering microbial fundamentals, biochemical engineering, microbial products, food and feed production with microorganisms, biotransformations, enzyme technology, and gene technology. Various medical topics are included, such as antibiotics, vaccines, tumors, cardiology, human genetic diseases, and bioelectronics.

Smith, George P. II. *The New Biology: Law, Ethics, and Biotechnology.* New York: Plenum Press, 1989. A review of legal and ethical concerns involved with the development of biomedical and biotechnical advances.

Trevan, M. D., et al. *Biotechnology: The Biological Principles.* New York: Taylor & Francis, 1987. Written for students familiar with biochemistry, microbiology, and molecular biology, this book explains the rationale and problems in specific areas such as microbial metabolism, the growth and culturing of microorganisms, genetic manipulation, and biocatalyst technology.

Vasil, Indra K. *Biotechnology: Science, Education, and Commercialization.* New York: Elsevier, 1990. Broad overviews of several areas of biotechnology, in particular the regional and international efforts to overcome problems in education and commercial development. Also includes a review of the Human Genome Project.

BIOPHYSICS

SPECIALTY

ANATOMY OR SYSTEM AFFECTED: All

SPECIALTIES AND RELATED FIELDS: Audiology, biotechnology, neurology, nuclear medicine, ophthalmology, optometry, radiology

DEFINITION: The scientific field that applies the laws, methods, and instrumentation of physics to study the structures, systems, and processes of biological organisms.

KEY TERMS:

atom: the smallest chemically and biologically active unit of matter; composed of electrons enclosing an atomic nucleus containing protons and neutrons

cell: the basic unit of living matter; composed of a cell membrane, a cell nucleus containing DNA, and many other specialized, complex units

charge: the quantity of electricity responsible for attraction and repulsion among atoms and molecules

current: the flow of electrical charges through space or a material

deoxyribonucleic acid (DNA): the helical genetic material of plants, animals, and many lower organisms

electron: the negatively charged, fundamental particle that gives atoms their structure and their chemical and biological activity

energy: a measure of a system's capacity to do work

momentum: the product of mass and velocity for a particle; inverse with wavelength (the distance between peaks of a wave)

photon: the smallest unit of an electromagnetic wave; energy increases with the frequency of wave peaks

quantum theory: the theory that energy, momentum, and other physical quantities appear in indivisible units of finite quantity

voltage: energy per unit charge; typical biological voltages range from hundredths to tenths of a volt

SCIENCE AND PROFESSION

A young boy skips a stone across a still pond, and a startled frog jumps into the water. Physics studies nature in the arc of the stone, the rippling of the water, the sound of the splash, and the surprising motions of the atoms and molecules within the stone and the water of the pond. Biology, on the other hand, studies the boy and the frog—their cells, nerves, muscles, and senses—which are very different from the dead mass of the stone and the still water of the pond. Despite their immense differences, the boy, the frog, the stone, and the pond have the same atoms and obey the same basic laws of nature. Biophysics enters, for example, when the boy hears the sound of the splash, one of many meeting grounds between biology and physics as they merge into one knowledge. Since biological systems are chemical and mathematics is the language of physics, biophysics has significant overlap with biochemistry and biomathematics.

Biology is the scientific investigation of the laws of life. In particular, biology studies both the structure and function of cells and organisms such as viruses, bacteria, plants, and animals, including their communities. It studies the means by which life nourishes and maintains itself and by which it perpetuates itself by genetic transmission, reproduction, and evolution. Medical science applies this knowledge in the service of humankind. Physics is the scientific investigation of the laws of nature. Physics has two major divisions, experimental and theoretical physics. Instruments are the tools of the experimental physicist, and mathematics are the tools of the theoretical physicist. Distinct from biology, physics restricts its investigations to inanimate objects. At the human level, nature appears as matter and waves; physics studies the properties of both and their interactions. For the arena of biophysics, the most useful branches of physics are atomic, energetic, fluid, and electromagnetic physics.

Broadly taken, atomic physics studies atoms and their nuclei and molecules (which are isolated atom groups) and their formation into solids, liquids, and gases. Atoms consist of electrons circulating around a tiny nucleus of protons and neutrons. Electrons have negative charges and give the atoms their distinctive shapes and chemical, biological, and medical properties. Protons and neutrons are similar except that protons have a positive charge and neutrons have no charge. The protons hold the electrons within the atoms by electrical forces, while nuclear forces bind protons and neutrons within the nucleus. The exchange of electrons between and among atoms determines the chemical properties of materials, including biological and medical materials.

Most atoms are neutral, with an equal number of electrons and protons. Hydrogen, with one electron and one proton, is the smallest atom and a common biological constituent, along with carbon, nitrogen, and oxygen, which possess six, seven, and eight electrons, respectively. When an electron is missing from an otherwise neutral atom, the atom becomes a positive ion. Adding an electron converts a neutral atom to a negative ion. Ions are abundant in biological fluids. The hydrogen positive ion, along with calcium, potassium, and sodium positive ions and the chlorine negative ion, are important biological atomic ions. In most electronic devices, electrons produce electrical activity, but in living organisms and humans, ions govern this activity.

Since atomic nuclei do not play a significant role within living organisms, the smallest matter particles of biological importance are atoms. Groups of atoms make biological molecules, deoxyribonucleic acid (DNA), carbon dioxide, water, and bones, for example. Some atomic nuclei are unstable and release energetic particles and waves. These radioactive products are usually damaging to cells and their DNA, but under controlled conditions, they are useful, for example, as radioactive tracers.

Energetic physics studies the basic forces of nature. The electromagnetic force, together with gravity and the nuclear forces, is one of the known fundamental forces of nature. In biological materials, other forces, such as the osmotic force, are complex manifestations of the electrical force. These forces allow matter to interact—to hold, pull, and push other matter and to exchange energy and momentum. While the prime biological interaction among matter is electrical, the major interaction between matter and waves is electromagnetic. An example is the absorption of the electromagnetic wave—light—by the eye to form visual images.

Fluids are groups of atoms or molecules that move easily; included in this definition are both liquids and gases. Biological fluids are important for the transportation of materials across cell membranes, for blood circulation, and for respiration. Fluid physics investigates fluid motions under the influence of various forces. Confined fluids develop pressures as a result of the forces between the fluid particles. Under a pressure difference, fluids flow toward the lower pressure. Thus, blood flows because of the blood pressure generated by the heart and arteries.

Electromagnetic physics studies electrical, magnetic, and electromagnetic fields in detail. Charge motion occurs when an electrical voltage acts across conducting materials, whether in an electronic device or in a biological system. In the body, biochemical activity generates voltages across nerve cell membranes, allowing the nerves to serve as the body's electronic network.

Oscillating electric charges produce electromagnetic waves. Thus nuclei produce gamma rays and atoms generate X rays and ultraviolet, visible, and infrared waves; electronic devices generate a variety of microwave and radio waves. Individual electromagnetic waves appear as packets, called photons, which carry both energy and momentum. Photon energy and momentum decrease dramatically in going from gamma rays to radio waves. Gamma rays and X rays carry high energy and momentum and are very destructive if encountered by molecules within cells. Both of these radiations easily penetrate soft tissues, so that their damage may permeate an entire organism. (Low X-ray dosages, however, give safe images of the body's structure.) Even ultraviolet rays carry sufficient energy to damage biological organisms. Since ultraviolet rays are not very penetrating, they mainly damage skin cells.

Visible photons carry enough energy to be useful to life as it has evolved on Earth and not too much to be damaging. Infrared photons produce heat. Individual microwave and radio photons have essentially no biological effects, but both can cause damage if the total energy that they carry creates excess heat, as with a defective microwave oven, or if the electric or magnetic fields in the waves produce undesirable biological effects. The level at which such effects occur has not been clearly established.

Senses are the means by which organisms know their surroundings. Light (an electromagnetic wave) and sound (a matter wave in air) are two physical stimuli. Vision and hearing are the biological responses to these stimuli. Biophysics of the senses studies vision, hearing, and other senses, including the orientational, chemical, somatic, and visceral senses.

Color vision is an extraordinary phenomenon. The human eye evolved under direct and reflected sunlight. Light absorbed differently by three color pigments in the retina signals to the brain the colors of an illuminated scene. Lack of one or two of the pigments produces different forms of color blindness. Normal humans can distinguish roughly twenty thousand different colors. The response of the eye peaks at yellow green, where sunlight has its maximum energy at the earth surface. Matching detector response to source output is characteristic of any efficient electronic detector. Indeed, evolution has made the eye so efficient that a dark-adapted eye can respond to perhaps only one visible photon. This superb detector is at the limit allowed by the laws of physics.

The ear is another exquisite sense organ fashioned by evolution. Hearing picks up sound waves. Speech is one prime source for sound, so human hearing matches the human vocal range. Although human hearing extends over a very wide range, from about 20 to 20,000 cycles per second, it is so precise that the ear can tune into single tones.

A possible explanation to this paradoxical behavior is that evolution has shaped the ear as a mechanical traveling wave amplifier.

Perceived sensations move from a sense organ, such as the eye, by electrical signals conducted over the nervous system to the animal brain. The response to these signals triggers other nerve impulses to the muscles which contract and move the animal, such as a frog jumping into a pond. This is the arena of electrical biophysics, which investigates the effects of electrical and magnetic fields in living organisms.

Nerve impulses are electrical signals within the nerve. A stimulus at the end of a nerve initiates chemical changes that produce the electrical motion of ions. Tunnel-like proteins on the membrane surface channel the ions across the membrane. The resulting local change in charge propagates along the length of the nerve; in this way, for example, sound in the ear sends signals to the brain. This electrical activity produces low-frequency electrical waves that can be detected in various parts of the body, such as by brain wave monitors and electrocardiograms (EKGs or ECGs).

Typical nerve voltages occur in pulses somewhat smaller than one hundredth of a volt, lasting several thousandths to hundredths of a second. These pulses involve the conduction of sodium and potassium positive ions across the membrane through the protein ion channels. The result is ionic communication in the nervous system. The human brain is part of that system and generates electrical waves with frequencies of about 0.5 to 50.0 cycles per second, with voltages of hundredths to tenths of a volt when picked up by external electrodes attached to the scalp.

Electrocardiograms pick up electrical activity in the heart. The beating heart displays time traces with narrow spikes of uniform height. These spikes represent electrical signals that trigger the heart muscle to contract at a continuous, seemingly rhythmic beat of about once a second. The electrical stimulus, however, is decidedly not rhythmic but is instead a staccato beating. A mathematical technique called Fourier analysis shows that such spikes have a wide range of rhythmic frequencies, from zero to about 10 cycles per second.

Danger would ensue if the electrical activity of the heart became a pure rhythm. If this happens, the frequency range collapses to around 6 cycles per second, too fast for the heart to follow. Deadly ventricular fibrillations may follow. The heart beats in shallow, spasmodic pulses, and sudden cardiac arrest results. Here medical physics saves lives in the form of heart pacemakers and defibrillators. A pacemaker delivers mild electrical current to speed up a chronically slow heart rate, while a defibrillator provides a sharp electrical jolt to restore the normal heartbeat when fibrillation threatens cardiac arrest. Without treatment, patients identified as candidates for sudden cardiac arrest have only a 60 percent change of living a full year. The odds rise to 90 percent, however, for those who receive jolts from a defibrillator.

The latest generation of defibrillators is quite sophisticated. They can coax ventricular tachycardia back to a slower, normal beat by delivering mild electrical currents but also deliver ever-stronger stimulation and, if needed, a sharp jolt to prevent cardiac arrest. Some devices deliver a positive pulse immediately followed by a negative one. This requires less energy from the power source and produces less tissue damage in the patient.

DIAGNOSTIC AND TREATMENT TECHNIQUES

Perhaps the most obvious example of the influence of physics upon biology and medicine is in instruments. Physicists and engineers continually fashion new instruments based on novel developments in physics, and many of these find important applications in biology and medicine. This area of biophysics changes continually. As the complexity of instrumentation is reduced to the routine, the necessity for the involvement of physicists disappears. Biology and medicine take over the new tool.

The optical microscope is an example of a valuable instrument taken into biology and medicine. E. B. Wilson (1856-1939) used a microscope to draw the first primitive pictures of the cell in 1922. Only six cell constituents were clearly shown. Today, advanced instruments such as the electron microscope have provided a more detailed picture of the cell, with its dozens of specialized structures. Microscopes have long been a staple of medicine and are now supplemented by fiberoptic technology. Thin fibers guide light inside the patient's body and allow a physician to heal lesions and diseased sections with lasers.

X-ray analysis is another valuable tool of the biophysicist. X rays have wavelengths that match the distances between atoms in molecules. Thus, molecules produce distinctive X-ray patterns. Computational analysis allows a scientist to determine molecular structure from these patterns. In 1953, James D. Watson and Francis Crick used X-ray analysis to determine the double helix structure of DNA, allowing the genetic codes to be cracked.

Sophisticated computer analysis of a patient's three-dimensional X-ray patterns provides startling and accurate imaging of the body's interior without intrusion. Magnetic resonance imaging (MRI) provides complementary three-dimensional internal images, using microwave resonance in a high magnetic field produced by superconducting magnets. MRI produces images by picking up radio signals from the hydrogen atoms that permeate all body tissues. The spinning hydrogen nuclei are aligned by the strong magnetic field. A pulse of radio waves disorients the nuclei, which emit a distinctive radio signal as they reorient to the magnetic field. In comparison, ultrasonography is a surprisingly simple tool, creating images with high-frequency sound.

The use of lasers in medicine has become widespread. A medical laser is created by choosing a suitable laser wavelength to offer desirable penetration and absorption within the human tissue involved in a given procedure, along with an effective beam delivery and tissue removal systems. A partial list of medical laser applications includes retinal attachment, corneal alterations to adjust vision, dental drilling, the removal of surface lesions and stains on the skin, pulsed lithotripsy to break kidney stones into fragments, laser angioplasty to repair and unclog blood vessels, gynecological surgery, and bloodless incision for all types of procedures. Of importance to the physician are ease of operation of the laser equipment, reliability, reasonable cost, and, above all, effectiveness.

Body tissues are mainly composed of water. The water molecule absorbs strongly in the infrared spectrum and is transparent to the visible spectrum. Hemoglobin (in the blood) and melanin (in the skin) play important roles in laser-tissue interactions. Both absorb strongly, but differently, in the visible and near infrared ranges. The bulk of medical procedures that use lasers rely on rapid, selective heating of the target body tissue. For example, bloodless laser surgery requires rapid heating and vaporization of body tissue in the cut. The pulse duration is adjusted so that a thin layer of nearby tissue is heated to cause coagulation and stop bleeding.

An exciting, but experimental, cancer treatment which involves lasers is photodynamic therapy. Safe, light-sensitive dyes, such as the porphyrins, are injected into animals that have tumors. The dyes are absorbed by the tumors, and the tumor is exposed to intense laser light. The dyes alter to a toxic form, and tumor destruction is produced.

Lasers also make possible many research activities. One extraordinary application is the use of the laser's intense beam to act as optical tweezers. The beam can capture one living cell for study and can move organelles within the cell.

A final application is within molecular biophysics, which deals with the molecular constituents of living cells. Here biophysics applies quantum physics to determine the physical structure and biological behavior of the molecules that make up the human body.

Individually, all the molecules studied are inanimate and dead. With the aid of modern computers, physics accurately describes the behavior of the smaller cell constituents. In principle, quantum theory appears to be capable of describing the most complex molecules, including DNA, the basis of the genetic code. This code instructs the assembly of amino acids and proteins, and therefore the structure of an organism. In this task, quantum theory appears to be limited only by computational complexity.

When these dead molecules assemble as a cell, life begins. Viruses are such an assembly, but they inhabit the border region between large, inanimate molecules and the smallest living cells. The *Escherichia coli* (*E. coli*) virus is about a hundred atoms across and contains approximately one hundred thousand atoms. With the virus, dead physics meets live biology and medicine has its most elementary protagonist. Here all the sciences are challenged with the unanswered question of how life arises from the dead and survives.

PERSPECTIVE AND PROSPECTS

Physics has both enriched biology and profited greatly from the discoveries of many scientists educated in medical colleges and universities. These pioneers include Copernicus, Galileo, and at least a dozen other noted scientists who practiced from the fifteenth century to the nineteenth century. During this period, medicine was the major scientific profession—and before the seventeenth century the only one—at universities.

Nicolaus Copernicus (1473-1543), who proposed that the sun was the center of the solar system; studied medicine briefly in Padua, Italy. Galileo Galilei (1564-1642) was a medical student at Pisa, Italy, but finished in Canon law. He used one of the first telescopes to help verify Copernicus' ideas, constructed some of the first microscopes, and laid the foundations for the present understanding of the laws of motion.

The list of medical doctors who made significant scientific contributions is long. William Gilbert (1544-1603), physician to Queen Elizabeth I, pioneered the study of electricity and magnetism. Luigi Galvani (1737-1798), for twenty years a doctor, investigated animal electricity. The physician William Wollaston (1766-1828) discovered palladium and rhodium and was the first to observe ultraviolet light. Thomas Young (1773-1829) practiced medicine unsuccessfully, but he made important contributions to the understanding of energy and developed the three-color theory of vision. Julius Robert Mayer (1814-1878), a medical practitioner for ten years, presented the law of energy conservation five years before its more widely known introductions by James P. Joule (1818-1889) and surgeon Hermann von Helmholtz (1821-1894). Helmholtz was the first to determine nerve pulse speed, and he developed the cochlea theory of hearing and did important work in electromagnetism.

The broad education favored by the early medical schools fostered pioneering scientific discoveries by its students and physicians, uniquely merging physics and biology at the beginnings of biophysics.   —*Peter J. Walsh, Ph.D.*

See also Anatomy; Audiology; Computed tomography (CT) scanning; Ears; Electrocardiography (ECG or EKG); Eyes; Imaging and radiology; Laser use in surgery; Magnetic field therapy; Magnetic resonance imaging (MRI); Microscopy; Nervous system; Neurology; Optometry; Physiology; Sense organs.

FOR FURTHER INFORMATION:

Ackerman, Eugene, Lynda B. Ellis, and Lawrence E. Williams. *Biophysical Science*. 2d ed. Englewood Cliffs, N.J.: Prentice Hall, 1979. An excellent introductory biophysics text. Contains some mathematics, but the general reader can ignore it in choosing among the topics.

Biological Sciences Curriculum Study. *Biological Science.* Rev. ed. Boston: Houghton Mifflin, 1968. An admirable high school biology text. Its excellent photographs and illustrations make it a pleasure to browse through.

Carlson, Anton J., Victor Johnson, and H. Mead Cavert. *The Machinery of the Body.* 5th rev. ed. Chicago: University of Chicago Press, 1961. An excellent text on body physiology which introduces physical principles as needed without mathematics. Presents the biology of biophysics.

Casey, E. J. *Biophysics: Concepts and Mechanisms.* New York: Reinhold, 1965. A standard in the field. An introductory text which provides the basics needed to understand biophysics.

Marion, Jerry B. *General Physics with Bioscience Essays.* New York: John Wiley & Sons, 1979. A physics text with twenty-seven simple, readable bioscience essays sprinkled throughout. The essays apply physics to biology using only elementary math.

Sybesma, Christiaan. *Biophysics: An Introduction.* Rev. ed. Boston: Kluwer Academic, 1989. An introductory text on biophysics tilted toward the theoretical side of the science. More abstract than the other references listed here, requiring a good science background.

BIOPSY

PROCEDURE

ANATOMY OR SYSTEM AFFECTED: Cells

SPECIALTIES AND RELATED FIELDS: Cytology, dermatology, general surgery, gynecology, histology, oncology, pathology, radiology

DEFINITION: The removal and examination of tissue and cells from the body, which is performed to establish a precise diagnosis and to determine proper treatment and prognosis.

KEY TERMS:

cytology: the study of cells, their morphologic changes, and pathology

endoscopy: the visual inspection of body cavities and hollow structures and organs through the use of a tubelike instrument which can be introduced through any body orifice (e.g. mouth, anus) or through small cuts into the skin leading to a cavity

excisional biopsy: biopsy by incision to excise and completely remove an entire lesion, including adjacent portions of normal tissue

frozen section: an extremely thin tissue section cut by a specially designed instrument called a microtome from tissue that has been rapidly frozen, for the purpose of microscopic evaluation and rendering a diagnosis

incisional biopsy: biopsy of a selected sample of lesion

needle biopsy: the obtaining of tissue fragments by the puncture of a tumor, through a larger caliber needle, syringe, and plunger; the tissue within the lumen of the needle is obtained through the rotation and withdrawal of the needle

oncology: the branch of medicine concerned with the study and treatment of cancer

pathology: the branch of medicine that treats the essential nature of disease, especially of the structural and functional changes in cells, tissues, and organs of the body which cause or are caused by disease

staining: the artificial coloring of tissue sections and cells to facilitate their microscopic study

surgical pathology: the branch of pathology that deals with the interpretation of biopsies

INDICATIONS AND PROCEDURES

Biopsy is one of the most common diagnostic tools in medicine. Illness or disease can be caused by biological agents (such as viruses, bacteria, fungi, and parasites), physical agents (such as radiation, heat, extreme cold, and trauma), by genetic and metabolic abnormalities (such as diabetes), or by cancer, which is a new, abnormal growth commonly called a tumor. Often, however, the cause of an illness or disease may not be known. Nevertheless, the structural changes caused by the disease are characteristic enough so that the study of these alterations can give a clear picture of the nature and course of the disease. Diseases may primarily affect one organ at a time, such as hepatitis (the inflammation of the liver), or may involve many organ systems at once, as in acquired immunodeficiency syndrome (AIDS).

The signs and symptoms of disease are not specific and are often shared by many conditions. For example, all diseases of the liver can result in jaundice, or yellowing of the skin, and abnormal blood tests. The clinician, who may be an expert in liver disease, may not be able to tell for certain whether the underlying liver condition is caused by a virus, by a toxic substance such as alcohol, or by both. A needle biopsy of the liver may then be obtained. The sample is examined by an expert surgical pathologist, and a specific diagnosis is rendered.

Similarly, a lump in the breast may be innocuous (benign) or cancerous (malignant). Only a biopsy of such a lesion can determine this conclusively. Such a biopsy can be obtained by fine needle aspiration, which is a simple procedure that can be performed in a clinic, or by excision in the operating room. A frozen section is then made for the purpose of rapid diagnosis and management.

Once a biopsy is obtained, it is placed in a special fixative, such as formalin. This solution will preserve—or fix—the internal structure of the tissue and its cells. Expert technicians in histology, called histotechnologists, will then embed the tissue in waxlike paraffin to obtain a "block." The tissue block is then placed in a microtome and extremely thin pieces (about 5 micrometers thick in width) are cut from it. The slices are placed on glass slides and stained with different dyes, the most common of which is hematoxylin and eosin (H & E), to delineate the cellular substructures. The slides are examined by a surgical pathologist, who renders a pathology report in which the gross and microscopic features are described, and a diagnosis is made. A differential diagnosis may also be made, in which other possible causes of disease that may give a similar histologic picture are discussed. In addition to the routine study described above, a much more extensive and expensive workup of the biopsy may be done, depending on the anticipated complexity of the condition and organ.

The study of a biopsy requires diligent preparation and staining of the tissue, which is the realm of histotechnologists. Staining refers to the application of artificial dyes to tissue sections and cells to facilitate their microscopic study. Certain tissues and cell parts have different chemical and biological affinities for dyes which, when properly applied, help demarcate and differentiate the properties of these cells. A huge battery of special stains exists that can be used to examine every aspect of cell function in both health and disease. For example, specific enzymes can be evaluated; this technique is called enzyme histochemistry.

Immunologic stains, which help evaluate the status of immune system cells, are expensive and extremely tedious, and their proper interpretation requires considerable expertise. A huge battery of antibodies are commercially available for such testing. When directed against specific antigenic cell markers, they form immune complexes that can be targeted with immunological stains. Such stains can then be evaluated by immunofluorescence or immunoperoxidase techniques. Both types employ as their principle of action the forming of complexes between antigens and antibodies and the staining of these complexes. Immunofluorescence staining techniques involve the use of special stains that cause the tissue to shine when it is viewed under a fluorescent microscope; such procedures are performed on frozen section tissues. With immunoperoxidase stains, fixed tissues are used, and the stains are permanent.

Tissue samples can also be studied with an electron microscope, in which electron beams greatly magnify subcellular structures. In this way, the alterations of specific cellular components such as cell membranes, mitochondria, and intracellular viruses can be visualized and analyzed. This ultrastructural study is especially valuable in needle biopsies of the kidneys, as well as in the study of certain unusual cancer cells.

Another highly sophisticated method used to evaluate tissue and cell function in a biopsy is the application of molecular genetics and molecular biopsy techniques. The polymerase chain reaction (PCR) involves the splitting (splicing) of a specific section of genetic material in a cell and its amplification through a chemical chain reaction into innumerable folds, so that it can be visualized through a light microscope. This type of evaluation allows for the ex-

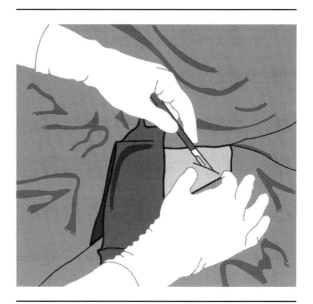

A biopsy is performed when diagnosis requires a sample of cells, tissue, or fluid for further analysis in the laboratory. The gathering of such a sample can be done with a scalpel (shown here), needle, curette, or syringe.

amination of specific microorganisms in a cell and can determine the presence of certain genetic markers of unusual diseases or cancer.

Another way to study the properties of cells is by examining their genetic makeup. Karyotyping is a technique in which the actual chromosomes in a cell are photographed during mitotic divisions; the chromosomes appear as patterns of bands. Genetic abnormalities can be identified by the number of chromosomes and their appearance. This procedure is often used in the study of cancer cells. An even more sophisticated study of cellular genetic makeup is called gene rearrangement, in which the order of gene stacking is examined for specific markers of certain cancerous growths, especially of white blood cells. Other techniques that are used to evaluate cell functions and morphology are cellular imaging, in which the contours of cell membranes and surfaces are compared using computers, and the use of flow cytometers, in which cells are targeted immunologically and then counted. Both techniques are employed in cancer studies and the second is also used for patients with abnormal immune systems, such as those with AIDS.

The aforementioned studies are expensive and available only at large medical centers and research institutes. The diagnostic workup in most hospitals, however, does not require the use of these sophisticated methods. Usually, routine H & E stains are applied. The Papanicolaou stain is commonly used with fine needle aspiration biopsies.

A department of pathology in a large medical center usually has one or more surgical pathologists, who are closely affiliated with the clinical and surgical departments and with their many branches and specialties. Interpreting biopsies obtained by any of the surgical or medical specialties is the most important duty of the surgical pathologist, and it requires great expertise and diligence. Because of the complexity of this task, specialized experts in pathology are becoming the norm. For example, a dermatopathologist is a surgical pathologist trained to interpret skin biopsies. Similarly, hematopathologists, neuropathologists, and nephropathologists are experts in the interpretation of blood-related, nerve and brain-related, and kidney-related biopsies, respectively.

In incisional biopsies, only a portion of the lesion is sampled, and the procedure is strictly of a diagnostic nature. In excisional biopsy, the entire lesion is removed, usually with a rim of normal tissue, and therefore the procedure serves both as a diagnostic and therapeutic function. The decision whether to perform an incisional or an excisional biopsy depends primarily on the size and location of the lesion; the smaller the lesion, the more logical it is to remove it completely. On the other hand, it is preferable to sample a deeply seated large tumor first because the type and extent of the excision varies considerably depending on the tumor type. For example, a small skin mole is usually excised completely, whereas a large soft tissue or bone tumor should be sampled.

Biopsies are also classified according to the instrument used to obtain them: cold knife versus cautery, needle, or endoscope. Of these the one usually least suitable for microscopic study is that obtained with a cautery, which uses a hot knife that burns, chars, and distorts tissue.

An endoscope is a tubelike fiberoptic instrument that is inserted into an orifice or small incision in order to view the contents of a body cavity. The instrument can be rigid or flexible and is equipped with a light source (usually a laser) and a small cutting tool at its tip to allow for the removal of small samples of tissue. Endoscopic biopsies are frequently used to obtain tissue and cell samples from the lungs and the airways, mainly to diagnose laryngeal and lung cancers; this procedure is usually done by a lung specialist. The endoscope is also used to sample lesions in the esophagus, stomach, intestines, and the rest of the intestinal tract, including the rectum. Such procedures are usually performed by a gastroenterologist, a specialist in the stomach and the gastrointestinal tract. Endoscopic biopsies of the urinary bladder and the prostate are done by urologists.

Needle biopsies are commonly used to obtain samples from superficial or deep-seated lumps. A slender, cylindrical core of tissue, corresponding to the open diameter of the needle, is obtained. The needle biopsy is commonly used to obtain tissue samples from kidneys, bone, and the deep viscera such as the liver. The modified technique of aspiration cytology, commonly called fine needle aspiration, employs a fine-caliber needle (0.6 to 0.9 millimeter in open diameter) and is widely used to obtain cytologic and minute tissue samples, especially for lesions of the lymph glands, breasts, thyroid gland, salivary glands, lungs, and prostate. Fine needle aspiration is often inexpensive, safe, quick, and, when performed and interpreted by experienced workers, quite accurate. Because of the ready availability and relative inexpense of the endoscopic and fine needle aspiration biopsy techniques, they have become popular; almost every part of the body is now within reach of one or another of these two techniques.

Frozen section biopsy requires great expertise because this biopsy is usually a form of consultation done during surgery. A tissue sample is instantly frozen, sectioned, stained, and examined—all within about fifteen minutes—in order to render a specific diagnosis. The implications of this diagnosis are far reaching and will influence the surgical procedure and the long-term therapy and outcome for the patient. A frozen section report, for example, may determine whether an organ such as a breast, lung, or kidney must be removed and whether long-term radiation therapy or chemotherapy will be administered; such would be the case if the diagnosis is read as malignant.

There are two indications, other than establishing a diagnosis, for performing a frozen section: determining the adequacy of the margins of surgical excision (for example, to remove a malignant tumor completely) and establishing whether the tissue obtained contains an ample diagnosable sample to carry out other specialized tissue studies.

USES AND COMPLICATIONS

The following examples illustrate the practical use of the various biopsy techniques.

An excisional biopsy is performed on a pigmented dark lesion on a sun-exposed surface of the body of a young man and is diagnosed as malignant melanoma, which is a tumor of the pigment-producing cells of the body. This diagnosis is confirmed through the use of specialized immunological stains employing specific antibodies against melanin. The pathologist also comments that surgical margins of excision of that tumor are safe and do not contain tumor, and that the tumor is only superficial in nature and does not show deep invasion into the tissue. These two points imply that the patient will probably have a complete cure.

A fine needle aspiration biopsy is applied on a lump on the breast of a young woman. The material obtained is spread on slides, stained with a Papanicolaou stain, and evaluated within hours of its removal. The lump is diagnosed as a fibroadenoma, which is a benign tumor that is completely innocuous and of no further consequence to the young patient.

An elderly patient has an endoscopic biopsy of a visualized mass in the colon, which proves to be cancer. The patient is taken to the operating room, and the colon is resected. A frozen section is performed on the margin on the surgical excision to make sure that it contains no tumor.

The stains used in this example are the simple and routine H & E stains.

A liver biopsy is performed on a patient with jaundice (yellowing of the skin), and a diagnosis of viral hepatitis B is made. This diagnosis was made following the study of the liver biopsy by routine stains and by stains that use immunological antibodies against the viral antigen. This is a specific and highly accurate diagnostic study.

A lymph gland excisional biopsy is performed on a patient who feels lumps all over his body. The biopsy is examined with routine and special stains, immunological marker studies, and gene rearrangement. Such extensive studies are performed to make sure that his condition is completely benign and is not neoplastic—that is, that he does not have malignant lymphoma (cancer of lymph tissue).

The biopsy, in its varied forms and techniques, has become an essential component of quality medical care. The biopsy report is both a medical and a legal document. Tissue slides and blocks are often stored for many years, in some places indefinitely. Peer slide reviews and consultations are common and are used as gauges for quality control and management. There are some limitations with histologic diagnosis, which mainly revolve around recognizing a specialist's own limitations and the need to seek a consultation by another expert pathologist as needed.

PERSPECTIVE AND PROSPECTS

The first attempts to affirm the role of biopsy in medical practice were made by Carl Ruge and Johann Veit of the University of Berlin, who in the 1870's introduced surgical biopsy as an essential diagnostic tool. Despite the inevitable controversies that followed, Johann F. A. von Esmarch, a professor of surgery and a leading military surgeon of his time, presented forceful arguments at the German Surgical Congress of 1889 on the need to establish a microscopic diagnosis before operating in suspected cases of malignant tumors requiring extensive mutilating procedures. Shortly thereafter, the freezing microtome was introduced for the purpose of creating frozen sections, which hastened the acceptance of this recommendation. In the United States, the specialty of surgical pathology, which deals with biopsy interpretations, was created by a collaboration between surgeons and a gynecologist.

It is said that the first full-fledged American surgical pathologist was Joseph Colt Bloodgood, in the division of surgical pathology created by W. S. Halsted of The Johns Hopkins Hospital in Baltimore, Maryland. The founders of modern American surgical pathology and biopsy interpretation are Arthur Purdy Stout of Columbia Presbyterian Hospital in New York, James Ewing and his successors Fred Stewart and Frank Foote of Memorial Hospital in New York City, and Pierre Masson of the University of Montreal, Canada.

The biopsy remains the cornerstone for modern medical management, especially in cancer therapy. It will continue to enjoy that role in diagnostics as more venues become established to obtain, study, and evaluate minute tissue and cytologic samples.   —*Victor H. Nassar, M.D.*

See also Breast biopsy; Breast cancer; Colon and rectal polyp removal; Colon cancer; Cyst removal; Cysts and ganglions; Cytology; Cytopathology; Dermatology; Dermatopathology; Endometrial biopsy; Endoscopy; Histology; Immunopathology; Invasive tests; Laboratory tests; Malignant melanoma removal; Mastectomy and lumpectomy; Oncology; Pathology; Skin; Skin cancer; Skin disorders; Skin lesion removal; Tumor removal; Tumors.

FOR FURTHER INFORMATION:

Ackerman, Lauren V., and Juan Rosai. *Ackerman's Surgical Pathology.* 2 vols. 7th ed. St. Louis: C. V. Mosby, 1989. This standard text on surgical pathology contains chapters on biopsy interpretation of all body organs. Written by a foremost authority on the subject matter and richly illustrated. A book found on the shelf of every surgical pathologist.

Bancroft, John D., and Alan Stevens, eds. *Theory and Practice of Histological Techniques.* 4th ed. Edinburgh, Scotland: Churchill Livingstone, 1996. A standard text on tissue preparation and the various methods of staining, used mostly by histologists and technicians. A somewhat technical book.

Koss, Leopold G., Stanislaw Woyke, and Wlodzimierz Olszewski. *Aspiration Biopsy: Cytologic Interpretation and Histologic Basis.* 2d ed. New York: Igaku-Shoin, 1992. The definitive treatise on the subject of fine needle aspiration biopsy.

Sternberg, Stephen S., ed. *Diagnostic Surgical Pathology.* New York: Raven Press, 1989. An authoritative treatise written by recognized experts on the various fields in biopsy interpretation. Frequently used by surgical pathologists and students of the discipline.

Yazdi, Hossein M., and Irving Dardick. *Diagnostic Immunocytochemistry and Electron Microscopy: Guides to Clinical Aspiration Biopsy.* New York: Igaku-Shoin, 1992. An up-to-date resource on highly technical and specialized methods in biopsy interpretation.

BIOSTATISTICS

PROCEDURE

ANATOMY OR SYSTEM AFFECTED: None

SPECIALTIES AND RELATED FIELDS: All

DEFINITION: The application of statistical concepts to biology and medicine in order to summarize the characteristics of samples and to test predictions about the populations from which the samples were taken.

KEY TERMS:

correlation: a number between −1 and +1 that describes the strength of the relationship between two variables

descriptive statistics: the use of numbers to summarize the characteristics of samples *inferential statistics:* the making and testing of numerical statements about populations

null hypothesis: a statement about a population that can be tested numerically

population: all the people, research animals, or other items of interest in a particular study

probability: a number varying between 0 (for an impossible event) to 1 (for an absolutely certain event)

random sample: a sample in which every member of the population has the same probability of being included

regression: an equation that allows one variable to be predicted from another

sample: the members of a population that are actually studied or whose characteristics are measured

variable: any quantity which varies, such as height or cholesterol level

THE METHODOLOGY OF STATISTICS

The aim of every study in the field of biostatistics is to discover something about a population—all patients with a particular disease, for example. Populations are usually much too large to be studied in their entirety: It would be very impractical to round up all the patients with diabetes in the world for a study, and the researcher would still miss those who lived in the past or who have yet to be born. For this reason, most research focuses on a sample drawn from the population of interest—for example, those diabetics who were studied at a particular hospital over a two-year period. Ideally, the sample would be a random sample, one in which each member of the population has an equal chance of being included. In practice, a random sample is hard to achieve: The patients with diabetes at a hospital in Chicago, for example, will differ in various ways from those at hospitals in London, Hong Kong, or rural Mexico.

Descriptive statistics are statistics that describe samples. The most commonly used statistics are mean, median, mode, and standard deviation. The mean of n values is simply the sum of all the values divided by n, or, symbolically,

$$\overline{X} = \text{S}x \, / n$$

where $\overline{X}$ (X with a bar over it, pronounced "x-bar") stands for the mean, n stands for the number of observations, and Σx *(pronounced "sum of x")* stands for the sum obtained when all the different values of x (n of them) are added together. The median of a series of values is the middle value; it must always be the case that half of the values are above the median and half are below. The mode is simply the most common value, the value that occurs most often.

The mean, median, and mode are all "typical" values that characterize the center of distribution of all the values. The standard deviation, which is always positive, is a measure of variation that describes how close all the values cluster about a central value. The formula for the standard deviation is

$$s = \sqrt{\frac{\Sigma (x - \overline{X})^2}{n - 1}}$$

The numerator is calculated by subtracting the mean ($\overline{X}$) from each value, squaring the difference, and adding together all these squared differences. After the sum is divided by $n - 1$, the square root of the entire quantity is taken to determine the standard deviation. A small standard deviation indicates that the values differ very little from one another; a large standard deviation indicates greater variability among the values.

When two quantities vary, such as height and weight, correlation and regression coefficients are also calculated. A correlation coefficient is a number between -1 and $+1$. A correlation near $+1$ shows a very strong relationship between the two variables: When either one increases, the other also increases. A correlation near -1 is also strong, but when either variable increases, the other decreases. A correlation of 0 shows independence, or no relationship, between the variables: An increase in one has no average effect on the value of the other. Correlations midway between 0 and 1 show that an increase in one variable corresponds only to an average increase in the other, but not a dependable increase in each value. For example, taller people are generally heavier, but this is not true in every case.

Regression is a statistical technique for finding an equation that allows one variable to be predicted from the value of the other. For example, a regression of weight on height allows a researcher to predict the average weight for persons of a given height.

Inferential statistics, the statistical study of populations, begins with the study of probability. A probability is a number between 0 and 1 that indicates the certainty with which a particular event will occur, where 0 indicates an impossible occurrence and 1 indicates a certain occurrence. If a certain disease affects 1 percent of the population, then each random sampling will be subject to a .01 probability that the next person sampled will have the disease. For a larger sample than only one individual, the so-called binomial distribution describes the probability that the sample will include no one with the disease, one person with the disease, two people with the disease, and so on.

A variable such as height is subject to so many influences, both genetic and environmental, that it can be treated mathematically as if it were the sum of thousands of small, random variations. Characteristics such as height usually follow a bell-shaped curve, or normal distribution (see figure on next page), at least approximately. This means that very few people are unusually tall or unusually short; most have heights near the middle of the distribution.

Each study using inferential statistics includes four major steps. First, certain assumptions are made about the populations under study. A common assumption, seldom tested, is that the variable in question is normally distrib-

Normal Distribution

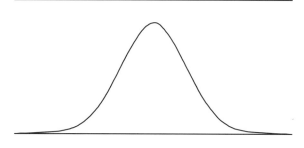

Table 1. A Comparison Between Diabetics and Nondiabetics

Diabetics		Nondiabetics
Height (cm)	*Weight (kg)*	*Height (cm)*
166	78	172
171	90	180
157	72	184
161	82	187
179	92	166
186	82	173

uted within the population. Second, one or more samples are then drawn from the population, and each person or animal in the population is measured and tested in some way. Most studies assume that the samples are randomly drawn from the populations in question, even though true randomness is extremely difficult to achieve. Third, a particular assumption, called the null hypothesis, is chosen for testing. The null hypothesis is always an assumption that can be expressed numerically and that can be tested by known statistical tests. For example, one might assume that the mean height of the population of all diabetics is 170 centimeters (5.525 feet). Fourth, each statistical procedure allows the calculation of a theoretical probability, often a calculated value from a table. If the calculated probability is moderate or high, the null hypothesis is consistent with the observed results. If the calculated probability is very small, the observed results are very unlikely to occur if the null hypothesis is true; in these cases, the null hypothesis is rejected.

Some common types of inferential statistics are t-tests, chi-square tests, and the analysis of variance (also called ANOVA).

THE APPLICATION OF STATISTICS TO MEDICINE

Nearly all medical research studies include biostatistics. Descriptive statistics are often presented in tables of data or in graphic form.

In the following example, height and weight data were gathered from a sample of six diabetic patients, and height was also measured in a sample of six nondiabetic patients (see table 1). The mean height of these diabetic patients is $(166 + 171 + 157 + 161 + 179 + 186) \div 6 = 1020 \div 6 = 170$ centimeters. In order to calculate the standard deviation, this mean is subtracted from each of the six values, to yield differences of -1, 1, -13, -9, 9, and 16. Squaring these differences and adding them up gives a numerator of $16 + 1 + 169 + 81 + 81 + 256 = 604$. Dividing this by $n - 1 = 5$ (n is 6) and taking the square root reveals that the standard deviation is 11.0 centimeters (rounded to the nearest tenth). Similar calculations show that the mean height of the nondiabetic sample is 177 centimeters, with a standard deviation of 8.0 centimeters.

In this example, the nondiabetic sample averaged 7 centimeters taller than the diabetic sample. Inferential statistics can be used to find out if this difference is a meaningful one. In this case, a technique known as a t-test can compare the means of two samples to determine whether they might have come from the same population (or from populations with the same mean value). The assumptions of this test (not always stated explicitly) are that the six diabetic patients were randomly drawn from a normally distributed population and that the six nondiabetic patients were randomly drawn from another normally distributed population. The null hypothesis in this case is that the populations from which the two samples were drawn have the same mean height. The value of t calculated in this test is 1.141; this value is looked up in a table to reveal that the probability is larger than .1 (or 10 percent). In other words, if the null hypothesis is true (and the diabetic and nondiabetic samples are drawn from these same population), then this value of t (or a larger value) is expected to arise by chance alone more than 10 percent of the time. Under the usual criterion of a test at the 5 percent level of significance, one would keep or accept the null hypothesis. This means that the difference between the above sample means is not large enough to demonstrate a difference between the two populations from which these samples are derived. There may in fact be an average difference in height between diabetic and nondiabetic populations, but samples this small cannot detect such a difference reliably. In general, when differences between populations are small, larger sample sizes are required to demonstrate their existence.

T-tests similar to the one above can also be used in drug testing. A drug is given to one set of patients, and a placebo (a fake medicine lacking the essential drug ingredient being tested) is given to a second group. Some relevant measurement (such as the level of an important chemical in the drug which the patients normally lacked) is then compared between the two groups. The null hypothesis would be that the groups are the same and that the drug makes no difference. Rejection of the null hypothesis would be the same as demonstrating that the drug is effective.

For the diabetic patients in the above sample, a correlation coefficient of .60 can be calculated. This moderate level of correlation shows that, on the average, the taller among these patients are also heavier, while the shorter patients are also generally lighter. Despite this average effect, however, individual exceptions are likely to occur. The square of the correlation coefficient, .36, indicates that about 36 percent of the variation in weight can be predicted from height. The equation for making the prediction in this case is

$$weight = 13.99 + .404 \ (height)$$

where the numbers 13.99 and .404 are called regression coefficients. The variable being predicted (weight in this example) is sometimes called the dependent variable; the variable used to make the prediction (in this case, height) is called the independent variable. A high positive correlation signifies that the regression equation offers a very reliable prediction of the dependent variable; a correlation near zero signifies that the regression equation is hardly better than assigning the mean value of the dependent variable to every prediction.

To illustrate another type of inferential statistics, consider the following data on the diseases present among elderly patients who own pets, compared to a comparable group who do not. This type of table is called a contingency table.

Table 2. A Contingency Table Comparing Pet Owners and Non-owners

	Pet owners	Non-owners	Totals
Arthritis	22	58	80
Heart disease	11	29	40
Cancer	21	9	30
Other	36	54	90
TOTALS	90	150	240

In this case, 90 ÷ 240, or three-eighths of the patients sampled, are pet owners. Thus, if there were no relationship between the diseases and pet ownership (which is the null hypothesis), one would expect three-eighths of the eighty arthritis patients (which = 30) to be pet owners and five-eighths of the eighty (which = 50) to be nonowners. Calculating all the expected frequencies in this way, one can compare them with the actual observations shown above.

The result is a statistic called chi-square, which in this problem has a value of 18.88. A table of chi-square values shows that, for a 2 × 4 contingency table, a chi-square value this high occurs by chance alone much less than 1 percent of the time. Thus, something has been observed (a chi-square value of 18.88) that is extremely unlikely under the

null hypothesis of no relationship between disease and pet ownership, so the null hypothesis is rejected and one must conclude that there is a relationship. This conclusion only applies to the population from which the sample was drawn, however, and it does not reveal the nature of the relationship. Further investigation would be needed to discover whether pet ownership protected people from arthritis, whether people who already had arthritis were less inclined to take on the responsibility of pet ownership, or whether people who had pets gave them up when they became arthritic. All these possibilities (and more) are consistent with the findings.

The analysis of variance (also called ANOVA) is a very powerful technique for comparing many samples at once. Suppose that overweight patients were put on three or four different diets; one diet might be better than another, but there is also much individual variation in the amount of weight lost. Analysis of variance is a statistical technique that allows researchers to compare the variation between diets (or other treatments) with the individual variation among the people following each diet. The null hypothesis would be that all the diets are the same and that individual variation can account for all the observed differences. Rejecting the null hypothesis would demonstrate that a consistent difference existed and that at least one diet was better than another. Further tests would be required to pinpoint which diet was best and why.

PERSPECTIVE AND PROSPECTS

The historical foundations of biostatistics go back as far as the development of probability theory by Blaise Pascal (1623-1662). Karl Friedrich Gauss (1777-1855) first outlined the characteristics of the normal (also called Gaussian) distribution. The chi-square test was introduced by Karl Pearson (1857-1936). The greatest statistician of the twentieth century was Ronald A. Fisher (1890-1962), who clearly distinguished descriptive from inferential statistics and who developed many important statistical techniques, including the analysis of variance.

Although medicine existed long before statistics, it has become a nearly universal practice for every research study to use statistics in some important way. New medical procedures and new drugs are constantly being evaluated by comparison with other procedures or older drugs, using statistical techniques. —*Eli C. Minkoff, Ph.D.*

See also Epidemiology; Screening.

FOR FURTHER INFORMATION:

Brase, C. H., and C. P. Brase. *Understandable Statistics.* 4th ed. Lexington, Mass.: D. C. Heath, 1991. A good introduction, with many helpful examples that are carefully explained.

Brook, R. J. *The Fascination of Statistics.* New York: Marcel Dekker, 1986. A very simple introduction.

Daniel, W. W. *Biostatistics: A Foundation for Analysis in the Health Sciences.* 5th ed. New York: John Wiley &

Sons, 1991. A good reference specific to problems of drug testing and similar medical applications.

Dietrich, F. H. *Basic Statistics: An Inferential Approach.* 3d ed. San Francisco: Dellen, 1989. A good introduction to inferential statistics.

Hays, William L. *Statistics.* 5th ed. Fort Worth, Tex.: Harcourt Brace, 1994. A basic, standard introduction with many examples.

Langley, Russell. *Practical Statistics for Non-mathematical People.* New York: Drake, 1971. An introduction to statistics for those readers with math anxiety.

Phillips, J. L. *How to Think About Statistics.* New York: W. H. Freeman, 1988. A very simple introduction.

Sokal, R. R., and F. J. Rohlf. *Biometry.* 2d ed. San Francisco: W. H. Freeman, 1981. A good advanced reference, especially with respect to various types of ANOVA.

Walpole, R. E. *Elementary Statistical Concepts.* New York: Macmillan, 1976. An introduction that gently eases the reader into some moderately advanced concepts.

Zar, J. H. *Biostatistical Analysis.* 2d ed. Englewood Cliffs, N.J.: Prentice Hall, 1984. A good, very thorough, but somewhat technical account.

BIOTECHNOLOGY. *See* BIONICS AND BIOTECHNOLOGY.

BIRTH. *See* CHILDBIRTH; CHILDBIRTH, COMPLICATIONS OF.

BIRTH DEFECTS
DISEASE/DISORDER

ANATOMY OR SYSTEM AFFECTED: All bodily tissues

SPECIALTIES AND RELATED FIELDS: Embryology, genetics, neonatology, obstetrics, pediatrics, perinatology

DEFINITION: Congenital malformations or structural anomalies and their accompanying functional disorders which originate during embryonic development; they are involved in up to 6 percent of human live births.

KEY TERMS:

deletion: the loss of a portion of a chromosome as a result of induced or accidental breakage

multifactorial inheritance: the interaction of genetic and environmental factors, which leads to certain congenital malformations

mutation: a change in the deoxyribonucleic acid (DNA) which may lead to the occurrence of congenital malformations

nondisjunction: the failure of chromosomes to separate during cell division, resulting in new cells that either lack a chromosome or have an extra chromosome

organogenetic period: the period of embryonic development, from approximately fifteen to sixty days after fertilization, during which most body organs form

spina bifida: a birth defect involving malformation of vertebrae in the lower back, often resulting in paralysis and lower-body organ impairment

teratogen: an environmental factor that can induce the formation of congenital malformations

teratology: the study of congenital malformations

translocation: the structural chromosomal defect that occurs when a piece of one chromosome attaches to another

CAUSES AND SYMPTOMS

As the human embryo develops, it undergoes many formative stages from the simple to the complex, most often culminating in a perfectly formed newborn infant. The formation of the embryo is controlled by both genetic factors and interactions between the various embryonic tissues. Because the genes play a vital role as the blueprint for the developing embryo, they must be accurate and the cellular mechanisms that allow the genes to be expressed must also work correctly. In addition, the chemical and physical communications between cells and tissues in the embryo must be clear and uninterrupted. The development of the human embryo into a newborn infant is infinitely more complex than the design and assembly of the most powerful supercomputer or the largest skyscraper. Because of this complexity and the fact that development progresses without supervision by human eye or hand, there are many opportunities for errors that can lead to malformations.

Errors in development can be caused by both genetic and environmental factors. Genetic factors include chromosomal abnormalities and gene mutations. Both can be inherited from the parents or can occur spontaneously during gamete formation, fertilization, and embryonic development. Environmental factors, called teratogens, include such things as drugs, disease organisms, and radiation.

Chromosomal abnormalities account for about 6 percent of human congenital malformations. They fall into two categories, numerical and structural. Numerical chromosomal abnormalities are most often the result of nondisjunction occurring in the germ cells that form sperm and eggs. During the cell division process in sperm and egg production deoxyribonucleic acid (DNA) is duplicated so that each new cell receives a complete set of chromosomes. Occasionally, two chromosomes fail to separate (nondisjunction), such that one of the new cells receives two copies of that chromosome and the other cell none. Both of the resulting gametes (either sperm or eggs) will have an abnormal number of chromosomes. When a gamete with an abnormal number of chromosomes unites with a normal gamete, the result is an individual with an abnormal chromosome number. The missing or extra chromosome will cause confusion in the developmental process and result in certain structural and functional abnormalities. For example, persons with an extra copy of chromosome number 21 suffer from Down syndrome, which often includes mental deficiency, heart defects, facial deformities, and other symptoms. Abnormal chromosome numbers may also result from an egg's being fertilized by two sperm, failure of cell division during gamete formation, and nondisjunction in one or more cells of the early embryo.

Structural chromosomal abnormalities result from chromosome breaks. Breaks occur in chromosomes during normal exchanges in material between chromosomes (crossing over). They also may occur accidentally at weak points on the chromosomes, called fragile sites, and can be induced by chemicals and radiation. Translocations occur when a broken-off piece of chromosome attaches to another chromosome. For example, an individual who has the two usual copies of chromosome 21 and, as the result of a translocation, carries another partial or complete copy of 21 riding piggyback on another chromosome will have the symptoms of Down syndrome. Deletions occur when a chromosome break causes the loss of part of a chromosome. The cri du chat syndrome is caused by the loss of a portion of chromosome number 5. Infants affected by this disorder have a catlike cry, are mentally retarded, and have cardiovascular defects. Other structural chromosomal abnormalities include inversions (in which segments of chromosomes are attached in reverse order), duplications (in which portions of a chromosome are present in multiple copies), and isochromosomes (in which chromosomes separate improperly to produce the wrong configuration).

Gene mutations (defective genes) are responsible for about 8 percent of birth defects. Mutations in genes occur spontaneously because of copying errors or can be induced by environmental factors such as chemicals and radiation. The mutant genes are passed from parents to offspring; thus certain defects may be present in specific families and geographical locations. Two examples of mutation-caused defects are polydactyly (the presence of extra fingers or toes) and microcephaly (an unusually small cranium and brain). Mutations can be either dominant or recessive. If one of the parents possesses a dominant mutation, there will be a 50 percent chance of this mutant gene being transmitted to the offspring. Brachydactyly, or abnormal shortening of the fingers, is a dominantly inherited trait. Normally, the parent with the dominant gene also has the disorder. Recessive mutations can remain hidden or unexpressed in both parents. When both parents possess the recessive gene, there is a 25 percent chance that any given pregnancy will result in a child with a defect. Examples of recessive defects are the metabolic disorders sickle-cell anemia and hemophilia.

Environmental factors called teratogens are responsible for about 7 percent of congenital malformations. Human embryos are most sensitive to the effects of teratogens during the period when most organs are forming (organogenetic period), that is, from about fifteen to sixty days after fertilization. Teratogens may interfere with development in a number of ways, usually by killing embryonic cells or interrupting their normal function. Cell movement, communication, recognition, differentiation, division, and adhesion

are critical to development and can be easily disturbed by teratogens. Teratogens can also cause mutations and chromosomal abnormalities in embryonic cells. Even if the disturbance is only weak and transitory, it can have serious effects because the critical period for development of certain structures is very short and well defined. For example, the critical period for arm development is from twenty-four to forty-four days after fertilization. A chemical that interferes with limb development such as the drug thalidomide, if taken during this period, may cause missing arm parts, shortened arms, or complete absence of arms. Many drugs and chemicals have been identified as teratogenic, including alcohol, aspirin, and certain antibiotics.

Other environmental factors that can cause congenital malformations include infectious organisms, radiation, and mechanical pressures exerted on the fetus within the uterus. Certain infectious agents or their products can pass from the mother through the placenta into the embryo. Infection of the embryo causes disturbances to development similar to those caused by chemical teratogens. For example, German measles (rubella virus) causes cataracts, deafness, and heart defects if the embryo is infected early in development. Exposure to large doses of radiation such as those released by the accident at the Chernobyl nuclear power plant in 1986 or by the atomic bombs dropped on Hiroshima and Nagasaki, Japan, during World War II, can result in death and damage to embryonic cells. There was an increase of about 10 to 15 percent in birth defects in children born to pregnant women exposed to atomic bomb radiation in Japan. Diagnostic X rays are not known to be a cause of birth defects. Some defects such as hip dislocation may be caused by mechanical forces inside the uterus; this could happen if the amnion is damaged or the uterus is malformed, thus restricting the movement of the fetus. About 25 percent of congenital defects are caused by the interaction of genetic and environmental factors (multifactorial), and the causes of more than half (54 percent) of all defects are unknown.

TREATMENT AND THERAPY

Because many birth defects have well-defined genetic and environmental causes, they often can be prevented. Preventive measures need to be implemented if the risk of producing a child with a birth defect is higher than average. Genetic risk factors for such defects include the presence of a genetic defect in one of the parents, a family history of genetic defects, the existence of one or more children with defects, consanguineous (same-family) matings, and advanced maternal age. Prospective parents with one or more of these risk factors should seek genetic counseling in order to assess their potential for producing a baby with such defects. Also, parents exposed to higher-than-normal levels of drugs, alcohol, chemicals, or radiation are at risk of producing gametes that may cause defects, and pregnant women exposed to the same agents place the developing embryo at risk. Again, medical counseling should be sought by such prospective parents. Pregnant women should maintain a well-balanced diet that is about 200 Calories higher than normal to provide adequate fetal nutrition. Women who become anemic during pregnancy may need an iron supplement, and the U.S. Public Health Service recommends that all women of childbearing age consume 0.4 milligram of folic acid (one of the B vitamins) per day to reduce the risk of spina bifida and other neural tube defects. Women at high risk for producing genetically defective offspring can undergo a screening technique whereby eggs taken from the ovary are screened in the laboratory prior to in vitro fertilization and then returned to the uterus. Some couples may decide to use artificial insemination by donor if the prospective father is known to carry a defective gene.

The early detection of birth defects is crucial to the health of both the mother and the baby. Physicians commonly use three methods for monitoring fetal growth and development during pregnancy. The most common method is ultrasound scanning. High-frequency sound waves are directed at the uterus and then monitored for waves that bounce back from the fetus. The return waves allow a picture of the fetus to be formed on a television monitor, which can be used to detect defects and evaluate the growth of the fetus. In amniocentesis, the doctor withdraws a small amount of amniotic fluid containing fetal cells; both the fluid and the cells can be tested for evidence of congenital defects. Amniocentesis generally cannot be performed until the sixteenth week of pregnancy. Another method of obtaining embryonic cells is called chorionic villus sampling and can be done as early as the fifth week of pregnancy. A tube is inserted into the uterus in order to retrieve a small sample of placental chorionic villus cells, identical genetically to the embryo. Again, these cells can be tested for evidence of congenital defects. The early discovery of fetal defects and other fetal-maternal irregularities allows the physician time to assess the problem and make recommendations to the parents regarding treatment. Many problems can be solved with therapy, medications, and even prenatal surgery. If severe defects are detected, the physician may recommend termination of the pregnancy.

Children born with defects often require highly specialized and intense medical treatment. For example, a child born with spina bifida may have lower-body paralysis, clubfoot, hip dislocation, and gastrointestinal and genitourinary problems in addition to the spinal column deformity. Spina bifida occurs when the embryonic neural tube and vertebral column fail to close properly in the lower back, often resulting in a protruding sac containing parts of the spinal meninges and spinal cord. The malformation and displacement of these structures result in nerve damage to the lower body, causing paralysis and the loss of some neural function in the organs of this area. Diagnostic procedures including X rays, computed tomography (CT) scans, and urinalysis

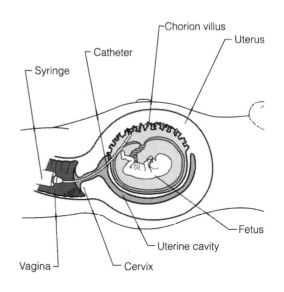

Chorionic villus sampling is one method of obtaining embryonic cells from a pregnant woman; examination of these cells helps physicians determine fetal irregularities or defects, which allows time to assess the problem and make recommendations for treatment.

are carried out to determine the extent of the disorder. If the sac is damaged and begins to leak cerebrospinal fluid, it needs to be closed immediately to reduce the risk of meningitis. In any case, surgery is done to close the opening in the lower spine, but it is not possible to correct the damage done to the nerves. Urgent attention must also be given to the urinary system. The paralysis often causes loss of sphincter muscle control in the urinary bladder and rectum. With respect to the urinary system, this lack of control can lead to serious urinary tract infections and the loss of kidney function. Both infections and obstructions must be treated promptly to avoid serious complication. Orthopedic care needs to begin early to treat clubfoot, hip dislocation, scoliosis, muscle weakness, spasms, and other side effects of this disorder.

The medical treatment of birth defects requires a carefully orchestrated team approach involving physicians and specialists from various medical fields. When the abnormality is discovered (before birth, at birth, or after birth), the primary physician will gather as much information as possible from the family history, the medical history of the patient, a physical examination, and other diagnostic tests. This information is interpreted in consultation with other physicians in order to classify the disorder properly and to determine its possible origin and time of occurrence. This approach may lead to the discovery of other malformations, which will be classified as primary and secondary. When the physician arrives at a specific overall diagnosis, he or she will counsel the parents about the possible causes and development of the disorder, the recommended treatment and its possible outcomes, and the risk of recurrence in a subsequent pregnancy. Certain acute conditions may require immediate attention in order to save the life of the newborn.

In addition to treating the infant with the defect, the physician needs to counsel the parents in order to answer their questions. The counseling process will help them to understand and accept their child's condition. In order to promote good parent-infant bonding, the parents are encouraged to maintain close contact with the infant and participate in its care. Children born with severe chronic disabilities and their families require special support. When parents are informed that their child has limiting congenital malformations, they may react negatively and express feelings of shock, grief, and guilt. Medical professionals can help the parents deal with their feelings and encourage them to develop a close and supportive relationship with their child. Physicians can provide a factual and honest appraisal of the infant's condition and discuss treatments, possible outcomes, and the potential for the child to live a happy and fulfilling life. Parents are encouraged to learn more about their child's disorder and to seek the guidance and help of professionals, support groups, family, and friends. With the proper care and home environment, the child can develop into an individual who is able to interact positively with family and community.

PERSPECTIVE AND PROSPECTS

Birth defects have been recognized and recorded throughout human history. The writer of the Old Testament book of 2 Samuel (21:20) describes the defeat of a giant with six fingers and six toes. Defects were recorded in prehistoric art, and the cuneiform records of ancient Babylon considered birth defects to be omens of great significance. Aristotle described many common human birth defects such as polydactyly. Superstitions about birth defects abounded during the Middle Ages. People believed that events occurring during pregnancy could influence the form of the newborn; for example, deformed legs could be caused by contact with a cripple. Mothers of deformed children were accused of having sex with animals. In a book written about birth defects in 1573, *Monstres et prodiges*, Ambroise Paré describes many human anomalies and attempts to explain how they occur. Missing body parts such as fingers or toes were attributed to a low sperm count in the father, and certain characteristics such as abnormal skin pigmentation, body hair, or facial features were said to be influenced by the mother's thoughts and visions during and after conception.

With advances in science and medicine these superstitions were swept aside. Surgery for cleft palate was per-

formed as early as 1562 by Jacques Honlier. William Harvey, the seventeenth century English physician, recognized that some birth defects such as cleft lip are normal embryonic features that accidentally persist until the time of birth. The study of embryology, including experiments on bird and amphibian embryos, blossomed as a science during the nineteenth century, leading to a better understanding of how defects arise. At the same time, physicians were developing improved ways to treat birth defects. By 1816, Karl von Graefe had developed the first modern comprehensive surgical method for repairing cleft palate. The modern technique for repairing congenital pyloric stenosis (narrowing of the junction between the stomach and small intestine) was developed by Conrad Ramstedt in 1912. The principles of genetic inheritance developed by Gregor Mendel in the mid-1800's were rediscovered by biologists at the beginning of the twentieth century and soon were applied to the study of human heredity, including the inheritance of birth defects. Geneticists realized that defects such as hemophilia and Down syndrome are inherited diseases. Beginning in the 1930's, other scientists began to show that congenital defects could be induced in experimental animals by such factors as dietary deficiencies, hormone imbalances, chemicals, and radiation. Many tragic accidental human experiments also led to a better understanding of environmentally caused birth defects. The tranquilizer thalidomide caused limb malformations in more than seven thousand children in Europe before it was withdrawn from the market in 1961. Pregnant women treated for cervical cancer in the 1960's with large doses of radiation bore children with defects and mental retardation.

Indeed, much of the medical and environmental health research today centers on the effects of drugs, toxic chemicals, radiation, and other factors on human health and development. Genetic counseling and testing of parents at risk for inherited defects has become an accepted part of medical practice. In addition, there have been many advances in the treatment of congenital defects since the 1950's. Modern orthopedic and plastic surgery is used to correct such problems as clubfoot and cleft palate. Transplants are used to correct deficiencies of the liver, kidneys, and other organs. Biomedical engineers have developed improved prosthetic devices to replace lost limbs and to aid in hearing, speaking, and seeing. An understanding of metabolic disorders such as phenylketonuria (PKU) has led to better treatment that utilizes special diets and medications. Because it is difficult to undo the damage of congenital defects fully, the most promise seems to be in the areas of prevention and protection. Prospective parents and their medical care providers need to be alert to potential hereditary problems, as well as to exposure to hazardous environmental agents. Pregnant women need to maintain a healthy diet and check with their physicians before taking any drugs. With advances in preventive medicine, diagnosis, and treatment, the future is much brighter for reducing the health toll of congenital malformations.

—*Rodney C. Mowbray, Ph.D.*

See also Amniocentesis; Cardiology, pediatric; Cerebral palsy; Childbirth; Childbirth, complications of; Chorionic villus sampling; Cleft lip and palate repair; Cleft palate; Color blindness; Congenital heart disease; Cystic fibrosis; Diabetes mellitus; DNA and RNA; Down syndrome; Dwarfism; Embryology; Endocrinology, pediatric; Enzymes; Fetal alcohol syndrome; Gene therapy; Genetic counseling; Genetic diseases; Genetics and inheritance; Gigantism; Hemophilia; Hydrocephalus; Mental retardation; Multiple sclerosis; Muscular dystrophy; Mutation; Obstetrics; Phenylketonuria (PKU); Porphyria; Pregnancy and gestation; Premature birth; Screening; Sickle-cell anemia; Spina bifida; Tay-Sachs disease; Thalassemia.

FOR FURTHER INFORMATION:

Bloom, Beth-Ann, and Edward Seljeskog. *A Parent's Guide to Spina Bifida*. Minneapolis: University of Minnesota Press, 1988. Designed to assist the parents of children with spina bifida. The book includes chapters on the nature of the disorder and how it is treated, the medical problems associated with spina bifida, and how to help the afflicted child while he or she is growing up. Also includes a useful glossary, a list of organizations and support groups, and an extensive bibliography.

Moore, Keith L., and T. V. N. Persaud. *The Developing Human*. 5th ed. Philadelphia: W. B. Saunders, 1993. An outstanding textbook on human embryonic development. Chapter 8 deals specifically with the causes of congenital malformations, and several other chapters include more detailed information about common defects occurring in each of the body's systems. The book is easy to understand and well illustrated.

Nixon, Harold, and Barry O'Donnel. *The Essentials of Pediatric Surgery*. 4th ed. Boston: Butterworth Heinemann, 1992. Describes in laypersons' terms the surgical treatment of many congenital abnormalities, including birth injuries, imperforate anus, spina bifida, hydrocephalus, pyloric stenosis, birthmarks, cleft lip and palate, hernias, urinary and digestive tract deformities, undescended testis, intersex problems, limb malformations, and congenital heart disease. The book is well illustrated with descriptive line diagrams and includes a thorough discussion of each procedure.

Stray-Gundersen, Karen, ed. *Babies with Down Syndrome*. Kensington, Md.: Woodbine House, 1986. A complete guide for parents with a Down syndrome child, written by doctors, nurses, educators, lawyers, and parents. The book includes a complete medical description of the disorder and extensive coverage of care concerns, child development, education, and legal rights. Contains an extensive glossary, reading list, and resource guide.

Warkany, Josef, Ronald J. Lemire, and Michael Cohen. *Mental Retardation and Congenital Malformations of the Central Nervous System*. Chicago: Year Book Medical Publishers, 1981. A medical reference book that gives complete descriptions of congenital malformations of the nervous system and their effects on the eyes, ears, heart, skeleton, and skin. The authors also include a thorough discussion of congenitally caused mental illness. The book is technical in nature but informative and authoritative. Well illustrated; includes extensive listings of technical articles.

BITES AND STINGS
DISEASE/DISORDER

ANATOMY OR SYSTEM AFFECTED: Heart, immune system, skin

SPECIALTIES AND RELATED FIELDS: Emergency medicine, immunology, toxicology

DEFINITION: Injuries from animals or insects.

Bites and stings cause four major types of damage to the victim's body: physical damage, the introduction of disease-causing organisms, the introduction of poisons (toxins, venoms), and allergic responses, including anaphylactic shock. Often, more than one form of damage is associated with a bite or sting. Alone or in combination, they can be life-threatening, but usually the damage from a bite or sting is minor. A wide variety of organisms can bite or sting, but the most important among them are mammals, reptiles (snakes and lizards), some fish (sharks, rays, moray eels), arthropods (including insects, centipedes, spiders, mites, ticks, and scorpions), and cnidarians (jellyfish, Portuguese man-of-wars, and their relatives).

Bites causing physical damage. Bites delivered by a mammal (most often a dog or cat) are likely to cause the most extensive physical damage. The specialized teeth of mammals, especially carnivores, in combination with powerful jaw muscles, can produce a serious wound. If wounding is in a vulnerable spot or is very extensive, or if the bleeding is not stopped, the physical damage can be fatal. A bite that causes physical damage is almost certain to introduce bacteria, viruses, or other infectious agents. An important example is the rabies virus, but many kinds of organism are dangerous if introduced into the bloodstream, or into the bone marrow of bones broken by the bite. Most mammalian bites do not introduce toxins into the victim. Some shrews have a venom in their saliva, but their small size and secretive habits minimize their threat to human health. Bites from mammals are also of minimal concern with respect to dangerous allergic responses. Physical damage is also the most serious problem in shark and moray eel bites.

Prevention, by avoiding animals prone to bite, is usually readily accomplished. Treatment involves stopping the bleeding, repairing the damage, and preventing infection.

Bites introducing infectious agents. Bites that cause serious physical damage are not the only ones that can introduce infectious agents. Any bite or sting can introduce infection to the victim because it penetrates the first line of defense, the skin. The arthropods are the most important disease vectors. Malaria is caused by a parasitic protozoan (single-celled, animal-type organism) transferred from one host to another by mosquitoes. Lyme disease is caused by a bacterium and is transported between hosts by ticks. Viruses cause yellow fever, and mosquitoes transport the virus to new hosts. Insects and ticks are vectors for a number of other diseases, most of which are introduced to the victim by a bite (including the stabs of blood-sucking arthropods such as mosquitoes).

Prevention of these diseases involves avoiding and/or eliminating the vectors; neither is always possible. Active immunization (stimulating the host to form antibodies against the disease-causing organism) is also used when available. Treatment involves drugs that destroy the disease organism or the use of passive immunization (the injection of preformed antibodies against the disease organism).

Bites and stings introducing toxins. Toxins or poisons are introduced to the victim most often by arthropods (scorpion stings, spider bites), cnidarians (stings), or reptiles (bites). Some mollusks—the cone shell snails, for example—can also inject toxins into a victim. The chemicals involved include enzymes that destroy tissue, neurotoxins that interfere with appropriate nerve cell responses (blocking or stimulating nerve cell signals), and others that interfere with the normal functions of the victim's body chemistry. Rattlesnakes and their relatives, coral snakes, and the Gila monster (a large lizard) are examples of poisonous reptiles. The brown recluse and black widow spiders are dangerous examples of their group. The sea wasp (a jellyfish) and the Portuguese man-of-war are the best known, but by no means the only, dangerous cnidarians in coastal waters off North America.

Prevention involves avoiding the animals that inject the toxin, which is easily accomplished much, but not all, of the time. Treatment involves injection of antivenin, a solution of antibodies that neutralize a specific toxin. Research on snake antivenin indicates that it might be possible to create a single antivenin which inactivates several snake venoms.

Bites and stings causing allergic reactions. Any bite or sting can cause an allergic response in the victim, because all introduce large foreign molecules, called antigens. These are often proteins, and they stimulate a response in the victim's immune system. If the response is more than that needed to destroy the antigen, it is called an allergic response and the foreign protein is called an allergen. The allergic response may simply be a nuisance causing minor inflammation, but it is exceptionally dangerous if it escalates into anaphylaxis. Anaphylaxis is a hyperreaction to a foreign substance in which the heart rate increases; bronchioles in the lungs constrict, making breathing difficult; and blood pressure drops. If symptoms continue, the victim may go into shock and even die. The toxins introduced by venomous arthropods, reptiles, cnidarians, and mollusks are often allergenic, even causing anaphylaxis, but even non-poisonous or minimally toxic materials such as the venom introduced in a bee or wasp sting can cause life-threatening anaphylactic shock in sensitive people. A painful sting for people not sensitized to the foreign material becomes a threat to the life of a sensitized, hypersensitive person.

Prevention, by avoiding the allergen, is the preferred defense against allergic reactions. If avoidance is not possible or cannot be assured, the injection of small amounts of the substance to which an individual is hypersensitive, followed by increasingly larger doses, is sometimes effective in desensitizing the individual. Treatment of severe anaphylactic reactions involves the injection of adrenaline. Antihistamines, taken orally or injected, are used in less severe situations.

—Carl W. Hoagstrom, Ph.D.

See also Allergies; Arthropod-borne diseases; Emergency medicine; Encephalitis; Epidemiology; Immune system; Infection; Leishmaniasis; Lice, mites, and ticks; Lyme disease; Malaria; Parasitic diseases; Plague; Poisoning; Rabies; Shock; Sleeping sickness; Snakebites; Toxicology; Tropical medicine; Yellow fever; Zoonoses.

FOR FURTHER INFORMATION:

"Bites and Stings: It's That Time of Year." *Patient Care* 26 (May 30, 1992): 79-110.

Caras, Roger A. *Dangerous to Man: The Definitive Story of Wildlife's Reputed Dangers.* Rev. ed. New York: Holt, Rinehart and Winston, 1975.

Foster, Steven, and Roger A. Caras. *A Field Guide to Venomous Animals and Poisonous Plants: North America, North of Mexico.* Boston: Houghton Mifflin, 1994.

Halstead, Bruce W., and Paul S. Auerbach. *Dangerous Aquatic Animals of the World: A Color Atlas.* Princeton, N.J.: Darwin Press, 1992.

Harvey, Alan L., ed. *Snake Toxins.* New York: Pergamon Press, 1991.

Tu, Anthony T., ed. *Reptile Venoms and Toxins.* New York: Marcel Dekker, 1991.

BLADDER INFECTIONS. *See* URINARY DISORDERS.

BLADDER REMOVAL. *See* CYSTECTOMY.

BLADDER STONES. *See* STONE REMOVAL; STONES.

BLEEDING

DISEASE/DISORDER

ANATOMY OR SYSTEM AFFECTED: Blood, blood vessels, circulatory system

SPECIALTIES AND RELATED FIELDS: Emergency medicine, family practice, hematology, internal medicine, vascular medicine

DEFINITION: Damage or disruption to hemostasis (the normal absence of bleeding)—the appropriate interactions among blood cells, proteins in the blood, and blood vessels—resulting in loss of blood or abnormal clotting.

KEY TERMS:

coagulation: the sequential process by which multiple, specific factors (predominantly proteins in plasma) interact, ultimately resulting in the formation of an insoluble clot made of fibrin

fibrin: the insoluble protein that forms the essential portion of a blood clot; the soluble protein in plasma converted to fibrin is called fibrinogen

fibrinolysis: the process of dissolving clots; the fibrinolytic system dissolves fibrin through enzymatic action

hemostasis: the arrest of bleeding from injured blood vessels, confining circulating blood to those vessels; blood vessels, platelets, the coagulation system, and the fibrinolytic system contribute to the process of hemostasis

plasma: the fluid portion of blood in which the particulate components are suspended; the majority of coagulation factors are proteins in plasma

platelets: disk-shaped structures in blood that are vital for the maintenance of normal hemostasis

vitamin K: a group of fat-soluble vitamins that play an integral role in the production of multiple, properly functioning coagulation factors by the liver

CAUSES AND SYMPTOMS

Patients with bleeding abnormalities are commonly encountered in medicine. Such patients may be evaluated because of previous bleeding episodes, a family history of bleeding, or sometimes abnormalities detected during preliminary studies before surgery or other invasive procedures. Bleeding episodes are often described as local (the source of bleeding is pinpointed to a specific part of the body) or generalized (abnormal bleeding occurring at multiple, distinct anatomic sites). It is important to distinguish between these two possibilities because treatment may differ markedly. Localized bleeding disorders may be correctable with surgery, while the treatment of generalized bleeding disorders may be more complex and long-term. The evaluation of patients with suspected bleeding disorders includes a detailed medical history, a thorough physical examination, and appropriate screening tests for hemostatic functioning. Subsequently, more specific laboratory tests are usually required to define the nature of a bleeding abnormality. Abnormal bleeding may result from blood vessel abnormalities (vascular defects), low platelet counts (thrombocytopenia), excessively high platelet counts (thrombocytosis), platelet function abnormalities, deficiencies or abnormalities of plasma coagulation factors, excessive breakdown of blood clots (excessive fibrinolysis), or a combination of these abnormalities. Bleeding disorders may be inherited or acquired.

Generalized bleeding abnormalities are suggested by several characteristics. Bleeding from multiple sites, bleeding in the absence of a known causative event (often termed spontaneous bleeding), and bleeding following trauma that is much more severe than expected for the degree of injury are all characteristics of generalized bleeding defects. An unexplained increase in bleeding severity may be a sign of a newly acquired generalized bleeding abnormality.

Inherited disorders. There are numerous inherited disorders of hemostasis. Fortunately, most are quite rare. The two most common inherited bleeding disorders are von Willebrand's disease and hemophilia A. Inherited bleeding disorders usually become evident in infancy or early childhood. There is often a family history of abnormal bleeding, and abnormal bleeding may have been experienced in association with surgery or trauma. Bleeding from the umbilical cord at birth or bleeding following circumcision may provide evidence of inherited hemostatic disorders. In contrast, a lack of abnormal bleeding following surgery such as tonsillectomy or dental procedures such as tooth extraction lowers the likelihood that even a mild inherited hemostatic disorder is present. There are, however, exceptions to such trends. Inherited disorders of hemostasis such as Ehlers-Danlos syndrome or hereditary hemorrhagic telangiectasia may not become evident until later in life. Idiopathic (or immune) thrombocytopenic purpura (ITP) is an acquired hemostatic abnormality which may occur in childhood, usually as a result of an infection. Hemorrhagic disease of the newborn is a short-lived bleeding abnormality caused by a transient deficiency of coagulation factors (known as the vitamin K dependent factors) in the newborn period.

Family history is helpful in the evaluation of hemostatic disorders because a pattern of bleeding among family members may be revealed. If only male members of a family are affected, this suggests an X-linked recessive pattern of inheritance (transmitted by the X sex chromosome). Such diseases are usually transmitted from females who are carriers of the trait. Hemophilia A, hemophilia B, and Wiskott-Aldrich syndrome are transmitted as X-linked recessive traits. Inherited bleeding disorders such as von Willebrand's disease occur in both sexes through non-sex-linked, or autosomal, transmission. Some bleeding disorders occur because of a gene mutation. Some individuals, therefore, are the first members of their family to have an inherited bleeding disorder.

Acquired disorders. These may first become evident in adulthood. A negative family history for bleeding may exist, and diseases may be present that are associated with bleeding abnormalities, such as kidney or liver disease. Liver disease may lead to abnormal bleeding for numerous reasons. Causes of abnormal bleeding include decreases in plasma coagulation factors (most coagulation factors are manufactured by the liver), low platelet counts, platelet function abnormalities, production of abnormal coagulation factors (such as abnormal fibrinogen), vulnerability to a condition called disseminated intravascular coagulation (DIC), and abnormal lysis (breakdown) of blood clots. Platelet function abnormalities are associated with kidney failure and many blood diseases (for example, dysproteinemias, leukemias, and myeloproliferative disorders). Vitamin K is necessary for the production of numerous functional plasma coagulation factors. A deficiency of vitamin K, therefore, may lead to abnormal bleeding. Poor nutrition or antibiotic therapy may lead to vitamin K deficiency, which may also occur in newborns. One source of vitamin K is bacteria located in the gastrointestinal (GI) tract. Because the newborn GI tract is sterile, newborns have no bacterial source of vitamin K. Some medical conditions, such as sprue or biliary obstruction, may lead to inadequate absorption of vitamin K from the GI tract.

Numerous drugs and medications may cause abnormal bleeding. Drugs or medications may cause low platelet counts or platelet dysfunction or may affect coagulation factors. Oral anticoagulant therapy (warfarin therapy), which is used in the treatment of blood clots in the legs, causes a reduction of functional vitamin K dependent coagulation factors and is a common cause of drug-induced bleeding.

Nutritional deficiency, a major problem in many parts of the world, may result in bleeding disorders. One example is severe protein deficiency, a syndrome known as kwashiorkor, which produces severe liver damage. Vitamin C deficiency may cause scurvy, which may result in skin hemorrhages, bleeding gums, and bleeding beneath the lining of the bones (subperiosteal bleeding).

Evaluating hemostatic functioning. Dental extractions are a good measure of hemostatic functioning because bleeding occurs over rigid bone. The bleeding sites, therefore, are not easily compressible. Persistent and excessive bleeding after incisor removal is more significant as a diagnostic indicator than such bleeding following molar removal. (Even patients with normal hemostasis may experience persistent bleeding after molar extractions.) Tonsillectomy is evaluated in a similar manner. Because tonsillectomy may lead to persistent bleeding in the setting of normal hemostasis, the significance of excessive bleeding following tonsillectomy may be difficult to interpret. The lack of bleeding following tonsillectomy, however, implies normal hemostasis.

Investigation of trauma-related bleeding is an important component of hemostatic evaluation. When considering trauma-related bleeding, it is important to determine other details related to the events: Were blood transfusions required? What methods were used to bring bleeding under control? How easily was bleeding brought under control? Was there clearly a local cause of bleeding? Were any medications being taken which could lead to abnormal bleeding? A lack of abnormal bleeding with prior trauma does not

First Aid for Trauma-Related Bleeding

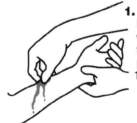

1. Press hard over the wound. If necessary, pinch the wound edges together with fingers and thumb. Maintain pressure for at least 10 minutes.

2. Lay the patient down to elevate the bleeding area (this reduces the area blood flow).

Never move a part which may be fractured.

3. Replace the hand pressure with pressure from a pad held firmly in place by a tight bandage or by whatever is at hand: stockings, belts, socks, handkerchiefs, ties.

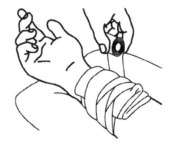

4. If blood appears to be oozing through, do not investigate by removing the bandage already applied; instead apply additional pressure with more padding and bandage. Continue this procedure until control is achieved.

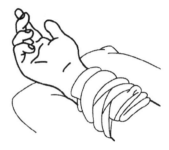

5. Apply antishock measures, as necessary. Get medical aid.

absolutely exclude inherited bleeding disorders. Patients with milder forms of hemophilia may only bleed abnormally following severe trauma. Oral contraceptives or pregnancy influence the hemostatic reaction to a degree that may mask von Willebrand's disease in women.

Diagnosis by type of bleeding. In diagnosis, the type of abnormal bleeding may provide important clues. In vascular or platelet abnormalities, bleeding typically occurs in the skin or mucous membranes. Bleeding usually starts within seconds of the time of injury and may continue for hours; however, once the bleeding stops it may not recur. Posttraumatic bleeding in coagulation disorders may be delayed for many hours after a traumatic episode; recurrent episodes of bleeding following trauma are also a characteristic of such disorders.

Petechiae, small, red spots about the size of a pinhead, represent tiny hemorrhages from small blood vessels, such as capillaries. These spots are a sign of platelet or vascular abnormalities. Petechiae caused by vasculitis (the inflammation of blood vessels) are often elevated lesions that are distinct to the touch (palpable) as well as being evident visually. Petechiae associated with low platelet counts or abnormalities of platelet function are not palpable and, while often widespread, may first appear on the lower extremities, such as the ankles, or on mucous membranes, such as in the mouth.

Ecchymoses (bruises) are larger lesions caused by the leakage of blood into tissue of the skin or mucous membranes, usually as the result of trauma. Ecchymoses can be seen with all hemostatic disorders. Spontaneous ecchymoses, bruises appearing in the absence of prior trauma, may be a sign of a hemostatic problem. The location of the ecchymoses may provide diagnostic information. Bruises occurring only on the limbs, which are at greater risk for minor trauma, are less indicative of a possible bleeding abnormality than bruising which occurs on the trunk. Women frequently have one or two bruises, which may be normal. More than a half dozen bruises on a woman, however, warrants further evaluation. Easy bruising in a man also warrants further study.

Hematomas are collections of blood that accumulate in organs, body spaces, or tissues. They produce deformity of the area in which they develop and may be quite painful. Hematomas tend to be associated with abnormalities in the coagulation mechanism, such as hemophilia. Bleeding into joint spaces is known as hemarthrosis. Hemarthroses are characteristic of severe coagulation disorders such as hemophilia. Telangiectases and angiomata, caused by vascular malformations, are red spots or patches caused by the presence of blood in abnormally dilated vessels. Unlike the other lesions previously discussed, these vascular lesions blanch with pressure.

Epistaxis (nose bleeding) is most frequently caused by mild trauma (for example, nose blowing) to dilated vessels

of the nose in individuals with normal hemostasis. Epistaxis in the setting of bleeding disorders is often associated with low platelet counts, the vascular abnormality called hereditary hemorrhagic telangiectasia, and von Willebrand's disease. Epistaxis consistently occurring on one side may be the result of a local abnormality, as opposed to a generalized hemostatic defect.

Abnormal bleeding may also be seen in other areas. Gingival bleeding (gum bleeding) may be caused by gum disease; however, it is also seen in association with low platelet counts, platelet dysfunction, scurvy, and in conditions where there are abnormally high levels of proteins in the blood (hyperviscosity syndrome). Hematuria (blood in the urine) may be caused by low platelet counts, platelet dysfunction, coagulation factor abnormalities, and oral anticoagulant therapy. Hematuria is a serious medical symptom that requires medical investigation to determine the cause. Bleeding from the GI tract can be seen with all types of hemostatic disorders. GI bleeding must be completely investigated to determine whether there is local cause for the bleeding or the bleeding is part of a generalized hemostatic defect. Menorrhagia (abnormal bleeding during menstrual periods) is associated with low platelet counts, platelet dysfunction, von Willebrand's disease, and coagulation factor abnormalities. Information such as the number and type of sanitary pads or tampons needed, period duration, the necessity of sanitary pad changes at night, the passage of clots, and the requirement of iron for anemia may be helpful in quantifying menstrual blood loss.

Laboratory tests. Laboratory evaluation of hemostatic functioning consists of screening tests, to aid in the detection of abnormalities, and confirmatory tests, to characterize the disorders. Microscopic examination of a blood smear is a simple screening procedure that may provide valuable information. A disease process associated with abnormal bleeding, such as leukemia, may be detected. Numerous red cell fragments may be present in hemostatic disorders such as DIC or thrombotic thrombocytopenic purpura (TTP). An estimate of the number of platelets and an evaluation of their size and shape can be made. Abnormally low and high platelet counts can lead to abnormal bleeding. Large platelets can be seen in conditions in which they are being destroyed rapidly, such as ITP. Large platelets are also seen in Bernard-Soulier syndrome, an inherited platelet function disorder.

The automated platelet count and bleeding time are screening tests for the evaluation of platelets. A normal interaction between platelets and damaged blood vessels is a necessary first step to control bleeding. This step is often termed primary hemostasis. An adequate number of normally functioning platelets are necessary to provide normal primary hemostasis. A representative normal range for the platelet count is 150,000 to 400,000 platelets per microliter of blood. In the absence of platelet dysfunction, spontaneous bleeding is rare when the platelet count is greater than 20,000 per microliter. The risk of life-threatening hemorrhage does not markedly increase until the platelet count drops below 10,000 per microliter. The bleeding time is primarily used to screen for platelet dysfunction, although it may also indicate some vascular abnormalities. The bleeding time measures the interval required for bleeding to cease following a standard skin incision on the forearm. A blood pressure cuff on the arm is inflated to a pressure of 40 millimeters of mercury during the procedure. A representative normal range for the bleeding time is four to seven minutes. A prolonged bleeding time may be a sign of a platelet or vascular abnormality.

The plasma coagulation system is composed primarily of a set of proteins that interact to produce clotting of blood (fibrin clots). This system is often referred to as secondary hemostasis. Most plasma coagulation factors are identified by a roman numeral (for example coagulation factor VIII). For ease of analysis, the plasma coagulation system has been divided into groups of proteins known as the intrinsic pathway, the extrinsic pathway, and the final common pathway. Screening tests for the plasma coagulation system include the thrombin time (TT), the prothrombin time (PT), and the activated partial thromboplastin time (aPTT). The screening tests detect significant deficiencies or abnormalities of plasma coagulation factors and help localize the defects within the pathways.

Specific, and often more complex, laboratory studies of hemostasis are performed based on information derived from the medical history, physical examination, and screening laboratory tests. The goal of specific tests is to pinpoint the diagnosis of hemostatic abnormalities.

Platelet disorders. Thrombocytopenia, a low platelet count in the blood, has numerous causes. Platelets are produced in the bone marrow and subsequently released into the blood. Bone marrow damage may result in inadequate numbers of platelets. Drugs, toxins, radiation, and infections may damage the bone marrow. Certain diseases, such as leukemia or other cancers, may lead to the replacement of bone marrow cells with abnormal cells or fibrous tissue. Some diseases result in inadequate release of platelets from the bone marrow. Inadequate platelet release may be the result of nutritional deficiencies, such as vitamin B_{12} or folic acid deficiencies, or it can be seen in some rare hereditary disorders, such as May-Hegglin anomaly or Wiscott-Aldrich syndrome. Individuals with an enlarged spleen may develop thrombocytopenia because of the pooling of platelets within the organ. Massive transfusion may result in thrombocytopenia when the blood volume is replaced with transfused solutions that do not contain platelets.

Certain disorders result in the rapid destruction or consumption of platelets. If the production of platelets by the bone marrow does not compensate for the rate of destruction, thrombocytopenia occurs. Platelet consumption with resultant thrombocytopenia is a component of DIC. Thrombocytopenia caused by accelerated destruction may also occur with prosthetic heart valves, blood infections (sepsis), and vascular defects called hemangiomas. The development of antibodies against one's own platelets (such as with ITP) causes platelet consumption. ITP can be a self-limited disorder with a complete return to normal (acute ITP) or a prolonged thrombocytopenic condition (chronic ITP). Acute ITP is seen most frequently in children between two and six years of age. The disease is preceded by a viral infection in about 80 percent of cases. The platelet count returns to normal within six months in more than 80 percent of patients; the usual period of thrombocytopenia is four to six weeks. Mortality from acute ITP occurs in about 1 percent of cases. Chronic ITP typically occurs in young and middle-aged adults, and the disorder is about three times more common in females than in males. As many as 50 percent of children born to mothers with ITP have thrombocytopenia at birth as a result of the transfer of antiplatelet antibodies across the placenta. Isoimmune neonatal thrombocytopenia and post-transfusion purpura are other conditions in which thrombocytopenia is caused by antiplatelet antibodies.

Numerous drugs have been associated with thrombocytopenia. Examples of such drugs include gold salts, quinine, quinidine, sulfonamide drugs, and heparin. Thrombocytopenia may occur within twenty-four hours following exposure to an offending drug. All nonessential medications should be discontinued in patients suspected of having drug-induced thrombocytopenia.

Platelet function defects may be inherited or acquired. They may occur without evidence of an associated disease or be secondary to a recognizable clinical disorder. Platelet function defects are suspected when there is abnormal skin or mucous membrane bleeding, a prolonged bleeding time, and a normal platelet count. Bleeding disorders caused by the inability of platelets to stick to damaged blood vessel walls in a normal manner are called platelet adhesion defects; Bernard-Soulier syndrome and von Willebrand's disease are examples of such defects.

Certain molecules necessary for normal platelet function are contained within platelets (that is, in the storage pool). Deficiencies or defects of these molecules lead to platelet dysfunction and are called storage pool defects. Examples of storage pool defects include gray platelet syndrome and dense granule deficiency. Platelet release defects occur when there is a failure to release storage pool contents normally. Hereditary deficiency of the enzymes cyclooxygenase or thromboxane synthetase causes platelet release defects. Aspirin causes a platelet release defect by inactivating cyclooxygenase.

Disorders that render platelets unable to interact with one another to form large clumps at the site of vascular injury are known as platelet aggregation defects. Ganzmann's thrombasthenia and hereditary afibrinogenemia are examples of such defects.

Platelets also play a key role in secondary hemostasis by providing a surface on which many coagulation factors can interact. A bleeding disorder results if the platelet surface is incapable of supporting secondary hemostasis. Hereditary bleeding disorders caused by this type of platelet defect are quite rare.

Arterial Pressure Points

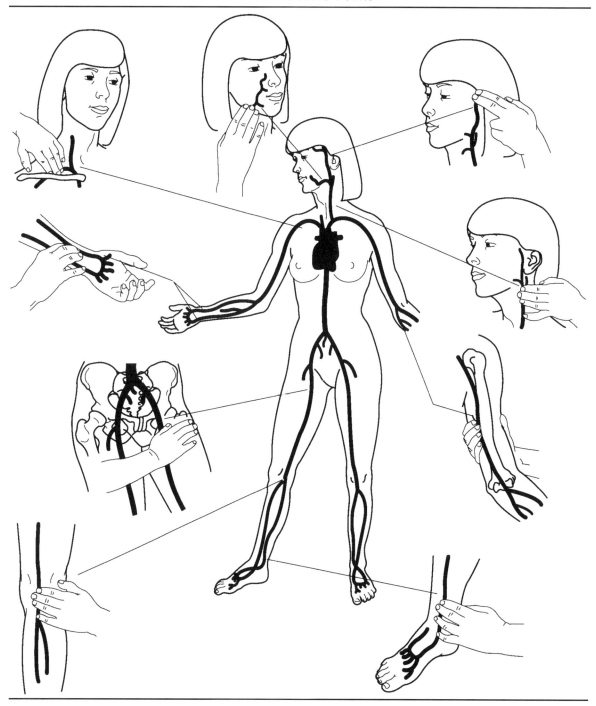

Acquired platelet dysfunction is quite common. Renal failure (uremia) may cause acquired platelet dysfunction. Liver disease can cause multiple bleeding abnormalities, including platelet dysfunction. A vast number of drugs and medications, such as aspirin and penicillin, cause platelet dysfunction. Acquired platelet function defects are seen with cardiopulmonary bypass procedures and in association with numerous blood diseases.

Coagulation disorders. The overall incidence of inherited coagulation factor disorders is about 1 in 10,000. In such conditions, there is either a failure to make a sufficient amount of a coagulation factor (quantitative disorder) or a dysfunctional factor is made (qualitative disorder). An inherited disorder exists for every coagulation factor, although most are quite rare. Symptoms range from serious spontaneous bleeding, which occurs in the severe forms of hemophilia A (factor VIII disorder) or hemophilia B (factor IX disorder), to an absence of abnormal bleeding in other inherited conditions (factors XII, prekallikrein, and high molecular weight kininogen). In general, for disorders which cause bleeding, the more profound the coagulation factor defect, either quantitatively or qualitatively, the more severe the bleeding. Severe disorders are usually easily identified. Moderate or mild disorders are more common and may go undetected until there is a significant hemostatic challenge, such as surgery.

Von Willebrand's disease is probably the most common inherited bleeding disorder. It is caused by deficiencies or defects in a vital group of hemostatic proteins known collectively as von Willebrand factor. Manifestations include epistaxis, menorrhagia, prolonged bleeding after trauma or surgery, frequent ecchymoses, and persistent gum bleeding. Severe episodes of epistaxis may occur during childhood, and such episodes may cease during puberty. In women, epistaxis may recur after the menopause. Important diagnostic clues include a family history of abnormal bleeding, affected members in every generation (males and females), and marked worsening of bleeding following the ingestion of aspirin or other drugs that impair platelet function. Von Willebrand's disease consists of a very diverse spectrum of abnormalities: At least twenty-one distinct subtypes of von Willebrand's disease have been recognized.

Hemophilia A and hemophilia B are clinically indistinguishable; laboratory testing is required for their diagnosis. Hemophilia A is illustrated here. Hemophilia A is an inherited disorder of a portion of coagulation factor VIII. Hemophilia A is typically seen in males, while females are carriers of the abnormal gene and can transmit the disease. Twenty percent of affected individuals have a negative family history and likely developed their disease because of a mutation of the factor VIII gene. Once the abnormal gene is established in a family, the severity of the disease is the same for all affected males. Hemophilia A is divided into severe, moderate, and mild subtypes based on the amount of functional factor VIII present. Bleeding in hemophiliacs may be spontaneous or post-traumatic. Spontaneous bleeding tends to occur only in severe hemophilia. It characteristically affects joints and muscles, and it may lead to crippling injury without prompt and adequate treatment. Post-traumatic bleeding may occur in mild, moderate, or severe hemophilia A. Such episodes are often prolonged and dangerous. Bleeding into the head (intracranial bleeding) remains a common cause of severe disability and death in hemophilia A. Modern treatment, however, has reduced the incidence of this severe complication. Antibodies (inhibitors) directed against factor VIII develop in approximately 12 to 15 percent of patients who require transfusions to provide factor VIII. The development of inhibitors is a serious complication which may compromise the effectiveness of therapy. Factor VIII inhibitors may occur in nonhemophiliacs, leading to serious bleeding in affected males and females.

Acquired coagulation factor disorders may be caused by reduced or absent factor production (for example, in liver disease), the production of defective or inactive factors (such as in liver disease or vitamin K deficiency), factor inhibitors, or accelerated consumption or clearance of factors. Examples in the latter group include DIC (accelerated consumption), kidney disease (factors lost in the urine), and the attachment of factors to abnormal tissue, which occurs in a disease called amyloidosis.

DIC is a hemostatic disorder which arises as part of a disease or medical condition. Examples of associated conditions include obstetrical accidents, abnormal destruction of red blood cells within blood vessels, infections, malignancies, burns, severe injuries, liver disease, and diseases of blood vessels. DIC may be an explosive, life-threatening syndrome (high-grade DIC) or a troublesome, less dramatic feature of a disease (low-grade DIC). Conditions associated with DIC cause abnormal activation of the hemostatic response, resulting in the widespread formation of blood clots in the vascular system. The clots obstruct the blood supply to vital organs (the kidneys, heart, lungs, and brain), leading to impaired organ function. Abnormal bleeding may develop if coagulation factors and platelets become depleted because of their incorporation into widespread blood clots. The breakdown of blood clots may also become inadequately controlled and contribute further to abnormal bleeding.

PERSPECTIVE AND PROSPECTS

The existence of bleeding disorders has been known for many centuries. Abnormal bleeding observed in the males of certain families was described in the Jewish Talmud in the second century. Interest in such disorders increased markedly with the discovery of hemophilia in the royal families of Europe. In 1853, Queen Victoria gave birth to her fifth son, Leopold. She was a carrier of hemophilia, and Leopold had the disease. He died of a brain hemorrhage following a minor blow to the head at the age of thirty-one.

Two of Victoria's daughters gave birth to affected sons. Her granddaughter, Alexandra, became the czarina of Russia, and Alexandra's only son, Alexis, suffered from hemophilia.

The transformation of fluid blood to a solid mass has fascinated investigators since ancient times. Aristotle noted that blood contained fibers and, upon cooling, solidified. He also observed that "diseased" blood did not solidify. The realization that blood clotting minimized blood loss from wounds occurred in the early eighteenth century. In the late eighteenth century, William Hewson described the clotting time of whole blood. He found it to be shortened in some diseases and infinite in one woman after delivering a baby. In 1863, work published by Lord Joseph Lister laid the foundation for the discovery of the intrinsic pathway of coagulation. In 1905, Paul Morawitz, aided by the discoveries of such investigators as Alexander Schmidt and Olof Hammarsten, proposed what is now called the classic theory of blood coagulation. This led to the characterization of the extrinsic pathway of coagulation. In 1964, the "cascade" (by Robert Macfarlane) and "waterfall" (by Earl Davie and Oscar Ratnoff) hypotheses of coagulation were proposed. These discoveries paved the way for much of the current understanding of coagulation.

Alfred Donné is credited with the first description of platelets, reported in 1842. In 1881, Giulio Bizzozero became the first author to use the term "blood platelets." Shortly thereafter, discoveries in the late nineteenth century highlighted the importance of platelets in normal hemostasis. In recent times, the study of platelets has intensified. A large volume of information on platelets and platelet function has accumulated since the 1960's.

The study of the cells lining blood vessels (endothelium) and their role in hemostasis is a relatively young discipline. Much has already been learned about these cells, and much more information is anticipated. The future promises great advances in the study of hemostasis and hemostatic disorders. Further definition of the interrelationships of endothelium, platelets, and coagulation factors in normal and abnormal hemostasis is expected. There is hope for a greater understanding of inherited hemostatic disorders. Additional studies on the processes that keep blood from clotting (anticoagulants) and those that break down clots (fibrinolysis) are expected. The effect of diseases such as cancer on hemostasis awaits clarification, as does the effect of hemostasis on other processes, such as the spread of cancer.

—*James R. Stubbs, M.D.*

See also Anemia; Blood and blood components; Circulation; Concussion; Ebola virus; Emergency medicine; Healing; Hematology; Hematology, pediatric; Hemophilia; Shock; Transfusion; Vascular medicine.

FOR FURTHER INFORMATION:

Colman, Robert W., et al., eds. *Hemostasis and Thrombosis: Basic Principles and Clinical Practice.* 3d ed. Philadelphia: J. B. Lippincott, 1993. This is the bible in the study of hemostasis. An extensive and comprehensive reference textbook that deserves a spot on the bookshelf of all those involved with hemostasis.

Hirsh, Jack, and Elizabeth A. Brain. *Hemostasis and Thrombosis: A Conceptual Approach.* 2d ed. New York: Churchill Livingstone, 1983. A fun book for learning the principles of hemostasis. The text is filled with easy-to-understand illustrations that succeed in making difficult concepts very straightforward.

Owen, Charles A., E. J. Walter, and John H. Thompson. *The Diagnosis of Bleeding Disorders.* 2d ed. Boston: Little, Brown, 1975. A classic in the field of hemostasis. Although this is a somewhat older work, much vital information on hemostasis can still be obtained from the text. The extensive chapter on the history of hemostasis is interesting reading.

Ratnoff, Oscar D., and Charles D. Forbes, eds. *Disorders of Hemostasis.* 2d ed. Philadelphia: W. B. Saunders, 1991. A comprehensive textbook edited by two giants in the field of hemostasis. Although this is a detailed textbook, the authors cover various aspects of hemostasis in an organized and understandable manner.

Thompson, Arthur R., and Laurence A. Harker. *Manual of Hemostasis and Thrombosis.* 3d ed. Philadelphia: F. A. Davis, 1983. This manual provides concise descriptions of the various aspects of hemostasis. It is well written and serves as a valuable "quick source" of information on bleeding disorders.

Triplett, Douglas A. *Hemostasis: A Case Oriented Approach.* New York: Igaku-Shoin, 1985. In a manner similar to the book by Jack Hirsh and Elizabeth A. Brain (above), Triplett has made learning hemostasis quite pleasant. Most of the material in this book is presented in the form of specific patient cases, and it is an effective teaching method.

BLEPHAROPLASTY. *See* FACE LIFT AND BLEPHAROPLASTY.

BLINDNESS

DISEASE/DISORDER

ANATOMY OR SYSTEM AFFECTED: Eyes

SPECIALTIES AND RELATED FIELDS: Geriatrics and gerontology, ophthalmology

DEFINITION: The absence of vision, or its extreme impairment to the extent that activity is limited; about 95 percent of all blindness is caused by eye diseases, the rest by injuries.

KEY TERMS:

glaucoma: excessive pressure inside the eye that can damage the optic nerve

laser: an intense light beam used in eye surgery

macular degeneration: a deterioration of vision in the most sensitive, central region of the retina

retina: a paper-thin membrane lining the inside surface of the eyeball, where light is transformed into nerve impulses

trachoma: a contagious eye infe~~ction~~ found in Third World countries

CAUSES AND SYMPTOMS

The major cause of blindness among older adults in the Western world is glaucoma. The aqueous fluid produced inside the eye fails to drain properly and causes pressure to build up. In extreme cases, the eyeball becomes hard. Without prompt treatment, the outer layer of the optic nerve starts to deteriorate. The patient can still see straight ahead, but not off to the side. When the cone of forward vision has narrowed to less that 20 degrees (called tunnel vision), the patient is considered legally blind.

Cataracts are another common defect of vision among the elderly. The lens of the eye develops dark spots that interfere with light transmission. Cataracts are not caused by an infection or a tumor but instead are a normal part of the aging process, like gray hair. There is no known treatment to retard or reverse the growth of cataracts.

Macular degeneration and diabetes mellitus can cause blindness as a result of hemorrhages from tiny blood vessels in the retina. The macula is a small region in the middle of the retina where receptor cells are tightly packed together to obtain sharp vision for reading or close work. With aging, blood circulation in the macula gradually deteriorates until the patient develops a black spot in the center of the field of view. Advanced diabetes also causes blood vessel damage in the eye. In serious cases, fluid can leak behind the retina, causing it to become detached. The resulting visual effect resembles a dark curtain that blacks out part of the scene.

Trachoma is a blinding eye disease that afflicts millions of people in poor parts of the world. It is a contagious infection of the eyelid similar to conjunctivitis (commonly known as pinkeye). If untreated, it causes scarring of the cornea and eventual blindness. Trachoma is caused by a virus that is spread by flies, in water, or by direct contact with tears or mucus.

Many kinds of injuries may cause blindness. Car accidents, sports injuries, chemical explosions, battle wounds, or small particles that enter the eye all can result in a serious loss of vision.

TREATMENT AND THERAPY

An indispensable tool in the treatment of serious eye problems is the laser. Its intense light focused into a tiny spot, the laser's heat can burn away a ruptured blood vessel or weld a detached retina back into place. For glaucoma patients, medication to reduce fluid pressure in the eye may be effective for a while. Eventually, a laser can be used to burn a small hole through the iris in order to improve fluid drainage. The laser can only be used to prevent blindness, however, and not to restore sight.

Cataracts formerly were a major cause of blindness among older people. Once the eye lens starts to become cloudy, nothing can be done to clear it. Cataract surgery to remove the defective lens and to insert a permanent, plastic replacement has become common. In the United States, more than a million cataract surgeries are performed annually, with a success rate that is greater than 95 percent.

The infectious eye disease called trachoma has been known for more than two thousand years. Effective modern treatment uses sulfa drugs taken orally, combined with antibiotic eyedrops or ointments. Unfortunately, reinfection is common in rural villages where most people have the disease and sanitation is poor. The World Health Organization has initiated a public health program to teach parents about the importance of cleanliness and frequent eye washing with sterilized water for their children.

PERSPECTIVE AND PROSPECTS

Various techniques have been developed for helping sightless people to live a self-reliant lifestyle. Using a white cane or walking with a trained dog allows a blind person to get around without assistance. Biomedical engineers have designed a miniature sonar device built into a pair of glasses that uses reflected sound waves to warn the wearer about obstacles.

The Braille system of reading, using patterns of raised dots for the alphabet, was invented in 1829 and is still widely used. For blind students, voice recordings of textbooks, magazines, and even whole encyclopedias are available on tape. A recent development is an optical scanner connected to a computer with a voice simulator that can read printed material aloud.

The National Federation of the Blind was founded in 1940. Its goals are to assist the blind to participate fully in society and to overcome the still-prevalent stereotype that the blind are helpless. Blind men and women hold jobs as engineers, teachers, musical performers, ministers, insurance agents, computer programmers, and school counselors. As society becomes more sensitive to all forms of disability, opportunities for blind people continue to expand.

—Hans G. Graetzer, Ph.D.

See also Cataract surgery; Cataracts; Color blindness; Diabetes mellitus; Eye surgery; Eyes; Glaucoma; Macular degeneration; Visual disorders.

FOR FURTHER INFORMATION:

Lerman, Sidney. "Glaucoma." *Scientific American,* August, 1959, 110-117. Describes how excess pressure can build up in the eye to cause blindness. Excellent illustrations with clear explanations.

Maurer, Marc. "Reflecting the Flame." *Vital Speeches of the Day* 57 (September 1, 1991): 684-690. A speech by the president of the National Federation of the Blind. He criticizes the media, government agencies, and educators for perpetuating false stereotypes of helplessness. Maurer is a forceful spokesperson for the blind.

Peninsula Center for the Blind. *The First Steps: How to Help People Who Are Losing Their Sight*. Palo Alto, Calif.: Peninsula Center, 1982. A pamphlet designed to help people cope with the emotional trauma of blindness and the process of adjustment. Highly recommended.

Werner, Georges H., Bachisio Latte, and Andrea Contini. "Trachoma." *Scientific American*, January, 1964, 79-86. Describes this infectious eye disease, which is prevalent in poor nations of the world. The efforts to develop effective treatment and a vaccine are reported.

BLOOD AND BLOOD COMPONENTS
BIOLOGY

ANATOMY OR SYSTEM AFFECTED: Blood vessels, circulatory system, immune system, liver, lymphatic system

SPECIALTIES AND RELATED FIELDS: Hematology, immunology, serology

DEFINITION: The fluid that circulates in the veins and arteries, carrying oxygen and nutrients through the body, transporting waste materials to excretory channels, and participating in the body's defense against infection.

KEY TERMS:

blood: the fluid that circulates through the cardiovascular system; composed of a fluid fraction and a cellular fraction consisting of erythrocytes, leukocytes, and thrombocytes

blood group system: a classification of individuals into groups on the basis of their possession or nonpossession of specific blood substances

blood typing: the identification of the blood group substances of an individual so as to classify him or her in a specific blood group

erythrocytes: red blood cells; the nonnucleated, disk-shaped blood cells that contain hemoglobin

hemoglobin: the oxygen-carrying red pigment present in red blood cells that is responsible for oxygen exchange in cells and tissues

leukocytes: white blood cells; any of the white or colorless nucleated cells occurring in blood

plasma: the protein-containing fluid portion of the blood in which the blood cells are normally suspended

serum: the clear, yellowish fluid obtained from blood after it has been allowed to clot

thrombocytes: platelets; small, irregularly shaped cells in the blood that participate in blood clotting

STRUCTURE AND FUNCTIONS

Blood provides a common communication channel for all organs in the body. It is responsible for the transport of oxygen, enzymes, hormones, drugs, and many other substances, as well as for the transfer of heat produced by chemical reactions in the body. The average-sized adult has about 10 pints of blood. At rest, 10 pints a minute (and up to 40 pints during exercise) are pumped by the heart via the arteries to the lungs and all other tissues. This blood then returns to the heart through the veins, in a continuous circuit.

About half the volume of blood consists of cells, which include red blood cells (erythrocytes), white blood cells (leukocytes), and platelets (thrombocytes). The remainder is a fluid called plasma, which contains dissolved proteins, sugars, fats, and minerals.

All types of blood cells are formed within the bone marrow by a series of divisions from a single type of cell called a stem cell. Red blood cells, or erythrocytes (from the Greek *eruthros*, "red"), are very small, have no nucleus, and consist almost completely of hemoglobin. Very little oxygen is needed for the survival of these cells. They have a large surface relative to their volume, which allows oxygen and carbon dioxide to diffuse in and out of the cell rapidly. This large surface also allows the cell to swell and shrink and to be squashed through narrow capillaries without its surface being subjected to shearing or bursting. Red blood cells cannot repair themselves, and after three or four months in the circulation they are eliminated and replaced. Their main function is to act as containers for hemoglobin; as such, they are among the most highly specialized cells in the body.

Hemoglobin, the red, iron-containing pigment responsible for the color of blood, has a great affinity for oxygen. It will release the oxygen in a situation where free oxygen is scarce, as it is among the live cells of working tissues. Hemoglobin gives blood an oxygen-carrying capacity eighty times greater than if the oxygen were merely dissolved in plasma. When hemoglobin gives up its oxygen, it becomes capable of taking up carbon dioxide, which it carries to the lungs. Thus this substance provides a sophisticated oxygen delivery system that provides the proper amount of oxygen to the tissues under a wide variety of circumstances. Hemoglobin occupies 33 percent of the volume of the red cell and accounts for 90 percent of its dry weight.

Leukocytes, or white blood cells (from the Greek *leukos*, meaning "clear" or "white"), are larger and less plentiful than red blood cells and can also be found outside the blood. Their purpose is to clean the system of wastes and foreign material and to act as defense against living germs. They travel through the circulatory system and can pass through the walls of blood vessels to do their work in the surrounding tissues. White blood cells play an important role in the defense against infection by viruses, bacteria, fungi, parasites, and inflammation of any cause. There are three main types: granulocytes, monocytes, and lymphocytes. Granulocytes, or polymorphonuclear leukocytes, contain granules and have an oddly shaped nucleus; they are themselves of three types: neutrophils, basophils, and eosinophils. The most important are the neutrophils, which are responsible for isolating and killing invading bacteria (pus consists largely of neutrophils). They are also called phagocytes ("engulfing cells") because of their capability to swallow bacteria and other foreign materials. They normally remain in the blood for only six to nine hours and then travel to the tissues, where they spend a few more days and then move to sites of infection. Eosinophils are involved in allergic reactions. Monocytes circulate in the blood for six to nine days and are also a type of phagocyte important in the immune system.

Lymphocytes are the entities responsible for immune response, such as the production of antibodies and the rejection of tissue grafts. They direct the activity of all other cells in the immune response. Many of them are formed in the lymph nodes rather than in the bone barrow. Their lifetime is between three months and ten years. Unlike granulocytes and monocytes, they do not engulf solid particles but instead play a part in antibody production. An antibody is a protein which may dissolve freely in the blood plasma or in other body fluids and may afix to other cells. Antibodies can be regarded as disinfectants, since they kill or specifically mark foreign material so that it is more readily noticed, caught, digested, or swept away by scavenger cells. There are many different types of lymphocytes, each of which has a different function. T lymphocytes are responsible for delayed hypersensitivity phenomena and produce substances called lymphokines, which affect the function of many cells. They also moderate the activity of other lymphocytes called B lymphocytes. These cells form the antibodies that protect against a second attack of a disease. Most of these cells are in a state of patrol, forming an early warning system which moves out of the circulation, into the tissue fluids, and back to the blood. If these cells encounter foreign material that fits a specific molecular pattern in their structure, or receive such material from another cell, they move to a lymph node or similar area. There they divide to produce a line of daughter cells, all of which manufacture an antibody specifically active against that foreign or irregular material.

Platelets, or thrombocytes, are the smallest cells in blood; they can survive there for about nine days. They circulate in the blood in an inactive state, but under certain circumstances they begin to adhere to blood vessels and one another, producing and releasing chemicals that begin the process of blood clotting. Thus they are critical in hemostasis (the arresting of bleeding).

Plasma is the straw-colored fluid in which blood cells are suspended. It is composed mainly of water (95 percent), with a salt content that is similar to salt water. Some of its other important constituents are nutrients, waste products, proteins, and hormones. Nutrients are transported to the tissues after absorption from the intestinal tract or following release from storage places such as the liver. They include sugars, fats, vitamins, minerals, and the amino acids required to make proteins. The main waste product of tissue metabolism is urea, which is transported in the plasma to the kidneys. The waste product from the destruction of hemoglobin is a yellow pigment called bilirubin, which is normally removed from the plasma by the liver and turned into bile. Among the proteins in plasma are substances such as

The Components of Blood

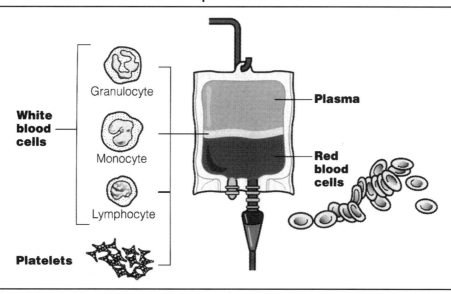

Blood consists of cells floating in a fluid called plasma. Red blood cells contain hemoglobin, an important substance that carries oxygen; platelets are involved in clotting mechanisms; and white blood cells, which are divided into granulocytes, monocytes, and lymphocytes, are responsible for the immune response to foreign matter.

fibrinogen (involved in the process of coagulation and clotting), immunoglobulins and its complements (bacteria fighters that are part of the immune system), and albumin. Hormones are chemical messengers transported from various glands to their target organs.

The term "blood group" refers to the classification of blood according to differences in the makeup of its red blood cells. The ABO system consists of three blood group substances, the A, B, and H antigens (substances that induce the production of an antibody when injected into an animal), which are components of erythrocyte surface substances. Individuals with type A cells carry anti-B antibodies in their serum; those with type B cells carry anti-A antibodies; those with type AB cells (which bear both A and B antigens) carry neither anti-A nor anti-B antibodies; and type O individuals, whose cells bear neither antigen, carry both anti-A and anti-B antibodies. The transfusion of type A blood into a type B individual, for example, clumps together the transfused erythrocytes and results in an often fatal blockage of blood vessels, which indicates the importance of blood typing before a transfusion is performed.

Another blood group system is based on the rhesus (or Rh) factor. The system involves several antigens, but the most important is called factor D. It is found in 85 percent of the population; those individuals are called Rh positive. If it is not present, the person is classified as Rh negative. Based on this system, individuals are therefore classified as O positive or AB negative, for example, on the basis of their ABO and Rh blood groups. The main importance of the Rh group is during pregnancy. An Rh-negative women who is pregnant with an Rh-positive baby may form antibodies against the baby's blood. Such women are given antibodies directed against factor D after delivery to prevent the development of anti-D antibodies, which would cause hemolytic disease of the newborn in successive Rh-positive infants. The transfusion of Rh-positive blood into an Rh-negative patient can cause a serious reaction if the patient has had a previous blood transfusion that contained the Rh antigen.

About four hundred other antigens have been discovered, but they are widely scattered throughout the population and rarely cause transfusion problems. Only the ABO and the Rh blood group systems have major clinical importance.

Blood typing is used to categorize blood for transfusion. Knowledge of blood group substances and of their inheritance has been useful for legal, historical, and medical purposes. The ABO blood groups are found in all people, but the frequency of each group varies with race and geographical distribution. This fact can aid anthropologists who are involved in investigating, for example, early population migrations. The blood group of an individual is determined by the genes inherited from his or her parents. Identification of a blood group can be used in a paternity case to establish that a man could not have been the father of a particular child, although it cannot be shown positively that a man is the father by blood grouping. Blood found at the scene of a crime can be typed and used to exclude suspects if the type does not match. Some blood groups are associated with particular disorders. For example, blood group A has been found to be more common in people suffering from cancer of the stomach, while group O is found more often in people suffering from peptic ulcers.

DISORDERS AND DISEASES

Blood tests can be used to check on the health of major organs as well as respiratory functions, hormonal balance, the immune system, and metabolism. They can reveal not only the blood cell abnormalities characteristic of some diseases but also healthy variations in blood induced by response to infections. Blood tests can be classified into three categories. Hematological tests involve studying the components of blood itself by looking at the number, shape, size, and appearance of its cells, as well as by testing the function of clotting factors. The most important tests of this type are the blood count, blood smear, and blood-clotting tests. Biochemical tests look at chemicals in the blood such as sodium, potassium, uric acid, area, vitamins, gases, and drugs. In microbiological tests, blood is examined for microorganisms, such as bacteria, viruses and viral particles, fungi, and parasites, and for antibodies that form against them.

Known causes of blood disorders include genetic reasons (an inherited abnormality in the production of some blood component), nutritional disorders (such as a vitamin deficiency), infections by microorganisms, tumors (such as bone marrow cancer), poisons (carbon monoxide, lead, and snake and spider venoms), drugs (which can produce blood abnormalities as a side effect), and radiation.

Abnormalities can occur in any of the components of blood, including some constituents of plasma. Leukemias are disorders in which the number of white blood cells is abnormally high. In acquired immunodeficiency syndrome (AIDS), the T lymphocytes are infected by a virus, resulting in dysfunction and an increased risk for certain types of infections and cancers. Abnormal platelets or the lack of platelets can lead to some types of bleeding disorders, such as hemophilia (an inability of the blood to clot properly). Unwanted clot formation (thrombosis) can occur from circumstances that overactivate the blood's clotting mechanisms. Anemia results from a deficiency of hemoglobin and a corresponding reduction in the blood's oxygen-carrying capacity; this is the most common blood disorder. Deficiencies of the proteins in blood plasma include albuminemia (albumin deficiency).

PERSPECTIVE AND PROSPECTS

Blood is a liquid of complex structure and vital functions that has been considered the essence of life for centuries. There is no shortage of irrational or unscientific ideas about the supposed properties of human blood—one can speak of "blood brotherhood," "blood feuds," "blood relations," and of someone being "bloodthirsty."

The present medical understanding of blood has developed over the past two or three thousand years. The study of blood began in Egypt and Mesopotamia, around 500 B.C., and it moved to the countries around the Mediterranean that had become intellectually active. Ancient Greek thinkers noted that there were differences between arteries and veins, and that the blood moved through them. According to whether the heart, the liver, or the brain was thought to be the prime organ controlling the rest of the body, various functions were tentatively ascribed to blood, such as its relation to sleep, the distribution of heat, and the animation of the body.

The Greek school of medicine became personified in Hippocrates. He denied the widely accepted theory of the existence of spirits and proposed that the body followed natural laws. He presented the concept of body juices, or humors. There were four of them: blood, lymph or phlegm, yellow bile (or choler), and black bile (or melancholy), with blood being the most important one. The philosopher Aristotle accepted the humoral hypothesis. One of his pupils was Alexander the Great, whose military conquests spread Greek influence widely. A notable medical school developed in Alexandria, Egypt, and the ideas of Hippocrates and Aristotle were taught there. There was, however, a variation in regard to blood; namely, the theory of plethora, in which it was postulated that an excess of blood in the circulatory system or one organ caused illness.

Four hundred years later, Galen, a product of the Alexandria School of Medicine, denied the doctrine of plethora and went back to the humoral approach. Health and disease were thought to occur as a result of an upset in the equilibrium of these humors. Bloodletting to restore the balance of the humors by purging the body of its contaminated fluids was practiced from the time of Hippocrates until the nineteenth century. During Galen's time, animal dissection was widely practiced and provided a better concept of blood and its functions. It was proposed that the liver changed food to blood, which was distributed to the body along the veins. At the same time, impurities from the body were thought to be absorbed into the venous blood and to be returned to the liver and then to the right side of the heart, where they supposedly ascended in the pulmonary artery to the lungs to be exhaled.

The weakening of medieval ideas set the stage for English doctor William Harvey's discovery of the circulation of blood. He used the analogy of the heart as a pump and veins and arteries as pipes, where blood is moving around and is being driven in some kind of continuous circuit. Four years after Harvey died in 1661, the Italian anatomist Marcello Malpighi observed the capillary blood vessels with the aid of the microscope. The cellular composition of blood was also recognized with the aid of this device, as

Antoni van Leeuwenhoek, a Dutch naturalist, accurately described and measured red blood cells. The discovery of white blood cells and platelets followed after microscope lenses were improved. William Hewson first observed leukocytes in the eighteenth century. He thought that these cells came from the nucleated cells in the lymph and that they eventually emerged from the spleen as red blood cells. In the nineteenth century, the interest in leukocytes intensified with studies on inflammation and microbial infection.

In 1852, Karl Vierordt published the first quantitative results of blood cell analysis, after several attempts were made to correlate blood cell counts with various diseases. The observation of crystalline hemoglobin was first reported in 1849. In 1865, Felix Hoppe-Seyler discovered the oxygen-carrying capacity of the red pigment (hemoglobin) in the cells. The early history of protein chemistry is essentially that of hemoglobin, as it was one of the first molecules to have its molecular weight accurately determined and the first to be associated with a specific physiological function (that of carrying oxygen).

In 1900, the German pathologist Karl Landsteiner began mixing blood taken from different people and found that some mixtures were compatible and others were not. This incompatibility resulted in illness and sometimes death after transfusions. He discovered two types of marker proteins, or antigens, on the surface of red blood cells, which he called A and B. According to whether a person's blood contains one or the other antigen, both, or neither, it is classified as type A, B, AB, or O. He also discovered the Rh factor in 1940 during experiments with rhesus monkeys. Improved methods of blood examination in the 1920's and the growth of knowledge of blood physiology in the 1930's allowed anemias and other blood disorders to be studied on a rational basis.

Modern hematology recognizes that alteration in the components of blood are a result of disease, and research is conducted continually for a better understanding of this relationship and of blood itself. —*Maria Pacheco, Ph.D.*

See also Anemia; Angiography; Bleeding; Blood bank; Blood testing; Bone marrow transplantation; Cholesterol; Circulation; Dialysis; Ebola virus; Fluids and electrolytes; Forensic pathology; Heart; Hematology; Hematology, pediatric; Hemophilia; Hypercholesterolemia; Hyperlipidemia; Hypoglycemia; Immunization and vaccination; Ischemia; Jaundice; Laboratory tests; Leukemia; Liver; Nephrology; Nephrology, pediatric; Pathology; Pharmacology; Rh factor; Septicemia; Serology; Sickle-cell anemia; Thalassemia; Thrombolytic therapy and TPA; Toxemia; Toxicology; Transfusion.

FOR FURTHER INFORMATION:

Clayman, Charles B., ed. *American Medical Association Encyclopedia of Medicine*. New York: Random House, 1989. An excellent presentation on blood—its components, illnesses, and treatments.

Hackett, Earle. *Blood: The Biology, Pathology, and Mythology of the Body's Most Important Fluid.* New York: Saturday Review Press, 1973. A good examination of historical and scientific perspectives of the study of blood.

Larson, David E., ed. *The Mayo Clinic Family Health Book.* 2d ed. New York: William Morrow, 1996. Good presentation of blood; concentrates on illnesses, their causes and treatments.

Seeman, Bernard. *The River of Life: The Story of Man's Blood from Magic to Science.* New York: W. W. Norton, 1961. Offers an interesting and entertaining historical perspective of the perceptions and beliefs surrounding blood.

Voet, Donald, and Judith G. Voet. *Biochemistry.* New York: John Wiley & Sons, 1990. An excellent general biochemistry book that contains a few sections on blood and blood components, their properties and functions.

Zeleny, R. O., ed. *The World Book Medical Encyclopedia.* Chicago: World Book, 1988. Provides a similar presentation to that in *The Mayo Clinic Family Health Book.*

Zucker-Franklin, D., et al. *Atlas of Blood Cells: Function and Pathology.* 2d ed. Philadelphia: Lea & Febiger, 1988. Great pictorial presentation of blood components in different stages of function and disease.

BLOOD BANK
ORGANIZATION

DEFINITION: A temporary storehouse of blood, kept at reduced temperatures, for transfusions into persons needing an additional supply; such transfers are vital in surgery and in unexpected emergency procedures.

KEY TERMS:

cardiology: the study of the heart and its action, as well as the diagnosis and treatment of its diseases

cardiovascular: relating to or involving the heart and blood vessels

corpuscle: a minute particle; a protoplasmic cell floating free in the blood

erythrocyte: a red blood cell

hematosis: the formation of blood

hemophilia: a tendency (usually hereditary) to profuse bleeding, even from slight cuts

leukocyte: a white or colorless blood corpuscle

phagocyte: any leukocyte active in ingesting and destroying waste and harmful material

phlebotomy: the act or practice of opening a vein for letting blood

serology: the science of serums, their reactions, preparation, and use

THE STUDY OF BLOOD THROUGHOUT HISTORY

For centuries, blood was thought to be a simple liquid, but it is actually a body tissue. The cells, instead of being joined together as in solid body tissues, are suspended in a fluid called plasma, which is more than half of blood composition. The cellular portion of blood is largely red blood cells and smaller numbers of white blood cells and platelets. Blood itself is the final functioning tool of the circulatory system, which helps to transport the blood to where it is needed in the body. Blood is an extremely complicated substance, and more things are being learned about it every year.

Some ancient civilizations, such as that of the Greeks, recognized that blood was an important fluid in the body, but they thought that it was motionless in certain areas. Between 300 and 250 B.C., some Egyptians were studying the anatomy of corpses. About 300 B.C., the Greek physician Praxagoras showed that there were tubes connected to the heart. Some were filled with blood; others were empty, filled with air. One of the physician's students, Herophilus, found that arteries gave a beat or pulse. When dissection was outlawed in Egypt, progress in learning about blood was stopped for a thousand years.

Galen, the Greek physician who served five Roman emperors over thirty years to 200 A.D., believed that the arteries originated in the heart and pumped blood. Contrary to later Egyptian medical thought, Galen theorized that the heart was one pump, not two. Around 1300, doctors in Italy began to dissect bodies again, and in 1316, Mondino de Luzzi wrote the first book dealing entirely with anatomy, in which he supported Galen's teachings. In 1543, Belgian anatomist Andreas Vesalius wrote a much-improved book on anatomy which did not improve, however, on Galen's theories about the heart.

In 1242, a Syrian surgeon named Ibn an-Nafīs had written a book in which he theorized about how blood moved from the right ventricle to the left and that a double pump was involved in moving it. Ironically, his writings were not discovered by Europeans until 1924.

Meanwhile, Spanish physician Michael Servetus published a treatise in 1553 describing how circulation of blood to the lungs and back (often called the lesser circulation) might occur. Unfortunately, because he also included religious views, all copies of his writings that could be found were destroyed, and he was burned at the stake. Eventually, in 1694, a copy of his book was found; his circulation theory matched later findings.

In 1559, an Italian anatomist, Realdo Colombo, also thought of lesser circulation and published a book on it. Colombo's work was so widely read that he is credited with discovering lesser circulation. In 1574, another Italian, Girolamo Fabrici, observed little valves on veins that opened in only one direction. The importance of this discovery was deducted by a student of Fabrici, the English doctor William Harvey, when he determined that blood in the leg veins could move only to the heart. His laboratory work proved that the heart pumped blood into the arteries and that the blood returned by way of the veins. Further, Harvey showed that the blood had a double circulation, returning to both ventricles. His continued experimentation showed that the same blood had to circulate and be used repeatedly.

All these medical pioneers were hampered by the inability to see more than the human eye would permit—until the development of lenses and microscopes. In 1661, Italian anatomist Marcello Malpighi was able to see, with the aid of a microscope, very fine blood vessels that connected the smallest arteries and veins: capillaries. With the discovery of capillaries, the concept of the circulation of blood was complete. In the eighteenth century, the English scientist Stephen Hales was the first to measure blood pressure.

The microscope also enabled scientists to observe some components of blood. Malpighi saw reddish objects in a clear, faintly yellow fluid. Dutch scientist Jan Swammerdam, with the aid of a microscope, was able to describe them further. In 1674, the renowned Dutch scientist Antoni van Leeuwenhoek, using the best of these early microscopes, was able to describe the red cells as flat disks with depressions in the center. He even tried to measure them; his calculations were refined in 1852 by German scientist Karl Vierordt. Leeuwenhoek was able to study the path of red blood cells in tadpoles, frogs, and other animals and determined that, without doubt, blood traveled in an entirely closed circle, proving Harvey's contention. Soon, in 1669, English doctor Richard Lower noted that blood coming through arteries was red and that blood flowing toward the heart in veins was bluish.

English chemist Joseph Priestley discovered the gas oxygen in 1774, and French chemist Antoine-Laurent Lavoisier was able to show in 1778 that air consisted (mainly) of two gases, oxygen (one-fifth) and nitrogen (four-fifths). A German chemist, Julius Lothar Meyer, showed in 1857 that oxygen did not generally mix with the liquid part of the blood, combining instead with red blood cells.

The scientific detective work on blood continued with the aid of improved microscopes. It was learned that the cells of the body contained complicated substances called proteins, each of which was made up of groups of atoms called molecules. German scientists were among the first to examine the composition of blood. Otto Funke obtained a protein from red blood cells in 1851. Then Felix Hoppe-Seyler purified it, studied it, and named it hemoglobin ("blood protein"). The secrets of this precious commodity continued to unfold. In 1747, Italian chemist Vincenzo Antonio Menghini found that there was a small quantity of iron in blood, apparently in red blood cells.

Gradually, these findings led to the transfusion of blood from one person to another. In the seventeenth century, blood transfusions were attempted between animals. In 1666, Richard Lower unsuccessfully tried to transfuse blood from an animal to a human being. Sometimes the operation helped, but occasionally people died after such a transfusion, so doctors largely abandoned the practice. Then, in 1818, James Blundell, an English physician who

theorized that the blood of a particular kind of animal would only help that particular kind, transfused blood from healthy human beings to other human beings who needed blood. While often successful, the procedure sometimes caused agglutination, in which red blood cells clumped together and would not function properly.

In 1901, an Austrian doctor named Karl Landsteiner solved the problem by observing that there were four kinds of blood cells. Depending on the chemical content, the blood was typed A, B, AB, and O. Continuing practice showed that not all blood types work well with each other; some tend to agglutinate when introduced to the wrong type.

Although red blood cells are by far the most numerous objects that float in the bloodstream, they are not the only ones. In 1850, French physician Casimir-Joseph Davaine noticed cells, pale and uneven in shape, that were much larger than red blood cells. By 1869, he noticed that these cells would absorb bits of foreign matter in the blood. In 1875, German doctor Paul Ehrlich, interested in using dyes on these white cells, found that he was able to classify them into different types.

In the late nineteenth century, Russian scientist Élie Metchnikoff (also known as Ilya Ilich Mechnikov), while studying bacteria, noticed that whenever there was a cut, white cells were carried to it in great numbers by the blood. So much blood went to the injured part that it grew red and inflamed and was painful from the pressure exerted by the blood on the vessel walls. Metchnikoff called the bacteria-eating cells phagocytes. He had become interested in the study of bacteria following the pioneering work of France's Louis Pasteur in the 1860's.

The clotting of wounds became more interesting to the medical community. In 1842, French scientist Alfred Donne had reported a new type of object floating in the bloodstream. An Italian physician, Giulio Cesare Bizzozero, concluded that the foreign objects had something to do with clotting. He called them platelets because their shape resembles tiny plates. What was to be learned about them much later is that they have a life span of about nine days and that they break down when exposed to air after bleeding starts. As they begin to break down, platelets release a substance that starts a long chain of chemical changes that ends in clotting.

While many scientists were concentrating on the study of red blood cells, white blood cells, and platelets, attention was also being paid to plasma, the colorless liquid that is a vehicle for objects floating in it. Eventually, it was learned that plasma carries red blood cells to the lungs to take up oxygen, and then to all the rest of the body to deliver the oxygen. Plasma carries white blood cells to any part of the body where they are needed to fight bacteria. It also carries platelets to any part of the body where blood loss must be stopped. Furthermore, the watery plasma absorbs heat at the liver and delivers it to the skin, so that the body stays warm.

More recent studies show that about 8 percent of plasma is composed of dissolved substances that are important in keeping conditions in the body even. Some chemicals in the plasma neutralize acids and bases, which could threaten cells. The plasma also carries glucose molecules and fatty acids to specific destinations in order to produce energy in the body. Furthermore, it dissolves wastes such as carbon dioxide and delivers urea to the kidneys for disposal. Hormones, which were first discovered in 1902, are also carried by the plasma to any part of the body where they are needed.

More than half the weight of substances dissolved in plasma are proteins. Proteins fall into two groups, albumins and globulins. Some proteins combine easily with substances that the body needs in small amounts. Gammaglobulins have the capacity to neutralize foreign molecules—viruses or the poisonous toxins produced by bacteria—by combining with them. Gammaglobulins that act in this way are called antibodies.

All these discoveries and many others (such as the existence of fibrinogen, fibrin, the Rh factor, and enzymes) have combined to improve the procedures for storing and transfusing blood. Safeguarding blood for transfusion has always been a problem. The precious liquid is unstable, and a fresh supply has always been needed in any emergency.

In the late 1930's, Russian scientists discovered that citrated blood can be stored if refrigerated at a temperature of about 4.5 degrees Celsius (40 degrees Fahrenheit). Then, in 1936, a Canadian doctor, Norman Bethune, made large-scale use of a blood bank with antifascist forces during the Spanish Civil War. During World War II, the noted American blood bank pioneer Charles Drew, who had made a special study of ways to store and ship blood plasma, organized a nationwide "Blood for Britain" campaign in which thousands of lives were saved.

Before blood banks could evolve, a number of additional discoveries had to be made. Before the discovery of agglutins and blood typing, blood was transfused directly from donor to patient. The two lay side by side, and the blood flowed from the artery of the donor to the vein of the recipient. There was no way of measuring the amount of blood being transfused. It became dangerous for the donor if he or she changed from rosy-colored and talkative to pale or unconscious. There was also danger that a blood clot in the tube might enter the patient's blood vessels. In addition, the blood might be flowing too fast and overload the patient's heart.

A new tube to facilitate blood transfusion more safely was developed in 1909. Then, in 1914, Argentine doctor Luis Agote discovered that sodium citrate could stop the clotting of blood, permitting blood to be kept in a bottle while it was slowly directed into a patient's vein. Physicians could finally control the amount and speed of transfusions.

The use of stored blood began in 1918 by Oswald H. Robertson, a World War I physician, who found it could be kept virtually intact for several days by storing it at low temperatures, from 2 to 4 degrees Celsius. The first large blood bank was established at the Cook County Hospital in Chicago in 1937.

THE ROLE OF BLOOD BANKS

A blood bank is an organizational unit responsible for collecting, processing, and storing blood to be used for transfusion and other purposes. It is usually a subdivision of a laboratory in a hospital and is often charged with the responsibility for all serologic testing. Although blood can be withdrawn from one person and transfused directly into another, the usual practice is for hospitals and authorized agencies to select donors, draw blood (phlebotomy), screen the specimens, arrange them into blood groups, and store the blood until it is needed.

The storage of blood was once short-lived because of clotting and too-high temperature levels. A blood bank can now store blood for much longer periods of time, sometimes a year or two. It is stored with an anticoagulant, generally an acid-citrate-dextrose (ACD) solution composed of trisodium citrate, citric acid, dextrose, and sterile water. Red blood cells from blood stored in an ACD solution will survive in the recipient for one hundred days. Blood banks consider blood unsuitable for transfusion if it is retained more than twenty-one days. After that, stored blood may be reduced to plasma by centrifuging it to eliminate the red blood cells.

All chemical changes in blood are slowed by refrigeration. It has been found that prolonged storage of blood can be achieved by freezing and maintaining it at extremely low temperatures—below −70 degrees Celsius (−94 degrees Fahrenheit). While freezing and thawing of whole blood does not harm plasma, it can damage red blood cells unless glycerol or dimethyl sulfoxide solutions are used to minimize the damage and permit red cells to be maintained in a frozen state for months without significant injury.

After Karl Landsteiner discovered that blood could be classified into four major blood groups, safer transfusions could be attempted. Landsteiner also worked with the American pathologist Alexander S. Wiener to discover another system of blood grouping known as the Rh system. The name was derived from the rhesus monkeys with which the scientists experimented.

It was found that a person with type A blood (having "A" agglutinogens in the red blood cells and "b" agglutinins in the blood plasma) cannot successfully give blood to a person with type B blood (having "B" agglutinogens and "a" agglutinins) because the clumping of blood cells will occur.

Successful blood transfusions depend on the type of agglutinogens in the donor's red blood cells, not on the type of agglutinin in the plasma, because the recipient's blood cells greatly outnumber the agglutinin in the donor's blood and serious clumping could not occur. A donor's red blood cells, however, are few enough in number that all of them can be agglutinated by the recipient's agglutinins. These clumps could then plug the capillaries, reducing and eventually cutting off the flow of blood. This reaction is serious and can cause death.

A person with type AB blood, who has both "A" and "B" agglutinogens in the red blood cells and no agglutinins in the plasma, can receive the red blood cells of any other group. A type O person (a universal donor) has no agglutinogens and can donate blood to any person but can only receive type O blood. In practice, however, physicians use donors having the same type as their recipients.

The ABO system of grouping blood types has led to further refinements. Ten major and minor blood groupings have been identified from the variety of proteins also found in blood cells. The most important is the Rh system. There are two Rh blood types, Rh positive and Rh negative. A person with the Rh-positive factor has the protein, while a person with Rh-negative blood does not have the protein. Infusing an Rh-negative person with Rh-positive blood causes special agglutinins to be formed in the blood of the recipient. A later transfusion of Rh-positive blood would result in the agglutination of the red blood cells received.

This reaction is especially important when incompatibility occurs between the blood of a pregnant woman and her baby. This happens only if the mother has Rh-negative blood and the baby has Rh-positive blood because it has inherited Rh-positive genes from the father. When such a baby is born, some of the baby's blood enters the mother's circulation system, causing her body to produce antibodies to combat the "foreign material." Since this intrusion of blood almost always happens as a delayed reaction after the baby is born, the first baby is probably unharmed, but a subsequent baby could be the victim of these antibodies, which the mother's body continues to produce. Such a developing baby could suffer the destruction of its red blood cells if it has Rh-positive blood, unless preventive steps such as a blood transfusion for the baby are taken. Another medical development is a serum for protective vaccination that has almost eliminated the dangers of Rh incompatibility.

Blood transfusions are regularly used in crises such as accidents or life-threatening illnesses. Most commonly, they are used to restore the volume of circulating blood lost by acute hemorrhaging. They are also used to restore the large volume of plasma that is often lost after severe burns. In acute or chronic anemia cases, such as with acquired immunodeficiency syndrome (AIDS), they are used to maintain hemoglobin and red blood cells at adequate levels. Transfusions are also used to provide platelets for coagulation in order to counteract various bleeding disorders or acute hemorrhaging.

The technique of blood transfusion has become routinely simple. Blood withdrawn by hypodermic needle from an arm vein of a healthy donor is passed through plastic tubing into a sterile glass bottle or plastic bag that contains sodium citrate or another solution that prevents coagulation. The blood is then transfused into the arm of the recipient through a second plastic tube connection which contains a gauze filter. About 500 milliliters (about 1 pint) are drawn and infused slowly, except in emergency cases.

Blood transfusions are being used more extensively—and more safely—than ever before. Many more surgeries are possible with transfusions: organ implants, heart repair, limb reconstruction, grafting for severe burn cases, and bone grafts. Blood transfusions are also important in the treatment of anemia and AIDS.

PERSPECTIVE AND PROSPECTS

In the United States, the work of blood banks comes under the ultimate supervision of the Food and Drug Administration (FDA) and federal agencies, as well as the Oversight and Investigations Subcommittee of the House Energy and Commerce Committee. Also interested in their function are the congressionally funded Public Health Service and the Centers for Disease Control. The largest United States blood bank is that of the Red Cross, which provides, through its local affiliates, about half of the 18 million units of blood donated each year. The Red Cross, as well as individual nonprofit and commercial agencies, is striving for improved health and safety procedures in blood donation.

The American Association of Blood Banks gathers and interprets data each year. It has found that there have been relatively few transfusion-induced cases of viral infection. Almost all the transfusion-related AIDS cases, for example, developed in 1985, before tighter screening of donors, safer procedures, and strict testing were instituted. Only fifteen cases of AIDS from blood transfusion were reported between 1985 and 1992. This contrasts with the pre-1985 figure of 3,425 transfusion-associated cases of AIDS reported to the Centers for Disease Control.

Concern for other viral infections transmitted through blood transfusions has increased vigilance against blood impurities and has improved sanitary procedures. Governmental agencies, the Red Cross, and private corporations have intensified their efforts to protect the quality of the blood supply. The International Society of Blood Transfusion continues to examine new threats.

Steps are continually reviewed to improve recordkeeping, blood collection, tracking, and distribution by all organizations. The FDA has a comprehensive inspection program which focuses on all phases of the collection-dispersal program of all blood banks, as well as on their training of workers and updating of procedures. It looks closely at procedures for donor screening, the testing for hepatitis and AIDS virus antibodies, and the quarantine and destruction of unsuitable blood products.

The American Red Cross complies with these regulations and works with the FDA to create the safest blood supply possible. It has a state-of-the-art computerized information system. It keeps track of all its donors and retains files on all persons disqualified from giving blood and the reasons. This information is available throughout the United States. The computerized program is also being expanded internationally because there is a growing import-export business between countries in need of new supplies. Data banks are being developed with lists of disqualified would-be donors, types and quantities of blood in storage, location of hospitals and distribution centers, and other information vital to the prompt, efficient, and safe distribution of blood.

The Blood Center, a nonprofit blood bank that serves eighty-five hospitals across a sixteen-country area, uses an automatic tracking software system to help send the right blood or blood components to those in need and to guard against contaminated blood entering the supply. The system collects 47,000 units a year.

Contrary to popular belief, donors are seldom paid for blood in the United States; this practice effectively came to an end in the early 1970's. Donors have no financial incentive to give blood.

Blood safety begins with screening. Only healthy individuals are allowed to give blood. Blood samples undergo extensive screening designed to detect any blood-borne infectious agent. Some collection agencies are developing lists of unwanted donors, persons with a high risk of having been exposed to the AIDS virus or to other dangerous viruses or bacteria, such as those that cause hepatitis or syphilis. The goal is to reduce the chance of contagion as much as possible.

Four million patients a year receive blood, largely in emergency cases. Many are in need of emergency surgery for an internal disorder, but many others are victims of social violence, earthquakes, and hurricanes. Large scale devastation often comes close to depleting the blood supply in an area. New and repeat donors, therefore, are always in demand. New ways of storing blood safely and for longer periods of time are constantly being researched. Some components can be frozen, for example, to give them a longer usable life.

Currently, there is a possible sequence of seven tests to screen blood donations. A polymerase chain reaction (PCR) test almost always amplifies and detects human immunodeficiency virus (HIV). Other tests are sophisticated efforts to detect HIV-1, HIV-2, and hepatitis C viruses. A test whose acronym ELISA, for enzyme-linked immunosorbent assay, is often supported by the Western blot, which conclusively demonstrates specific antibodies to specific viral proteins. It is an expensive set of procedures, and hospitals, clinics, and other medical institutions are working on how to reduce these costs.

Many viruses are elusive, including the dreaded HIV, which takes time to develop. To hasten its identification, scientists have developed the technique of "pooling" by combining blood known to contain infected cells with sam-

ples of blood with uninfected normal lymphocytes in an effort to stimulate HIV replication and make the HIV come to light faster. It has been found that the most reliable mix is a pool of fifty donors. The concept of pooling is scientifically valid and economically feasible.

While the risk of acquiring a hepatitis infection has been reduced from a possibility of 33 percent to less than 1 percent, there is growing concern among the public that individuals might be susceptible to specific blood diseases.

—Walter Appleton

See also Bleeding; Blood and blood components; Blood testing; Cytology; Emergency medicine; Hematology; Hematology, pediatric; Rh factor; Screening; Serology; Transfusion.

FOR FURTHER INFORMATION:

"American Association of Blood Banks." *NCI Cancer Weekly* 19 (November, 1990): 12. A definition of how infectious agents pose challenges for international blood supply safety.

Asimov, Isaac. *How Did We Find Out About Blood?* New York: Walker, 1986. Describes the scientific knowledge that exists about functions of blood in the body, from the beliefs held by the ancient Greeks to discoveries in more modern times.

Beard, Jonathan, and Andy Coghlan. "Filters Provide Traps for Catching Viruses." *New Scientist* 131 (July 20, 1991): 20. A report of how membrane filters are being used to purge blood plasma of contaminants.

Contreras, Marcela, et al. "Low Incidence of Hepatitis Confirmed by Virus Serology Testing." *The Lancet* 337 (March 30, 1991): 753-757. Relates the discovery of a non-A and non-B hepatitis virus following blood transfusions in Western nations and Japan, leading to newly developed immunological techniques to detect it.

Jones, Laurie. "Blood Safety Questioned." *American Medical News*, May 6, 1991, 3-4. A citation of deficiencies in the Red Cross blood supply system.

Leitman, Susan F., et al. "Clinical Implications of Positive Tests for Antibodies to HIV-1." *The New England Journal of Medicine* 321, no. 14 (October 5, 1989): 917-924. A description of the monitoring of discrepancies between positive immunoassay results and negative or indeterminate Western blot results.

Margolis, Neil. "Technology Gets Blood to Those in Need." *Computerworld* 23 (April 17, 1989): 17. A description of modern blood bank automation—how it can get rare specimens to emergency situations and how it can alleviate shortages in various parts of the United States.

Riedman, Sarah R. *Your Blood and You.* 2d ed. New York: Abelard-Schuman, 1963. A broad overview of the circulatory system, including the structure and function of the heart and the blood vessels.

Schwartz, J. Sanford, et al. "Strategies for Screening Blood for HIV Antibody." *The Journal of the American Medical*

Association 264, no. 13 (October 3, 1990): 1704-1710. A detailed analysis of the costs and risks of each strategy for screening blood donations. In addition to extensive testing, the authors consider reducing unnecessary transfusions, recruiting blood donors from low-risk groups, and decreasing the general incidence of HIV infection.

Surgenor, Douglas M., Edward L. Wallace, and Steven H. S. Hao. "Collection and Transfusion of Blood in the United States, 1892-1988." *The New England Journal of Medicine* 322, no. 23 (June 7, 1990): 1646-1650. A review of a study of the effects of blood collection and transfusion during a six-year period by the American Red Cross from data acquired from the American Association of Blood Banks.

"Transfusion Nursing." *American Journal of Nursing* 91 (June, 1991): 42-56. Describes trends and practices for the 1990's, including choosing blood components and equipment, performing autologous transfusion, preventing and managing transfusion reactions, and building a safe community blood supply.

BLOOD POISONING. *See* SEPTICEMIA.

BLOOD TESTING

PROCEDURE

ANATOMY OR SYSTEM AFFECTED: Blood, blood vessels, circulatory system, skin

SPECIALTIES AND RELATED FIELDS: Cytology, forensic medicine, hematology, pathology, public health, serology, toxicology

DEFINITION: The withdrawal of blood from an individual and its analysis for one of the many purposes, including blood typing and a search for acquired or genetic disease indicators.

KEY TERMS:

antibody: a protein synthesized in response to a specific antigen; antibodies physically combine with antigens as part of the immune process

antigen: a molecule which induces the production of antibodies

antiserum: the fluid portion of blood that contains specific antibodies

Rh factor: a specific antigen present on 85 percent of an individual's red blood cells; also called Rhesus factor

INDICATIONS AND PROCEDURES

Most blood tests require a substantial sample of blood. A sample of several milliliters or more is withdrawn from a vein using a syringe. The sample is transported to a diagnostic laboratory for the appropriate analysis.

Red blood cells are marked on their surface with the protein antigens designated A, B, AB (both A and B), or O (no antigen). Individuals possess antibodies, found in the liquid or serum portion of the blood, to the antigens that they themselves do not possess. In ABO typing, red blood

cells are isolated from the blood sample and mixed with antisera with a known antibody type. Cells marked with antigen A will clump when mixed with antibody A, cells with B antigen will clump when exposed to antibody B, AB antigens clump with either, and O clumps with neither. The type of positive clumping reaction determines blood type. Rh type is determined in the same manner, with Rh-positive blood exhibiting a clumping reaction with Rh antibodies. Histocompatibility leukocyte antigen (HLA) typing is performed similarly but uses white blood cells as the antigenic material. HLA typing is more complex and time consuming because more than forty different HLAs are known to exist.

Deoxyribonucleic acid (DNA) analysis requires isolating DNA from white blood cells and amplifying certain regions with a procedure called polymerase chain reaction (PCR). The amplified DNA is cut with enzymes and run through an electric field in a gel matrix, thus separating the pieces of DNA by size. Specific patterns are visually analyzed. When this technique is repeated across many different regions of a person's DNA, a pattern unique to that individual can be obtained. This information can be used to answer questions of paternity and relatedness or to help convict or exonerate suspects in murder and rape cases. A similar analysis is used to determine the presence of certain genetic diseases or the possibility of transmitting a genetic disease.

The use of blood tests to diagnose diseases covers a wide range, and the test is matched to the analysis requested. Abnormal levels of red blood cells can indicate anemia, while abnormal white cell counts may suggest a severe infection. Inappropriate enzyme levels could signal organ malfunction, and abnormal hormone levels indicate an endocrine disease. High levels of particular antibodies herald an infection with the corresponding antigenic agent.

USES AND COMPLICATIONS

Blood testing may be performed for a variety of reasons. If an individual has suffered a large loss of blood and/or requires surgery that may necessitate a blood transfusion, ABO and Rh factor blood typing is performed. Pregnant women need to know their own Rh status and that of their fetus in order to prevent gestational complications from Rh incompatibility. If an organ transplant is required, the HLAs present on all cells except red blood cells must be matched as closely as possible to prevent graft rejection. In the event of paternity determination or forensic analysis, the DNA sequences found in white blood cells can be analyzed for proper identification. Some genetic diseases in an affected individual, a fetus, or unaffected individuals who may transmit the genetic disease to their offspring can be detected with blood DNA analysis. Many types of disorders and diseases are diagnosed through a determination of the presence of abnormal levels of blood cell types, enzymes, hormones, and electrolytes (sodium, potassium, phosphate, magnesium, and calcium) or the presence of infectious agents in the blood, such as bacteria and viruses. Not all genetic diseases can be tested using DNA analysis. A partial list of those that can be detected includes hemophilia, Huntington's disease, cystic fibrosis, and sickle-cell anemia. Others, such as Tay-Sachs disease, can be detected with an enzyme test of the blood.

Should proper ABO typing not be performed and an individual be given an incompatible blood transfusion, the antibodies in the individual's blood would destroy the newly transfused cells, causing a life-threatening condition. Failure to diagnose and treat an Rh incompatible pregnancy could result in death of the fetus or a baby born with severe hemolytic disease of the newborn and jaundice because of the destruction of fetal blood cells by the mother's immune system.

In modern hospitals with standard precautions, there are only minor side effects to blood withdrawal with a syringe. Some pain from puncturing the vein wall may occur, as well as localized bruising. If the procedure is done under unsanitary conditions or if needles are used repeatedly, the risk of transmitting bacterial infections or viral infections such as hepatitis and acquired immunodeficiency syndrome (AIDS) increases dramatically.

PERSPECTIVE AND PROSPECTS

DNA analysis is rapidly providing new and better diagnostic tools for the identification of genetic disease and its carriers as well as for the prediction of an individual's tendency to develop certain cancers, such as of the breast and colon, and heart disease. Such predictive tests could save millions of lives through close monitoring and early treatment.

Such advances of technology, however, are not without consequences. Since genetic testing became routine in the 1980's, there has been great concern about the access of employers and insurance companies to such potentially damaging information. For many years, lack of regulation of DNA testing laboratories frequently resulted in incorrect or ambiguous test results. Movements toward regulation and licensing of these laboratories are alleviating these problems. —*Karen E. Kalumuck, Ph.D.*

See also Acquired immunodeficiency syndrome (AIDS); Anemia; Blood and blood components; Blood bank; Cholesterol; Circulation; Dialysis; DNA and RNA; Endocrine disorders; Forensic pathology; Genetic counseling; Genetic diseases; Genetics and inheritance; Grafts and grafting; Hematology; Hematology, pediatric; Hormones; Human immunodeficiency virus (HIV); Immune system; Laboratory tests; Pathology; Pregnancy and gestation; Rh factor; Screening; Serology; Transfusion.

FOR FURTHER INFORMATION:

Pierce, Benjamin A. *The Family Genetic Sourcebook.* New York: John Wiley & Sons, 1990.

Youngson, Robert M. "Blood Transfusion." In *The Surgery Book.* New York: St. Martin's Press, 1993.

BLOOD TRANSFUSION. *See* TRANSFUSION.

BONE CANCER
DISEASE/DISORDER

ANATOMY OR SYSTEM AFFECTED: Bones, musculoskeletal system

SPECIALTIES AND RELATED FIELDS: Immunology, oncology, orthopedics, radiology

DEFINITION: Cancer of the bone, which may have originated there or have spread from another site in the body.

KEY TERMS:

adjuvant therapy: the use of multiple treatments for cancer, such as chemotherapy following surgery to prevent metastasis

biopsy: the removal of tissue from a suspected cancer site, in order to identify abnormal cells under microscopic examination by a pathologist

bone scan: a diagnostic technique using a radioactive tracer which is strongly absorbed by a tumor, whose location then can be detected by radiation counters

computed tomography (CT) scanning: a method of displaying the outline of a tumor, utilizing a computer to combine information from multiple X-ray beams

magnetic resonance imaging (MRI): a diagnostic technique used to see the outline of an internal organ or a tumor without using X rays

medullary cavity: the interior of a bone, where new blood cells are formed by the bone marrow, surrounded by a hard outer cortex

metastasis: the spread of cancer cells from an original tumor site to other parts of the body

palliative treatment: the use of drugs or radiation to suppress a tumor and to provide relief from pain when a cure is not possible

sarcoma: a malignant tumor originating in bone or connective tissue

staging: a numerical classification system used by physicians to describe how far a cancerous growth has advanced

CAUSES AND SYMPTOMS

Out of about one million new cancers that are diagnosed annually in the United States, less than 1 percent are primary bone cancer. Most of these cases arise in children under the age of twenty. If diagnosis is made before the bone cancer has spread to the lungs or other sites in the body, prompt treatment by surgery, radiation, or chemotherapy can provide a good prognosis for recovery.

In older adults, most cases of so-called bone cancer actually are secondary tumors that have spread from other parts of the body, especially from the breast, prostate, thyroid, lung, or kidney. Such metastasized tumors consist of cells that are characteristic of their original, primary site. Secondary bone cancers are far more common than those which start in the bone.

The first symptom of bone cancer in children usually is a localized swelling followed by persistent, dull pain. It is easily mistaken for a sprain or a bruise that might come from a minor injury. Additional symptoms are fatigue, fever, loss of appetite, and other signs of general illness. Unfortunately, early symptoms may be ignored until the disease has already spread to other parts of the body. Before chemotherapy became available in the 1970's, the spread of bone cancer to the lungs occurred within two years for about 80 percent of patients.

A variety of diagnostic techniques are available to the physician if the examination of a patient arouses the suspicion of bone cancer. Blood tests, including a study of liver and kidney functions, have become increasingly useful because of improvements in analytical procedure. X-ray photography and computed tomography (CT) scanning will give pictorial evidence of any lesions or excess bony growth. Magnetic resonance imaging (MRI) provides the best visualization of tumors extending into soft tissue. Finally, the most important diagnostic procedure is biopsy. Usually, the bone is opened surgically and a sample of tissue is taken. Sometimes, a hollow needle inserted through the bone cortex can be used to withdraw a small sample. A pathologist who specializes in oncology examines the tissue under a microscope to confirm if cancer cells are present and to identify their type.

Magnetic resonance imaging as a diagnostic technique was developed in the 1980's, giving remarkable picture clarity for soft tissue. A strong magnetic field and radio waves are used to determine the concentration of hydrogen in a region of the body. Since tissue is mostly water (which contains hydrogen) and bone is dry, the image will show bright areas for tissue or soft organs against a dark background. Also, MRI shows contrast between normal tissue and a denser, tumorous mass.

Another diagnostic technique, the bone scan, is used to investigate whether a tumor has metastasized to other bones in the body. A small amount of radioactive tracer, usually technetium, is injected into the patient. It circulates in the bloodstream and gradually accumulates in the bone marrow. After several hours, radiation counters are used to scan the entire skeleton from head to foot. Regions of rapid cell growth, which may signal a tumorous mass, are indicated by a relatively high counting rate. If secondary tumors are detected by the bone scan, their shape and size can be investigated further using MRI.

Several kinds of bone cancer have been identified. One type is called osteosarcoma. It occurs most frequently during puberty, when a child's bones are growing rapidly. The tumor is likely to develop inside the long bones of the arms, in the legs near the knee, or in the pelvis. As its size increases and the surrounding bone material becomes soft, the bone may fracture because of internal pressure in the bone. Osteosarcomas also may grow on the exterior surface of bones, producing hard spikes that radiate outward. Another type of bone cancer is called Ewing's sarcoma. MRI and CT scans commonly exhibit a "moth-eaten" appearance where bone destruction has taken place. Both the inner (medullary) cavity and the outer cortex of the bone can be affected. Subsequently, a tumorous mass develops within the covering of tissue that surrounds the bone. This abnormal growth tends to form concentric layers, like the skin of an onion. The localized swelling expands in size, causing soreness and eventually impeding motion at the joints.

Bone cancer can take a variety of other forms. For example, a tumor may invade the bone from the outside and then penetrate into the medullary cavity. In order to make an accurate diagnosis and institute the best possible treatment for bone cancer, particularly for children, it is important for patients and their families to find an oncologist and supporting staff with specialized experience in this relatively rare condition. In general, the orthopedic surgeon who does the biopsy should be a specialist who is trained to do the ultimate bone surgery, so that any cancer cell contamination at the site of the biopsy will be completely removed.

TREATMENT AND THERAPY

In order to develop an appropriate treatment plan for a patient with bone cancer, all the relevant diagnostic information must be brought together. A medical team consisting of a radiologist, pathologist, radiation therapist, orthopedic surgeon, and medical oncologist will assess how far the cancer has advanced. This is called staging, that is, classifying its stage of growth.

Three designations commonly are used to characterize a cancer: G for its grade (based on the microscopic tissue analysis), T for tumor size and penetration, and M for evidence of metastasis. For example, (G1) (T2) (M0) would describe a low grade tumor (G1) that has broken out of its bone compartment (T2) but has not metastasized (M0) to the lungs or elsewhere.

Before 1970, treatment of a cancerous bone normally meant amputation. The prognosis for recovery was less than 20 percent, however, because microscopic, invisible metastases to the lungs and other organs usually were already present. The experimental search for drugs that can fight cancer cells started in the 1930's. Dr. Charles B. Huggins discovered that the female sex hormone estrogen could halt the growth of prostate cancer in men. He received the Nobel Prize in Medicine in 1966 for his work. Since that pioneering success, several hundred thousand drugs have been tested, with less than a hundred showing any substantial benefit. The anticancer drugs also can have severe side effects on healthy cells. Fortunately, a rapidly growing tumor has a higher rate of metabolism, so drugs will kill the cancer cells at a lower dose and spare most normal cells.

An effective method of treating bone cancer in children is to use chemotherapy or radiation even before surgery, in order to shrink the size of a tumor. Instead of complete amputation, the surgeon may need to remove only part of a bone, thus saving the limb. Even when a bone joint must be amputated, it may still be possible to salvage the limb by inserting an artificial joint or one from an organ donor.

In older adults, cancer of the bone almost invariably is caused by metastasis from another location in the body. The tumor in the bone may be very painful. Radiation to the affected area can provide palliative treatment, while more aggressive action is taken against the primary cancer site.

A wide range of medications is available to help control pain and to counteract the disagreeable side effects of radiation or chemotherapy. Special attention is given to the diet of cancer patients to prevent weight loss and to maintain body strength. Loss of appetite and digestion problems are common symptoms during therapy. Strong painkilling drugs such as codeine and morphine sometimes are necessary. The dose should be limited, however, so that the patient's ability to interact socially is not completely lost.

Vigorous research to find more effective therapies for cancer is widely supported. The goal is to find procedures that are less mutilating, less expensive, and less painful for the patient. Promising new drugs must be tested to determine how large a dose is needed and how serious the side effects are. Therefore, patients may be asked to become volunteers in clinical trial of an experimental treatment. Although people have a justified sense of reluctance to become "guinea pigs" in an untested therapy, clinical trials with human subjects have been essential in the development of successful medical procedures. Firm guidelines have been established for testing new therapies, such as the requirement to obtain the informed consent of patients and their families. In addition, doctors in the United States are responsible to a medical oversight committee and are obligated to submit their results for professional review. Cancer treatment can make progress through willing participation by patients in the carefully planned clinical trials.

PERSPECTIVE AND PROSPECTS

Bone cancer first came to the attention of the American public in the 1920's through a notorious case of industrial poisoning. A manufacturing company in New Jersey was utilizing radioactive radium to make watch dials that would glow in the dark. The women workers who were hired to apply the luminous paint would twirl the paint brushes between their lips to make a fine tip. The ingested radium, being chemically similar to calcium, became concentrated in bones, especially of the jaw and neck. Eventually, more than forty workers died of bone cancer, including the company's chief chemist.

After this incident, it became clear that radiation has a particularly damaging effect on bone marrow. In fact, any rapidly dividing cells in the body are especially radiosensitive. This would include hair, skin, and the reproductive system. It is unfortunate that it took until the 1950's before X-ray fluoroscopes were removed from shoe stores. Parents were fascinated to see the bones of their child's foot inside a new shoe without realizing that the radiation was harmful.

Until 1970, the outlook for a child who developed bone cancer was very poor. In spite of amputation of the affected limb, 80 percent of the young patients died within two years. In 1972, Norman Jaffe and Emil Frei in Boston made a major breakthrough in therapy by giving their patients large doses of a drug called methotrexate after limb surgery. It was a new approach in chemotherapy to stop the cancer from spreading even though no metastasis was visible yet. The experimental drug was so powerful that other antidote drugs were given to control side effects. The first trial with seventeen children was very successful, with all of them still surviving after twenty-one months.

Yet an article written in 1994 by Tim Beardsley summarizing the status of cancer in the United States came to a rather pessimistic conclusion. The cancer rate was higher and the likelihood of cure had not improved for most types of adult cancer since the "war on cancer" was initiated by President Richard M. Nixon in 1971. The cumulative effects of smoking, poor diet, and continuing exposure to harmful chemicals may help to explain this lack of progress. The good news was that the death rate from childhood cancer fell by almost half in that period. Early diagnosis and improved therapy have helped greatly. The family of a child with cancer can now look forward with substantial hope for a cure without recurrence. —*Hans G. Graetzer, Ph.D.*

See also Bone disorders; Bones and the skeleton; Cancer; Chemotherapy; Fracture and dislocation; Fracture repair; Hip fracture repair; Malignancy and metastasis; Nuclear radiology; Oncology; Orthopedic surgery; Orthopedics; Orthopedics, pediatric; Radiation therapy; Sarcoma; Tumors.

FOR FURTHER INFORMATION:

Beardsley, Tim. "A War Not Won: Trends in Cancer Epidemiology." *Scientific American* 270, no. 1 (January, 1994): 130-138. A summary of factual data about the prevalence of cancer in the United States. In spite of $25 billion spent by the National Cancer Institute, the overall death rate from cancer continues to increase. Critics suggest redirecting funds from expensive cures to prevention.

Brody, Jane E., and Arthur I. Holleb. *You Can Fight Cancer and Win*. New York: Quadrangle-New York Times, 1977. A hopeful and informative book about cancer for the general reader. Symptoms, treatment, possible causes, prevention, and family adjustment to cancer are discussed. Highly recommended.

Cady, Blake, ed. *Cancer Manual*. 7th ed. Boston: American Cancer Society, 1986. A collection of forty essays on various aspects of cancer management, written for health care professionals. The article that discusses sarcomas of the bone requires some knowledge of medical terminology. One interesting chapter deals with worthless cures.

Dollinger, Malin, Ernest H. Rosenbaum, and Greg Cable et al. *Everyone's Guide to Cancer Therapy.* Rev. 2d ed. Kansas City, Mo.: Andrews and McMeel, 1994. An excellent source of medical information about cancer, written for the general public. Various cancer sites in the body are described, and one essay focuses on sarcomas of the bone. A helpful glossary of medical terminology is provided.

Editors of Time-Life Books. *Fighting Cancer.* Alexandria, Va.: Time-Life Books, 1981. A brief overview of cancer diagnosis and therapy, containing many photographs and color diagrams. How abnormal cancer cells differ from healthy cells can be explained in pictures much more easily than in words. Informative and readable.

Holleb, Arthur I., ed. *The American Cancer Society Cancer Book: Prevention, Detection, Diagnosis, Treatment, Rehabilitation, Cure.* Garden City, N.Y.: Doubleday, 1986. An authoritative reference book on all aspects of cancer, written by forty leading specialists and carefully edited to avoid technical jargon. Contains chapters on chemotherapy, radiation, pain management, and childhood cancer. Clearly written and highly recommended.

Morra, Marion, and Eve Potts. *Choices: Realistic Alternatives in Cancer Treatment.* New York: Avon Books, 1987. A comprehensive reference book written for cancer patients and their families. Uses a question-and-answer format, with explanations given in nontechnical language. Offers good information at an introductory level.

Murphy, G., L. Morris, and D. Lange. *Informed Decisions: The Complete Book of Cancer Diagnosis, Treatment, and Recovery.* New York: Viking Press, 1997. This text from the American Cancer Society is intended for the layperson. It is exemplary in its discussion of cancer.

BONE DISORDERS
DISEASE/DISORDER

ANATOMY OR SYSTEM AFFECTED: Back, bones, legs, musculoskeletal system

SPECIALTIES AND RELATED FIELDS: Geriatrics and gerontology, oncology, orthopedics, rheumatology

DEFINITION: The various traumatic events that can occur to the bones and the tissues surrounding them, such as fractures, dislocations, degenerative processes, infections, and cancer.

KEY TERMS:
acute: referring to the sudden onset of a disease process

cartilage: connective tissue between bones that forms a pad or cushion to absorb weight and shock

chronic: referring to a lingering disease process

pathogen: any disease-causing microorganism

CAUSES AND SYMPTOMS

Bones are usually studied in combination with their surrounding structures because many of the disorders to which bones can be subjected also involve muscular, cartilaginous,

and other tissues to which they are connected. Hence, a common term for this medical category is "musculoskeletal and connective tissue disorders."

There are 206 bones in the human body that serve three functions. Some form protective housing for body organs and structures; these include the skull, which encloses the brain, and the rib cage, which encloses the heart and lungs. Some support the body's posture and weight, including the spine and the bones of the hip and legs. The third function is motion: Most of the bones in the body are involved in movement. These bones include those of the hands, wrists, arms, hips, legs, ankles, and feet.

Bone consists of three sections: an outer layer called the periosteum; the hard bony tissue itself, consisting of mineral compounds that form rigid skeletal structures; and the interior, a spongy mass of cancellous (chambered) tissue, where blood marrow is manufactured and some fat cells are stored. Bone is living tissue. It is a depository for calcium, phosphate, and other minerals that are vital to many body processes. Calcium and phosphate in particular are constantly being deposited in and withdrawn from bone tissue to be used throughout the body.

Bones can be attacked in many ways: They can be broken or dislocated; the processes by which they form, grow, and maintain themselves can be compromised; they can be attacked by pathogens; they can be subject to a series of degenerative diseases that impede function and even destroy bone tissue; and they can become cancerous.

Dislocations take place when the bones of a joint are forced out of alignment. They may occur in the elbows of young children whose arms are forcibly pulled. Fractures are more common. They arise from sports activities, accidents, falls, or hundreds of possible causes, including various disease conditions.

Osteoporosis and other diseases can destroy bone structure to the point where fractures occur with minimal stress. This condition is common in elderly women. The supply of calcium within the bones is gradually drained, leaving the bones porous and brittle. Hip fractures occur often in these people. Also, compression fractures occur in the vertebrae (the bones of the spine), causing the spine to bend forward. A hump develops, and the patient may not be able to raise his or her head.

Osteomalacia is similar to osteoporosis. Called rickets in children, this disease is caused by a deficiency in vitamin D, which impairs the absorption of calcium by the bone. In this condition, bones become soft and pliable. In children, leg bones do not develop correctly and may become bowed. The chest and stomach may protrude.

Bone infection is called osteomyelitis; it occurs most often in children. Infection can be introduced to the bone by fracture or other exposure, or it can be carried to the bone in the blood.

By far the most prevalent long-term bone disorders are

those in the general class of diseases called arthritis. Osteoarthritis, a common form, is sometimes called "wear-and-tear arthritis" because it usually surfaces in older people after years of work have constantly challenged certain joints. It occurs often in contact sports such as football, where its progression can be accelerated by years of rough-and-tumble activity. Joints are cushioned by pads of cartilage. Eventually, this cartilage can wear down and become rough. It cannot protect the bones of the joint, and little nodes form at the ends of the bones. Bones of the neck and back are often affected, as are the hips and knees.

Osteoarthritis is painful and debilitating, but it is rarely crippling. More painful and far more serious is rheumatoid arthritis, a progressive disease. It often starts with inflammation in the joints of the hands or feet and is usually bilateral, for example affecting both hands, both feet, or both knees. While rheumatoid arthritis may start with relatively mild inflammation, it can progress to severe deformity and even total destruction of the joint. Fingers and toes can become grossly twisted; the joint can become completely fused and immobile.

There are other relatively common forms of arthritis. People with the skin condition psoriasis can develop psoriatic arthritis. Reiter's syndrome is a form of arthritis that can be transmitted through sexual contact. Ankylosing spondylitis is a form of arthritis that can affect any of the joints in the torso, such as the shoulders and hips, but is most often found in the neck and spine. Patients with inflammatory bowel disease (IBD) may also develop a concomitant arthritis in the joints of the hands or feet.

The bone condition called gout can affect many joints, but it appears most often in the big toe. The body produces a substance called uric acid. If, for any reason, too much is produced, or if it is not properly eliminated, uric acid crystals can form around joints and trigger inflammation. Gout is extremely painful, and an attack may last for weeks.

The spine is subject to a wide range of disorders. One of the most common is the prolapsed (slipped) disk. The individual vertebrae of the spine are separated and cushioned by pads of cartilage called disks. For various reasons, a disk can bulge out and impinge on the nerves of the spinal column. The result can be severe pain, numbness, and loss of movement. In some individuals, the spine fails to grow correctly or becomes misaligned, or curved. This condition is called scoliosis. The curvature of the spine can cause the ribs on one side of the body to separate as those on the other side are pushed together. Over time, this separation can cause severe heart and lung problems.

Many cases of joint pain are attributable to inflammation of the tissues surrounding the bony structures. An example is bursitis, in which the bursa, a saclike membrane enclosing many joints, becomes inflamed. Repetitive activities, such as throwing a baseball, hitting a tennis ball, or scrubbing the floor on one's knees, can irritate the membrane and cause inflammation.

Bone cancers or tumors can be benign or malignant. Cancer rarely begins in the bone; it usually spreads there from a tumorous site elsewhere in the body. Of the cancers that arise directly within bone tissue, the most common are multiple myeloma and osteosarcoma.

TREATMENT AND THERAPY

In treating a fractured bone, the most important thing is to realign the segments and keep them immobile until they can fuse. Most often, the physician will X-ray the fracture, set the bones correctly, and immobilize the limb in a cast. If injury to the spinal column is suspected, the physician may also order computed tomography (CT) scanning. Surgery is sometimes required in order to set the bones, and the surgeon may join the bone segments together with pins, plates, or screws. In some cases, it is possible to cement bone fragments together with a special glue. Broken arms, legs, fingers, and toes can usually be easily immobilized with appropriate casts or splints. In cases of accidents, falls, or other trauma, if there is any suspicion of injury to the spinal column, it is critical not to move the patient. Movement can worsen the injury and even cause permanent paralysis.

Dislocations, like fractures, should be X-rayed. If the spinal column appears to be involved, CT scanning may be required. The misaligned bones are put back in their proper positions, and the joint is immobilized, often with a splint.

Osteoporosis requires both preventive and therapeutic care. If the physician recognizes that an individual, usually a postmenopausal woman, is at high risk for osteoporosis, supplementary calcium will be prescribed and, in some patients, estrogen replacement therapy. When osteoporosis has begun, supplementary calcium, vitamin D, and hormone therapy may check the progress of the disease.

A patient may suffer from acute back pain because of crushed vertebrae in the spine. Pain relievers such as aspirin may be required, and the patient may need orthopedic support. Gentle exercise is recommended to strengthen back muscles.

In osteomalacia, vitamin D, phosphorus, and calcium supplements are the mainstays of therapy. In osteomyelitis, antibiotics will usually eradicate the infection, but in some cases, surgery is required in order to remove infected tissue. In other cases, amputation is the only option.

The first line of therapy for osteoarthritis and rheumatoid arthritis is the relief of pain and inflammation. The physician may recommend rest and immobilization of the joint; heating pads and hot baths may give some relief. Exercise can maintain motility in the joints and help the patient avoid stiffness. Most patients are given over-the-counter pain relievers such as aspirin, ibuprofen, or acetaminophen. In a large number of patients, however, these drugs are either not adequate to manage the pain or, as in the case of aspirin, ibuprofen, and others, may be irritating to the gastrointestinal tract. Gastrointestinal disturbances are also common with the drugs proscribed for arthritis. Gastric and duodenal ulcers are often reported and are sometimes so severe that the patient requires surgery. In a small but significant number of patients who develop such ulcers, the outcome is fatal.

Because rheumatoid arthritis is a crippling disease that worsens over the years, the physician has an additional goal: to prevent the progress of the disease, avoiding bone deterioration and degeneration. In these patients, a group of drugs called disease-modifying antirheumatic drugs (DMARDs) may be used in conjunction with pain relievers. Corticosteroids are also used to alleviate acute episodes of pain and inflammation. They can be very effective, but they cannot be used over the long term and may have severe side effects.

Surgery is often required for arthritis patients. Synovectomy is a procedure in which part or all of the synovial membrane that surrounds the diseased joint is removed. It gives temporary relief in inflammation and may help preserve joint function. When a joint has deteriorated severely, the physician may recommend joint replacement therapy. In this procedure, the degenerated bone and joint structures are surgically removed and replaced with an orthopedic device of metal and/or plastic. This procedure is most effective in hip replacement, although it is also used in the knee.

Relief of pain is the main goal of therapy in other arthritic conditions such as psoriatic arthritis and Reiter's syndrome. In ankylosing spondylitis, exercise is also an important facet of treatment, to help avoid stiffening of the spine.

Gout has a tendency to recur. Therefore there are medications for acute episodes, such as pain relievers, and others to control levels of uric acid and prevent attacks.

Benign bone tumors sometimes require surgery. Malignant tumors can be treated surgically and may also require radiation and chemotherapy.

PERSPECTIVE AND PROSPECTS

Radical new therapies for bone disorders are evolving, with exciting possibilities: bone regeneration, bone cements, and glues to knit fractures and replace bone destroyed by disease.

Osteoarthritis, rheumatoid arthritis, and other forms of arthritis continue to afflict vast populations around the world. Current medical treatment is significantly flawed by the incidence of side effects, especially gastrointestinal effects, from the medications used. The search for safer medications is ongoing, as is the search for treatment modalities that will halt the degenerative processes of rheumatoid arthritis.

Orthopedic implants are now quite successful in the hip, sometimes successful in the knee, but otherwise not universally useful in elbows, fingers, toes, and other joints that can be destroyed by disease. This is an area that is being addressed.

Operating techniques and instrumentation improve constantly. Many procedures are now done with the aid of arthroscopic instruments. Rather than an extensive incision to reveal the joint and surrounding tissues, the surgeon works through a tiny hole, through which he or she can inspect the inflamed joint and even perform minor surgery.

Operations on prolapsed spinal disks once entailed long incisions and laborious, careful removal of disk tissue. Fusion of the involved vertebrae was often necessary, limiting spinal movement. Healing time could be extensive. Today, simpler, less painful procedures may be as successful and far less traumatic. In one procedure, an enzyme is injected into the prolapsed disk, causing it to shrink and reducing pressure on nearby nerves. In another procedure, disk material is removed with a needle inserted through the skin into the disk.

Overall, progress in the treatment of bone disorders has been significant: Many people who would have lived with deformities and disability are being helped with modern medical and surgical techniques, medications, and instrumentation.
—*C. Richard Falcon*

See also Amputation; Arthritis; Bone cancer; Bone grafting; Bone marrow transplantation; Bones and the skeleton; Cerebral palsy; Chiropractic; Feet; Foot disorders; Fracture and dislocation; Fracture repair; Hammertoe correction; Head and neck disorders; Heel spur removal; Hip fracture repair; Jaw wiring; Kneecap removal; Lower extremities; Orthopedic surgery; Orthopedics; Orthopedics, pediatric; Osgood-Schlatter disease; Osteoporosis; Paget's disease; Rheumatology; Rickets; Sarcoma; Scoliosis; Slipped disk; Spina bifida; Spinal disorders; Spine, vertebrae, and disks; Upper extremities.

FOR FURTHER INFORMATION:

Cooper, Kenneth H. *Preventing Osteoporosis*. New York: Bantam Books, 1989. As the title suggests, Cooper's main interest is to advise women on how to avoid developing the brittle bones of osteoporosis. His text is clear, and the recommendations reflect contemporary practice.

Larson, David E., ed. *Mayo Clinic Family Health Book*. 2d ed. New York: William Morrow, 1996. Bones, muscles, and connective tissues are discussed, with disease conditions, symptoms, treatment, and outlook clearly explained. The text and illustrations are complete and easy to understand.

Schommer, Nancy. *Stopping Scoliosis*. Garden City, N.Y.: Avery Publishing Group, 1991. Schommer covers the condition of scoliosis with thoroughness and clarity.

Yates, George, and Michael B. Shermer. *Meeting the Challenge of Arthritis*. Los Angeles: Lowell House, 1990. A good treatment of the arthritic diseases, covering their causes and treatment. Concentrates on helping patients to help themselves.

BONE FRACTURES. *See* **FRACTURE AND DISLOCATION.**

BONE GRAFTING
PROCEDURE
ANATOMY OR SYSTEM AFFECTED: Bones, immune system, musculoskeletal system
SPECIALTIES AND RELATED FIELDS: Hematology, immunology, orthopedics
DEFINITION: The transplantation of a section of bone from one part of the body to another, or from one individual to another.

INDICATIONS AND PROCEDURES
Ideally, the grafting procedure involves the transfer of bone tissue from one site to another on the same individual, which is termed an autogenous graft. This method eliminates the chance of rejection, allowing the transplantation of entire functional units of tissue: arteries, veins, and even nerves, as when a toe is used to replace a finger or thumb (toe-digital transfer). Autogenous rib or fibula grafts may be utilized for the reconstruction of the face or extremities.

Often, bone grafts are used during situations in which a bone fracture is not healing properly. A fracture that fails to heal in the usual time is considered to be a delayed union. Cancellous material from the bone (the spongy inner material), usually obtained from the iliac crest of the pelvis or from the ends of the long bones, is placed around the site. The fracture must then be immobilized for several months, allowing the grafted material to infiltrate and repair the fracture.

USES AND COMPLICATIONS
The grafting of bone tissue is carried out to correct a bone defect, to provide support tissue in the case of a severe fracture, or to encourage the growth of new bone. The source of the skeletal defect may be congenital malformation, disease, or trauma. For example, reconstruction may be necessary following cancer surgery, particularly for the jaw or bones elsewhere in the face.

If the autogenous bone supply is inadequate to fill the need, allogeneic bone grafts, the transplantation of bone from an individual other than an identical twin, may be necessary. Such foreign tissue is more likely to undergo rejection, reducing the chance of a successful procedure; the more closely the tissues of the two persons are matched, the less likely rejection will be a problem.

If the graft is able to vascularize quickly and to synthesize new tissue, the procedure is likely to be successful. The graft itself may provide structural support, or it may gradually be replaced by new bone at that site, completing the healing process. —*Richard Adler, Ph.D.*

See also Amputation; Bone cancer; Bone disorders; Bones and the skeleton; Fracture and dislocation; Fracture repair; Grafts and grafting; Lower extremities; Oncology; Orthopedic surgery; Orthopedics; Transplantation; Upper extremities.

BONE MARROW TRANSPLANTATION
PROCEDURE
ANATOMY OR SYSTEM AFFECTED: Back, blood, bones, immune system, musculoskeletal system
SPECIALTIES AND RELATED FIELDS: General surgery, genetics, hematology, immunology, oncology
DEFINITION: The replacement of diseased or inadequate bone marrow with healthy marrow.
KEY TERMS:
bone marrow: the material in the center of bones which produces red blood cells (which carry oxygen), platelets (which stop bleeding), and white blood cells (which are the functional units of the immune system)
stem cell: a master cell from which other blood cells develop; these cells are primarily located in the bone marrow

INDICATIONS AND PROCEDURES
Bone marrow transplantation is used when the immune and blood-forming systems of the body are malfunctioning or have been severely damaged. Without adequate white blood cells, a person will soon die from infection. Transplantation is an attempt to cure or arrest diseases such as leukemia, cancer, and sickle-cell anemia and conditions such as brain tumors and hereditary diseases. Bone marrow transplantation is used when all other methods of treatment have failed. The procedure is usually performed on patients who are younger than fifty years old, with the greatest success rates found in children.

Before the procedure can be performed, a suitable donor must be found. The donor can be the patient (autologous transplantation) or someone else (allogeneic transplantation). Once the donor is identified, the bone marrow is harvested. This procedure is usually done under general anesthesia and takes one to two hours. A needle is inserted in the hip, and marrow is sucked out from different locations in the pelvic bone. Approximately 1 to 3 pints of marrow are taken. The donor usually stays overnight in the hospital and may be sore for one or two weeks following the operation.

The marrow, which contains the stem cells necessary to reestablish the blood-producing and immune systems of the patient, is processed and stored until the patient is prepared for the transplantation. During the hospital stay, the patient is kept in a sterile room to prevent infection. If the surgery is being performed on a cancer patient, the patient receives extensive chemotherapy and/or radiation before the donor marrow is transplanted; this action destroys any cancer cells in the patient, as well as his or her immune system.

The patient then receives the bone marrow transplantation in a manner similar to a blood transfusion: The donor cells are introduced through the veins and into the bloodstream. Until the transplanted cells begin to function (usually two to four weeks), the patient receives blood and platelet transfusions, as well as antibiotics to fight infection. The patient is usually discharged from the hospital in a month but must take antibiotics and antiviral medications for six months to two years after the transplantation because the recovery of the immune system is slow.

USES AND COMPLICATIONS

Bone marrow transplantation is a risky procedure with a success rate that ranges from 10 to 90 percent. One of the greatest obstacles is finding a suitable donor. The best possible match is between siblings, but even here the probability of a correct match is only 25 percent. Unrelated donor and patient matches made with marrow from donor banks increase the risk of a mismatch.

Finding a suitable donor is imperative because of the risk of graft-versus-host disease (GVHD). GVHD occurs when the donor cells recognize the host's body as foreign and react against it. This reaction may occur within a hundred or more days after the transplant and can vary in severity from a mild rash to the fatal destruction of tissue and organs. For correctly matched donors and recipients, the risk of life-threatening GVHD is 10 to 20 percent. For mismatched donors and recipients, the risk rises to 80 percent. In some cases, especially with leukemia and cancerous blood diseases, patients who suffer mild GVHD have an improved chance of survival because part of GVHD is a graft-versus-leukemia (GVL) effect. In these cases, the transplanted immune system acts against any remaining leukemia cells.

When the patient does not have a condition that damages the bone marrow, transplantation can be performed with his or her own marrow. After marrow has been collected from the patient, radiation and/or chemotherapy can be used to destroy the remaining immune system. Autologous transplantation eliminates the need to find a compatible donor and the risk of GVHD. This method can be used for treating solid tumors and has shown promise in curing brain tumors that were once considered fatal, with a success rate of 20 percent.

PERSPECTIVE AND PROSPECTS

Research on bone marrow transplantation began in the early 1950's, with the first successful transplantations performed on children in 1968. By the 1990's, more than five thousand bone marrow transplantations were being performed worldwide every year. The development of drugs that work to suppress the immune system have increased the chances for survival for these patients.

Several areas of research promise even better results in the future. A growing understanding of disease at the genetic level offers the possibility of separating unhealthy bone marrow cells from healthy ones. Methods of growing cells outside the body for use in transplantation are being developed. Progress has also been made in increasing the donor pool. National and international programs actively seek potential donors. Healthy people may begin storing their own bone marrow for a possible need in the future.

Perhaps one of the most promising potential sources of donor bone marrow is umbilical cord blood, which is rich in stem cells. Transplants using umbilical cord blood were first used in 1989 and have proven very successful. If established, umbilical cord blood banks could greatly increase the quantity of available donor marrow.

—*Virginia L. Salmon*

See also Blood and blood components; Blood banks; Bones and the skeleton; Cancer; Chemotherapy; Immune system; Immunology; Immunopathology; Leukemia; Oncology; Radiation therapy; Sickle-cell anemia; Transfusion; Transplantation.

FOR FURTHER INFORMATION:

Bone Marrow Transplantation and Peripheral Blood Stem Cell Transplantation. Rev. ed. Bethesda, Md.: U.S. Department of Health and Human Services, Public Health

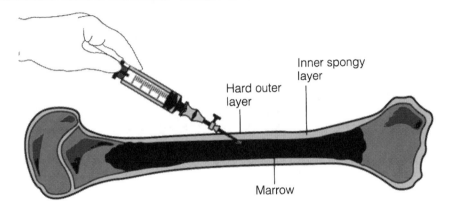

Bone marrow transplantation is used to treat several types of cancer. Marrow can be extracted from a donor or from the patient and reintroduced at a later time, usually after chemotherapy or radiation therapy.

Service, National Institutes of Health, 1994. A research report from the NIH that includes bibliographic references.

Golde, David W. "The Stem Cell." *Scientific American* 265 (December, 1991): 86-93. A good overview of stem cells and their use in treating blood and immune system diseases.

Kline, Ronald. "New Marrow for Old." *Technology Review* 96, no. 8 (November/December, 1993): 43-49. A well-written article with an overview of the procedures involved in bone marrow transplantation, as well as future challenges and ethical considerations.

Marget, Madeline. *Life's Blood.* New York: Simon & Schuster, 1992. Presents basic information on bone marrow transplantation, supplemented by interviews with doctors and the stories of patients and their families.

Swerdlow, Joel L. "A New Kind of Kinship." *National Geographic* 180, no. 3 (September, 1991): 64-92. This article addresses advances in transplantation and research, as well as the need for organ and tissue donors.

BONES AND THE SKELETON

ANATOMY

ANATOMY OR SYSTEM AFFECTED: Back, feet, hips, legs, musculoskeletal system

SPECIALTIES AND RELATED FIELDS: Exercise physiology, orthodontics, orthopedics, osteopathic medicine, podiatry, sports medicine

DEFINITION: Bones are hard tissues that form the skeleton, the structure underlying the softer tissues of the body; they provide support while allowing flexibility.

KEY TERMS:

calcitonin: a hormone made and released by the thyroid gland that lowers the level of calcium in the blood by stimulating the formation of bone

collagen: a protein found in bone and other connective tissues; collagen fibers are well suited for support and protection because they are sturdy, flexible, and resist stretch

hormones: molecules made in the body and released into the blood that act as chemical messengers for the regulation of specific body functions

matrix: in bone, the matrix is a solid nonliving material that is a composite of protein fibers and mineral crystals

osteoblast: a bone cell that can produce and form bone matrix; osteoblasts are responsible for new bone formation

osteoclast: a large bone cell that can destroy bone matrix by dissolving the mineral crystals

osteocyte: the primary living cell of mature bone tissue

tissue: a collection of similar cells that perform a specific function

STRUCTURE AND FUNCTIONS

Bones are active throughout life: The 206 bones of the skeleton establish the size and proportions of the body and interact with all other organ systems. Disorders of the skeleton can have profound effects on the other organ systems and serious health consequences for the organism.

Bone, or osseous tissue, contains specialized cells and a solid, stony matrix. The unique hardened quality of the matrix results from layers of calcium salt crystals such as calcium phosphate, which is responsible for about two-thirds of a bone's weight, and calcium carbonate. The living cells found in bone account for less than 2 percent of the total bone mass.

Despite the great strength of the calcium salts, their inflexible nature means that they can fracture when exposed to sufficiently great bending or twisting forces, or to sharp impacts. Because the calcium crystals exist as minute plates positioned on a framework of collagen protein fibers, the resulting composite structure does lend a certain degree of flexibility to the bone matrix.

Based on the internal organization of its matrix, bone is classified as either compact (dense) bone or cancellous (spongy) bone. Compact bone is internally more solid, while cancellous bone is made from bony filaments (trabeculae) whose branching interconnections form a three-dimensional network. The cavities of the cancellous bone network are filled usually by bone marrow, the primary location for blood cell formation in adults.

Both types of bone contain bone cells (osteocytes) living in small chambers called lacunae, found periodically between the plates of the matrix. Microscopic channels (canaliculi) connect neighboring lacunae and permit the exchange of nutrients and wastes between osteocytes and accessible blood vessels. Osteocytes provide the collagen fibers and the conditions for proper maintenance of the mineral crystals of the matrix.

A typical skeletal bone has a central marrow cavity that is bordered by cancellous bone. This is enclosed by compact bone, and the outer surface is covered by periosteum. Periosteum consists of a fibrous outer layer and a cellular inner layer. The periosteum plays an important part in the growth and repair of bone, and it is the attachment site for muscles. Collagen protein fibers from the periosteum interconnect with the collagen fibers of the bone.

The marrow cavity inside the bone is lined by endosteum. Endosteum is an incomplete layer covering the trabeculae of cancellous bone and contains a variety of different types of cells. The endosteum also plays important roles during bone growth and repair.

The bone matrix is not an unchanging, permanent structure. During the life of a person, the bone matrix is being constantly dissolved while new matrix is synthesized and deposited. Approximately 18 percent of the protein and mineral constituents of bone are replaced each year. Such bone remodeling can result in altered bone shape or internal rearrangement of the trabeculae. It may also result in a change in the total amount of minerals stored in the skeleton. These processes of bone demineralization (osteolysis) and new bone production (osteogenesis) are precisely regulated in the healthy individual.

The type of bone cell responsible for dissolving the mineralized matrix is called an osteoclast. The cells that produce the materials that later become the bony matrix are called osteoblasts. The activities of these cells are influenced by several hormones as well as by the physical stress forces to which a bone may be exposed, such as when a particular muscle becomes stronger as the result of weight training and pulls more strongly on the bones to which it is attached. Increased stress forces on a bone result in that bone becoming thicker and stronger, thereby allowing the bone to withstand better the stresses and reducing the risks of bone fracture. When bones are not subjected to ordinary stresses, such as in persons confined to bed or in astronauts living in microgravity conditions during space flight, there is a corresponding loss of bone mass, with the unstressed bones becoming thinner and more brittle. After several weeks in an unstressed state, a bone can lose nearly a third of its mass. Following the resumption of normal loading stresses, the bone can regain its mass just as quickly.

The skeleton has five major functions: support for the body; protection of the soft tissues and organs; leverage to change the direction and size of the muscular forces; blood cell production, which occurs within the red marrow residing in the marrow cavities of many bones; and storage of both minerals (to maintain the body's important reserves of calcium and phosphate) and fats (in yellow marrow to serve as an important energy reserve for the body).

The Major Bones of the Human Skeleton

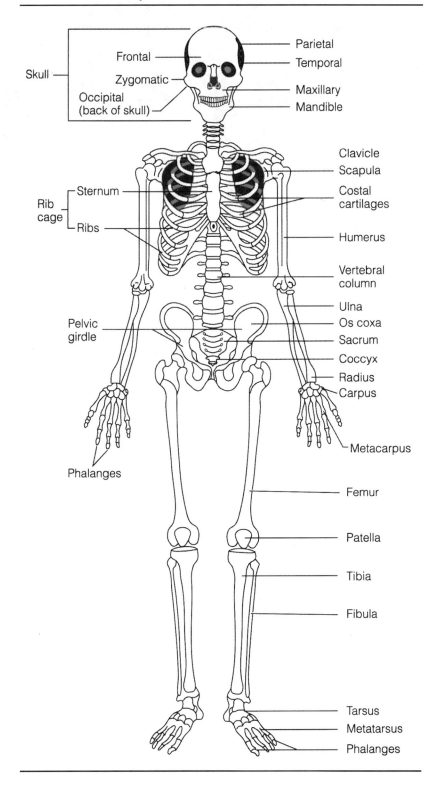

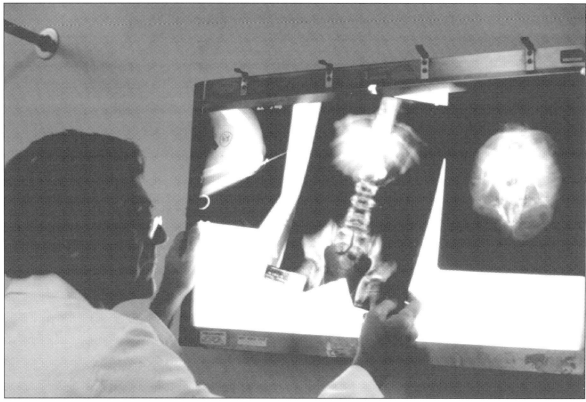

The use of X rays is one of the best ways to evaluate the health and structure of the skeleton. (Tom and Dee Ann McCarthy/Rainbow)

The human skeleton contains 206 bones. These are distributed between two subdivisions of the skeleton: the axial skeleton and the appendicular skeleton. The axial skeleton contains 80 bones distributed among the skull (29 bones), the chest, or thoracic, cage (25 bones), and the spinal (vertebral) column (26 bones). The remaining 126 bones are found in the appendicular skeleton's components: 4 bones in the shoulder (pectoral) girdles, 60 bones in the arms (including the 54 bones located in both of the hands and wrists), 2 bones in the hip (pelvic) girdle, and 60 bones in the legs (including the 52 bones found in the ankles and feet).

Skeletal bones are classified according to their shape. Long bones occur in the upper arm, the forearm, the thigh, the lower leg, the palm, the fingers, the sole of the foot, and the toes. Short bones are cuboid in shape and are found in the wrist and the ankle. Flat bones form the top of the skull, the shoulder blade, the breastbone, and the ribs. Sesamoid bones are typically small, round, and flat. They are found near some joints, such as the kneecap on the front of the knee joint. Irregular bones have shapes that are difficult to describe because of their complexity. Examples of irregular bones are found in the spinal column and the skull.

Learning to name the bones solely by their appearance is made somewhat easier by the fact that each one has a definitive form and distinctive surface features. The places where blood vessels and nerves enter into a bone, or lie along its surface, are commonly discernible as indentations, grooves, or holes. The locations where muscles are connected to bones by tendons, or where a bone is tethered to another bone by ligaments, are often clearly visible as elevations, projections, or ridges of bony matrix, or as roughened areas on the surface of the bone. Finally, the areas of the bone that are involved in forming joints (articulations) with other bones have characteristic shapes that impart particular properties to the joint. Various specialized terms are used to name these features.

Articulations are found wherever one bone meets another. The amount of motion permitted between the bones forming an articulation ranges from none (for example, between the skull bones) to considerable (as at the shoulder joint). The anatomy of the joint determines its functional capability, and the parts of the bones that form the joint have distinctive structural features.

DISORDERS AND DISEASES

Among the disorders of the skeleton, a number of them occur during the growth and development of the bones. The problems usually result in abnormal (most often decreased) stature or abnormal shape of the bones. The aberrations may alter the entire skeleton or be restricted to a portion of it. The basis of the pathology is to be found in a disruption of the normal, orderly sequence of events that take place during the growth and remodeling of the bones.

Osteopetrosis belongs to this class of disturbance. It is an inherited condition in which abnormal remodeling results in increased bone density. This seems to result from a reduced level of activity by the cells responsible for dissolving the bone matrix—the osteoclasts. In healthy, normal individuals, there is a precisely regulated relationship between osteoclast and osteoblast activity. Depending on the current needs of the body, or merely those of a single bone, the rate of bone matrix formation by osteoblasts may be greater than, equal to, or less than the rate of bone resorption by osteoclasts.

Osteoclasts are derived from cells that are made in the bone marrow. For this reason, bone marrow transplantation has been tried as a treatment for osteopetrosis; however, only a few patients have been successfully cured by this approach. There has also been some improvement in the condition of at least one osteopetrosis patient following treatment with a hormone related to vitamin D. This particular hormone can increase bone resorption and thereby may prevent the increase in bone density that characterizes this condition.

Another member of this category of disturbance is commonly referred to as cretinism. The basic problem in cretinism is underactivity of the thyroid gland during the development of the fetus, resulting in a decrease in the production of thyroid hormones in the fetus. This condition can be caused by an insufficient supply of the element iodine in the pregnant mother, or it may result from inherited errors in the production of the thyroid hormones.

Among the organ systems seriously impacted by this condition is the skeleton. The bones do not develop correctly and show retarded growth in length. Consequently, the bones are shorter and thicker than normal, with corresponding changes in the appearance of the child. Early diagnosis of the condition and timely treatment with drug forms of the thyroid hormones can halt the disease. Otherwise, the adult skeleton has the form referred to as a dwarf, with stubby arms and legs, a somewhat flattened face, and disproportionately large chest and head.

A disorder of the pituitary gland can result in skeletal development abnormalities that are opposite to those observed in cretinism: namely, excessive growth in the length of bones. This condition is called giantism (or gigantism) and results from the overproduction of growth hormone by the pituitary gland before normal adult stature has been achieved. The most common cause of this situation is a tumor in the pituitary gland. Cases are known of people attaining heights of more than eight feet tall. Unfortunately, because of complications involving other organ systems as a result of the excessive production of growth hormone, the persons suffering from this disorder usually die before the age of thirty.

Surgical removal of the pituitary tumor is often attempted. If the tumor is successfully removed, then the overproduction of growth hormone will be stopped. In other cases, radiation treatments are used to destroy the tumor. It is also possible to combine both of these treatment techniques. Drug therapy is also possible. Because of the high doses necessary and the accompanying side effects of high drug dosages, however, the reduction of growth hormone levels through drug treatment is usually applied only in conjunction with one or both of the other therapies.

There are also disorders which afflict adult bone. Most of the remodeling disorders involve a loss of bone mass. The group of disorders known as osteoporosis (porous bone) is a rather common example which affects approximately 29 percent of women and 18 percent of men between the ages of forty-five and seventy-nine in the United States. The reduction in bone mass is sufficient to result in increased fragility and ease of breakage. There is also slower healing of bone fractures. In advanced cases, bones have been known to break when the person sneezes or simply rolls over in bed.

Loss of bone mass is a normal feature of aging, becoming quite marked after the age of seventy-five, particularly in the hip and leg bones. Because of the normal decrease in bone mass with aging, there is not a clear distinction to be made between normal, age-related skeletal changes and the clinical condition of osteoporosis. The occurrence of excessive fragility at a relatively early age is an indication that osteoporosis is developing. Normally, between the ages of thirty and forty, the activity of the osteoblast cells (those that form bone matrix) begins to decrease while the osteoclast cells (those that dissolve the matrix) maintain their previous level of activity. This results in the loss of about 8 percent of the total bone mass each decade for women and about 3 percent for men. Because of unequal loss in the different regions of the skeleton, the outcome is a gradual reduction in height, the loss of teeth, and the development of fragile limbs.

Osteoporotic bones are indistinguishable from normal bones with respect to their bone composition. The problem is simply too little of the strength-imparting matrix, with both compact and spongy bone being affected.

There are multiple causes of osteoporosis. Some cases have no known cause (idiopathic osteoporosis), some are inherited, and others are brought about as a result of hormonal (endocrine) disorders, vitamin or mineral deficiency, or effects of the long-term use of certain drugs.

The fact that women are more often affected than men, and that the process is most conspicuous in women beyond the age of the menopause, has implicated the female sex hormones (and, specifically, their decreased production) in the initiation of the osteoporotic process. One form of therapy is the administration of certain female sex hormones (specifically estrogens) to postmenopausal women (who have decreased production of estrogens). This treatment slows their loss of bone mass.

Other treatments of osteoporosis include administering the hormone calcitonin and increasing the dietary intake of the mineral calcium. The hormone calcitonin, produced by the thyroid gland, is sometimes used to treat osteoporosis because it stimulates the production of bone matrix by increasing the activity of the osteoblasts. At the same time, calcitonin inhibits the breakdown of bone by decreasing the activity of osteoclasts. Although this treatment theoretically should produce the desired result of preventing the accelerated loss of bone mass characteristic of osteoporosis, actual clinical results are not always positive.

For those cases of osteoporosis that are the result of endocrine gland disturbances, the appropriate treatment depends on the specific glandular disorder that is present. In some instances, hormone replacement therapy can produce improvement in the patient's condition.

Regular exercise is a means both of preventing the onset of osteoporosis and of slowing its progression. Because muscular activity is critical for the maintenance of bone mass, extended periods of inactivity or immobilization can actually induce osteoporosis. For women, it is known that the amount and regularity of their exercise during the teenage years is strongly associated with their chances of developing osteoporosis thirty and more years later. The exercise need only be of moderate intensity in order to decrease significantly the risk of developing osteoporosis. Indeed, exercise that is at a level of intensity so high that it interferes with the normal female menstrual cycle (stopping the occurrence of menstruation completely or causing irregular cycle lengths) can actually increase the risk of developing osteoporosis later in life.

PERSPECTIVE AND PROSPECTS

Bone has, as one of its primary functions, the protection of softer, more vulnerable tissues and organs. The physical properties of bone—it is as strong as cast iron but only weighs as much as an equally large piece of pine wood—make it ideally suited for this job. This combination of strength and lightness derives from the bony matrix of mineral crystals and the architecture of the bone, which unites compact and spongy bone.

The physical and chemical properties of the mineral crystals also result in the permanency of bone following death. Often the only trace of a dead body is the skeleton. Because of the resistance of bone to the processes of decomposition that befall the other tissues of the body following death, investigators are often able to determine the sex of the person whose skeleton has been found even though all other tissues have long since disappeared. This is possible because of the characteristic differences between male and female adult skeletons. Racial differences in the detailed structure of the skull and pelvis, age-related changes in the skeleton, signs of healed bone fractures, and the prominence of ridges where muscles attach (giving clues about the degree of muscular development) are also valuable sources of information when attempting to identify skeletal remains.

The sexual differences in the human skeleton are most obvious in the adult pelvis. These are genetically determined differences that are structural adaptations for childbearing. For example, the pelvis is smoother and wider in the female than in the male. Other differences include a lighter and smoother female skull, a more sloping male forehead, a larger and heavier male jawbone, and generally heavier male bones that also typically possess more prominent markings.

Among the common age-related changes found in skeletons are a general reduction in the mineral content and less prominent bone markings, both of which become more obvious after about age fifty. Various bones in the skull fuse together at characteristic ages ranging from one to thirty years of age. Other bones throughout the body can also be examined to achieve more accurate estimates of the age of a skeleton at the time of death.

Another consequence of the permanent nature of bone is that it provides a record of the changes in the skeletal anatomy of humans that have occurred during the hundreds of thousands of years of human evolution. Expert examination of skeletal remains can actually reveal an amazing wealth of information concerning the health and even the lifestyle of the deceased.   —*John V. Urbas, Ph.D.*

See also Amputation; Anatomy; Arthritis; Arthroplasty; Arthroscopy; Bone cancer; Bone disorders; Bone grafting; Bone marrow transplantation; Bunion removal; Cerebral palsy; Chiropractic; Cleft lip and palate repair; Cleft palate; Disk removal; Dwarfism; Feet; Foot disorders; Fracture and dislocation; Fracture repair; Gigantism; Hammertoe correction; Head and neck disorders; Heel spur removal; Hip fracture repair; Jaw wiring; Kneecap removal; Laminectomy and spinal fusion; Lower extremities; Orthopedic surgery; Orthopedics; Orthopedics, pediatric; Osgood-Schlatter disease; Osteopathic medicine; Osteoporosis; Paget's disease; Physical rehabilitation; Podiatry; Rheumatology; Rickets; Sarcoma; Scoliosis; Slipped disk; Spinal disorders; Spine, vertebrae, and disks; Sports medicine; Temporomandibular joint (TMJ) syndrome; Tendon disorders; Tendon repair; Upper extremities.

FOR FURTHER INFORMATION:

Goldberg, Kathy E. *The Skeleton: Fantastic Framework.* Washington, D.C.: U.S. News Books, 1982. A wonderful book for the general reader that presents introductory information on almost any topic related to the skeleton. Features many color photographs, excellent artwork, X-ray pictures, and historically interesting figure reproductions. The book also contains a good glossary and an extensive index. The writing style is easy and informal, yet very informative.

Joyce, Christopher, and Eric Stover. *Witnesses from the Grave: The Stories Bones Tell.* Boston: Little, Brown, 1991. This book presents a fascinating account of the work of Clyde Snow, a forensic anthropologist. Snow has reported on new findings about what lies under the ground at Custer's Last Stand at the Little Bighorn. He has also identified the victims of serial killer John Wayne Gacy. Information is presented relating to bone and the skeleton, but only to the extent required for appreciation of the story. Intended for the general reader.

Marieb, Elaine N. *Human Anatomy and Physiology.* 3d ed. Redwood City, Calif.: Benjamin/Cummings, 1995. Nonscientists at the advanced high school level or above will be able to understand this fine textbook. Chapters 6 ("Bones and Bone Tissue"), 7 ("The Skeleton"), and 8 ("Joints") are very well illustrated and include many applications in the fields of physical education and medical science. The book includes a complete glossary, index, pronunciation guide, and other helpful features. Each chapter features a chapter outline and learning objectives, as well as a chapter summary and review questions.

Seeley, Rod R., Trent D. Stephens, and Philip Tate. *Anatomy and Physiology.* St. Louis: Mosby Year Book, 1992. A beautifully illustrated text for readers at the advanced high school level and above. Three chapters (6, 7, and 8) are concerned with bone, skeleton, and joints. There are numerous essays on sports medicine, pathologies, clinical applications, and more, as well as a complete index, glossary, and pronunciation guide.

Van De Graaff, Kent M., and Stuart Ira Fox. *Concepts of Human Anatomy and Physiology.* 4th ed. Dubuque, Iowa: Wm. C. Brown, 1995. Chapters 8 through 11 present a first-rate introduction to bones, the skeleton, and joints. The many clear illustrations, photographs, clinical commentaries, and X rays, as well as a pronunciation guide, a complete index, and a glossary, make this a very accessible book for the nonspecialist reader at the advanced high school level and above. Each chapter begins with an interesting case study and related questions pertaining to the subject of the chapter.

BOTULISM
DISEASE/DISORDER
ANATOMY OR SYSTEM AFFECTED: Gastrointestinal system, muscles, musculoskeletal system, nervous system, stomach

SPECIALTIES AND RELATED FIELDS: Emergency medicine, neurology, public health, toxicology

DEFINITION: Botulism is food poisoning caused by eating incompletely cooked or contaminated canned foods; such foods may contain bacteria which produce a toxin that

is absorbed by the digestive tract and spread to the central nervous system. Symptoms, which usually occur eighteen to thirty-six hours after eating the contaminated food, include blurred vision, drooping eyelids, dry mouth, slurred speech, vomiting, diarrhea, and weakness leading to paralysis; no fever or disturbance of mental ability occurs. In infants, symptoms may also include severe constipation, feeble cry, and an inability to suck. Botulism may require hospitalization and antitoxin injections; if left untreated, it can prove fatal.

—*Jason Georges and Tracy Irons-Georges*
See also Bacterial infections; Bacteriology; Food poisoning; Toxicology.

BRAIN
ANATOMY
ANATOMY OR SYSTEM AFFECTED: Head, nerves, nervous system, psychic-emotional system

SPECIALTIES AND RELATED FIELDS: Neurology, psychiatry, psychology

DEFINITION: The most complex organ in the body, which is used for thinking, learning, remembering, seeing, hearing, and many other conscious and subconscious functions.

KEY TERMS:
action potential: an electrochemical event that nerve cells use to send signals along their cellular extensions in the nervous system

axon: a nerve cell extension used to carry action potentials from one place to another in the nervous system

dendrite: a branching nerve cell extension that receives and processes the effects of action potentials from other nerve cells

dyskinesia: a neurologic disorder causing difficulty in the performance of voluntary movements

nucleus: in reference to brain structure, a collection of nerve cell bodies separable from other groups by their cellular form or by surrounding nerve cell extensions

soma: the body of a cell, where the cell's genetic material and other vital structures are located

synapse: an area of close contact between nerve cells that is the functional junction where one cell communicates with another

tract: a collection of nerve fibers (axons) in the brain or spinal cord that all have the same place of origin and the same place of termination

STRUCTURE AND FUNCTIONS
The human brain is a complex structure that is composed of two major classes of individual cells: nerve cells (or neurons), and neuroglial cells (or glial cells). It has been estimated that the adult human brain has around one hundred billion neurons and an even larger number of glial cells. An average adult brain weighs about 1,400 grams and has a volume of 1,200 milliliters. These values tend to vary

directly with the person's body size; therefore, males have a brain that is typically 10 percent larger than that of females. There is no correlation of intelligence with brain size, however, as witnessed by the fact that brains as small as 750 milliliters or larger than 2,000 milliliters still show normal functioning.

Neurons process and transmit information. The usual structural features of a neuron include a cell body (or soma), anywhere from several to several hundred branching dendrites that are extensions from the soma, and a typically longer extension known as the axon with one or several synaptic terminals at its end.

The information that is processed and transmitted in the brain takes the form of very brief electrochemical events (with a typical duration of less than 2 milliseconds) called action potentials or nerve impulses. These impulses most often originate near the point at which the axon and soma are joined, and then travel at speeds of up to 130 meters per second along the axon to the synaptic terminals.

It is at the synaptic terminals that one neuron communicates its information to other neurons in the brain. These specialized structural points of neuron-to-neuron communication are called synapses. Most synapses are found on the dendrites and soma of the neuron that is to receive the nerve signal. A neuron may have as many as fifty thousand synapses on its surface, although the average seems to be around three thousand. It is thought that as many as three hundred trillion synapses may exist in the adult brain.

The neuroglia function as supporting cells. They have a variety of important duties that include acting as a supporting framework for neurons, increasing the speed of impulse conduction along axons, acting as removers of waste or cellular debris, and regulating the composition of the fluid environment around the neurons in order to maintain opti-

The Anatomy of the Brain

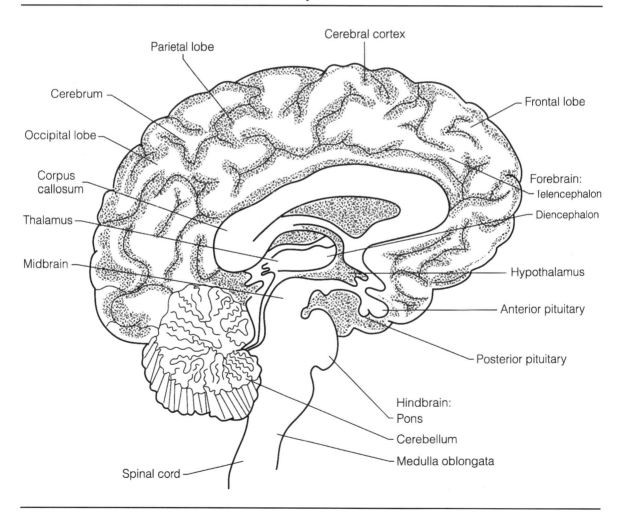

mal working conditions in the brain. Neuroglia actually make up about half of the brain's total volume.

The brain can be divided into two major components: gray matter and white matter, both named for their general appearance. The gray matter is composed primarily of neural soma, dendrites, and axons that transmit information at relatively slow speeds. The white matter is made of collections of axons that have layers of specialized glial cells wrapped around them. This enables much faster information transfer along these axons.

The brain has six major regions. Beginning from the top of the spinal cord and moving progressively upward, these regions are the medulla oblongata, the pons, the cerebellum, the mesencephalon (or midbrain), the diencephalon, and the cerebrum.

The initial lower portion of the medulla oblongata resembles the spinal cord. The medulla has a variety of functions besides the simple relaying of various categories of sensory information to higher-brain centers. Within the medulla there are a number of centers that are important for the execution and regulation of basic survival and maintenance duties. These duties are called visceral functions and include jobs such as regulating the heart rate, breathing, digestive actions, and blood pressure.

The term "pons" comes from the Latin word meaning bridge. The pons serves as a bridge from the medulla oblongata to the cerebellum, which is actually situated on the backside of the brain stem. The pons contains tracts and nuclei that permit communication between the cerebellum and other nervous system structures. Some pontine nuclei facilitate the control of such voluntary and involuntary muscle actions as chewing, breathing, and moving the eyes; other nuclei process information related to the sense of balance.

The cerebellum is a small brain in itself. The two main functions of the cerebellum are to make adjustments to the muscles of the body, quickly and automatically, that assist in maintaining balance and posture, and to coordinate the activities of the skeletal muscles involved in movements or sequences of movements, thereby promoting smooth and precise actions. These functions are possible because of the input of sensory information to the cerebellum from position sensors in the muscles and joints; from visual, touch, and balance organs; and even from the sense of hearing. There are also many communication channels to and from the cerebellum and other brain areas concerned with the generation and control of movements. While the cerebellum is not the origin of commands that initiate movements, it does store the memories of how to perform patterns of muscle contractions that are used to execute learned skills, such as serving a tennis ball.

The mesencephalon, or midbrain, is located just above the pons. The midbrain contains pathways carrying sensory information upwards to higher-brain centers and transmitting motor signals from higher regions down to lower-brain and spinal cord areas involved in movements.

Two important pairs of nuclei, the inferior and superior colliculi, are found on the backside of the mesencephalon. They coordinate visual and acoustic reflexes involving eye and head movements, such as eye focusing and orienting the head and body toward a sound source. The nucleus known as the substantia nigra operates with nuclei in the cerebrum to generate the patterns and rhythms of such activities as walking and running. Additional mesencephalic nuclei are important for the involuntary control of muscle tone, posture maintenance, and the control of eye movements.

The diencephalon, located above the midbrain, contains the two important brain structures known as the thalamus and hypothalamus. The thalamus is the final relay for all sensory signals (except the sense of smell) before these arrive at the cerebral cortex (the cerebrum's outer covering of gray matter). The hypothalamus is important for regulating drives and emotions, and it serves as a master link between the nervous and endocrine systems.

The thalamus is a collection of different nuclei. Some cooperate with nuclei in the cerebrum to process memories and generate emotional states. Other nuclei have complex involvement in the interactions of the cerebellum, cerebral nuclei, and motor areas of the cerebral cortex.

The relatively small hypothalamus plays many crucial roles that help to maintain stability in the body's internal environment. It regulates food and liquid intake, blood pressure, heart rate, breathing, body temperature, and digestion. Other significant duties encompass the management of sexual activity, rage, fear, and pleasure.

The final major brain region is the cerebrum, which is the largest of the six regions and the seat of higher intellectual capabilities. Sensory information that reaches the cerebrum also enters into a person's conscious awareness. Voluntary actions originate in the cerebral neural activities.

The cerebrum is divided into two cerebral hemispheres, each covered by the gray matter known as the cerebral cortex. Below the cortex is the white matter, which consists of massive bundles of axons carrying signals between various cortical areas, down from the cortex to lower areas, and up into the cortex from lower areas. Embedded in the white matter are also a number of cerebral nuclei.

The cerebral cortex has areas that are the primary sensory areas for each of the senses, and other areas whose major duties deal with the origin and planning of motor activities. The association areas of the cortex integrate and process sensory signals, often resulting in the initiation of appropriate motor responses. Cortical integrative centers receive information from different association areas. The integrative centers perform complex analyses of information (such as predicting the consequences of various possible responses) and direct elaborate motor activities (such as writing).

The cerebral nuclei, also called the basal nuclei or basal ganglia, form components of brain systems that have complex duties such as the regulation of emotions, the control of muscle tone and the coordination of learned patterns of movement, and the processing of memories.

The electrochemical signal that constitutes an action potential in a neuron, and that is sent along the neuron's axon to the synaptic contacts formed with other neurons in the brain, is the basic unit of activity in neural tissue. Although the electrical voltage generated by a single action potential is very small and difficult to measure, the tremendous number of neurons active at any moment results in voltages large enough to be measured at the scalp with appropriate instruments called electroencephalographs. The recorded signals are known as an electroencephalogram (EEG).

Although interpreting an EEG can be compared to standing outside of a football stadium filled with screaming fans and trying to discern what is happening on the playing field by listening to the crowd noises, it still provides clinically useful information and is used regularly in clinics around the world each day. The typical EEG signal appears as a series of wavy patterns whose size, length, shape, and location of best recording on the head provide valuable indications concerning the conditions of brain regions beneath the recording electrodes placed on the scalp.

DISORDERS AND DISEASES

One of the most useful applications of the EEG is in the diagnosis of epilepsy. Epilepsy is a group of disorders originating in the brain. There are multiple possible causes. Epilepsy is characterized by malfunctions of the motor, sensory, or even psychic operations of the brain, and there are often accompanying convulsive movements during the attack.

The most common type is known as idiopathic epilepsy, so called because there is no known cause of the attacks. The usual episode occurs suddenly as a large group of neurons begins to produce action potentials in a very synchronized fashion (called a seizure), which is not the typical mode of action in neural tissue. There may be no impairment of consciousness or a complete loss of consciousness, and the seizure may be restricted to a localized area of brain tissue or may spread over the entire brain. When areas of the brain that generate or control movements become involved, the patient will exhibit varying degrees of involuntary muscle contractions or convulsions.

Some cases of epilepsy can be traced to definite causes such as brain tumors, brain injuries, drug abuse, adverse drug reactions, or infections that have entered the brain. Regardless of the cause, the diagnosis is often made through examination of the EEG whereby a trained examiner can quickly identify the EEG abnormalities characteristic of epilepsy.

The usual treatment is directed toward preventing the synchronized bursts of neural activity. This is most often achieved by administering anticonvulsive drugs such as phenobarbital or phenytoin. These agents block the transmission of neural signals in the epileptic regions, and thereby suppress the explosive episodes of synchronized neuronal discharges that induce the seizures. Many epileptics are successfully treated by this approach and are able to lead normal, productive lives, free from the uncontrollable seizures. In some cases, the medication can eventually be discontinued and the patient will never again suffer a seizure.

Unfortunately, there are also cases where even the strongest medications do not prevent the seizures, or only do so at the expense of debilitating drug effects. In the most severe cases, the patients may have dozens of seizures each day, making any form of normal existence impossible. In addition, the large number of seizures eventually can lead to permanent brain damage. For some of these patients, the most drastic form of treatment has been used: surgical removal of the brain tissue responsible for the seizures. This technique is accompanied by great risk because of the danger that removing a portion of brain tissue may leave the patient unable to speak or to speak intelligently, unable to understand spoken words, unable to interpret visual information, or suffering from any of a wide variety of behavioral disturbances, depending on the precise area of the brain that has been removed.

Although this approach is not appropriate in all cases, it has been successful in many. For these patients, success is usually defined as the possibility, following surgery, to control or prevent future seizures through the use of anticonvulsive drugs, and to resume a normal life or a life that is much more normal than it was before surgery.

A varied group of disorders known as dyskinesias causes difficulty in the performance of voluntary movements. The movements actually look like normal body movements or portions of normal movements. Dyskinesia often results from problems involving the basal nuclei. When the basal nuclei are affected, the dyskinesic movements usually do not occur during sleep and are reduced during periods of emotional tranquility. Anxiety, emotional tension, and stressful conditions, however, cause the dyskinesia to become worse. These observations can be explained by the fact that neural pathways are known to connect the brain centers involved with the generation of emotional states to the basal nuclei.

One example of a dyskinesia affecting the basal nuclei is the inherited condition of Huntington's disease (or Huntington's chorea), for which no treatment exists. A chorea is a dyskinesia in which the patient's movements are quick and irregular. Huntington's chorea first makes its appearance when the patient is in middle age. It results in the progressive degeneration of the basal nuclei, known as the corpus striatum, that are located in the cerebrum. Some of the common symptoms are involuntary facial grimacing, jaw and tongue movements, twisting and turning movements of the torso, and speaking difficulties. As the brain atrophy (degeneration) progresses, the patients become totally disabled. Death usually results ten to fifteen years following the appearance of the first symptoms.

A category of generalized disturbances of higher-brain function is known as dementia, more commonly referred to as senility. The term "senile" is derived from the Latin word meaning "old age," and its use reflects the fact that senility was previously considered to be an inevitable consequence of aging. Senility, or dementia, is characterized by a generalized deficiency of intellectual performance (often referred to as being "feeble-minded"), mental deterioration, memory impairment, and limited attention span. These are often accompanied by changes in personality such as increased irritability and moodiness.

Various diseases can cause dementia. One of the most frequently observed is known as Alzheimer's disease, which is progressive and usually develops between the ages of forty and sixty. The disease is marked by the death of neurons in the cerebral cortex and the deep cerebral regions known as the nucleus basalis and the hippocampus. The exact cause of neural death in Alzheimer's disease is unknown. While some cases are inherited, other instances seem to appear without any family history of the disease. Death usually occurs within ten years after the appearance of the first symptoms, and no cure exists.

The areas of the brain showing neural degeneration also have abnormal collections of a specific type of protein. The appearance of this protein in the blood and the fluids that surround the brain is a clinical sign for Alzheimer's disease. The areas of the brain that deteriorate during the progression of this disease illustrate the functional roles played by these regions. The hippocampus, in particular, is crucial for learning, the storage of long-term memories, memory of recent events, and the sense of time. Therefore, the death of hippocampal neurons helps to explain the memory disturbances and related behavioral changes seen in Alzheimer's disease patients.

PERSPECTIVE AND PROSPECTS

Given the complexity of the human brain, understanding its structure and function is the ultimate challenge to medical science. The challenge exists because, in order to rationally treat brain disorders, it is necessary to know how a normal brain functions. An appreciation of this can be gleaned by studying the history of some approaches used through the ages to treat brain disorders.

For example, in the Middle Ages it was a common practice to treat people suffering from epilepsy by cutting open the patient's scalp and pouring salt into the wound (all of which was performed without anesthesia, since anesthetics were not yet known). The purpose of this treatment was to poison the spirits possessing the patient, forcing them to leave.

As modern science discovered the cellular basis of life, such draconian measures were gradually replaced with treatments directed toward the biochemical imbalances, infections, or interruptions of blood flow that were found to be the cause of many brain disorders. The development of nonsurgical techniques permitting the visualization of the brain regions that are active, or inactive, during various tasks or illnesses greatly advanced the understanding of brain function and improved diagnosis, the planning of effective treatments, and the tracking of either the improvement or the deterioration of patients.

Late in the 1970's, the disease known as acquired immunodeficiency syndrome (AIDS) attracted the attention of the world's scientists. AIDS is caused by the human immunodeficiency virus (HIV). Nearly 60 percent of AIDS patients experience various neurological problems, including difficulties of movement, loss of memory, and cognitive disturbances. In some cerebral cortical areas, as many as half of the neurons may die. In order to understand how the AIDS virus causes these effects, it is necessary to analyze how the brain's components function when infected by the virus, and then to form a clear explanation of the consequences of viral infection.

HIV actually infects certain classes of neuroglial cells. Infection of these glial cells causes them to release distinct types of chemicals that can be toxic to neurons. One type of glial cell, known as the astrocyte, can begin to appear in abnormally large numbers as a result of these chemicals being released. In turn, the presence of large numbers of astrocytes provokes the release of even more of the toxic chemicals. This sort of effect is referred to as a positive feedback loop. The significance of this cascade of mutually stimulating events (neurotoxic chemicals causing astrocytes to appear in greater numbers, and increased numbers of astrocytes causing more production of neurotoxic chemicals) is that only a few HIV-infected cells can trigger extensive neural damage.

Additionally, a protein part of the virus, called gp120, can stimulate release of the same neurotoxic chemicals and can disrupt the normal functioning of the astrocytes. One important function of astrocytes is to regulate the chemical environment of neurons by removing certain types of chemicals. One of these chemicals, called glutamate, is normally present and used by some neurons to send signals to other neurons at their synaptic contacts. When glutamate is not promptly removed from the environment of the target neurons, however, it becomes toxic to the neurons and kills them. The HIV protein gp120 disrupts the ability of astrocytes to remove glutamate, thereby increasing the death of neurons in the brain as they become exposed to toxic levels of glutamate. —*John V. Urbas, Ph.D.*

See also Abscess drainage; Abscesses; Addiction; Alcoholism; Altitude sickness; Alzheimer's disease; Amnesia; Anatomy; Aneurysmectomy; Aneurysms; Angiography;

Aphasia and dysphasia; Biofeedback; Brain disorders; Cluster headaches; Coma; Computed tomography (CT) scanning; Concussion; Craniotomy; Dementia; Dizziness and fainting; Dyslexia; Electroconvulsive therapy; Electroencephalography (EEG); Embolism; Emotions, biomedical causes and effects of; Encephalitis; Endocrinology; Endocrinology, pediatric; Epilepsy; Fetal tissue transplantation; Hallucinations; Head and neck disorders; Headaches; Hydrocephalus; Hypnosis; Learning disabilities; Light therapy; Memory loss; Meningitis; Mental retardation; Migraine headaches; Narcolepsy; Narcotics; Neurology; Neurology, pediatric; Neurosurgery; Parkinson's disease; Positron emission tomography (PET) scanning; Psychiatric disorders; Psychiatry; Psychiatry, child and adolescent; Psychiatry, geriatric; Psychology; Seizures; Shunts; Sleep disorders; Strokes and TIAs; Systems and organs; Thrombosis and thrombus; Toxicology; Trembling and shaking; Tumor removal; Tumors; Unconsciousness.

FOR FURTHER INFORMATION:

Davis, Joel. *Mapping the Mind: The Secrets of the Human Brain and How It Works.* New York: Carol, 1997. An easy-to-read book on the brain and mind that gives details about different structures and functions.

Edelman, Gerald M. *Bright Air, Brilliant Fire.* New York: Basic Books, 1992. The author is a winner of the 1972 Nobel Prize in Physiology or Medicine and a leading brain scientist. This book is accessible to the nonscientist because of the importance that the author places on the subject of understanding the brain and how it gives rise to the mind. At the end of the book, there is an excellent collection of suggested additional sources to consult for each chapter.

Marieb, Elaine N. *Human Anatomy and Physiology.* 3d ed. Redwood City, Calif.: Benjamin/Cummings, 1995. Non-scientists at the advanced high school level or above will be able to understand this fine textbook. Chapters 11 ("Fundamentals of the Nervous System and Nervous Tissue"), 12 ("The Central Nervous System"), and 15 ("Neural Integration"), as well as parts of several other chapters dealing with additional aspects of the nervous system, are well illustrated and include many applications in the fields of physical education and medical science. The book includes a complete glossary, index, pronunciation guide, and other features. Each chapter includes an outline and learning objectives.

Scientific American 267 (September, 1992). A special issue entitled *Mind and Brain.* This outstanding collection of articles by leading scientists, edited by Jonathan Piel, presents information on a wide range of topics such as the development of the brain, age-related changes in the brain, sex differences in the brain, major disorders of the brain and the mind, and others. The high-quality illustrations and easily understood text of the articles make this issue an excellent source of information about the brain.

Seeley, Rod R., Trent D. Stephens, and Philip Tate. *Anatomy and Physiology.* St. Louis: Mosby Year Book, 1992. A beautifully illustrated text with drawings, photographs and summary tables. Four chapters (12, 13, and parts of 15 and 16) are concerned with the brain and nervous tissue. Included in the text are numerous interesting essays on pathologies, clinical applications, and more, as well as a complete index, a glossary, and a good pronunciation guide. For readers at the advanced high school level and above.

Van De Graaff, Kent M., and Stuart Ira Fox. *Concepts of Human Anatomy and Physiology.* 4th ed. Dubuque, Iowa: Wm. C. Brown, 1995. Chapters 14 and 15 present a first-rate introduction to the brain and nervous tissue. Other aspects of the nervous system are treated in chapters 16 through 19. The many clear illustrations, photographs, clinical commentaries, summary tables, pronunciation guide, and complete index and glossary make this a very accessible book for the nonspecialist at the advanced high school level and above. Each chapter begins with an interesting case study and related questions that pertain to the subject of the chapter.

BRAIN DISORDERS

DISEASE/DISORDER

ANATOMY OR SYSTEM AFFECTED: Brain, head, nervous system, psychic-emotional system

SPECIALTIES AND RELATED FIELDS: Embryology, geriatrics and gerontology, neurology, psychiatry

DEFINITION: Disorders of the brain can interfere with its role in the control of body functions, behavior, learning, and expression, while defects can also threaten life itself.

KEY TERMS:

anencephaly: a fatal congenital condition in which tissues that should have differentiated to form the brain failed to do so

coma: a condition of unconsciousness that may or may not be reversible; various degrees of coma are assessed by the presence or absence of reflex responses, such as pupil dilation when a light is shone into the eyes

dementia: a diseased state in which intellectual ability is ever decreasing; personality changes, decreased interest or ability to care for one's self, and long-term and short-term memory loss can indicate dementia

embolus: a clot or other piece of matter that may travel through the circulatory system to tiny blood vessels (as in the brain) and block the path that normally allows blood flow

hydrocephalus: a painful condition caused by excess cerebrospinal fluid within the spaces of the brain

ischemia: an inadequate blood flow to a region; may be caused by an incomplete blockage in or constriction of a blood vessel (as may occur with atherosclerosis or a blood clot)

seizure: a misfiring of cortical neurons that alters the patient's level of consciousness; the seizure may or may not involve muscular convulsions

stroke: a complete loss of blood flow to a region of the brain that is of sudden onset and causes abrupt muscular weakness, usually to one side of the body

thrombus: a blood clot that is attached to the interior wall of a blood vessel

CAUSES AND SYMPTOMS

The cerebral cortex acts as a processor for sensory information and as an integrator of memory, interpretation, creativity, intellect, and passion. Disorders of the brain or brain defects can disrupt these processing or integrating functions. Disorders of the brain include such commonly heard terms as stroke, ischemia, dementia, seizure, and coma. Brain disorders may also occur as a result of infection, various tumors, traumas leading to blot clots (hematomas) or lack of oxygen (hypoxia), and cancer. Brain defects include anencephaly, a congenital defect in which a newborn lacks a brain, and hydrocephaly, commonly called "water on the brain."

A stroke is any situation in which the blood supply to a region of the brain is lost. This can occur as a result of a cerebral hemorrhage, during which blood escapes from blood vessels to surround and compress brain tissue; cerebral thrombosis, whereby a clot attached to the wall of a blood vessel restricts the amount of blood flowing to a particular region; or an embolus, a foreign substance which may be a clot that migrates in the bloodstream, often to lodge in a smaller vessel in the brain. The embolus will block blood flow to some area. An embolus can originate from substances other than a blood clot, which is why health care staff often squirt fluid out of a needle before administering a shot or other therapy: to ensure that no air embolus, which could induce a stroke or prove fatal if it enters the brain, is injected.

Transient ischemic attacks (TIAs) are often thought of as small strokes, but, technically, ischemia simply means that oxygen is not reaching the cells within a tissue. Basically, the mechanism is similar to a stroke, in that blood flow to a portion of the brain is compromised. Although blood actually reaches the brain tissue during ischemia, there is not a sufficient flow to ensure that all cells are receiving the oxygen necessary to continue cellular life. This condition is called hypoxia (low oxygen). If hypoxia is sustained over a sufficient period of time, cellular death occurs, causing irreversible brain damage.

The important differences between a stroke and a TIA are the onset and duration of symptoms, as well as the severity of the damage. Persons with atherosclerosis actually have fat deposits along the interior walls of their blood vessels. These people are vulnerable to experiencing multiple TIAs. Many TIAs are small enough to be dismissed and ignored; others are truly inapparent, causing no symp-

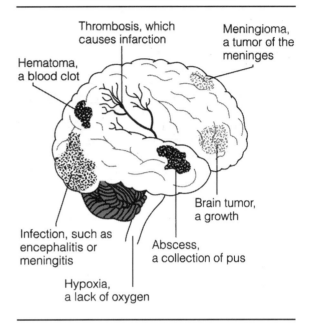

Common Brain Disorders

toms. This is unfortunate because TIAs often serve as a warning of an impending full-scale stroke. Action and treatments could be implemented, if medical advice is sought early, to decrease the likelihood of a stroke. Repeated TIAs also contribute to dementia.

Dementia is not the normal path for the elderly, nor is it a sign of aging. Dementia is a sign of neurological chaos and can be caused by diseases such as Alzheimer's disease or acquired immunodeficiency syndrome (AIDS). Although most elderly are not afflicted with dementia, nearly all have a slowing of reaction and response time. This slowing is believed to be associated with chemical changes within nerve cell membranes as aging occurs; slowing of reaction times is not necessarily indicative of the first steps on a path to dementia. In addition, forgetfulness may not be a sign of dementia, since it occurs at all ages. Forgetfulness is such a sign, however, if it is progressive and includes forgetting to dress or forgetting one's name or date of birth.

While it is incorrect to say that dementia is caused by aging, it is correct to say that dementia is age-related. It may first appear in a person any time between the late thirties and the mid-nineties, but it usually begins to appear in the late seventies. Patients with Alzheimer's disease are believed to account for about 20 percent of all cases of dementia. Other diseases cause dementia, including an autosomal-dominant genetic disease called Huntington's disease. Huntington's disease manifests itself with a distinct chorea, or dance, of the body that is neither solicited nor controlled. This genetic disease is particularly cruel in that its symptoms appear in midlife, often after the adult has had offspring and passed on the gene. The disease continues to alter the intellect and personality of the afflicted one and progresses to the point of complete debilitation of the body and mind.

A seizure occurs when a collection of neurons misfires, sending nerve impulses that are neither solicited nor controllable. In the everyday use of the term, seizure describes a condition of epilepsy or convulsion. Medically speaking, a seizure is a sign of an underlying problem within the gray matter of the brain; it is the most common neurological disorder. Epilepsy is a term used to describe a condition of repeated seizures, while convulsion is a term generally applied to describe an isolated seizure. A seizure may occur as a consequence of extreme fever or a violent blow to the head. Seizures are also associated with metabolic disorders, such as hypoglycemia (low blood sugar); trauma causing a loss of blood or oxygen to a region, such as in a newborn after a traumatic birth; toxins, as seen in drug abuse or withdrawal; or bacterial or viral encephalitis or meningitis. In addition, about one-third of those persons who survive a gunshot wound to the head will experience seizures afterward. In closed head trauma, which can occur in a sporting or automobile accident, there is a 5 percent chance of post-trauma seizures.

Loss of consciousness can be caused by a violent impact to the head, a lack of oxygen or blood flow to the head, a metabolic imbalance, or the presence of a toxin such as alcohol. Usually, this is a transient event, but it may become a permanent condition. When this happens, a person is said to be in a coma. A comatose person exists in a nonresponsive state and may be assessed for brain death. Brain death is a legally defined term which means that no electrical activity in the brain is seen on an electroencephalogram (EEG). Thus some comatose patients may be determined to be brain-dead, particularly if the condition is deemed irreversible.

Brain defects are not common, but they do occur. One particularly tragic defect is the absence of a brain in a newborn, called anencephaly. Death usually occurs within a few hours of birth. Although anencephaly is rare and generally associated with a genetic factor, there have been cases in population clusters, such as one in the Rio Grande area of south Texas, suggesting that an environmental factor may contribute to these defects.

Another defect that may appear in newborns or in an infant's first months of life is hydrocephalus. Although the descriptive term "water on the brain" is often used, the condition does not involve a collection of water in the cranium; rather, it involves an accumulation of cerebrospinal fluid (CSF). CSF is the fluid that insulates the brain and allows it to "float" under the bony cranial encasement. As the ventricles, or spaces, in the brain fill with CSF, bulging occurs and pressure builds to the point of compressing the surrounding brain tissue. This can be very painful and is fatal if untreated. Hydrocephalus can be caused by an overproduction of CSF or a blockage of the CSF drainage from the ventricles of the brain. The symptoms often include a protrusion or abnormal shape of the cranium. In newborns, the skull bones have not yet sutured (fused) to one another, so the soft bones are pushed apart, causing unusual head shapes. This is a warning sign. Another sign is observed if a newborn's head has a circumference greater than 35.5 centimeters (14 inches); if that is the case, the newborn must be immediately checked for hydrocephalus. Adolescents and adults may also experience hydrocephalus. This can be a response to head trauma, infection, or the overproduction of CSF. The symptoms include lethargy, headache, dullness, blurred vision, nausea, and vomiting.

Treatment and Therapy

TIAs can progress to strokes. In fact, about 30 percent of those diagnosed with TIA will have a major stroke within the subsequent four years. One of the most prevalent causes of TIAs is hypertension. Hypertension is known as the "silent killer" because many persons with this problem ignore the subtle symptoms of fatigue, headache, and general malaise. Hypertension is also known as a good predictor of major strokes if left untreated. Thus, hypertensive persons need to be diagnosed as such in order to control their blood pressure. This allows them to avoid or delay either a major stroke or multiple TIAs. Management for the hypertensive's blood pressure may include taking diuretics and hypotensive drugs (to lower the blood pressure). If taken diligently, these drugs offer longevity and quality of life to the sufferer. Aside from hypertension, TIAs may be induced in some metabolic disorders, which should be corrected if possible, or by constricted blood vessels. Sometimes, surgery on such vessels can stop the ischemic attacks and prevent or delay the onset of a stroke.

Although TIAs lead to strokes, strokes are not necessarily preceded by a TIA. Nearly 90 percent of all major strokes occur without a TIA warning. Sadly, hypertension is the main contributor to this number. Measures can be taken to avoid strokes. This includes maintaining cardiovascular health by exercising, not smoking, and managing hypertension, diabetes mellitus, or other problems that may place stresses on the body's chemical balance.

Dementia is so poorly understood in terms of causes that a rational probe of drug therapy or a cure is nearly impossible. The drugs most often used in dementia treatment, the ergoloid mesylates, are used to manage the symptoms; namely, the confused mind. These drugs, however, do not stop or prevent the unexplained cellular degeneration associated with dementia. It is interesting to note that a tiny subgroup within those persons suffering from Alzheimer's disease have greatly improved in mental status with the drug tacrine. It is unfortunate that all patients are not responsive to this drug—a fact which suggests that Alzheimer's disease is a complex condition.

Seizures are treated pharmacologically according to type.

Carbamazepine, phenobarbitol, phenytoin, and valproate are some of the drugs available to treat seizure disorders. Barbiturates may also be used in certain cases. Most of these drugs are highly effective when taken as prescribed, and patient noncompliance is the main cause of drug failure. Sometimes, two drugs are combined in therapy. It should be mentioned that pregnant women with epilepsy are urged to continue taking antiepilepsy drugs during pregnancy since a maternal seizure may be more damaging to the fetus than the drug itself.

Some forms of hydrocephalus can be corrected surgically by performing a CSF shunt from the cranium to the peritoneal (abdominal) region, where the fluid can be eliminated from the body as waste. This is not without risk, and the introduction of infection into the brain is a major concern.

PERSPECTIVE AND PROSPECTS

The therapies in use for brain diseases and disorders have been derived from the practical experience of physicians, the laboratory research of scientists, and the hopes of multitudes of doctors, patients, families, and friends. Medical science has done much to improve the lives of those who suffer with seizures, to reduce the risk of strokes to the hypertensive person and those with TIAs, and is making great progress in treating certain kinds of dementia. Yet much remains to be done.

While one can argue that much is known about the human brain, it would be erroneous to argue that the human brain is fully understood. Despite centuries of research, the brain, as it functions in health, remains largely a mystery. Since the healthy brain is yet to be understood, it is not surprising that the medical community struggles to determine what goes wrong in dementia, seizure, or mental illness or to discover drug therapies that can cross the blood-brain barrier. Thus, the human brain is the uncharted frontier in medicine. As technology improves to support researchers and medical practitioners in their pursuits of cures and treatments for brain diseases and disorders, one can only remain hopeful for the future ability to restore health to the damaged human brain.   —Mary C. Fields

See also Abscess drainage; Abscesses; Alzheimer's disease; Amnesia; Aphasia and dysphasia; Brain; Cerebral palsy; Cluster headaches; Concussion; Dementia; Dyslexia; Electroconvulsive therapy; Embolism; Encephalitis; Epilepsy; Guillain-Barré syndrome; Hallucinations; Headaches; Hemiplegia; Hydrocephalus; Lead poisoning; Learning disabilities; Memory loss; Meningitis; Migraine headaches; Motor neuron diseases; Multiple sclerosis; Nervous system; Neuralgia, neuritis, and neuropathy; Neurology; Neurology, pediatric; Neurosurgery; Numbness and tingling; Palsy; Paralysis; Parkinson's disease; Seizures; Tics; Unconsciousness.

FOR FURTHER INFORMATION:
Bannister, Roger. *Brain and Bannister's Clinical Neurology.* 7th ed. Oxford, England: Oxford University Press, 1992. Several chapters are dedicated to the topics of seizures, dementia, hydrocephalus, and loss of consciousness. Because the writing can be fairly technical, it is best used by someone with a background in human anatomy and physiology.

Clayman, Charles B., ed. *The American Medical Association Family Medical Guide.* 3d rev. ed. New York: Random House, 1994. An excellent reference for the beginner. The scientific accuracy of the text is not compromised by its accessibility.

Parsons, Malcolm. *Colour Atlas of Clinical Neurology.* 2d ed. St. Louis: Mosby Year Book, 1993. An excellent atlas that allows the pictures to tell the story. The color photographs and brief descriptions capture the essence of brain disorders and remind the reader that people are suffering from these maladies.

BREAST AUGMENTATION, REDUCTION, AND RECONSTRUCTION

PROCEDURES

ANATOMY OR SYSTEM AFFECTED: Breasts

SPECIALTIES AND RELATED FIELDS: General surgery; plastic, cosmetic, and reconstructive surgery; psychiatry

DEFINITION: Procedures performed for aesthetic enhancement of the breasts, which may be undertaken on an elective basis, following surgery to correct defects resulting from a pathological process such as cancer, or to correct genetic deformities.

KEY TERMS:

areola: the pigmented tissue immediately surrounding the nipple

augmentation: an increase in the volume of the breast; also an improvement in breast contour and softness

debridement: the removal of all foreign material and contaminated and devitalized tissues from or adjacent to a traumatic or infected lesion until healthy surrounding tissue is exposed

ptosis: downward drooping or sagging of tissue, caused by the influence of gravity or the loss of muscular or other support

reduction: a decrease in the total volume or mass of breast tissue; this usually corrects undesirable ptosis

silicone: a plastic made primarily of silicon polymer

INDICATIONS AND PROCEDURES

Breast augmentation, reduction, and reconstruction are procedures that are undertaken for different but related reasons. These procedures are almost always performed using general anesthesia. Augmentation procedures increase the size of breasts and are performed electively to correct hypomastia (abnormally small breasts). Reduction procedures decrease the size and shape of breasts. This is called reductive mammoplasty. Most commonly, reductions are performed on an elective basis for aesthetic reasons, but they can be indicated to relieve back, shoulder, and neck pain.

Such abnormally large breast size is called mammary hyperplasia. Reconstruction involves the use of tissues from other parts of the body or prosthetic devices to restore a normal shape and contour.

Some breast augmentation can be achieved through exercises designed to increase the size of underlying muscle tissue. Hypertrophy of the pectoralis major muscle can enhance existing breast tissue, increasing the apparent size of the breast without surgery. Greater increases in breast size require the use of a prosthesis. These are available in two basic designs. The first is a thin-walled, smooth Silastic shell with a second, seamless interior envelope filled with silicone gel or saline solution. A variant is similar in design but made of polyurethane. A second type has a microscopically textured outer shell with an interior envelope and is available in both Silastic and polyurethane.

There are alternative sites for incisions to augment breasts. The site selected depends on the size and shape of the implant to be used. The safest surgical approach is from the underside of the breast (inframammary), with the incision being made in the skin fold formed by the bottom margin of the breast. A small scar will result. A second incision site is around the outer edge of the areola of the nipple (circumareolar). Scarring is minimal and hardly noticeable. A third approach is through an incision under the armpit (axillary). This leaves no scar on the breast but is technically more difficult.

The underlying pectoralis major muscle is separated from the fascia beneath it, creating a pocket for the implant. The implant is inserted and attached to adjacent tissue. The pocket is closed with sutures that will dissolve and do not have to be removed; the skin is carefully closed. The patient is seen approximately a week after surgery for a check-up and removal of any skin sutures.

Limited breast reduction can be achieved through dietary restrictions. Once a normal weight for body height is achieved, however, additional breast reduction through dieting is undesirable. Surgical reduction involves the removal of tissue. The amount and location of tissue to be removed depends on the initial size of the breast. Commonly, tissue is removed from the most dependent (lowest) portion of the breast. It is important to preserve the nipple and immediately underlying structures: the nerves and lactic ducts.

Vertical incisions are made in the underside of the breast. The excess tissue is removed, preserving the nipple, areola, nerves, and connecting ducts. A wedge-shaped portion of skin is also removed. After all bleeding is stopped, the remaining breast tissue is sutured together and the skin carefully closed. Care in closure and immediate postoperative

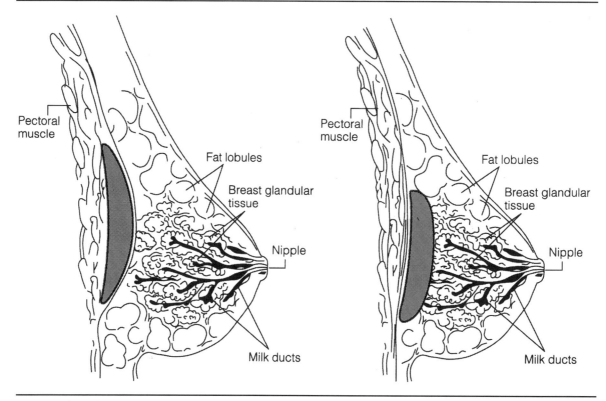

Breast implants for augmentation or reconstruction can be placed behind the pectoral muscle (left) or in front of it (right).

activity will minimize scarring. The breast should be adequately supported, and stretching should be avoided for the first few weeks after surgery. The patient returns in a week so that the surgeon can monitor healing and remove skin sutures.

Reconstruction of breast tissue for reasons other than those described above is similar. In cases of trauma, damaged tissue is debrided, underlying tissues are replaced and sutured together, and the skin is carefully closed. The nipple, areola, and nerves are protected and preserved to the greatest extent possible. Skin closure may require assistance from a plastic surgeon to minimize scarring.

USES AND COMPLICATIONS

Breast surgery is useful to correct breast ptosis (sagging). Sagging occurs with normal aging and the influence of gravity. The extent and severity of this condition are functions of the size of the breast, the adequacy of undergarment support, and position of the nipple. With minimal ptosis, a prosthesis can be inserted to provide internal support. With severe ptosis, a combination of tissue removal and relocation of the nipple and areola are performed simultaneously. These procedures can usually be done using local anesthesia on an outpatient basis.

Two potential complications of all breast surgery are infection and scarring. Infections are infrequent but must be treated aggressively when they occur. If a prosthesis is involved, it is usually removed and reinserted three to six months later. Scarring is of concern because breast surgery is most often undertaken for cosmetic or aesthetic reasons. The placement of incisions along skin folds and careful skin closure help to minimize scarring. Restricting immediate postoperative activities, especially those that require stretching, also reduces untoward scarring.

Two potential problems exist with the use of prostheses: contracture and leakage. Contracture occurs when the tissue immediately surrounding the prostheses shrinks and pulls the prosthesis out of position, detracting from the normal appearance of the breast. This condition formerly occurred in approximately 25 percent of cases but has been largely eliminated through the use of a textured outer envelope. Microscopic surface variations provide anchoring points for tissue and deter contracture formation. When both inner and outer envelopes rupture, the implant material can reach adjacent tissues. Silicone is irritating and can lead to the formation of nodules. Saline is now the material of choice for filling breast prostheses. Such leaks have received widespread attention in the media, but they are uncommon. In recent years, the legal climate has led to the virtual withdrawal of all silicone-based products from use in North America. Saline implants have been widely and safely used.

PERSPECTIVE AND PROSPECTS

With the exception of repairing the effects of unexpected trauma, most breast surgery is undertaken for cosmetic or aesthetic reasons. Individuals are influenced by those around them and by messages received from the media concerning what breast size and shape are desirable. Although these values change over time, it is more difficult to alter breast tissue. Aging plays a role. Supportive elements within tissues break down with age, resulting in unwanted but inevitable sagging of tissues.

Breast size, shape, and integrity are intimately related to feelings of self-worth and confidence. Reduction is indicated for massively oversized breasts. Augmentation is indicated in instances of pathology that require removal of a portion of breast tissue. Augmentation is an uncommon medical reason for enlarging genetically small breasts.

While what constitutes "massive" or "small" is ultimately a personal decision, the media, peers, and family members all exert pressures. Because most people would like to improve or alter their appearance, they are susceptible to the messages that reach them. Some women who are dissatisfied with their breasts may benefit from noninvasive approaches such as altering their eating and exercise habits. Others may need to improve their general self-image in order to accept their bodies as they are. Thus, only a relatively few remain as true candidates for breast surgery. The surgical techniques and procedures are available, but it is unusual that the hand of a skilled surgeon can improve on natural endowments over the longer term of a lifetime.

—*L. Fleming Fallon, Jr., M.D., M.P.H.*

See also Aging; Breast biopsy; Breast cancer; Breast disorders; Breasts, female; Grafts and grafting; Mammography; Mastectomy and lumpectomy; Oncology; Plastic, cosmetic, and reconstructive surgery; Sex change surgery.

FOR FURTHER INFORMATION:

Bostwick, John. *Aesthetic and Reconstructive Breast Surgery*. St. Louis: Matthew Medical Books, 1990. This textbook presents an excellent discussion of cosmetic and reconstructive breast surgery.

Georgiade, Nicholas G., ed. *Aesthetic Breast Surgery*. 7th ed. Philadelphia: W. B. Saunders, 1990. This book describes procedures for cosmetic breast surgery. It is written by internationally recognized authorities and well illustrated.

Guthrie, Randolph, and Doug Podolsky. *The Truth About Breast Implants*. New York: John Wiley & Sons, 1994. This book helps to clear away the confusion and anxiety surrounding the silicone implant controversy. The author is a plastic surgeon who details the safest techniques now available to women, tells how to find the right doctor, and explains what women should expect at every step for both breast reconstruction and enlargement.

BREAST BIOPSY

PROCEDURE

ANATOMY OR SYSTEM AFFECTED: Breasts (female)
SPECIALTIES AND RELATED FIELDS: General surgery, gynecology

DEFINITION: The surgical removal of a lump or tissue from the breast to determine whether it is malignant.

INDICATIONS AND PROCEDURES

Among American women, breast cancer is the most common malignancy. (While men can have breast cancer, such cases are relatively rare.) Women have learned the importance of regular self-examination of their breasts and the need to report suspicious lumps and other changes to a physician. Women finding suspicious lumps is the most common indication for breast biopsy to be done. Mammography (an X ray of the breasts) is also used as a cancer screening tool, and suspicious findings often lead to biopsy. Some physicians use breast ultrasound to determine whether biopsy is needed.

Many techniques are used to conduct a breast biopsy. The physician can use a thin needle and syringe to collect cells from suspicious areas (fine needle aspiration). Often, draining a cyst (a fluid-filled sac) is the only treatment needed. Surgeons can conduct a core needle biopsy, using a needle with a cutting edge to cut out a small piece of tissue. Small lumps are often removed in an excisional biopsy (lumpectomy). When lumps are larger, the surgeon may do an incisional biopsy to remove part of the lump for further examination. When no lump is present but suspicious tissue has been revealed by mammography, the surgeon can use the X ray to place small needles in order to remove tissue samples.

Pathologists examine the lump, tissue, or cells removed from the breast to determine whether cancer is present. If cancer is found, the patient has several treatment options, including removal of part or all of the breast, lumpectomy with radiation therapy, chemotherapy, or hormone therapy.

—*Russell Williams, M.S.W.*

See also Biopsy; Breast augmentation, reduction, and reconstruction; Breast cancer; Breast disorders; Breasts, female; Cancer; Cyst removal; Cysts and ganglions; Gynecology; Mammography; Mastectomy and lumpectomy; Mastitis; Oncology; Pathology; Plastic, cosmetic, and reconstructive surgery; Tumor removal; Tumors.

FOR FURTHER INFORMATION:

DeVita, Vincent, et al., eds. *Cancer: Principles and Practice of Oncology*. 5th ed. Philadelphia: J. B. Lippincott, 1997.

Greenfield, Lazar, ed. *Surgery: Scientific Principles and Practice*. Philadelphia: J. B. Lippincott, 1993.

U.S. Department of Health and Human Services, Public Health Service, and National Institutes of Health. *Breast Biopsy: What You Should Know*. Bethesda, Md.: Author, 1990.

BREAST CANCER

DISEASE/DISORDER

ANATOMY OR SYSTEM AFFECTED: Breasts, glands, lymphatic system

SPECIALTIES AND RELATED FIELDS: Genetics; gynecology; oncology; plastic, cosmetic, and reconstructive surgery

DEFINITION: Malignancy occurring in breast tissue and possibly involving the associated lymph nodes.

KEY TERMS:

adjuvant therapy: therapy used in addition to surgery in order to control the growth of remaining cancer cells

benign: not cancerous

BRCA1, BRCA2: genes associated with hereditary forms of breast cancer

chemotherapy: adjuvant therapy which uses drugs to kill cancer cells

malignant: cancerous

metastasis: the spread of cancer cells from a tumor to other sites in the body

CAUSES AND SYMPTOMS

Genetic and familial risk factors. Some families have a clear history of breast cancer. It is estimated that nearly 10 percent of the 180,000 diagnosed cases of breast cancer in the United States have developed because of some hereditary defect. Research efforts have intensified to isolate the genes associated with this form of cancer. In 1994, the first such gene association with hereditary forms, BRCA1, was isolated; shortly afterward, a second gene, BRCA2, was also shown to be linked to hereditary forms of breast cancer. Clinicians may be able to use a simple blood test to screen women for the presence of the defective gene and therefore identify those with an increased risk of developing breast cancer. Any clustering of breast cancer within a family, especially among immediate family members, is probably indicative of hereditary or familial breast cancer. This is especially true when family members develop breast cancer at an early age, particularly at or before the mid-forties. Women with a family history of breast cancer should seek regular screening and counseling regarding the best-known methods of prevention and therapy. Current preventive methods include modification of diet and lifestyle, hormonal treatment with antiestrogens such as tamoxifen, and prophylactic (preventive) mastectomies.

Diet. Although the exact role that diet may play in the development of breast cancer is still unclear, there is evidence to indicate that factors such as dietary fat may increase the risk for the development of this disease. Comparison of the rates of breast cancer in different countries throughout the world show that certain populations, such as women in Japan and China, tend to have much lower rates of breast cancer than Caucasians in the United States. Not only is their total intake of fat much lower than that of American women (15 percent versus 40 percent of total calories), but as their intake of fat increases (as seen in Asian families that have moved to the United States and adopted Westernized diets) so have their rates of breast cancer. Since fat has also been linked to an increased risk for the development of colon cancer and heart disease, it has been recommended that the overall consumption of fat in the diet be limited to less than 30 percent of total calo-

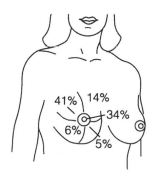

Breast cancer sites
and incidence of
occurrence

Common sites of breast cancer.

ries. Vitamins and certain minerals may also be effective in helping to prevent breast cancer. Vitamins A, C, and E are antioxidants that have been shown to protect cells from cancer-causing chemicals. Some minerals such as selenium and zinc also appear to have a protective effect on cells. Adequate amounts of these nutrients should be included in the diet, either through consumption of vegetables, fruits, and grains, which supply these nutrients, or through supplements. Several studies have demonstrated a link between alcohol consumption and breast cancer. Alcohol consumption, even in moderate amounts, can increase a woman's risk for breast cancer, an effect which is even more evident in women who consumed alcohol at a young age. This causal relationship does not, however, appear to affect women who are close to the menopause. It seems that the main effect of alcohol, as with fat, may be during the period of a woman's reproductive lifetime, when breast cells are most vulnerable to genetic damage.

Reproductive and hormonal factors. Three major reproductive-related events influence a woman's risk for the development of breast cancer: the age when menstruation begins (menarche), the age at first full-term pregnancy, and the age when the menopause occurs. An increased risk of breast cancer has been found in women who have started menstruation before the age of twelve, who have had their first full-term pregnancy after the age of thirty, and/or who enter the menopause after the age of fifty-five. These findings indicate that reproductive hormones such as estrogen may play a role in the development of breast cancer. The apparent association between reproductive hormones and breast cancer raises concerns about potential risks associated with birth control pills (oral contraceptives) or postmenopausal estrogen replacement pills. Studies to date show some evidence that the use of oral contraceptives slightly increases the risk of developing breast cancer, but the risks depend upon many factors, including type of birth

control pill used, age when use is started, and overall duration of use. The potential risk of using oral contraceptives must be weighed against other risks associated with alternative contraceptives, unwanted pregnancies, or abortion. Postmenopausal women have been treated with ovarian hormones (estrogen with or without progesterone) to alleviate the symptoms of the menopause and, more recently, to reduce the risks of osteoporosis and ischemic heart disease. There are few definitive data to establish a clear association between such hormone replacement therapy and an increased risk for the development of breast cancer. Again, the potential risk associated with the use of these hormones, even by women who have had breast cancer or who are at high risk for the development of breast cancer, must be weighed against such factors as a potential high risk for osteoporosis or heart disease or against the severity of menopausal symptoms.

Psychosocial aspects. Findings from a number of studies have suggested an association between psychological factors and disease outcome in breast cancer patients. It has been shown that women who are described by their physicians as having a "fighting spirit" live significantly longer than more passive women. Recent studies have also demonstrated that participation of cancer patients in psychosocial support groups significantly increases survival time. These and other findings suggest that suppression of negative feelings, severe stress, and lack of social support predict a poorer outcome with cancer. Conversely, patient assertiveness and sense of control, especially when enhanced by social support, appear to improve the course of this disease. How these psychological factors influence the immune system is being investigated.

Mammography and breast self-examination. Two methods of screening for breast cancer are mammography (an X ray of the breast) and breast self-examination. Routine use of both of these screening methods can help to detect breast cancer at earlier stages, where surgery and chemotherapy have been shown to be highly effective. It is recommended that a breast self-examination be done once a month. If the woman is menstruating, the best time to perform the examination is two or three days after the end of the cycle, when the breasts are not swollen or tender. If a woman is not menstruating, she should pick one day per month, such as the first or last day of the month, to do a breast self-examination. Women learning how to examine their breasts may want to perform the examination once a week until they learn how their breast tissue changes over time. Once familiar with the changes in their breasts, they can check the tissue only once a month. In addition, doctors should examine the breasts during routine medical checkups. Although there is some controversy surrounding mammograms before the age of fifty, it is currently recommended that routine mammograms be scheduled between the ages of forty and fifty. After the age of fifty, women

Breast Self-Examination

Visual exam

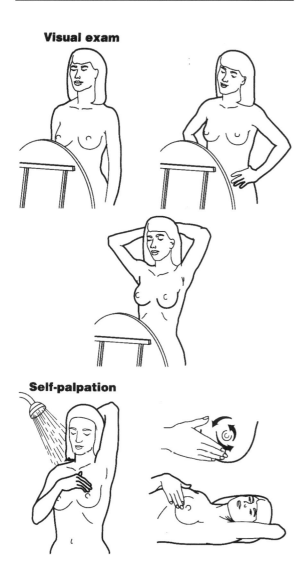

Self-palpation

Women should examine their breasts both visually, to detect any changes in appearance, such as size, asymmetries (one breast suddenly, as opposed to historically, larger than the other), "peau d'orange"—the appearance of dimpled skin resembling orange peel—and other unusual features. Women should also apply pressure to their breasts, working circularly from the nipple to the far periphery of the breast (including the underarms), to determine the presence of any lumps or other unusual nodules. Self-exam should be combined with routine visits to a physician and regular mammograms, which can detect cancer long before it develops into a palpable lump.

should have mammograms scheduled every year or every other year, coinciding with their routine physicals.

Following an unusual mammogram reading or the discovery of a suspicious lump, a biopsy is required to evaluate fully whether cancer is present. A biopsy may be done by one of the following techniques: a fine-needle aspirate (the collection of cells within a lump by a small needle, done on an outpatient basis); a needle biopsy (the removal of a core of tissue with a needle, done on an outpatient basis); an incisional biopsy (the removal of a wedge of tissue, done on an outpatient basis); or an excisional biopsy (the removal of the entire lump, which may require general anesthesia).

Most breast cancers (86 percent) begin within the ducts of the breast. A much smaller percentage (12 percent) develops within the lobules, with the remainder (2 percent) developing in surrounding tissue. A ductal or lobular cancer that has not grown outside the duct is called ductal or lobular carcinoma in situ, noninvasive carcinoma, or simply intraductal (intralobular) carcinoma. A ductal or lobular cancer that has grown outside the duct is called invasive or infiltrating carcinoma.

TREATMENT AND THERAPY

Treatment for breast cancer depends upon the age of the woman (premenopausal or postmenopausal), the extent of the local tumor invasion, the size of the tumor, the aggressiveness of the cancer cells, the number of regional lymph nodes involved, and whether cancer is detected in distant organs (metastasis). Standard treatment options include surgery, radiation therapy, and adjuvant therapy (chemotherapy and/or hormonal therapy).

Surgical options include lumpectomy (the removal of the tumor mass only), partial mastectomy (the removal of a wedge of breast tissue), quandrantectomy (the removal of at least 2 to 3 centimeters of normal tissue around the tumor and the excision of the overlying skin of that quadrant), mastectomy (the removal of all breast tissue, surrounding skin, and regional lymph nodes), and radical mastectomy (the removal of all breast tissue, skin, underlying pectoral muscle, and lymph nodes). New studies are indicating that the timing of surgery relative to the stage of the menstrual cycle in premenopausal women may affect long-term survival. It appears that having surgery during the luteal phase (the second half of the woman's menstrual cycle) favorably influences survival.

Radiation therapy is designed to treat a specific area (unlike chemotherapy, which travels through the bloodstream and affects the entire body). Radiation therapy is administered by a linear accelerator, which shoot radioactive particles directly at a clearly defined region of the body (the breast area and possibly the lymph nodes). Radiation therapy is usually administered one day a week for a given number of weeks. Breast conservation therapy, consisting of excision of the primary tumor and a limited amount of adjacent breast tissue followed by radiation therapy, has been proven to be as effective as mastectomy for early stage breast cancer.

Adjuvant therapy, including chemotherapy and/or hormonal therapy, is indicated for all node-positive patients. Chemotherapy is the use of drugs designed to kill actively dividing cancer cells. More than one kind of drug is typically used because different drugs interfere with the process of cell division in different ways, making the overall treatment more effective. Since these toxic drugs act on dividing cells, they also kill actively dividing normal cells such as hair cells and bone marrow cells. It is important that the bone marrow, which gives rise to red blood cells and white blood cells (immune cells), be allowed to recover from the effects of chemotherapy. Giving chemotherapy in cycles rather than all at once not only helps the bone marrow to recover but also kills cancer cells that may be actively dividing at different times. Hormonal therapy is designed to alter the growth of hormone-sensitive cancer cells. Some cancer cells need estrogen to grow. It has been shown that either removing endogenous sources of estrogen (by removing the ovaries) or giving antiestrogens such as tamoxifen helps to control the growth of these cancer cells. Tamoxifen is frequently used in postmenopausal women, and the drug is being tested in a large clinical trial to help prevent breast cancer in healthy, but high-risk, women.

PERSPECTIVE AND PROSPECTS

Breast cancer is on the rise throughout the Western world. In the United States, it is the second leading cause of cancer deaths: In 1994, it was estimated that 180,000 women would be diagnosed with breast cancer and that nearly 50,000 would die from the disease that year. The overall lifetime risk of developing breast cancer in the United States is 11 percent, which means that one out of nine women will develop breast cancer by the age of eighty-five. Multiple environmental, lifestyle, and genetic factors are believed to be involved in the development of this disease, and the increase in risk has been associated with changing environmental and lifestyle patterns.

The Isolation of BRCA1 and BRCA2

Epidemiological studies among breast cancer patients carried out by Mary-Claire King during the early 1980's suggested a genetic basis for some forms of the disease. While most of the nearly 180,000 cases diagnosed each year appear randomly, from 10 to 20 percent of cases appear to be clustered within families. While similar observations had previously been reported, King suggested that the clustering was consistent with a role played by a single gene; in 1990, she mapped the gene to chromosome 17.

In 1994, a team led by Mark Skolnick determined the precise location of the gene, which they named BRCA1. Mutations in the BRCA1 gene were found in approximately 12 percent of women with early-onset forms of breast cancer, those diagnosed before the age of thirty. Mutations associated with the same gene were also linked to certain forms of familial ovarian cancers.

Mutated forms of the BRCA1 gene, however, could be found in only half of all cases of familial breast cancer, suggesting the presence of an additional gene or genes associated with this form of the disease. In 1994 and 1995, a team led by Michael Stratton pinpointed a second gene, located on chromosome 13, which also predisposed women to hereditary forms of the disease; they named the gene BRCA2. Mutations in BRCA2 also appear to predispose men to a rare form of hereditary breast cancer.

The actual function of the products of the BRCA1 and BRCA2 genes, and the role that they play in cancer, is uncertain. Both protein products appear to interact with enzymes that function in the repair of damaged DNA. If so, the absence of BRCA1 or BRCA2 function may predispose certain tissues to greater risk of environmental damage or mutation, leading to cancer development.

Germline mutations (those present at birth) in either of the two genes appear to account for nearly all forms of hereditary breast cancers. The mutations are found in disproportionate numbers of Jewish women of Ashkenazi ancestry. More than 1 percent of these women carry mutations in the BRCA1 gene, accounting for 20 percent of breast cancers among young Jewish women. Approximately 80 percent of these women are at risk of developing cancer over the course of their life span; while the risk of cancer among women in the general population carrying similar mutations is uncertain, women with the mutations clearly have a genetic predisposition toward the disease.

With the isolation of the genes associated with hereditary forms of breast (and ovarian) cancer, it is now possible actively to screen women who are most at risk. For women who are determined to carry a mutated form of one of the genes, the benefits are clear. Counseling these women is still a matter of contention, however, and is an area of growing concern among both patients and their physicians. Furthermore, the implications of a negative test are still less than clear; nonhereditary forms of the disease are still far more common. There is also the question of insurance coverage for women at risk, including coverage for procedures that might fall in the category of preemptive treatment, such as breast removal. Similar arguments have been posed in screening for other forms of hereditary diseases. —*Richard Adler, Ph.D.*

Clinicians and researchers are constantly evaluating new methods to control the growth of cancer cells. New treatments that are being tested in clinical trials throughout the United States include the use of monoclonal antibodies, the use of paclitaxel (Taxol), and the administration of cancer vaccines. Monoclonal antibodies are made in laboratories. These antibodies are similar to those that the body makes against foreign invaders (bacteria and viruses), except that monoclonal antibodies can be made to bind specifically to cancer cells. Monoclonal antibodies that have been tagged with chemicals detectable by a scanner can be used to find cancer cells in the body. Monoclonal antibodies can also be tagged with radioactive substances or poisons which directly kill cancer cells and spare normal cells. Taxol is a drug which has been isolated from the yew tree. This drug acts by preventing cancer cells from dividing and is being tested in patients with recurrent breast cancer. Several centers in the United States and Canada are testing vaccines designed to fight cancer cells. Specific molecules that are found on tumor cells and not on normal cells are being used as injectable vaccines to stimulate the production of antibodies against cancer cells.

—*Sylvia Adams Oliver, Ph.D.*
updated by Richard Adler, Ph.D.

See also Breast augmentation, reduction, and reconstruction; Breast biopsy; Breast disorders; Breasts, female; Cancer; Chemotherapy; Gynecology; Malignancy and metastasis; Mammography; Mastectomy and lumpectomy; Oncology; Radiation therapy.

FOR FURTHER INFORMATION:

Boston Women's Health Collective. *The New Our Bodies, Ourselves.* New York: Touchstone-Simon & Schuster, 1992.

Davies, Kevin. *Breakthrough: The Race to Find the Breast Cancer Gene.* New York: John Wiley & Sons, 1996.

Love, Susan, and Karen Lindsey. *Dr. Susan Love's Breast Book.* 2d ed. Reading, Mass.: Addison-Wesley, 1995.

Murphy, G., L. Morris, and D. Lange. *Informed Decisions: The Complete Book of Cancer Diagnosis, Treatment, and Recovery.* New York: Viking Press, 1997.

Varmus, Harold, and Robert Weinberg. *Genes and the Biology of Cancer.* New York: W. H. Freeman, 1993.

BREAST DISORDERS

DISEASE/DISORDER

ANATOMY OR SYSTEM AFFECTED: Breasts, glands, lymphatic system

SPECIALTIES AND RELATED FIELDS: Genetics; gynecology; plastic, cosmetic, and reconstructive surgery

DEFINITION: A variety of noncancerous breast conditions. "Fibrocystic condition or disease" is an umbrella term which has been used to define these disorders, which include swelling and tenderness, cysts, mastalgia (breast pain), infections and inflammations (mastitis), nipple dis-

charge, fibroadenomas, and epithelial proliferation of varying degrees. These conditions are known to occur in approximately 90 percent of women. Although a diagnosis of fibrocystic disease was previously thought to increase a woman's risk for the development of breast cancer, further studies and the reevaluation of older data have shown that only a small percentage of these women later develop carcinoma in either breast. The following are brief descriptions of commonly occurring, benign breast conditions.

Mastalgia. Also commonly termed mastodynia, mastalgia is defined as breast pain. Cyclic mastalgia has been associated with reproductive hormones such as estrogen and progesterone since breast tenderness and pain tend to occur just before menstruation with the symptoms becoming less intense once bleeding starts. The most promising therapies include hormonal treatment (birth control pills or progesterone ointments) and the modification of diet (avoiding fatty and fried foods, reducing the consumption of caffeine-containing beverages, and taking vitamin supplements, especially of vitamins E and B). Noncyclical pain occurs much less frequently than cyclical pain. The occurrence of this type of breast pain does not vary with the menstrual cycle and typically occurs in a single, localized spot. The cause of this pain is not fully understood.

Fibroadenomas. Lumps that typically develop during the teenage years through the twenties and that do not fluctuate during the menstrual cycle are called fibroadenomas. These benign lumps are smooth and round, and they move freely within the breast tissue. Although the lumps may last throughout a woman's lifetime once they appear, they can easily be removed surgically. The conditions that cause the growth of fibroadenomas are unknown.

Cysts. Breast cysts are found in approximately 60 percent of premenopausal women. They occur most often in women who are approaching the menopause, but they also develop when a woman is in her thirties and forties. Cysts are fluid-filled sacs, much like blisters, that develop within the breast tissue. Cysts may feel pliable if they are near the surface of the breast or may feel hard, much like a lump, if they are located deep within the breast tissue. The fluid within the cyst can easily be removed by needle aspiration in a doctor's office. Cysts are almost never malignant and do not increase a woman's risk of developing breast cancer.

Infections and inflammations. The breast may become inflamed or infected because of lactational mastitis, nonlactational mastitis, or chronic subareolar abscesses. Lactational mastitis is the result of a localized bacterial infection which occurs most often within a blocked duct. Nonlactational mastitis typically occurs in a woman whose immune system is depressed; it is an infection which usually involves the skin of the breast and therefore covers a larger area of the breast than lactational mastitis. Both of these conditions can be treated with antibiotics. Chronic subareolar abscesses are infections of the small, dead-end glands

Common Breast Disorders

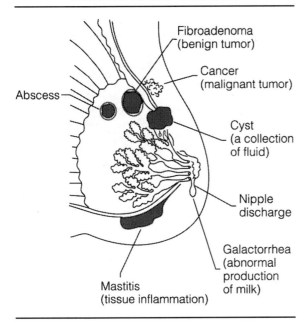

Abscess

Fibroadenoma (benign tumor)

Cancer (malignant tumor)

Cyst (a collection of fluid)

Nipple discharge

Galactorrhea (abnormal production of milk)

Mastitis (tissue inflammation)

that surround the nipple. These abscesses appear as localized hot areas on the border of the nipple, much like a boil. If caught early, they can be treated with antibiotics; if not, the abscess and gland must be surgically removed.

Nipple discharge. Discharge from the nipple is a common occurrence in women of all ages and reproductive histories. Although naturally occurring, nipple discharge should be checked if it is unilateral (occurring in one breast), spontaneous, and persistent. These symptoms could be attributable to intraductal papilloma (wartlike growths), intraductal papillomatosis, intraductal carcinoma in situ, or invasive cancer. Only about 4 percent of spontaneous unilateral bloody discharges are the result of cancer. In galactorrhea, an increase in prolactin production causes the abnormal discharge of breast milk in a woman who is not lactating. Each of these conditions requires a different treatment, which can be discussed with a physician.

Epithelial dysplasia and hyperplasia. The abnormal, but benign, growth of the epithelial cells that form the ductal branching of the breast tissue is termed epithelial dysplasia, while epithelial hyperplasia refers to an abnormal increase in the number of nonmalignant cells in a normal tissue arrangement. The degree of abnormality of these cells can be determined through the histological (microscopic) examination of breast tissue obtained during a biopsy. Epithelial dysplasia can be divided into three main categories: nonproliferative (mild hyperplasia, cysts, epithelial-related calcifications, fibroadenomas), proliferative (mild-to-moderate hyperplasia, papillomas, sclerosing adenosis), and atypical hyperplasia. Biopsy-proven atypical hyperplasia of the

breast tissue has been shown to increase a woman's risk of developing breast cancer significantly, especially if the woman has a family history of breast cancer.

—*Sylvia Adams Oliver, Ph.D.*

See also Breast biopsy; Breast-feeding; Breasts, female; Cyst removal; Cysts and ganglions; Mastitis.

FOR FURTHER INFORMATION:

Boston Women's Health Collective. *The New Our Bodies, Ourselves.* New York: Touchstone-Simon & Schuster, 1992.

Epps, R., and the American Medical Women's Association, eds. *The Women's Complete Handbook.* New York: Dell Books, 1995.

Love, Susan, and Karen Lindsey. *Dr. Susan Love's Breast Book.* 2d ed. Reading, Mass.: Addison-Wesley, 1995.

BREAST-FEEDING

BIOLOGY

ANATOMY OR SYSTEM AFFECTED: Breasts, glands, reproductive system

SPECIALTIES AND RELATED FIELDS: Gynecology, nutrition, obstetrics, perinatology

DEFINITION: The preferred feeding method for infants, providing optimal nutrition for the infant (including immunologic protection), mother-infant bonding, and enhanced maternal health.

KEY TERMS:

alveoli: the milk-producing cells of the mammary gland

bifidus factors: factors in colostrum and breast milk that favor the growth of helpful bacteria in the infant's intestinal tract

bonding: a process in which a mother forms an affectionate attachment to her infant immediately after birth

colostrum: the secretion from the breast before the onset of milk

foremilk: the milk released early in a nursing session, which is low in fat and rich in nutrients

hindmilk: the milk released late in a nursing session, which is higher in fat content

lactoferrin: a breast milk factor that binds iron, preventing it from supporting the growth of harmful intestinal bacteria; it may also promote the ability to absorb dietary iron

let-down reflex: the reflex that forces milk to the front of the breast

oxytocin: the hormone secreted from the posterior pituitary gland that stimulates the mammary glands to eject milk; it also stimulates the uterus to contract after birth

prolactin: a hormone secreted from the anterior pituitary gland that signals the breast to start and sustain milk production

PROCESS AND EFFECTS

The terms "breast-feeding," "nursing," and "lactation" all refer to the best-known method of infant feeding. Although there are a few rare exceptions, almost every mother can breast-feed and thereby provide low-cost, nutritional support for her infant. Although it is often thought otherwise, the size of the mother's breast has no relationship to successful lactation. In fact, the physiology of successful lactation is determined by the maturation of breast tissue, the initiation and maintenance of milk secretion, and the ejection or delivery of milk to the nipple. This physiology is dependent on hormonal control, and all women have the required anatomy for successful lactation unless they have had surgical alteration of the breast.

Hormonal influence on breast development begins in adolescence. Increased estrogen causes the breast ducts to elongate and duct cells to grow. (The ducts are narrow tubular vessels that run from the segments of the breast into the tip of the nipple.) More fibrous and fatty tissue develops, and the nipple area matures. As adolescence progresses, regular menstrual cycle hormones cause further development of the alveoli, which are the milk-producing cells.

The elevated levels of estrogen present during pregnancy promote the growth and branching of milk ducts, while the increase in progesterone promotes the development of alveoli. Throughout pregnancy and especially during the first three months, many more milk ducts are formed. Clusters of milk-producing cells also begin to enlarge, while at the same time placental hormones promoted breast development.

Shortly before labor and delivery, the hormone prolactin is produced by the pituitary gland. Prolactin, which is necessary for starting lactation and sustaining milk production, reaches its peak at delivery. Another hormone, oxytocin, which is also produced by the pituitary, stimulates the breast to eject milk. This reaction is called the "let-down reflex," which causes the milk-producing alveoli to contract and force milk to the front of the breast. Oxytocin serves an important function after delivery by causing the uterus to contract. Initially, the let-down reflex occurs only when the infant suckles, but later on it may be initiated simply by the baby's cry. An efficient let-down reflex is critical to successful breast-feeding. Emotional upset, fatigue, pain, nervousness, or embarrassment about lactation can interrupt this reflex; these psychological factors, rather than breast size or physiology, are predictive of successful lactation.

Not only is breast-feeding a natural response to childbirth, but the nutrient content is tailor-made for the human infant as well. More than one hundred constituents of breast milk, both nutritive and nonnutritive, are known. Although the basic nutrient content is a solution of protein, sugar, and salts in which fat is suspended, those concentrations vary depending on the period of lactation and even within a given feeding.

Colostrum, often called "first milk," is produced in the first few days after birth. It is lower in fat and Calories

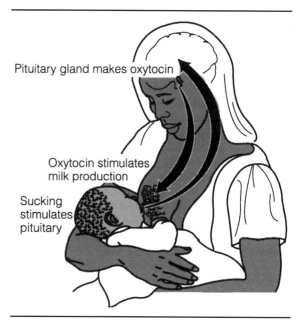

Breast-feeding involves a hormonal feedback loop that encourages milk production.

(kilocalories) and higher in protein and certain minerals than is mature breast milk. Colostrum is opaque and yellow because it contains a high concentration of the vitamin A–like substances called carotenes. It also has a high concentration of antibodies and white blood cells, which pass on immunologic protection to the infant.

Within a few days after birth, the transition is made from colostrum to mature milk. There are two types of mature milk. Foremilk is released first as the infant begins to suckle. It has a watery, bluish appearance and is low in fat and rich in other nutrients. This milk accounts for about one-third of the baby's intake. As the nursing session progresses, the draught reflex helps move the hindmilk, with its higher fat content, to the front of the breast. It is important that the nutrient content of breast milk be determined from a sample of both types of milk in order to make an adequate assessment of all nutrients present.

Breast milk best meets the infant's needs and is the standard from which infant formulas are judged. Several nutrient characteristics make it the ideal infant food. Lactose, the carbohydrate content of breast milk, is the same simple sugar found in any milk, but the protein content of breast milk is uniquely tailored to meet infant needs. An infant's immature kidneys are better able to maintain water balance because breast milk is lower in protein than cow's milk. Most breast milk protein is alpha-lactalbumin, whereas cow's milk protein is casein. Alpha-lactalbumin is easier to digest and provides two sulphur-containing amino acids that are the building blocks of protein required for infant growth.

The fat (lipid) content of breast milk differs among women, and even from the same woman, from day to day. The types of fatty acids that make up most of the fat component of the milk may vary in response to maternal diet. Mothers fed a diet containing corn and cottonseed oil produce a milk with more polyunsaturated fatty acids, which are the predominant fatty acids in those oils. Breast milk is higher in the essential fatty acid called linoleic acid than is cow's milk, and it also contains omega-3 fatty acids. About 55 percent of human milk Calories come from fat, compared to about 49 percent of Calories found in infant formulas. In addition, enzymes in breast milk help digest fat in the infant's stomach. This digested fat is more efficiently absorbed than the products that result from digesting cow's milk.

Breast milk contains more cholesterol than cow's milk, which seems to stimulate development of the enzymes necessary for degrading cholesterol, perhaps offering protection against atherosclerosis in later life. Cholesterol is also needed for proper development of the central nervous system.

The vitamin and mineral content of breast milk from healthy mothers supplies all that is needed for growth and health except for vitamin D and fluoride, and these are easily supplemented. Breast milk and the infant's intestinal bacteria also supply all the necessary vitamin K, but since no bacteria are present at birth, an injection of vitamin K should be given to prevent deficiencies.

Breast milk mineral content is balanced to promote growth while protecting the infant's immature kidneys. Breast milk has a low sodium content, which helps the immature kidneys to maintain water balance. No type of milk is a good source of iron. Although breast milk contains relatively small amounts of iron, about 50 percent of this iron can be absorbed by the body, compared to only 4 percent from cow's milk. This phenomenon is called bioavailability. Because of the high bioavailability of breast milk iron, the introduction of solids, which are given to replace depleted iron stores, can be delayed until six months of age in most infants; this delay may help to reduce the incidence of allergies in susceptible infants. There is also evidence that zinc is better absorbed from breast milk.

The vitamin content of milk can vary and is influenced by maternal vitamin status. The water-soluble vitamin content of breast milk (the B vitamins and vitamin C) will change more because of maternal diet than the fat-soluble vitamin content (vitamins A, E, and K). If women have diets that are deficient in vitamins, their levels in breast milk will be lower. Yet even malnourished mothers can breast-feed, although the quantity of milk is decreased. As the maternal diet improves, the level of water-soluble vitamins in the milk increases. There is a level, however, above which additional diet supplements will not increase the vitamin content of breast milk.

There are many nonnutritive advantages to breast-feeding. A major advantage is the immunologic protection and resistance factors that it provides to the infant. Bifidus factors, found in both colostrum and mature milk, favor the growth of helpful bacteria in the infant's digestive tract. These bacteria in turn offer protection against harmful organisms. Lactoferrin, another resistance factor, binds iron so that harmful bacteria cannot use it. Lysozyme, lipases, and lactoperoxidases also offer protection against harmful bacteria.

Immunoglobulins are present in large amounts in colostrum and in significant amounts in breast milk. These protein compounds act as antibodies against foreign substances in the body called antigens. Generally, the resistance passed to the infant is from environmental antigens to which the mother had been exposed. The concentration of antibodies in colostrum is highest in the first hour after birth. Secretory IgA is the major immunoglobulin that provides protection against gastrointestinal organisms. Breast milk also contains interferon, an antiviral substance which is produced by special white blood cells in milk. Protection against allergy is another advantage of breast-feeding. It is not known, however, whether less exposure to the antigens found in formula or some substance in the breast milk itself provides this protection. Normally, a mucous barrier in the intestine prevents the absorption of whole proteins, the root of an allergic reaction. In the newborn, this barrier is not fully developed to allow whole immunologic proteins to be absorbed. The possibility that whole food proteins will be absorbed as well is greater if cow's milk or early solids are given, and this absorption increases the potential for allergic reactions.

Other possible benefits of breast-feeding are protection against the intestinal disorders Crohn's disease and celiac sprue and insulin-dependent diabetes. The reasons for this protection are not clear.

Breast-feeding encourages infant bonding, a process in which the mother forms an affectionate attachment to her baby. It is a matter of controversy whether breast-feeding mothers bond better than bottle-feeding mothers. If a mother has early and prolonged contact with her baby, however, the mother is more likely to breast-feed and to nurse her baby for more months.

Milk from mothers delivering preterm infants is higher in protein and nonprotein nitrogen, calcium, IgA, sodium, potassium, chloride, phosphorus, and magnesium. It also has a different fat composition and is lower in lactose than mature milk of mothers delivering after a normal term. These concentrations support more rapid growth of a preterm infant.

Breast-feeding is not only good for the baby but also good for the mother. There is an association between reduced breast cancer rates and breast-feeding, although the reason is not known. In addition, the hormonal influences caused by suckling the infant help to contract the uterus, returning it to prepregnancy size and controlling blood loss. Breast-feeding also helps to reduce the mother's weight. Calories required to make milk are drawn from the fat stores that were deposited during pregnancy. Nevertheless, breast-feeding should be viewed not as a quick weight loss program but as a healthful, natural weight loss process.

If a woman breast-feeds completely, which means that no supplements or solid foods are given until the baby is six months of age, often she will not menstruate. Many women find this lack of menstrual periods psychologically pleasant while not realizing the physiological benefit of restoring the iron stores that were depleted during pregnancy and delivery. An important advantage to breast-feeding in developing countries is that it can help to space pregnancies naturally. Most infant malnutrition occurs when the second child is born, because breast-feeding is stopped for the first child. The first child is weaned to foods that do not supply enough nutrients. By spacing pregnancies out, the first child has a chance to nurse longer.

Breast-feeding is very convenient and does not require time to mix and prepare formula or sterilize bottles. Breast milk is always sterile and at the proper temperature. The money needed for the extra food required to produce breast milk is much less than that required to purchase commercial formula. This can be a major benefit for women with low incomes and is critically important for the health of those babies born in developing countries.

COMPLICATIONS AND DISORDERS

Some special problems or circumstances can make breast-feeding difficult. The breasts may become engorged—so full of milk that they are hard and sore—making it difficult for the baby to latch onto the nipple. Gentle massaging of the breasts, especially with warm water or a heating pad, will allow release of the milk and reduce pain in the breast. This situation is common during the first few weeks of nursing but will occasionally recur if a feeding is missed or a schedule changes.

Sometimes a duct will become plugged and form a hard lump. Massaging the lump and continuing to nurse will remedy the situation. If influenza-like symptoms accompany a plugged duct, the cause is probably a breast infection. Since the infection is in the tissue around the milk-producing glands, the milk itself is safe. The mother must apply heat, get plenty of rest, and keep emptying the breast by frequent feedings. Stopping nursing would plug the duct further, making the infection worse.

Of concern to many mothers are reports of contaminants in breast milk. Drugs, environmental pollutants, viruses, caffeine, alcohol, and food allergens can be passed to the infant through breast milk. Drug transmission depends on the administration method, which influences the speed with which it reaches the blood supply to the breast. Whether that drug can remain functional after it is subjected to the

acid in the baby's digestive tract varies. Large amounts of caffeine in breast milk can produce a wakeful, hyperactive infant, but this situation is corrected when the mother stops her caffeine consumption. Large amounts of alcohol produce an altered facial appearance which is reversible; however, some psychomotor delay in the infant may remain even after the mother's drinking has stopped. Nicotine also enters milk, but the impact of secondhand smoke may pose more of a health threat than the nicotine content of breast milk. Since the human immunodeficiency virus (HIV), the virus that causes acquired immunodeficiency syndrome (AIDS), can also pass through breast milk, HIV-positive mothers should not breast-feed their infants.

Of greater concern is the presence of contaminants that cannot be avoided, such as pesticide residues, industrial waste, or other environmental contaminants. Polychlorinated biphenyls (PCBs) and the pesticide DDT have received the most attention. Long-term exposure to contaminants promotes their accumulation in the mother's body fat, and the production of breast milk is one way to rid the body of these contaminants. Concentrations present in the breast milk vary. Ordinarily, these substances are in such small quantities that they pose no health risk. Women who have consumed large amounts of fish from PCB-contaminated waters or have had occupational exposure to this chemical, however, need to have their breast milk tested. It is also possible for these substances to enter the infant's food supply from other sources.

PERSPECTIVE AND PROSPECTS

Although breast-feeding is the best method of infant feeding, many women choose not to breast-feed. Before the 1700's, human milk was the only source for infant feeding. If a mother did not breast-feed, a woman called a wet nurse fed her baby. At the end of the nineteenth century, formula feeding became popular when bottles were developed and water sanitation improved. Breast-feeding declined to less than 20 percent by 1970 but dramatically increased to 60 percent in the early 1980's.

Breast-feeding used to be more prevalent among more-educated, higher-income mothers. Increased employment of women outside the home, however, has dramatically altered trends in breast-feeding. Although mothers may opt to breast-feed in the hospital, many quit because they are returning to work and believe that it would be too difficult to continue. A working mother needs four to six weeks at home to establish successful breast-feeding.

Formula use has increased in developing countries. Because formula is very expensive, it is often diluted with water and therefore does not provide enough nutritional support to the infant. The quality of water is often so poor in these countries that the infant is exposed to disease-causing organisms. In addition, formula-fed infants do not receive the immunologic protection of breast milk. The result is a higher infant mortality rate.

There are very few instance in which a woman should not breast-feed her infant. Babies with a rare genetic disorder called galactosemia cannot nurse since they lack the enzyme to metabolize milk sugar. Phenylketonuria (PKU), another genetic disorder, requires close monitoring of the infant's blood phenylalanine level, but the infant can be totally or at least partially breast-fed. Breast-feeding is contraindicated for women suffering from AIDS, alcoholism, drug addiction, malaria, active tuberculosis, or a chronic disease that results in maternal malnutrition. The presence of other conditions, from diabetes to the common cold, are not reasons to avoid breast-feeding.

Lactation, the secretion of milk, is a physiological process, but breast-feeding is a learned practice, a philosophy about nurturing an infant that goes beyond nutritional support. Society needs to foster this practice. Unfortunately, the etiquette of nursing in public areas is not clearly defined, often resulting in embarrassment that inhibits mothers from nursing their babies. The only remedy is for society to recognize that the normal function of breasts is to nurture infants. Breast-feeding represents a vital resource that improves the health and nutritional status of children, especially in underdeveloped countries.

—*Wendy L. Stuhldreher, Ph.D., R.D.*

See also Breast disorders; Breasts, female; Glands; Hormones; Mastitis; Nutrition; Perinatology; Phenylketonuria (PKU); Pregnancy and gestation.

For Further Information:

Bennett, Peter N., Allan Astrup-Jensen, et al., eds. *Drugs and Human Lactation*. New York: Elsevier, 1996. This book on the health aspects of breast-feeding is subtitled *A Comprehensive Guide to the Content of Consequences of Drugs, Micronutrients, Radiopharmaceuticals, and Environmental and Occupational Chemicals in Human Milk*.

Huggins, Kathleen. *The Nursing Mother's Companion*. Boston: Harvard Common Press, 1986. This personable book provides comprehensive information about breast-feeding. Topics include preparation, special situations, returning to work, and nursing the older infant.

Mason, Diane, and Diane Ingersoll. *Breastfeeding and the Working Mother*. Rev. ed. New York: St. Martin's Griffin, 1997. This book, written by women who have personal experience in the area, provides a host of practical tips for the working mother who wishes to breast-feed her baby. How-to basics as well as suggestions for practically every job situation are addressed.

Price, Anne, and Nancy Dana. *The Working Woman's Guide to Breastfeeding*. Deephaven, Minn.: Meadowbrook, 1987. This book provides information about pumping and storing milk and selecting a breast pump. Presents the nursing mother with several choices about the work situation and explains her legal rights.

Pryor, Karen. *Nursing Your Baby*. Rev. ed. New York: Harper & Row, 1973. This long-standing reference is considered to be a classic work on breast-feeding. Information about establishing successful nursing, the advantages of breast-feeding, and extensive chronicling of the breast-feeding experience throughout the infant's first year of life is laced with warmth and understanding toward women facing obstacles to nursing.

Raphael, Dana. *The Tender Gift: Breastfeeding*. New York: Schocken Books, 1976. Although this book provides basic information on breast-feeding, its unique feature is a survey of breast-feeding in many cultures. Emphasizes the need to give support to the mother who breast-feeds. Historical and cultural influences on infant feeding practices are documented.

Rolfes, Sharon Rady, and Linda Kelly DeBruyne. *Life Span Nutrition: Conception Through Life*. Edited by Eleanor Noss Whitney. St. Paul, Minn.: West, 1990. Chapter 5 of this textbook contains a comprehensive section on breast-feeding. Covers societal support, special medical conditions, physiology, the nutritional characteristics of breast milk, and the nutrient requirements for nursing mothers. An easy-to-read text with illustrations of the physiology of breast-feeding.

Stanway, Penny, and Andrew Stanway. *Breast Is Best*. London: Pan Books, 1980. Written by two doctors who are also parents, this book provides practical, yet medically sound information about many aspects of breast-feeding. Chapters on etiquette, working, special situations, and readers' questions and answers cover issues not discussed in other books.

The Womanly Art of Breastfeeding. 3d rev. ed. Franklin Park, Ill.: La Leche League International, 1981. This bible of breast-feeding covers preparation, the advantages of breast-feeding, and how to overcome problems. This illustrated manual provides the most up-to-date, comprehensive information, supported by an advisory board of medical experts. A must-read for all nursing mothers.

BREASTS, FEMALE

Anatomy

Anatomy or system affected: Endocrine system, glands, muscles, musculoskeletal system, reproductive system

Specialties and related fields: Endocrinology; gynecology; obstetrics; oncology; plastic, cosmetic, and reconstructive surgery

Definition: The female mammary glands and their surrounding muscles and tissues.

Key terms:

alveolar cell: also known as an acinar cell; the fundamental secretory unit of the mammary glandular tissue

colostrum: thin, yellow milky secretions of the mammary gland just a few days before and after childbirth; it contains more proteins and less fat and carbohydrates than does milk

Cooper's ligament: projections of breast parenchyma covered by fibrous connective tissue that extend from the skin to the deep layer of superficial fascia

lactiferous duct: a single excretory duct from each lobe of mammary glandular tissue that converges yet opens separately at the tip of nipple; the mammary gland has fifteen to twenty lactiferous ducts

milk line: a line that originates as a primitive milk streak on each front side of the fetus; it extends from axilla to vulva, where rudimentary breast tissues or nipples could be located

myoepithelial cell: a cell that is anatomically located next to the alveolar cells and contractile in nature to aid in the movement of milk from the alveoli into the ducts

STRUCTURE AND FUNCTIONS

Mammogenesis—the growth and differentiation of the mammary gland—begins early in fetal life. By the sixth week of fetal development, the primitive milk streak can be identified as an ectodermal thickening along the ventrolateral aspect on each side of the fetus. In the ensuing weeks, this milk streak regresses, leaving normally only one pair of mammary glands in the thoracic region; however, multiple nipples and breast tissue may occasionally continue to develop anywhere along the milk line, extending from the armpit to the groin.

During the second trimester, projections of the ectoderm from the primary sprouts—usually between fifteen and twenty—will eventually elongate and arborize (branch out) to form the lactiferous ducts. Canalization of the ducts occurs late in fetal life and requires placental hormones for stimulation. Once the ducts canalize, two layers of epithelial cells are identified: the inner layer of cells, which forms the secretory component, and the outer layer of cells, which forms the myoepithelium, constituting the contractile elements for the expulsion of milk.

Between approximately four and seven days after birth, 80 to 90 percent of newborns have breast secretions (so-called witches' milk). Such secretions have been noted with equal frequency in male and female infants, and they usually last for three or four weeks. After the first neonatal month, the breast tissue reverts to an undifferentiated state and remains quiescent until puberty. Minimal ductal growth occurs during childhood, and there is no lobuloalveolar development.

At puberty, the surge of female hormones initiates lactiferous duct proliferation, along with deposition of fat and connective tissue. These changes produce a rapid increase in the size and density of the breast and are coordinated by the action of multiple hormones (prolactin, cortisol, growth hormone, insulin, and thyroxin) in addition to estrogen and progesterone. Estrogen encourages ductal proliferation and maturation, while progesterone stimulates lobuloalveolar growth. Ovarian steroids appear necessary for mammary development, as breast enlargement fails to occur at puberty in girls with gonadal dysgenesis. By the time of breast enlargement, the areola becomes more pigmented and the nipple enlarges. In adult women, size, density, and nodularity of the breast are dependent on the build of the individual, because much of the breast tissue consists of fat.

During the menstrual cycle, the breasts undergo a cyclic change. The rising estrogen and progesterone levels cause an increase in blood flow and interlobular edema. The engorgement, along with increase in density and nodularity, is particularly noticeable late in the menstrual cycle. In the week preceding menstruation, hormonal changes can bring about breast discomfort, tenderness, and a sensation of fullness. This increased sensitivity, often accompanied by marked nodularity, makes the clinical breast examination difficult. It is therefore important to examine the breasts seven to ten days following the onset of menstruation, as only during this time can tumors be differentiated from physiological nodularity. At menses, the breast decreases in size, the result of a reduction in the number and size of glandular cells with loss of edema.

During pregnancy, the breast undergoes final maturation in preparation for lactation. In the early weeks, the breast begins to enlarge, and marked histological changes take place. There is concurrent enlargement, pigmentation, and increased vascularity of the nipple. The earliest histological

The Anatomy of the Female Breast

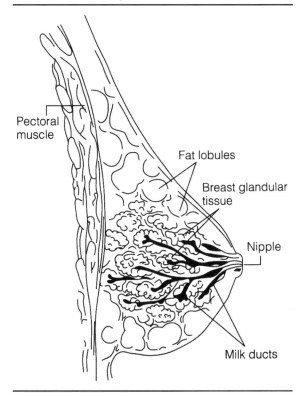

Pectoral muscle

Fat lobules

Breast glandular tissue

Nipple

Milk ducts

change within the acinar epithelial cells is cytoplasmic vacuolation. Lymphocytes, plasma cells, and eosinophils collect in the interstitial spaces. During the second trimester, the lobules enlarge and there is increase in the number and size of the constituent acini. The mammary blood supply is enhanced by increasing vascular luminal diameters and by formation of new capillaries around the lobules. During the last trimester, the secretory cells fill with fat droplets, and the alveoli are distended with a proteinaceous secretion termed colostrum.

Within three to four days postpartum, estrogen and progesterone levels rapidly decline. Prolactin can now, unrepressed by estrogen and progesterone, activate lactation, which is maintained by the infant's suckling. This stimulates further release of prolactin and oxytocin, which activate the myoepithelial cells, leading to expulsion of the alveolar secretion. During the first few days of lactation, only colostrum is produced. Once the colostrum has been expelled, normal production of milk ensues. Prolactin sustains milk production. Each nursing episode makes prolactin increase fivefold to tenfold, but, as weeks go by, prolactin levels gradually return to normal until even the nursing-induced rise is negligible. For unknown reasons, however, successful lactation can be maintained for months.

Changes of involution occur in the breast with increasing age and also after lactation. Between the ages of thirty-five and forty-five, the glandular tissue begins to disappear and alveoli and lobules shrink. These changes are not uniform throughout the breast; some lobules remain prominent, while others become more atrophic. At the menopause, the breasts decrease in size and become less dense. There is an increase in the elastic tissue component of the breast.

Anatomically, the extent of the normal female breast is approximately from the second to the sixth rib. The medical border touches the sternum, and the lateral border extends to the mid-portion of the armpit (axilla). The majority of the glandular tissue is in the upper outer quadrant and often extends deep into the axilla. The most important factor controlling the variation in breast size, shape, and density is obesity.

The mammary gland is enclosed between the superficial and deep layers of the superficial fascia. The superficial layer is a thin and delicate structure that is thicker at the inferior portion of the breast and becomes thinner as it approaches the clavicle. The deeper layer splits off the superficial fascia and extends deep into the mammary gland. Between this deep layer and the pectoral fascia, there is a well-defined space, termed retromammary space, that contains loose tissue, allowing the breast to glide freely over the chest wall. Portions of the deep layer of the superficial fascia form connective tissue extensions that pass through the retromammary space and join with the pectoral fascia. These extensions help support the breast. The breast is firmly fixed to the skin in the area of the nipple, and the

remainder of the lobules are attached to the skin by dense fibrous bands termed Cooper's ligaments. Involvement of these ligaments with cancer gives rise to the physical sign of skin dimpling.

The breast is composed of glandular tissue, blood vessels, nerves, lymphatics, and varying amounts of fat. The glandular tissue is composed of between fifteen and twenty lactiferous ducts radially arranged around the nipple, each separated by fibrous septa. The terminal portion of the lactiferous duct dilates, forming the lactiferous sinus before it empties into the nipple. The functional unit of the breast is the terminal duct lobular unit, which consists of between ten and one hundred alveoli with the intralobular terminal duct and extralobular terminal duct.

The arteries supplying the breast are derived from the thoracic branches of the internal mammary artery, the axillary artery, and the intercostal arteries. The chief blood supply to the breast is from perforating branches of the internal mammary artery. The venous drainage of the breast is through the superficial subcutaneous veins, which drain either through the superficial veins into the lower neck or via medical connections into the internal mammary veins. There are also three groups of deep venous drainage. Although there appears to be some cross-drainage from one breast to the other, it is highly unlikely that this is a significant route for metastatic spread of carcinoma to the opposite breast.

Innervation of the breast skin is separated by quadrants. The upper quadrants receive their innervation from the third and fourth branches of the cervical plexus, while the lower quadrants are supplied by the thoracic intercostal nerves. The nipple's sensitivity is derived from the lateral cutaneous branch of the fourth intercostal nerve.

Lymphatic drainage of the breast can be divided into a superficial system draining the skin and a deeper system draining the lobules. The drainage from the upper quadrants passes to the axilla, as does drainage from the lower medial quadrant and adjacent abdominal wall. The breast's lymphatic drainage is primarily to the axilla, with lesser drainage occurring along the internal mammary chain.

DISORDERS AND DISEASES

Congenital anomalies of the breast are relatively rare. The most common are accessory breast tissue (polymastia) and accessory nipples (polythelia) along the milk line. A complete lack of one or both breasts (amastia) or nipples (athelia) is very rare; however, underdeveloped rudimentary breasts are not uncommon. Accessory breasts or nipples occur in approximately 2 percent of the population. Their most frequent location is just below the normal breast. This accessory breast tissue is of little clinical significance, although it is subject to the same disease processes that occur in normal breasts.

Hypertrophy, or overgrowth, of the breast is another development variation that affects young women, especially adolescents. The most frequent type of true hypertrophy of the breast occurs in adolescence following a normal puberty. The breasts fail to cease enlargement as they reach their normal limits. The excessive growth is the result of increased deposition of fibrous and adipose tissue. Little abnormality is to be found in the glandular elements of the breast. The breasts may gain massive size and require surgical reduction.

The pathology of benign breast lesions can be broadly categorized into inflammatory, hyperplastic, and neoplastic groups. The inflammatory conditions of the breast may be acute or chronic and can be caused by various factors, including infectious agents, foreign bodies, or trauma. Acute mastitis is usually the result of spread of microorganisms from the nipple, particularly during lactation. The breast shows acute inflammation with swelling, warmness, and redness. An abscess, or collection of pus, may form in the subareolar or deep glandular tissue. Diffuse cellulitis occasionally develops as the infection spreads into the adjacent soft tissue. Acute mastitis usually resolves following appropriate antibiotic treatment. Chronic mastitis may follow acute mastitis, or its onset may be insidious. The causative organisms are similar to those responsible for acute mastitis.

Fat necrosis within the breast tissue may follow trauma or a breast augmentation procedure using silicone or other materials. It may also be associated with necrosis developing in a malignant tumor. A history of trauma with surrounding bruises and pain is found in only about half the cases. Fat necrosis often manifests itself as a small, firm nodular mass of insidious onset. The consistency, adhesion to skin, and lack of pain, as well as the presence of calcifications on mammography, add to the confusion with carcinoma. In chronic cases, extensive fibrosis is seen. Careful microscopic sampling of different areas of the lesion is necessary, since malignant tumors could be associated with the foci of fat necrosis.

Almost all women are affected by a benign condition called fibrocystic change of breast at some time in their lives. Many other terms have been used for fibrocystic change in the medical literature, such as mammary dysplasia, fibrocystic disease, and chronic cystic mastitis, but these terms are no longer considered appropriate. This condition primarily affects women between twenty and forty-five years of age. Symptoms include nodularity in the breasts that may be associated with pain and tenderness, particularly around menses. Although the pathogenesis is not clear, fibrocystic changes appear to be the result of a hormonal imbalance of estrogen and progesterone. Oral contraceptives reduce the incidence of some types of fibrocystic changes. Genetic makeup, age, parity, and lactational history, as well as psychosomatic factors, may also play a role. The majority of fibrocystic changes are not premalignant.

The most common benign neoplasm of the breast is fibroadenoma, with most cases occurring between fifteen and thirty years of age. It is estimated that 10 to 25 percent of women have one or more of these tumors, which are thought to be of lobular origin. These neoplasms are estrogen-dependent, are often associated with menstrual irregularities, and can enlarge significantly during pregnancy. Clinically, fibroadenomas are usually well-defined, rounded lesions that have a firm or rubbery consistency. They are freely mobile, since there are no attachments between the tumor and the adjacent tissue. Fibroadenomas vary in size, with the majority being between 1 and 3 centimeters in diameter. Some tumors, however, can be as large as 10 to 12 centimeters and are termed giant fibroadenoma; these are more common in adolescents, particularly blacks in their second decade of life. The large size of these tumors may be intimidating, but they have no malignant potential. Local excision with nipple preservation is adequate and allows subsequent normal development of the breast.

Breast cancer has been the major cause of death for several decades among women in the United States. In 1991 alone, 175,000 women were afflicted with breast cancer. It is the second leading cause of cancer mortality after lung carcinoma. As of 1992, it was estimated that one out of nine American women has a lifetime risk of developing breast cancer. The incidence of this disease has increased at a 2 to 4 percent rate per year since 1980. The underlying reason for this continual growth in breast cancer cases remains unclear.

The initial physical signs and symptoms of breast carcinoma are varied. The most common clinical manifestation is a discrete lump. Swelling, nipple retraction, skin dimpling, axillary lumps, and occasionally bloody nipple discharge make up the remainder of the local physical signs. In general, nipple discharge is not often associated with cancer. When it is, it is usually a persistent, spontaneous bloody discharge. In women less than fifty years of age, the presence of a bloody discharge is usually associated with an intraductal papilloma, which is not a malignant breast lesion. Skin retraction is caused by shortening of the Cooper's ligaments; its presence classically raises strong suspicion of a breast carcinoma. Other benign breast lesions can produce similar changes, however, the most common of which are plasma cell mastitis, fat necrosis, and Mondor's disease. Women with distant metastasis may experience general malaise, weight loss, bone pain, and headaches.

The site of the breast lump is most cases is in the upper outer quadrant or in the retroareolar area, just beneath the nipple. This is likely attributable to the fact that the majority of mammary glandular tissue occupies the upper outer quadrant of the breast. Approximately 5 percent of breast cancers occur in both breasts.

There are several different histopathological subtypes of

breast cancer. Their recognition by the pathologist is crucial, since some have different prognostic implications. Most breast malignancies are primarily epithelial in origin, with only a small number of sarcomas and metastatic tumors reported. Although the terminal duct lobular unit is probably the location of origin of almost all cancers, neoplasms are traditionally classified into ductal and lobular carcinomas.

The most common malignant neoplasm of the breast is a nonspecific type of infiltrating ductal carcinoma, which is reported in 75 percent of breast cancer cases. It is presumed to be ductal in origin, and there may be coexistent areas of intraductal carcinoma, although this component is not always obvious. There is a poorly defined area of firmness that can often be palpated within the breast. At the time of surgical biopsy, most of these cancers range between 1 and 3 centimeters in diameter. Tumors less than 1 centimeter in diameter are not usually detected, although the increased use of screening mammography has brought some of these early lesions to light. Other tumors may reach a massive size, greater than 10 centimeters, before the patient seeks medical advice, often because of the patient's denial or lack of knowledge. The mass has a hard consistency and gives a gritty resistance when the specimen is cut. The outer margin of the mass is irregular with numerous fibrous bands, which can cause retraction of the nipple and dimpling of the overlying skin. The neoplasm may also be fixed to the underlying chest wall. Ulceration of the nipple or other parts of the skin is uncommon, except in advanced cases.

Invasive lobular carcinoma is the second most common breast malignancy, accounting for less than 10 percent of all breast cancers. These tumors tend to be multifocal and bilateral. When the opposite or "uninvolved" breast is sampled, about one-third show areas of carcinoma. Nodules of invasive lobular carcinoma are frequently difficult to localize, and occasionally no masses are encountered.

PERSPECTIVE AND PROSPECTS

Perhaps the diseases and treatment of no other organ have had more significance for human culture than those of the breast. Breast cancer has been described in many cultures and can even be found recorded in early Egyptian hieroglyphics. Breast cancer is important not only because of its frequency but also because of its psychosocial implications. In certain contexts, the breast symbolizes motherhood and nourishment, while in others it represents beauty and femininity.

In recent years, the investigation of breast diseases has blossomed. The normal physiological conditions of the breast, various benign diseases, and breast cancer have been clearly separated. The significance, prognosis, relation to breast cancer, and treatment of these diseases have been elucidated. Epidemiological studies have shown marked differences in the incidence of breast cancer within popula-

tions. These findings have suggested hypotheses as to the etiology and natural history of breast cancer. Increased patient awareness and continued advancement of screening mammography have resulted in earlier diagnosis of the disease.

Throughout the nineteenth century and in the early twentieth century, the prognosis for breast cancer was dismal because of the advanced stage of the disease at the usual time of its initial manifestation. In 1894, William Halsted and Willy Meyer each published, independently and for the first time, a description of the radical mastectomy procedure, including the resection of the entire breast, pectoral muscles, axillary lymph nodes, and associated skin and subcutaneous tissue. It was not until the late 1930's, however, that the Halsted radical mastectomy was beginning to be questioned by other surgeons. Enthusiasm for more conservative management—simple mastectomy with adjuvant radiation therapy—was ignited.

In the early 1950's, newer concepts emerged for the management of benign and malignant breast diseases. For example, the concept that breast cancer was a systemic disease and potentially unaffected by local treatment had risen. For the first time, a staging system was devised. Several studies confirmed that the most important prognostic indicator was the presence or absence of axillary nodal metastasis. In the 1960's and 1970's, hormonal therapy and adjuvant chemotherapy gradually gained acceptance.

Developments in the understanding of breast diseases and the variety of treatments available have provided major roles for the surgeon, medical oncologist, radiation oncologist, diagnostic radiologist, and pathologist. The multidisciplinary approach necessitates a coordinated, multidisciplinary team of experts to achieve the most optimal outcome of patient care.

—*Stan Liu, M.D., and Lawrence W. Bassett, M.D.*

See also Anatomy; Biopsy; Breast augmentation, reduction, and reconstruction; Breast biopsy; Breast cancer; Breast disorders; Breast-feeding; Cancer; Cyst removal; Cysts and ganglions; Glands; Gynecology; Mammography; Mastectomy and lumpectomy; Mastitis; Muscles; Oncology; Pathology; Plastic, cosmetic, and reconstructive surgery; Reproductive system; Sex change surgery; Systems and organs; Tumor removal; Tumors.

FOR FURTHER INFORMATION:

Isaacs, John H. *Textbook of Breast Disease*. St. Louis: Mosby Year Book, 1992. This text, a summation of significant efforts from multiple physicians predominantly in the field of obstetrics and gynecology, offers a concise and clear description of the management of breast problems. There is also information on the effect of breast disease on sexual function and a detailed description of clinical and self-examination of the breast.

Love, Susan M., and Karen Lindsey. *Dr. Susan Love's Breast Book*. 2d ed. Reading, Mass.: Addison-Wesley,

1995. This easy-to-read paperback is one of the most influential books in women's health written for a general audience. The splendidly well-written guide explains breast development, changes with age, and breast cancer detection and treatment with exceptional clarity and detail.

Marchant, Douglas J., Nathan G. Kase, and Richard L. Berkowitz, eds. *Contemporary Issues in Obstetrics and Gynecology: Breast Disease.* New York: Churchill Livingstone, 1986. This monograph, briefly and simply, provides a concise overview of breast disorders and therapy. Marchant offers a gynecologist's view of diagnosis and treatment. One of the chapters is dedicated to the important discussion of risk factors and hypotheses that attempt to explain the etiology of breast cancer.

Mitchell, George W., Jr., and Lawrence W. Bassett, eds. *The Female Breast and Its Disorders.* Baltimore: Williams & Wilkins, 1990. This comprehensive text offers the expertise of multiple representatives from diverse fields—including obstetrics and gynecology, diagnostic radiology, pathology, surgery, medicine, therapeutic radiology, and psychiatry—in discussing many facets of breast function, disease, diagnosis, and treatment. It is intended not only for physicians but also for nonmedical personnel who provide health care for women and are actively involved in the management of breast problems.

Oktay, Julianne S., and Carolyn A. Walter. *Breast Cancer in the Life Course: Women's Experience.* New York: Springer, 1991. This superbly written book deals with the emotional and psychological impact of having breast cancer at different phases of adulthood. Using multiple case studies and vignettes, the authors provide readers with easy-to-understand discussions of how women of different ages adapt to and cope with breast cancer.

Rogers, Kenneth, and A. J. Coup. *Surgical Pathology of the Breast.* London: Butterworth, 1990. This book contains multiple histopathologic illustrations of both malignant and benign breast diseases. In addition, many color photographs are provided to highlight the important physical signs of malignancy. It is aimed at medical students and junior trainees in the fields of surgery, pathology, radiotherapy, and medical oncology.

BREATHING DIFFICULTY. *See* HEART ATTACK; PULMONARY DISEASES; RESPIRATION.

BRONCHITIS

DISEASE/DISORDER

ANATOMY OR SYSTEM AFFECTED: Chest, lungs, respiratory system

SPECIALTIES AND RELATED FIELDS: Family practice, internal medicine, pulmonary medicine

DEFINITION: An inflammation of the bronchial tree of the lungs.

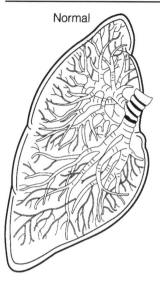

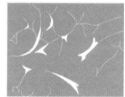

Chronic obstructive lung disease

Normal vs. obstructed bronchioles.

CAUSES AND SYMPTOMS

The inflammation associated with bronchitis may be localized or diffuse, acute or chronic, and it is usually caused by infections or physical agents. In its infectious form, acute bronchitis is part of a general, acute upper-respiratory infection, sometimes brought on by the common cold. It can also develop from a virus infection of the nasopharynx, throat, or tracheobronchial tree. Acute bronchitis is most prevalent in winter. Factors contributing to the onset of the disease include exposure, chilling, malnutrition, fatigue, or rickets. The inflammation may be serious in debilitated patients and those with chronic pulmonary disease, and the real danger rests in the development of pneumonia. Certain physical and chemical irritants can bring on acute bronchitis. Such agents as mineral and vegetable dusts, strong acid fumes, volatile organic compounds, and tobacco smoke can trigger an attack.

The disease causes thickening of the bronchi and a loss of elasticity in the bronchial tree. Changes in the mucous membranes occur, leukocytes infiltrate the submucosa, and a sticky, mucopurulent exudate is formed. The normally sterile bronchi are invaded by bacteria and cellular debris. A barking cough is often present, and this serves as an essential mechanism for eliminating bronchial secretions.

Chronic bronchitis is characterized by swollen mucous membranes, tenacious exudate, and spasms in the bronchiolar muscles. The result is dyspnea, the ventilatory insufficiency known as shortness of breath.

TREATMENT AND THERAPY

Acute bronchitis is treated with bed rest and medication to counteract the symptoms of inflammation. The room air should be kept warm and humid. Steam inhalation and cough syrup sometimes give relief from the severe, painful cough.

All surveys have demonstrated a high incidence of bronchitis in cigarette smokers when compared with nonsmokers, thus providing a good reason for the cessation of smoking.

—Jane A. Slezak, Ph.D.

See also Coughing; Inflammation; Lungs; Pneumonia; Pulmonary diseases; Pulmonary medicine; Pulmonary medicine, pediatric; Respiration.

FOR FURTHER INFORMATION:

Bennett, J. Claude, et al., eds. *Cecil Textbook of Medicine.* 20th ed. Philadelphia: W. B. Saunders, 1996. A comprehensive textbook covering the diagnosis and treatment of diseases.

Berland, Theodore, and Gordon Snider. *Living with Your Bronchitis and Emphysema.* New York: St. Martin's Press, 1972. A reference for those with lung disease. Includes suggestions for clearing airways and helping oneself breathe.

Petty, Thomas, and Louise Nett. *For Those Who Live and Breathe with Emphysema and Chronic Bronchitis.* Springfield, Ill.: Charles C Thomas, 1967. A book written for patients suffering from emphysema and bronchitis. The book covers medical facts, rehabilitation programs, and includes an extensive glossary.

Shayevitz, Myra, and Berton R. Shayevitz. *Living Well with Emphysema and Bronchitis.* Garden City, N.Y.: Doubleday, 1985. A book written to help those suffering from chronic lung disease. Provides an agenda for living with the disease.

BULIMIA

DISEASE/DISORDER

ANATOMY OR SYSTEM AFFECTED: Gastrointestinal system, psychic-emotional system, stomach, throat

SPECIALTIES AND RELATED FIELDS: Gastroenterology, nutrition, pediatrics, psychiatry, psychology

DEFINITION: Bulimia is a compulsive eating disorder in which the patient (usually a young woman) goes on food binges and then intentionally purges herself, either through self-induced vomiting or by using laxatives. As with anorexia nervosa, the patient has a fear of gaining weight, but unlike anorectics, bulimics may or may not experience a significant weight loss. Nevertheless, there are medical dangers: Chronic laxative use can result in dehydration and other gastrointestinal disorders, and repeated vomiting may cause severe tooth decay from the gastric acids found in bile. Counseling is necessary to address the patient's underlying psychological illness.

—Jason Georges and Tracy Irons-Georges

See also Anorexia nervosa; Eating disorders; Malnutrition; Nausea and vomiting; Nutrition; Obesity; Poisoning; Psychiatry, child and adolescent; Psychology; Weight loss and gain.

BUNION REMOVAL

PROCEDURE

ANATOMY OR SYSTEM AFFECTED: Bones, feet

SPECIALTIES AND RELATED FIELDS: Family practice, general surgery, orthopedics, podiatry

DEFINITION: The removal of an enlargement which develops on the joint of the big toe.

INDICATIONS AND PROCEDURES

Bunions are usually found as abnormal enlargements around the joint of the big toe. They generally form when a bursa, one of the fluid-filled sacs at regions of friction such as between bones and tendons, becomes inflamed near the joint at the base of this toe. Bunions are characterized by inflammation and swelling in the region, and they often result in lateral displacement of the big toe.

The specific cause of bunions is not always known and at times may be related to certain anatomical features of the foot. Nevertheless, a common cause of bunion formation is improper footwear, particularly among women. Shoes that push the toes together, particularly pointed footwear and high heels, frequently place inward pressure on the large toe, forcing it over the adjacent toe. The tendon associated with the toe may itself become weakened from the displacement, aggravating the problem. The result is that with prolonged use of such shoes, the large toe may become permanently displaced, and the region may become inflamed. The bursa may also expand over the joint, intensifying the pain.

Treatment initially involves the selection of more comfortable footwear; this may itself reduce pain and inflammation. Splinting of the big toe, forcing it into its proper position, may be helpful if the displacement has not progressed too far. Often, such splinting is carried out at night. If the problem does not correct itself, surgery may be considered.

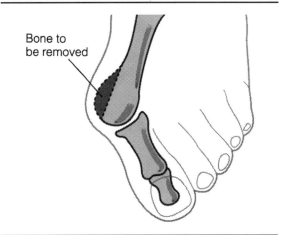

Bone to be removed

A bunion, a bony overgrowth of the big toe, can be removed surgically by cutting off the excess segment of bone, thus reshaping the foot.

5

Surgery generally involves a bunionectomy, the removal of a portion of the joint. The tension associated with the tendon holding the joint in place may also be relieved during the surgery.

USES AND COMPLICATIONS

Relatively few complications are associated with the surgery. The bunion may recur, particularly if improper footwear continues to be worn. Release of tension as the tendon is excised or altered may result in overcorrection. The toe may be immobilized for several weeks, though the patient is usually able to walk a few days after the surgery.

—*Richard Adler, Ph.D.*

See also Bones and the skeleton; Feet; Foot disorders; Orthopedic surgery; Orthopedics; Podiatry.

BURNS AND SCALDS
DISEASE/DISORDER

ANATOMY OR SYSTEM AFFECTED: Skin, other tissues in severe cases

SPECIALTIES AND RELATED FIELDS: Critical care; dermatology; emergency medicine; physical therapy; plastic, cosmetic, and reconstructive surgery

DEFINITION: Injury to skin and other tissues caused by contact with dry heat (fire), moist heat (steam or hot liquid), chemicals, electricity, lightning, or radiation.

KEY TERMS:

burn: an injury to tissues caused by contact with dry heat (fire), moist heat (steam or a hot liquid), chemicals, electricity, lightning, or radiation

burn degrees: system of classification for burns based on the depth of damage to the skin

major (or severe) burn: a burn covering more than 20 percent of the body and any deep burn of the hands, face, feet, or perineum

minor burn: a superficial burn of less than 5 percent of the body that can be treated without hospitalization

moderate burn: a burn that requires hospitalization but not specialized care

rule of nines: a system used to designate areas of the body, represented by various body parts; used in determining the extent of a burn

skin graft: a surgical graft of skin from one part of the body to another or from one individual to another

CAUSES AND SYMPTOMS

Burns are injuries to tissues caused by contact with dry heat (fire), moist heat (steam or a hot liquid, also called scalds), chemicals, electricity, lightning, or radiation. The word "burn" comes from the Middle English *brinnen* or *brennen* (to burn) and from the Old English *byrnan* (to be on fire) combined with *baernan* (to set afire). Each year in the United States, more than two million people are burned or scalded badly enough to need medical treatment, and about 70,000 require admission to a hospital. Burns are most common in children and older people, and many are caused

by accidents in the home that are usually preventable.

The depth of the injury is proportional to the intensity of the heat of the causative agent and the duration of exposure. Burns can be classified according to the agent causing the damage. Some examples of burns according to this classification are brush burns, caused by friction of a rapidly moving object against the skin or ground into the skin; chemical burns, caused by exposure to a caustic chemical; flash burns, caused by very brief exposure to intense radiant heat (the typical burn of an atomic explosion); radiation burns, caused by exposure to radium, X rays, or atomic energy; and respiratory burns, caused by inhalation of steam or explosive gases.

Burns can also be classified as major or severe (involving more than 20 percent of the body and any deep burn of the hands, face, feet, or perineum), minor (a superficial burn involving less than 5 percent of the body that can be treated without hospitalization), and moderate (a burn that requires hospitalization but not specialized care, as with burns covering 5 to 20 percent of the body but without deep burns of hands, face, feet, or perineum).

While many domestic burns are minor and insignificant, more severe burns and scalds can prove to be dangerous. The main danger for a burn patient is the shock that arises as a result of loss of fluid from the circulating blood at the site of the burn. This loss of fluid leads to a fall in the volume of the circulating blood in the area. The maintenance of an adequate blood volume is essential to life, and the body attempts to compensate for this temporary loss by withdrawing fluid from the uninjured areas of the body into the circulation. In the first forty-eight hours after a severe burn is received, fluid from the blood vessels, salt, and protein pass into the burned area, causing swelling, blisters, low blood pressure, and very low urine output. The body loses fluids, proteins, and salt, and the potassium level is raised. Such low-fluid levels are followed by a shift of fluid in the opposite direction, resulting in excess urine, high blood volume, and low concentration of blood electrolytes. If carried too far, this condition begins to affect the viability of the body cells. As a result, essential body cells such as those of the liver and kidneys begin to suffer, eventually causing the liver and kidneys to cease proper function. Liver and renal failure are revealed by the development of jaundice and the appearance of albumin in the urine. In addition, the circulation begins to fail, with a resultant lack of oxygen in the tissues. The victim becomes cyanosed, restless, and collapsed, and in some cases death ensues. Other possible problems related to burns include collapse of the circulatory system; shutdown of the digestive and excretory systems, shock, pneumonia, and stress ulcers.

In addition, particularly with severe burns, there is a strong risk of infection. This type of burn can leave a large area of raw skin surface exposed and extremely vulnerable to any microorganisms. The infection of extensive burns may cause fatal complications if effective antibiotic treatment is not given. The combination of shock and infection can often be life-threatening unless expert treatment is immediately available.

The immediate outcome of a burn is more determined by its extent (amount of body area affected) than by its depth (layers of skin affected). The "rule of nines" is used to assess the extent of a burn in relation to the surface of a body. The head and each of the arms cover 9 percent of the body surface; the front of the body, the back, and each leg cover 18 percent; and the crotch accounts for the remaining 1 percent. The greater the extent of a burn, the more seriously ill the victim will become from loss of fluid. The depth of the burn (unless it is very great) is mainly of importance when the question arises as to how much surgical treatment, including skin grafting, will be required. An improvement over the rule of nines in the evaluation of the seriousness of burns is the Berkow formula, which takes into account the age of the patient.

A burn caused by chemicals differs from a burn caused by fire only in that the outcome of the chemical burn is usually more favorable, since the chemical destroys the bacteria on the affected part and reduces the chance of infection. Severe burns can also be caused by contact with electric wires. As current meets the resistance in the skin, high temperatures are developed and burning of the victim takes place. Exposure to 220 volts burns only the skin, but higher voltage can cause severe underlying damage to any tissue in its path. Electrical burns normally cause minimal external skin damage, but they can cause serious heart damage and require evaluation by a physician. Explosions and the action of acids and other chemicals also cause burns. Severe and extensive fire burns are most frequently produced by the clothes catching fire.

TREATMENT AND THERAPY

General treatment of a burn injury includes pain relief, the control of infection, the maintenance of the balance of fluids and electrolytes in the system, and a good diet. A high-protein diet with supplemental vitamins is prescribed to aid in the repair of damaged tissue. The specific treatment depends on the severity of the burn. Major burns should be treated in a specialized treatment facility, while minor burns can be treated without hospitalization. A moderate burn normally requires hospitalization but not specialized care.

In the case of minor burns or scalds, all that may be necessary is to hold the body part under cold running water until the pain is relieved, as cooling is one of the most effective ways of relieving the pain of a burn. If the burn involves the distal part of a limb—for example, the hand and forearm—one of the most effective ways of relieving the pain is to immerse the burned part in lukewarm water and add cold water until the pain disappears. If the pain does not return when the water warms up, the burn can be dressed in the usual way (a piece of sterile gauze covered by cotton with a bandage on top). The part should be kept at rest and the dressing dry until healing takes place. Blisters can be pierced with a sterile needle, but the skin should

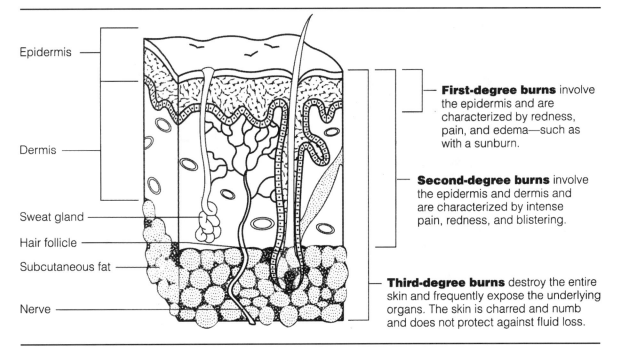

Epidermis

Dermis

Sweat gland

Hair follicle

Subcutaneous fat

Nerve

First-degree burns involve the epidermis and are characterized by redness, pain, and edema—such as with a sunburn.

Second-degree burns involve the epidermis and dermis and are characterized by intense pain, redness, and blistering.

Third-degree burns destroy the entire skin and frequently expose the underlying organs. The skin is charred and numb and does not protect against fluid loss.

Burns are measured by the layer(s) of skin affected.

not be cut away. No ointment or oil should be applied, and an antiseptic is not always necessary. Even this type of burn can be serious if it covers as much as two-thirds of the body area. On a child, such burns are dangerous on an even smaller area of the skin, and special attention should be given to the patient.

In the case of moderate burns or scalds, it is advisable to use antiseptics (such as chlorhexidine, bacitracin, and neomycin), and the patient should be taken to a doctor. Treatment may consist of using a dressing impregnated with a suitable antibiotic or of applying a cream containing antiseptic and pain-relieving creams and covering the burn with a dressing sealed at the end. This dressing is left on for four to five days and removed if there is evidence of infection or if pain occurs.

For severe burns and scalds, the only sound rule is to go to the hospital. Unless there is a need for resuscitation, or attention to other injuries, nothing should be done on the spot except to make sure that the patient is comfortable and warm and to cover the burn with a clean or sterile cloth. Clothing should be removed from the burned area only if this does not traumatize the skin further. Burned clothing should be sent to the burn center, as it may help determine the chemicals and other substances that either caused or entered the wound. Once the victim is in the hospital, the first thing to check is the extent of the burn and whether a transfusion is necessary. If the burn covers more than 9 percent of the body surface, a transfusion is required. It is essential to prevent infection or to bring it under control. A high-protein diet with ample fluids is needed to compen-

Rule of Nines

Anterior head and neck 4$\frac{1}{2}$%

4$\frac{1}{2}$%

Anterior and posterior head and neck 9%

Posterior head and neck 4$\frac{1}{2}$%

4$\frac{1}{2}$%

Anterior and posterior upper extremities 18%

Anterior trunk 18%

Posterior trunk 18%

Posterior upper extremities 9%

Anterior upper extremities 9%

4$\frac{1}{2}$%

4$\frac{1}{2}$%

Anterior and posterior trunk 36%

4$\frac{1}{2}$%

4$\frac{1}{2}$%

Perineum 1%

9%

9%

9%

9%

Posterior lower extremities 18%

Anterior lower extremities 18%

Anterior and posterior lower extremities 36%

(a)

100%

(b)

The "rule of nines" specifies the extent and hence seriousness of a burn in relation to the body's surface area.

sate for the protein that has been lost along with the fluid from the circulation. The process of healing is slow and tedious, including careful nursing, physiotherapy, and occupational therapy. The length of hospital stay can vary from a few days in some cases to many weeks in the case of severe and extensive burns.

In some cases depending on the extent of the burn, it will be necessary to consider skin grafting, in which a graft of skin from one part of the body (or from another individual) is implanted in another part. Skin grafting is done soon after the initial injury. The donor skin is best taken from the patient, but when this is not possible, the skin of a matched donor can be used. Prior to grafting, or in some cases as a substitute for it, the burn may be covered with either cadaver or pig skin to keep it moist and free from exogenous bacterial infection. Newly developed artificial skin holds great promise for treating severe burns.

In the case of chemical burns, treatment can be specific and depends on the chemical causing the burn. For example, phenol or lysol can be washed off promptly, while acid or alkali burns should be neutralized by washing with sodium bicarbonate or acetic acid, respectively, or with a buffer solution for either one. In many cases, flushing with water to remove the chemical is the first method of action.

Victims who have inhaled smoke may develop swelling and inflammation of the lungs, and they may need special care for burns of the eyes. People who have suffered an electrical burn may suffer from shock and may require artificial respiration; which should begin as soon as contact with the current has been broken.

PERSPECTIVE AND PROSPECTS

Burns have been traditionally classified according to degree. The French surgeon Guillaume Dupuytren divided burns into six degrees, according to their depth. A first-degree burn is one in which there is simply redness; it may be painful for a day or two. This level of burn is normally seen in cases of extended exposure to X rays or sunlight. A second-degree burn affects the first and second layers of skin. There is great redness, and the surface is raised up in blisters accompanied by much pain. Healing normally occurs without a scar. A third-degree burn affects all skin layers. The epidermis is entirely peeled off, and the true skin below is destroyed in part, so as to expose the endings of the sensory nerves. This is a very painful form of burn, and a scar follows on healing. With a fourth-degree burn, the entire skin of an area is destroyed with its nerves, so that there is less pain than with a third-degree burn. A scar forms and later contracts, and it may produce great deformity in the affected area. A fifth-degree burn will burn the muscles as well, and still greater deformity follows. In a sixth-degree burn, a whole limb is charred, and it separates as in gangrene.

In current practice, burns are referred to as superficial (or partial thickness), in which there is sufficient skin tissue left to ensure regrowth of skin over the burned site; and deep (or full thickness), in which the skin is totally destroyed and grafting will be necessary. It is difficult to determine the depth of a wound at first glance, but any burn involving more than 15 percent of the body surface is considered serious. As far as the ultimate outcome is concerned, the main factor is the extent of the burn—the greater the extent, the worse the outlook.

Unfortunately, burns are most common in children and older people, those for whom the outcome is usually the worst. Many of the burns are caused by accidents in the home, which are usually preventable. In fact, among the primary causes of deaths by burns, house fires account for 75 percent of the incidents. Safety measures in the home and on the job are extremely important in the prevention of burns. Severe and extensive burns most frequently occur when the clothes catch fire. This rule applies especially to cotton garments, which burn quickly. Particular care should always be exercised with electric fires and kettles or pots of boiling water in houses where small children or elderly people are present.

In the United States, most severely burned patients are given emergency care in a local hospital and are then transferred to a large burn center for intensive long-term care. The kind of environment provided in special burn units in large medical centers varies, but all have as their main objective avoiding contamination of the wound, as the major cause of death in burn victims is infection. Some special units use isolation techniques and elaborate laminar air flow systems to maintain an environment that is as free of microorganisms as possible.

The patient who has suffered some disfigurement from burns will have additional emotional problems in adjusting to a new body image. Burn therapy can be long and tedious for the patient and for family members. They will need emotional and psychological support as they work their way through the many problems created by the physical and emotional trauma of a major wound.

—*Maria Pacheco, Ph.D.*

See also Critical care; Critical care, pediatric; Dermatology; Electrical shock; Emergency medicine; Grafts and grafting; Healing; Heat exhaustion and heat stroke; Radiation sickness; Shock; Skin; Wounds.

FOR FURTHER INFORMATION:

Clayman, Charles B., ed. *American Medical Association Encyclopedia of Medicine.* New York: Random House, 1989. A concise presentation of numerous medical terms and illnesses. A good general reference.

Glanze, Walter D., Kenneth N. Anderson, and Lois E. Anderson, eds. *The Mosby Medical Encyclopedia.* Rev. ed. New York: Plume, 1992. Excellent general reference for the layperson. Offers a concise but clear presentation of numerous medical topics.

Landau, Sidney, ed. *International Dictionary of Medicine*

and Biology. New York: John Wiley & Sons, 1986. Contains a brief presentation of medical and biological terms. A good, easy-to-comprehend general reference.

Macpherson, Gordon, ed. *Black's Medical Dictionary.* 38th ed. London: A & C Black, 1995. An excellent presentation of the topic can be found in this general medical reference work.

Miller, Benjamin, and Claire B. Keane. *Encyclopedia and Dictionary of Medicine, Nursing, and Allied Health.* 5th ed. Philadelphia: W. B. Saunders, 1992. A good, concise presentation of the topic of burns.

BURSITIS

DISEASE/DISORDER

ANATOMY OR SYSTEM AFFECTED: Hands, joints, knees, legs

SPECIALTIES AND RELATED FIELDS: Internal medicine, rheumatology

DEFINITION: An inflammation of a bursa, one of the membranes that surround joints.

CAUSES AND SYMPTOMS

Bursas are flattened, fibrous sacs that minimize friction on adjacent structures during activity involving a joint. The most well known bursas are around the knees, elbows, and shoulders. These protective joint sacs are lined with a fluid-producing membrane called the synovial membrane. Bursas are common in sites where ligaments, muscles, skin, or tendons overlie and may rub against bone. Most bursas are present at birth, but false bursas may develop at any site where there is excessive motion.

Bursitis is inflammation of a bursa, causing it to become warm, painful, and often swollen. Bursitis is usually caused by the inappropriate or excessive use of a joint. For example, pressure, friction, infections, or injury to a joint and surrounding tissues can cause membranes of the bursa to become inflamed.

Bursitis of the kneecap (prepatellar bursitis, or "housemaid's knee") is commonly caused by prolonged kneeling on a hard surface such as the floor. Similarly, olecranon bursitis ("student's elbow") is caused by pressure of the elbow against a table or desk. Perhaps the most common type of bursitis is of the shoulder joint, called subdeltoid bursitis.

TREATMENT AND THERAPY

The treatment for bursitis caused by overuse is usually rest and avoidance of the activity that resulted in the condition. Several days of rest is typically all that is needed for the swelling to subside. Ice packs may help relieve some of the minor pain and inflammation. If the inflammation does not subside after a few days, a physician may prescribe anti-inflammatory drugs such as ibuprofen or naproxen to reduce the inflammation and pain. Occasionally, a doctor will inject the inflamed bursa with a corticosteroid such as triamcinolone. In rare cases, where the symptoms are re-

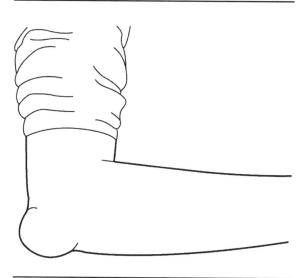

Bursitis produces a painful, fluid-filled swelling around a joint; bursitis may occur in the bursa at any joint, such as the elbow.

current, a physician may remove the bursa (bursectomy). If the bursitis is caused by an infection, the most appropriate treatment is antibiotic therapy. During and after medical or surgical treatment, physical therapy may be recommended to improve the strength and mobility of the joint.

—*Matthew Berria, Ph.D.*

See also Arthritis; Gout; Inflammation; Osteoarthritis; Rheumatoid arthritis; Rheumatology.

FOR FURTHER INFORMATION:

Clayman, Charles B., ed. *The American Medical Association Encyclopedia of Medicine.* New York: Random House, 1989.

Marieb, Elaine N. *Human Anatomy and Physiology.* 3d ed. Redwood City, Calif.: Benjamin/Cummings, 1995.

BYPASS SURGERY

PROCEDURE

ANATOMY OR SYSTEM AFFECTED: Abdomen, blood vessels, chest, circulatory system, gastrointestinal system, heart, intestines, stomach

SPECIALTIES AND RELATED FIELDS: Cardiology, gastroenterology, general surgery

DEFINITION: A procedure used to change the flow through a tubular structure (generally a blood vessel or section of intestine) to detour an area of blockage or to shorten the path.

KEY TERMS:

angina: chest pain caused by coronary artery disease

angioplasty: a medical procedure used to widen narrowed arteries, especially in the heart

ischemia: decreased blood flow to an organ

morbid obesity: a condition characterized by the excessive accumulation of fat (in which the patient is more than 100 pounds overweight or 100 percent overweight)

INDICATIONS AND PROCEDURES

Bypass surgery can be divided into two general types: that related to the heart and cardiovascular system and that related to the intestines and digestive system.

In the cardiovascular system, bypass surgery is intended to detour the flow of blood around an area which is blocked by fat deposits and cholesterol. Although bypass surgery can be used in many areas of the cardiovascular system to bypass a block, most surgeries involve the coronary arteries, which surround the heart and provide the heart muscle with oxygen and nutrients. When the coronary arteries are blocked, insufficient blood flow to the heart muscle may occur. If there is insufficient blood flow to maintain normal function of the heart, ischemia results and the individual typically will feel pressure and burning pain in the chest, back, neck, jaw, or arms. This pain is called angina. If there is insufficient blood flow to maintain the life of the heart muscle, a heart attack or myocardial infarction occurs. The heart muscle that is deprived of enough oxygen dies.

In coronary artery bypass surgery, the chest is opened to expose the heart. Blood flow through the heart is diverted through an oxygenator and a pump to continue the flow of oxygenated blood throughout the body. Then the surgeon removes the saphenous vein from one of the legs of the patient. This vein is sutured to the heart from the aorta to a coronary artery. Upon completion of the surgery, the blood will flow from the aorta through the grafted vessel

Coronary Bypass Graft

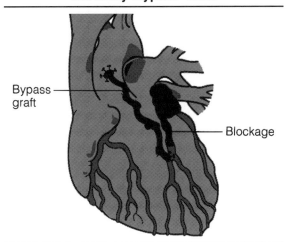

Bypass graft

Blockage

Bypass surgery can be performed in any part of the body where a blood vessel has become blocked; a common location for such a procedure is the heart, where from one to four arteries may require the placement of bypass grafts.

to a coronary artery, bypassing the portion of the coronary artery where the blockage exists.

Intestinal bypass surgery is used for people who are morbidly obese. It is intended to shorten the length of the small intestine in order to decrease the area where nutrients (and calories) are absorbed, making it easier for the patient to lose weight.

There are several types of intestinal bypass surgeries. What they all have in common is that the small intestine is cut and sutured to another part of the intestine that is closer to the point where it meets the colon (large intestine). The effect of the surgery is to decrease the distance that food travels through the small intestine.

Another form of bypass in the digestive system involves the stomach. The stomach is cut, stapled, or sutured to make it smaller, and a portion of the small intestine is stapled or sutured to the stomach. This staple or suture area is where food leaves the stomach and proceeds through the shortened small intestine. In addition to decreasing the distance that food travels through the small intestine, the purpose of decreasing the size of the stomach is to make the patient feel satisfied when consuming less food.

USES AND COMPLICATIONS

The success rate of coronary artery bypass surgery is excellent, and the death rate is very low. After successful bypass surgery, the patient should have good blood flow through the coronary arteries and sufficient blood and oxygen available to the heart muscle. The biggest problem with bypass surgery is the tendency for blockages to reform from deposits of fat and cholesterol on the grafted vessel. To minimize further blockages, these patients are encouraged to make changes in their lifestyles. Cessation of smoking, low-fat diets, and exercise are some of the methods recommended.

The success rate of intestinal bypass surgery has been marginal. Although fatal complications have been few, major problems can occur. Because of the lack of absorption of all nutrients ingested, patients can develop nutritional deficiencies. For example, B complex vitamins and iron deficiencies are possible. Additionally, ulcers, liver damage, infections, and chronic diarrhea are common. One of the worst problems is that despite the surgery, the patient may not lose a substantial amount of weight.

PERSPECTIVE AND PROSPECTS

The concept of coronary artery bypass surgery was studied in the late 1950's and early 1960's by Rene Favaloro, Donald Effler, Mason Sones, and Laurence Groves at the Cleveland Clinic in Ohio. In 1967, Favaloro developed the procedure using the saphenous vein graft. This procedure was further developed by several surgical teams until it became a widely used technique in the early 1970's. According to the American Heart Association, 265,000 individuals had bypass surgery in 1991. With the development of new drugs and angioplasty, however, the future of bypass surgery is questionable. In angioplasty, a catheter is inserted into the blocked artery and a balloon on the end of the catheter is inflated. The inflated balloon flattens the fatty deposits against the arterial wall, allowing the blood to flow freely.

Intestinal bypass surgery as treatment for morbid obesity was also initiated in the mid-1950's. Working independently, two surgical teams, one headed by John H. Linner and the other by Richard Varco, developed similar but different methods of bypass surgery. These procedures have been used and modified continually. When it comes to weight loss for the morbidly obese, different procedures, both surgical and nonsurgical, work more effectively with different people. Therefore, intestinal bypass is not recommended for many morbidly obese individuals. When good surgical techniques are used on the appropriate individual, however, bypass surgery can be very effective.

—*Bradley R. A. Wilson, Ph.D.*

See also Angina; Angioplasty; Arteriosclerosis; Cardiology; Cholesterol; Circulation; Gastrectomy; Gastroenterology; Gastrointestinal system; Gastrostomy; Heart; Heart disease; Heart valve replacement; Ileostomy and colostomy; Intestines; Obesity; Vascular medicine; Vascular system.

FOR FURTHER INFORMATION:

Bradley, Rebecca L. "Alterations in Nutrition." In *Principles and Practices of Adult Health Nursing*, edited by Patricia Gauntlett Beare and Judith L. Myers. 2d ed. St. Louis: Mosby Year Book, 1994.

Brammell, H. L., et al. *Cardiac Rehabilitation*. Denver: Webb-Waring Lung Institute, 1979.

Richmond, Caroline. "The Body's Transport Systems." In *Health, Medicine, and the Human Body*, edited by Bernard Dixon. New York: Macmillan, 1986.

CALCULI. *See* STONES.

CANCER

DISEASE/DISORDER

ANATOMY OR SYSTEM AFFECTED: All

SPECIALTIES AND RELATED FIELDS: Cytology, histology, immunology, oncology, orthopedics, radiology

DEFINITION: Inappropriate and uncontrollable cell growth within one of the specialized tissues of the body, threatening normal cell and organ function and in serious cases traveling via the bloodstream to other areas of the body.

KEY TERMS:

carcinogen: a cancer-causing substance; usually a chemical that causes mutations

cell: the basic functional unit of the body, each of which contains a set of genes and all the other materials necessary for carrying out the processes of life

cell cycle: a stepwise process whereby one cell duplicates itself to form two cells; it is the way in which most growth occurs, and the cycle leads to cancer if it becomes defective

gene: a master molecule that encodes the information needed for the body to carry out one specific function; many thousands of genes working together are needed to sustain normal human life

initiation: the first abnormal change that starts a cell along the pathway to cancer

metastasis: the process whereby tumor cells spread from one part of the body to another

mutation: damage to a gene that changes how it works

oncogene: a gene that functions normally to allow cells to progress through the cell cycle; when mutated, such genes can cause cancer

promotion: the second step in tumor development, which causes initiated cells to begin growing into tumors

tumor suppressor genes: genes that normally keep cell division in check, orderly and properly timed; when mutated, they can cause cancer

CAUSES AND SYMPTOMS

Cancer is a disease of abnormal growth. Growth is an important feature in the development of all living things, but it must be precisely controlled for life processes to occur properly. Much is known about how growth occurs and how it is regulated with such precision.

All growing cells pass through a strictly regulated series of events called the cell cycle. Most structures of the cell are duplicated during this sequence. At the end of the cycle, one cell is separated into two "daughter cells," each of which receives one copy of the duplicated cellular structures. The most important structures that must be exactly duplicated are the genes, the master blueprints that govern all cellular activities. Human life starts with a single microscopic cell—a fertilized egg. This cell divides again and again; the adult human body is composed of more than a

trillion cells, each with a very specific job to perform.

After adulthood is reached, most cells of the body stop duplicating themselves. Some cell types, however, do need to continue dividing to replace worn-out cells; these include cells of the blood, skin, intestine, and some other tissues. Such growth is very accurately controlled so that excess cells are not produced. It is in these cell types, those that normally grow in the adult body, that cancer most often occurs. A small defect arises in one gene so that the cells are able to progress through the cell cycle even though more cells are not needed. This is the start of cancer. Such cancer cells do not need to grow faster than do their normal neighbors; their key feature is simply that they continue growing when no more cells should be produced. At first, these cells very closely resemble their neighbors. For example, newly altered blood cells still look very much like normal blood cells, and in most respects they are.

The first defect that gets cancer started is called initiation. It is typically the result of a mutation in one of the genes whose job it is to control some feature of the cell cycle. There are probably several hundred such genes, each of which regulates a different aspect of the cell cycle. These genes have perfectly normal jobs in the life of the cell until they become damaged. When there is a mutation in a controlling gene, the gene functions improperly: It does not govern the cell cycle quite right, and the cell cycle therefore proceeds when it should instead be halted. Such cancer-causing genes are called oncogenes.

After the initiation of cancer, additional mutations and other defects begin to pile up, and the defective cells become increasingly abnormal. Tumor suppressor genes, which normally function to keep cell division from becoming disorganized, are the site of these second-stage mutations. Those cells whose cell division and growth genes have mutated (oncogenes) and whose cell division and growth inhibitor genes (tumor suppressor genes) have also been mutated will become cancer cells. Typically, a second change, called promotion, must take place before cancer cells begin really growing freely. The promotion step typically allows the initiated cell to escape some policing activity of the body. For example, various hormones provide cells with instructions about how to behave; a promotion-type change may allow a cell to ignore such instructions. Both initiation and promotion occur randomly. Many cells that are initiated, however, fail to grow into tumors. It is only those relatively few cells that happen to acquire both defects that become a problem. Fortunately, very few cells will have both their oncogenes turned "on" and their tumor suppressor genes turned "off."

At this point, the new cancer cell is dividing and collecting in large numbers. These excess cells make up a mass called a tumor (except in the blood and lymph cancers, in which the cancer cells circulate individually). Nevertheless, all these cells are fairly "normal." Indeed, at this early stage, cancer is relatively easy to control using methods such as surgery. The excess cells may not cause much harm—warts, for example, are excess numbers of growing cells. Such relatively harmless tumors are called benign. If the cancer is detected at this early stage, while it is still relatively harmless, effective treatment and even a cure are still quite possible, which is why early diagnosis is so important in cancer medicine.

Unfortunately, more and more defects accumulate in these cells as they grow, and some of these defects (again by chance) will be particularly harmful. The most harmful changes make the growing cells capable of causing damage to other parts of the body. For example, cancer cells may acquire the ability to digest their way through nearby tissues, a process called invasion. Eventually, the functions of organs containing such cells become impaired. Such an invasion of body parts can be extremely painful as well. Other cancer cells may come loose from the tumor and travel to other parts of the body in the circulatory or lymphatic system: This process is called metastasis. In advanced stages of cancer, a patient may actually have dozens or hundreds

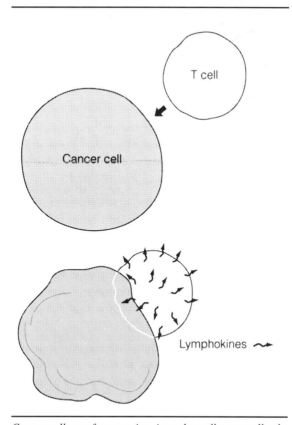

Cancer cells are fast-growing, irregular cells; normally, the body releases killer T cells that interact with antigens on the surface of the cancer cell, releasing lymphokines that are toxic to the cancer cell.

of tumors, all of which have developed from a single parent tumor. Cells that can invade or metastasize are called malignant. It becomes increasingly difficult to eradicate cancer cells as they become more malignant. Pathologists are highly skilled at distinguishing benign from malignant cancer cells based on their appearance in a microscope and can provide accurate diagnosis of how far a case of cancer has progressed. Such information is crucial for deciding how best to treat the cancer.

Most kinds of cancer typically occur during old age. Because each of the events that leads to tumor development is rather uncommon, it takes years for the several required mistakes to accumulate in a single cell, which then grows into a tumor. A few kinds of cancer occur most commonly in children. Such children usually have inherited one or more of the genetic defects that lead to cancer (already mutated oncogenes or tumor suppressor genes) from their parents. It then takes less time before the additional required defects are likely to occur. Thus, a tendency toward certain kinds of cancer can be inherited in families, as with other genetic traits (such as hair and eye color, height, and nose shape).

Cancer occurs when anything causes oncogenes and tumor suppressor genes to function abnormally, allowing cells to continue growing when they should not. The delicate genes in an individual's cells can be modified chemically by a number of different highly active and dangerous chemicals known collectively as carcinogens. Several kinds of radiation also pose a threat to genes. The best-known example is ultraviolet radiation from the sun, which can damage genes of the skin and lead to skin cancer. Finally, certain kinds of viruses can cause oncogenes to function improperly.

TREATMENT AND THERAPY

Most people who live to an advanced age can expect to be faced with cancer. Because cancer is such a serious and widespread health problem, enormous efforts have gone into learning how the disease develops and then applying those discoveries to cure and prevent cancer.

The cancer treatments used most commonly are of three kinds: surgery, chemotherapy, and radiation therapy. First, and most straightforward, is the surgical removal of tumors. If done at an early stage, before cancer has spread, this method can be highly successful. Even so, surgery is much easier and less dangerous for some cancers (for example, skin cancer) than for others (such as brain tumors, which can be difficult to reach and remove safely). Naturally, surgery is much less successful with widely spread cancers such as leukemia (a cancer of blood cells) and in more advanced stages of cancer.

The second type of cancer treatment is chemotherapy. Patients are treated with chemicals that prevent cells from duplicating themselves, or at least limit or slow that process. Such drugs, which are usually injected, reach all parts of the body and so are much more effective than surgery when cancer has reached a later stage of spreading. Different kinds of chemicals work in very different ways to achieve this result. These chemicals can be roughly divided into four categories. First are chemicals that react directly with the substances required for cells to survive and function. Many such agents directly attack a cell's genes, preventing them from passing along information required for a cancer cell to stay alive. Second are antimetabolites, which prevent the chemical reactions that allow cells to produce energy (energy must also be available for cells to stay alive). The third category consists of steroid hormones. Cancer cells in some organs of the body respond to these hormones, which can therefore be used to regulate their growth. Thus estrogens, the female sex steroid hormones, are often used for treatment of breast cancer, whereas the male sex steroids, or androgens, may influence prostate cancer. Fourth are miscellaneous drugs, a few other chemicals that affect cancer cells in some different way. For example, drugs called vinca alkaloids stop the mechanical process of one cell dividing into two, in this way preventing growth. A derivative of the insecticide DDT (dichloro-diphenyl-trichloroethane) prevents unwanted steroid-hormone production and has been useful for treating tumors of the adrenal gland.

The most common and difficult problem with the chemotherapeutic approach to cancer management is that normal cells that happen to be growing are also affected by the same drugs that halt the growth of cancer cells. This reaction causes many difficulties for patients, some serious and some less so. Probably the most serious problems are in the immune system. The growth of blood cells that make antibodies, called lymphocytes, is necessary before antibodies can be produced in response to an infectious disease. Because these cells cannot grow, patients in chemotherapy are much more vulnerable to illnesses caused by bacteria and viruses. Other blood cells, including those that carry oxygen, are also affected, causing additional problems. Skin cells and cells lining the digestive tract stop dividing, causing additional difficulties for the patients. A less serious problem for such patients is hair loss, as hair cells also are prevented from growing.

Designing drug treatments that kill cancer cells while minimizing these problems is a demanding and precise task for oncologists (physicians who specialize in cancer research and treatment). Some drugs affect different cell types in somewhat different ways, allowing normal cells to continue their functions while killing tumor cells. Doses and timing of treatments can be adjusted to maximize the effect of the drugs. It is typical for several drugs that act in different ways to be given in the same treatment, to assure that all cancer cells are halted; this approach is called combination chemotherapy. It is of critical importance that all cancer cells be stopped because a single unaffected cancer cell at any place in the body can begin growing after che-

motherapy and develop into a cancer, a process known as relapse.

Another useful approach for improving chemotherapy is drug targeting. The chemical structure of tumor cells is subtly different from that of normal cells, and it is sometimes possible to make use of this difference. For example, a drug can be attached to an antibody molecule that reacts with a tumor protein (antigen) that is not found on normal cells. In this way, most of the drug will be directed to the tumor cells, while normal cells will receive a much lower dose. Hormones and other molecules also attach to specific molecules on cells, and this fact can sometimes be exploited to target drugs if the tumor cells have a particularly high number of such molecules.

Another problem with drug delivery is that the most effective drugs are rapidly degraded by the body's defense systems and secreted from the body. The actual period of exposure to an active drug in the body can be quite brief (a few minutes) for this reason. Methods have been developed for hiding or disguising drugs so they are not removed so rapidly. For example, some drugs can be placed inside fat droplets, and in this way they can escape detection by the immune system and breakdown in the liver.

Because of the great importance of effective chemotherapy, thousands of new compounds are screened each year for their effectiveness against cancer. The first step in this process is the careful and extensive testing of such compounds on animals, usually mice and rats. Both the effectiveness of the drug against cancer and its effects on normal bodily functions are carefully measured. Drugs that pass the animal tests are then tried out in cautious human tests. Often, the first patients tested are those with advanced cancer conditions who volunteer for such treatment. Three further levels of human testing then follow before a new drug can be marketed. Only about one in five thousand drugs tested reaches clinical trials; one in fifty thousand becomes available for general use. The testing process is lengthy and expensive, but thousands of lives are saved each year because of the careful testing and development of new chemotherapies.

The third type of cancer treatment is radiation therapy. The radiation of choice is X rays, which can penetrate the body to reach a tumor and which can be produced at very high dosages using modern equipment. X rays can be focused on a specific small area or can be given over the whole body in the case of metastasized cancer. Therapeutic radiation damages genes to such an extent that they become physically fragmented and nonfunctional, ending the life of the target cell.

Radiation therapy has some of the same drawbacks as chemotherapy. Again, the most serious problem is that normal cells in the pathway of the radiation will also be killed. Bone marrow, the source of blood cells, is destroyed by whole-body cancer treatments. This problem can be overcome after radiation therapy by transplanting new bone marrow to the patient from close relatives, so that a treated patient can begin to remanufacture blood cells. Ironically, radiation designed to kill cancer cells can also turn normal cells into new cancer cells. Some normal cells may receive a reduced exposure of X rays. The dosage may be just sufficient to damage oncogenes of normal cells, causing them to become cancerous. Thus radiation therapy must be carried out with great care and precision.

PERSPECTIVE AND PROSPECTS

Cancer has plagued humankind for thousands of years. Fossils of humanoid ancestors show evidence of cancer, bone cancer is identifiable in Egyptian mummies, and the ancient Greek physician Hippocrates described many kinds of cancer that were common during his time. Animals and even plants develop abnormal growths comparable to cancer in people—the curse of cancer is inherent in the way that all organisms grow.

The first major insight into why cancer occurs was made by Percivall Pott, a British physician. In 1775, he reported his observations on scrotal cancer in young chimney sweeps. This cancer was unusually frequent in these boys. Pott suggested that repeated exposure to the irritating soot in chimneys was what started this cancer. He is credited with the first description of cancer initiation.

During the next 150 years, the major advances in fighting cancer were safer and more effective surgery procedures. These important improvements were made much easier by the development of effective anesthetics and antibiotics. Also, by the end of the nineteenth century, the principles of radiation therapy and chemotherapy were being established, based on fundamental research in physics and chemistry.

Progress in the battle against cancer was steady in the first half of the twentieth century. The principles of initiation and promotion became firmly established, and the features of most kinds of cancer were thoroughly described. It became clear that cancer is not a single disease, that each type has its own causes and potential cures. Cancer epidemics, for example among asbestos workers, drove home the lesson that substances in the environment can cause cancer and must be carefully monitored.

In the 1940's and 1950's, research on genes started a revolution in the understanding of biology and how the human body functions. These new advances were quickly related to cancer, and it was understood that defective genes could lead to abnormal growth. The exciting implication of this insight was that a solution to the cancer problem seemed within grasp: It was necessary either to prevent mutations in cancer-causing genes or to correct such errors after they happened.

In the 1970's and 1980's, the intense effort of scientists and physicians around the world resulted in the oncogene and tumor suppressor gene concept. Finally, cancer cell growth was understood as resulting from defects in genes that have a perfectly normal function in the economy of the body. Meanwhile, new advances made it possible to analyze and manipulate genes in ways only dreamed of previously. Gene therapy became another weapon in the arsenal available to physicians. Immunotherapy is another important area of cancer research. It attempts to use the body's own defenses (white blood cells, antibodies, and natural toxins such as interferon) to kill cancer cells.

Because of its nature and importance, the fight against cancer has involved an unusually broad spectrum of medical and scientific specialties. As a result, people are becoming increasingly protected from this disease. Cancer-causing agents are closely regulated, and new diagnostic procedures can detect abnormal cells at the earliest stages.

—Howard L. Hosick, Ph.D.
updated by Connie Rizzo, M.D.

See also Biopsy; Bone cancer; Bone marrow transplantation; Breast biopsy; Breast cancer; Carcinoma; Cells; Cervical, ovarian, and uterine cancers; Chemotherapy; Colon and rectal polyp removal; Colon and rectal surgery; Colon cancer; Colonoscopy; Cystectomy; Cytology; Cytopathology; Dermatopathology; Endometrial biopsy; Gastrectomy; Hodgkin's disease; Hysterectomy; Imaging and radiology; Immunology; Immunopathology; Kaposi's sarcoma; Laryngectomy; Leukemia; Liver cancer; Lung cancer; Lung surgery; Lymphadenopathy and lymphoma; Malignancy and metastasis; Malignant melanoma removal; Mammography; Mastectomy and lumpectomy; Oncology; Plastic, cosmetic, and reconstructive surgery; Prostate cancer; Prostate gland removal; Radiation therapy; Sarcoma; Screening; Skin cancer; Skin lesion removal; Stomach, intestinal, and pancreatic cancers; Terminally ill, extended care for the; Tumor removal; Tumors.

FOR FURTHER INFORMATION:

Cairns, John. *Cancer: Science and Society*. San Francisco: W. H. Freeman, 1978. Cairns is a prominent molecular biologist who has turned his attention to cancer. He writes eloquently but nontechnically about the biology and medical implications of cancer. Several chapters are designed specifically to introduce concepts to individuals with little background in science. An excellent and accessible overview of the basic features of this disease.

Levenson, Frederick B. *The Causes and Prevention of Cancer*. New York: Stein & Day, 1985. A very personal attempt to give an overview of cancer and how it fits into health maintenance in general. Presented as a storylike narrative with the emphasis ultimately on the author's unproved ideas about cancer prevention and its relationship to human life.

Levitt, Paul M., and Elissa S. Guralnick. *The Cancer Reference Book: Direct and Clear Answers to Everyone's Questions*. New York: Facts on File, 1983. A different format, structured as a series of specific questions and answers dealing mostly with practical, medically oriented questions about cancer. Contains a simple glossary, an honest discussion of treatments, and facts about many individual kinds of cancer.

Maugh, Thomas H., II, and Jane L. Marx. *Seeds of Destruction*. New York: Plenum Press, 1975. This book is by two science writers who are skilled at explaining complex facts and ideas. Although the book is not up to date on more recent findings, it is still an accurate and unusually clear summary of the basic biology of cancer.

Murphy, G., L. Morris, and D. Lange. *Informed Decisions: The Complete Book of Cancer Diagnosis, Treatment, and Recovery*. New York: Viking Press, 1997. This text from the American Cancer Society is intended for the layperson. It is exemplary in its discussion of cancer.

Oppenheimer, Steven B. *Cancer: A Biological and Clinical Introduction*. Boston: Allyn & Bacon, 1982. A more rigorous treatment of the characteristics of cancer than are the other books listed. It is unusually well written, however, and those willing to expend the extra effort required will be rewarded with a deeper understanding of the characteristics of cancer.

Prescott, D. M., and Abraham S. Flexer. *Cancer: The Misguided Cell*. Sunderland, Mass.: Sinauer Associates, 1986. The authors focus primarily on how cells change during cancer. This book describes more basic biology than most of the other publications listed.

Siegel, Mary-Ellen. *The Cancer Patient's Handbook: Everything You Need to Know About Today's Care and Treatment*. New York: Walker, 1986. Siegel is a physician who explains concepts in simple terms. A very practical discussion of medical procedures related to cancer, including diagnosis and therapy. Provides descriptions of the various kinds of cancer and a useful glossary.

Tierney, Lawrence M., Jr., et al., eds. *Current Medical Diagnosis and Treatment*. 37th ed. Norwalk, Conn.: Appleton and Lange, 1998. This text, updated yearly, is the point of reference for physicians and other health care practitioners. It incorporates each year's biomedical research discoveries that have immediate, relevant, and applicable use for the patient.

CANDIDIASIS

DISEASE/DISORDER

ANATOMY OR SYSTEM AFFECTED: Abdomen, bladder, blood, gastrointestinal system, genitals, immune system, mouth, reproductive system, skin, urinary system

SPECIALTIES AND RELATED FIELDS: Family physicians, immunologists, infectious disease physicians, internists

DEFINITION: An acute or chronic fungal infection of humans and animals that can be superficial or deep-seated, caused by a species of the fungus *Candida*.

KEY TERMS:

acquired immunodeficiency syndrome (AIDS): a severe and usually fatal disease caused by infection with the human immunodeficiency virus (HIV); infection results in progressive impairment of the immune system

antifungal agents: drugs that can result in the inhibition of growth or killing of fungi; these drugs may be topical or systemic in application

cell-mediated immunity: protection mediated by thymus-derived lymphocytes; this type of immunity is particularly important for certain types of pathogenic organisms such as *Candida*

chlamydoconidia (chlamydospores): budding organisms that form directly from vegetative mycelia (molds); they differ from true spores, which are the result of sexual reproduction

culture: the propagation of organisms, such as fungi, on artificial media; *Candida* organisms grow in many kinds of media in both the yeast and mold forms

dimorphism: the ability of a fungus to exist in two forms, yeasts and molds; yeasts are unicellular round, oval, or cylindrical cells, and molds are branching tubular structures called hyphae

germ tube test: an initial laboratory test used to identify unknown yeasts and performed by microscopically examining a colony of yeast inoculated into rabbit or human plasma

histopathology: the study of the appearance and structure of abnormal or diseased tissue under the microscope

phagocytosis: the progress of ingestion and digestion by cells that are part of the immune system; this process is one of the ways that mammals use to defend themselves against infectious invaders, including *Candida* organisms

CAUSES AND SYMPTOMS

Candida is a genus of dimorphic fungi found widely in nature. This fungus may be found in soil, inanimate objects, plants, and most important, as a harmless parasite of humans and other mammals. It can exist in two forms: as a yeast and as a mold. In the yeast phase, this fungus exists as a normal inhabitant in and on human bodies. Nearly all infections are of such endogenous origin, but human-to-human transmission may occasionally occur from mother to newborn or between sexual partners. The yeasts reproduce asexually by budding, and a sexual stage has been recognized only in a few species. Pseudohyphae develop when yeasts and their progeny adhere to one another, forming chains. Hyphae, the branching tubular structures of molds, are formed in tissue invaded by the fungus.

Identification of *Candida* as the causative agent in clinical infections depends largely on the microscopic examination of infected tissue or secretions and on a culture of *Candida* prepared from infected material. Histopathological examination may reveal yeast forms and/or hyphal or pseudohyphal forms. The microscopic appearance of these organisms is similar to those of some other fungi, and a culture is necessary to confirm this fungus as the respon-

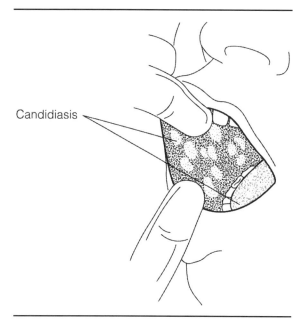

Candidiasis of the mouth is a fungal infection characterized by white patches and commonly called "thrush mouth."

sible pathogen. *Candida* will grow on many types of artificial microbiologic media and can usually be grown on the same media used to grow bacteria. With some types of infection, however, the use of special media or techniques may lead to a higher yield from cultures. After an unknown yeast is grown on artificial media, tests must be performed to determine its identity. Most laboratories initially use the germ tube test, in which yeast is introduced into rabbit or human plasma at 35 degrees Celsius for one to two hours. In this test, a structure called a germ tube is observed if the yeast is *Candida albicans*, *Candida stelloidea*, or rare strains of *Candida tropicalis*. If this test is positive (a germ tube is produced), then most laboratories assume that the microorganism is *C. albicans*—it is by far the most common species causing disease—and conduct no further, and usually more expensive, tests. Simple cultural tests may also be used to identify *C. albicans*, including the formation of spiderlike colonies on eosin methylene blue agar or the production of chlamydoconidia on cornmeal agar. The identification of *Candida* antigens in the serum of patients with widespread or disseminated infection is sometimes used to assist in the diagnosis of candidiasis, but this test is neither sensitive nor specific.

The bodies of humans and other mammals possess multiple defense mechanisms against candidiasis. The skin and mucous membranes provide a protective wall, but breaks in the mucocutaneous barrier may occur in many ways, including trauma, surgery, and disease. A balanced microbial flora in the gastrointestinal tract prevents the overgrowth of *Candida* organisms, which can lead to penetra-

tion of this fungus into the lining of the gastrointestinal tract and its entrance into the bloodstream. When invasion occurs, phagocytic cells (including monocytes, neutrophils, and eosinophils) further protect the body by ingesting and killing *Candida* organisms. Phagocytosis is assisted by serum proteins called opsonins. Lymphocytes are also important defenders against this fungus and are part of the cell-mediated immune system. Candidiasis may result when cell-mediated immunity is defective, as is the case with the hereditary condition of chronic mucocutaneous candidiasis or with acquired immunodeficiency syndrome (AIDS). Approximately 80 percent of healthy people exhibit delayed hypersensitivity reactions to *Candida* antigens, indicating the presence of a previously induced cell-mediated immunity directed against such an infection.

Candidiasis may be divided into superficial mucocutaneous and deep-seated, tissue-invasive types. There are more than one hundred fifty species of this fungus, but only ten are recognized as human pathogens, and *C. albicans* is the most important. Oral candidiasis, or thrush, is a common infection characterized by white patches on the tongue and oral mucosal surfaces (oropharyngeal infection). Scrapings taken from these patches contain masses of yeasts, pseudohyphae, and hyphae. Culturing is not as useful as clinical appearance and microscopic examination, since *Candida* organisms can be grown from normal mouths. Thrush is particularly common when the immune system is impaired, as in patients with cancer or AIDS or in asthmatics treated with inhaled steroids. Infection of other parts of the gastrointestinal tract, especially the esophagus, may occur in patients with a variety of underlying conditions, including an impaired immune system, gastrointestinal surgery, and antibiotic treatment. Esophageal involvement often results in difficult or painful swallowing. Only about half of patients with esophageal candidiasis will also have the more easily diagnosed oropharyngeal infection. Some patients with gastrointestinal candidiasis will develop systemic or disseminated infection.

Vaginal candidiasis, the most common type of vaginitis, is a common form of the infection associated with an overgrowth of *Candida* organisms in the vagina followed by mucocutaneous invasion. The patient will have a thick, curdlike vaginal discharge and itching of the surrounding skin areas. Antibiotic therapy, pregnancy, birth control pills, diabetes, and AIDS all predispose women to this form of infection. Recurrent or chronic infection can occur and may be associated with tissue invasion or impaired response of lymphocytes to the infection in some patients.

Cutaneous infection is common with candidiasis. This fungus is often the cause of diaper rash in infants; the condition often results from infection of skin under wet diapers by *Candida* organisms from the gastrointestinal tract. Intertrigo is another skin condition produced by candidiasis in the warm, moist area of skin folds, and similar environments result in perianal or scrotal infections that cause intense itching (pruritus). A widespread eruption of infection involving the trunk, thorax, and extremities is occasionally seen in both children and adults. Disseminated candidiasis, usually in association with persistent candidemia (the presence of the fungus in the bloodstream), may be associated with widely distributed, nodular skin lesions. Candidiasis of the skin, mucous membranes, hair, and nails beginning early in life and associated with defective cell-mediated immunity has been called chronic mucocutaneous candidiasis. This disease is often associated with a variety of endocrine diseases, including diabetes mellitus and decreased function of the parathyroid, thyroid, and adrenal glands.

Deep-organ involvement with candidiasis is serious and often life-threatening. The placement in the body of foreign material used for medical therapy may provide the initial breeding ground for the infection. Examples of these devices are vascular catheters, artificial heart valves, artificial vascular grafts, and artificial joints and other orthopedic implants. The environment created by these foreign materials makes it impossible for the normal defense mechanisms of the body to function.

Urinary tract infection with *Candida* organisms is seen in association with urinary catheters, especially when usage is chronic. Colonization of the urine with *Candida* organisms may also occur following a course of antibiotics or in diabetic patients. Infection of the kidney can result if the candidiasis spreads upward from the bladder through the ureter or via the bloodstream. Renal involvement has been reported in up to 80 percent of patients with disseminated candidiasis. In disseminated disease, infection is spread to the kidney through the bloodstream, with the formation of renal abscesses. Primary renal infection occurs when the kidney is invaded directly without concomitant invasion through the blood. Such direct infection may occur in association with urinary catheters or following surgical procedures involving the genital and urinary tracts. A particularly severe form of ascending renal infection, more frequent in diabetic patients, causes necrosis of the renal papillae and renal failure.

Ocular candidiasis (endophthalmitis) may occur when the eye is infected with *Candida* organisms either by direct invasion or through the bloodstream. Virtually any portion or structure of the eye may be involved. Examination of the retina using an ophthalmoscope can reveal white spots, resembling cotton balls, indicating *Candida* organisms in the blood vessels of the eye. This finding may also be a clue to infection elsewhere in the body that has spread through the bloodstream to the eye.

Endocarditis (inflammation of the lining of the heart) occurs when a native or artificial heart valve becomes infected. Candidiasis is an increasingly frequent cause of endocarditis of the native valves of intravenous drug abusers and artificial valves of all varieties. Such endocarditis is presumptively diagnosed when the organism is grown from blood specimens in the presence of a heart murmur. Abnormal growth on the heart valves, called vegetation, can usually be demonstrated using echocardiography. Fragments of vegetation may break off and circulate in the bloodstream, leading to the obstruction of vessels in many organs of the body including the brain, eyes, lungs, spleen, and kidneys. Without treatment, this disease is uniformly fatal.

Disseminated candidiasis is seen in the most susceptible patients, including those with cancer, prolonged postoperative illness, and extensive burns. In these patients, further risk is associated with the use of central venous or arterial catheters, broad-spectrum antibiotic therapy, artificial feeding, or abdominal surgery. Dysfunction of neutrophils, or neutropenia, may increase the susceptibility of the patient to widespread infection with *Candida* organisms and can also be seen with AIDS. The kidney, brain, heart, and eye are the most common organs to be involved. Despite severe and extensive disease, specific diagnosis of disseminated candidiasis is difficult during life and is often only made at the time of postmortem examination.

TREATMENT AND THERAPY

Candidiasis may be prevented by avoiding or ameliorating the underlying predisposing factor or disease state and by decreasing or halting growth of the fungi. Dry or cracked skin can be treated with dermatologic lubricants. Invasive devices used for medical treatment should be placed in the body under the most sterile conditions and only employed when absolutely necessary. Care of these devices, including urinary catheters, intravascular lines, and peritoneal renal dialysis catheters must be performed by skilled personnel using the most sterile approach possible. If antibacterial therapy is used excessively, fungal overgrowth may occur; *Candida* organisms can grow with ease in the gastrointestinal tract and vagina when bacteria are inhibited or killed by antibiotics, and overgrowth can lead not only to local infection but also to bloodstream invasion and secondary infection elsewhere in the body. Moreover, the treatment of underlying disease states such as diabetes mellitus, neoplasia, and AIDS will lessen the detrimental effects of candidiasis on the immune system.

Growth of *Candida* organisms can be decreased by altering the local conditions that favor their proliferation. For example, changing a baby's diaper frequently and applying a drying powder can avoid the wet and warm conditions that can result in diaper rash. Obese patients can lose weight, which will minimize skin fold infections. Wearing nonocclusive clothing, especially cotton fabrics, is often helpful in discouraging candidiasis.

Antifungal agents are often used to prevent candidiasis. Hospitalized patients recovering from surgery who have received antibacterial agents are given nystatin, an oral, nonabsorbed antifungal, to prevent the overgrowth of *Candida* organisms in the gastrointestinal tract. For cancer patients receiving chemotherapy, systemic antifungal drugs are often employed during the period when the cancer chemotherapy has had the most deleterious effects on the immune system.

Antifungals are employed by the topical, oral, parenteral (through a blood vessel or muscle), or irrigation routes for treatment of candidiasis. Among the many antifungal agents, nystatin, flucytosine, amphotericin B, and a variety of imidazole agents are the most commonly used. Antifungals utilize a number of different mechanisms that impede the metabolic activities of the organism or disrupt the integrity of the cell membrane on the outer surface of the fungus. Amphotericin B and fluconazole are useful in the treatment of systemic or deep-organ disease. Amphotericin B is produced by the fungus *Streptomyces nodosus* and is administered intravenously for systemic and deep-organ disease and by bladder irrigation for lower urinary tract infection (cystitis). When administered intravenously, amphotericin B has serious side effects, including fever, chills, kidney failure, liver abnormalities, and bone marrow suppression. Fluconazole has fewer adverse effects and can be administered by the oral or intravenous routes; for these reasons, it is now commonly used as the initial therapy for candidiasis. Amphotericin B remains the treatment of choice for serious or life-threatening infection or when a *Candida* species isolated from a patient has been demonstrated by laboratory testing to be resistant to other antifungal agents.

In addition to antifungals, removal of foreign material or infected tissue is often necessary to treat severe candidiasis. Catheters, vascular grafts, artificial heart valves, artificial joints, and other devices must be removed and then replaced, if necessary, while the patient is receiving antifungal therapy or after the infection is cured. In some cases, such as with endocarditis, the infected tissue must be surgically removed to ensure a cure.

As with prevention, treatment of the underlying disease state greatly assists other measures directed against candidiasis. Gaining control of hyperglycemia in diabetes mellitus patients, viral infection in AIDS patients, and bone marrow suppression in cancer patients will aid in the treatment of candidiasis when it is present.

PERSPECTIVE AND PROSPECTS

More than two thousand years ago, the Greek physicians Hippocrates and Galen described oral lesions that were probably thrush, but it was not until 1839 that fungi were found in such lesions. Deep-seated infection was first described in 1861, and endocarditis was identified in 1940. Candidiasis was recognized as an indicator disease in the 1987 surveillance definition for AIDS by the Centers for Disease Control in the United States. *Candida* ranks among the most common pathogens in hospital-acquired infections.

Candidiasis is on the increase largely because of increasingly sophisticated medical therapies and the worldwide epidemic of AIDS. Medical devices, immunosuppressive medical therapies, and organ transplantation are all becoming more common, and it is anticipated that candidiasis will increase in a corresponding manner. Likewise, as the number of patients infected with human immunodeficiency virus (HIV) progress to clinical illness, the cases of candidiasis are expected to rise dramatically.

More effective preventive and therapeutic measures will be necessary to combat such an increase in cases of candidiasis. New antifungal agents will need to be developed to treat resistant strains of *Candida*. Laboratory testing to determine whether various antifungal agents can kill or inhibit the growth of *Candida* species isolated from patients will need to be more widely available and more frequently performed if organisms resistant to antifungals are to be identified. Early identification of resistant organisms will benefit patients by providing more effective antifungal therapy early in the course of treatment. Testing procedures will need to employ better methodology that is standardized to enable laboratories in different locations to compare results and determine regional or national trends in antifungal resistance. —*H. Bradford Hawley, M.D.*

See also Endocarditis; Fungal infections; Rashes.

FOR FURTHER INFORMATION:

Biddle, Wayne. *Field Guide to Germs*. New York: Henry Holt, 1995. This comprehensive book is easily accessible to the nonspecialist and includes a discussion of nearly every virus, bacterium, and fungus known to cause human and nonhuman animal disease. The history of the microbe and the treatment of diseases are included.

De Vita, Vincent T., Jr., Samuel Hellman, and Steven A. Rosenberg. *AIDS: Etiology, Diagnosis, Treatment, and Prevention*. 3d ed. Philadelphia: J. B. Lippincott, 1992. The definitive reference text concerning acquired immunodeficiency syndrome. Contains excellent chapters describing the clinical types of candidiasis in these patients and their treatment.

Holmberg, Kenneth, and Richard D. Meyer, eds. *Diagnosis and Therapy of Systemic Fungal Infections*. New York: Raven Press, 1989. This specialized text offers a thorough review of the various types of systemic fungal infections and appropriate preventive and therapeutic measures; the majority of this text concerns candidiasis.

Koneman, Elmer W., et al. *Color Atlas and Textbook of Diagnostic Microbiology*. 4th ed. Philadelphia: J. B. Lippincott, 1992. A practical text with excellent tables, charts, and photographs of microorganisms, including *Candida*. Also contains information on the collection of specimens from patients, the processing of cultures, and the interpretation of laboratory data.

Kwon-Chung, K. J., and John E. Bennett. *Medical Mycology*. Philadelphia: Lea & Febiger, 1992. A fine text concerning fungal diseases. All aspects of these diseases, including their diagnosis and treatment, are covered.

Ledger, William J. *Infection in the Female.* 2d ed. Philadelphia: Lea & Febiger, 1986. An excellent treatise on gynecologic and obstetric infections. Offers information about the aspects of candidiasis in the female patient.

Mandell, Gerald L., R. Gordon Douglas, Jr., and John E. Bennett, eds. *Principles and Practice of Infectious Diseases.* 4th ed. New York: Churchill Livingstone, 1995. An outstanding textbook in infectious diseases, with chapters on the various diseases caused by Candida, illnesses and conditions associated with this fungus, and antifungal agents.

Reese, Richard E., and Robert F. Betts, eds. *A Practical Approach to Infectious Diseases.* 3d ed. Boston: Little, Brown, 1991. A well-written and very popular text. This clinically oriented, multiauthor book on infectious diseases, including candidiasis, contains carefully chosen, annotated references at the end of each of the twenty-eight chapters. Offers a very good section on antifungal chemotherapy.

CARCINOMA
DISEASE/DISORDER
ANATOMY OR SYSTEM AFFECTED: All

SPECIALTIES AND RELATED FIELDS: Cytology, dermatology, histology, immunology, oncology

DEFINITION: A carcinoma is a malignant neoplasm, or cancer, arising from the epithelial cells that make up the surface layers of skin or other membranes; by contrast, sarcomas are malignant neoplasms that arise from the mesodermal cells of connective tissue, bone, and muscle. Carcinomas commonly occur in the skin, the large intestine, the lungs, the breasts and cervix in women, and the prostate gland in men. The term "carcinoma" is often used as a synonym for "cancer."

—*Jason Georges and Tracy Irons-Georges*

See also Biopsy; Bone cancer; Bone marrow transplantation; Breast biopsy; Breast cancer; Cancer; Cervical, ovarian, and uterine cancers; Chemotherapy; Colon cancer; Endometrial biopsy; Immunology; Immunopathology; Liver cancer; Lung cancer; Malignancy and metastasis; Malignant melanoma removal; Mammography; Mastectomy and lumpectomy; Oncology; Prostate cancer; Radiation therapy; Sarcoma; Skin cancer; Skin lesion removal; Stomach, intestinal, and pancreatic cancers; Tumor removal; Tumors.

CARDIAC REHABILITATION
PROCEDURE
ANATOMY OR SYSTEM AFFECTED: Chest, circulatory system, heart

SPECIALTIES AND RELATED FIELDS: Cardiology, exercise physiology, nursing, nutrition, occupational health, physical therapy, psychology

DEFINITION: The activities that ensure the physical, mental, and social conditions necessary for returning cardiac patients to good health.

KEY TERMS:

aerobic exercise: exercise that requires oxygen for energy production and that can be sustained for prolonged periods of time; involves large muscle groups, increases the heart rate and breathing rate, and is rhythmic and continuous

atherosclerosis: a buildup of fatty deposits or plaques which effectively reduces the inner diameter of the arteries, thus obstructing the normal flow of blood

cardiovascular disease: any of a group of diseases that affect the heart, including coronary artery disease, hypertension, congestive heart failure, congenital heart defects, and valvular heart disease

coronary artery bypass graft (CABG): a surgical procedure in which a blocked coronary artery is bypassed using a vein or artery; this intervention provides a blood supply to areas beyond the distal attachment of the graft

coronary artery disease (CAD): a disease which results in a narrowing of the coronary arteries and a concomitant reduction of oxygen supply to the heart muscle

electrocardiogram (EKG or ECG): a mechanical representation of the electrical activity generated by the heart and recorded on paper or displayed on a cathode-ray tube

invasive testing: techniques involving the puncture or incision of the skin or the insertion of an instrument or foreign material into the body

MET: a measure of human energy expenditure; 1 MET is equal to the amount of energy expended at rest (approximately 3.5 milliliters of oxygen per kilogram of body weight per minute)

myocardial infarction: irreversible damage to heart muscle tissue caused by insufficient oxygen supply to that tissue

percutaneous transluminal coronary angioplasty (PTCA): a procedure undertaken to increase the internal diameter of a coronary artery by inflating a small balloonlike device at the site or sites where the artery has narrowed because of plaque buildup

risk factors: those habits or conditions that increase the likelihood of developing a disease or disorder

target heart rate range: a heart rate range that is to be maintained during exercise training

INDICATIONS AND PROCEDURES

Cardiovascular disease (CVD), or heart disease, is the leading cause of death and disability in most of the industrialized nations of the world. For those persons who survive a cardiac event, discharge from a hospital or medical setting without further assistance may lead to financial, physical, and mental incapacity.

Just as interventional procedures and medical care are important for the initial treatment of acute cardiac events, such as a myocardial infarction (heart attack) or angina (chest pain), cardiac rehabilitation influences long-term morbidity and mortality. Such preventive cardiology assists persons with CVD in three main areas: education, behavior modification, and patient and family support. The two primary goals of the rehabilitation program are to help increase the patient's functional capacity (the ability to perform activities of daily living) and to counteract or arrest the patient's disease process using a multidisciplined educational approach.

In order to provide direction in prevention and rehabilitation, research studies have clearly defined several modifiable risk factors for heart disease, which are presented to patients. Among the most significant are smoking, high serum cholesterol, hypertension, and physical inactivity. Assistance with education about and modification of these risk factors, through risk factor counseling and participation in physical activity, is provided in modern cardiac rehabilitation programs.

Methods for providing education on risk factor modification can vary greatly from program to program, but include such means as didactic lecturing, slide presentations, printed material for patients to read, demonstrations (such as cooking and stress reduction techniques), providing loaner books, and one-on-one counseling.

The exercise portion of the cardiac rehabilitation is most often the time-consuming element of the program. It involves controlling and monitoring four major variables: mode (type of activity, such as bicycling, walking, or stair-stepping), duration (length of time the patient exercises), frequency (number of times per week that exercise is performed), and intensity (exertion level of the patient, usually assessed by the heart rate response).

To become involved in the cardiac rehabilitation program, a patient is initially screened by a physician, nurse, or other clinical specialist and directed to the appropriate level (or phase) of intervention.

There are three to four clinical phases involved with cardiac rehabilitation, as various groups categorize them differently. The Exercise and Cardiac Rehabilitation Committee of the American Heart Association outlines three phases; the American Association of Cardiovascular and Pulmonary Rehabilitation (AACVPR) outlines four phases.

Phase 1 occurs while the patient is still in the hospital. It begins when the patient's condition is stabilized, sometimes as soon as forty-eight hours after the coronary event or procedure. This phase can begin in the coronary care unit (CCU) or the intensive care unit (ICU). Phase 1 incorporates several disciplines, including physical therapy, nursing, psychiatry, dietetics, occupational therapy, and exercise science. It is designed to prevent the deleterious physiological effects of bed rest.

The physical components of this phase include maintaining a range of motion and gradually returning to activities of daily living. Patients gradually advance through stages until they are able to walk up to 200 or 400 feet. Before discharge, patients are encouraged to walk up and down one flight of stairs. Stair climbing is done while accompanied by a physical therapist or other clinician who monitors heart rate and blood pressure. The level of exertion during the early portion of this phase is normally 1 to 2 METs. Thus, in phase 1, the mode of exercise focuses on motion (sitting, standing, and finally walking), the frequency is seven days per week, the duration of exercise is usually five to ten minutes at a time, and the intensity of activity should not cause the heart rate to exceed twenty beats above the resting rate while standing.

For coronary artery bypass graft (CABG) patients who have not experienced a myocardial infarction, progress during this phase is usually faster than for heart attack patients. Percutaneous transluminal coronary angioplasty (PTCA) patients may receive only a few days of rehabilitation, as they are usually discharged from the hospital sooner than heart attack or CABG patients.

The mental components of phase 1 include risk factor modification education and an introduction to rehabilitation concepts. Risk factor education at this point provides a good foundation for the basic concepts that will be explained during the education program in phase 2. For those patients who are appropriate candidates for a phase 2 program, information on that phase is then provided.

Phase 2 customarily begins within three weeks of discharge from the hospital and lasts for four to twelve weeks. During phase 2, patients are exposed to a level of exertion commensurate with several criteria: the patient's clinical status (stable or unstable, depending on whether the patient is experiencing problems related to the disease); the patient's functional capacity, or fitness level; orthopedic limitations, such as muscle or joint problems; the goals for functional capacity (what tasks the patient wants to be able to perform); and any other special circumstances or situations.

In a given phase 2 program, there are a variety of patients, all with varying levels of physical fitness. Through variations in the mode, duration, frequency, or intensity of exercise, these differing levels of fitness can be accommodated. A variety of exercise modes are presented in the phase 2 program, including walking, stationary cycling, stationary rowing, simulated stair-climbing, water aerobics, swimming, and upper-body ergometry. The exercise for this phase frequency is three to six days per week, the duration consists of twenty to forty-five minutes of continuous aerobic activity, and the intensity should produce a heart rate that is 60 to 85 percent of the symptom-limited maximal heart rate. Exercises are monitored by an exercise specialist (one of a number of clinician titles described by the American College of Sports Medicine) and a cardiovascular fitness nurse. Exercise intensity is determined in most cases by heart rate and may be monitored by electrocardiogram (EKG or ECG) telemetry on a number of patients simultaneously.

One of the interesting psychological components to phase 2 cardiac rehabilitation is that most programs are arranged so that new participants are coming into the program

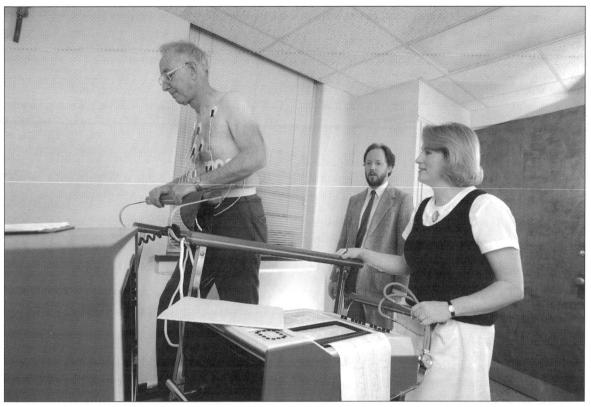

An elderly patient undergoes a cardiac stress test to evaluate heart function. (Digital Stock)

as participants who have been in the program for several sessions are leaving. Newer participants are able to identify with those already in the program as a result of similarities in cardiac experiences. It has been suggested that this identification decreases the anxiety level of a patient who is just becoming involved in the program.

Patients move into phase 3 of cardiac rehabilitation, a community-based outpatient program, when cardiovascular and physiological responses to exercise have been stabilized and the patient has achieved the goals initially set. Phase 3 is generally considered to be an extended, supervised program which usually lasts from four to six months but which can continue indefinitely.

Participants in phase 3 programs become more involved in and in charge of their own exercises. Typically, these programs do not include EKG monitoring. Individuals are given more responsibility with respect to maintaining their own heart rates in their training heart rate range. Usually, an exercise specialist, nurse, or physician is available to oversee the exercises. The mode, frequency, duration, and intensity of exercise in this phase is similar to that of phase 2.

Phase 4 is a maintenance program. Although many rehabilitation settings label this a phase 3 program, the phase 4 program is considered to be the longest-term, on-going phase and is of indefinite length. Many phase 2 cardiac rehabilitation program graduates remain in phase 3 or phase 4 programs for years. The mode, frequency, duration, and intensity of the exercise program for phase 4 is also similar to that of phase 2.

USES AND COMPLICATIONS

Traditionally, cardiac rehabilitation has been recommended for individuals convalescing from myocardial infarctions or heart surgery (CABG, PTCA, or valve replacement). More recently, the eligibility for cardiac rehabilitation has been extended to include heart transplant recipients and others with cardiac-related illnesses.

Improvement of work capacity is one of the goals of cardiac rehabilitation. The mechanisms involved in increasing work capacity (aerobic capacity and maximal oxygen consumption) normally include increases in both central (cardiac output, stroke volume, and heart rate) and peripheral (muscle changes, atrioventricular oxygen difference) adaptations. Nevertheless, this does not preclude patients with reduced left ventricular (LV) function from participation in a medically supervised exercise program. For the reduced LV function patient, improvement in exercise tolerance can occur; this improvement may be attributable mainly to peripheral adaptations.

For the low-risk patient, cardiac rehabilitation may seem

unnecessary since unsupervised exercise programs have been demonstrated to be safe and effective and to improve exercise capacity. For healthy lifestyle modification to take place, however, the educational component of cardiac rehabilitation may provide the patient with invaluable knowledge. In order to reduce the chance of recurrence or severity of a myocardial infarction in an effective manner, a healthy lifestyle is encouraged. Additional potential benefits of participation include improved self-esteem, positive mental attitude, and decreased anxiety and depression.

Low-risk patients, who account for about one-third to one-half of heart attack patients and about three-quarters of CABG patients, have a first-year mortality of less than 2 percent. Moderate-risk patients have a first-year mortality rate of between 10 percent and 25 percent. High-risk patients' mortality rates are greater than 25 percent. While cardiac rehabilitation is not effective in all circumstances, proper assessment of an individual's clinical situation and competent administration of the program can optimize the outcome for participants.

Increasing numbers of cardiac rehabilitation programs are accepting unconventional patient populations. These patients now include heart transplant recipients, congestive heart failure patients, individuals suffering from ischemic heart disease, and those with arrhythmias and/or pacemakers.

Although most of the prescribed exercise regimens for these patients parallel those for the conventional cardiac patient, there are subtle differences. In the heart transplant population, for example, heart rate response differs from nontransplant patients. The adjustment of heart rate to various workloads lags in acute heart transplant recipients; that is, the heart rate does not increase as rapidly as it does for normal patients. To accommodate this difference, researchers have suggested that, in place of heart rate response, clinicians use a "rating of perceived exertion" scale to monitor the patients' responses to exercise.

Even patients who have orthopedic limitations, such as arthritis or chronic injuries, may be accommodated in the exercise portion of the cardiac rehabilitation program. Exercises can be adjusted to allow participants to derive cardiovascular benefits without causing them unnecessary discomfort.

Although cardiac rehabilitation is safe in general, several factors may emerge during graded exercise testing (a screening for entry into a cardiac rehabilitation program) that can identify those patients who may be at increased risk. These factors include a significant depression or elevation of the S-T wave segment from a resting EKG, angina, extensive left ventricular dysfunction and severe myocardial infarction, ventricular dysrhythmias, inappropriate blood pressure response to exercise, achieving a peak heart rate of less than 120 beats per minute (if not taking a negative chronotropic medication, which slows down the heart rate), and a functional exercise capacity of less than 4 to 5 METs. Inclusion

in one of these categories does not preclude participation in a cardiac rehabilitation program, but it may warrant specific exercise guidelines and close monitoring.

Among the criteria for exclusion from a cardiac rehabilitation program are unstable angina, acute systemic illness, uncontrolled arrhythmias, tachycardia, diabetes, symptomatic congestive heart failure, a resting systolic blood pressure over 200 millimeters of mercury (mm Hg) or a resting diastolic blood pressure over 110 mm Hg, third-degree heart block without a pacemaker, and moderate to severe aortic stenosis.

For those who meet the criteria for inclusion in a cardiac rehabilitation program, risk stratification (low, moderate, or high) may be employed. This allows an appropriate amount of supervision to be in place based on each patient's goals and condition. Clinical observations and tests allow each patient to be assessed individually. Within each phase, levels of risk may be established. Various proposals have been made for risk stratification prior to entry into a cardiac rehabilitation program, including stratification based on several factors: the degree of left ventricular dysfunction, presence or absence of myocardial ischemia, extent of myocardial injury, and presence of ventricular arrhythmias.

Some of the most widely examined noninvasive assessment tools include the extent of QRS wave abnormalities on a resting EKG and the results of exercise stress testing, twenty-four-hour ambulatory EKG monitoring, radionuclide ventriculography, and echocardiography. A combination of these test results may be used to determine the course of action provided to an individual.

As with any effective therapy, exercise as a form of cardiac rehabilitation is neither without hazard nor always beneficial. If appropriate clinical guidelines are utilized, however, the benefit-risk ratio can be very favorable. In a 1986 study of 51,303 patients from 142 outpatient cardiac rehabilitation programs in the United States (representing 2,351,916 patient-hours of exercise), the incidence rate for fatal and nonfatal cardiac events was 1 in 111,996. This low incidence of cardiac-related events during participation in programs is probably attributable to improved risk stratification, the use of appropriate medical and surgical therapies, and improved exercise guidelines. On the rare occasions when cardiac events occur, reports have indicated that up to 90 percent of all patients with exercise-related cardiac arrest are successfully resuscitated when the patient experiences the event in a properly equipped and supervised program.

PERSPECTIVE AND PROSPECTS

Until the 1940's, patients recovering from acute myocardial infarctions met with restriction of physical activity, bed rest, and psychological apprehension about exertion. Over the next two decades, the deleterious physiological effects of prolonged bed rest began to be described. During this time, a few investigators were beginning to encourage early treatment of the patient who has experienced an acute heart attack, including armchair work and walking within four weeks of the acute event.

In the 1950's, British physician Jeremy Morris and his colleagues conducted research that initiated interest in the relationship between coronary artery disease (CAD) and a sedentary lifestyle. In this study, he found that London bus drivers had twice the risk of developing CAD than their more physically active bus conductor counterparts. In addition, among those drivers and conductors who had experienced a heart attack, the drivers were twice as likely as the conductors to die either during or within two months of their heart attack.

During the 1960's, the beginnings of what are now considered cardiac rehabilitation programs incorporated exercise training on a somewhat limited basis. Restricted exercise regimens began a few weeks after cardiac events and increased in intensity on a very gradual basis. Generally, the patient population considered appropriate for such programs consisted of those individuals who had experienced uncomplicated myocardial infarctions. Some risk factor modification education was initiated, but not on a large scale primarily because data supporting improved patient outcomes were not proven.

Soon afterward, the "On Ward" program, designed to begin on the tenth day following a heart attack, was introduced based on work by William P. Blocker, Jr., and colleagues. In 1971, J. M. Kaufman suggested that rehabilitation of uncomplicated myocardial infarction patients could begin as early as two days after the heart attack. At this time, many hospitals had some form of cardiac rehabilitation program; most of them, however, consisted almost exclusively of exercise training. This approach addressed the physiological changes necessary for improving the functional capacity of the patients but did not address long-term behavior modification and education.

In 1986, Ralph S. Paffenbarger, Jr., published the most prominent exercise and heart disease study to date. In his study using 16,936 Harvard University alumni from thirty-five to seventy-four years of age, he validated the concept that physical inactivity is independently related to CAD. In the next seven years, various research on a total of more than 32,000 people was done confirming that hypothesis.

Also in 1986, another group of physicians and researchers described some of the deleterious effects of bed rest, including decreased physical work capacity, decreased cardiac output, skeletal muscle wasting, orthostatic hypotension (abnormally low blood pressure upon standing), decreased blood volume, loss of muscular strength, and reduced pulmonary function. Exercise was shown to be beneficial in reducing some of these effects.

Based on the information outlined above, a multifactorial approach to cardiac rehabilitation has been undertaken in order to provide patients with the information and skills necessary to alter their lifestyles. This approach includes education, in the form of lectures, handouts, videotapes, and informal discussions; behavior modification, by way of regularly scheduled, supervised aerobic exercise programs and nutritional counseling; and support, by means of cardiac rehabilitation classroom meetings and support groups. With this increased scope of care for the cardiac patient, some institutions are providing cardiac patients with access to a broader base of clinicians. This group may include physicians, nurses, exercise specialists or physiologists, dietitians, physical therapists, social workers, psychologists, and occupational therapists. Even with all these components in place, however, exercise training remains the focal point of most contemporary cardiac rehabilitation programs.

Recent studies using meta-analysis have substantiated the hypothesis that exercise-based cardiac rehabilitation programs that include risk factor/behavior modification significantly decrease mortality. Decreasing the number and/or magnitude of the known risk factors for heart disease has been shown to effect a significant improvement in the cardiovascular risk profile for these patients. Research has demonstrated the fact that, although various degrees of CAD may remain after participation in a cardiac rehabilitation program, patients can achieve a sense of well-being. For some patients, this benefit alone may improve health and reduce the financial burden often associated with postinfarction convalescence. —*Frank J. Fedel*

See also Angina; Arrhythmias; Bypass surgery; Cardiology; Cardiology, pediatric; Circulation; Congenital heart disease; Electrocardiography (ECG or EKG); Exercise physiology; Heart; Heart attack; Heart disease; Heart transplantation; Heart valve replacement; Ischemia; Pacemaker implantation; Physical rehabilitation; Preventive medicine; Stress reduction.

FOR FURTHER INFORMATION:

American Association of Cardiovascular and Pulmonary Rehabilitation. *Guidelines for Cardiac Rehabilitation Programs.* 2d ed. Champaign, Ill.: Human Kinetics Books, 1995. This short text is laid out well, with many citations of research studies and books on cardiac rehabilitation. A broad-based book that provides information for existing rehabilitation programs and proposes new programs.

Blocker, William P., and David Cardus, eds. *Rehabilitation in Ischemic Heart Disease.* New York: SP Medical & Scientific Books, 1983. Thoroughly researched, this text is almost a bible for any cardiac rehabilitation program. Provides a broad base of background information, in addition to the history and philosophy of the rehabilitation process.

Comoss, Patricia McCall, E. A. Smith Burke, and Susan Herr Swails. *Cardiac Rehabilitation: A Comprehensive Nursing Approach.* Philadelphia: J. B. Lippincott, 1979.

This well-outlined text provides five major areas of discussion in each phase of cardiac rehabilitation: patient assessment and program background, planning, implementation, and evaluation. Aimed at clinicians and provides a framework for a cardiac rehabilitation program.

Gordon, Neil F., and Larry W. Gibbons. *The Cooper Clinic Cardiac Rehabilitation Program.* New York: Simon & Schuster, 1990. Focused on the philosophy of the Cooper Clinic's founder, Kenneth H. Cooper, this primer provides a wide array of anecdotes for the layperson, as well as a good foundation for the clinician. Includes personal stories from former cardiac patients regarding the intimate process of cardiac rehabilitation, lending credibility to the book. Written by clinicians who care about their patients, one of the intangible attributes of cardiac rehabilitation.

Kavanagh, Terence. *The Healthy Heart Program.* Toronto: Van Nostrand Reinhold, 1980. An expanded and updated version of the author's 1976 book *Heart Attack? Counterattack!* This text covers myriad topics ranging from the global perspective of heart disease to preparing to compete in a marathon. Although not geared for use as a clinical teaching aid, the book covers the topic of heart disease very well. Kavanagh wrote the book after working at the Toronto Rehabilitation Centre with more than one thousand CAD patients. The author, a physician and avid exerciser, tries to encourage those with CAD to look ahead to positive results.

McGoon, M. *The Mayo Clinic's Heart Book.* New York: William Morrow, 1993. The most respected text for laypeople on heart disease. Covers all aspects of anatomy, physiology, diagnosis, treatment, and prevention.

CARDIOLOGY

SPECIALTY

ANATOMY OR SYSTEM AFFECTED: Chest, circulatory system, heart

SPECIALITIES AND RELATED FIELDS: Emergency medicine, preventive medicine, vascular medicine

DEFINITION: The branch of medicine concerned with the diagnosis and treatment of diseases of the heart and the coronary arteries, including arteriosclerosis, hypertension, and congenital defects.

KEY TERMS:

acute: referring to the onset of a disease process

chronic: referring to a lingering disease process

coronary arteries: the two arteries that surround the heart and supply the heart muscle with oxygen and nutrients

heart attack: the common term for a myocardial infarction

heart failure: a condition in which the heart pumps inefficiently, allowing fluid to back up into the lungs or body tissue

sudden cardiac death: a situation in which the heart stops beating or beats irregularly, stopping blood flow

SCIENCE AND PROFESSION

Cardiology is the study of the heart and its various diseases: inflammation of the heart muscle, diseases of the heart valves, atherosclerosis and arteriosclerosis (*athero* meaning "deposits of soft material," *arterio* meaning "pertaining to the arteries," and *sclerosis* meaning "hardening"), and congenital defects. This field also concerns related diseases, such as hypertension (high blood pressure) and certain renal, endocrine, and lung disorders.

The heart contains four chambers, the right and left atria on top and the right and left ventricles below. The walls of the heart are three layers of tissue: the outer layer, the epicardium; the middle layer, the myocardium; and an inner layer, the endocardium, which includes the heart valves. The heart is contained in a protective sac, called the pericardium.

The pumping of the heart is a coordinated contraction. The right atrium receives blood from the veins and contracts, pumping blood through the tricuspid valve into the right ventricle. The right ventricle then contracts, pumping blood through the pulmonary valve into the lungs, where it gives up carbon dioxide and receives oxygen. Blood then enters the left atrium, which contracts and sends blood through the mitral valve to the left ventricle. It pumps the blood through the aortic valve into the arterial system, which consists of the aorta and progressively narrower arteries and arterioles. The blood arrives finally in the capillaries, where it delivers nourishment and oxygen to tissues throughout the body and picks up waste products and carbon dioxide. The blood then enters the venous system, first into the venules (tiny veins that lead to larger veins) and finally to one of the two branches of the vena cava: the superior vena cava from the upper part of the body, and the inferior vena cava from the lower. They connect outside the heart and bring blood back into the right atrium.

The heartbeat, the rhythmic contraction of the heart muscle, is controlled by the conduction system. Electrochemical impulses cause muscle fibers to contract, pumping blood through the chambers, and relax, letting the chambers fill again. The contractions are initiated by specialized "pacemaker" tissues in the sinoatrial (S-A) or sinus node, in the junction of the superior vena cava and the right atrium. The pacemaker signal travels to the atrioventricular (A-V) node, near the tricuspid valve. The impulse crosses the A-V node and travels to the bundle of His, specialized fibers that carry it to the ventricles.

Virtually every part of the heart is subject to disease: each layer of the heart muscle, each valve, each chamber, and the coronary arteries. The coronary arteries are quite small and are subject to the accumulation of plaque on their inner walls, a condition known as atherosclerosis. This plaque can be cholesterol, scar tissue, clotted blood, or calcium. As the plaque accumulates, the artery narrows, reducing the flow of blood into the heart muscle. The reduction in blood flow reduces the heart's supply of oxygen, causing myocardial ischemia (lack of blood). There is usually a signal of pain called angina pectoris (*angina* meaning "choking pain" and *pectoris* meaning "of the chest"). Often, the patient feels tightening in the chest with sharp pain behind the sternum. The pain can radiate into either arm or the jaw. It is usually caused by overexertion, exposure to cold, stress, or overeating.

As a rule, an attack of angina pectoris lasts only a few minutes and is relieved by rest, but it can signal the beginning of a heart attack. In addition, coronary arteries contain muscle fibers that can go into spasm and tighten, reducing blood flow into the heart. This condition, too, can cause anginal pain, heart attack, and death. Some patients who have myocardial ischemia do not have anginal pain. This is known as silent ischemia, and it is usually discovered only with an electrocardiogram (ECG) or exercise stress test.

There are four major classes of angina pectoris: stable angina, in which pain begins when the heart's need for oxygen exceeds the amount that it receives; unstable angina, which is significantly more serious than stable angina; variant angina, which is characterized by chest pain at rest and may be caused by spasm of the coronary arteries; and postinfarction angina, unstable angina that appears after acute myocardial infarction.

When atherosclerotic plaque builds up in the coronary arteries, the inner lining of the vessel becomes rough. As a result, a blood clot (thrombus) can form on the plaque, making the vessel even narrower or clogging it completely (coronary thrombosis). When this occurs, blood flow to parts of the heart is stopped, and heart cells die from lack of oxygen. This condition is medically known as myocardial infarction (from *infarct*, meaning "an area of dead cells") and commonly known as a heart attack.

The prognosis for patients who survive a heart attack is variable. In two-thirds of patients, spontaneous thrombolysis (the dissolution of the blood clot) starts to occur within twenty-four hours. About half of heart attack patients, however, will go on to develop postinfarction angina, which usually indicates severe, multivessel coronary artery disease.

Diseases of the conduction system can result in arrhythmias, or disturbances in the regularity of the heartbeat. Arrhythmias can be relatively benign or can severely restrict the patient's physical activity. They can also cause sudden cardiac death. The most common arrhythmias are bradycardia, slowing of the heartbeat, and tachycardia, quickening of the heartbeat.

Normally, the chambers beat in synchronization with each other. In some arrhythmias, the chambers of the heart beat out of synchronization. These arrhythmias include atrial fibrillation, paroxysmal atrial tachycardia, ventricular tachycardia, and ventricular fibrillation. In atrial fibrillation,

the atria beat very rapidly (three hundred beats per minute), out of synchronization with the ventricles. When the condition is prolonged, blood clots may form in the atria and may cause a stroke, or the stoppage of blood flow in a blood vessel. With paroxysmal atrial tachycardia, a disturbance in the conduction of the A-V node causes the heart to beat up to two hundred fifty times a minute. The condition is usually not serious, but if it persists, fainting or heart failure could develop. Ventricular tachycardia exists when ectopic, or irregular, beats develop in the ventricular muscle; if they go on, blood pressure falls. In ventricular fibrillation, which is the leading cause of sudden cardiac death, ventricular contractions are weak, ineffective, and uncoordinated. Blood flow stops, and the patient faints. If the condition is not corrected, the patient can die in minutes.

Heart block can be another consequence of conduction disease. If, for various reasons, all the impulses from the sinus node do not pass through the A-V node and the bundle of His, the result is one of three degrees of heart block. First-degree heart block, which is not apparent to the patient, appears on the ECG as a delay in the impulse from the atria to the ventricles. Second-degree heart block occurs when some of the impulses from the atria fail to reach the ventricles. Often, the result is an irregular pulse. This condition can be attributable to a certain heart drug and may disappear when the drug is discontinued. In third-degree heart block, impulses from the pacemaker tissues fail to reach the ventricles. A lower pacemaker assumes the function of stimulating contractions of the ventricles in an "escape rhythm." When this occurs in third-degree heart block, the heart rate often slows down so precipitously that blood flow to the brain and other organs is severely restricted. Dizziness and loss of consciousness may follow. Heart failure can also be the result of a congenital defect, inflammation, myocardial infarction, or other causes.

Disorders in the valves of the heart are most often caused by congenital defects or the effects of rheumatic fever. Rheumatic fever is caused by streptococcal bacteria and usually begins with a throat infection. If this "strep throat" is not treated, rheumatic fever may develop. Acute rheumatic fever is associated with mitral or aortic valve insufficiency (leakage). Chronic rheumatic heart disease can include mitral or aortic stenosis (narrowing). Valves are scarred with fibrous tissue and/or calcific (calcium-containing) deposits that cause the valve openings to become narrower.

Mitral stenosis usually develops slowly. Ten to twenty years after rheumatic fever, the valve narrows so much that blood flow from the atrium into the ventricle is impeded. As blood accumulates in the left atrium, pressure within the atrium increases, and the chamber becomes enlarged. Blood is forced back into the lungs, resulting in pulmonary edema (fluid in the lungs). Blood vessels in the lungs become engorged; the increased pressure forces fluid into the air sacs. Symptoms of mitral stenosis include shortness of breath, fatigue, feelings of suffocation, wheezing, agitation, and anxiety. In severe cases, fluid may also accumulate in the lower extremities. Mitral stenosis can also cause atrial fibrillation, which in turn can generate potentially lethal blood clots.

Mitral "regurgitation," another mitral valve disorder, can also be caused by rheumatic fever. The valve fails to close completely during left ventricle contraction. Blood leaks back into the left atrium, and blood flow into the aorta is reduced. The heart has to work harder to pump blood into the body. Mitral regurgitation may lead to enlargement of the left atrium and left ventricle. Pulmonary edema, shortness of breath, fatigue, and palpitations are late symptoms of severe disease.

Still another disorder is mitral valve prolapse, or mitral insufficiency. The mitral valve consists of two leaflets of tissue that fall apart to open and come together to close. Prolapse occurs when either or both of these leaflets bulge into the left atrium. Some patients experience palpitations and chest pain. In rare cases, significant valve leakage occurs, requiring surgery.

The aortic valve consists of three leaflets or "cusps" that can become fused, calcified, or otherwise compromised because of rheumatic fever or a congenital heart defect. The opening narrows, and blood flow into the aorta is reduced. Pressure increases inside the left ventricle, causing it to pump harder. The wall of the left ventricle thickens, a condition called ventricular hypertrophy. Aortic stenosis may not be evident until it is quite advanced. Symptoms include heart murmur, weakness, fatigue, anginal pain, breathlessness, and fainting.

Tricuspid stenosis and regurgitation occur but are rare, as is pulmonary regurgitation. Pulmonary or pulmonic valve stenosis, however, is a common congenital heart defect. There is a characteristic heart murmur produced by turbulence of blood through the narrow pulmonary valve. Pressure increases in the right ventricle. Fainting and heart failure are possible in severe cases.

In congestive heart failure, the heart pumps inefficiently, failing to deliver blood to the body and allowing blood to back up into the veins. It may occur on the left or the right side, or both. If the left side of the heart is pumping inefficiently, blood flows back into the lungs, causing pulmonary edema. If the right side of the heart is inefficient, blood seeps back into the legs, resulting in edema of the extremities. Blood can also back up into the liver and the kidneys, resulting in engorgement and reduced arterial flow that prevent these organs from getting the nutrition and oxygen they need to function.

Cardiomyopathy refers to diseases of the myocardium. There are many possible causes, including "end-stage" coronary artery disease; infectious agents such as fungi, viruses, and parasites; overconsumption of alcohol; or genetic defects. The three main classes of cardiomyopathy are dilated congestive cardiomyopathy, hypertrophic cardiomyopathy, and restrictive cardiomyopathy. In dilated congestive cardiomyopathy, either all the heart chambers are involved (diffuse), or some but not all chambers are involved (nondiffuse). The cause of this class of cardiomyopathy is usually a viral infection (in which case it is called myocarditis), but drugs, alcohol, and nonviral diseases may be responsible. The heart pumps inefficiently, causing fatigue, breathlessness, and edema in the lower extremities. The heart chambers may enlarge, and blood clots may form. With hypertrophic cardiomyopathy, the myocardium thickens and reduces the cavity of the left ventricle so that blood flow into the aorta is reduced. The condition is usually chronic, with fainting, fatigue, and breathlessness as symptoms. Restrictive cardiomyopathy is rare. With this condition, the heart muscle loses elasticity and cannot expand to fill with blood between contractions. Symptoms include edema, breathlessness, and atrial and ventricular arrhythmias.

The endocardium and the pericardium can become inflamed because of infection or injury, resulting in endocarditis or pericarditis. Bacterial endocarditis usually affects abnormal valves and heart structures that have been damaged by rheumatic fever or congenital defects. Fulminant (sudden and severe) infections can destroy normal heart valves, especially with intravenous drug abuse. The symptoms of bacterial endocarditis are fever, weight loss, malaise, night sweats, fatigue, and heart murmurs. The condition can be fatal if the invading organism is not eradicated. Nonbacterial thrombotic endocarditis or noninfective endocarditis arises from the formation of thrombi on cardiac valves and endocardium caused by trauma, immune complexes, or vascular disease. Pericarditis often occurs concomitantly with, or as a result of, viral respiratory infection. The inflamed pericardium rubs against the epicardium, causing acute pain. Large amounts of fluid may develop and press on the heart in "cardiac tamponade." This condition can impede heart action and blood flow and can be life-threatening. In constrictive pericarditis, the pericardium becomes thicker and contracts. This action prevents the heart chambers from filling, decreasing the amount of blood drawn into the heart and pumped out to the body.

Primary cardiac tumors, those originating in the heart, are rare. While usually benign, they can have fatal complications. Malignant tumors also occur, and metastasis (movement of cancer cells throughout the body) may bring malignancies to the heart.

Congenital heart defects occur in about 0.8 percent of births. Ventricular septal defect, a hole in the wall between the ventricles, is the most common. It is detected by a loud murmur. Atrial septal defect is common but rarely leads to symptoms until the third decade of life.

DIAGNOSTIC AND TREATMENT TECHNIQUES

The stethoscope, ECGs, and the X ray are basic tools that the cardiologist uses for the diagnosis of heart conditions. By listening to heart sounds through the stethoscope, the physician can learn much about the status of heart function, particularly heart rhythm, congenital defects, and valve dysfunction.

ECG patterns of electrical impulses help the physician discover chamber enlargement and other cardiac abnormalities. In a stress test, the ECG is attached to a patient who is running on a treadmill or riding a bicycle-like apparatus. The test assesses the exercise tolerance of patients with coronary artery disease and other conditions.

The chest X ray provides a picture of the size and configuration of the heart, the aorta, the pulmonary arteries, and related structures. It can detect enlarged chambers and vessels and other disorders. In some cases, radioactive isotopes are injected into the patient, and the patterns that they form in the heart and surrounding arteries are "read" by a scanner to help the physician make a diagnosis. The echocardiogram uses ultrasound to outline heart chambers and detect abnormalities within them and in the myocardium. It is also used to analyze patterns of blood flow.

Newer, more sophisticated instruments the cardiologist uses include fast-computed tomography, called cine-CT because it gives the physician a visualization of heart activity. Magnetic resonance imaging (MRI), MR spectroscopy, and positron emission tomography (PET) scanning help the cardiologist investigate heart function and anatomy.

These techniques and procedures are conducted outside the body. Sometimes it is necessary, however, to go into the body. One such technique is diagnostic catheterization with angiography. A thin flexible tube (catheter) is inserted into a blood vessel in the groin or arm and threaded into a coronary artery or the heart. Pressures and blood oxygen are measured in the heart chambers. A radio-opaque dye is then injected through the catheter. The inside of the artery or the heart becomes visible to the X ray and is recorded on film (a process sometimes called cineangiography). Angiography can also be used with radioactive isotopes. The radiation detected by a scanner can help the physician discover abnormalities in the coronary arteries and the heart.

Diagnosis of angina pectoris is usually based upon the patient's complaint of chest pain. An ECG can help confirm the diagnosis. Yet many patients with coronary artery disease have normal ECGs at rest, so stress testing with the ECG is considered more reliable. Patients may be given pharmacologic stress tests if they are unable to do physical exercise.

Drug therapy for coronary artery disease and angina pectoris is directed at keeping the coronary arteries open and avoiding myocardial ischemia. Primary among the drugs used is nitroglycerin, taken under the tongue or in a transdermal (through-the-skin) patch—or, in emergencies, intravenously. There are many nitrate compounds that fulfill similar functions. Beta-adrenergic blocking agents, or beta-blockers, decrease heart rate and blood pressure, reducing the heart's oxygen requirement and workload, thus reducing the incidence of angina. Some serious arrhythmias are also suppressed. Calcium-channel blockers dilate coronary arteries and maintain coronary blood flow while decreasing blood pressure, reducing heart work, and stabilizing heart rhythm.

If coronary artery disease progresses to the point where there is risk of myocardial infarction, various catheter and surgical procedures may be considered. Coronary angioplasty is used to open a clogged artery mechanically. The cardiologist threads a catheter with a tiny balloon into the clogged artery and inflates the balloon at the site of the blockage. This procedure is repeated until the vessel is open. Another procedure used when coronary arteries are blocked is coronary artery bypass surgery. The surgeon takes sections of vein or artery from another part of the body and implants them between the aorta and the heart, creating new coronary arteries and bypassing those that are clogged.

When clogged coronary arteries cause a myocardial infarction, the patient should be treated in a special medical facility, preferably in a coronary care unit (CCU). Heart attacks rarely begin in the hospital, however, so the medical team must keep the patient alive on the way to the CCU. Primary ventricular fibrillation is the greatest danger, and it must be corrected immediately by medication or electrical defibrillation. Sometimes heart block and profound bradycardia occur, which could cause a drop in blood pressure that could in turn cause cardiac arrest.

The aims of emergency myocardial infarction treatment are to ease discomfort, minimize the mass of infarcted myocardial tissue, reduce heart work, stabilize heart rhythm, and maintain oxygen perfusion throughout the body by regulating blood pressure. Treatment and medications used in the CCU include continuous ECG monitoring (both during and after the heart attack), oxygen, nitroglycerin, antiarrhythmia agents, analgesics for pain, thrombolytic agents to dissolve clots, diuretics, agents to treat shock, and sedatives. Beta-blockers, calcium-channel blockers, anticoagulants, and antianxiety drugs may also be used.

About 60 percent of patients who have suffered from myocardial infarction develop congestive heart failure. In treating congestive heart failure from heart attacks or other causes, the cardiologist uses both dietary instruction and medication. Salt restriction is recommended to reduce edema. The three most commonly prescribed drugs are diuretics to reduce edema, digitalis (digoxin or digitoxin) to increase the force of the heart's contraction, and vasodilators to reduce the resistance of blood vessel walls, to facilitate blood flow, and to reduce heart work. Intractable congestive heart failure may be a reason for a heart transplant.

The main goals of therapy for cardiac arrhythmias are to improve heart function and to prevent sudden cardiac death. Drug therapy must be individualized to correct the particular arrhythmia. Digitalis, quinidine, procainamide, tocainamide, and atropine are often used. Beta-blockers and calcium-channel blockers are also helpful in stabilizing heart rhythm.

If heart block becomes severe, an artificial pacemaker is implanted in the chest to regulate the heartbeat.

Disorders of the heart valves are not usually treated with drugs. While awaiting surgery, it may be necessary to treat heart failure, or the effects of valve disease in other parts of the body. For example, diuretics may be required to reduce edema, an antiarrhythmia agent may be needed to control atrial fibrillation, or anticoagulants may be used to prevent blood clots. Some stenotic valves can be opened using a modification of the balloon catheter technique, or surgical reconstruction may be possible. Often, it is necessary to replace the valve with a new one made of human or porcine tissue, or with a mechanical valve.

Pulmonary edema is a severe form of heart failure and is life-threatening. In emergencies, oxygen is given, in severe cases by inserting a breathing tube into the patient's trachea. Medications are given to relieve pulmonary congestion, and if the pumping action of the heart is compromised, digitalis or another medication can strengthen the contractility of the heart.

In treating dilated cardiomyopathy, the cardiologist uses appropriate medications that may include diuretics, vasodilators, antiarrhythmia agents, and digitalis. Alcohol restriction is required.

If bacteria or other microorganisms are involved, appropriate antibiotic therapy must be instituted to eradicate the cause. Patients with congenital or valvular heart disease are high risks for cardiac and valve infection. They are given preventive antibiotic therapy before undergoing surgical or dental procedures.

In acute pericarditis, if excessive fluid builds up, a procedure called pericardiocentesis may be performed to drain the fluid between the pericardium and the heart wall. In cardiac tamponade, pericardiocentesis may be lifesaving. In chronic constrictive pericarditis, an operation may be necessary to remove tissue that has stiffened and strangled the heart.

PERSPECTIVE AND PROSPECTS

Cardiology is a major medical specialty in the United States because heart disease is the major killer of Americans. Today's cardiologist turns increasingly to preventive medicine as a means of reducing morbidity (the relative incidence of a disease) and mortality. These measures include programs against smoking and programs advocating cholesterol reduction, stress reduction, exercise, and other measures that have been found useful in preventing heart disease.

There is much more to be learned about heart disease. It appears to be a consequence of highly industrialized societies, but there are questions that have to be answered, such as why heart disease is so prevalent in the United States but significantly less frequent in other, equally industrial societies.

Ongoing studies continue to accumulate data on increasingly large populations in more and more countries. Links between behavior, habits, nutrition, and ecology may be found that will give a clearer picture of why heart disease became a major killer in the twentieth century. Increased knowledge will improve diagnosis and treatment, improving patient care and the quality of life for sufferers of heart disease.
—*C. Richard Falcon*

See also Aneurysmectomy; Aneurysms; Angina; Angiography; Angioplasty; Arrhythmias; Arteriosclerosis; Biofeedback; Bypass surgery; Cardiac rehabilitation; Cardiology, pediatric; Chest; Cholesterol; Circulation; Congenital heart disease; Electrocardiography (ECG or EKG); Endocarditis; Exercise physiology; Heart; Heart attack; Heart disease; Heart failure; Heart transplantation; Heart valve replacement; Hypercholesterolemia; Hypertension; Ischemia; Mitral insufficiency; Pacemaker implantation; Palpitations; Rheumatic fever; Sports medicine; Thoracic surgery; Thrombolytic therapy and TPA; Thrombosis and thrombus; Transplantation; Vascular medicine; Vascular system.

FOR FURTHER INFORMATION:

Dranov, Paula. *Heart Disease*. New York: Random House, 1990. Dranov's book is readable and covers the state of cardiologic practice in the United States. The style is excellent for the layperson.

Kowalski, Robert E. *Eight Steps to a Healthy Heart*. New York: Warner Books, 1992. The author describes heart disease prevention, details what happens to a heart attack victim in the CCU, and discusses bypass surgery and the steps that lead to recovery.

Lamb, Lawrence E. *Your Heart and How to Live with It*. New York: Viking Press, 1969. This patient-oriented text is useful for understanding how heart patients cope with the disease. It is valuable for helping the patient understand how to cooperate with therapy to get the maximum benefit from his or her physician's regimen.

Larson, David E., ed. *Mayo Clinic Family Health Book*. 2d ed. New York: William Morrow, 1996. Perhaps the best general medical text for the layperson, this book covers the entire medical field. While the information is derived from a wide variety of highly technical sources, the articles are written to be easily understood by a general audience.

Zaret, Barry L., et al., eds. *Yale University School of Medicine Heart Book*. New York: William Morrow, 1992. This book is devoted entirely to the heart, so it is more thorough than Larson's. Of particular interest are techniques for prevention and control of heart disease.

CARDIOLOGY, PEDIATRIC
SPECIALTY

ANATOMY OR SYSTEM AFFECTED: Chest, circulatory system, heart

SPECIALTIES AND RELATED FIELDS: Emergency medicine, neonatology, pediatrics, vascular medicine

DEFINITION: The medical field concerned with the diagnosis and treatment of heart diseases in newborns, infants, and children.

KEY TERMS:

echocardiograph: an instrument that uses ultrasound to record activities within the heart and great arteries

electrocardiograph: an instrument for recording heart function

inpatient: one who is treated while held in a medical facility (versus an outpatient, who comes to the facility for treatment as needed)

noninvasive: referring to a procedure that does not require entering the body

stethoscope: an instrument for listening to sounds in the body, such as the heartbeat

valves: structures that close periodically to allow the passage of blood, such as those that connect heart chambers to each other and to the great arteries

SCIENCE AND PROFESSION

It is imperative that pediatric cardiologists be connected to large, extensive medical facilities in order to have available all the special facilities, instruments, and personnel that are required to treat heart diseases in children. The medical center should have full nursery facilities, including a neonatology section for the care of newborns and premature babies. It should have a surgical facility competent to deal with the special heart problems of children: Most children with heart disease will be treated surgically. It should have a wide range of specialized instruments and skilled personnel for diagnosis and treatment.

Heart disease in adults usually involves the coronary arteries and defects in heart rhythms. It usually surfaces in late youth, middle age, or old age, and is usually attributable to or associated with lifestyle (a high-cholesterol diet, smoking, and/or stress) and disease (diabetes mellitus or high blood pressure). In children, however, the most common heart diseases are congenital (present at birth) or caused by infections such as rheumatic fever or Kawasaki disease. About 0.8 percent of newborns have some form of congenital heart defect. Such defects may become manifest in the womb, at birth, in infancy or childhood, or later in life.

In the hospital, the pediatric cardiologist has three major patient groups: inpatient neonates and infants; older inpatient children, who are usually in the hospital for surgery; and outpatient infants and children whose disease conditions are being monitored.

DIAGNOSTIC AND TREATMENT TECHNIQUES

Proper diagnosis of the child's condition is paramount to successful treatment. The cardiac examination begins with the physician's first glance at the patient in which he or she looks for signs of respiratory difficulty or cyanosis (a bluish tinge to the lips or fingertips). The physician will also measure the child's heart rate and rhythm, blood pressure, and growth pattern.

The pediatric cardiologist has an array of diagnostic tools, including electrocardiography, echocardiography, and stress testing. The main instrument, however, is the stethoscope because many pediatric heart problems are most readily detectable through auscultation, listening to sounds of the body. The pediatric cardiologist must develop extraordinary expertise in detecting and analyzing heart sounds. He or she must learn to differentiate between abnormalities in heart sounds that are functional and benign and those that indicate a disease condition. Through the stethoscope, the physician will hear the heartbeat, murmurs, clicks, and other sounds. Differences in loudness, pitch, variability, and timing are among the factors that must be considered in the diagnosis.

The electrocardiogram, echocardiogram, and other instruments will confirm the diagnosis and help the pediatric cardiologist determine the best course of therapy for the child. Many surgical procedures are used to correct defects in the child's heart: Valves can be repaired or replaced, tissue can be repaired, narrow passages can be opened, and gross abnormalities can be corrected. The success rate of these procedures is excellent, but any heart operation is a major surgery with significant risks. The child who undergoes heart surgery must face a wide range of additional perils. Children with severe heart disease who are cured or significantly helped through surgery must be carefully monitored because there are sometimes postoperative residua (conditions that are partially or wholly uncorrected) or postoperative sequelae (conditions that develop as a result of surgery) and other complications of surgery.

This surveillance by the pediatric cardiologist and other members of the medical team must continue for years. Often, long after the operation, the patient may develop significant arrhythmias and other anomalies. Some of these patients will require implanted pacemakers to avoid sudden death. Some will develop new valvular problems, and some patients who were given prosthetic (artificial) valves may develop infections, blood clots, or obstructions at the site.

PERSPECTIVE AND PROSPECTS

Pediatric heart diseases have existed perhaps since the dawn of the human era. Many children lived as well as they could with their infirmities—some more or less normally, some with moderate or severe restriction on their activities, and some dying in their youth.

Pediatric cardiology has made great strides in maintaining life and improving the physical status of these children. As medical specialists, pediatric cardiologists are relative newcomers, the specialty being less than half a century old. Nevertheless, through their efforts and accomplishments, hundreds of thousands of men, women, and children are alive and well, who might be dead, impaired, or debilitated.

There is still a long way to go. Pediatric heart disease, involving as it often does the physical structure of the heart, would appear comparatively mechanical and straightforward. In fact, these conditions are enormously challenging because of the wide range of anatomic, hemodynamic, and electrophysical problems that they may entail.

Also challenging are the new avenues that have opened for the pediatric cardiologist. Infant heart transplantation, unheard-of a generation ago, is now possible, if not yet commonplace. The dramatic increase in the number of premature babies who are being kept alive involves the pediatric cardiologist as a vital part of the neonatal team. There are also constant, persistent efforts to improve the quality of care both for children requiring surgery and for those who can be helped by other means.

—*C. Richard Falcon*

See also Aneurysmectomy; Aneurysms; Angina; Angiography; Arrhythmias; Biofeedback; Bypass surgery; Cardiac rehabilitation; Cardiology; Chest; Circulation; Congenital heart disease; Electrocardiography (ECG or EKG); Endocarditis; Exercise physiology; Genetic counseling; Genetics and inheritance; Heart; Heart attack; Heart disease; Heart failure; Heart transplantation; Heart valve replacement; Ischemia; Mitral insufficiency; Pacemaker implantation; Palpitations; Pediatrics; Rheumatic fever; Sports medicine; Thoracic surgery; Thrombolytic therapy and TPA; Thrombosis and thrombus; Transplantation; Vascular medicine; Vascular system.

FOR FURTHER INFORMATION:

Dranov, Paula. *Random House Personal Medical Handbook: For People with Heart Disease.* New York: Random House, 1991.

Larson, David E., ed. *Mayo Clinic Family Health Book.* 2d ed. New York: William Morrow, 1996.

Zaret, Barry L., et al., eds. *Yale University School of Medicine Heart Book.* New York: William Morrow, 1992.

CARIES, DENTAL
DISEASE/DISORDER

ANATOMY OR SYSTEM AFFECTED: Gums, mouth, teeth

SPECIALTIES AND RELATED FIELDS: Dentistry

DEFINITION: Commonly known as tooth decay or cavities, dental caries are disintegrations of tooth enamel, allowing injury to the dentin below the enamel and eventually allowing injury to the pulp, which contains nerves and blood vessels. Dental caries are caused by bacteria in the mouth that produce acid. Food debris and sugars provide the fuel for bacteria development. Risk of dental caries increases with poor nutrition and improper diet, as well as with poor dental hygiene. Existing caries can be stopped by a dentist by removing all decay and filling the space left with a metal or ceramic substance.

—*Jason Georges and Tracy Irons-Georges*

See also Dental diseases; Dentistry; Endodontic disease; Gingivitis; Periodontal surgery; Periodontitis; Root canal treatment; Teeth; Tooth extraction; Toothache.

CARPAL TUNNEL SYNDROME
DISEASE/DISORDER

ANATOMY OR SYSTEM AFFECTED: Arms, hands, joints, nerves, tendons

SPECIALTIES AND RELATED FIELDS: Neurology, occupational health

DEFINITION: A common disorder that causes discomfort and decreased hand dexterity via excessive pressure on the median nerve at the wrist, often caused by repetitive wrist and hand movements.

KEY TERMS:

carpal tunnel: a narrow tunnel formed by a U-shaped cluster of eight bones called carpals at the base of the palm

Development of Dental Caries

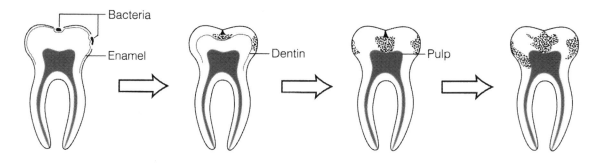

Bacteria enter tooth after acid used in food digestion destroys enamel.

Untreated tooth decay spreads to dentin, beneath enamel, allowing bacterial invasion.

Advanced stage is reached once bacteria reach pulp of tooth.

Pulp will die, destroying tooth, if a dentist does not intervene.

and the inelastic transverse carpal ligament that lies across the arch

median nerve: a nerve running through the carpal tunnel that carries sensory impulses from the thumb, index and middle fingers, and half of the ring finger to the central nervous system; it has a motor branch that supplies the thenar muscles on the thumb side of the hand

CAUSES AND SYMPTOMS

Carpal tunnel syndrome, also known as median nerve palsy, is caused by the transverse carpal ligament compressing the median nerve. This nerve passes through the carpal tunnel alongside nine tendons attached to the muscles that enable the hand to close and the wrist to flex. The tendons have a lubricating lining called the synovium, which normally allow the tendons to smoothly glide back and forth through the tunnel during wrist and hand movements. The median nerve is the softest component within the tunnel and becomes compressed when the tendons are stressed and become swollen. Median nerve compression most often results when the synovium becomes thick and sticky as a result of the wear and tear of aging or repeatedly performing stressful motions with the hands while holding them in the same position for extended periods. Entrapment of the median nerve is less commonly caused by rheumatoid arthritis, diabetes mellitus, poor thyroid gland function, excessive fluid retention such as during pregnancy or by medications, vitamin B_6 or B_{12} deficiency, or bone protruding in the tunnel from previous dislocations or fractures of the wrist.

Initial symptoms of carpal tunnel syndrome include tingling and numbness in the hands, often beginning in the thumb and index and middle fingers, that causes the hand to feel as though it were asleep and shooting pain from the thenar region radiating as far up as the neck. Later symptoms include burning pain from the wrist to the fingers, changes in touch or temperature sensation, clumsiness in the hands, and muscle weakness creating an inability to grasp, pinch, and perform other thumb functions. Swelling of the hands and forearms and changes in sweat gland functioning in the hands may also be noted. Symptoms can be intermittent or constant and often progress to the point of regularly awakening the patient at night. Temporary relief is sometimes available by elevating, massaging, and shaking the hand. Although very treatable if diagnosed early, carpal tunnel syndrome can escalate into persistent pain, which can become so crippling that workplace duties and such simple tasks as holding a cup, writing, and buttoning a shirt are compromised.

A clinical examination for confirmation of median nerve impingement includes wrist examination, an X ray for previous injury and arthritis, assessment of swelling and sensitivity to touch or pinpricks, and the reproduction of symptoms by tapping of the median nerve (Tinel's test) and holding the wrist in a flexed position for several minutes

Carpal Tunnel Syndrome

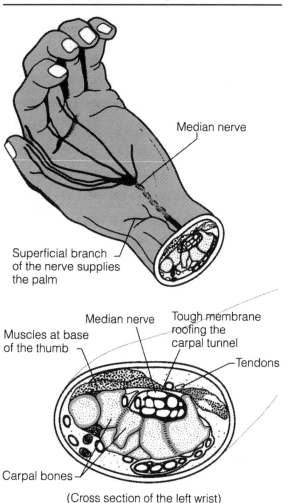

Median nerve

Superficial branch of the nerve supplies the palm

Median nerve

Muscles at base of the thumb

Tough membrane roofing the carpal tunnel

Tendons

Carpal bones

(Cross section of the left wrist)

Repetitive wrist motion such as typing may put excessive pressure on the median nerves and cause numbness and tingling in the hands, a condition known as carpal tunnel syndrome. If rest, wrist splints, and painkillers do not alleviate the problem, surgery may be needed to relieve the pressure.

(Phalen's test). Nerve conduction tests, which measure nerve transmission speed by electrodes placed on the skin, and electromyogram evaluation, which notes muscle function abnormalities, may also assist in a diagnosis.

TREATMENT AND THERAPY

Early diagnosis and the taking of appropriate preventative measures, such as ergonomic modifications in the way that upper extremity movements are performed, often reduce the risk of developing advanced carpal tunnel syndrome. The need to compensate for weak muscles with an inappropriate wrist position can be reduced by maintaining a neutral (straight) wrist position instead of a flexed, extended, or twisted wrist position; utilizing the entire hand and all the fingers to grasp and lift objects, instead of gripping solely with the thumb and index finger; minimizing repetitive movements; allowing the upper extremities regular rest periods; using power tools, instead of hand tools; alternating work activities; switching hands; reducing movement speed; and stretching and using strengthening exercises for the hand, wrist, and arm. Keeping the hands warm to maintain good blood circulation and avoiding smoke-filled environments, which reduce peripheral blood flow, are also recommended.

Treatment generally begins with splinting of the wrist and medication, but surgery may be required if symptoms do not subside within three months. Both nocturnal splints and job-specific occupational splints can effectively keep the wrist in a neutral position, thus avoiding the extreme wrist flexion or extension that narrows the carpal tunnel. Wrist supports lying on the desk in front of a computer keyboard are often helpful, but the benefit of strapping on wrist splints while typing is controversial because disuse atrophy may result, potentially creating a muscle imbalance. Aspirin and other oral nonsteroidal anti-inflammatory drugs (NSAIDs) may reduce swelling and inflammation, relieving some nerve pressure. Corticosteroids and cortisone-like medications injected directly into the carpal tunnel can help confirm diagnosis if the symptoms are relieved. Diuretics and vitamin supplementation may also be beneficial. If initial symptoms do not subside, pain increases, or the risk of permanent nerve and muscle damage exists, then surgery may be necessary, with subsequent rehabilitation and ergonomic counseling with a physical or occupational therapist. An outpatient surgical procedure called carpal tunnel release involves dividing the transverse ligament to open the carpal tunnel to relieve pressure and removing thickened synovial tissue, with recovery expected in six to ten weeks.

PERSPECTIVE AND PROSPECTS

The historic roots of carpal tunnel syndrome can be traced back to the 1860's, when meatpackers complained of pain and loss of hand function, which physicians initially attributed to reduced circulation. Modern occupations that require repetitive motions for extended periods—such as typing on a computer keyboard, construction and assembly-line work, and jackhammer operation—have caused a dramatic rise in cumulative trauma disorders such as carpal tunnel syndrome, while other workplace injuries have leveled off. A new endoscopic procedure utilizing a much smaller incision and a fiber-optic camera holds considerable promise for alleviating the median nerve pressure that causes carpal tunnel syndrome.   *—Daniel G. Graetzer, Ph.D.*

See also Nervous system; Neuralgia, neuritis, and neuropathy; Neurology; Neurosurgery; Occupational health; Pain management; Upper extremities.

FOR FURTHER INFORMATION:
Katz, R. T. "Carpal Tunnel Syndrome: A Practical Review." *American Family Physician* 51, no. 1 (1995): 48-57.
Kulick, R. G. "Carpal Tunnel Syndrome." *Orthopaedic Clinics of North America* 27, no. 2 (1996): 345-354.
Rosenbaum, Richard B., and Jose L. Ochoa. *Carpal Tunnel Syndrome and Other Disorders of the Median Nerve.* Boston: Butterworth-Heinemann, 1993.

CAT SCANS. *See* COMPUTED TOMOGRAPHY (CT) SCANNING.

CATARACT SURGERY
PROCEDURE
ANATOMY OR SYSTEM AFFECTED: Eyes
SPECIALTIES AND RELATED FIELDS: General surgery, geriatrics and gerontology, ophthalmology
DEFINITION: The removal of an eye lens with cataracts and the implantation of a plastic replacement using microsurgery.

KEY TERMS:
cornea: the transparent, curved front surface of the eye
microsurgery: surgery done while looking through a microscope
retina: a thin membrane at the back of the eyeball where light is converted into nerve impulses that travel to the brain
ultrasonic: referring to high-frequency sound waves above the range of human hearing

INDICATIONS AND PROCEDURES
Cataracts are dark regions that develop in the eye lens, causing a decrease in light transmission to the retina. They are a common medical problem among older adults. Cataract removal is the most frequently performed surgery in the United States and gives rise to the single largest expenditure of Medicare funds.

Some misconceptions about cataracts should be refuted. Cataracts are not an infection, a growth, or a film on the surface of the lens. They do not cause pain, redness, teardrops, or other discomforts. The formation of cataracts is a normal part of the aging process, like gray hair or wrinkled skin. The initial symptom is a gradual deterioration of vision, usually in one eye at a time. There is no known treatment other than to remove the lens surgically.

Certain factors increase the probability of early cataract formation. For example, medications such as cortisone (used in arthritis treatment) increase the risk of getting cataracts. A diet deficient in protein has been linked to cataracts. A blow to the eye from an accident can start cataract growth. Diabetics are more likely to develop cataracts than the general public. Some studies have shown that exposure to X rays, ultraviolet radiation, and environmental pollutants can also cause early cataracts.

In preparation for cataract surgery, the patient is given

an injection to produce drowsiness. Eyedrops are administered to dilate the pupil, thus providing easier access to the eye lens. Local anesthetic is used to keep the eyelid from closing and to deaden the sensitive surface of the cornea. A microscope is positioned above the eye.

The surgeon makes a small, semicircular incision in the cornea. An ultrasonic probe then is inserted through the pupil into the lens capsule. Ultrasonic sound waves break up the lens into small fragments, which are suctioned out while fluid is washed into the opening. The surgeon must operate the microscope, the ultrasonic generator, and the suction apparatus by means of foot pedals while manipulating the probe by hand.

After the defective eye lens has been extracted, an artificial lens is inserted in its place. The implant is made of clear plastic, about the size of an aspirin tablet. Two metal loops embedded in the plastic are used to center the implant and to keep it there permanently. Finally, the incision in the cornea is closed with tiny sutures. During recuperation, the patient is instructed to avoid strenuous exercise and to protect the eye from any hard contact. Normally, there is little pain, although some eye irritation should be expected during the healing process.

USES AND COMPLICATIONS

The plastic lens implanted during cataract surgery has a fixed focal length, with no power of accommodation for different distances. It acts like a box camera that gives a good picture at a set distance, while near and far objects are blurry. After the surgery has healed, the patient has to be fitted with glasses, for reading and for distant vision, respectively.

A number of complications can result from cataract sur-

The Removal of Cataracts

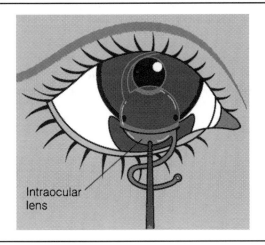

Intraocular lens

The presence of a cataract, cloudiness of the eye lens that obscures vision, often requires the removal of the entire lens and its replacement with an artificial lens (shown here), which is held in place with loops.

gery. Some patients develop so-called secondary cataracts, which produce a cloudiness of the eye membrane behind the implant. This condition is routinely corrected using a laser beam.

Another potential complication is increased astigmatism. During surgery, the spherical symmetry of the corneal surface can become distorted if some sutures are tighter than others. If the curvature of the cornea is not uniform, part of the image formed on the retina will be out of focus. Astigmatism can be corrected with prescription glasses.

All operations have some risks, and a small percentage of cataract surgeries can have serious complications. Among these are a detached retina, glaucoma, and hemorrhage from blood vessels in the retina. Such problems, however, are rare.

PERSPECTIVE AND PROSPECTS

Surgery for cataracts was known in Roman times. The physician would insert a needle through the white of the eye directly into the defective lens and push the lens out of the line of vision, leaving it in the eyeball. The procedure must have been very painful, with a high chance for infection.

The complete removal of a lens from the eyeball was done for the first time in 1745. A French physician, Jacques Daviel, made a small cut in the cornea through which he was able to extract the lens. A major advance in eye surgery was the discovery of local anesthetic by Karl Koller in 1884. He found that a drop of cocaine solution applied directly to the eye deadened all sensation there. Synthetic substitutes such as novocaine were developed, thereafter making eye surgery virtually painless.

Before 1950, a cataract patient had to wear extremely thick eyeglasses to replace the focusing action of the natural lens that was removed. Plastic lens implants are now a safe and reliable method to restore good vision. In the 1960's, the ultrasonic probe was developed to replace forceps for removing the eye lens. The size of the required incision was much smaller and the healing time correspondingly shorter.

In the future, drugs may be found to delay the onset of cataracts so that surgery will not be necessary. Further research is needed to obtain a better understanding of the biochemical changes in the eye lens with aging.

—*Hans G. Graetzer, Ph.D.*

See also Aging; Aging, extended care for the; Astigmatism; Cataracts; Corneal transplantation; Eye surgery; Eyes; Glaucoma; Laser use in surgery; Microscopy, slitlamp; Ophthalmology; Optometry.

FOR FURTHER INFORMATION:

Eden, John. *The Physician's Guide to Cataracts, Glaucoma, and Other Eye Problems.* Yonkers, N.Y.: Consumer Reports Books, 1992.

Kelman, Charles D. *Cataracts: What You Must Know About Them.* New York: Crown, 1982.

Shulman, Julius. *Cataracts.* Rev. ed. New York: St. Martin's Griffin, 1995.

CATARACTS

DISEASE/DISORDER

ANATOMY OR SYSTEM AFFECTED: Eyes

SPECIALTIES AND RELATED FIELDS: Geriatrics and gerontology, ophthalmology, optometry

DEFINITION: Dark regions in the lens of the eye that cause gradual loss of vision.

KEY TERMS:

artificial lens implant: a plastic lens inserted permanently into the eye to replace a defective natural lens that has been removed

cornea: the transparent front surface of the eye; its curvature produces about 60 percent of the focusing power needed to produce an image on the retina

extracapsular cataract extraction: a procedure in which the lens is emulsified (broken up) with an ultrasonic probe and the pieces are suctioned out

intracapsular cataract extraction: a procedure in which the faulty lens is removed in one piece while still inside its capsule

iris: the colored portion of the eye that regulates the amount of light entering the pupil at its center

laser: an intense light beam, used in eye surgery to reattach a detached retina or to open a secondary cataract

microsurgery: surgery performed with the aid of a microscope

retina: the dark membrane on the inside rear surface of the eye, where light is converted into nerve signals sent to the brain

CAUSES AND SYMPTOMS

Cataracts are imperfections in the clarity of the eye lens that reduce its ability to transmit light. They are a very common medical problem. In the United States, cataract removal is the most frequently performed surgery and the largest line-item cost in the Medicare budget. There are many misconceptions about cataracts. Cataracts are not an infection, a growth, a disease, or a film on the surface of the lens. They do not cause pain, redness, teardrops, or other discomforts of the eye. The initial symptom is a gradual deterioration of vision, usually in one eye at a time. There is no known treatment other than to remove the lens surgically. After surgery, neither the lens nor the cataracts can grow back. The formation of cataracts is a normal part of aging, like gray hair or hardening of the arteries. All people would develop cataracts eventually if they lived long enough.

In a discussion of cataracts, it is helpful to review the structure of the human eye. The eye is often compared to a camera, with its lens and film. The camera lens, however, can be moved back and forth slightly to focus on objects at different distances, whereas the eye lens is squeezed into a thicker shape by muscular action to change its focus. Both camera and eye have a variable-size diaphragm to regulate the amount of light that is admitted.

When light enters the eye, it first encounters a transparent, tough outer skin called the cornea. There are no blood vessels in the cornea, but many nerve cells make it sensitive to touch or other irritation. Immediately behind the cornea is the clear aqueous fluid that carries oxygen and nutrients for cell metabolism. Next comes the colored portion, the iris of the eye, with a variable-size opening at its center called the pupil. The pupil has no color, but looks black, like the opening of a cave. A person looking at his or her own eye in a mirror and then shining a flashlight on it can see the black pupil quickly shrink in size.

Next comes the lens of the eye, surrounded by an elastic membrane called the capsule. The lens is suspended by short strands, or ligaments, which are attached to a sphincter muscle. When the muscle contracts, the lens becomes thicker in the middle, thus increasing its focusing strength. The transparent lens has no blood vessels, so its metabolism is provided by the aqueous fluid. Behind the lens is the vitreous fluid, which fills about two-thirds of the eyeball and maintains its oval shape. At the back of the eye is the retina, where special visual cells convert light into electrical signals that travel to the brain via nerve fibers.

The lens of the eye is not simply a homogeneous fluid, but has a unique, internal structure and growth pattern. It continues to grow larger throughout the life of the individual. New cells originate at the front surface of the lens, just inside the capsule enclosure. These cells divide and grow into fibers that migrate toward the middle, or nucleus, of the lens. The whole structure has been compared to the layers of an onion, with the oldest cells at the center. The protein molecules in the nucleus are less soluble and more rigid than those in the outer part of the lens. By the age of forty, in most people the firm nucleus has enlarged until the lens has lost much of its elasticity. Even with considerable muscular strain, the curvature of the lens surface will no longer bulge enough to focus on nearby objects. The eye loses its power of accommodation, and reading glasses will be needed.

The mechanism by which cataracts form in the lens is not yet clearly understood. Like the loss of accommodation, however, it is a normal part of the aging process. One proposed biochemical explanation is the Maillard reaction, in which glucose and protein molecules combine when heated to form a brown product. The Maillard reaction is responsible for the browning of bread or cookies during baking. The same process is thought to occur even at body temperature, but very slowly over a period of years. Some scientists have theorized that wrinkled skin, hardening of the arteries, and other normal features of aging may be caused by this reaction. The biochemistry of aging is an active area of research, in which the deterioration of the eye lens is only one example.

The most common symptom of cataracts is a loss of clear vision that cannot be corrected with eyeglasses. Brighter lighting can partially help to overcome the blockage of light transmission. There is one paradoxical situation reported by some patients, however, whose vision becomes worse in bright light. The explanation for this problem is that brightness causes the pupil to become smaller. If the cataract is centered right in the middle of the lens, it will block a larger fraction of the incoming light. In dimmer light, the pupil opening is larger, so light can pass through the clear periphery of the lens.

By far the most common cataracts are those attributable to normal aging, called senile cataracts. (This has nothing to do with the common use of the term "senility" to describe declining mental ability.) So-called secondary cataracts can also develop in special circumstances. For example, exposure to X rays or nuclear radiation will increase the probability of cataracts, and the eye lens seems to be particularly sensitive to the effects of ionizing radiation. Certain medications such as cortisone, which is used in arthritis treatment, increase the risk of cataracts. A diet deficient in protein, especially in developing countries, has been associated with cataract formation. A blow to the eye from a sports injury or an accident can lead to a cataract. Diabetics are more likely to develop cataracts than the general public. Some studies have suggested that electric shock, ultraviolet rays, or certain environmental pollutants may be other causes.

Some babies are born with cataracts. These are called congenital and are frequently associated with the mother having had German measles (rubella) during the first three months of pregnancy. Surgery on the infant's eye must be done with little delay. Otherwise, the nerve connections between eye and brain will not develop, and permanent blindness can result.

Cataracts are much more prevalent in Israel and India than in Western Europe. It is not clear yet whether race or different diets and life habits are the determining factors. Some ophthalmologists believe that cataracts run in families, suggesting a genetic influence. The evidence is not conclusive, and further studies are needed. What causes cataracts is much less understood than how to treat them surgically.

TREATMENT AND THERAPY

When cataracts begin to form in the eye lens, no medication can remove them and they will not get better on their own. The patient's vision will continue to deteriorate as the cataracts mature, although the process may be quite

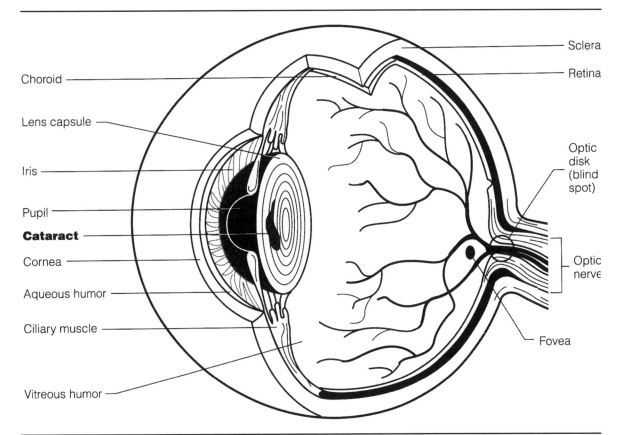

Cataracts are dark regions in the eye lens that lead gradually to obscured vision and blindness.

slow. Fortunately, modern techniques of surgery for cataract removal have a success rate of better than 95 percent.

Consider a typical middle-aged man who believes that his vision is getting worse. When he goes to an optometrist, he is informed that his eye examination has revealed the onset of senile cataracts (as a result of aging). He is referred to an ophthalmologist, who finds no need for surgery at this time, but recommends more frequent, semiannual checkups. The patient is told that reading or other eye-straining activities will not accelerate cataract growth, but that brighter lighting will help him to see more clearly. During the next several years, the cataracts slowly darken and increase in size. Eventually, distant vision in one eye (even with glasses) may deteriorate to 20/160, which means that what he is able to see at 20 feet can be seen by a normal person at 160 feet. The ability of the patient to drive a car is seriously impaired, and surgery is indicated. It is not a medical emergency, but operating on one eye while the other one is still fairly clear is recommended.

Once the decision has been made to go ahead with surgery, it is necessary for the patient to have a thorough physical examination. The doctor checks for possible health problems that could complicate cataract surgery. Among these are diabetes, high blood pressure, kidney disease, anemia, and glaucoma (excess pressure in the eye). Normally, extracting the cataractous lens and implanting an artificial, plastic one are done at the same time. Before proceeding with surgery, the ophthalmologist must determine what the proper strength of the implant lens should be, so that light will focus properly on the retina. An accurate measurement is made by reflecting a beam of high-frequency sound waves (ultrasound) from the back of the eye. Measuring the time for an echo to return gives the needed data for calculating the strength of the implant lens.

On the day of the surgery, the patient is given an injection to make him drowsy and eyedrops to dilate the pupil. Gradually, more eyedrops are administered to produce a large dilation, so that access to the lens is easier. In the operating room, local anesthetic is injected to keep the eyelids from closing and to deaden the normally very sensitive surface of the cornea. To prepare for surgery, a microscope is moved into place above the eye. Making an incision in the cornea, removing the defective lens, inserting and fastening the artificial lens, and finally closing the incision with a very fine needle and thread are all performed by the surgeon while looking through the microscope. Its magnification and focus controls are operated using foot pedals, so that both of the surgeon's hands are free.

There are three basic types of cataract extraction. Each method has its advantages and disadvantages. The first method is called intracapsular extraction. The capsule is the membrane that surrounds the lens. Intracapsular means that the lens and capsule are removed together, that is, with the lens still inside its capsule. The advantage of this method

is that no part of the lens is left behind to cause possible problems with infection or swelling later. The disadvantage is that the incision at the edge of the cornea must be fairly large to allow the lens and capsule to be pulled out together. Five to ten stitches are needed to close the incision. The patient must avoid strenuous activity for about a month to permit thorough healing. Before 1962, forceps were used to bring the lens and capsule out of the eye. Then Charles D. Kelman introduced the cryoprobe, which uses a freezing process. When the rather slippery lens is touched by the cold probe, it freezes to the probe and can be pulled out in one piece. Most eye surgeons have adopted the cryoprobe for intracapsular extraction.

A second method of cataract surgery is called extracapsular extraction, in which the lens is removed, while the capsule is left in the eye. The advantage is that the unbroken back surface of the capsule can prevent leakage of fluid from the rear of the eye and therefore can decrease the chances for damage to the retina. A disadvantage is that small fragments of the lens may remain behind, causing infection or irritation. The size of the incision and the recuperation period are about the same as for the intracapsular method.

The third method of cataract surgery is an improvement of extracapsular extraction, first developed by Kelman in 1967. An ultrasonic probe is used to emulsify, or break up, the lens. The small pieces are then suctioned out of the capsule while fluid is washed into the opening. The main advantage of emulsification is that the incision can be very small, because the lens is brought out in fragments, not as a whole. The incision may be only 3 millimeters long, and a single suture to close it would heal rapidly. This method requires very specialized training, however, because surgeons must learn to operate the microscope, the ultrasonic generator, and the suction apparatus with their feet while manipulating the probe with their hands.

After the eye lens has been extracted, an artificial lens is inserted in its place. The implant is made of clear plastic, about the size of an aspirin tablet. Two spring loops embedded in the plastic are used to center the implant and to keep it there permanently. A variety of different spring loop attachments has been designed by ophthalmologists. In the United States, if a particular design is prone to failure, the Food and Drug Administration (FDA) has the authority to ban its use.

To complete the surgery, the incision in the cornea is closed. During the recuperation period, the patient is instructed to avoid strenuous exercise and to protect the eye from any hard contact. Normally there is little pain, although some eye irritation should be expected during the healing process. A plastic implant lens has a fixed focal length, with no power of accommodation for different distances. It is like a box camera that gives a good picture at a set distance, while near and far objects are somewhat blurry. After the eye has healed thoroughly, the patient is fitted with prescription glasses for reading and for distant vision, respectively.

A number of minor complications can develop after cataract surgery. About one-third of the patients develop a so-called secondary cataract, which is a clouding of the capsule membrane just behind the implant. This condition is easily corrected with a laser beam to open the membrane, requiring no surgery. Another potential complication is astigmatism. The eye is squeezed and flattened slightly, and the curvature of the surface will differ between the flattened and the more rounded regions. During surgery, the symmetry of the corneal surface can be distorted if some sutures are tighter than others. Astigmatism is relatively easy to correct with prescription glasses.

All operations have some risks, and a small percentage of cataract surgeries can lead to serious complications. Among these are a detached retina, glaucoma caused by scar tissue, and hemorrhage into the vitreous fluid in front of the retina. Fortunately, such problems are rare, and the percentage of successful eye surgeries continues to improve.

PERSPECTIVE AND PROSPECTS

In the history of medicine, surgery for cataracts has been traced back to Roman times. The method was called "couching." The physician would insert a needle through the white of the eye into the lens and he would try to push the lens down out of the line of vision, leaving it in the eyeball. The procedure must have been painful, with a high chance for infection. The complete extraction of a lens from the eye was done for the first time in 1745. A French ophthalmologist named Jacques Daviel was performing a couching operation, but was unable to push the lens out of the line of sight. On the spur of the moment, he decided to make a small cut in the cornea, through which he was able to extract the lens. The operation was successful. During the following ten years, he repeated his procedure more than four hundred times with only fifty failures, a much better result than with couching.

A major advance in eye surgery was the discovery of local anesthesia by Carl Koller in 1884. Together with the famous psychiatrist Sigmund Freud, Koller had been investigating the psychological effects of cocaine. He noticed that his tongue became numb from the drug and wondered if a drop of cocaine solution locally applied to the eyes might work as an anesthetic. He tried it first on a frog's eye and then on himself, and the cocaine made his eye numb. He published a short article, and the news spread to other physicians. Synthetic substitutes such as novocaine were developed and came into common use, thereafter making eye surgery virtually painless.

When the lens of the eye is surgically removed, it becomes impossible to focus light on the retina. A strong replacement lens is needed. For example, the French painter Claude Monet had cataract surgery in the 1920's, and pho-

tographs show him with the typical thick cataract glasses of that time. Today, contact lenses or artificial lens implants are much better alternatives to restore good vision.

The recovery period after cataract surgery used to be several weeks of bed rest, with the head kept absolutely still, because the cut in the cornea had to heal itself without any stitches. The development of microsurgery made it possible for the surgeon to see the extremely fine thread and needle that can be used for closing the cut. With stitches in place, the patient can usually carry on normal activities within a day after surgery.

In the 1960's, the cryoprobe and the ultrasound probe were developed to replace forceps for removing an eye lens. The size of the required incision was smaller and the healing time correspondingly shorter. In the 1980's, reliable lens implants became available, making near-normal vision possible again. In the future, perhaps drugs can be found that will prevent or delay the onset of cataracts, so that surgery will not be necessary. Further research is needed to obtain a better understanding of biochemical changes in the eye lens that occur with aging.

—*Hans G. Graetzer, Ph.D.*

See also Aging; Blindness; Cataract surgery; Eye surgery; Eyes; Ophthalmology; Optometry; Visual disorders.

FOR FURTHER INFORMATION:

Eden, John. *The Physician's Guide to Cataracts, Glaucoma, and Other Eye Problems.* Yonkers, N.Y.: Consumer Reports Books, 1992. The author, an ophthalmologist, describes the medical history of a typical cataract patient in her sixties: the original diagnosis, gradually deteriorating vision, surgery with the insertion of an artificial lens implant, postoperative care, and the fitting of prescription glasses. Informative and reassuring.

Houseman, William. "The Day the Light Returned." *New Choices for Retirement Living* 32 (April, 1992): 54-58. A personal account of a patient who had successful cataract surgery. Under local anesthetic, his faulty eye lens was removed and a plastic lens was inserted. The whole procedure took only half a day. The initial eye examination and follow-up care after surgery are described.

Kelman, Charles D. *Cataracts: What You Must Know About Them.* New York: Crown, 1982. The author is one of the world's leading cataract surgeons. In the 1960's, he invented the cryogenic probe and later the ultrasonic procedure for removing a faulty lens. This book describes cataract formation, eye surgery, lens implantation (with enlarged photographs), and possible medical complications. Highly recommended.

Lerman, Sidney. "Cataracts." *Scientific American* 206 (March, 1962): 106-114. An informative, basic article on the structure of the normal eye and the formation of cataracts as a result of aging, radiation exposure, or other factors. Excellent illustrations and accompanying explanations.

Ravin, James G. "Monet's Cataracts." *Journal of the American Medical Association* 254 (July, 1985): 394-399. Monet was a famous French painter who had cataract surgery in 1922. The article gives interesting details about the operation, his recovery (lying immobilized with sandbags for ten days), and his difficulty with the thick eyeglasses of that era. A fascinating story.

Shulman, Julius. *Cataracts*. Rev. ed. New York: St. Martin's Griffin, 1995. A well-written book by an ophthalmologist to educate patients who may need cataract surgery. Using nontechnical language and helpful diagrams, Shulman explains several methods for extracting the eye lens. Authoritative and highly recommended.

Van Heyningen, Ruth. "What Happens to the Human Lens in Cataract." *Scientific American* 233 (December, 1975): 70. The structure of the human eye is described, with a labeled cutaway drawing. Mechanical stress, a high blood sugar level, and other factors are identified as potential causes for the deteriorating transparency within the lens. Offers good explanations.

CATHETERIZATION

PROCEDURE

ANATOMY OR SYSTEM AFFECTED: Bladder, blood vessels, circulatory system, genitals, heart, reproductive system, throat, urinary system

SPECIALTIES AND RELATED FIELDS: Anesthesiology, cardiology, critical care, emergency medicine, general surgery, pulmonary medicine, radiology, urology

DEFINITION: The insertion of a tube into a cavity of the body to withdraw fluids from or introduce fluids into that cavity.

KEY TERMS:

bladder: the organ that stores urine until it is discharged from the body

urethra: the tube that transfers urine from the bladder to the outside of the body

INDICATIONS AND PROCEDURES

Many different types of catheters exist, and they can be used for many different purposes. What they all have in common is the placement of a tube (catheter) into a body cavity. The tube is used to draw a gas or liquid from the cavity or to inject a gas or liquid into the cavity. The most common uses of catheterization are the opening of an airway for breathing, the withdrawal of urine from the bladder, and the injection of dye or other substances such as an intravenous (IV) drip into blood vessels.

Catheterization can be used to assist in the breathing process. This procedure may be necessary when the patient's airway is blocked, the patient is unconscious and unable to breathe, or the patient needs help to breathe. The tube or catheter is placed into the mouth, nose, throat, or lungs. Oxygen passes through the tube and into the lungs, where it can be absorbed by the blood. Catheters can also be used to remove secretions from these same areas to open the airway and improve breathing. They are also necessary in many emergency situations to open and maintain breathing. At times, a catheter must be introduced directly into the lungs through an incision in the neck, near the Adam's apple; this procedure is known as a tracheostomy. A catheter may also be introduced into the patient's nose to transport oxygen into the lungs. Catheterization is important for maintaining breathing during surgery under general anesthesia, when the body's breathing mechanisms are shut down.

Another common catheterization procedure involves the introduction of a urethral catheter. This type of catheter is inserted into the urethra to drain urine from the bladder. Such a procedure may be necessary when the urethra is blocked in order to empty the bladder, or it may be used to collect urine when the person is unable to control his or her own bladder.

An area where catheters are being used more frequently is heart diagnosis and surgery. In cardiac catheterization, a catheter is inserted into a large blood vessel (a vein or artery) in the upper arm or groin area. The physician then maneuvers the catheter into the heart and uses it to inject a dye directly into the organ. An X ray can show the distribution of the dye within the heart, allowing the physician to see if and where any coronary arteries are blocked. In addition, cardiac catheters can be used to determine blood pressures within the heart, the amount of oxygen in the blood in the heart, and how the valves are functioning. More recently, cardiac catheters have been developed to perform some types of surgery. A good example is balloon angioplasty. Using similar procedures to insert the catheter, the cardiologist guides a specialized catheter into the coronary artery to the area of the blockage. A small balloon on the end of the catheter is inflated, pushing the fatty material blocking the artery against the blood vessel wall and opening the artery to allow for the normal flow of blood.

USES AND COMPLICATIONS

Catheterization has been used safely and successfully for many years. When a person is unable to breathe on his or her own, airway catheters have been instrumental in saving lives and making such patients more comfortable. Such procedures have been widely used on a daily basis, with few complications.

Likewise, urethral catheters are routinely employed to control the flow of urine from the bladder. This type of catheterization can be seen in many clinical settings. Although caution must be used to prevent the introduction of bacteria into the bladder and subsequent infection, this procedure is considered to be safe and effective.

The overall success rate of cardiac catheterization has been good, with few deaths resulting from the procedure. It is a valuable tool for the diagnosis of heart diseases and disorders because a major incision in the chest is avoided.

This procedure is performed many times each day in all cardiac care units. Angioplasty has also been successful, but it is useful for only some types of blockages. A major risk of angioplasty is rupture of the artery if the balloon is inflated too much. When this happens, open heart surgery is necessary to prevent death. The death rate from angioplasty is less than 1 percent, however, and the success rate exceeds 90 percent. Another problem with balloon angioplasty is that in 33 percent of the cases, the blockages reform within six months. Nevertheless, this procedure offers a good alternative to coronary artery bypass surgery.

PERSPECTIVE AND PROSPECTS

The use of catheterization for airway management was first tried in 1871 by Friedrich Trendelenburg. Through the years, such procedures have been improved. Catheters continue to be instrumental for airway management and will be for a long time to come.

The cardiac catheterization of a living human being was done by Werner Forssmann in the 1920's: He performed the procedure on himself. His techniques were further developed by André Frédéric Cournand in the 1940's, for which he won the Nobel Prize in Physiology or Medicine in 1956. Continued advances in the procedure and improved technology have increased the applications of cardiac catheterization. New and better procedures, which will continue to replace some types of open heart surgery, are expected in the future. —*Bradley R. A. Wilson, Ph.D.*

See also Amniocentesis; Anesthesia; Anesthesiology; Angiography; Angioplasty; Biopsy; Blood testing; Cardiology; Circulation; Heart; Lumbar puncture; Pharmacology; Radiopharmaceuticals, use of; Respiration; Resuscitation; Surgical procedures; Tracheostomy; Transfusion; Urinary system; Urology; Vascular medicine; Vascular system.

FOR FURTHER INFORMATION:

Finucane, Brendan T., and Albert H. Santora. *Principles of Airway Management.* 2d ed. St. Louis: C. V. Mosby, 1996.

Karch, Amy Morrison. *Cardiac Care: A Guide for Patient Education.* New York: Appleton-Century-Crofts, 1981.

CELL THERAPY

PROCEDURE

ANATOMY OR SYSTEM AFFECTED: Cells, immune system, joints, skin

SPECIALTIES AND RELATED FIELDS: Alternative medicine, cytology

DEFINITION: Cell therapy, also known as live cell or fresh cell therapy, is the injection of fetal lamb cells for the purpose of rejuvenation; it was invented by Swiss surgeon Paul Niehaus. Cells derived from fetal lambs whose mothers have been slaughtered are injected into the patient. One series of treatments requires the cells from six lambs, and treatments must be repeated periodically. Claims of positive effects of this treatment include a gen-

eralized greater fitness, increased libido, better skin quality, improved well-being, relief from arthritis, and other antiaging phenomena. Practitioners believe that the injections reverse cellular damage. Cell therapy has also be promoted as being of great benefit to children with Down syndrome; clinical studies indicate no improvement in the intelligence or motor skills of children receiving the therapy. Potential side effects of cell therapy include fatigue and pain at the injection site and the possible transmission of viruses from sheep to human. Treatments are extremely expensive, and the scientific community has yet to document any actual physical benefit from this therapy. —*Karen E. Kalumuck, Ph.D.*

See also Alternative medicine; Cells; Immunology.

CELLS

BIOLOGY

ANATOMY OR SYSTEM AFFECTED: Bones, immune system, musculoskeletal system, nerves, nervous system, skin

SPECIALTIES AND RELATED FIELDS: Bacteriology, cytology, histology

DEFINITION: The fundamental structural and functional units of all living organisms.

KEY TERMS:

chromosome: one DNA molecule of the cell nucleus, held in combination with chromosomal proteins

cytoskeleton: a network of filaments (including microtubules, microfilaments, and intermediate filaments) that supports the cytoplasm and extensions of the cell surface

endoplasmic reticulum: a system of cytoplasmic membrane-bound sacs that, with attached ribosomes, synthesize proteins destined to enter membranes or to be stored or secreted

gene: a segment of DNA encoding a protein; RNA molecules such as messenger and ribosomal RNA

Golgi complex: a system of membrane sacs in which proteins are chemically modified, sorted, and routed to various cellular destinations

membrane: a thin layer of lipid and protein molecules that controls transport of molecules and ions between the cell and its exterior and between membrane-bound compartments within the cell

mitochondrion: a membrane-bound cytoplasmic organelle that constitutes the primary location of oxidative reactions providing energy for cellular activities

nucleolus: a nuclear structure formed through the activity of chromosome segments in the production of ribosomal RNA and the assembly of ribosomal subunits

peroxisome: a membrane-bound organelle that contains reaction systems linking biochemical pathways taking place elsewhere in the cell; also called a microbody

ribosome: a cytoplasmic particle assembled from ribosomal RNA and ribosomal proteins that uses messenger RNA molecules as directions for synthesizing proteins

STRUCTURE AND FUNCTIONS

Cells contain complex biochemical systems that can use energy sources to power cellular activities such as growth, movement, and reaction to environmental changes. The information required to assemble the enzymatic and structural molecules involved in these activities is stored in cells and is duplicated and passed on in cell division.

Cells are divided into two major internal regions, nucleus and cytoplasm, which reflect a fundamental division of labor. In the nucleus are the deoxyribonucleic acid (DNA) molecules that store the hereditary information required for cell growth and reproduction. The nuclear region also contains enzymes that copy the hereditary information into ribonucleic acid (RNA), which is used as instructions for making proteins in the cytoplasm. Enzymes within the nucleus also duplicate the DNA in preparation for cell division. The cytoplasm makes proteins according to the directions copied in the nucleus and also synthesizes most other molecules required for cellular activities. The cytoplasm carries out several additional vital functions, including motility and the conversion of fuel substances into usable forms of chemical energy.

Cells are organized by membranes. These layers of lipid and protein molecules, not much more than 7 to 8 nanometers thick, form an outer boundary, the plasma membrane, which separates the cell contents from the exterior. Several internal membrane systems divided the cell interior into specialized compartments called organelles. The lipid part of membranes consists of a double layer of molecules called a bilayer. The lipid bilayer provides the structural framework of membranes and acts as a barrier to the passage of water-soluble substances. Membrane proteins, which are suspended in the lipid bilayer or attached to its surfaces, carry out the specialized functions of membranes.

The plasma membrane forming the outer cell boundary has a variety of functions. The most significant is the transport of substances between the cytoplasm and the cell's exterior, which is carried out by proteins forming channels in the membrane. These channels pass specific water-soluble molecules or ions. The plasma membrane also contains proteins functioning as receptors, which recognize and bind to specific molecules from the surrounding medium. On binding to their target molecules, which include peptide hormones, many receptors trigger internal cellular responses that coordinate the activities of cells in tissues and organs. Other plasma membrane proteins recognize and adhere to molecules on the surfaces of other cells or to extracellular structures such as collagen. These adhesive functions are critical to the development and maintenance of tissues and organs. Other plasma membrane proteins identify cells as

The Structure of a Cell

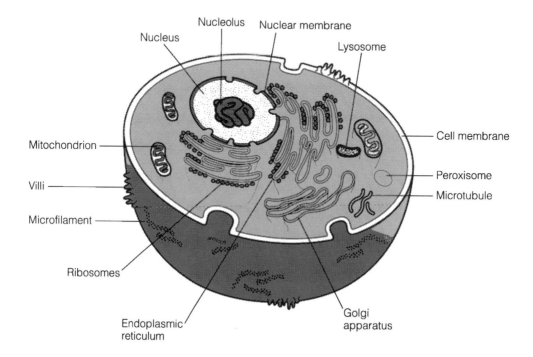

part of the individual or as foreign.

The nucleus is separated from the cytoplasm by two concentric membranes, one layered just inside the other, forming a system known as the nuclear envelope. At closely spaced intervals, the envelope is perforated by pores, about 70 to 90 nanometers in diameter, which form channels between the nuclear interior and the surrounding cytoplasm. The pores are filled by a ringlike mass of proteins that controls the movement of large molecules, such as proteins and RNA, through the nuclear envelope.

Within the nucleus are chromatin fibers containing the nuclear DNA, held in association with two major types of proteins, the histone and nonhistone chromosomal proteins. The histones are primarily structural molecules that pack DNA into chromatin fibers. The nonhistones include proteins that regulate gene activity. The hereditary information of the human nucleus is subdivided among forty-six linear DNA molecules. Each individual DNA molecule, with its associated histone and nonhistone proteins, is a chromosome of the nucleus.

Each segment of a chromosome containing the information used to make an RNA copy constitutes a gene. One type of gene encodes messenger RNA (mRNA) molecules, which contain information required to make proteins. Another type of gene encodes ribosomal RNA (rRNA) molecules. Ribosomal RNA forms part of ribosomes, complex RNA-protein particles in the cytoplasm that assemble proteins according to the directions carried in mRNA molecules. The regions of the chromosomes active in making rRNA are collected into structures called nucleoli. Within nucleoli, rRNAs are assembled with proteins into subunits of ribosomes.

The cytoplasm surrounding the nucleus is packed with ribosomes and a variety of organelles. The boundary membranes of the organelles set them off as distinct chemical and molecular environments, specialized to carry out different functions. Ribosomes may be either freely suspended in the cytoplasm or attached to the surfaces of a system of flattened, membranous sacs called the endoplasmic reticulum. Freely suspended ribosomes make proteins that enter the cytoplasmic solution as enzymes, structural supports, or motile elements. Ribosomes attached to the endoplasmic reticulum assemble proteins that become part of membranes or eventually enter small, membrane-bound sacs for storage or release to the cell exterior.

Proteins made in the rough endoplasmic reticulum—those sacs with ribosomes—are modified chemically in another system of membranous sacs, the Golgi complex or apparatus. This system usually appears as a cup-shaped stack of flattened, ribosome-free sacs. The modifications carried out in the Golgi complex may include the addition of chemical groups such as sugars, and the clipping of surplus segments from proteins. Following modification, proteins are sorted into small, membrane-bound sacs that pinch off from the Golgi membranes. These sacs may be stored in the cytoplasm or may release their contents to the cell exterior.

One type of membrane-bound sac containing stored proteins, the lysosome, is particularly important to cell function. Lysosomes contain a group of enzymes collectively capable of breaking down all major molecules of the cell. Many substances taken into cells are delivered to lysosomes, where they are digested by the lysosomal enzymes. Lysosomes may also release their enzymes into the cytoplasm or to the cell exterior. Release within the cell causes cell death, which may be part of pathological conditions or may occur as part of normal development.

Most of the chemical energy required for cellular activities is produced by reactions taking place in another cytoplasmic organelle, the mitochondrion. Mitochondria are surrounded by two separate membranes, one enclosed within the other. Within mitochondria occur most of the oxidative reactions that release energy for cellular activities. Fuel for these reactions is provided by breakdown products of all major cellular molecules, including carbohydrates, fats, proteins, and nucleic acids.

The oxidative functions of mitochondria are supplemented by the activities of peroxisomes (also called microbodies). These structures, which consist simply of a boundary membrane surrounding a solution of enzymes, carry out reactions that link major oxidative pathways occurring elsewhere in the cytoplasm. Microbodies are particularly important to the oxidation of fatty acids.

Almost all cell movements are generated by either of two cytoplasmic structures, microtubules or microfilaments. Microtubules form the motile elements of sperm tails; microfilaments are responsible for the movements of skeletal, cardiac, and smooth muscle. Microtubules are fine, hollow cylinders about 25 nanometers in diameter, assembled from subunits of a protein known as tubulin. Microfilaments are thin, solid fibers 5 to 7 nanometers in diameter, assembled from subunits of a different protein, actin. Both structures produce motion through protein crossbridges that work as transducers converting chemical energy to mechanical energy. One end of a crossbridge attaches to the surface of a microtubule or microfilament; the opposite, reactive end attaches to another microtubule or microfilament or to other cell structures. The crossbridge produces motion by making an attachment at its reactive end, forcefully swiveling a short distance, and then releasing. Distinct proteins form the swiveling crossbridges for the two motile elements.

In addition to their functions in cell motility, both microtubules and microfilaments form supportive networks inside cells collectively called the cytoskeleton. Another group of supportive fibers with diameters averaging about 100 nanometers, the intermediate filaments, also forms parts of the cytoskeleton. Intermediate filaments assemble from a large family of related proteins that is distinct from the tubulins and actins forming microtubules and microfilaments.

DISORDERS AND DISEASES

Because cell structure and function underlie the totality of bodily functions, all aspects of health and disease reflect normal and abnormal cellular activities. Perhaps the most critical and important of these activities to contemporary medical science is the conversion of normal to abnormal activity responsible for cancer. In cancer, cells grow and divide uncontrollably, break free from their normal cell contacts, and migrate to other regions of the body.

The cell transformations occurring in the development of cancer involve changes at several levels. Most of these changes reflect an alteration of one or more genes in the cell nucleus from normal to aberrant forms called oncogenes. Most oncogenes prove to encode proteins involved in a relatively small number of activities. These include nonhistone proteins regulating gene activity, growth hormones, receptors in the plasma membrane for peptide hormones, and proteins taking part in internal cellular response systems triggered by receptors. Directly or indirectly, the altered proteins encoded in oncogenes induce internal changes that lead to uncontrolled cell division and loss of normal adhesions to neighboring cells.

For example, the oncogene *src* encodes a protein that adds phosphate groups to other proteins as a cellular control measure. In many types of cancer cells, the *src* gene or its product is hyperactive. One of the targets of the enzyme encoded in the gene is a receptor protein of the plasma membrane. In some cancer cells, uncontrolled addition of phosphate groups to the receptor causes it to lose its attachment to extracellular structures that hold the cells in place. This loss contributes to the tendency of the tumor cells to break loose and migrate to other parts of the body.

In some cases, movement of DNA segments from one chromosome to another is involved in the transformation of cells from normal to cancerous types, including several types of leukemias. For example, in many leukemias, breaks occur in chromosomes 8 and 14 of the human set in cell lines producing leukocytes, and segments are exchanged between the chromosomes. The exchange moves the gene *myc* from its normal location in chromosome 8 to a region of chromosome 14 that encodes a major segment of antibody proteins. In its normal location, the *myc* gene encodes a chromosomal regulatory protein that controls genes involved in cell division. When translocated to chromosome 14, *myc* comes under the influence of DNA sequences that promote the high activity of the antibody gene. As a result, *myc* becomes hyperactive in triggering cell division and contributes to the uncontrolled division of white blood cells characteristic of leukemias.

Alterations in cytoplasmic organelles are also directly responsible for some human diseases. The enzymes contained in lysosomes are abnormally secreted in many human diseases. The degenerative changes of arthritis, for example, are suspected to be caused in part by the abnormal release of enzymes from the lysosomes of bone or lymph cells into the fluids that lubricate joints. Some of the damage to lung tissues caused by inhalation of silica fibers in silicosis is also related to lysosomal function. Microscopic silica fibers are taken in by macrophages and other cells in the lungs; these fibers are delivered to lysosomes for breakdown, as are many other substances. The fibers accumulate in the lysosomes, causing lysosomal enlargement and eventually breakage, with destructive release of lysosomal enzymes into the cytoplasm. Some human diseases related to lysosomes are caused by inherited mutations destroying the activity of lysosomal enzymes. For example, an inherited deficiency in one lysosomal enzyme, hexosaminidase, interferes with reactions clipping carbohydrate segments from molecules removed from the cell surface. As a result, the subparts of these molecules accumulate in lysosomes and cannot be recycled. Their concentration on cell surfaces is diminished; loss of these molecules from nerve cells, particularly a group called gangliosides, can lead to seizures, blindness, loss of intellect, and early death.

Human disease has also been linked to inherited changes in mitochondria. The mutations interfere with the oxidative reactions inside the organelle or have detrimental effects on the transport of substances through the mitochondrial membranes. The mutations cause the most severe problems in locations where the energy supplied by mitochondria is highly critical, particularly in the central nervous system and skeletal and cardiac muscle. Mitochondrial deficiencies in these locations are typically responsible for symptoms such as muscular weakness, irregularities in the heartbeat, and epilepsy.

Deficiencies in motile systems based on microtubules and microfilaments are also associated with human disease. For example, a group of inherited defects known as the immotile cilia or Kartagener's syndrome is characterized by acute bronchitis, sinusitis, chronic headache, male sterility, and reversal of the position of the heart from the left to the right side of the body. In individuals with the disease, the cyclic crossbridges driving microtubule-based motion are missing. Male sterility results from loss of motility by sperm tails; other deficiencies result from the immotility of cilia on cells lining the respiratory system and the cavities of the brain. (Cilia are microtubule-based cellular appendages that beat like sperm tails to maintain the flow of fluids over cell surfaces.) In the respiratory system, loss of ciliary beating stops the flow of mucus that normally removes irritating and infectious matter from the lungs and respiratory tract. This deficiency explains the sinusitis and bronchitis. Presumably, an insufficient flow of fluids in the ventricles of the brain, normally maintained by ciliated cells lining these cavities, produces the headaches. The reversed position taken by the heart remains unexplained.

Even the cytoskeleton has been associated with human disease. For example, deficiencies in intermediate filaments of the cytoskeleton have been implicated in the hereditary disease epidermolysis bullosa. In this disease, skin cells are fragile, and slight abrasions that would cause little or no problem in normal individuals lead to severe blistering, ulceration, and scarring.

PERSPECTIVE AND PROSPECTS

Knowledge of cell structure and function developed gradually from the first morphological descriptions of cells in the seventeenth century. By the 1830's, enough information had accumulated for Theodor Schwann and Matthias Schleiden to propose that all living organisms are composed of one or more cells and that cells are the minimum functional units of living organisms. Their conclusions were supplemented in 1855 by a third postulate by Rudolf Virchow: that all cells arise only from preexisting cells by a process of division. Further work established that the cell nucleus contains hereditary information and that the essential feature of cell division is transmission of this information from parent to daughter cells.

The study of cell chemistry and physiology began in the late eighteenth and early nineteenth centuries. By the end of the nineteenth century, investigators had isolated, identified, and synthesized many organic substances found in cells and worked out the structural components of proteins and nucleic acids. This chemical work was complemented by biochemical studies leading to the discovery of enzymes. The gradual integration of cell structure, physiology, and biochemistry continued; by the 1930's, the field had shifted from morphological observations to biochemical and molecular studies of cell function. Crucial to this shift was the research of George Beadle and Edward Tatum, who concluded from their studies that mutant genes encode a faulty form of an enzyme necessary to produce a substance needed for normal growth. On this basis, they proposed that each gene codes for a single enzyme—the famous "one gene-one enzyme" hypothesis.

Further biochemical work revealed the oxidative reactions providing chemical energy for cell activities. This research was integrated with structural studies of cytoplasmic organelles by Albert Claude, who developed a technique for isolating and purifying cell parts by cell fractionation and centrifugation. Claude and his associates successfully isolated ribosomes, endoplasmic reticulum, Golgi complexes, lysosomes, microbodies, and mitochondria by these methods, which allowed biochemical analysis of the fractions. This work was facilitated by development of the electron microscope, allowing elucidation of the ultrastructure of many of the organelles studied biochemically in cell fractions.

Experiments in the 1940's implicating DNA as the hereditary molecule sparked an intensive effort to work out the three-dimensional structure of this molecule, culminating in the discovery of DNA structure in 1953 by James D. Watson and Francis Crick. Their discovery led to an effort to determine the molecular structure of genes and their modes of action, which was greatly facilitated by the development of rapid methods for nucleic acid sequencing. Using these methods, many genes have been completely sequenced; the sequences, in turn, allowed deduction of the amino acid sequences of many proteins. The comparisons of gene and protein sequences and structure in normal and mutant forms made possible by these developments provided fundamental insights into the mechanisms controlling and regulating genes and the molecular functions of proteins, revolutionizing biology and medicine.   —*Stephen L. Wolfe, Ph.D.*

See also Amniocentesis; Antibiotics; Bacteriology; Biopsy; Cancer; Cell therapy; Cholesterol; Chorionic villus sampling; Cloning; Cytology; Cytopathology; DNA and RNA; Enzymes; Gene therapy; Genetic engineering; Genetics and inheritance; Glycolysis; Gram staining; Immunology; Immunopathology; Laboratory tests; Microbiology; Microscopy; Mutation; Oncology; Pathology.

FOR FURTHER INFORMATION:

Alberts, Bruce, et al. *Molecular Biology of the Cell.* 3d ed. New York: Garland, 1994. Describes the evolution of cells and introduces cell structure and function. The text is clearly written at the college level and is illustrated by numerous diagrams and photographs. An extensive bibliography of technical and scientific articles appears at the end of each chapter.

Campbell, Neil A. *Biology.* 4th ed. Redwood City, Calif.: Benjamin/Cummings, 1997. This classic introductory textbook provides an excellent discussion of essential biological structures and mechanisms. Its extensive and detailed illustrations help to make even difficult concepts accessible to the nonspecialist. Of particular interest are the five chapters comprising the unit entitled "The Cell."

Darnell, James, Harvey Lodish, and David Baltimore. *Molecular Cell Biology.* 2d ed. New York: Scientific American Books, 1990. An excellent textbook written at the college level. The introduction, "The History of Molecular Cell Biology," and chapter 4, "The Study of Cell Organization and Subcellular Structure," outline the evolution of cells and basic cell structure and function and describe technical approaches used in the study of cells. Many highly illustrative diagrams and photographs are included. A very extensive bibliography of technical articles and books is included at the end of each chapter.

Fawcett, Don W. *The Cell.* 2d ed. Philadelphia: W. B. Saunders, 1981. This book, an atlas of mammalian cell structure, presents electron microscope pictures of all aspects of human and other mammalian cells, accompanied by a brief but informative description of cell organelles and structures. The micrographs are of exceptional quality; one of the most useful books available as an introduction to cell structure and function.

Lewin, Benjamin. *Genes.* 4th ed. Cambridge, Mass.: Cell Press, 1990. A college textbook that discusses the entire field of molecular biology and genetics, with many references to the structure and activity of the cell nucleus. Although written at the college level, it is readable and accessible to a general audience. Many highly informative illustrations and diagrams are included.

Watson, James D. *The Double Helix.* New York: Atheneum, 1968. An entertaining and informative account of the events leading to the discovery of DNA structure by Watson and Francis Crick. The book not only outlines the scientific events leading to the discovery—which stands as one of the most important findings of biology—but also describes, with humor and insight, interpersonal relationships among the scientists involved. The book provides a rare glimpse of the inner workings of scientific investigation at the highest levels.

Wolfe, Stephen L. *Molecular and Cellular Biology.* Belmont, Calif.: Wadsworth, 1993. Chapter 1, "Introduction to Cell and Molecular Biology," presents cell structure and function and outlines the history of developments in cell biology, biochemistry, and molecular biology. The book, written at the college level, is readable and illustrated with many useful and informative diagrams and photographs.

CEREBRAL PALSY

DISEASE/DISORDER

ANATOMY OR SYSTEM AFFECTED: Back, bones, hands, legs, muscles, musculoskeletal system, nervous system, spine

SPECIALTIES AND RELATED FIELDS: Embryology, neurology, physical therapy, speech pathology

DEFINITION: Cerebral palsy is a term applied to a variety of nonprogressive muscular and nervous system disorders caused by brain damage occurring to a child during pregnancy or birth. Risks to the newborn increase with prematurity and the mother's alcohol consumption during pregnancy. The symptoms of cerebral palsy include lack of muscle tone, slow development, unusual body posture, stiffness, and muscle spasms. More severe cases include widespread loss of muscular control, seizures, and mental retardation, as well as deficiencies in speech, vision, and hearing. Treatment may include orthopedic braces, sur-gical correction of some deformities, physical and speech therapy, and medication to control seizures and relieve spasms. —*Jason Georges and Tracy Irons-Georges*

See also Birth defects; Mental retardation; Muscle sprains, spasms, and disorders; Muscles; Nervous system; Neurology; Neurology, pediatric; Palsy; Seizures.

CERVICAL, OVARIAN, AND UTERINE CANCERS

DISEASE/DISORDER

ANATOMY OR SYSTEM AFFECTED: Gentials, lymphatic system, reproductive system, uterus

SPECIALTIES AND RELATED FIELDS: Gynecology, immunology, obstetrics, oncology

DEFINITION: The primary cancers of the female reproductive system.

KEY TERMS:

benign: referring to a tumor made of a mass of cells which do not leave the site where they develop

cancer: one of a group of diseases in which cells divide uncontrollably; cancerous tissues do not contribute to the function of the body

cervix: the narrowest part of the uterus, which opens into the vagina

endometrium: the inner lining of the uterus, which normally thickens and then is sloughed off during each menstrual cycle; estrogens cause its growth and development, and progesterone prepares it for possible pregnancy

malignant: referring to a tumor which is capable of losing cells, which can travel via blood or lymph fluid to other sites

metastasis: the process by which malignant tumors invade other tissues either locally or distally

neoplasm: the new and abnormal formation of a tumor

ovary: the female gonad located in the pelvic cavity, where egg production occurs; the principal organ that produces the hormones estrogen and progesterone

tumor: a mass of cells characterized by uncontrolled growth; it can be either benign or malignant

uterus: the female organ in which the embryo develops; it is located in the pelvic cavity and is connected to the ovaries by the uterine tubes

---

Spastic Cerebral Palsy

 Diplegia: Both legs and arms affected, with legs worse than arms.

 Hemiplegia: One leg, one arm affected, on same side of body.

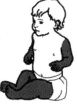 **Quadriplegia:** All four limbs are severely, if unequally, affected.

CAUSES AND SYMPTOMS

Although people commonly talk about cancer as a single disease, it actually includes more than one hundred different diseases. These diseases do appear to have a common element to them. All cancer cells divide without obeying the normal control mechanisms. These abnormal cells have altered deoxyribonucleic acid (DNA) that causes them to divide and form other abnormal cells, which again divide and eventually form a neoplasm, or tumor.

If the neoplasm has the potential to leave its original site and invade other tissues, it is called malignant. If the tumor stays in one place, it is benign. One major difference between these tumors is that malignant cells seem to have lost the cellular glue that holds them to one another. Therefore, they can metastasize, leaving the tumor and infiltrating nearby tissues. Metastatic cells can also travel to distant sites via the blood or lymph systems.

Medical scientists do not know exactly what causes a cell to become cancerous. In fact, it is likely that several different factors in some combination cause cancer. Genetic, viral, hormonal, immunological, toxic, and physical factors may all play a role. Whatever the cause, cancer is a common disease, resulting in one out of five deaths in the United States. Tumors of the reproductive tract occur in relatively high rates in women. Cervical cancer accounts for 6 percent, ovarian cancer 5 percent, and cancer of the lining of the uterus (endometrial cancer) 7 percent of all cancers in women.

Cervical cancer is most frequently found in women who are between forty and forty-nine years of age, but the incidence has been steadily increasing in younger women. Several factors appear to be involved in initiating this cancer: young age at first intercourse, number of sexual partners (as well as the number of the partner's partners), infection with sexually transmitted diseases such as herpes simplex type 2 and human papilloma virus, and cigarette smoking. Since most patients do not experience symptoms, regular checkups are necessary. The Pap (Papanicolaou) smear performed in a physician's office will detect the presence of cervical cancer. In this procedure, the physician obtains a sample of the cervix by swabbing the area and placing the cells on a microscope slide for examination.

Ovarian cancer accounts for more deaths than any other cancer of the female reproductive system. While the cause of ovarian cancer is unknown, the risk is greatest for women who have not had children. Ovarian cancer does not appear to run in families, and its incidence is slightly decreased in women who use oral contraceptives for many years. Ovarian tumors generally affect women over fifty years of age.

There are two major types of ovarian cancer: epithelial and germ cell neoplasms. About 90 percent of ovarian cancers are epithelial and develop on the surface of the ovary. These tumors often are bulky and involve both ovaries.

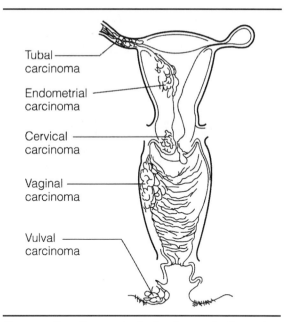

Common sites of cancer in the female reproductive system.

Germ cell tumors are derived from the eggs within the ovary and, if malignant, tend to be highly aggressive. Malignant germ cell neoplasms tend to occur in women under the age of thirty.

Ovarian cancer is generally considered a silent disease, as the signs and symptoms are vague and often ignored. Abdominal pain is the most obvious symptom, followed by abdominal swelling. Some patients also report gastrointestinal disorders such as changes in bowel habits. Abnormal vaginal bleeding may occur but like the other symptoms is not specific for the disease. Diagnosis is made using imaging techniques such as ultrasound, computed tomography (CT) scanning, and magnetic resonance imaging (MRI).

Uterine cancer, also known as endometrial cancer, most frequently affects women between the ages of fifty and sixty-five. Like most cancers, the cause of endometrial cancer is not clear. Nevertheless, relatively high levels of estrogens have been identified as a risk factor. For example, obese women, women who have an early onset of their first period (menarche), and women who never became pregnant tend to have high estrogen levels for longer durations than those without these conditions. Medical scientists believe not only that it is estrogens that are important but also that the other ovarian hormone, progesterone, must be lower than normal for the cancer to develop. Therefore, progesterone appears to have a protective effect in endometrial cancer. Detection of endometrial cancer is accomplished by having a physician take a small tissue sample (biopsy) from the lining of the uterus. The sample can be examined under the microscope to determine if the cells are cancerous.

TREATMENT AND THERAPY

A variety of treatments are available for patients with cancers of the reproductive tract: surgical removal of the organ, hormonal therapy, chemotherapy, or radiation therapy.

The treatment of cervical cancer depends on the size and location of the tumor and whether the cells are benign or malignant. If the patient is no longer capable of or interested in childbearing, then she may choose to have her uterus, including the cervix, removed in the procedure known as hysterectomy. The physician may also use a laser, cryotherapy (use of a cold instrument), or electrocautery (use of a hot instrument) to destroy the tumor without removing the uterus. Malignant tumors may require a total hysterectomy and removal of associated lymph nodes, which can trap metastatic cells. This surgery may be followed by radiation or chemotherapy if there is a possibility that all cancer cells have not been removed.

Cervical cancer diagnosed in a pregnant patient can complicate the treatment. Fortunately, only about 1 percent of cervical cancers are found in pregnant women. If the cancer is restricted to the cervix (that is, it has not metastasized), treatment is usually delayed until after childbirth. It is interesting to note that a normal vaginal delivery may occur without harming the mother or the infant. Malignant cervical cancer must be treated in a similar way as in nonpregnant women. If the cancer is found in the first trimester, a hysterectomy or radiation therapy or both is used to help eradicate the malignancy. Obviously, these approaches terminate the pregnancy. During the second trimester, the uterus must be emptied of the fetus and placenta, followed by radiation therapy or removal of the affected reproductive organs. In the third trimester, the physician will typically try to delay treatment until he or she believes that the fetus has developed sufficiently to stay alive when delivered by cesarean section. A vaginal delivery is not recommended, as it has been shown to lower the cure rate of malignant cervical cancer. Treatment after delivery consists of surgery, radiation therapy, and chemotherapy.

The prognosis in patients who have elected surgical removal of the tumor is a five-year survival rate of up to 90 percent. Cure rates for patients undergoing radiation therapy are between 75 and 90 percent. Chemotherapeutic agents have not had as much effect, as they significantly reduce only 25 percent of tumors. It is important to note that the best outcomes are achieved with early diagnosis.

Ovarian cancers are treated with a similar approach. Surgery may involve the removal of the ovaries, uterine tubes, and uterus, as well as associated lymph nodes depending upon the extent of malignancy. Radiation and chemotherapy are usually employed but oftentimes are not effective. The drug taxol is a relatively new agent which shows some promise in treating ovarian cancers. This drug was isolated from the bark of the yew tree and shows some specificity for ovarian tumors. Taxol prevents cell division in ovarian tumors, slowing the progression of the disease.

The outcome for ovarian cancer is usually not as good as for cervical and endometrial cancers, since the disease is usually in an advanced stage by the time that it is diagnosed. The overall survival rate without evidence of recurrence in patients with epithelial ovarian cancers is between 15 and 45 percent. The more uncommon germ cell ovarian cancers have a much more variable prognosis. With early diagnosis, aggressive surgery, and the use of newer chemotherapeutic agents, the long-term survival rate for all ovarian cancer patients approaches 70 percent.

Surgery is often the treatment of choice for endometrial cancer. As with cervical cancer, however, treatment depends upon the extent of the disease and the patient's wishes relative to reproductive capabilities and family planning. A hysterectomy—removal of the uterine tubes, ovaries, and surrounding lymph nodes—is usually indicated. Chemotherapy and radiation therapy are occasionally utilized as adjunctive therapy, as is progesterone. Progesterone (medroxyprogesterone or hydroxyprogesterone) may benefit patients with advanced disease, as it seems to cause a decrease in tumor size and regression of metastases. In fact, progesterone therapy in patients with advanced or recurrent endometrial cancer leads to regression in about 40 percent of cases. Progesterone therapy also has produced regression in tumors that have metastasized to the lungs, vagina, and chest cavity.

The outcome of endometrial cancer is influenced by the aggressiveness of the tumor, the age of the woman (older women tend to have a poorer prognosis), and the stage at which the cancer was detected. Almost two-thirds of all patients live without evidence of disease for five or more years after treatment. Unfortunately, 28 percent die within five years. For cancer identified and treated early, almost 90 percent of patients are alive five years after treatment.

PERSPECTIVE AND PROSPECTS

Even though medical science has advanced the ability to detect and treat cancers much earlier, many lives are still lost to cancer each year. Therefore, as with most diseases, prevention may be a significant way to reduce one's chances of getting cancer, as well as of reducing the effects of cancer itself.

The National Institutes of Health and the American Cancer Society have made several suggestions which can be followed to reduce the risk of cancer. The dietary guidelines include reducing fat intake to less than 30 percent of total calories, eating more high-fiber foods such as whole-grain breads and cereals, and eating more fruits and vegetables in general and in particular those high in vitamins A, C, and E.

Scheduling regular checkups with a health care provider may increase the likelihood of detecting cervical, ovarian, and uterine cancers early, even if no symptoms are present. Pelvic examinations should be performed every three years for women under the age of forty and yearly thereafter. Pap smear tests for cervical cancer should be undertaken yearly from the time that a woman becomes sexually active. Some physicians will take an endometrial tissue biopsy from women at high risk and at the time of the menopause.

Some data suggest that modifying lifestyle may help reduce the incidence of cervical cancer. The cervix is exposed to a variety of factors during intercourse, including infections and physical trauma. Multiple sexual partners increases the risk of sexually transmitted diseases which may predispose the cervix to cancer. This factor is compounded by the fact that infectious agents and other carcinogens can be transmitted from one individual to another. Therefore, theoretically the cervix can be exposed to carcinogens from a partner's sexual partners. Regular intercourse begun in the early teens also predisposes one to cervical cancer, as the tissue of the cervix may be more vulnerable at puberty. Barrier methods of contraception, mainly the condom, reduce the risk of developing cervical cancer by reducing the exposure of the cervix to potential carcinogens. Smoking also increases the risk of cervical cancer, perhaps because carcinogens in tobacco enter the blood which in turn has access to the cervix. Thus, such lifestyle changes as safer sexual practices, quitting smoking, and dietary changes would be beneficial to someone wanting to reduce the chance of having cervical cancer.

Women who are twenty or more pounds over ideal body weight are twice as likely to develop endometrial cancer, and the risk increases with increased body fat. Some estrogens are produced in fat tissue, and this additional estrogen may play a role in the development of endometrial cancer. Therefore, reduction of excess body fat through diet and exercise would be important for a woman who wished to reduce her chances of developing uterine cancer.

—*Matthew Berria, Ph.D.*

See also Biopsy; Cancer; Cervical procedures; Chemotherapy; Cryotherapy and cryosurgery; Endometrial biopsy; Genital disorders, female; Gynecology; Hysterectomy; Malignancy and metastasis; Radiation therapy; Reproductive system; Screening.

FOR FURTHER INFORMATION:

Clayman, Charles B., ed. *The American Medical Association Encyclopedia of Medicine.* New York: Random House, 1989. This encyclopedia lists in alphabetical order medical terms, diseases, and medical procedures. It does an excellent job of explaining the different types of cancer and their treatments.

Epps, R., and the American Medical Women's Association, eds. *The Women's Complete Handbook.* New York: Dell Books, 1995. This book by the oldest organization of female physicians in the United States is an invaluable guide for the layperson on female-specific diseases.

Fox, Stuart I. *Perspectives on Human Biology.* Dubuque, Iowa: Wm. C. Brown, 1991. Chapter 14 provides the

nonscientist with a basic understanding of cancer biology. Fox explains how oncogenes are thought to act in the formation of neoplasms and how antioxidant vitamins may protect against certain forms of cancer.

Hales, Dianne. *An Invitation to Health.* 5th ed. Redwood City, Calif.: Benjamin/Cummings, 1992. This text should be read by anyone who wishes an overview of health topics. Particularly important reading for those interested in the prevention of cancer.

Mader, Sylvia S. *Human Biology.* 3d ed. Dubuque, Iowa: Wm. C. Brown, 1992. Chapter 20 is devoted to a discussion of cancer and provides an excellent overview of cancer biology. This text was written for the nonscientist yet details contemporary theories on cancer formation and treatment.

Murphy, G., L. Morris, and D. Lange. *Informed Decisions: The Complete Book of Cancer Diagnosis, Treatment, and Recovery.* New York: Viking Press, 1997. This text from the American Cancer Society is intended for the layreader. It is exemplary in its discussion of cancer.

Rosenfeld, Isadore. *Modern Prevention: The New Medicine.* New York: Linden Press/Simon & Schuster, 1986. An easy-to-read book. The author is a practicing physician with the ability to communicate to patients in a down-to-earth style. Rosenfeld addresses the causes and prevention of cancer in chapter 23.

CERVICAL PROCEDURES
PROCEDURE
ANATOMY OR SYSTEM AFFECTED: Genitals, reproductive system, uterus
SPECIALTIES AND RELATED FIELDS: Gynecology
DEFINITION: Such procedures as biopsy, conization, cryosurgery, and electrocauterization, which are performed to analyze cervical tissue for abnormal cell development and/or to remove abnormal or cancerous tissue from the cervix.

INDICATIONS AND PROCEDURES

Surgical procedures performed on the cervix (the opening of the uterus into the vagina) such as biopsy, conization, cryosurgery, and electrocauterization are used to diagnose and treat cervical abnormalities. The first indication of a potential problem is usually a routine gynecological examination that reveals inflammation of the cervix or an abnormal Pap smear. In the Pap smear, a cell sample is scraped from the surface of the cervix and analyzed microscopically. Abnormal results range from slightly abnormal cell growth (dysplasia) to invasive cancer. If the Pap smear results indicate a condition more serious than dysplasia, further tests are conducted.

The first step in the diagnosis of a cervical abnormality is colposcopy and cervical biopsy. The colposcope is a lighted magnifying instrument similar to a pair of binoculars. When placed at the vaginal opening, it permits detailed viewing of the cervix. Abnormal areas are visualized, and a tissue sample of cervical cell layers is punched out for further analysis. Cervical biopsy is performed in a doctor's office and does not require anesthesia.

In cases of severe dysplasia or cancer localized to the cervix, a cone biopsy may be performed. Conization is conducted in a hospital under general anesthesia. A circular incision is made around the cervical opening with a knife or laser and is extended up at an angle to obtain a cone of tissue, including some from the cervical canal. The edges of the incision are sutured or cauterized. Examination of the cone can determine the severity and extent of cancer. In some cases, excision of the cone may have eliminated all the cancerous cells from the cervix.

Cryosurgery, also known as cryotherapy, freezes and destroys abnormal tissue with liquid nitrogen. This procedure can be done in a doctor's office and takes only a few minutes to perform. It can be used successfully to treat dysplasia, localized cancer cells, and reddened areas that sometime develop around the cervical opening, called cervical erosions. Anesthesia is unnecessary because there are no nerve cells in the cervix.

Dysplasia, cancer, and cervical erosions are also treated with electrocauterization. An electrically heated instrument is used to destroy abnormal cells. This procedure is performed in a doctor's office, without anesthesia, just after a woman's menstrual period. A speculum is used to open the vagina, and the tip of the electrocautery device is applied to the abnormal tissue. A scab forms and allows new healthy tissue to grow. Healing is complete in seven to eight weeks.

USES AND COMPLICATIONS

Mild dysplasias typically revert to a normal state spontaneously and are merely monitored for possible slow progression to a more serious state. When Pap smears and/or punch biopsy indicates more serious development of abnormal cells, cryotherapy or electrocauterization are used to destroy the suspicious tissue. While colposcopy is nearly painless, a punch biopsy may cause some cramping. Side effects of electrocauterization include cervical swelling, discharge for up to three weeks, and rarely, infection or infertility caused by the removal of too many cervical mucous glands. Scarring may occur, making future Pap smears difficult to interpret. Cryotherapy causes much less damage to the cervical opening than electrocauterization, but it may produce a temporary watery discharge and changes in cervical mucus.

If repeated colposcopies or Pap smears confirm severe dysplasia or localized cancer, and if the abnormal tissue extends into the cervical canal, a cone biopsy is performed. If analysis of the cone reveals that the abnormal tissue extends beyond the borders of the biopsied tissue, a second, larger conization may be performed. Conization is major surgery performed under general anesthesia, and bleeding and infection are common complications. Removal of too many cervical mucous glands may lead to infertility. Removal of cervical muscle may lead to an incompetent cervix, an inability of the cervix to maintain a pregnancy to term. There are surgical interventions, however, than can eliminate this problem.

If tests indicate that the cancer has become invasive and has spread beyond the borders of the cervix, a hysterectomy and possible removal of the lymph nodes is performed. This serious surgery renders the woman infertile and carries the same risks as any major surgery.

PERSPECTIVE AND PROSPECTS

In the 1940's, George Papanicolaou discovered that premalignant as well as malignant changes caused the cervix to shed cells that could be analyzed microscopically. Simultaneously, the colposcope was developed. Together Pap smears and colposcopies caused a revolution in the early detection and prevention of cervical cancer.

Advances in the classification of abnormalities from mild to severe, and the discovery that exposure to genital herpes virus, multiple sexual partners or mates with a history of multiple partners, smoking, and environmental toxins all contribute to the development of cervical malignancies, have led to this type of cancer being a more preventable and easily monitored disorder. Public education may lead to a decrease in the incidence of this disease.

New surgical techniques have improved the efficiency of abnormal tissue destruction, with fewer side effects. Loop electrosurgical excision procedure (LEEP) uses a low-voltage, high-frequency radio wave which runs through a thin wire loop to scoop our abnormal tissue from the cervix in a matter of seconds. Carbon dioxide laser treatment uses a laser beam to destroy cells in a small area, without damaging healthy tissue. Little bleeding occurs, and healing is rapid. Future advances in deoxyribonucleic acid (DNA) analysis may help to identify those who may be at risk for developing cervical cancer so that they may take preventive action and be closely monitored for early, successful treatment.

—*Karen E. Kalumuck, Ph.D.*

See also Biopsy; Cervical, ovarian, and uterine cancers; Cryotherapy and cryosurgery; Electrocauterization; Gynecology; Hysterectomy; Infertility in females; Oncology.

FOR FURTHER INFORMATION:

Carlson, Karen J., Stephanie A. Eisenstat, and Terra Ziporyn. *The Harvard Guide to Women's Health.* Cambridge, Mass.: Harvard University Press, 1996.

Clark, Adele. "Cervix." In *The New Our Bodies, Ourselves,* edited by the Boston Women's Health Book Collective. New York: Simon & Schuster, 1992.

Epps, R., and the American Medical Women's Association, eds. *The Women's Complete Handbook.* New York: Dell Books, 1995.

Gray, Mary Jane, et al., eds. *The Woman's Guide to Good Health.* Yonkers, N.Y.: Consumer Reports Books, 1991.

CESAREAN SECTION

PROCEDURE

ANATOMY OR SYSTEM AFFECTED: Abdomen, reproductive system, uterus

SPECIALTIES AND RELATED FIELDS: Anesthesiology, emergency medicine, general surgery, gynecology, neonatology, obstetrics, perinatology

DEFINITION: The surgical procedure used to remove a fetus by incisions into the mother's abdominal and uterine wall.

KEY TERMS:

amniotic fluid: the liquid that surrounds the fetus to protect it from injury and to help maintain a stable temperature

breech: a commonly encountered abnormal fetal presentation in which the buttocks is first delivered, rather than the head

cervix: the lower part of the uterus, which is continuous with the vaginal canal; it must enlarge significantly prior to vaginal delivery

incision: a cut made with a scalpel during a surgical procedure

labor: the physiological process by which the fetus and placenta are expelled from the uterus; labor involves strong uterine contractions

placenta: the oval, spongy tissue containing blood vessels that provides the fetus with nutrients and oxygen from the mother via the umbilicus

umbilicus: the cord that contains the blood vessels connecting the fetus to the placenta

INDICATIONS AND PROCEDURES

Cesarean section is performed when it is impossible or dangerous to deliver a baby vaginally. For example, the operation is necessary if the baby is unable to fit through the mother's pelvis or if it shows signs of fetal distress. Fetal distress is detected by abnormal changes in the fetal heart rate, which may indicate that the baby is not receiving adequate oxygen from the placenta. Other reasons for the procedure include a placenta that is lying over the cervix, which blocks the opening to the birth canal (placenta previa); scarring of the uterus from other surgical procedures (or previous cesarean section), which reduces the ability of the uterus to contract; unsuccessful induction of labor with oxytocin (Pitocin); breech presentation, in which the legs and buttocks present first; and postmaturity in which gestation and fetal development indicate that labor should have begun yet is delayed.

A cesarean section allows the delivery of a baby through a horizontal or vertical incision through the mother's abdominal and uterine walls. Prior to surgery, an anesthesiologist gives the mother an epidural or spinal anesthetic so that she can remain conscious but free of pain during the procedure. Occasionally, under certain emergency conditions such as severe fetal distress, a general anesthetic is given. The use of epidural anesthesia, however, is preferred in the majority of deliveries. The anesthesiologist adminis-

Delivery by Cesarean Section

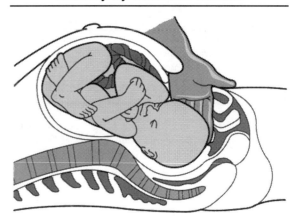

Several conditions may necessitate the delivery of a baby through an incision in the lower abdomen instead of through the birth canal, including fetal distress or the inability of the baby's head to fit through the mother's pelvis.

ters epidural anesthesia by injecting a locally acting anesthetic into the space that surrounds the spinal cord. This space is known as the epidural space, and when it is filled with anesthetic agents, the nerves to the abdominal and pelvic cavities are blocked.

A catheter is inserted into the urinary bladder to empty it prior to making an incision into the abdomen. Typically, a horizontal incision is made just above the pubic bone, as this type of cut heals more readily and is more cosmetically acceptable. Once the pregnant uterus is exposed, a second transverse incision is made in the lower region of the uterus. The amniotic fluid is drained off by suction, and the baby is delivered. Once the infant's head is exposed, its mouth and nose are cleared of any fluid that may hinder respiration. After completely removing the baby from the uterine cavity, the physician clamps the umbilical cord, cuts and ties it, and hands the baby to the parents or a member of the surgical team. Ten to twenty minutes following delivery, the uterus continues to contract and delivers the placenta. After the placenta is delivered, the physician sutures the uterine and abdominal walls and provides postoperative care to the patient. A drug known as ergonovine can be used after delivery of the infant to stimulate uterine contractions and to aid in preventing postpartum bleeding. A patient in pain or discomfort may be given analgesics such as meperidine or morphine as needed. The medical staff closely monitors the patient's vital signs, such as her heart rate, blood pressure, urine flow, and the status of the uterus, including abnormal bleeding.

USES AND COMPLICATIONS

The major adverse effects to women undergoing cesarean section have been complications caused by anesthesia, infection, hemorrhaging, and blood-clotting disorders, such as thromboembolic episodes in which a blood clot breaks loose from a vessel and causes a stroke, heart attack, or pulmonary embolism. One of the most frequent complications from cesarean section is postoperative fever. Physicians can reduce the incidence of fever, however, by administering antibiotics prophylactically. Risks to the fetus include entrapment of a fetal head or limb in the uterine incision, which may result in injury to the head or spine and limb fractures, and wounding of the fetus when the incision is made in the uterine wall.

Patients and their health care providers must weigh these potential adverse effects against the benefits of cesarean sections. Very rarely is a cesarean section performed when a normal vaginal delivery is possible. When an obstetrician recommends a cesarean section, he or she believes the benefits outweigh the potential complications. For most patients who are failing to progress in labor or whose baby is in the breech position or in distress, a cesarean section is indicated. It is not always necessary, however, for a cesarean section to be performed on a patient who has had a previous cesarean section.

PERSPECTIVE AND PROSPECTS

Cesarean section was first performed in ancient Rome when the law required physicians to examine the fetus in the event of a mother's death. Some medical historians have proposed that Julius Caesar was delivered in this way; the term for the procedure is derived from his name. Whether this story is truth or legend, however, is still a matter of debate. In the eighteenth century, many women attempted to perform the procedure as a method of abortion. These self-surgeries were usually unsuccessful and resulted in the mother's death.

Today, cesarean sections are safe for both the mother and the child when they are performed in a medical facility. The rate for delivery by cesarean section has increased in the United States since the 1960's. In 1965, 4.5 percent of babies were born via cesarean section, whereas 23 percent were delivered surgically in 1990. This latter rate has remained stable.

—*Matthew Berria, Ph.D., and Douglas Reinhart, M.D.*
See also Childbirth; Childbirth, complications of; Emergency medicine; Obstetrics; Reproductive system.

FOR FURTHER INFORMATION:

Clayman, Charles B., ed. *The American Medical Association Encyclopedia of Medicine.* New York: Random House, 1989.

Cunningham, F. Gary, et al. *Williams Obstetrics.* 20th ed. Stamford, Conn.: Appleton and Lange, 1997.

MacKay, Trent, and Arthur T. Evans. "Gynecology and Obstetrics." In *Current Medical Diagnosis and Treatment,* edited by Lawrence M. Tierney, Jr., et al. 37th ed. Norwalk, Conn.: Appleton and Lange, 1998.

CHEMOTHERAPY

PROCEDURE

ANATOMY OR SYSTEM AFFECTED: All

SPECIALTIES AND RELATED FIELDS: Oncology, pharmacology

DEFINITION: The treatment of a disease by the use of drugs (especially cancer).

KEY TERMS:

alkylating agents: drugs that introduce alkyl groups to biologically important cell constituents whose function is then impaired

antimetabolites: chemotherapeutic agents that act by inhibiting enzymes in the DNA synthetic pathway or by incorporating in the DNA itself

antitumor antibiotics: compounds obtained from microbial entities that show antitumor properties

immune modulation: cancer treatment based on a change in the relationship between the malignancy and the host

platinum analogues: platinum complexes that have shown antitumor activity

vinka alkaloids and epipodophyllotoxins: natural products derived from the periwinkle and mandrake plants, respectively, that exhibit antitumor activity

INDICATIONS AND PROCEDURES

The term "chemotherapy" is used to refer to the use of chemical agents in the treatment of any disease. It is employed most often, however, in reference to the treatment of cancer. Some drugs are capable either of stopping the undesirable spreading of cancer cells or of preventing cancer from occurring at all. These drugs, called chemotherapeutic agents, destroy cells by interfering with their life-sustaining functions. For example, one type of drug prevents cells from forming the proteins and enzymes that keep them alive. Another type kills by disrupting a step in the process of cell division, while a third type upsets the balance of hormones in a patient's body, creating conditions unsuitable for cancer survival. Unfortunately, all drugs that kill cancer cells also kill normal cells. On the other hand, they selectively kill more cancer cells than normal cells.

Chemotherapy is used when cancerous cells have spread through the body, so that their location cannot be precisely determined. Neither surgery nor radiation therapy can destroy widespread cancer, but drugs can circulate throughout the entire body and kill the cells that surgery and radiotherapy miss. Typically, a cancer cell develops resistance or spreads so extensively that an effective drug dose would kill the patient. Even when a cure is not achieved, however, chemotherapeutic agents can be useful in extending the life of patients, in sensitizing a tumor to radiation treatment, and as an adjuvant or precautionary method when doctors cannot determine whether a cancer has spread.

Immediately after a malignancy is diagnosed, it must be appropriately classified before therapy can be delivered. Out of classification comes an appropriate treatment prescription. The crucial decision in pretreatment planning is whether a cure is feasible. If a cure is possible, aggressive therapy is indicated and certain risks are worth taking. If a cure is not possible, then the therapeutic goal is the prolongation of life, the relief of symptoms, and the maintenance of as near-normal function as possible.

The route of administration is an important variable in the delivery of the required dose of chemotherapy. Administration can be oral, intravenous, by continuous infusion, or by intracavity instillation. The optimum drug dosage is also a critical variable. The objective is to provide the patient with the maximum therapeutic benefit and the minimum side effects. For the large majority of anticancer drugs, administered singly or in combination, bone marrow suppression represents the most important dose-limiting factor, and close monitoring of the patient is critical.

The choice of drugs to be used is dependent on the primary site of origin of the malignancy. Over the years, a database has been established that links specific primary tumor types with drugs that have demonstrated reproducible clinical activity. If combination therapy is chosen, the choice of drugs follows the following empirical guidelines: Each drug should be active when used alone against the disease in question; the drugs should have different postulated or known mechanisms of action; and the drugs should not have overlapping toxicity patterns.

TYPES OF CHEMOTHERAPY

Alkylating agents are reactive organic compounds that transfer alkyl groups in chemical reactions. Their effectiveness as anticancer drugs is attributable to the transfer of these alkyl groups to biologically important cell constituents whose function is then impaired. One example is the alkylation of guanine, one of the bases in deoxyribonucleic acid (DNA). The presence of the alkyl group in the guanine moiety blocks base pairing and prevents DNA replication, which stops cell division. The so-called nitrogen mustard compounds follow this mechanism of action. Examples of alkylating agents are cyclophosphamide, a nitrogen mustard compound, used in the treatment of lymphomas, different types of leukemia, and lung cancer; chlorambucil and melphalan, used in the treatment of multiple myeloma and ovarian cancer; and the nitrosoureas (derivatives of N-methyl-N-nitrosourea, or MNU), such as carmustine (BCNU) and lomustine (CCNU), which are useful in the treatment of brain neoplasms, gastrointestinal carcinomas, and malignant melanomas.

Antimetabolites are structurally similar to the naturally occurring compounds required for synthesis of purines, pyrimidines, and nucleic acids. They interfere with DNA synthesis by inhibiting key enzymes in the purine or pyrimidine synthetic pathways or by misincorporation in the DNA, leading to strand breaks or premature chain termination and slow cell division. An example of antimetabolites is 5-fluorouracil, which inhibits the formation of a thymine-containing nucleotide necessary for DNA synthesis; it is used in the treatment of breast cancer. Methotrexate is another antimetabolite; it binds to the enzyme responsible for the reduction of folic acid in the first step of the synthesis of nucleic acids, and is commonly used to treat leukemia. Other antimetabolites used for the treatment of leukemia are 6-thioguanine and 6-mercaptopurine.

Antitumor antibiotics are natural products of microbial metabolism. The singular purpose of these compounds is to afford these microbial organisms a selective advantage in hostile environments by interfering with the growth or proliferation of competing life-forms—therefore their usefulness in destroying cancer cells. Some of these antibiotics have been synthesized, but the naturally occurring ones have proven to be more effective. Antitumor antibiotics are effective against leukemia, lymphomas, sarcomas, carcinomas of most organs, and germ cell tumors. They are normally used as part of a multiagent chemotherapy regimen and also as part of adjuvant protocals. These compounds show a wide array of structures because of the variety of fungal organisms that are their source. They also exhibit a great diversity in mechanisms of action. For example, doxorubicin has been reported to have at least seven different mechanisms of action, and it is very difficult to determine which is the most effective. Daunorubicin acts by inhibition of DNA and ribonucleic acid (RNA) enzymes, idarubicin acts by the generation of oxygen-free radicals, and mitoxantrone's mechanisms of action include single-strand and double-strand DNA breaks, the peroxidation of cell membranes, and cell surface action.

Vinka alkaloids represent natural or semisynthetic drugs derived from the periwinkle plant, and the epipodophyllotoxins are semisynthetic products derived from the roots of the mayapple or mandrake plant. Of the vinka alkaloids, the most important are vincristine and vinblastine. Their general mechanism of action is the binding to dimers of tubulin, a protein subunit of microtubules. Microtubules perform many critical functions in the cell, such as the maintenance of cell shape, mitosis, meiosis, secretion, and intracellular transport. The binding of vinka alkaloids to tubulin causes the microtubule structures to disappear and the cell to die. They are useful in the treatment of Hodgkin's lymphomas and leukemia. Etoposide and teniposide, two of the epipodophyllotoxins, show good clinical activity, although their mechanism of action is not fully understood. Apparently involved in the mechanism are the breakage of single-strand and double-strand DNA and DNA protein cross-links. These compounds are useful in treating pediatric malignancies.

Hormonal therapy is an important and effective means to treat hormonally sensitive tumors, such as breast, endometrium, prostate, ovarian, and renal tumors. Although it is very hard to explain the mechanism of action, it is assumed that the initial step is the binding to a specific cell surface receptor. This can result in the inhibition of the production of factors necessary for tumor growth, the induction of growth inhibitory proteins, or the inhibition of oncogene expression. Examples of compounds employed in this type of therapy are the adrenocorticoids, used to treat leukemia; estrogens, used in breast cancer therapy; progestins, used for breast and endometrial cancer treatment; and androgens, used against breast cancer.

Immune modulation, or biological response modification against malignant disease, has been a long-sought goal. Developments in molecular biology and immunology and refinements in recombinant methodologies have set the stage for this approach to cancer treatment. It involves the modification of the relationship between the tumor and the host, primarily by modifying the host's response to tumor cells, with resultant therapeutic benefit. Among the substances studied is interferon, a simple glycoprotein with profound immunomodulatory, antiviral, and antiproliferative characteristics. There are three types of interferons, which attach themselves to receptors in the cell surface. This receptor-interferon complex initiates a variety of processes that affect DNA synthesis; it may also render a cell as foreign, facilitating the immune system's job of getting rid of it. In adoptive immunotherapy, immune-activated cells (or tumor killer cells) are administered to a host with advanced cancer in an attempt to mediate tumor regression. Tumor necrosis factor also exhibits antitumor activity and has also shown a synergistic effect with interferon.

Platinum analogues such as cisplatin produce high response rates in patients with small cell carcinoma of the lung, bladder cancer, and ovarian cancer. Most of the data are consistent with the hypothesis that the major target of the drug is DNA, although the type of lesions produced in the DNA structure is not clearly established.

USES AND COMPLICATIONS

All cancerous cells are descended from a normal cell that became malignant as a result of a genetic change. Cancer cells, which do not serve a useful function, live longer than normal cells, invade neighboring tissue, and tend to leave the original site of the cancer and spread to distant parts of the body. Cancer kills by causing a general weakening of the body until it fails; crippling particular organs so that they cannot function; exerting pressure on the skull and brain; obstructing air passages or major blood vessels; destroying blood coagulants; or blocking the immune system so that the body cannot fight disease. Surgery cannot be used in cases of widespread cancer or cancer involving vital parts of the body. Radiation therapy is best suited for treating cancers that are considerably more sensitive than normal tissue to the destructive effects of radiation, such as cancer of the lymph nodes, testicular cancer, and childhood cancers. All cancer chemotherapy is tedious and has its risks. In addition to being highly toxic, most of the useful chemotherapy agents are themselves carcinogenic. Often,

very high doses are necessary for effective treatment. As a result, combination therapy has increased in use because of the success of additive or even synergistic effects when two or more drugs are used, allowing the use of lower doses and reducing side effects.

Side effects of chemotherapy include nausea, vomiting, and diarrhea resulting from damage to the stomach and intestines; dryness and soreness of the mouth from damage to the mucous membranes; and partial loss of hair from damage to the hair follicles. When damage to the bone marrow occurs, the marrow ceases to supply the blood with a normal amount of white blood cells, platelets, and red blood cells, so that the body cannot properly control infection, bruising, or fatigue. Patients may also experience muscular weakness, loss of appetite, rashes, discoloration of the skin, irregular menstrual periods, and sterility. Most of these effects disappear when chemotherapy ends.

Unfortunately, cancer chemotherapy fails to cure most cancer patients because of the growth of resistant cells. Tumor cells are either intrinsically resistant or become resistant to individual drugs. A given chemotherapy regimen is followed until indication of the overgrowth of resistant cells, at which point treatment is ineffective. The development of effective drugs for treating cancer has been a landmark achievement of medical research. The hope for the eventual cure and prevention of malignancy rests with the development of safer agents with enhanced antitumor spectrums, as well as in the study of the synergistic effect of chemotherapy and biological response modifiers.

PERSPECTIVE AND PROSPECTS

As early as the time of the ancient Egyptians, people have attempted to cure cancer with drugs. During World War I, the toxic effect of a class of the chemical warfare gases called mustard gases was recognized. These gases were found to cause damage to the bone marrow and to be mutagenic. Beginning around 1935, other mustards of the nitrogen family were synthesized; they too caused mutations and cancer in some laboratory animals. Effective use of chemotherapy, however, dates only from World War II, when an American ship loaded with poisonous mustard gas was bombed and sunk off the coast of Italy. The sailors who died in the attack were found to have suffered a radical change in their blood, as the mustard gas had destroyed the lymph cells. After World War II, the secrecy surrounding the mutagenic nature of these chemicals was lifted, and it occurred to cancer researchers that cancers might be treated with chemicals that selectively destroy unwanted cells. This approach led to the development of a drug (a derivative of mustard gas) that is used to treat cancer of the lymph nodes. Later, additional drugs were developed to treat a wide variety of cancers. Approximately fifty different cancer-treating drugs are currently in use.

New antitumor chemicals may be developed by synthetic procedures, from natural sources, or by examining new synthetic compounds made for other purposes. The development and production of chemotherapeutic drugs may be divided into five steps: selection of materials to be used; bioassay of the selected material in appropriate experimental tumor systems (also known as screening); preclinical pharmacologic studies; quality production to meet clinical needs and pharmaceutical formulation; and clinical evaluation. Screening is based on the assumption that a drug that is useful in destroying an animal tumor will destroy a human tumor, although it is also possible to use human tumors grown in culture. Preclinical studies involve the determination of a safe dosage, mechanism of action, and the rates of drug disposition, biotransformation, and elimination. The clinical trial is the methodology by which new cancer treatments are evaluated. The goal of clinical trials is to demonstrate that new therapeutic approaches offer an improvement over existing treatments. In the United States, the Food and Drug Administration has published guidelines for the approval of new anticancer drugs. Approval of any new drug requires a minimum of two independent, well-controlled clinical studies demonstrating the drug's safety and efficacy for each proposed indication.

—Maria Pacheco, Ph.D.

See also Cancer; Cells; Drug resistance; Immune system; Immunology; Malignancy and metastasis; Oncology; Pharmacology; Radiation therapy; Tumor removal; Tumors.

FOR FURTHER INFORMATION:

Carter, Stephen K., Mary T. Bakowski, and Kurt Hellmann. *Chemotherapy of Cancer.* 3d ed. New York: John Wiley & Sons, 1987. A good reference book with sections on general cancer treatment, clinical trials, drug development, anticancer drugs, treatment of specific types of cancer. Very complete.

Chabner, Bruce A., and Jerry M. Collins, eds. *Cancer Chemotherapy: Principles and Practice.* Philadelphia: J. B. Lippincott, 1990. A compilation of works by more than thirty expert authors in the field of cancer chemotherapy. The book provides both an in-depth reference and a rapid source of critical information. An excellent reference work.

Joesten, Melvin D., David O. Johnston, John Netterville, and James L. Wood. *The World of Chemistry.* Philadelphia: W. B. Saunders College, 1991. A basic chemistry book with a good section on cancer and its treatments. Good for a quick reference.

Levitt, Paul M., Elissa S. Guralnick, A. Robert Kagan, and Harvey Gilbert. *The Cancer Reference Book.* New York: Facts on File, 1983. An excellent reference work that provides direct and clear answers to cancer-related questions. Presented in a question-and-answer format. Easy to read and informative.

Murphy, G., L. Morris, and D. Lange. *Informed Decisions: The Complete Book of Cancer Diagnosis, Treatment, and Recovery.* New York: Viking Press, 1997. This text from the American Cancer Society is intended for the layperson. It is exemplary in its discussion of cancer.

Perry, Michael C., ed. *The Chemotherapy Source Book.* Baltimore: Williams & Wilkins, 1992. A compilation of essays by experts in this field. Deals with the practical principles of chemotherapy, commercially available drugs by class (emphasizing their mechanisms of action), chemotherapy drug toxicity, combination therapy programs, and the therapy methods for specific tumors. A complete, thorough reference.

CHEST

ANATOMY

ANATOMY OR SYSTEM AFFECTED: Circulatory system, lungs, muslces, musculoskeletal system, respiratory system

SPECIALTIES AND RELATED FIELDS: Cardiology, pulmonary medicine

DEFINITION: The region of the body from the diaphragm to the neck, both within the rib cage (heart and lungs) and in front of it (breasts and muscles).

KEY TERMS:

breast: the mammary gland, along with the nipple in front of it and the surrounding fatty tissue

diaphragm: a curved muscular sheet that separates the chest cavity from the abdominal cavity

heart: a muscular pump that propels the blood through the circulatory system

lungs: the air sacs that are the principal respiratory organs; located in the chest

ribs: the bones that support the chest and define its outline

thoracic: pertaining to the chest

thorax: another name for the chest region

STRUCTURE AND FUNCTIONS

The chest, or thorax, consists of those parts of the body lying between the diaphragm and the neck. Included here are the rib cage, diaphragm, heart, lungs, chest muscles, and breast.

The skeletal support of the chest consists of the thoracic vertebrae and rib cage. In humans, there are usually twelve pairs of ribs and twelve thoracic vertebrae. Each thoracic vertebra consists of a cylindrical portion, the centrum or body, and a neural arch attached to the dorsal side of the centrum. The neural arch surrounds and protects the spinal column. A spinous process extends dorsally from the neural arch of each thoracic vertebra and serves as a site for muscle attachment. Near the base of each neural arch are two pairs of articular processes (zygapophyses). The superior pair of one vertebra face toward each other and articulate with the inferior articular processes of the adjacent vertebrae.

Attached to each thoracic vertebra is a rib. There are usually twelve pairs of ribs, but this number occasionally varies. Each rib consists of a bony portion and a cartilaginous extension, the costal cartilage. At its vertebral end, each rib has two articulating processes, the head (capitulum) and the tubercle (tuberculum). The costal cartilages of the first seven ribs (the number occasionally varies) extend all the way to the sternum. The next two or three ribs have costal cartilages that attach to the costal cartilage above them. The remaining ribs have costal cartilages that are "floating" and have no attachments. Together, the ribs make up a cagelike structure called the rib cage, which shapes the chest and protects the heart and lungs from injury.

The sternum, or breastbone, runs along the front of the chest in the midline of the body. It consists of a flattened top portion called the manubrium, a long, extended body (corpus), and an extension called the xiphoid process, which is made mostly of cartilage. The manubrium has notches for the attachment of the clavicle and the first rib on either side. The attachment for the second rib lies between the manubrium and corpus and is shared by both bones. The corpus of the sternum is formed by the fusion of five individual parts called sternebrae. The costal cartilages of the second through seventh ribs articulate with the corpus of the sternum and mark the boundaries between the individual sternebrae. Beyond the notch for the attachment of the seventh costal cartilage, the xiphoid process extends downward along the midline.

A muscular diaphragm marks the boundary between the chest cavity and the abdominal cavity. Although it is located at the lower end of the chest cavity, it originates in the neck region and derives its nerve supply, the phrenic nerve, from within the neck. The diaphragm is the principal muscle used in breathing. Normally dome-shaped and bowed upward, the diaphragm flattens when its muscles contract, expanding the chest cavity and resulting in the inhalation of air. Relaxation of the diaphragm returns the curvature of the dome upward, compressing the chest cavity and resulting in the exhalation of air. The diaphragm has openings for the passage of the esophagus and the major blood vessels, especially the descending aorta and inferior vena cava.

The heart and major blood vessels lie within the chest cavity and are protected by the rib cage. The heart is a muscular pump that has four chambers (two atria and two ventricles) in all adult mammals. The right atrium receives oxygen-poor blood from the body's organs via the superior vena cava (from the head and upper extremities) and the inferior vena cava (from the abdominal region, pelvic region, and lower extremities). Blood from the right atrium passes through the tricuspid valve to the right ventricle, from which it is pumped into the pulmonary artery. The pulmonary artery then divides in two branches that run separately to each lung. Oxygen-rich blood from the lungs returns to the heart by means of the pulmonary veins, which empty into the left atrium. Blood from the left atrium passes

The Organs and Structures of the Chest

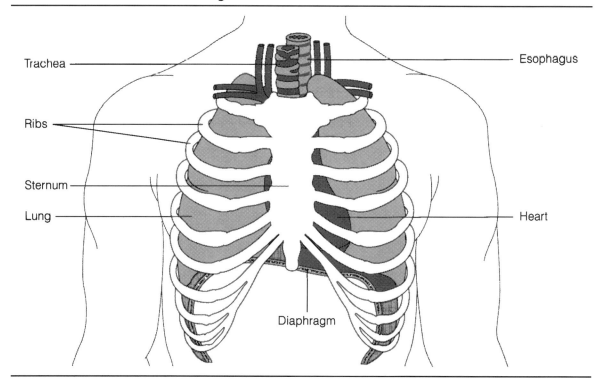

through the bicuspid valve and empties into the left ventricle, which has an extremely thick, muscular wall. Contraction of the left ventricle propels the blood out of the aorta and through the body via the arteries.

Contractions of the heart originate in a location known as the sinoatrial node, located on the surface of the right atrium. From this point, contractions spread to the atrioventricular node, located at the point where all four chambers meet. The wave of contraction then spreads rapidly down the septum between the two ventricles and up the side walls of each ventricle. A specialized bundle called the bundle of His, composed of modified muscle fibers (Purkinje fibers), is responsible for this rapid conduction.

Except for the pulmonary arteries, the arteries of the chest region are all branches of the aorta, the major artery that flows out from the left ventricle of the heart in an upward direction. The aorta can be subdivided into an initial portion (the ascending aorta), an aortic arch, and a longer descending aorta which extends from the thoracic region into the pelvis. The coronary arteries are small but important branches that arise from the ascending aorta as it leaves the heart. These arteries supply blood to the muscular wall of the heart itself. From the arch of the aorta, the most common pattern of branching is that of a brachiocephalic trunk, which then splits into a right common carotid and right subclavian artery, followed by a left common carotid artery and then a left subclavian artery. There is considerable variation, however, in this pattern of branchings. The carotid arteries run up the sides of the neck to supply blood to the head and neck.

The subclavian arteries of either side run first upward and then laterally through the chest cavity, continuing toward the upper extremity as the axillary artery. Along its course, each subclavian artery gives off the following branches: vertebral artery, thyrocervical trunk, internal thoracic artery, costocervical artery, and descending scapular artery. The vertebral artery, the largest branch, supplies blood to the vertebrae of the neck region and ultimately to the base of the brain. The short thyrocervical trunk divides almost immediately into three branches: an inferior thyroid artery to the larynx, trachea, esophagus, and the surrounding muscles; a suprascapular artery to the subclavius and sternocleidomastoid muscles and to the overlying skin; and a transverse cervical artery to the muscles of the shoulder region.

The right and left internal thoracic arteries (also called internal mammary arteries) run along the ventral side of the chest, just beneath the costal cartilages and just to either side of the sternum. Each internal thoracic artery gives off branches to the diaphragm, the pleura, the pericardium, the thymus, the transverse thoracic muscle, the ribs and intercostal muscles, the pectoral muscles, and the mammary glands. Beyond the sixth rib, each internal thoracic artery divides into a musculophrenic branch to the last six ribs and the diaphragm and a superior epigastric artery, which descends along the abdominal surface, supplying the muscles of this region before meeting the inferior epigastric artery that ascends from the pelvic region.

The veins of the chest region include the external and internal jugular veins, draining the head and neck, and the subclavian veins, draining the upper extremities. These veins come together to form the right and left brachiocephalic veins, which then drain into the superior vena cava. The superior vena cava also receives several smaller tributaries, including the azygos vein, the paired internal thoracic and inferior thyroid veins, the highest intercostal vein, and several smaller veins of the vertebral column. The azygos vein (on the right) and the hemizygous vein (on the left) run parallel to each other on either side of the vertebral column along the dorsal or rear wall of the chest cavity, draining blood from the muscles of the back, the bronchi, the ribs, and the mediastinum. The right and left internal thoracic veins receive tributaries from the ribs and intercostal muscles as well as the diaphragm, pericardium, and mediastinum. The highest intercostal veins drain the first two or three intercostal spaces on either side, also receiving smaller tributaries from the bronchi and the upper portion of the diaphragm. The inferior thyroid veins drain the thyroid gland, esophagus, trachea, and larynx. In addition to the above, the veins of the heart muscle all drain into a coronary sinus, which runs between the left atrium and ventricle, then drains directly into the right atrium near the inferior vena cava.

The lungs, the principal organs of respiration, consist of several lobes. The right lung has superior, medial, and inferior lobes; the left lung has superior and inferior lobes only. Inhalation of air, or inspiration, is brought about by the lowering (contraction) of the diaphragm and by the raising and outward expansion of the rib cage. Exhalation of air, or expiration, in brought about by the raising (relaxation) of the diaphragm and by the relaxation of the intercostal muscles, lowering and contracting the rib cage. Under most conditions, inspiration is an active process requiring muscular contraction, while expiration takes place passively as the muscles relax.

Together, the heart, lungs, and the thoracic portion of the esophagus occupy the thoracic cavity, or chest cavity. Each of these organs is surrounded by a thin membrane, the visceral pleura. This membrane is continuous with the parietal pleura, another thin membrane that lines the outer walls of the chest cavity. The right and left visceral pleura come together to form a septum called the mediastinum, which separates the bulk of the thoracic cavity into right and left pleural cavities, each containing one of the lungs. The pericardial cavity, containing the heart, is inserted between the layers of the mediastinum. Also occupying part of the thoracic cavity is a large mass of lymphoid tissue, the thymus body. The thymus is irregular in shape and occupies the highest portion of the thoracic cavity above the heart.

Muscles of the chest region may be divided into those associated developmentally with the upper extremity and those that are associated instead with the trunk of the body. One muscle, the trapezius, is a modified gill muscle that belongs developmentally to neither group. Fibers of the trapezius muscle originate from the cervical and thoracic vertebrae, including the adjoining ligaments and the adjacent part of the skull. These fibers converge onto the spine and acromion of the scapula and onto the clavicle. The muscles associated with the trunk of the body are called axial muscles. Of those in the chest or thoracic region, four are responsible primarily for movements of the shoulder blade (scapula), twelve for movements of the rib cage, and another eleven for movements of the vertebral column.

The levator scapulae runs from the transverse processes of the first four cervical vertebrae to the vertebral border of the scapula; by contracting, it raises and rotates the scapula. The two rhomboid muscles run from the vertebral column to the vertebral border of the scapula. The rhomboideus minor originates from the spinous processes of the seventh cervical and the first thoracic vertebra and from the nuchal ligament that runs from these spinous processes to the skull. The rhomboideus major originates from the spinous processes of the second through fifth thoracic vertebrae. Both rhomboideus muscles run diagonally from the vertebral column to the vertebral border of the scapula, including the base of the scapular spine. The serratus anterior, also called serratus ventralis, is a sheetlike muscle that lies between the scapula and the rib cage. Its fibers originate from the ribs as a series of strips that converge slightly; they all insert onto the vertebral border of the scapula. The attachments of this muscle to the ribs resemble a series of angular saw-teeth (serrations) that give the muscle its name. The four preceding muscles all share a common embryological origin, and all have a common nerve supply from the dorsal scapular nerve.

The axial muscles associated with movements of the rib cage include the scalenus anterior, scalenus medius, scalenus posterior, intercostals, subcostals, levatores costarum, transversus thoracis, serratus posterior superior, serratus posterior inferior, rectus abdominis, and diaphragm. The three scalene muscles, as their name implies, are all shaped like elongated scalene triangles. The scalenus anterior arises from the transverse processes of the third through sixth cervical vertebrae and inserts (attaches) onto the first rib. The largest of the scalene muscles is the scalenus medius, which runs from the transverse processes of the last six cervical vertebrae to an insertion on the first rib. The scalenus posterior arises from the transverse processes of the last two or three cervical vertebrae and inserts onto the second rib.

The intercostal muscles run between the ribs in two sets of fibers. The external intercostals run from each rib to the next in a diagonal direction; the upper end of each fiber is situated closer to the vertebral column than is the lower end. The internal intercostals also run diagonally from each rib to the next, but deep to the fibers of the external intercostals and perpendicular to them, so that the lower end of each fiber is closer to the vertebral end of each rib than is the upper end. Both sets of intercostals are broad, extending nearly along the entire extent of each rib, but the fibers are in each case short, extending only from one rib to the next. The subcostals are similar in position and orientation to the internal intercostals, except they are usually confined to the last few ribs and they span two or three intercostal spaces at a time. The levatores costarum are a continuation of the external intercostals onto the transverse processes of the vertebrae, from the last cervical vertebra to the eleventh thoracic vertebra. Each levator costarum is a triangular slip located in the angle between one of the ribs and the vertebra in front of it, running from the transverse process of the vertebra onto the rib.

The transversus thoracis is a flat muscle which covers part of the inside of the rib cage. Its fibers originate from the corpus and xiphoid process of the sternum; these fibers radiate both horizontally and diagonally upward to insert on the deep surfaces of the second through sixth ribs. The serratus posterior superior arises from the spinous processes of the first few thoracic vertebrae and the seventh cervical vertebra, as well as from the ligaments connecting these spinous processes with one another and with the skull. The fibers converge only slightly and are inserted in four separate slips onto the superior margins of the second through fifth ribs. The serratus posterior inferior is a similar but broader muscle located further down the spine. It arises from the spinous processes of the last two thoracic and first few lumbar vertebrae, runs diagonally upward, and divides into four separate slips that insert onto the inferior margins of the last four ribs. The rectus abdominis, obliquus externus, obliquus internus, and transversus abdominis are abdominal muscles that pull down on the chest and particularly on the rib cage. The rectus abdominis consists of a strip of muscle fibers running vertically along the ventral midline. The other abdominal muscles are sheetlike and cover the majority of the abdominal surface. Contractions of these muscles generally pull downward on the ribs and oppose the expansion of the rib cage.

The diaphragm is also an axial muscle of the chest cavity. Its muscle fibers originate from the inside of the xiphoid process of the sternum (the sternal portion), from the inner surfaces of the last six ribs and their costal cartilages (the costal portion), and from two muscular arches and two tendinous crura that make up the lumbar portion. The medial lumbocostal arch forms a passage for the greater psoas muscle, while the lateral lumbocostal arch forms a passage for the lumbar quadrate muscle. The right and left crura arise from the ventral surfaces of the first few lumbar vertebrae. Together, the sternal, costal, and lumbar portions of the diaphragm converge upon a sheetlike central tendon, which is divided into large left and right leaflets and a small middle leaflet.

The axial muscles concerned with movements of the thoracic vertebrae include the longus and splenius muscles and the muscles of the erector spinae complex. The longus colli arises from the centra of the last few cervical and first few thoracic vertebrae along their ventral surfaces; it runs upward to insert onto the bodies of the first four cervical vertebrae and the transverse processes of the fifth and sixth cervical vertebrae. The splenius capitis originates from the spinous processes of the last cervical and the first three or four thoracic vertebrae and from the ligaments connecting these processes to one another and to the back of the skull. The muscle inserts onto the occipital and temporal bones on the back of the skull, including the mastoid process. The splenius cervicis arises from the spinous processes of the third through sixth thoracic vertebrae and runs to an insertion on the transverse processes of the first few cervical vertebrae. The muscles of the erector spinae complex include the iliocostalis, longissimus, spinalis, semispinalis, multifidius, rotatores, and intertransverarii. Collectively, these muscles are responsible for dorsal movements (extension) of the vertebral column throughout the lumbar, thoracic, and cervical regions.

The muscles associated developmentally with the extremities are called appendicular muscles. Appendicular muscles of the chest region include the pectoralis, latissimus dorsi, and subclavius. The pectoralis major is triangular in shape; it originates from the sternum, costal cartilages, and a portion of the clavicle, from which its fibers converge toward an insertion onto the greater tuberosity of the humerus. The pectoralis minor originates from the third through fifth ribs and inserts onto the coracoid process of the scapula. The latissimus dorsi is a broad, flat muscle that originates from the lower half of the vertebral column (and part of the ilium) by way of a tough tendinous sheet (the lumbar aponeurosis); it inserts high on the humerus. The subclavius muscle runs from the bottom surface of the clavicle diagonally onto the first rib. Upon contraction, this muscle helps pull the shoulder inward and the rib cage upward.

Each of the paired breasts consists of a mammary gland, nipple (papilla), areola, and surrounding fat tissue. The breasts are small in children and remain small in most adult men, but they become larger during puberty in women and enlarge even more during late pregnancy and throughout lactation. Toward the end of pregnancy, the gland begins to secrete milk, a white, nutritive fluid containing lactose (milk sugar), proteins, and some fats (more sugar and less fat than in cow's milk). The secretion of milk is known as lactation. During lactation, the mammary gland continues to secrete milk as long as the baby continues nursing. When the child is weaned, the mammary gland undergoes a process of involution (shrinkage). The smaller ducts of the mammary gland collect into larger ducts, each draining a wedge-shaped section of the breast. These larger ducts converge toward a raised nipple (papilla) from which the milk exudes. The nipple is surrounded by a circular area, the areola, characterized by thin skin which is a bit more heavily pigmented (usually redder) than the remainder of the breast.

DISORDERS AND DISEASES

A wide variety of medical problems can occur in the chest region, including a number of diseases and traumatic injuries. Because of the presence of the heart and lungs, injuries and diseases of the chest region are often life-threatening and may be fatal. These include diseases of the heart and major vessels, diseases of the lungs and bronchi, and cancer of the breast. Common heart disorders include myocardial infarction, coronary artery disease, and chest pain (angina pectoralis); less common disorders include arrhythmias and heart murmurs. Disorders of the lungs and bronchi include lung cancer, pulmonary emphysema, and such infectious diseases as tuberculosis, lobar pneumonia, and bronchial pneumonia.

Thoracic specialists include heart specialists (cardiologists), respiratory specialists (pulmonologists), cancer specialists (oncologists), neuromuscular specialists, and neurologists. Thoracic surgeons specialize in the surgery of the chest. Thoracotomy is a cutting into the thoracic cavity, usually for the repair of the heart, the lungs, or both. Thoracotomy is the first step in open heart surgery, coronary bypass surgery, pacemaker implantation, and heart or lung transplants.

Disorders of the breast are so distinctive that many different specialists are involved. The most feared and most fatal of these diseases is breast cancer, often treated by surgical removal of the tumor or of the entire breast. Other breast disorders include mastitis, an inflammation of the breast in women. Rare conditions include the presence of extra (supernumerary) breasts in either sex. Also rare are the hormonal or reproductive disorders that result in the premature enlargement of the female breast or in its failure to develop during adolescence. Enlargement of the breast in males is a condition known as gynecomastia; it often results from abnormal levels of steroid hormones associated with marijuana abuse, but it may arise from other causes. Usually only the fat tissue enlarges in this condition (and never as much as in women); the mammary gland, nipple, and areola remain underdeveloped. Much less common is a condition called Klinefelter's syndrome, in which a tall, thin male develops breasts comparable in size to those of a thirteen-year-old girl. This condition is controlled by a chromosomal defect (XXY). The opposite chromosomal defect (XO) results in Turner's syndrome, in which a short, web-necked female has breasts that enlarge only slightly and that never develop fully. Both Klinefelter's and Turner's syndromes result in a degree of mental retardation and in sterility.

Breast surgery may be performed by several types of surgeons, including general surgeons, thoracic surgeons, cancer surgeons, and plastic surgeons. Common surgical operations include the removal of a breast tumor (lumpectomy) or of the entire affected breast (mastectomy) in cases of breast cancer. In addition, plastic surgeons may perform such cosmetic operations as breast augmentation (using implants) or breast reduction.

PERSPECTIVE AND PROSPECTS

The heart, lungs, breasts, and the major muscles and bones of the chest region were studied by the ancients. The Latin names that are used today are derived in large measure from the writings of Galen, or Caius Galenus, physician to the Roman army in the second century. Renaissance artists such as Leonardo da Vinci (1452-1519) and Michelangelo (1475-1564) dissected human corpses illegally in order to gain further knowledge of the anatomical structures visible on the body's surface. These studies were followed by the well-illustrated anatomical texts of Andreas Vesalius (1514-1564), who corrected many of Galen's errors.

Good medical understanding of the circulatory system began with the studies of the Renaissance physician William Harvey (1578-1657), who examined the veins in the arms of many patients. It was Harvey who discovered the valves in the veins and who proved that the blood circulates outward from the heart and then back. Anatomists who have described the finer details of the structure of the heart include Jan Evangelista Purkinje (1787-1869) and Wilhelm His, Jr. (1863-1934).   —*Eli C. Minkoff, Ph.D.*

See also Anatomy; Asthma; Bones and the skeleton; Breasts, female; Bronchitis; Bypass surgery; Cardiac rehabilitation; Cardiology; Cardiology, pediatric; Choking; Common cold; Congenital heart disease; Coughing; Cystic fibrosis; Electrocardiography (ECG or EKG); Embolism; Emphysema; Heart; Heart transplantation; Heart valve replacement; Heartburn; Interstitial pulmonary fibrosis (IPF); Legionnaires' disease; Lung cancer; Lungs; Pacemaker implantation; Pertussis; Pleurisy; Pneumonia; Pulmonary diseases; Pulmonary medicine; Pulmonary medicine, pediatric; Respiration; Resuscitation; Thoracic surgery; Tuberculosis.

FOR FURTHER INFORMATION:

Agur, Anne M. R., and Ming J. Lee. *Grant's Atlas of Anatomy.* 9th ed. Baltimore: Williams & Wilkins, 1991. Contains many excellent, detailed illustrations.

Anson, Barry J. *An Atlas of Human Anatomy.* 2d ed. Philadelphia: W. B. Saunders, 1963. Excellent color-coded illustrations with little explanatory text.

Crouch, James E. *Functional Human Anatomy.* 4th ed. Philadelphia: Lea & Febiger, 1985. A very readable book with good explanations; a very good beginning reference.

Gray, Henry. *Gray's Anatomy.* Edited by Peter L. Williams et al. 38th ed. New York: Churchill Livingstone, 1995.

A classic work with the most thorough descriptions. Most of the excellent color illustrations offer realistic detail, and the rest emphasize well-selected highlights.

King, Barry G., and Mary Jane Showers. *Human Anatomy and Physiology.* 6th ed. Philadelphia: W. B. Saunders, 1969. Excellent functional explanations of the workings of most organs, although muscle actions are not as thoroughly explained as in the other works cited here.

Rosse, Cornelius, and Penelope Gaddum-Rosse. *Hollinshead's Textbook of Anatomy.* 5th ed. Philadelphia: Lippincott-Raven, 1997. A very thorough, modern, detailed reference with good descriptions and illustrations.

CHEST PAIN. *See* HEART ATTACK; PAIN, TYPES OF.

CHICKENPOX

DISEASE/DISORDER

ANATOMY OR SYSTEM AFFECTED: Respiratory system, skin

SPECIALTIES AND RELATED FIELDS: Dermatology, family practice, internal medicine, public health, virology

DEFINITION: Chickenpox is a very contagious though mild disease caused by the herpes zoster virus. Affecting all

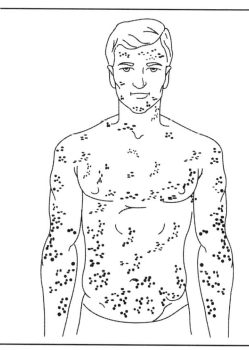

Chickenpox causes skin eruptions that form blisters and itch; although children are the most common victims of the disease, adults may also catch it (often if they did not have it as children), and the results can be more serious, including longer recovery periods and greater risk of complications, such as male sterility.

ages, but mostly children between the ages of five and ten, chickenpox causes fever, abdominal pain, and skin eruptions almost anywhere on the body, including the scalp, mouth, nose, throat, penis, or vagina. Blisters erupt every three to four days and collapse within twenty-four hours, forming scabs. Recovery for children usually occurs in seven to ten days. Adults take longer to recover, have more severe symptoms, and are more likely to develop complications, such as sterility in men and pneumonia. Symptoms may be treated with wet compresses and a cool environment to reduce itching; bed rest, fluids, and medication may be used to reduce fever.

—*Jason Georges and Tracy Irons-Georges*
See also Childhood infectious diseases; Herpes; Infertility in males; Rashes; Shingles; Viral infections.

CHILD ABUSE. *See* DOMESTIC VIOLENCE.

CHILDBIRTH
BIOLOGY
ANATOMY OR SYSTEM AFFECTED: Reproductive system, uterus

SPECIALTIES AND RELATED FIELDS: Gynecology, neonatology, obstetrics, perinatology

DEFINITION: The process whereby a fetus moves from the uterus to outside the mother's body—a natural event that normally requires no, or minimal, medical intervention.

KEY TERMS:

birth canal: the passageway from the uterus to the outside of the mother's body formed by the fully opened cervix in continuity with the vagina

cervix: a ring of tissue at the lowest and narrowest part of the uterus forming a canal that opens into the vagina

contraction: a squeezing action of the uterus that results in birth

dilation: the opening of the cervix to allow passage of the fetus through the birth canal

hormone: a chemical carried in the blood that acts as a messenger between two or more body parts

labor: the period in the birth process in which forceful and rhythmic uterine contractions are present

parturition: the process or action of giving birth

placenta: a structure located inside the uterus during pregnancy that provides oxygen to the fetus, removes fetal wastes, and produces hormones; also known as the afterbirth

prostaglandins: chemical messengers that are not carried in the blood and that function only locally

uterus: the organ in the female pelvis that supports the fetus during pregnancy and expels it during birth; also known as the womb

vagina: the stretchy tubular structure that leads from the uterus to the outside of the mother's body; part of the birth canal

PROCESS AND EFFECTS

In humans, pregnancy lasts an average of forty weeks, counting from the first day of the woman's last menstrual cycle. Actually, ovulation, and therefore conception and the start of pregnancy, does not normally occur until about two weeks after the beginning of the last menstrual period, but because there is no good external indicator of the time of ovulation, obstetricians typically count the weeks of pregnancy using the easily observed last period of menstrual bleeding as a reference point. Because of the uncertainty about the actual time of ovulation and conception, the calculated due date for an infant's birth may be inaccurate by as much as two weeks in either direction.

There is incomplete understanding of the processes that determine the timing and initiation of childbirth. Near the end of pregnancy, the uterus undergoes changes that prepare it for the birth process: The cervix softens and becomes stretchy, the cells in the uterus acquire characteristics that enable them to contract in a coordinated fashion, and the uterus becomes more responsive to hormones that cause contractions.

A number of substances are involved in the preparation of the uterus for birth, including the hormones estrogen and progesterone (produced within the placenta), the hormone relaxin (from the maternal ovary and/or uterus), and prostaglandins (produced within the uterus). The fetus participates in this preparation, since it provides precursors necessary for the uterine synthesis of estrogens. In addition, the amnion and chorion, two membranes surrounding the fetus, are capable of producing prostaglandins that assist in the preparation of the uterus.

Once labor begins, the hormone oxytocin (from the maternal pituitary gland) and uterine prostaglandins cause uterine contractions. It is not known what triggers the onset of labor or how the preparatory hormones and prostaglandins work together.

In humans, the onset of labor is indicated by one or more of three signs: the beginning of regular, rhythmic uterine contractions; the rupture of the amniotic membrane, a painless event that is usually accompanied by the leakage of clear fluid from the vagina; and the expulsion of a slightly bloody mucus plug from the cervix, which is an indication that the cervix is beginning to dilate. These signs may appear in any order, or occasionally one sign may be absent or unnoticed. For example, the amniotic membrane may fail to rupture spontaneously; in this case, the attendant will usually pierce the membrane in order to facilitate the birth.

Uterine contractions are the most prominent indication of labor, which is divided into three stages. In the first stage of labor, the contractions have the effect of dilating the cervix from its initial size of only a few millimeters to full dilation of 10 centimeters, large enough to permit the passage of the fetus. When the first stage of labor starts, the contractions may be up to twenty minutes apart, with each contraction of relatively short duration. As the first stage progresses, the contractions become longer and closer together, so that by the end of the first stage there may be only a minute between contractions. There is no downward movement of the fetus during the first stage of labor, but the contractions do force the fetus against the cervix, and this force is important in causing cervical dilation. This first stage lasts for an average of eleven hours in women giving birth for the first time, but up to twenty hours is considered normal. The average length of the first stage of labor in women who have previously delivered is reduced to seven hours, with a norm of up to fourteen hours.

In the second stage of labor, the fetus moves downward through the fully dilated cervix and then into the vagina as a result of the force exerted by the continuing uterine contractions. Voluntary contractions of the abdominal muscles by the mother can help shorten this stage of labor by ap-

plying additional force, but in the absence of voluntary contractions (as with an anesthetized mother), the uterine contractions are usually sufficient to cause delivery. In 96 percent of human births, the fetus is situated so that the head is downward and thus is first to pass through the birth canal. Because the vagina does not lie in the same line as the cervix and uterus, the head of the fetus must flex and rotate as the fetus progresses downward past the mother's pelvic bones. The final barrier to the birth of the fetus is the soft tissue surrounding the vaginal opening; once the head of the fetus passes through and stretches this opening, the rest of the body usually slips out readily. The average duration of this second stage of labor in women delivering for the first time is slightly more than one hour; the average duration is shortened to twenty-four minutes in women who have previously delivered. Most women agree that the actual birth of the child during the second stage is less un-

Stages of Childbirth

Stage one

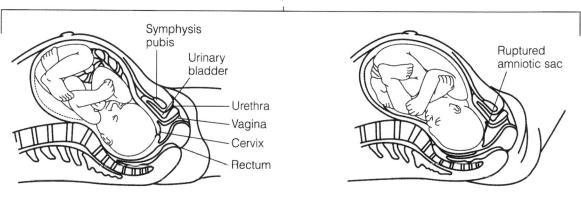

Symphysis pubis
Urinary bladder
Urethra
Vagina
Cervix
Rectum

Ruptured amniotic sac

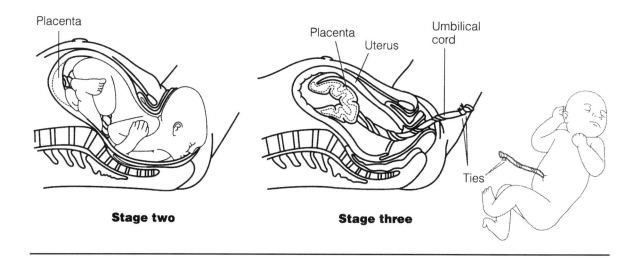

Placenta

Stage two

Placenta
Uterus
Umbilical cord

Stage three

Ties

comfortable than the strong uterine contractions that occur at the very end of the first stage of labor, when the cervix is dilating the last centimeter or so.

Most infants begin to take regular, deep breaths immediately upon delivery. These breaths serve to inflate the lungs with air for the first time. The infant now becomes dependent on breathing to supply oxygen to the blood, whereas oxygen had been supplied to the fetal blood by circulation through the placenta.

Following delivery of the infant, the mother enters the third stage of labor, during which continued uterine contractions serve to reduce the size of the uterus and expel the placenta. The placenta usually separates from the uterus and is expelled five to fifteen minutes after the birth of the infant.

Uterine contractions do not end with the delivery of the placenta; they continue, with decreasing frequency and intensity, for as long as six weeks following childbirth. These later contractions, known as afterpains, serve to reduce bleeding from the site of placental attachment and to return the uterus and cervix to their prepregnancy condition.

Another significant process that occurs in the mother's body following delivery is the onset of milk production. During pregnancy, the breasts are prepared for later milk production by a number of hormones, but actual milk production does not begin until about the second day after delivery. It appears that the decrease in progesterone levels caused by the removal of the placenta at birth allows milk production to commence.

Most obstetrical attendants agree that the ideal childbirth situation is a labor and delivery with a minimum of medical intervention. If all goes well, the role of the attendant will be primarily that of a support person. Most women are admitted to a hospital or birthing center during the first stage of labor. The mother's blood pressure and temperature will be frequently checked. In addition, the strength and timing of contractions will be assessed either by a hand placed lightly on the abdomen or by an electronic monitor that detects uterine activity through a sensor belt placed around the abdomen. The fetal heart rate will be measured with a stethoscope or by an electrical lead placed on the fetus' scalp through the cervix. Cervical dilation can be assessed by a vaginal examination: The attendant will insert one or more fingers into the cervix to determine its state of dilation. It is also important that the attendant provide emotional support and reassurance to the mother throughout the delivery.

During the second stage of labor, the attendant will monitor the progress of the fetus through the birth canal. By inserting a hand into the vagina and feeling for the fetal skull bones, the attendant can determine the exact placement of the fetus within the birth canal. As the infant's head appears at the vaginal opening, an incision called an episiotomy is usually performed to prevent accidental tearing of these tissues. Many physicians believe that episiotomy should be done to prevent possible vaginal tearing, since a planned incision is easier to repair than an accidental tear. Another advantage of episiotomy is that it tends to speed the expulsion of the infant, which may be an advantage to both the mother and the child at this stage. The episiotomy incision is made after the injection of a local anesthetic to numb the area, and the incision is stitched closed following the delivery of the placenta.

Once the infant's head has emerged from the vagina, the attendant uses a suction device to clear the infant's nose and mouth of fluid. As the rest of the infant emerges, the attendant supports the body; a quick examination is conducted at this time to determine whether the infant has any major health problems. The umbilical cord that joins the infant to the placenta is usually cut within a few minutes after birth. When the placenta is delivered, the attendant will examine it for completeness and then will perform a thorough examination of the mother and child to ensure that all is well.

COMPLICATIONS AND DISORDERS

If the labor and delivery do not progress normally, the attendant has available a number of medical interventions that will promote the safety of both the mother and the baby. For example, labor may be induced by administration of oxytocin through an intravenous catheter. Such induction is performed if the amniotic membrane ruptures without the spontaneous onset of uterine contractions or if the pregnancy progresses well beyond the due date. The induction of labor has been found to be safe, but careful monitoring of the progress of labor is required.

Another fairly common procedure is the use of forceps to assist delivery. These tonglike instruments have two large loops that are placed on the sides of the fetal head when the head is in the birth canal. Forceps are not used to pull the fetus from the birth canal; instead, they are used to guide the fetus through the birth canal and to assist in the downward movement of the fetus during contractions. The use of forceps can help to speed the second stage of labor, and injury to the fetus or the mother is minimal when the forceps are not applied until the fetal head is well within the birth canal, as is the convention. Some type of anesthesia is always used with a forceps delivery. In some areas, vacuum extraction of the fetus is preferred. As the name implies, vacuum extraction makes use of a suction cup on the end of a vacuum hose; the suction cup is affixed to the fetal scalp.

Many women require some type of pain relief during labor, although this need can be reduced by thorough education and preparedness during the pregnancy. A wide range of pain-reducing drugs (analgesics), sedatives, and tranquilizers is available for use during the first stage of labor. These are typically administered by injection; they work at the level of the brain to alter the perception of pain and to promote relaxation. The goal is to use the minimum drug dose that allows the woman to be comfortable. The main danger is that these drugs reach the fetus through the placental circulation; side effects in the infant, which can persist for many hours after delivery, may include depressed respiration, irregular heart rhythm or rate, and sleepiness accompanied by poor suckling response.

Anesthetics that numb pain-carrying nerves in the mother may also be used during the first and second stages of labor. Two routes of delivery are in common use: epidural and spinal, both of which involve the injection of anesthetic drugs into or near the membranes around the mother's spinal cord. The epidural route of injection places the anesthetic in a space that lies outside the spinal cord membranes; with spinal anesthesia, the injection is made slightly deeper into the membranous layers. An advantage of both methods is that the mother remains awake during the delivery and can assist by pushing during the second stage.

Although the disadvantages of both anesthetics, and especially of epidurals, has been downplayed, these procedures do impose restrictions on the mother. Once an epidural has been given, for example, a woman must stay in bed because it will be difficult for her to move her legs; some hospitals do offer "mobile epidurals," which use a type of drug that blocks the pain while still allowing the woman to walk around, but these are the exception, not the rule. Because walking helps to stimulate labor, the use of epidurals can be counterproductive. The use of epidurals is also associated with a prolongation of the second stage of labor and with increased need for forceps to assist delivery. Headaches, backaches, low blood pressure, nausea, and other side effects may result in the mother following the use of anesthetics. Moreover, contrary to past evidence, recent studies have suggested that the drugs in epidurals cross the placenta to the baby, causing health risks.

General anesthesia refers to the use of drugs that induce sleep; they may be administered by inhalation or by injection. Because of profound side effects in both the mother and child, most physicians use general anesthesia only in an emergency situation requiring an immediate cesarean section.

Cesarean section refers to the delivery of the fetus through an incision made in the mother's abdominal and uterine walls. (The name derives from an unsubstantiated legend that Julius Caesar was delivered in this way.) Cesarean deliveries may be planned in advance, as when a physician notes that the fetus is in a difficult-to-deliver position, such as breech (buttocks downward) or transverse (sideways). Multiple fetuses may also be delivered by cesarean section in order to spare the mother and her infants excessive stress. Alternatively, cesarean delivery may be performed as an emergency measure, perhaps after labor has started. One indication of the need for emergency cesarean delivery is fetal distress, a condition characterized by an abnormal fetal heart rate and rhythm. Fetal distress is thought to be an indication of reduced blood flow to the placenta, which may be life-threatening to the fetus. Cesarean section may be performed using spinal or epidural anesthesia, as well as general anesthesia. A woman who delivers one child by cesarean section does not necessarily require a cesarean for later deliveries; each pregnancy is evaluated separately.

PERSPECTIVE AND PROSPECTS

Prior to 1800 in the United States, most women were attended during childbirth by female midwives. In some areas, a midwife was provided a salary by the town or region; her contract might stipulate that she provide services to all women regardless of financial or social status. In other areas, midwives worked for fees paid by the clients. Midwives of this time had little, if any, formal training and learned about birth practices from other women. Because birth was considered a natural event requiring little intervention on the part of the attendant, the midwife's medical role was limited and the few doctors available were consulted only in difficult cases. Although birth statistics were not kept at the time, anecdotal accounts from the diaries of midwives and doctors suggest that the births were most often successful, with rare cases of maternal or infant deaths.

The nineteenth century saw a gradual shift away from the use of midwives to a preference for formally trained male doctors. This shift was made possible by the establishment of medical schools that provided scientific training in obstetrics. Because these schools were generally closed to women, only men received this training and had access to the instruments and anesthesia that were coming into use.

Maternity hospitals came into being during the 1800's but were at first used primarily by poor or unmarried women. Women of higher social status still preferred to deliver their children in the privacy of their homes. Indeed, home birth was safer than hospital birth, since the building of hospitals had outpaced the knowledge of how to sanitize them. Rates of infection and maternal and infant death were higher in hospitals than in homes.

By the 1930's, the situation had reversed: Hospital births had become safer than home births, because sanitation and surgical procedures had improved. There followed an increasing trend for women to enter hospitals for delivery, so that the percentage of women giving birth in hospitals increased from about 25 percent in 1930 to almost 100 percent by 1960. In the same period, maternal and infant mortality showed a dramatic reduction. The shift to hospital birth had coincided with an interventionist philosophy: Most women were anesthetized during delivery, and forceps deliveries and episiotomy became more common.

By the 1960's, the older idea of "natural" childbirth—that is, a birth which encourages active labor and the use of drug-free types of pain relief with as little medical intervention as possible—had regained popularity. This change in attitude was brought about in part by recognition that analgesic and anesthetic drugs often had profound effects on the infant and often prevented strong mother-infant bonding in the immediate hours after delivery.

It was also brought about by the Lamaze method of childbirth, conceived by French doctor Fernand Lamaze and introduced to the United States with Marjorie Karmel's book *Thank You, Dr. Lamaze* (1959). In this method, women learn controlled breathing techniques to relax and to cope with contractions during labor. A labor coach, who is often the baby's father, helps to initiate and facilitate these techniques. Because natural childbirth must be learned, usually through childbirth classes offered in hospitals during the last trimester of pregnancy, it is also called prepared childbirth.

By the latter part of the twentieth century, a compromise between the more radical approaches of the past seemed to have been reached, with common practice in obstetrics being to allow the birth to proceed naturally when possible, but with the advantage of having refined drugs, diagnostics, and surgical techniques available if needed. The midwife had been reinstated as a specially trained nurse who could supervise normal births and provide educated assistance at difficult ones. —*Marcia Watson-Whitmyre, Ph.D. updated by Cassandra Kircher*

See also Amniocentesis; Birth defects; Breast-feeding; Cesarean section; Childbirth, complications of; Chorionic villus sampling; Conception; Ectopic pregnancy; Embryology; Episiotomy; Fetal alcohol syndrome; Gynecology; In vitro fertilization; Miscarriage; Multiple births; Neonatology; Obstetrics; Perinatology; Postpartum depression; Pregnancy and gestation; Premature birth; Reproductive system; Stillbirth; Ultrasonography.

FOR FURTHER INFORMATION:

Chestnut, David H., ed. *Obstetric Analgesia and Anesthesia*. Philadelphia: Harper & Row, 1987. Noteworthy for its completeness, this volume contains individual chapters covering specialized aspects of obstetric anesthesia. One chapter covers prepared childbirth as a technique for pain management.

Creasy, Robert K., and Robert Resnik, eds. *Maternal-Fetal Medicine: Principles and Practice*. 3d ed. Philadelphia: W. B. Saunders, 1994. This complete text covers all aspects of pregnancy and delivery, from conception to medical care of the newborn. Chapters cover normal physiology as well as problems and their treatment.

Cunningham, F. Gary, et al. *Williams Obstetrics*. 20th ed. Stamford, Conn.: Appleton and Lange, 1997. This standard medical school text is still named in honor of its first author, J. Whitridge Williams, who was a professor of obstetrics at The Johns Hopkins Medical School at the beginning of the twentieth century. Although written for the medical specialist, this work is fairly easy to read.

Karte, Diana, and Roberta M. Scaer. *A Good Birth, a Safe Birth*. 3d ed. Boston: Harvard Common Press, 1991. Written to educate expectant women on how to take control of their own birth experience, this book candidly discusses the options available during childbirth at the end of the twentieth century.

Lieberman, Adrienne B. *Giving Birth*. New York: St. Martin's Press, 1987. Written by an instructor in natural childbirth, this guide for expectant parents contains twelve firsthand accounts of birth experiences. Medical issues are well explained. Contains a chapter on home birth.

Quilligan, Edward J., and Frederick P. Zuspan, eds. *Current Therapy in Obstetrics and Gynecology*. 4th ed. Philadelphia: W. B. Saunders, 1994. Short sections cover the treatment of most reproductive and infant health problems. This compact book contains a wealth of information, such as charts showing fetal weight at different points in pregnancy, the responsibilities of various members of the obstetrical team, and the criteria used in determining specific treatments.

Reynolds, Karina, Christoph Lees, and Grainne McCarten. *Pregnancy and Birth: Your Questions Answered*. New York: DK, 1997. Written by two obstetricians and a midwife, this easy-to-read question-and-answer book covering pregnancy and childbirth is illustrated with numerous photographs, drawings, and charts.

Simkin, Penny, Janet Whalley, and Ann Keppler. *Pregnancy, Childbirth, and the Newborn: A Complete Guide for Expectant Parents*. Rev. ed. Deephaven, Minn.: Meadowbrook Books, 1991. This comprehensive guide is written in easy-to-understand language and is medically accurate and up to date. Contains many excellent illustrations and charts. The authors are associated with the Childbirth Education Association of Seattle.

Wertz, Richard W., and Dorothy C. Wertz. *Lying-in: A History of Childbirth in America*. Expanded ed. New Haven, Conn.: Yale University Press, 1989. Written in a style accessible to the general reader, this book charts the social history of childbirth practices in the United States. The authors suggest reasons for all the major changes that have occurred in obstetrical practice. Well illustrated with pictures showing instruments and procedures of bygone times.

CHILDBIRTH, COMPLICATIONS OF
DISEASE/DISORDER

ANATOMY OR SYSTEM AFFECTED: Reproductive system, uterus

SPECIALTIES AND RELATED FIELDS: Gynecology, neonatology, obstetrics

DEFINITION: The difficulties that can occur during childbirth, either for the mother or for the baby.

With medical monitoring and diagnostic tests, about 5 to 10 percent of pregnant women can be diagnosed as high-risk pregnancies, and appropriate precautions and preparations for possible complications can be made prior to labor. Yet up to 60 percent of complications of labor, childbirth, and the postpartum period (immediately after birth) occur in women with no prior indications of possible complications. Difficulties in childbirth can be placed into two general categories—problems with labor and problems with the child—and encompass a wide range of causes and possible treatments.

Complications of labor. Cesarean birth (also called cesarean section, C-section, or a section) is the surgical removal of the baby from the mother. About one in ten infants is delivered by cesarean birth. In this procedure, one incision is made through the mother's abdomen and a second through her uterus. The baby is physically removed from the mother's uterus, and the incisions are closed. This type of surgery is very safe but carries with it the general risks of any major surgery and requires approximately five days of hospitalization. In some cases, diagnosed preexisting conditions suggest that a cesarean birth is necessary and can be planned; in the majority of cases, unexpected difficulties during labor dictate that an emergency cesarean section be performed.

Some conditions leave no question about the necessity of a cesarean section. These absolute indications include a variety of physical abnormalities. Placenta previa is a condition in which the placenta has implanted in the lower part of the uterus instead of the normal upper portion, thereby totally or partially blocking the cervix. The baby could not pass down the birth canal without dislodging or tearing the placenta, thereby interrupting its blood and oxygen supply. Placenta previa is frequently the cause of bleeding after the twentieth week of pregnancy, and it can be definitively diagnosed by ultrasound. For women with this condition, bed rest is prescribed, and the baby will be delivered by cesarean birth at the thirty-seventh week of pregnancy.

Placental separation, also known as placenta abruptio, is the result of the placenta partially or completely separating from the uterus prior to the normal separation time after birth. This condition results in bleeding, with either mild or extreme blood loss depending on the severity of the separation. If severe, up to four pints of blood may be lost, and the mother is given a blood transfusion. If the pregnancy is near term, an emergency cesarean section will deliver the child.

Occasionally, as the baby begins traveling down the birth canal, the umbilical cord slips and lies ahead of the baby. This condition, called prolapsed cord, is very serious because the pressure of the baby against the cord during a vaginal delivery would compress the cord to the extent that the baby's blood and oxygen supply would be cut off. This condition necessitates an emergency cesarean section.

Some conditions that occur during labor are judged for their potential for causing harm to either the mother or the

Breech Birth

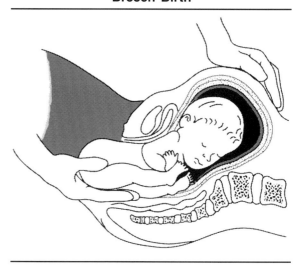

Breech birth, one of several complications that may occur during childbirth, is the emergence of the infant buttocks-first rather than head-first; such a birth is risky for the child, and often birth is accomplished by cesarean section, a surgical procedure to eliminate that risk.

baby. The physician's decision to proceed with vaginal delivery will be based on the severity of the complication and consideration of the best option for the mother and baby. A few of the more common indicators for possible cesarean section which occur during labor include a fetal head size that is too large for the mother's birth canal; fetal distress, evidenced by insufficient oxygen supply reaching the baby; rupturing of the membranes without labor commencing or prolonged labor after membranes burst (usually twenty-four hours); and inelasticity of the pelvis in first-time mothers over forty years of age.

Other maternal conditions are diagnosed prior to the onset of labor, and the physician may or may not recommend a cesarean birth based on the severity of the complication. These include postmaturity, in which the onset of labor is at least two weeks overdue and degeneration of the placenta may compromise the health of the baby; maternal diseases, such as diabetes mellitus and toxemia, in which the stress of labor would be highly risky to the mother; and previous cesarean section.

Complications with the baby. Premature labor can occur between twenty and thirty-six weeks gestation, and a premature infant is considered to be any infant whose birth weight is less than 5.5 pounds. Certain maternal illnesses or abnormalities of the placenta can lead to premature birth, but in 60 percent of the cases there is no identifiable cause. If labor begins six weeks or more prior to the due date, the best chance of infant survival is to be delivered and cared for at a hospital with a perinatal center and specialized intensive care for premature infants. Prior to twenty-four weeks development, a premature infant will not survive as a result of inadequate lung development. The survival rate of premature infants increases with age, weight, and body system maturity.

In about 4 percent of births, the baby is in the breech position—buttocks first or other body part preceding the head—rather than in the normal head-down position. Delivery in this position is complicated because the cervix will not dilate properly and the head may not be able to pass through the cervix. Other complications of breech position are prolapse or compression of the umbilical cord and trauma to the baby if delivered vaginally. Manual techniques may be used to rotate the baby into the correct position. Vaginal delivery may be attempted, frequently aided by gentle forceps removal of the baby. Breech babies are frequently born by cesarean section.

Cephalopelvic disproportion is a condition in which the baby's head is larger than the pelvic opening of the mother. This can only be determined after labor has begun, because the mother's muscles and joints expand to accommodate the baby's head. If at some point during labor the doctor determines that the baby will not fit through the mother's pelvic opening, a cesarean section will be performed.

—*Karen E. Kalumuck, Ph.D.*

See also Birth defects; Cesarean section; Childbirth; Diabetes mellitus; Eclampsia; Episiotomy; Multiple births; Obstetrics; Pregnancy and gestation; Postpartum depression; Premature birth; Reproductive system; Stillbirth.

FOR FURTHER INFORMATION:

Carlson, Karen J., Stephanie A. Eisenstat, and Terra Ziporyn. *The Harvard Guide to Women's Health.* Cambridge, Mass.: Harvard University Press, 1996.

Gonik, Bernard, and Renee A. Bobrowski. *Medical Complications in Labor and Delivery.* Cambridge, Mass.: Blackwell Scientific, 1996.

Hotchner, Tracie. *Pregnancy and Childbirth.* Rev. ed. New York: Avon Books, 1997.

Sears, William, and Martha Sears. *The Birth Book.* Boston: Little, Brown, 1994.

Stoppard, Miriam. *Conception, Pregnancy, and Birth.* London: Dorling Kindersley, 1993.

CHILDHOOD INFECTIOUS DISEASES
DISEASE/DISORDER

ANATOMY OR SYSTEM AFFECTED: Gastrointestinal system, immune system, lungs, muscles, musculoskeletal system, nose, respiratory system

SPECIALTIES AND RELATED FIELDS: Bacteriology, epidemiology, family practice, immunology, internal medicine, pediatrics, public health, virology

DEFINITION: A group of diseases including diphtheria, tetanus, measles, polio, rubella (German measles), mumps, and pertussis (whooping cough).

KEY TERMS:

anorexia: diminished appetite or aversion to food

conjunctivitis: inflammation of the conjunctiva, which lines the back of the eyelid, extends into the space between the lid and the globe of the eye, and goes over the globe to the transparent tissue covering the pupil

erythematous: related to or marked by reddening

malaise: a general feeling of discomfort, of being "out of sorts"

nuchal rigidity: stiffening of the back of the neck

oophoritis: inflammation of the ovary

orchitis: inflammation of the testis

photophobia: dread or avoidance of light

prodrome: a forewarning symptom of a disease

rhinitis: inflammation of the nasal mucous membrane

salivary glands: the glands that produce saliva

CAUSES AND SYMPTOMS

Acute communicable diseases occur primarily in childhood because most adults have become immune to such diseases, either by having acquired them as children or by having been inoculated against them. For example, prior to the use of vaccine for measles—a highly contagious disease found in most of the world—the peak incidence of the disease was in five- to ten-year-olds. Most adults were immune. Before a vaccine was developed and used against measles, epidemics occurred at two- to four-year intervals in large cities. Today, most cases are found in nonimmunized preschool children or in teenagers or young adults who have received only one dose of the vaccine.

A person infected with red measles (also known as rubeola) becomes contagious about ten days after exposure to the disease virus, at which time the prodromal stage begins. Typically, the infected person experiences three days of slight to moderate fever, a runny nose, increasing cough, and conjunctivitis. During the prodromal stage, Koplik's spots appear inside the cheeks opposite the lower molars. These lesions—grayish white dots about the size of sand particles with a slightly reddish halo surrounding them that are occasionally hemorrhagic—are important in the diagnosis of measles.

After the prodrome, a rash appears, usually accompanied by an abrupt increase in temperature (sometimes as high as 104 or 105 degrees Fahrenheit). It begins in the form of small, faintly red spots and progresses to large, dusky red confluent areas, often slightly hemorrhagic. The rash frequently begins behind the ears but spreads rapidly over the entire face, neck, upper arms, and upper part of the chest within the first twenty-four hours. During the next twenty-four hours, it spreads over the back, abdomen, entire arms, and thighs. When it finally reaches the feet after the second or third day of the rash, it is already fading from the face. At this point, the fever is usually disappearing as well.

The chief complications of measles are middle-ear infections, pneumonia, and encephalitis (a severe infection of the brain). There is no correlation between the severity of the case of measles and the development of encephalitis, but the incidence of the infection of the brain runs to only one or two per every thousand cases. Measles can also exacerbate tuberculosis.

The incubation period for rubella (German measles) lasts between fourteen and twenty-one days, and the disease occurs primarily in children between the ages of two and ten. Like the initial rash of measles, the initial rash of rubella usually starts behind the ears, but children with rubella normally have no symptoms save for the rash and a low-grade fever for one day. Adolescents may have a three-day prodromal period of malaise, runny nose, and mild conjunctivitis; adolescent girls may have arthritis in several joints that lasts for weeks. The red spots begin behind the ears and then spread to the face, neck, trunk, and extremities. This rash may coalesce and last up to five days. Temperature may be normal or slightly elevated. Complications from rubella are relatively uncommon, but if pregnant women are not immune to the disease and are exposed to the rubella virus during early pregnancy, severe congenital anomalies may result. Because similar symptoms and rashes develop in many viral diseases, rubella is difficult to diagnose clinically. Except in known epidemics, laboratory confirmation is often necessary.

The patient with mumps is likely to have fever, malaise, headache, and anorexia—all usually mild—but "neck swelling," a painful enlargement of the parotid gland near the ear, is the sign that often brings the child to a doctor. Maximum swelling peaks after one to three days and begins in one or both parotid glands, but it may involve other salivary glands. The swelling pushes the earlobe upward and outward and obscures the angle of the mandible. Drinking sour liquids such as lemon juice may increase the pain. The opening of the duct inside the cheek from the affected parotid gland may appear red and swollen.

The painful swelling usually dissipates by seven days. Abdominal pain may be caused by pancreatitis, a common complication but one that is usually mild. The most feared complication, sterility, is not as common as most believe. Orchitis rarely occurs in prepubertal boys and occurs in only 14 to 35 percent of older males. In 30 percent of patients with orchitis, both testes are involved, and a similar percentage of affected testes will atrophy. Surprisingly, impairment of fertility in males is only about 13 percent; absolute infertility is rare. Ovary involvement in women, with pelvic pain and tenderness, occurs in only about 7 percent of postpubertal women and with no evidence of impaired fertility.

Measles, rubella, and mumps are all viral illnesses, but *Hemophilus influenzae* type B is the most common cause of serious bacterial infection in the young child. It is the leading cause of bacterial meningitis in children between the ages of one month and four years, and it is the cause of many other serious, life-threatening bacterial infections in the young child. Bacterial meningitis, especially from *Hemophilus influenzae* and pneumococcus, is the major cause of acquired hearing impairment in childhood.

Poliomyelitis (polio), an acute viral infection, has a wide range of manifestations. The minor illness pattern accounts for 80 to 90 percent of clinical infections in children. Symptoms, usually mild in this form, include slight fever, malaise, headache, sore throat, and vomiting but do not involve the central nervous system. Major illness occurs primarily in older children and adults. It may begin with fever, severe headache, stiff neck and back, deep muscle pain, and abnormal sensations, such as of burning, pricking, tickling, or tingling. These symptoms of aseptic meningitis may go no further or may progress to the loss of tendon reflexes and asymmetric weakness or paralysis of muscle groups. Fewer than 25 percent of paralytic polio patients suffer permanent disability. Most return in muscle function occurs within six months, but improvement may continue for two years. Twenty-five percent of paralytic patients have mild residual symptoms, and 50 percent recover completely. A long-term study of adults who suffered the disease has documented slowly progressive muscle weakness, especially in patients who experienced severe disabilities initially.

Tetanus is a bacterial disease which, once established in a wound of a patient without significant immunity, will build a substance that acts at the neuromuscular junction, the spinal cord, and the brain. Clinically, the patient experiences "lockjaw," a tetanic spasm causing the spine and extremities to bend with convexity forward; spasms of the facial muscles cause the famous "sardonic smile." Minimal stimulation of any muscle group may cause painful spasms.

Diphtheria is another bacterial disease that produces a virulent substance, but this one attacks heart muscle and nervous tissue. There is a severe mucopurulent discharge from the nose and an exudative pharyngitis (a sore throat accompanied by phlegm) with the formation of a pseudomembrane. Swelling just below the back of the throat may lead to stridor (noisy, high-pitched breathing) and to the dark bluish or purplish coloration of the skin and mucous membranes because of decreased oxygenation of the blood. The result may be heart failure and damaged nerves; respiratory insufficiency may be caused by diaphragmatic paralysis.

Clinically, pertussis (whooping cough) can be divided into three stages, each lasting about two weeks. Initial symptoms resembling the common cold are followed by the characteristic paroxysmal cough and then convalescence. In the middle stage, multiple, rapid coughs, which may last more than a minute, will be followed by a sudden inspiration of air and a characteristic "whoop." In the final stage, vomiting commonly follows coughing attacks. Almost any stimulus precipitates an attack. Seizures may occur as a result of hypoxia (inadequate oxygen supply) or brain damage. Pneumonia can develop, and even death may occur when the illness is severe.

Varicella (chickenpox) produces a generalized itchy, blisterlike rash with low-grade fever and few other symptoms. Minor complications, such as ear infections, occasionally occur, as does pneumonia, but serious complications such as infection in the brain are thankfully rare. It is a very inconvenient disease, however, requiring the infected person to be quarantined for about nine days or until the skin lesions have dried up completely. Varicella, a herpes family virus, may lie dormant in nerve linings for years and suddenly emerge in the linear-grouped skin lesions identified as herpes zoster. These painful skin lesions follow the distribution of the affected nerve. Herpes zoster is popularly known as "shingles."

Hepatitis type B is much more common in adults than in children, except in certain immigrant populations in which hepatitis B viral infections are endemic. High carrier rates appear in certain Asian and Pacific Islander groups and among some Inuits in Alaska, in whom perinatal transmission is the most common means of perpetuating the disease. Having this disease in childhood can cause problems later in life. An estimated five thousand deaths in the United States per year from cirrhosis or liver cancer occur as a result of hepatitis B. Carrier rates of between 5 and 10 percent result from disease acquired after the age of five, but between 80 and 90 percent will be carriers if they are infected at birth. The serious problems of hepatitis B occur most often in chronic carriers. For example, 50 percent of carriers will ultimately develop liver cancer. The virus is fifty to one hundred times more infectious than human immunodeficiency virus (HIV), the virus that causes acquired immunodeficiency syndrome (AIDS). Health care workers are at high risk of contracting hepatitis B, but virtually everyone is at risk for contracting this disease because it is so contagious.

TREATMENT AND THERAPY

The Immunization Practices Advisory Committee of the U.S. Public Health Service recommends immunizing all infants and some adolescents against hepatitis B, but the Committee on Infectious Diseases of the American Academy of Pediatrics recommends extending hepatitis B immunization to all adolescents, if possible. Based on field trials, the hepatitis B vaccine appears to be between 80 and 90 percent effective. The plasma-derived vaccine is protective against chronic hepatitis B infection for at least nine years. Newer, yeast-derived vaccines appear to be safe for administration to all, including pregnant women and infants: Both the vaccine and a placebo evoke the same incidence of reactions. These yeast-derived vaccines will be monitored to see if a booster dose is needed.

The incidence of infection with hepatitis B increases rapidly in adolescence, but teenagers are less likely to comply with immunization than are infants. Asking adolescents to participate in a three-dose immunization program over a six-month period is likely to result in high dropout rates. Therefore, the American Academy of Pediatrics' committee has recommended combining vaccination at birth with vaccination of teenagers. Two states, Alaska and Hawaii, have implemented universal immunization of infants with hepatitis B vaccine, and so have twenty nations.

Primary vaccination with DPT (diphtheria, pertussis, and tetanus) vaccine is recommended at two months, four months, and six months of age, followed by boosters with a new vaccine, DTaP, at fifteen months and upon entry into school (at four to six years of age). The last two vaccinations once used the DPT vaccine. The newer DTaP vaccine includes an acellular pertussis component manufactured in Japan, as well as the traditional diphtheria and tetanus toxoids. This Japanese acellular pertussis component contains various pertussis antigens but much less of the pertussis toxic products than the older, whole-cell vaccine. The substitution of the DTaP for the older DPT vaccine decreases the incidence of local and febrile reactions, but its effectiveness for the primary vaccinations has yet to be established.

Once a child reaches fifteen months of age, only one dose of the *Hemophilus influenzae* type B vaccine is necessary, but vaccination should begin at two months of age. Two vaccines are licensed for use in infants, HbOC and PRP-OMP. HbOC is given on a four-dose schedule at two, four, six, and fifteen months of age, whereas PRP-OMP is given on a three-dose schedule at two, four, and twelve months of age. These vaccines are safe and at least 90 percent effective in preventing serious illness, such as sepsis and meningitis, from influenza B.

At two and four months of age, infants should receive an oral polio vaccination, with boosters at fifteen months and upon entry into school (four to six years of age). TOPV, the polio vaccine, contains a live virus that is excreted and may infect close contacts. Therefore, children who have close contact with someone who is immunocompromised (or who are themselves immunocompromised) should receive EIPV, an enhanced, inactivated polio virus vaccine.

MMR (measles, mumps, rubella) vaccination should take place at fifteen months and at four to six years of age. If the infant lives in a high-risk area, the first dose should occur at twelve months of age. While women who are pregnant or plan to become pregnant in the next three months should not receive MMR vaccination, children may receive the vaccine even if the mother is pregnant, since the viruses are not shed by immunized individuals.

In the 1990's, researchers announced that they had developed a vaccine to prevent chickenpox. Preliminary trials show the vaccine to be safe and effective even in immunocompromised patients.

Other available vaccines to prevent serious infections in children are recommended only in special circumstances.

These include vaccines to prevent classic viral flu and pneumococcal disease. (The viral flu is to be distinguished from the bacterial vaccine to prevent influenza B.) Vaccination with the viral influenza vaccine is recommended especially for elderly and high-risk persons, their household contacts, and health care personnel who may come in contact with such patients. Any child who has a heart disease, lung disease, diabetes, or other serious chronic disease should receive the vaccine. This includes the child who is immunocompromised, even if he or she is HIV-positive.

Pneumococcal vaccine is not routinely given to children and is not recommended for use in children under two years of age, but it is given to children who are at risk of overwhelming pneumococcal infections. For example, children without spleens and children with sickle-cell anemia should be considered for vaccination against pneumococcal disease.

Some parents refuse to have their children vaccinated against pertussis because of concerns about the vaccine's safety. Media focus on the safety of pertussis vaccines, as well as legal suits, has frightened many physicians as well, the result being that they may be overly cautious in interpreting vaccine contraindications. Yet primary care physicians have also been sued for failing to give timely immunizations, which may result in complications from preventable disease. The Tennessee Medicaid Pertussis Vaccine Data should reassure them of the vaccine's safety. Other pertussis vaccine safety information is also available, including reports from the American Academy of Pediatrics' Task Force on Pertussis and Pertussis Immunization.

The means exist to prevent many serious illnesses from infectious diseases in childhood, but both parents and health care professionals must make the effort to vaccinate all children at the appropriate times in their lives.

PERSPECTIVE AND PROSPECTS

Some vaccines are more protective than others; effectiveness may hinge on a number of factors. In 1989, for example, 40 percent of people who developed measles had been vaccinated correctly under the old guidelines of one dose. Recommendations were therefore revised to include a booster dose. In the case of the hepatitis B vaccine, initial recommendations for administration of the vaccine established no injection site (only intramuscular), but studies revealed that there were fewer vaccine failures in recipients who were vaccinated in the deltoid region of the arm as opposed to the buttocks. The recommendation for injection site was therefore revised.

In the United States, vaccine coverage became woefully inadequate during the 1980's: One state's department of health, in a 1987 study, discovered that only 64 percent of children who were two years old were adequately vaccinated with DPT, oral polio, and MMR vaccines. Undoubtedly, multiple and interacting factors have inhibited adequate vaccine coverage, including physicians' attitudes and practice behaviors. For parents, the cost of vaccination, lack of health insurance, and other barriers to health care frustrate their efforts to get their children immunized. Some parents, for ideological or other reasons, may even be disinterested in or opposed to vaccination. In today's highly mobile society, however, all persons should keep a standard personal immunization record to facilitate immunization coverage. —*Wayne R. McKinny, M.D.*

See also Bacterial infections; Bacteriology; Chickenpox; Common cold; Epidemiology; Family practice; Hepatitis; Herpes; Immunization and vaccination; Infection; Influenza; Measles, red; Microbiology; Mononucleosis; Mumps; Pediatrics; Pertussis; Poliomyelitis; Rabies; Rheumatic fever; Rhinitis; Roseola; Roundworm; Rubella; Rubeola; Scarlet fever; Smallpox; Strep throat; Tapeworm; Tetanus; Tonsillitis; Tuberculosis; Typhoid fever and typhus; Viral infections; Worms.

FOR FURTHER INFORMATION:

Behrman, Richard E., ed. *Nelson Textbook of Pediatrics.* 15th ed. Philadelphia: W. B. Saunders, 1996. This standard pediatrics textbook contains complete discussions of all common (and uncommon) causes of infectious disease in children. Many chapters are well written and easily understood by the nonspecialist.

Berkow, Robert, and Andrew J. Fletcher, eds. *The Merck Manual of Diagnosis and Therapy.* 16th ed. Rahway, N.J.: Merck Sharp & Dohme Research Laboratories, 1992. Published since 1899, this classic work is well indexed and easy to use. Discussions of the various infectious diseases of childhood are usually brief but thorough.

Burg, Fredric D., ed. *Treatment of Infants, Children, and Adolescents.* Philadelphia: W. B. Saunders, 1990. One can quickly find specific information about vaccine dosages and other valuable information in this text.

Korting, G. W. *Diseases of the Skin in Children and Adolescents.* Philadelphia: W. B. Saunders, 1970. An older textbook that contains color photographs of skin lesions in many childhood infectious diseases, matched by brilliant discussions of clinical patterns and signs.

Robbins, Stanley L., Ramzi S. Cotran, and Vinay Kumar, eds. *Robbins' Pathologic Basis of Disease.* 5th ed. Philadelphia: W. B. Saunders, 1994. An excellent textbook that combines the clinical and the pathological beautifully.

CHIROPRACTIC

SPECIALTY

ANATOMY OR SYSTEM AFFECTED: Back, bones, hips, musculoskeletal system, nervous system, spine

SPECIALTIES AND RELATED FIELDS: Neurology, orthopedics, preventive medicine

DEFINITION: The art and science of adjusting the spine and other bony articulations of the body in order to restore and maintain normal structure and function in the nervous system.

KEY TERMS:

adjustment: a thrust delivered into the spine or its articulations with the purpose of reestablishing normal joint and nerve function

nerve interference/pressure: chiropractic term that refers to a disturbance of normal nerve impulse transmission, usually via compression, stretch, or chronic irritation

neuromusculoskeletal: pertaining to the interrelationship between the nerves, muscles, and skeletal aspects of the body

palpation: the act of feeling with the hand; the application of the fingers with light pressure to the surface of the body for the purpose of determining the consistence of the parts beneath for physical diagnosis

subluxation: an incomplete or partial dislocation of a joint, which creates abnormal neurological and physiological symptoms in neuromusculoskeletal structures and/or other body systems via interference with nerve impulse transmission

SCIENCE AND PROFESSION

In the United States, chiropractic has the second largest patient base in the health care system. Licensed in every state, chiropractors are acknowledged as physicians along with medical doctors and osteopathic doctors, dentists, podiatrists, optometrists, and psychologists. Patients can consult with chiropractic physicians without referral. The scope of chiropractic practice varies from state to state, and reference must be made to specific state laws for exact information. The major premise of this field states that vertebrae of the spine can, and frequently do, become misaligned, causing interference in normal conduction of nerve impulses from the brain to the organs and tissues of the body. Although most spinal misalignments are corrected naturally through normal body movement, some become fixated. As a result, normal nerve transmission is impaired for long periods, and health suffers.

What distinguishes doctors of chiropractic from other health care professions is that they work primarily to identify, analyze, and adjust the vertebrae and pelvis back to their correct positions. Treatment is directed at restoring and maintaining normal structure and mechanical function of the spine to reduce irritation of the spinal cord and spinal nerves. These irritations lead to pain and distress of the muscles and joints of the body. Less acknowledged and still in want of collaborating research is the relationship between the subluxation, the neuromusculoskeletal system, and internal organ dysfunction. Contrary to popular belief, the scope of chiropractic is recognized for its ability to promote the total health and integration of the body from the inside out. In addition to spinal adjusting, chiropractors encourage those whom they treat to take personal responsibility for their lives by teaching ways to preserve health rather than wait until symptoms of disease appear.

Doctors of chiropractic may examine, diagnose, analyze, and use X rays for diagnostic purposes according to generally recognized procedures taught in accredited chiropractic colleges. Clinical practice generally encompasses consultation and taking a history of the patient; physical, neurological, orthopedic, and chiropractic examinations; X-ray analysis of the spine and articulating structures; the administration of adjustments; physiotherapy; nutritional support; and the use of orthopedic supports. In most states, chiropractic practice does not include the prescription or administration of medicine or drugs, performance of surgery, practice of obstetrics, administration of radiation therapy, treatment of infectious or sexually transmitted diseases, performance of internal exams, reduction of fractures, or administration of anesthetics. Historically, chiropractic physicians practice either solo or in a group setting with other chiropractors and do not have hospital privileges. This is changing as some chiropractic physicians are entering into group practice settings with other health care specialists and gaining admittance to hospitals in a limited capacity.

Chiropractic history dates back to 1895 when D. D. Palmer experimented with a spinal adjustment on Harvey Lillard. Lillard, a janitor, had experienced a "popping sensation" in his upper spine caused by heavy lifting and subsequently had a loss of hearing. After treatment, Lillard's hearing improved and Palmer formulated early chiropractic scientific premise and philosophy: that illness is essentially functional in nature and becomes organic only as an end process. His son, B. J. Palmer, is credited with refining and promoting the work of his father. Chiropractic lays claim to a colorful and compelling history into its first century. From its humble beginnings, it has survived as a viable alternative health care system in America and has emerged as the second largest health care entity in the industry. The early educational program organized by D. D. Palmer was admittedly crude, abbreviated, and inadequate. As the profession grew and matured, however, so did the educational standards to the current level, which is beyond reproach.

Chiropractic colleges are sanctioned as degree-granting institutions by the same regional accrediting agencies that regulate all other colleges and universities. Chiropractic colleges are accredited by the Council on Chiropractic Education, which is in turn approved by the United States Office of Education. Programs of study in chiropractic colleges parallel those in medical colleges except that chiropractic theory and practice replace surgery and medical theory. The medical curriculum is designed to prepare the medical student to diagnose and combat systemic diseases, with great emphasis on the use of drugs and surgery. The chiropractic curriculum, on the other hand, is designed to prepare the chiropractic student to evaluate and manage conservatively conditions from a holistic point of view, in which the various factors that affect a person's health are taken into consideration, including diet, nutritional supplementation, exercise, stress, and lifestyle.

Chiropractors have a full medical curriculum enabling them to make diagnoses. The education of a chiropractor begins with two years of preprofessional college study, with concentration in the human sciences. Although this prerequisite of two years is all that is required, the majority of students entering chiropractic college possess at least a bachelor's degree. The student then begins the Doctor of Chiropractic (D.C.) course of study at an accredited chiropractic college. The D.C. program is composed of four academic years of study most often divided into semesters or trimesters. The initial phase of study is much like any curriculum in the medical, dental, or veterinary schools consisting of courses in the basic sciences: organic chemistry, biochemistry, anatomy of the musculoskeletal system (including limbs, trunk, and head), anatomy of the internal structures of the body (including all the organs, blood vessels, and internal systems), neuroanatomy (the anatomy of the brain, spinal cord, and entire nervous system), physiology (the study of how these systems function), neurophysiology, pathology (the study of disease), bacteriology, histology (the microscopic study of body tissues), and microbiology. The remainder of the courses are concentrated on the clinical sciences: X-ray physics, positioning, and interpretation; laboratory diagnosis (blood and urine studies); physical examination and diagnosis; neurology; orthopedics; cardiology; obstetrics and gynecology; pediatrics; geriatrics; dermatology; gastrointestinal and genitourinary systems; physical therapy nutrition; and chiropractic adjustment techniques.

During the later part of the student chiropractor's matriculation, he or she will see patients in a college-affiliated clinic as an "extern," which prepares the future doctor for patient care and management. In addition to the basic chiropractic curriculum, there are residencies available in both radiology and orthopedics. A chiropractic graduate may apply to study an additional three years in order to become either a chiropractic radiologist or a chiropractic orthopedist. The training received in these programs is highly specialized, and both of these chiropractic specialists are the equal of their medical counterparts in terms of diagnostic abilities. In addition, comprehensive 360-hour programs of study in orthopedics, neurology, radiology, and sports medicine exist; doctors completing such programs are eligible to sit for an examination to be awarded Diplomate status by chiropractic boards in the corresponding specialties. Postgraduate education for the practicing chiropractor includes seminars and workshops in soft tissue injuries, disk syndromes, low back pain, and other common and difficult conditions. Interdisciplinary seminars and conferences in nutrition, fitness, biochemical imbalances, and numerous other areas of common interest allow physicians from every discipline the opportunity to exchange views and perspectives.

The licensing procedure for the graduate chiropractic doctor varies from state to state. During the formal educational process, chiropractic students are exposed to thorough written examinations in all basic science and clinical subjects which are administered by the National Board of Chiropractic Examiners. Successful completion of these written tests is a prerequisite to licensure in many states. Otherwise, completion of a written and practical examination administered by the respective state board is required, and in some states completion of the National Board Examinations and a state-administered written board are both required. The majority of states require doctors to attend certified educational seminars for continued licensure. The chiropractic profession is generally organized on a state basis through professional state associations and on a national basis through national organizations.

DIAGNOSTIC AND TREATMENT TECHNIQUES

To understand fully how chiropractic health care works, it is necessary to understand the spine and the role that it plays in overall body function. The nervous system—consisting of the brain, cranial nerves (nerves that originate in the head), the spinal cord, and thirty-one pairs of spinal nerves that branch out much as the limbs of a tree do—generates and regulates all activities in the body. While no one knows exactly how the nervous system functions, it is known that signals, or impulses, travel along the nerve fibers conveying information between the brain and the rest of the body. Since every tissue and organ of the body is connected to and controlled by nerves from the spinal cord and brain, removal or nerve interference can bring dramatic results. Interference with the transmission of these impulses results in alteration of normal body function. The cranium (skull) and spinal column, composed of twenty-four bones called vertebrae, house the brain and spinal cord. In addition to protecting the spinal cord, the spine is the core of the skeletal framework that supports upright posture, provides for organ and muscle attachment, and allows for the dynamics of human movement. Given this monumental job, the spine and its connecting framework are subject to much activity and abuse.

In order for the mechanics of body motion to occur properly, there must be full, free, and harmonious movement in every one of the spinal joints. The working unit of the spine is referred to as the motor unit. The motor unit is composed of two vertebrae joined by cartilage cushions called disks and four posterior joints called facet joints, two located to attach the superior vertebra and two to attach the inferior vertebra. The disks separate the vertebrae while allowing flexibility and shock absorption for the spine. They also maintain openings between the vertebrae that are necessary for the passage of the spinal nerves. The facet joints provide additional movement and are limited in their range of motion by ligaments. Restriction in any of them can only be compensated for by the other joints and adjoining structures (such as ribs, muscles, or tendons), thus producing strain in the compensating structures.

It is at the location of the facet joints of the spine where subluxation occurs—an alteration of the alignment and proper movement of the spinal joint resulting in irritation of the exiting spinal nerve via compression, stretch, or chronic (constant) irritation—and leads to alteration of normal body functions. Subluxations can result from various factors, including trauma, toxic irritation, muscular imbalance caused by disuse and/or repetitive tasks, ligamental weakening, organic dysfunction, and stress. The altered nerve impulse transmission, left uncorrected, results in accumulative dysfunction in the tissue cells of the body.

Spinal biomechanics, the basis of the chiropractor's evaluation, refers to the manner in which the spine works in movement. Restoration of spinal motion is the primary treatment on which chiropractors depend to alleviate patients' symptoms. The single most unique element of chiropractic procedures is the spinal adjustment. This chiropractic adjustment is a technique of physically moving the spine by hand or by instrument with the objective of mobilizing a fixated joint. It is a gentle but dynamic thrust applied to a specific joint in a way that generates joint movement in a specific direction. Basically, it is a way to "coax" a restricted joint into moving. Applied repeatedly over a period of time, spinal adjustments are capable

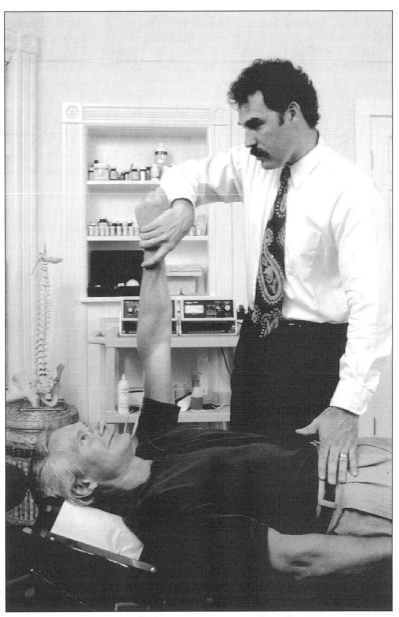

A chiropractor gives a manual muscle test to a patient. (T. J. Florian/Rainbow)

of restoring mobility to even the most chronic spinal subluxations. Deep-rooted subluxations that have existed for several years typically require months of care. Fixations of lesser duration and severity respond in less time, often the mildest in one treatment. The procedure works because the restoration of the proper mechanics of spinal motion via the spinal adjustment improves joint function, corrects specific joint problems, and helps prevent injury through increased spinal strength brought about by spinal joints that function properly.

Chiropractic health care can be useful for the detection and correction of existing health problems and/or for preventative purposes. In lieu of concentrating on bacterial or viral infections or treating the end-symptoms of disease processes, chiropractors look for the reason that a patient's symptom developed, including such contributing factors as environmental conditions, lifestyle, systemic stress, and malfunction. For example, instead of giving medication to stop the pain of headache, the chiropractor analyzes possible irritating factors, including subluxation, that may be causing the headache and addresses that factor first. Thus, in many cases, the prescription of medication can be avoided.

PERSPECTIVE AND PROSPECTS

Chiropractic originated in the second half of the nineteenth century during a time when many theories of healing were being promulgated. Chiropractic and osteopathy shared their early beginnings amid the emergence of several alternatives to the regular school of healing (medicine), including the Thomsonian system (the use of botanicals), the Hygienic movement (the use of fresh fruits and vegetables, fresh air, exercise, and better food preparation), and homeopathy. Daniel David Palmer, born in 1845 in Canada, was involved in making and losing several small mercantile fortunes when he made his way to Iowa in 1886 to become a magnetic healer. Over the next decade, he would attract patients from throughout the Midwest until one day in September, 1895, a janitor named Harvey Lillard came into his office, received an "adjustment," and regained his lost hearing. Soon afterward, the term "chiropractic" (Greek meaning "done by hand") was coined by Samuel Weed, a Palmer patient. D. D. Palmer began giving instruction at Dr. Palmer's School and Cure, later becoming Palmer Institute and Chiropractic Infirmary and finally Palmer Chiropractic College.

Brian Inglis, a distinguished British historian, commentator, and author of the two-volume work *The History of Medicine* (1965) has declared: "The rise of chiropractic . . . has been one of the most remarkable social phenomena in American history . . . yet it has gone virtually unexplored." In spite of its humble origins and formulative years, chiropractic has had a decided impact on the evolution of health care attitudes in the United States and to some degree in other parts of the Western world. For more than three-quarters of a century, it fought for its very survival, overcoming a strong medical lobby in 1977 when the American Medical Association (AMA) reversed its long-standing policy against professional interrelationships between medical doctors and chiropractors. In March, 1977, the AMA's Judicial Council announced:

> A physician may refer a patient for diagnostic or therapeutic services to another physician, a limited practitioner, or any other provider of health care services permitted by law to furnish such services, whenever he believes that this may benefit the patient. As in the case of referrals to physician-specialists, referrals to limited practitioners should be based on their individual competence and ability to perform the services needed by the patient.

Despite the AMA's policy change toward chiropractic, however, complete acceptance by the medical profession has not occurred. This reluctance has not been attributable solely to the attitudes of the medical profession. Rather, it is the result of a combination of the continued opposition of the medical profession and the resistance of chiropractors to subordinate themselves to medical prescription, as with physical therapists who practice under medical supervision. Chiropractors have been independent practitioners for too long, functioning at a high level in the diagnosis and treatment of illness, for them to be willing to regress in status.

It is likely that the chiropractic profession will continue on its present course of becoming a health profession with parallels to medicine. Emphasizing the uniqueness of chiropractic treatment and the contrasting philosophical approaches of health maintenance and therapy, chiropractic has not only survived but also flourished. Whether used as a preventive means to ensure good health or as a way to help the body cure itself of disease, chiropractic has sometimes succeeded where other health care measures have failed.

—*Cindy Nesci, D.C.*

See also Alternative medicine; Anxiety; Bone disorders; Bones and the skeleton; Muscle sprains, spasms, and disorders; Muscles; Pain, types of; Pain management; Physical rehabilitation; Spine, vertebrae, and disks; Spinal disorders; Stress; Stress reduction.

FOR FURTHER INFORMATION:

Altman, Nathaniel. *Everybody's Guide to Chiropractic Health Care.* New York: St. Martin's Press, 1990. A consumer's handbook written to inform the layperson who is searching for an alternative to traditional, medical health care.

DeRoeck, Richard E. *The Confusion About Chiropractors.* Danbury, Conn.: Impulse, 1989. A handbook for those wanting to understand the chiropractor's orientation and perspective.

Haldeman, Scott, ed. *Principles and Practice of Chiropractic.* Rev. 2d ed. Norwalk, Conn.: Appleton and Lange, 1992. A series of articles by leading authorities in the fields of history, sociology, neurophysiology, spinal biomechanics, and clinical chiropractic. Written with the purpose of presenting an accurate overview of the latest developments in the field.

Schafer, R. C. *Chiropractic Health Care: A Conservative Approach to Health Restoration, Maintenance, and Disease Resistance.* 3d ed. Des Moines, Iowa: Foundation for Chiropractic Education and Research, 1978. A general guide to chiropractic treatment. Discusses the philosophy behind this type of health care, as well as the methods that it employs.

Tousley, Dirk. *The Chiropractic Handbook for Patients.* 3d ed. Independence, Mo.: White Dove, 1985. This popular work on chiropractic is written with the general reader in mind. Contains information that will help patients understand their treatment.

CHLAMYDIA

DISEASE/DISORDER

ANATOMY OR SYSTEM AFFECTED: Eyes, genitals, joints, reproductive system

SPECIALTIES AND RELATED FIELDS: Family practice, gynecology, neonatology, puublic health, urology, virology

DEFINITION: Chlamydia is a common sexually transmitted disease caused by the transfer of viruslike intracellular parasites during vaginal, rectal, or oral sexual intercourse, or by vaginal infection during the delivery of a newborn, which may infect the baby's eyes. Following infection through sexual contact, there is an incubation period of five to twenty-eight days. Vaginal and urethral discharges as well as anal swelling, pain, and reddening of the vagina or tip of the penis may occur. Elsewhere in the body, the infection leads to fever, joint pain, blisters, and conjunctivitis in infants. Early treatment with medication cures the infection and prevents further complications.

—*Jason Georges and Tracy Irons-Georges*

See also Conjunctivitis; Genital disorders, female; Genital disorders, male; Gynecology; Reproductive system; Sexually transmitted diseases.

CHOKING
DISEASE/DISORDER
ANATOMY OR SYSTEM AFFECTED: Chest, lungs, neck, respiratory system, throat

SPECIALTIES AND RELATED FIELDS: Emergency medicine

DEFINITION: A condition in which the breathing passage (windpipe) is obstructed.

CAUSES AND SYMPTOMS
A person who is choking may cough, turn red in the face, clutch his or her throat, or any combination of the above. If the choking person is coughing, it is probably best to do nothing; the coughing should naturally clear the airway. The true choking emergency occurs when a bit of food or other foreign object completely obstructs the breathing passage. In this case, there is little or no coughing—the person cannot make much sound. This silent choking calls for immediate action.

TREATMENT AND THERAPY
An individual witnessing a choking emergency should first call for emergency help and then perform the Heimlich maneuver. The choking person should never be slapped on the back. The Heimlich maneuver is best performed while the choking victim is standing or seated. If possible, the person performing the Heimlich maneuver should ask the victim to nod if he or she wishes the Heimlich maneuver to be performed. If the airway is totally blocked, the victim will not be able to speak and may even be unconscious.

The individual performing the Heimlich maneuver positions himself or herself behind the choking victim and places his or her arms around the victim's waist. Making a fist with one hand and grasping that fist with the other hand, the rescuer positions the thumb side of the fist toward the stomach of the victim—just above the navel and below the ribs. The person performing the maneuver pulls his or her fist upward into the abdomen of the victim with several quick thrusts. This action should expel the foreign object from the victim's throat, and he or she should begin coughing or return to normal breathing.

Heimlich Maneuver

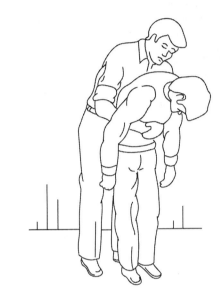

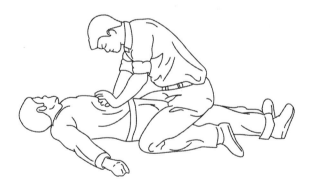

The Heimlich maneuver is ideally performed on a standing or seated victim who has indicated consent that this maneuver be performed by nodding or another gesture of affirmation; if unconscious, the victim may be lying on his or her back, and abdominal thrusts are administered using the heel of the hand. NOTE: *The illustration depicts only part of the procedure, which is not fully detailed above; for full information on the protocols for first aid for persons with obstructed airways, such as CPR, refer to the American Heart Association's Heartsaver Manual, which is periodically updated.*

The Heimlich maneuver is not effective in dislodging fish bones and certain other obstructions. If the airway is still blocked after several Heimlich thrusts, a finger sweep should be tried to remove the obstruction. First the mouth of the victim must be opened: The chin is grasped, and the mouth is pulled open with one hand. With the index finger of the other hand, the rescuer sweeps through the victim's throat, pulling out any foreign material. One sweep should be made from left to right, and a second sweep from right to left. The Heimlich maneuver may then be repeated if necessary.   —*Steven A. Schonefeld, Ph.D.*

See also Asphyxiation; Coughing; Respiration; Resuscitation; Unconsciousness.

FOR FURTHER INFORMATION:

Anderson, Kenneth N., et al., eds. *Mosby's Medical, Nursing, and Allied Health Dictionary.* 4th ed. St. Louis: C. V. Mosby, 1994.

Castleman, Michael. "Emergency! Fifty-four Ways to Save Your Life." *Family Circle* 107, no. 4 (March 15, 1994): 37.

Heimlich, H. J., and E. A. Patrick. "The Heimlich Maneuver: The Best Technique for Saving Any Choking Victim's Life." *Postgraduate Medicine* 87, no. 6 (May 1, 1990): 38-48, 53.

Stern, Loraine. "Your Child's Health: Mom, I Can't Breathe!" *Woman's Day* 57, no. 6 (March 15, 1994): 18.

CHOLECYSTECTOMY

PROCEDURE

ANATOMY OR SYSTEM AFFECTED: Abdomen, gallbladder, gastrointestinal system

SPECIALTIES AND RELATED FIELDS: General surgery

DEFINITION: The surgical removal of a diseased gallbladder.

INDICATIONS AND PROCEDURES

Cholecystectomy is indicated when the patient exhibits nausea, vomiting, and abdominal pain and examination reveals gallstones. Gallstones, which consist mostly of crystallized cholesterol and bile, form in the gallbladder and may lodge in the bile duct. The stones can be dissolved with medication or broken up with ultrasound and passed from the body. They can (and often do) form again, however, with renewed symptoms. Removal of the gallbladder is the method of choice to prevent the recurrence of symptoms. Surgery is performed under general anesthesia.

In open surgery, the abdomen is cleaned and a 7.5- to 15-centimeter (3- to 6-inch) incision made with a scalpel through the skin and abdominal tissues. The gallbladder is isolated from the liver. A duct and artery are tied off with surgical staples or sutures, and they are cut in order to free the gallbladder. The organ is removed, and the tissues are closed with sutures or staples.

In laparoscopic surgery, the surface is cleaned and the surgeon makes four small holes. A 1.3-centimeter (0.5-inch) cut is made at or near the navel, another just below the

breastbone, and two small punctures to the right of the incisions. The laparoscope, with a video camera and light, is inserted into the navel incision. Long, thin dissecting instruments are passed through the three punctures, and the gallbladder is cut free as in open surgery. The organ is removed through the navel incision, which is then closed with sutures or staples. The punctures are closed with small adhesive bandages.

USES AND COMPLICATIONS

Open surgery for cholecystectomy requires a hospital stay of five to eight days and a recovery time of four to six weeks. Complications occur in 1.0 to 9.4 percent of the surgeries and range from postoperative bleeding and diarrhea to intestinal obstruction. The mortality rate is low: 0.2 to 0.6 percent.

Laparoscopic surgery usually requires an overnight stay and a recovery period of five to seven days. Complications occur in 5.1 percent of the surgeries and are similar to those in open surgery, but they may also include severing the common bile duct that connects the liver and small intestine and puncturing major blood vessels, including the largest one, the aorta. Laparoscopy is relatively new, and the preliminary mortality rate is 0.1 percent.   —*Albert C. Jensen*

Cholecystectomy

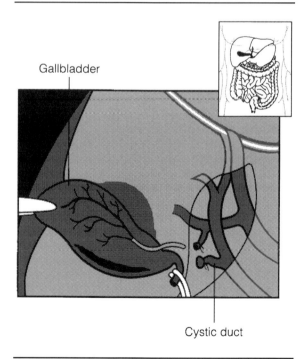

Gallbladder

Cystic duct

The removal of the gallbladder may be indicated with severe infection of the organs or with repeated attacks of biliary colic caused by the presence of gallstones; the inset shows the location of the gallbladder.

See also Cholecystitis; Gallbladder diseases; Gastroenterology; Gastroenterology; Gastrointestinal system; Laparoscopy; Stone removal; Stones.

CHOLECYSTITIS

DISEASE/DISORDER
ANATOMY OR SYSTEM AFFECTED: Gallbladder
SPECIALTIES AND RELATED FIELDS: Bacteriology, family practice, gastroenterology, internal medicine

Cholecystitis

A normal gallbladder and one inflamed by cholecystitis.

DEFINITION: Cholecystitis is the inflammation or bacterial infection of the gallbladder, which is usually caused by gallstones or blockage of the bile ducts. Signs may include an indigestion-like cramping pain in the upper-right abdomen, symptoms in the chest resembling a heart attack, or pain in the upper-right back and shoulder following fatty meals. More severe cases include abdominal spasms and tenderness, nausea and vomiting, fever, and sometimes jaundice, pale stools, and skin irritation. Cholecystitis can be prevented by avoiding foods that trigger indigestion or by having gallstones surgically removed. Surgery to remove an infected gallbladder may be necessary in chronic cases.

—*Jason Georges and Tracy Irons-Georges*
See also Cholecystectomy; Gallbladder diseases; Gastroenterology; Internal medicine; Stone removal; Stones.

CHOLERA

DISEASE/DISORDER
ANATOMY OR SYSTEM AFFECTED: Gastrointestinal system

SPECIALTIES AND RELATED FIELDS: Bacteriology, environmental health, epidemiology, gastroenterology, pediatrics, public health
DEFINITION: An infection of the small intestine caused by *Vibrio cholerae*, a comma-shaped bacterium.

CAUSES AND SYMPTOMS

The symptoms of cholera begin one to three days after the patient has ingested contaminated food or water. In mild cases, the patient experiences a brief episode of diarrhea. In severe cases, the symptoms progress quickly to include vomiting and a profuse watery diarrhea. The effects of *Vibrio cholerae* are caused by the production of a toxin that attacks the cells of the small intestine. Up to one liter of water and essential electrolytes such as sodium, potassium, and bicarbonate can be lost each hour.

TREATMENT AND THERAPY

The patient with cholera must be treated quickly with fluid and electrolyte replacement. A solution of salts, bicarbonate, and sugar in water can be given orally or intravenously. Antibiotic treatment shortens the duration of the disease. Without treatment, death can occur within twenty-four hours, and the death rate has exceeded 60 percent in some epidemics. With treatment, however, the death rate is less than 1 percent. A patient who recovers from cholera has some immunity in subsequent epidemics.

PERSPECTIVE AND PROSPECTS

The disease is often called Asiatic cholera because it was first reported in India. As travel increased, cholera spread to other areas of the world. During one epidemic in 1854, British physician John Snow systematically mapped the cases of cholera in London and determined that a single water pump was the source of the epidemic. Robert Koch discovered *Vibrio cholerae* as the cause of the disease in 1884. It was also determined that drinking water contaminated by human waste was the most common source of the disease. Modern sewer and water purification systems have virtually eliminated cholera in developed areas of the world.

Epidemics are still possible, especially when sanitary systems break down. In the early 1990's, an epidemic occurred in seven South American countries, resulting in more than 342,000 cases and 3,600 deaths. *Vibrio cholerae* occurs naturally in the Gulf of Mexico, and each year several cases in the United States result from eating shellfish taken from those waters. To avoid becoming ill, travelers to areas where cholera occurs are warned to eat only cooked food and drink only sterilized beverages. —*Edith K. Wallace, Ph.D.*
See also Bacterial infections; Bacteriology; Diarrhea and dysentery; Environmental health;

FOR FURTHER INFORMATION:
Barua, Dhiman, and William B. Greenough III, eds. *Cholera*. New York: Plenum Medical, 1992.
Berkow, Robert, ed. "Cholera." In *The Merck Manual of Diagnosis and Therapy*. 16th ed. Rahway, N.J.: Merck Sharp & Dohme Research Laboratories, 1992.

Jensen, Marcus M., and Donald N. Wright. *Introduction to Microbiology for the Health Sciences*. 3d ed. Englewood Cliffs, N.J.: Prentice Hall, 1993.

McNeill, William H. *Plagues and Peoples*. Garden City, N.Y.: Anchor Press, 1976.

CHOLESTEROL

BIOLOGY

ANATOMY OR SYSTEM AFFECTED: Blood vessels, cells, circulatory system, gastrointestinal system

SPECIALTIES AND RELATED FIELDS: Biochemistry, cytology, family practice, internal medicine, nutrition, preventive medicine, vascular medicine

DEFINITION: A lipid substance that is a structural component of cell membranes and which makes up the surface of lipoproteins.

KEY TERMS:

cholesterol: a lipid substance that is a component of cell membranes and the surface of circulating lipoproteins

cholesteryl ester: cholesterol linked to a fatty acid; it is stored in lipid droplets in the cytoplasm of cells and circulates in the core of lipoproteins

lipids: substances that are poorly soluble in water; in animal tissues, the principal lipids are triglycerides (fat), phospholipids, cholesterol, and cholesteryl esters

lipoproteins: lipid aggregates that transport fat and cholesteryl esters in the circulation; associated apolipoproteins determine how rapidly they are taken up by the liver or other tissues

sterols: a class of chemically related lipids; cholesterol is the principal sterol in vertebrates, but in plants its functions are served by related substances

STRUCTURE AND FUNCTIONS

Living cells are bounded by a cell membrane composed of a double layer of phospholipid, associated with and traversed by proteins that have catalytic, transportation, and signaling functions. Variable amounts of sterol are interspersed among the molecules of phospholipid in each membrane layer. Sterols are essential components in the membranes of fungal, plant, and animal cells (but not in bacteria). In vertebrates, the predominant sterol is cholesterol. There is little or no cholesterol in plant cell membranes; its place is taken by chemically related substances, chiefly sitosterol. This fact is of nutritional significance; only animal products add cholesterol to the diet.

In mammals, cholesterol is the precursor of steroid hormones, which are essential for mineral balance, adjustment of the body to stress, and normal reproductive function. It is also the precursor of bile acids, which are required for the absorption of dietary lipids. Bile acids play a role in cholesterol balance, since their formation and secretion by the liver, along with some free cholesterol, is the only significant pathway for removal of cholesterol from the body.

Cholesterol itself is required for normal functioning of the mammalian cell membrane. Cholesterol alters the membrane's fluidity—the ease with which proteins embedded in the membrane can move about and interact with one another—and also affects the activity of enzymes and transport proteins embedded in the membrane. Cultured cells that are prevented from making their own cholesterol will not grow unless it is provided in the medium.

Free cholesterol is confined to cellular membranes. Cholesterol content is highest (about one molecule of cholesterol for every one or two molecules of phospholipid) in the outer cell membrane that forms the boundary between a cell and its environment. It is much lower in intracellular membranes. Although cholesterol synthesis is completed within the endoplasmic reticulum, the ration of cholesterol to phospholipid in this membrane is less than one to twenty. In a typical cell, it is estimated that between 80 and 90 percent of the total free cholesterol is located in the outer cell membrane.

Cholesterol in excess of normal proportions is coupled (esterified) to long-chain fatty acids. The resulting cholesteryl ester accumulates, along with triglyceride, in lipid droplets in the cytoplasm. The activity of the enzyme catalyzing this esterification is increased when cholesterol is imported into the cell in excess of its needs. The ability to esterify and sequester cholesterol defends the cell against excessive membrane concentration of the free sterol.

Free cholesterol and cholesteryl ester are carried in plasma in lipoproteins. Lipoproteins are aggregates of several thousand molecules of lipid and one or more molecules of specific proteins (apolipoproteins). Each lipoprotein particle consists of a core of triglyceride and cholesteryl ester surrounded by a single layer of phospholipid and free cholesterol. The apolipoproteins are embedded in the surface of the particle. Liproproteins differ in size and relative lipid composition. In humans, about two-thirds of circulating cholesterol is contained in low-density lipoprotein (LDL), a core of cholesteryl ester with a single molecule of apolipoprotein B on the surface. LDL transports cholesterol from the liver to peripheral tissues. Most of the remaining circulating cholesterol is carried in high-density lipoprotein (HDL), which transports cholesterol from peripheral tissues back to the liver for disposal. Under normal conditions, LDL is the principal source of exogenous cholesterol available to a cell.

Uptake of LDL is mediated by a specific protein on the cell's surface, the LDL receptor, which is concentrated in pockets in the cell membrane termed coated pits. LDL receptors bind apolipoprotein B and particles such as LDL that contain this protein. Coated pits continually pinch off to form sealed vesicles (endosomes) inside the cell. At the same time, new coated pits form on the cell surface. When a coated pit pinches off, it carries with it LDL receptors and associated LDL. The fluid within the endosome is acidified, which causes LDL to dissociate from its receptor and float free. The LDL is transferred to lysosomes, where cholesteryl ester is cleaved to liberate cholesterol; along with the free cholesterol that formed part of the LDL surface, this liberated cholesterol is now available for use within the cell. The LDL receptor is returned to the cell surface, where it can again become associated with a coated pit and participate in a new round of LDL uptake.

The rate at which LDL is removed from the circulation depends on the concentration of LDL receptors in cells of the liver and other tissues. (Although there are other mechanisms for removing LDL, these are less efficient than uptake via the LDL receptor.) This process is subject to feedback regulation. When a cell contains an adequate supply of cholesterol, the synthesis of new LDL receptors is inhibited. This inhibition occurs at the transcriptional level: The rate at which the gene for the LDL receptor is copied into messenger ribonucleic acid (mRNA) is reduced. With less mRNA for this protein reaching the cytoplasm, the rate at which new copies of the protein are made also falls. Following normal turnover of existing receptors, the concentration of LDL receptors at the cell surface declines and the uptake of cholesterol is accordingly reduced.

The gene for the LDL receptor contains short stretches of deoxyribonucleic acid (DNA), termed sterol response elements (SREs), that make transcription sensitive to cholesterol-induced "down-regulation." These can be spliced out and inserted into another gene that codes for a bacterial protein. The foreign gene can be inserted into a mammalian cell, which will then begin to produce the corresponding protein. If the foreign gene does not contain an SRE, the rate of synthesis of the coded protein is unaffected by the cholesterol content of the recipient cell. When an SRE has been inserted into the gene in an appropriate location, however, excess cholesterol down-regulates transcription of the foreign gene just as it does that for the LDL receptor.

The signal that causes down-regulation of the cholesterol receptor has not been clearly identified. It is possible that an internal "regulatory" pool of cholesterol—such as the cholesterol content of certain internal membranes or the concentration of individual cholesterol molecules bound to some cytoplasmic protein carrier—is responsible. Some evidence, however, points to oxysterol analogs of cholesterol, rather than to cholesterol itself, as mediators of down-regulation. These analogs arise as minor metabolites of cholesterol and as intermediates and by-products of cholesterol synthesis. They are much more potent than cholesterol itself in inhibiting the synthesis of LDL receptors. A cytoplasmic oxysterol-binding protein has been identified whose affinity for different oxysterols parallels their relative potency in down-regulating the transcription of LDL receptor genes.

Mammalian cells also have the capacity to synthesize their own cholesterol. The enzymes catalyzing the successive reactions along this pathway are located in the cytoplasm and in the membranes of the endoplasmic reticulum.

The starting material from which cholesterol is made is acetic acid in the form of acetyl-coenzyme A (acetyl-CoA). This material is generated in mitochondria as an intermediate in the oxidation of glucose and of fatty acids. To be utilized for synthesis of cholesterol, it must first be transported from the mitochondria to the cytoplasm; a specific shuttle exists for this purpose. The synthesis of fatty acids from acetyl-CoA also takes place in the cytoplasm, and more of the translocated precursor is used for this purpose than to make cholesterol.

An early step on the pathway to cholesterol is the reduction of hydroxymethylglutaryl-coenzyme A (HMG-CoA) to mevalonic acid, catalyzed by HMG-CoA reductase. The enzymatic capacity to catalyze this reaction is substantially lower than that for other steps on the pathway, so that the overall rate of cholesterol synthesis is largely determined by the activity of this enzyme. Both amount and activity are regulated to match the rates of cholesterol synthesis to the needs of the cell. When the cell has adequate supplies of cholesterol, HMG-CoA reductase activity is low and, simultaneously, uptake via the LDL receptor is reduced. Conversely, when more cholesterol is needed, HMG-CoA reductase activity and overall cholesterol synthesis is increased, as is expression of the LDL receptor and the uptake of cholesterol.

HMG-CoA reductase activity is regulated at several points, including transcription of the gene, efficiency with which its mRNA is translated into protein, turnover of the enzyme protein, and inactivation by chemical modification. Regulation of the transcription of the HMG-CoA reductase gene and regulation of the LDL receptor gene appear to have the same fundamental mechanism. The gene for HMG-CoA reductase contains an SRE similar in sequence to those in the gene for the LDL receptor. Oxysterols that repress transcription of the LDL receptor exert the same effect on transcription of the gene for HMG-CoA reductase, and with the same relative potency. Mutant cells that have lost the capacity to respond to oxysterols by repressing the synthesis of LDL receptors also fail to respond by repressing the synthesis of HMG-CoA reductase.

Excess cholesterol also increases the rate at which HMG-CoA reductase is broken down. This might be a response to changes in cholesterol concentration in the internal membranes in which HMG-CoA reductase is embedded. When the gene for HMG-CoA reductase is altered to remove the sequences that anchor it to the membrane and the altered gene is inserted into a recipient cell, the mutant protein is located unattached in the cytoplasm. In contrast to the native enzyme, the rate of turnover of the altered gene product is not affected by the cholesterol content of the recipient cell.

Phosphorylation (attachment of a phosphate to specific amino acid residues) of HMG-CoA reductase is a third mechanism by which the synthesis of cholesterol is altered. This is best documented in the liver (which is also the principal site within the body for the synthesis of cholesterol). Liver cells contain an enzyme that phosphorylates and inactivates HMG-CoA reductase; the same enzyme also phosphorylates and inactivates the enzyme catalyzing the rate-determining step in the synthesis of fatty acids, acetyl-CoA carboxylase. The phosphorylation of both enzymes is promoted, and the synthesis of fatty acids and cholesterol is correspondingly inhibited, under fasting conditions. In the fed state, the reverse is true. These changes appear to be a response to circulating levels of the hormone insulin.

Most of the mevalonic acid that is produced by HMG-CoA reductase activity is converted to cholesterol. Since its formation is the rate-determining step on the pathway, the addition of mevalonic acid itself to the cell results in much higher rates of cholesterol synthesis than can be achieved with acetyl-CoA as starting material. Moreover, the synthesis of cholesterol from mevalonic acid is not controlled by feedback inhibition. Under these circumstances, expression of HMG-CoA reductase and expression of the LDL receptor are maximally repressed.

Mevalonic acid is also the precursor of other substances needed by the cell. These include dolichol (a coenzyme needed for the addition of carbohydrate residues to proteins), ubiquinone (a participant in electron transport reactions in mitochondria), and isoprenyl side chains that are attached to specific proteins. Although their synthesis consumes only a minor portion of the mevalonic acid produced by HMG-CoA reductase, these substances are essential to normal cell function. When HMG-CoA reductase is inhibited by lovastatin, a drug that competes with the substrate HMG-CoA for binding to the enzyme, cell growth is inhibited even when supplies of cholesterol in the medium are adequate. Resumption of cell growth requires the addition of small amounts of mevalonic acid as well as cholesterol. Mutant cell lines have been obtained that, even without lovastatin, are unable to grow unless mevalonic acid is present. The requirements of these cells can be met with a large amount of mevalonic acid in the medium or with a small amount of mevalonic acid plus a large amount of cholesterol.

The multiple roles of mevalonic acid are also reflected in the way that HMG-CoA reductase activity is regulated. Although transcription of the HMG-CoA reductase gene is reduced when cholesterol levels in the cell are high, some transcription continues to allow enough mevalonic acid to be produced to meet other needs of the cell. Adding small amounts of mevalonic acid further decreases the synthesis of HMG-CoA reductase by decreasing the rate at which its mRNA is translated into protein. In contrast, expression of the LDL receptor is not under dual regulation; maximal suppression can be obtained with cholesterol alone.

DISORDERS AND DISEASES

Excessive levels of LDL cholesterol are associated with an increased risk of coronary heart disease and stroke. Ef-

forts to reduce LDL cholesterol through changes in diet or through drugs take advantage of what is known about cholesterol balance in individual cells and in the body as a whole. The latter is determined by three factors: the dietary intake of cholesterol, the rate of cholesterol synthesis within the body (principally by the liver), and the rate of cholesterol disposal (also principally by the liver, through secretion of free sterol into the bile and by the conversion of cholesterol to bile acids). Accordingly, levels of LDL cholesterol can be diminished by limiting the intake and synthesis of new cholesterol, reducing cholesterol secretion by the liver (in the form of an LDL precursor particle), promoting LDL uptake by the liver (mediated by the LDL receptor), and increasing the formation and secretion of bile acids and free cholesterol.

The body can meet its need for cholesterol through synthesis; there is no dietary requirement. Cholesterol deficiency does not arise in humans even on a purely vegetarian (cholesterol-free) diet. The average Western diet, rich in meat and dairy products, contains between 250 to 500 milligrams of cholesterol per day. Small amounts of cholesterol in the diet are fairly well absorbed, but efficiency declines with larger quantities; on average, about half of the cholesterol consumed per day is assimilated. Absorption of cholesterol and other lipids in the small intestine requires the presence of bile acids. These mix with cholesterol and partially degraded dietary triglyceride to form small droplets that facilitate the absorption of lipids by the cells lining the small intestine. In the process, most of the bile acid (as well as cholesterol secreted in the bile) is reabsorbed and returned to the liver. The absorbed cholesterol is esterified and secreted into the lymph, along with triglyceride, in the core of chylomicrons. These large lipoproteins are reduced in size by removal of triglyceride in capillary beds, and the remnants, containing all the original cholesteryl ester, are taken up by the liver. Thus, the cholesterol absorbed in the intestine passes initially to the liver.

The liver, along with the small intestine, is also the most important site for cholesterol synthesis within the body. As explained above, hepatic synthesis of cholesterol is under feedback control. HMG-CoA reductase activity and cholesterol synthesis are suppressed when large amounts of dietary cholesterol reach the liver and are augmented when the diet is cholesterol-free. Drugs such as lovastatin that inhibit HMG-CoA reductase are useful in reducing cholesterol levels in the circulation, since they limit the ability of the liver to respond by making more cholesterol when the dietary intake is reduced.

Cholesterol within the liver may be incorporated into very low-density lipoprotein (VLDL) and secreted into the circulation. VLDL is secreted primarily to transport triglyceride to other tissues for use as a metabolic fuel or for storage. After serving this function, most of the VLDL remnants return to the liver. Those that escape hepatic reabsorption are transformed in the circulation into LDL. LDL is also taken up by the liver (and elsewhere), but at a much slower rate than VLDL remnant particles, so that this lipoprotein accumulates in the circulation. It is deposition of LDL in the lining of blood vessels that initiates the formation of atherosclerotic plaques—the beginning of atherosclerotic disease. Since cholesterol is required for the secretion of VLDL, HMG-CoA reductase inhibitors that cause a partial depletion of cholesterol in liver cells reduce the rate at which it enters the bloodstream. By the same means, they also increase expression of LDL receptors in liver cells, which results in a more rapid removal of LDL from the circulation. Both mechanisms reduce circulating levels of LDL cholesterol.

Cholesterol in the liver may also be converted to bile acids and secreted in the bile. Although most of the secreted bile acid comes back to the liver, some escapes reabsorption in the small intestine. The bile acid that is lost must be replaced by the metabolization of more cholesterol. Bile acid sequestrants such as cholestyramine are also used to reduce circulating cholesterol. They act by forming complexes with bile acids in the small intestine and interfere with their reabsorption. A larger fraction of the secreted bile acid is thus lost by excretion, and the rate of conversion of cholesterol to bile acid in the liver is correspondingly increased.

The liver secretes a large amount of free cholesterol into the bile. Most of this biliary cholesterol is reabsorbed and returned to the liver. Since bile acids are required for the intestinal uptake of cholesterol, a second beneficial action of bile acid sequestrants is to increase the fraction of biliary cholesterol that escapes reabsorption and is excreted. The combination of bile acid sequestrant and HMG-CoA reductase inhibitor is especially effective in lowering blood levels of LDL cholesterol by limiting the uptake of cholesterol from the diet, limiting the synthesis of cholesterol in the liver, increasing the clearance of cholesterol from the blood by the liver, and increasing the conversion of hepatic cholesterol to bile acids.

Other drugs used to reduce circulating LDL cholesterol levels include nicotinic acid, fibiric acid derivatives, and probucol. Nicotinic acid (niacin) is also a vitamin, but the amounts required to affect plasma cholesterol levels are far in excess of the daily requirement for this compound as an essential nutrient. At these pharmacologic doses, side effects such as itching, facial flushing, and gastric distress are common. Nicotinic acid decreases the formation of VLDL triglyceride in the liver and therefore reduces the formation of LDL; it also promotes the uptake of LDL through LDL receptors and increases the concentration of HDL cholesterol (cholesterol being returned to the liver for disposal). The underlying mechanisms for these actions have not been determined. Fibric acid derivatives, such as gemfibrazole, also reduce VLDL secretion and promote LDL uptake by the liver; again the mechanism of drug ac-

tion is uncertain. Probucol acts primarily to prevent chemical modification of LDL in the circulation that makes it more likely to be deposited in the walls of blood vessels.

Although high circulating levels of LDL cholesterol call for drug intervention, the risk of atherosclerotic disease can be reduced in most adults by attention to the dietary factors that affect cholesterol balance. Dietary studies have had a controversial history because of frequently contradictory findings. A few principles are, however, well supported by the data. First, eliminating cholesterol from the diet, with no other intervention, produces a significant drop in the levels of cholesterol in circulating LDL. Second, intake of calories beyond actual energy needs raises serum cholesterol. Excess fuel is stored as triglycerides, which to a large extent are formed in the liver and exported in VLDL. Since VLDL contains cholesterol, and since it is the precursor of LDL, high rates of triglyceride formation in the liver promote the accumulation of cholesterol in plasma LDL—which is especially likely to occur if the calories are ingested in the form of triglyceride. Not only does this increase the requirement for the liver to secret VLDL, but also the fatty acids derived from triglyceride stimulate cholesterol synthesis. Third, saturated fatty acids have the strongest tendency to elevate plasma cholesterol levels. This is the case even when these fatty acids are consumed as vegetable oils (such as palm oil and coconut oil) unaccompanied by cholesterol. The basis for this effect is not well understood but appears to result from decreased expression of LDL receptors in the liver. The American Heart Association recommends that not more than 200 milligrams per day of cholesterol be consumed in a diet which is matched to caloric need and in which not more than 30 percent of calories are consumed as fat (and not more than 10 percent as saturated fat).

PERSPECTIVE AND PROSPECTS

The average adult body contains about 150 grams of cholesterol. Less than 5 percent of this cholesterol is in circulating lipoproteins or trapped in atherosclerotic lesions. The remainder performs essential functions as a structural component of membranes and as the precursor of other vital substances. Although researchers have learned much about the subcellular distribution, the pathway for biosynthesis, and the mechanisms for transport of cholesterol, important questions remain. It is not known how cholesterol is transported within the cell or what determines its relative distribution among different cellular membranes. It is not known what signals suppress the synthesis of HMG-CoA reductase and LDL receptors or how the message is transmitted to the nucleus to diminish transcription of these genes. Some product of mevalonic acid metabolism other than cholesterol also regulates the expression of HMG-CoA reductase, but this factor has not yet been identified. It is not known why cholesterol is an absolute requirement for functioning of mammalian cell membranes. It is not known what determines the fraction of dietary cholesterol that is absorbed across the intestinal lining. Finally, there is much to learn about factors that regulate the secretion and reuptake of lipoproteins by the liver and that control the return to the liver of cholesterol in HDL.

These questions are of practical as well as academic interest. Coronary heart disease and other complications of atherosclerosis are the leading causes of death in the United States. Controlling and reversing this process is a serious medical challenge. While other factors such as hypertension, smoking, and diabetes mellitus contribute to the risk of atherosclerosis, reducing the level of cholesterol that circulates as a component of LDL and increasing the level transported in HDL have been shown to provide significant protection. Knowledge of how cholesterol is normally produced and assimilated has contributed to the design of drugs that reduce circulating levels by interfering with the absorption and synthesis of cholesterol and promoting its metabolism and excretion. This field of investigation continues to be a major concern of both basic and pharmaceutical scientists. —*Lauren M. Cagen, Ph.D.*

See also Arteriosclerosis; Blood and blood components; Blood testing; Cells; Digestion; Food biochemistry; Heart disease; Hypercholesterolemia; Hyperlipidemia; Metabolism; Nutrition; Preventive medicine; Strokes and TIAs.

FOR FURTHER INFORMATION:

Brown, Michael S., and Joseph L. Goldstein. "How LDL Receptors Influence Cholesterol and Atherosclerosis." *Scientific American* 251 (November, 1984): 58-66. The authors received the 1985 Nobel Prize in Physiology or Medicine for their pioneering studies of the LDL receptor and its role in the cellular uptake of cholesterol. Although more has been learned since the publication of this article, much of it as a result of the authors' further investigations. This article remains an excellent introduction to the subject.

_____. "A Receptor-Mediated Pathway for Cholesterol Homeostasis." *Science* 232 (April 4, 1986): 34-47. A more complete description of the subject discussed by the authors in their article in *Scientific American* (above).

Dietschy, John M. "Physiology in Medicine: LDL Cholesterol: Its Regulation and Manipulation." *Hospital Practice* 25 (June 15, 1990): 67-78. An excellent nontechnical introduction to the subject of cholesterol balance and its regulation by another major contributor to the field. The article discusses the effect of diet and drug interventions.

Goldstein, Joseph L., and Michael S. Brown. "Regulation of the Mevalonate Pathway." *Nature* 343 (February 1, 1990): 425-430. This article reviews the regulation of cholesterol synthesis. It is a lucid and brief summary, although written at a more advanced level than the authors' article in *Scientific American* (above).

Grundy, Scott M. *Cholesterol and Atherosclerosis*. Philadelphia: J. P. Lippincott, 1990. The author provides a general overview of cholesterol balance, elevated plasma cholesterol, and its management by diet and drugs. Although intended for physicians, the book is written in a simple and direct style and is profusely illustrated. The diagrams are exceptionally clear and cover systematically all the major points in the text.

Yeagle, Philip L. *Understanding Your Cholesterol*. San Diego: Academic Press, 1991. This popular work explains cholesterol and the risk factors that can lead to atherosclerosis. Includes a bibliography.

CHORIONIC VILLUS SAMPLING
PROCEDURE

ANATOMY OR SYSTEM AFFECTED: Reproductive system, uterus

SPECIALTIES AND RELATED FIELDS: Embryology, genetics, obstetrics, perinatology

DEFINITION: The collection of a small sample of chorionic villi tissue from a fetus, which is examined for genetic and chromosomal abnormalities.

INDICATIONS AND PROCEDURES

Chorionic villus sampling can be performed between the tenth and twelfth weeks of pregnancy to detect genetic and chromosomal abnormalities. The procedure is recommended when there is increased risk of genetic disorders in the fetus such as Down syndrome, sickle-cell anemia, and muscular dystrophy.

Chorionic villus sampling involves collecting a small sample of the chorionic villi, the fingerlike projections on the developing placenta that delivers food and oxygen to the fetus. A sample of chorionic villi can be obtained either by inserting a needle through the abdomen or by entering the cervix with a small flexible catheter through the vagina. The choice of approach depends on the position of the placenta. Ultrasound is used to locate the fetus and the placenta and its villi.

A 10 to 25 milligram sample is collected using a syringe, which is then purified and sometimes cultured. Since the chorionic villi originate from the same cell as the fetus, they normally have the same genetics. Results are available within days.

USES AND COMPLICATIONS

Along with exposing genetic and chromosomal disorders, chorionic villus sampling can be used to determine the sex of the embryo. Testing can be done early in the pregnancy. Therefore, if the woman should choose to terminate her pregnancy, an easier first-trimester abortion can be performed. If the results from the test are favorable, the parents have an early peace of mind.

Possible complications from chorionic villus sampling include vaginal bleeding and cramping. More serious risks involve spontaneous abortion and even possible fetal injury. The rate of miscarriage is about 1 percent higher with chorionic villus sampling.

Some studies suggest that chorionic villus sampling itself may cause some birth defects; others do not. Also, the procedure can be inaccurate. Abnormalities may occur in some placental cells but not in the fetus. This might lead to aborting a healthy fetus. With the guidance of a physician, the risks and benefits should be compared with other available procedures. —*Paul R. Boehlke, Ph.D., and Pavel Svilenov*

See also Abortion; Amniocentesis; Birth defects; Down syndrome; Embryology; Genetic counseling; Genetic diseases; Miscarriage; Muscular dystrophy; Obstetrics; Perinatology; Pregnancy and gestation; Reproductive system; Sickle-cell anemia; Ultrasonography.

CHROMOSOMAL ABNORMALITIES. *See* BIRTH DEFECTS; GENETIC DISEASES.

CHRONIC FATIGUE SYNDROME
DISEASE/DISORDER
ANATOMY OR SYSTEM AFFECTED: Immune system, muscles, musculoskeletal system, psychic-emotional system

SPECIALTIES AND RELATED FIELDS: Family physicians, hematologists, immunologists, internists, psychiatrists

DEFINITION: Chronic fatigue syndrome is a multifaceted disease state characterized by debilitating fatigue.

KEY TERMS:

adenopathy: the enlargement of any gland (often the lymph gland)

Burkitt's lymphoma: a tumor in the lower jaw of children that is believed to be caused by the Epstein-Barr virus, usually occurring in Africa

cell-mediated immune response: an immune response that involves cells rather than antibodies, particularly T lymphocytes rather than B lymphocytes

delayed hypersensitivity: an abnormal cell-mediated immune reaction caused by an exogenous agent and resulting in tissue destruction

infectious mononucleosis: acute self-limiting infection of lymphocytes by the Epstein-Barr virus

interleuken II: a protein messenger that regulates T cell activity and differentiation during the immune response

lymphocytes: agranular leukocytes that differentiate into B lymphocytes and T lymphocytes and play a fundamental role in the immune response

polymerase chain reaction: a laboratory method used to increase the amount of DNA found in small quantities

Spumavirus: a virus found in humans, primates, and cats that gives a foamy appearance to the lymphocyte tissue culture

suppressor T cell: a type of T lymphocyte that is believed to modulate the immune response

CAUSES AND SYMPTOMS
Chronic fatigue syndrome is a heterogenous disease state that has been difficult to define, diagnose, and treat because of poorly understood cause-and-effect relationships. The

disease can be best described in terms of long-lasting and debilitating fatigue, the etiology of which has been linked to such external factors as microbial agents, stress, and lifestyle as well as such internal factors as genetic makeup and the body's immune response. The fact that it is a physical disease with psychological components has also caused confusion in the medical community.

Among the many names that have been used for the disease, the three that demonstrate the many factors that contribute to chronic fatigue syndrome are chronic Epstein-Barr virus syndrome, chronic fatigue immune dysfunction syndrome, and "Yuppie flu." Because of the marked immunological aspects of the disease and the fact that different viruses have been found in patients with chronic fatigue, the disease is referred to as chronic fatigue immune dysfunction syndrome by many involved in the study. The Centers for Disease Control (CDC) continues to refer to it as chronic fatigue syndrome (CFS).

Although the disease is not specific by race, sex, or age group, there is demographic evidence that young white females make up two-thirds of the known cases. It is estimated by the CDC that between 1 and 10 of every 10,000 people in the United States have CFS. The disease has also been identified as a problem in Europe and Australia.

CFS can manifest itself in acute and chronic phases, although some patients do not remember an acute phase presentation. Acute phase symptoms are general and flulike, with a low-grade fever, sore throat, headache, muscle pain, painful lymph nodes, and overall fatigue. Unlike with a bout of influenza, the symptoms do not subside with time, instead intensifying into a chronic phase. The fatigue can become disabling, with severe muscle and joint pain, swollen and painful lymph nodes, and the inability to develop proper sleep patterns. Some researchers blame psychological and emotional stress, with a viral infection having triggered the initial acute phase. Although the psychological description does not fit all cases, problems of concentration, attention, and depression have been implicated to the point that researchers recognize both psychological and physical components. The working definition from both a research and a clinical perspective requires that the fatigue cause at least 50 percent incapacitation and last at least six months. The ineffectiveness of treatment, compounded by the inability to provide a concrete diagnosis, further complicates the psychological aspects of the disease for the patient.

Although the environment provides an array of agents that could trigger the physical condition of CFS, the hypothesis for a viral cause is supported by the flulike symptoms, occasional clustering of cases, and the presence of antiviral antibodies in the patient's serum. The involvement of the Epstein-Barr virus in CFS seems likely because of its role as the etiological agent of mononucleosis and Burkitt's lymphoma, which are similar diseases. In both of these diseases, the Epstein-Barr virus has a unique and harmful effect on the immune system because it directly invades B lymphocytes, the antibody-producing cells of the body, using them to grow new virus particles while disrupting the proper functioning of the immune system. Like CFS, mononucleosis is characterized by flulike symptoms and fatigue, but the disease is self-limiting and the patient eventually recovers.

Despite this seeming difference in outcome, the Epstein-Barr virus can cause a chronic condition. The viruses that infect humans can become dormant within the cells that they infect. The nucleic acid of a virus can become incorporated into the DNA of its host cell, and the body no longer shows physical signs of their presence. A virus can become active at times of physical or emotional stress and can once again trigger the physical symptoms of disease. For example, herpes simplex virus 1 remains dormant in its host cell but periodically, in response to environmental factors, causes a cold sore lesion.

Some patients with CFS have also been infected with two retroviruses, human T-cell lymphotropic virus type II (HTLV-II) and a Spumavirus. Both are related to the human immunodeficiency virus (HIV), the causative agent of acquired immunodeficiency syndrome (AIDS). Retrovirus genes are made of ribonucleic acid (RNA) rather than deoxyribonucleic acid (DNA), as are the genes of herpes-type viruses such as Epstein-Barr and herpes simplex virus 1. Retroviruses must convert their RNA into complementary DNA (cDNA) when they infect a host cell in order to incorporate their genes into the host cell genes. Although the two viruses are associated with some CFS patients, diagnostic tests developed to detect their presence have not confirmed that the CFS condition depends on their presence. This same finding is true of herpesvirus 6 and other viruses. Although viruses may play a role in CFS, they are not the only factors involved and are not substantive evidence to define a clinical or research case.

Immunological dysfunction has been observed in CFS patients because they demonstrate increased allergic sensitivity to skin tests when compared to normal individuals. Cells and cellular chemicals directly involved with protective immunity and the regulation of the immune response have been found in these patients in abnormal concentrations. For example, they have abnormal numbers of the natural killer cells and suppressor T cells that are essential to cell-mediated immunity. Cellular chemicals such as gamma interferon and interleuken II that regulate the activities of the cells in the cell-mediated and humeral immune responses are seen in abnormal concentrations in some CFS patients. Infectious agents, bacteria, viruses, yeasts, parasites, and even cancer cells are eliminated from the body when humeral and cell-mediated immune systems are operating properly. When the immune system is not working properly, however, not only is the body more susceptible to a variety of infectious agents but the immune system can actually begin to destroy normal body tissues, such as the thyroid gland and other vital organs, as well. Such disease states are referred to as autoimmune diseases. Allergic reactions are also examples of uncontrolled immune responses. The component immune dysfunction of CFS is thought to be significant enough for some researchers to recommend that new and worsening allergies be added as minor criteria to the case definition for the disease.

The psychological and emotional aspects of CFS are also in question. Some studies indicate that the brain is physically affected by inflammation and hormonal changes. Other studies demonstrate that some of the known viral infective agents can have neurological effects. Psychiatric studies give ample evidence that depression, memory loss, and concentration are significant problems for some CFS patients. The extent to which stress is a factor in the disease is unknown.

TREATMENT AND THERAPY

Defining and treating chronic fatigue syndrome has been difficult because it manifests itself as a systemic disease with confusing cause-and-effect relationships involving external factors such as infectious viruses, internal factors such as the immune response, and a psychological component that is difficult to assess in the light of the biological changes occurring in the body. The symptoms, provided by patient histories, physical examinations, and laboratory findings, involve neuromuscular, psychoneurological, and immunological changes that vary between patients. The variety of factors to consider has caused difficulty in establishing diagnostic criteria for primary care in a clinical setting or further definition of the disease and treatments in a research setting.

In 1988, the CDC established diagnostic criteria that are divided into two major criteria, eleven minor symptom criteria, and three minor physical criteria. The first major criterion defines chronic fatigue as lasting at least six months and causing debilitation to 50 percent of the patient's normal activity. The second major criterion requires that all other disease conditions that could fit the patient history, physical examination, and appropriate laboratory tests be ruled out. The categories of disease that might be similar to CFS are cancers, chronic degenerative disease, autoimmune disorders, microbial and parasitic disease, and chronic psychiatric disease. Combinations of some minor criteria that would fit a general flulike condition must be demonstrated.

In 1993, a meeting at the CDC attempted to evaluate what had been learned over the previous five-year period and to make recommendations regarding a case definition. It was suggested that the case definition format involve inclusion and exclusion criteria that would increase the number and range of cases being studied because of the heterogenous nature of the disease. The cases should also be subcategorized to provide a homogeneity that would allow for subgroup identification and comparison. The inclusion evidence should be simple, with a descriptive interpretation of the fatigue being essential and having objective criteria to define a 50 percent reduction of physical activity. Symptoms that are specific to unexplained fatigue should be used, while the physical exam information should not be included. It was also suggested that exclusion of any cases should involve an in-depth history (both medical and psychiatric), a physical examination, and standardized testing that would involve medical, laboratory, and psychiatric information.

Because it appears that CFS overlaps with many other medical and psychiatric conditions that can be identified and treated, there is debate as to how to interpret CFS as it relates to patient care and research. Some believe that an in-depth history is fundamental to the understanding of CFS and that CFS could be the final pathway that occurs from a variety of biological and psychosocial insults to the body.

The minor criteria used to define CFS involve both symptom and physical criteria that have not been proved adequate to validate or define the condition. In fact, the conflicting data have only served to emphasize further the clinical heterogeneity of the disease and suggest a heterogeneity of cause. Suggestions have been made to drop the concept of minor criteria, use symptoms that are specific for the unexplained fatigue, and drop all physical examination criteria. The argument for eliminating physical criteria is that more specific criteria exist for a case definition. Because physical symptoms are inconsistent or periodic, it is believed that a documented patient history would provide more case-specific information.

Although symptom criteria have widespread support in the case definition of CFS, symptoms with the greatest sensitivity and specificity are also being debated. Night sweats, cough, gastrointestinal problems, and new and worsening allergies are not presently considered and are believed by some to be more specific than fever or chills and sore throat. Others have proposed that symptoms should be reduced to chills and fever, sore throat, neck or axilla adenopathy, and sudden onset of a main symptom complex. The most prevalent symptoms are believed to be muscle weakness and pain, problems in concentration, and sleep disturbance.

The importance of the psychiatric component in CFS continues to be a problem in case definition. Some believe that the neurological component is a major criterion in case definition and that behavior symptoms, including stress and psychiatric illness, must be emphasized in clinical diagnosis as well as in therapy. It has been recommended that objective neuropsychological testing be used to determine cognitive dysfunction and depression. There is agreement that CFS patients have impaired concentration and attention, but forgetfulness and memory problems are questioned. There is also evidence that the duration and severity of myalgia are closely associated with psychological distress and that psychotherapy improves physical symptoms. Finally, it has been argued that the psychiatric component of the case definition is essential because there is evidence that the disease directly affects the brain and that CFS can cause both isolation and limitation of the patient's normal lifestyle.

Whatever the case definition, the second major criterion will be expressed in some form. Proper patient care necessitates extensive evaluation in order to identify the biological or psychological reasons for the problem. Proper CFS patient care demands the elimination of other serious disease possibilities that may appear superficially similar. Primary care physicians may find it difficult to make a diagnosis without a team of specialists in the areas of hematology, immunology, and psychiatry. Numerous laboratory tests must be made available. Although there are no specific recommended tests, those that must be performed should be tailored to specific patients and used by the team of specialists for their care.

The possibility of infectious disease, either as part of CFS (as in the case of certain viral agents) or as an autonomous infection having no relation to CFS, requires a variety of antibody tests to detect such viruses as Epstein-Barr or HIV. Skin tests such as the purified protein derivative (PPD) test for tuberculosis are used. Polymerase chain reaction and tissue culture for cytopathic effects have been developed to detect certain retroviruses for ultimate use in diagnosis at the clinical level.

The immune system is so intimately interactive with the entire body that most disease conditions are affected by or affect its function. The measure of its components provides a clue to the identity of the disease that is operating because they indicate whether normal protection activity or immune dysfunction (or a combination) is occurring in the patient.

The components of the immune system can be measured in numerous ways, from methodologies used in standard clinical laboratory procedures to research protocols used to study immune function and disease treatment. Tests are available that can measure total antibody concentration and the various subgroups IgG, IgM, IgA, IgE, IgD; cytokines such as interleuken II and gamma interferon; cellular components such as T cells and their subtypes (such as suppressor T cells and natural killer cells), and B cells.

Autoimmune diseases and allergies are immune dysfunction diseases in their own right. Because there is an immune dysfunction component to CFS, tests for these conditions are important considerations. An antinuclear antibody (ANA) test determines the presence of antibodies that attack the tissues of the patient, as in systemic lupus erythematosus. The type and extent of allergic reactions can be measured using the radioimmunosorbent (RIST) tests for total IgE concentration and radioallergosorbent (RAST) tests for IgE concentration for particular antigens.

Systemic disease states, including CFS, often involve generalized inflammation that is considered part of the body's protective response. While inflammation is important to the elimination of various infective agents, it is also involved in neurological and muscle tissue damage. C-reactive protein (CRP) and the erythrocyte sedimentation rate (ESR) tests measure the intensity of the inflammatory response. A variety of other tests provide information that indicates the extent of muscle, liver, thyroid, and other vital organ damage.

Although a diagnosis can be made for CFS, there is no standard treatment. Clinical treatment essentially takes the form of alleviating the symptoms. Antidepressants such as doxepin (Sinequan) are useful in the treatment of depression and are also used to control muscle pain, lethargy, and sleeping problems. Nonsteroidal anti-inflammatory drugs (NSAIDs) provide relief for headache and muscle pain. Two drugs that have demonstrated antiviral activities are acyclovir and ampligen; ampligen can also modulate the immune response.

An example of research to develop therapies that might alleviate other symptoms of CFS involves the treatment of a number of patients with dialyzable leukocyte extract and psychologic treatment in the form of cognitive-behavioral therapy. The patients' cell-mediated immune response after therapy was evaluated by peripheral blood T cell subset analysis and delayed hypersensitivity skin testing. Psychologic analysis was performed using numerous cognitive tests. Both therapies proved to be inconclusive.

Because of the systemic nature of the disease, including its psychoneurological component, consideration must be given to holistic medical treatment. Any treatment protocol must be able to address the interactive factors of CFS that are still being defined in terms of cause and effect. Some researchers believe that therapeutic treatment should comprise diet, exercise, vitamins, and homeopathic medicine. They further believe that psychoemotional treatment should allow patients to be responsible for their own recovery and help them to develop a personal lifestyle that provides general good health.

PERSPECTIVE AND PROSPECTS

It is believed that chronic fatigue syndrome is not a new phenomenon but a disease condition that is in the process of being defined. For several centuries, the medical community has described a disease condition involving fatigue, with fever, neuromuscular, and brain involvement. The condition was called little fever, vapors, neurasthenia or nervous exhaustion, and benign myalgic encephalomyelitis. The infectious nature of the condition resulted in names such as chronic brucellosis, chronic Epstein-Barr virus infection, chronic candidiasis, and postviral fatigue syndrome.

Since being linked with the Epstein-Barr virus, CFS has been the subject of many studies that support its definition as a heterogenous illness. The case definition provided by the CDC in 1988 has allowed the disease to be diagnosed and treated at the clinical level and to be identified and compared at the research level. The disease state has proven

to be elusive, however, and the case definition too complex and open to interpretation. It is believed that the refinement of the case definition proposed by the CDC in 1993 will promote greater understanding of the problem at both clinical and research levels, particularly because more objective criteria to validate and define CFS have not emerged.

As indicated by its very definition, CFS has presented the health care system with a challenge whereby the primary care physician receives information provided by a team of specialists. Continued technological advances and research into both the immune system and the nature of viral infection will provide new insights into more traditional treatment protocols. Nevertheless, the multicausal nature of CFS may require holistic medical treatment that can only be provided by personalized patient care. The neuropsychological components of the disease, as well as evidence demonstrating intimate ties between these components and the immune system, require a personal, active approach by the patient to achieving a healthy state. CFS provides a challenge to the patient to adapt to a personal lifestyle that will create a healthy mind and body.

CFS must also be considered in terms of the society in which it is manifest as a serious and genuine illness. Medical treatment and diagnostic testing can be costly as well as useless, particularly as the health care community continues to refine its understanding of the condition. Patients must remain vigilant regarding phony or trendy treatments that have no correlation to acceptable research findings; such treatments not only can be expensive but also could lead to deteriorating health. Furthermore, the definition and diagnosis of CFS have legal ramifications that have an impact on insurance and other forms of medical care compensation.   —*Patrick J. DeLuca, Ph.D.*

See also Fatigue; Immune system; Immunology; Mononucleosis; Stress.

FOR FURTHER INFORMATION:

Collinge, William. *Recovering from Chronic Fatigue Syndrome: A Guide to Self-Empowerment.* New York: Body Press/Perigee, 1993. An excellent book written for the general public that speculates on the multifaceted nature of the disease. Offers information for those who have CFS, such as suggested diets and treatments. Also provides addresses for support groups.

Holmes, Gary P., et al. "Chronic Fatigue Syndrome: A Working Case Definition." *Annals of Internal Medicine* 108, no. 3 (March, 1988): 387-389. An article of historical significance that gave credibility to the disease. Served as a starting point for organized data collecting about CFS in both research and clinical settings.

National Institutes of Health. *Chronic Fatigue Syndrome: Information for Physicians.* Bethesda, Md.: Author, 1997. A brief, concise description of what is known about CFS. Although printed for physicians, this pamphlet can be read and understood by nonspecialists.

Stoff, Jesse A., and Charles Pellegrino. *Chronic Fatigue Syndrome*. Rev. ed. New York: HarperPerennial, 1992. An excellent book describing the biological aspects of the disease in layperson's terms. Essential reading for anyone suffering from the disease because of its diary-like accounts, anecdotal data, emphasis on holistic treatment, and inspirational tone.

Yehuda, Shlomo, and David I. Mostofsky, eds. *Chronic Fatigue Syndrome*. New York: Plenum Press, 1997. Provides an updated description of CFS, the medical conditions from which it must be distinguished, and current treatment approaches.

CHRONOBIOLOGY

SPECIALTY

ANATOMY OR SYSTEM AFFECTED: All

SPECIALTIES AND RELATED FIELDS: Alternative medicine, endocrinology, neurology, preventive medicine

DEFINITION: The study of the biological cycles in the functioning of organisms; in humans, knowledge of such cycles as circadian rhythms may aid in the diagnosis and treatment of diseases.

KEY TERMS:

circadian rhythm: a cyclical variation in a biological process or behavior that has a duration of slightly greater than twenty-four hours

jet lag: the malaise, headache, fatigue, gastrointestinal disorders, and other symptoms that may result from traveling across several time zones within a few hours

melatonin: a hormone produced by the pineal gland within the epithalamus of the forebrain; it is usually released into the blood during the night phase of the light-dark cycle

period: the length of one complete cycle of a rhythm; ultradian rhythms are about twenty-four hours (twenty to twenty-eight hours), and infradian rhythms are longer than twenty-eight hours

seasonal affective disorder (SAD): a manic depression which undergoes a seasonal fluctuation as a result of various factors, both unknown and known

suprachiasmatic nuclei (SCN): two clusters of nerve cell bodies located in the hypothalamus of the forebrain; these structures display circadian rhythms and seem to be the source of rhythmicity for many of the body's other cycles

SCIENCE AND PROFESSION

Chronobiology refers to the study of various cycles or rhythms that are fundamental to living organisms, including human beings. Many of the early observations were made on plants and nonhuman animals, but the basic concepts also apply to human biology and medicine. In the twentieth century, early findings about cyclical changes in symptoms, body weight, pulse rate, and body temperature were substantiated and broadly expanded to include numerous aspects of human biology and medicine. Well-informed physicians now expect rhythms in their patients' behavior, physiology, and response to therapy. The extensive research on biological rhythms in diverse organisms makes up the specialized field called chronobiology. The presence of circadian, menstrual, weekly, seasonal (circannual), and other rhythms in humans necessitates a consideration of these cycles in any comprehensive approach to medical practice.

Despite their importance, the exact nature of these rhythms has not been resolved. Living organisms behave as though they have internal oscillators or biological clocks that time their activities. Some research provides evidence that many of the body's cells each have such internal timers. Until the exact causes for the various biological rhythms have been identified, there will be some limitations to the benefits derived from knowledge of their characteristics. An unsettled dispute concerns whether the actual timing information for circadian and other rhythms comes from within the organism (endogenous) or from the environment (exogenous). It is expected that travel to space beyond the moon may ultimately answer this question. Astronauts may have sufficient internal timing information to survive, or it may be necessary to create a rhythmic environment of change in light-dark cycles and perhaps magnetic field variations to provide vital timing information. In the meantime, there is much that is known in chronobiology.

In mammals, an important circadian timing mechanism resides in a cluster of cells called the suprachiasmatic nuclei, or SCN, which are located in the hypothalamus of the forebrain. From studies on laboratory mammals, it has been learned that removal of the SCN abolishes many of the body's circadian rhythms. In humans, chance tumors in this area are often found to disrupt the circadian rhythms of the patient. In laboratory mammals, it has been shown that there is a separate pathway from the eyes to the SCN that allows information about changes in the light-dark schedule to reach this part of the brain. Therefore, there is intense interest in learning more about the SCN and how it regulates circadian rhythms.

Additionally, the pineal gland, a small gland attached to the epithalamus of the forebrain, receives information from the SCN about the light-dark schedule. A hormone produced by the pineal gland called melatonin is released into the bloodstream at night and suppressed during daylight. Melatonin plays a significant role in the timing of body rhythms and sleep cycles. When melatonin levels rise, the brain interprets this as bedtime, a factor that has led to its increasing use as a treatment for jet lag.

The general physiology of the other tissues of the body are organized according to rhythmic processes. The exact question of whether such rhythms are dependent on the SCN is still a point of controversy. Nevertheless, the greater application of chronobiology to medicine does not have to await the solution of such theoretical questions. Even now, a wide variety of examples can be cited of the utility of chronobiologic principles in medicine.

Diagnostic and Treatment Techniques

Four medical applications of chronobiology will be discussed. One area from psychiatry is the treatment of seasonal affective disorder. Three from other areas of medicine are the chronobiological treatment of asthma, cancer, and jet lag.

Seasonal affective disorder, or SAD, is characterized by depression beginning each year as daylight shortens and fully remitting when days start to lengthen, sometimes switching to mania. The condition is related to where people live and the corresponding hours of sunlight; the condition remits in a few days when sufferers travel to sunnier climes and worsens as they travel to areas where the days are shorter. As many as one in four persons in the northern latitudes may suffer from SAD, and female sufferers outnumber male ones. Although the disorder has been recognized only recently, for years writers and poets have noted seasonal depression in themselves and others.

Some patients take a mid-winter vacation to a sunny climate to alleviate the condition. For those who cannot travel, the use of artificial lights has been introduced. Glow lights are placed in the homes of SAD patients and used early in the morning as well as after sunset to lengthen daylight hours. Morning lights appear to bring particularly prompt relief. Relapses have been reported when light is withdrawn. Research is currently underway to determine when during the day light is most effective, how much light it needed, the the mechanisms by which light works to fight SAD.

Some details are emerging about this process. The human forebrain contains a small organ about the size of a pea that produces the hormone melatonin according to a circadian schedule. Melatonin is usually released into the bloodstream during the night. The use of bright light therapy seems to inhibit the release of melatonin and thereby cause other changes in the brain chemistry. In some mammals, this mechanism may be important in regulating their seasonal behavior. In humans, the situation is more complex, and an adequate theory for the neurochemical basis of SAD and other mental disorders has yet to be advanced.

Asthma sufferers have long known that their symptoms worsen at night. This increase in coughing, wheezing, and breathlessness at night has only been recently identified with circadian rhythms rather than environmental factors. At first, some researchers thought that asthma was worse at night because the patients were lying down. It has been shown, however, that the symptoms show their circadian periodicity whether the person is lying down or not. The normal nightly decrease in airway passage diameter in the lungs of normal persons is exaggerated in the asthmatic. The most dangerous hours for the asthmatic are the very early morning hours, a time when there are more deaths among asthmatics. Interestingly, asthmatics who become adapted to a nighttime work schedule shift their most severe asthma symptoms to the daytime sleep period.

Experts in the field such as Michael H. Smolensky of the University of Texas contend that much more research needs to be done on the role of circadian rhythms in asthma and its treatment. For example, adrenocortical hormones, which are powerful anti-inflammatory agents, have been used successfully to treat asthmatics. It was discovered that the time of day when the hormones were given was of great importance. If the hormones are given in the evening, the patient's own adrenal gland is inhibited. Therefore, the best time to give such hormones is in the early morning, near the time when they are normally released in the body.

Theophylline is a drug that has been very successful in ameliorating the symptoms of asthmatics. It has been found that certain types of sustained-release theophylline are effective in reducing the early morning symptoms if the drug is taken the night before. In the study of asthma, the benefit of considering chronobiology has become obvious, and any new products to treat asthma need to be evaluated chronobiologically before they are made available to the general public.

Cancer diagnosis and treatment are aspects of medicine that are receiving increased consideration by chronobiologists. The normal growth of tissues occurs by cell division, or mitosis, a rhythmic process that is normally precisely regulated. Cancer is essentially unregulated mitosis, resulting in the growth of a tumor that is no longer subject to the control mechanisms of the body. Yet even this breakdown in regulation has its seasons. In human males, some types of testicular cancer are more often diagnosed in the winter, and in females some types of cervical cancer have a peak occurrence in the summer.

The treatment of cancer involves the use of surgery, radiation, or chemotherapy in an attempt to remove or kill the cancerous cells without substantial damage to the normal tissues. Early studies in animal models demonstrated that there are often specific times of the day that these types of cancer treatment can be most effective. In a few cases, the tumor may have a rhythm of mitosis that is no longer synchronized to the rhythm of the surrounding tissue. In these cases, it may be possible to administer drugs or radiation that inhibits mitosis according to a schedule that will affect the cancer cells but will not harm the host tissue. More often, there will be a mixed effect of the timed treatment, so that some suppression of mitosis occurs along with some side effects.

The application of chronobiology to the treatment of breast cancer has raised hopes that there can be a marked improvement for survival rates of women who undergo breast surgery. William J. M. Hrushesky of Albany Medical College found that women who had breast surgery near to the time of menses had a more than fourfold higher risk of recurrence and death than those patients who had surgery near the middle of the menstrual cycle. These findings are under review, and the final conclusions await the evaluation of more cases. It has also been observed that the diagnosis of breast cancer in the United States has a two-peaked seasonal rhythm in the spring and the fall. There is also evidence that the body temperature of the breast in normal women has a circadian rhythm along with perhaps an additional seven-day periodicity, whereas breasts with tumors have abnormal temperature rhythms of about twenty hours. This information may help in the early diagnosis of breast cancer if suitable automatic monitoring devices are used to measure breast temperature.

Jet lag may appear to be more of an inconvenience than a serious medical problem until one considers the disastrous consequences of a plane crash caused by pilot error or a poorly made decision by a diplomat in an international crisis. Wiley Post and Harold Gatty, on their 1931 plane trip around the world, were the first persons to suffer from this disorder. Essentially, the body is subjected to a shift in the day-night schedule, with sleep and meal times shifted earlier or later depending on the number of time zones crossed and the direction of the flight. The symptoms are general malaise, headaches, fatigue, disruptions of the sleep-wake cycle, and gastrointestinal disorders. There are individual differences in the time required to overcome jet lag. In general, younger and healthier people are better able to cope with such change.

A shift of six hours, such as a flight between New York and Paris, requires a substantial reorganization of one's circadian rhythms. It can take from two days to two weeks to resynchronize. Adaptation is slowest when one stays indoors and continues on a "home-time" schedule. Eastward flights are less easily tolerated than westward flights; the delays in resynchronization can take almost twice as long. The reason for the difference is that when one flies east, the sun comes up earlier relative to "home-time." It is easier for most people to "advance" than to shift "backward"—that is, to go from day to night than to go backward from night to day. For this reason, it is suggested that travelers fly early in the day when flying east and later in the day when flying west.

Unfortunately, little consideration has been given to chronobiology in scheduling work time and time off. Pilots, diplomats, business persons, and other time zone travelers often perform poorly when their body rhythms are disturbed by jet lag. Similarly, people who must change their work shift every few weeks often find their performance level dropping. The rate at which work shifts should be rotated forward to increase worker effectiveness is now coming under considerable study.

It should be realized that the living body has myriad hormones, enzymes, and other important constituents that have rhythms of several different periods. Maintaining the correct time relationship between the rhythms can be critical for normal health. In the diagnosis of disease, chronobiology has to be taken into account. Erhard Haus of the St. Paul-Ramsey Medical Center has spent many years detailing the circadian and other rhythms that must be considered. What is normal for the morning hours may be pathological for the evening hours. These rhythmic values are yet to be determined for many important diagnostic measurements.

PERSPECTIVE AND PROSPECTS

One of the earliest written observations of a biological cycle was by Androsthenes, a soldier marching with Alexander the Great in the fourth century B.C., who recorded that the tamarind tree opens its leaves during the day and closes them at night. In experiments on similar leaf movements in other plants, the astronomer Jean Jacques d'Ortous de Mairan in 1729 found that plants held in the dark continued to open and close their leaves on a roughly twenty-four-hour schedule. Thus, circadian rhythms were shown not to be simple responses to the rising and setting of the sun but rather internal oscillations.

Early observers more interested in humans also identified rhythms. In the fifth century B.C., Hippocrates reported that his patients had twenty-four-hour fluctuations as well as longer-term rhythms in their symptoms. Herophilus of Alexandria in the third century B.C. observed a daily change in the human pulse rate. The Italian scientist Sanctorius in 1711 made repeated measurements of his own body weight and the turbidity of his urine, both of which he found to vary during the month. Later, he went to the extreme measure of constructing a giant scale and living on its huge pan so that a frequent record could be made of his changing weight. The French scientists A. Seguin and A. L. Lavoisier in 1790 did research that revealed circadian rhythms in the body weight of men. These researchers suggested that men who did not show such circadian rhythms in body weight should be suspected of being ill. The British scientist J. Davy in 1845 reported that he had found both circadian and circannual (yearlong) rhythms in his own body temperature.

Yet the historical citations of persons taking an interest in chronobiology in past centuries were only of passing concern and did not, in most cases, help to establish this field. Chronobiology as a discipline has received attention from the medical community only since about the 1970's, and many of its contributions to improving health are yet to be realized. The foremost student of chronobiology as applied to medicine has been Franz Halberg of the University of Minnesota. He has repeatedly called the attention of the medical community to the importance of biological rhythms in maintaining health and in the diagnosis and treatment of disease. Halberg has promoted the use of "autorhythmometry," or the self-measurement of one's physiological variables to monitor one's changing health.

It has been shown that this method can be used effectively even by groups of schoolchildren.

The phase or the timing of the peaks and troughs of circadian rhythms is germane in both diagnosis and treatment. The advent of portable automatic recording devices that store physiological data on computer chips is opening up a means of documenting a patient's circadian rhythms around the clock for weeks at a time. Eventually, when patients visit physicians there will then be a complete record of body temperature, blood pressure, and other physiological variables. This database will provide a much better basis for decisions than the limited data normally taken during an infrequent medical visit.

The diagnosis of diabetes mellitus has been shown to depend to an extent on the time of day that the various tests, such as the glucose tolerance test, are administered. Some diabetics are "matinal" diabetics and do not have trouble regulating their blood glucose levels until the afternoon. These persons need to have glucose tolerance tests administered in the afternoon in order to reveal their diabetes. Many additional examples of the importance of chronobiology in diagnosis and treatment exist. As more physicians and health professionals become familiar with the concepts and application of chronobiology, the effectiveness of health care will be enhanced.

—*John T. Burns, Ph.D.*
updated by Miriam Ehrenberg, Ph.D.

See also Asthma; Cancer; Chemotherapy; Depression; Hormones; Light therapy; Melatonin; Metabolism; Physiology; Psychiatry; Sleep disorders; Stress; Stress reduction.

FOR FURTHER INFORMATION:

Campbell, Jeremy. *Winston Churchill's Afternoon Nap.* New York: Simon & Schuster, 1986. One of the more popular introductions to circadian rhythms, particularly in humans. Sleep, dreams, and other phenomena of widespread interest are emphasized. The book reads like a novel, but it still gives a good overview of the field.

Coleman, Richard M. *Wide Awake at 3:00 A.M.: By Choice or by Chance?* New York: W. H. Freeman, 1990. A popular presentation of the essentials of human chronobiology. Coleman is a former director of the Stanford University Sleep Disorders Clinic, and his coverage of this subspecialty is noteworthy. Shift work and jet lag are also discussed. The appendix supplies a questionnaire so that readers can determine if they are "owls" or "larks." Contains a glossary of technical terms.

Hayes, Dora K., John E. Pauly, and Russel J. Reiter, eds. *Chronobiology: Its Role in Clinical Medicine, General Biology, and Agriculture.* 2 vols. New York: Wiley-Liss, 1990. The proceedings of the Nineteenth International Conference of the International Society for Chronobiology that was held in Besthesda, Maryland, from June 20 to June 24, 1989. A wide range of research papers are included in these two volumes. Much of the information,

especially in "Part A," can be expected to influence the future practice of medicine.

Reinberg, Alain, and Michael H. Smolensky. *Biological Rhythms and Medicine: Cellular, Metabolic, Physiopathologic, and Pharmacologic Aspects.* New York: Springer-Verlag, 1983. An excellent source of detailed information about medical chronobiology, although written at the college or graduate student level. This volume helped to interest more physicians in applying chronobiology to their practices. Includes extensive lists of references.

Rosenthal, Norman E. *Winter Blues: Seasonal Affective Disorder—What It Is and How to Overcome It.* New York: Guilford Press, 1993. Written at the popular level, this book gives the layperson an overview of the symptoms and treatment of seasonal affective disorder.

Touitou, Yvan, and E. Haus, eds. *Biological Rhythms in Clinical and Laboratory Medicine.* New York: Springer-Verlag, 1992. An encyclopedic compilation of the recent research on medical chronobiology. Those readers who start here will have an exceptional, though advanced, introduction to the subject.

Waterhouse, J. M. *Your Body Clock.* New York: Oxford University Press, 1990. This text presents detailed, updated information on human chronobiology.

CIRCULATION

BIOLOGY

ANATOMY OR SYSTEM AFFECTED: Blood, blood vessels, circulatory system, liver

SPECIALTIES AND RELATED FIELDS: Cardiology, hematology, vascular medicine

DEFINITION: The flow of blood throughout the body; the circulatory system consists of the heart, lungs, arteries, and veins.

KEY TERMS:

aneurysm: a localized enlargement of a vessel, usually an artery

atherosclerosis: accumulation of plaque within the arteries

calcification: the deposit of lime salts in organic tissue, leading to calcium in the arterial wall

capillaries: hairlike vessels that connect the ends of the smallest arteries to the beginnings of the smallest veins

claudication: muscle cramps that occur when arterial blood flow does not meet the muscles' demand for oxygen

diastole: the period of relaxation in the cardiac cycle

hypertension: a blood pressure higher than what is considered to be normal

lumen: the space within an artery, vein, or other tube

stenosis: the constriction or narrowing of a passage

systole: the period of contraction in the cardiac cycle

thrombus: a blood clot that, commonly, obstructs a vein but may also occur in an artery or the heart

vasoconstriction: a decrease in the diameter of a blood vessel

vasodilation: an increase in the diameter of a blood vessel

STRUCTURE AND FUNCTIONS

The cardiovascular system is made up of the heart, arteries, veins, and lungs. The heart serves as a pump to deliver blood to the arteries for distribution throughout the body. The veins bring the blood back to the heart, and the lungs oxygenate the blood before returning it to the arterial system.

Contraction of the heart muscle forces blood out of the heart. This period of contraction is known as systole. The heart muscle relaxes between each contraction, which allows blood flow into the heart. This period of relaxation is known as diastole. A typical blood pressure taken at the upper arm provides a pressure reading during two phases of the cardiac cycle. The first number is known as the systolic pressure and represents the pressure of the heart during peak contraction. The second number is known as the diastolic pressure and represents the pressure while the heart is at rest. A typical pressure reading for a young adult would be 120/80. When blood pressure is abnormally elevated, it is commonly referred to as high blood pressure, or hypertension.

The heart is separated into two halves by a wall of muscle known as the septum. The two halves are known as the left and right heart. The left side of the heart is responsible for high-pressure arterial distribution and is larger and stronger when compared to the right side. The right side of the heart is responsible for accepting low-pressure venous return and redirecting it to the lungs.

Because of these pressure differences from one side of the heart to the other, the vessel wall constructions of the arteries and the veins differ. Strong construction of the arterial wall allows tolerance of significant pressure elevations from the left heart. The arterial wall is made up of three major tissue layers, known as tunics. Secondary layers of tissue that provide strength and elasticity to the artery are known as elastic and connective tissues. As with the artery, the wall of the vein is made up of three distinct tissue layers. Compared to that of an artery, the wall of a vein is thinner and less elastic, which allows the walls to be easily compressed by surrounding muscle during contraction.

While the heart is at rest, between contractions, newly oxygenated arterial blood passes from the lungs and enters the left heart. Each time the heart contracts, blood is forced from the left heart into a major artery known as the aorta. From the aorta, blood is distributed throughout the body. Once depleted of nutrients and oxygen, arterial blood passes through an extensive array of minute vessels known as capillaries. A significant pressure drop occurs as blood is dispersed throughout the immense network of capillaries. The capillaries empty into the venous system, which carries the blood back to the heart.

The primary responsibility of the venous system is to return deoxygenated blood to the lungs and heart. Much more energy is required from the body to move venous

The Circulatory System

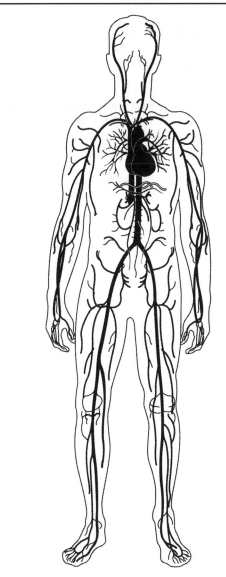

flow compared to arterial flow. Unlike the artery, the vein does not depend on the heart or gravity for energy to move blood. The venous system has a unique means of blood transportation known as the "venous pump," which moves blood toward the heart.

The components making up the venous pump include muscle contraction against the venous wall, intra-abdominal pressure changes, and one-way venous valves. Compression against the walls of a vein induces movement of blood. Muscle contraction against a vein wall occurs throughout the body during periods of activity. Activity includes every movement, from breathing to running. Variations in respiration cause fluctuations in the pressure within the abdomen, which produces a siphonlike effect on the veins, pulling venous blood upward. Valves are located within the veins of the extremities and pelvis. A venous valve has two leaflets, which protrude inward from opposite sides of the vein wall and meet one another in the center. Valves are necessary to prevent blood from flowing backward, away from the heart.

The venous system is divided into two groups known as the deep and superficial veins. The deep veins are located parallel to the arteries, while the superficial veins are located just beneath the skin surface and are often visible through the skin.

DISORDERS AND DISEASES

Numerous variables may affect the flow of blood. The autonomic nervous system is connected to muscle within the wall of the artery by way of neurological pathways known as sympathetic branches. Various drugs and/or conditions can trigger responses in the sympathetic branches and produce constriction of the smooth muscle in the arterial wall (vasoconstriction) or relaxation of the arterial wall (vasodilation). Alcohol consumption or a hot bath are examples of conditions which produce vasodilation. Exposure to cold and/or cigarette smoking are examples of conditions that produce vasoconstriction. Various drugs used in the medical environment are capable of producing similar effects. The diameter of the inner wall (lumen) of an artery influences the pressure and the flow of blood through it.

Another condition that alters the arterial diameter is atherosclerosis, a disease primarily of the large arteries, which allows the formation of fat (lipid) deposits to build on the inner layer of the artery. Lipid deposits are more commonly known as atherosclerotic plaque. Plaque accumulation reduces the diameter of the arterial lumen, causing various degrees of flow restriction. Plaque is similar to rust accumulation within a pipe which restricts the flow of water. A restriction of flow is referred to as a stenosis. The majority of stenotic lesions occur at the place where arteries divide into branches, also known as a bifurcation. In advanced stages of plaque development, plaque may become calcified. Calcified plaque is hard and may become irregular, ulcerate, or hemorrhage, providing an environment for new clot formation and/or release of small pieces of plaque debris downstream.

An arterial wall may become very hard and rigid, a condition commonly known as "hardening of the arteries." Hardened arteries may eventually become twisted, kinked, or dilated as a result of the hardening process of the arterial wall. A hardened artery which has become dilated is known as an aneurysm.

Normal arterial flow is undisturbed. When blood cells travel freely, they move together at a similar speed with very little variance. This is known as laminar flow. Nonlaminar (turbulent) flow is seen when irregular plaque or kinks in the arterial wall disrupt the smooth flow of cells. Plaque with an irregular surface may produce mild turbulence, while a narrow stenosis produces significant turbulence immediately downstream from the stenosis.

Many moderate or severe stenoses can be heard with the use of a standard stethoscope over the vessel of interest. A high-pitched sound can be heard consequent to the increased velocity of the blood cells moving through a narrow space. (A similar effect is produced when a standard garden hose is kinked to create a spray and a hissing sound is heard.) Medically, this sound is often referred to as a bruit. The term *bruit* (pronounced "broo-ee") is a French word meaning noise.

Patients with significant lower extremity arterial disease will consistently experience calf and occasionally thigh discomfort with exercise, which is relieved when the patient stands still for a few moments. This is known as vascular claudication and occurs from a pressure drop as a consequence of a severely stenotic (greater than 75-percent-diameter reduction) or occluded artery. If the muscle cannot get enough oxygen as a result of reduced blood flow, it will cramp, forcing the patient to stop and rest until blood supply has caught up to muscle demand. Alternate pathways around an obstruction prevent pain at rest, when muscle demand is low. Alternate pathways are also referred to as collateral pathways. Small, otherwise insignificant branches from a main artery become important vessels when the body uses them as collateral pathways around an obstruction. Time and exercise help to collateralize arterial branches into larger, more prominent arterial pathways. If collateral pathways do not provide enough flow to prevent the patient from experiencing painful muscle cramps while performing a daily exercise routine or to heal a wound on the foot, it may be necessary to perform either a surgical bypass around the obstruction or another interventional procedure such as angioplasty, atherectomy, or laser surgery.

Claudication may also occur in the heart. The main coronary arteries lie on the surface of the heart and distribute blood to the heart muscle. Patients suffering from coronary artery disease (CAD) may experience tightness, heaviness, or pain in the chest subsequent to flow restriction to the heart muscle as a result of atherosclerotic plaque within the coronary arteries. These symptoms are known as angina pectoris, or simply angina, usually occurring with exercise and relieved by rest. Intensity of the symptoms is relative to the extent of disease. A myocardial infarction (heart attack) is the result of a coronary artery occlusion.

Unlike the arteries, the venous system is not affected by atherosclerosis. The primary diseases of the veins include blood clot formation and varicose veins. A varicose vein is an enlarged and meandering vein with poorly functioning valves. A varicosity typically involves the veins near the skin surface, the superficial veins, and is often visualized as a irregular and/or raised segment through the skin surface. Varicosities are most common in the lower legs.

Valve leaflets are common sites for development of a thrombus. Thrombosis is the formation of a clot within a vein, which occurs when blood flow is delayed or obstructed for many hours. Several conditions that may induce venous clotting include prolonged bed rest (postoperative patients), prolonged sitting (long airplane or automobile rides), and use of oral contraceptives. Cancer patients are at high risk of clot formation secondary to a metabolic disorder which affects the natural blood-thinning process.

Because numerous tributaries are connected to the superficial system, it is easy for the body to compensate for a clot in this system by rerouting blood through other branches. The deep venous system, however, has fewer branches, which promotes the progression of a thrombus toward the heart. A thrombus in the deep venous system is more serious because the risk of pulmonary emboli, commonly known as blood clot to the lung, is much higher when compared to superficial vein thrombosis. The further a thrombus propagates, the higher the risk to the patient.

Lower extremity venous return must take an alternate route via the superficial venous system when the deep system is obstructed by a thrombus. This is known as compensatory flow around an obstruction.

PERSPECTIVE AND PROSPECTS

Historically, the vasculature of the human body was evaluated by placing one's fingers on the skin, palpating for the presence or absence of a pulse, and making note of the patient's symptoms. Prior to the 1960's, treatment of the circulatory system was very limited or nonexistent, resulting in a high death rate and large numbers of amputations, strokes, and heart attacks. The development of arteriography (the angiogram), a procedure in which dye is injected into the vessels while X rays are obtained, revealed more about the vasculature and the nature of disease involving it. In conjunction with arteriography came corrective bypass surgery.

This period of development was followed by vast improvements in diagnostics, treatment, and knowledge of preventive maintenance. Today, synthetic bypass grafts are commonplace and are used to reroute flow around an obstruction. In many cases, procedures such as atherectomy and angioplasty, in which plaque or a thrombus is removed through a catheter inserted into the vessel, are often performed as outpatient procedures without the need of surgery.

Diagnostic imaging of the cardiovascular system and the study of hemodynamics with the use of ultrasound have been useful for patient screening, the monitoring of disease progression, and the postoperative evaluation of surgical/interventional procedures. Ultrasound is a particularly valuable diagnostic tool because, compared to X rays or arteriography, it is less expensive, quick, painless, and noninvasive (no radiation, needles, or dye is required).

In addition to technological advances, new medications have been made available to reduce the risk of graft rejection, hypertension, and clotting and to lower blood cholesterol. Preventive measures, however, constitute the most effective approach to good health. Much new information has been made available to improve the knowledge of the general public regarding diet, exercise, and the avoidance of unhealthy habits as the way to create and maintain a healthier cardiovascular system. —*Bonnie L. Wolff*

See also Aneurysmectomy; Aneurysms; Angina; Angiography; Angioplasty; Arteriosclerosis; Biofeedback; Bleeding; Blood and blood components; Blood testing; Bypass surgery; Catheterization; Chest; Cholesterol; Claudication; Diabetes mellitus; Dialysis; Eclampsia; Edema; Embolism; Endarterectomy; Exercise physiology; Heart disease; Heart; Heat exhaustion and heat stroke; Hematology; Hematology, pediatric; Hemorrhoid banding and removal; Hemorrhoids; Hormones; Hypercholesterolemia; Hypertension; Ischemia; Kidneys; Lymphatic system; Phlebitis; Shock; Shunts; Strokes and TIAs; Systems and organs; Thrombolytic therapy and TPA; Thrombosis and thrombus; Transfusion; Varicose vein removal; Varicosis; Vascular medicine; Vascular system; Venous insufficiency.

FOR FURTHER INFORMATION:

Guyton, A. C. *Human Physiology and Mechanisms of Disease*. 6th ed. Philadelphia: W. B. Saunders, 1997. A well-written text for medical students interested in learning the physiological effects of disease. Although moderately detailed, most chapters are written in understandable terms and provide useful illustrations. Parts 3 and 4 pertain to the heart and circulation.

Hole, John W., Jr. *Human Anatomy and Physiology*. 6th ed. Dubuque, Iowa: W. C. Brown, 1993. A basic introductory anatomy and physiology text. Chapters on the blood and the cardiovascular system offer a basic understanding of hemodynamics in simple terms and using thoughtful illustrations.

Strandness, D. E., Jr. *Duplex Scanning in Vascular Disorders*. New York: Raven Press, 1990. This book is written for medical vascular specialists and is somewhat technical in nature; however, it is well written. The beginning of each chapter defines the importance of that particular subject and the clinical presentation, treatment, and typical course of the vascular disease involved. Chapters of interest are "Hemodynamics of the Normal Arterial and Venous System," "Hemodynamics of Arterial Stenosis and Occlusion," and "Hemodynamics of Venous Occlusion and Valvular Incompetence."

Zaret, Barry L., Marvin Moser, and Lawrence S. Cohen, eds. *Yale University School of Medicine Heart Book*. New York: William Morrow, 1992. A detailed medical text written to educate patients and medical students about the heart, cerebral, and peripheral vascular systems. This text is well written and easy to understand. Topics of interest include normal cardiovascular anatomy and physiology, major cardiovascular disorders, and methods of treatment.

CIRCUMCISION, FEMALE, AND GENITAL MUTILATION

PROCEDURE

ANATOMY OR SYSTEM AFFECTED: Genitals, reproductive system

SPECIALTIES AND RELATED FIELDS: General surgery; gynecology; plastic, cosmetic, and reconstructive surgery; psychiatry

DEFINITION: The partial or complete surgical removal of the clitoris, labia minora, and labia majora for cultural reasons.

KEY TERMS:

clitoridectomy: the removal of the entire clitoris, the prepuce, and adjacent labia

deinfibulation: an anterior episiotomy

episiotomy: the incision of the labia

infibulation: a clitoridectomy followed by the sewing up of the vulva

pharaonic circumcision: another term for infibulation

prepuce: the covering of the clitoris

sunna circumcision: the removal of the tip of the clitoris and/or the prepuce

INDICATIONS AND PROCEDURES

The various forms of female circumcision, although not universal to all cultures, have been practiced in numerous societies of the world for nearly two thousand years. Recorded evidence cites that female circumcision predates the advent of both Christianity and Islam and that early Christians, Muslims, and the Jewish group Falashas practiced circumcision on young girls. Historically, during the nineteenth century and until the 1940's, clitoridectomies were performed in Europe and America as a procedure to "cure" female masturbation, nervousness, and other specific types of perceived psychological dysfunction.

The 1989-1990 Demographic Health Survey of Circumcision stated that circumcision is still performed annually on an estimated 80 to 114 million women; 85 percent of these procedures involve clitoridectomy, while approximately 15 percent involve infibulation. Certain contemporary cultures of Africa, the Middle East, and parts of Yemen, India, and Malaysia continue these practices. Contemporary Middle Eastern countries practicing female circumcision and genital mutilation are Jordan, Iraq, the two Yemens, Syria, and southern Algeria. In Africa, it is practiced in the majority of the countries, including Egypt, Ivory Coast, Kenya, Mali, Mozambique, Sudan, and Upper Volta. It has been estimated that 99 percent of northern Sudanese women, aged fifteen to forty-nine, are circumcised. In and around Alexandria, Egypt, 99 percent of rural and lower income urban women are circumcised.

Cross-culturally, there are essentially four types of female genital circumcision and female genital mutilation. Circumcision or sunna circumcision is removal of the prepuce or hood of the clitoris, with the body of the clitoris remaining intact. Sunna means "tradition" in Arabic. Excision circumcision or clitoridectomy is the removal of the entire clitoris (both prepuce and glans) and all or part of the adjacent labia majora and the labia minora.

Intermediate circumcision is the removal of the clitoris, all or part of the labia minora, and sometimes part of the labia majora.

Infibulation or pharaonic circumcision is the removal of the clitoris, the labia minora, and much of the labia majora; on occasion, the remaining sides of the vulva are stitched together to close up the vagina, except for a small opening maintained for the passage of blood and urine.

All types of female genital mutilation frequently create severe, long-term effects, such as pelvic infections that usually lead to infertility; chronic recurrent urinary tract infections; painful intercourse; obstetrical complications; and, in some cases, surgically induced scars that can cause tearing of the tissue, and even hemorrhaging, during childbirth. In fact, it is not unusual for women who have been infibulated to require surgical enlargement of the vagina on their wedding night or when delivering children. Unfortunately, babies born to infibulated women frequently suffer brain damage because of oxygen deprivation (hypoxia) caused by a prolonged and obstructed delivery. The baby may die during the painful birthing process because of a damaged birth canal. Other physical and psychological difficulties for the circumcised woman may be sexual dysfunction, delayed menarche, and genital malformation.

From a cultural perspective, there are numerous reasons for these surgical procedures. It is a rite of passage and proof of adulthood. It raises a woman's status in her community, because of both the added purity that circumcision brings and the bravery that initiates are called upon to demonstrate. It is also thought to confer maturity and inculcate positive character traits, such as the ability to endure pain and to be submissive. In some cultures, the circumcision ritual is a positive one in which the girl is the center of attention and receives presents and moral instruction from her elders. It creates a bond between the generations, as all women in the society must undergo the procedure and thus have shared an important experience.

It is thought that a girl who has been circumcised will not have her conscience troubled by lustful thoughts or sensations or by physical temptations such as masturbation. Therefore, there is less risk of premarital relationships that can end in the stigma and social difficulties of illegitimate birth. The bond between husband and wife may be closer because one or both of them will never have had sex with anyone else. The relationship may be motivated by love rather than lust because there will be no physical drive for the wife, only an emotional one. There is little incentive for extramarital sex for the wife; hence, the marriage may be more secure. Children may be better cared for because the husband can be more confident that they are his. Generally, a girl who is not circumcised is considered "unclean" by local villagers and therefore unmarriageable. In some societies, a girl who is not circumcised is believed to be dangerous, even deadly, if her clitoris touches a man's penis.

Unfortunately, female genital circumcision and female genital mutilation surgeries are invariably conducted in unsanitary conditions in which a midwife or close female relative uses unsterile sharp instruments, such as pieces of glass, razor blades, kitchen knives, or scissors. The induction of tetanus, septicemia, hemorrhaging, and even shock are not uncommon. Human immunodeficiency virus (HIV) can be transmitted. No anesthesia is used. These procedures usually are experienced by the child at approximately three years of age, although the actual age depends upon the customs of the particular society or village. In order to minimize the risk of the transmission of viruses, countries such as Egypt have made it illegal for female genital mutilation to be practiced by anyone other than trained doctors and nurses in hospitals.

Treatment and Therapy

There is no information regarding the surgical restoration of severed or damaged genitals. Because of severe cultural sanctions by the participating groups, which continue to hold tenaciously to such practices, female genital circumcision is seldom discussed with outsiders. Those who follow these customs do not report their occurrence. Consequently, there are few data concerning the frequency of female genital circumcision and female genital mutilation within the United States, despite the knowledge that some immigrant groups from Africa, the Middle East, and Asia continue to practice these surgeries. Health care workers estimate that, within the United States, approximately ten thousand girls undergo these surgical procedures each year. Usually, the procedure is conducted in the home. Those who can pay physicians to perform the surgery may do so; in these cases, local anesthesia is used and the risk of infection is less.

Perspective and Prospects

Because of the high number of female genital mutilations and the deaths that this procedure has caused, it is now prohibited in Great Britain, France, Sweden, Switzerland, and some countries of Africa, such as Egypt, Kenya, and Senegal. The National Organization of Circumcision Information Resource Centers (NOCIRC) are opposed to the procedures, as well as to male circumcision. The United Nations Children's Fund (UNICEF) and the World Health Organization (WHO) consider female genital mutilation to be a violation of human rights, recommending its eradication. In the United States, former Congresswoman Patricia Schroeder introduced a bill that would outlaw female geni-

tal mutilation. The bill, called the Federal Prohibition of Female Genital Mutilation of 1995, was passed in 1996. The Canadian Criminal Code was enacted to protect children who are ordinarily residents in Canada from being removed from the country and subjected to female genital mutilation.

Both female genital circumcision and female genital mutilation perpetuate customs that seek to control female bodies and sexuality. It is hoped that with increasing legislation and attitude changes regarding bioethical issues, fewer girls and young women will undergo these mutilating surgical procedures. One problem in this campaign is the conflict between cultural self-determination and basic human rights. Feminists, physicians, and ethicists must work respectfully with, and not independently of, local resources for cultural self-examination and change. —*John Alan Ross*

See also Bleeding; Childbirth; Childbirth, complications of; Circumcision, male; Episiotomy; Ethics; Genital disorders, female; Gynecology; Infertility in females; Menstruation; Psychiatry; Reproductive system; Septicemia; Sexual dysfunction; Sexuality; Stillbirth.

For Further Information:

Elchala, U., B. Ben-Ami, R. Gillis, and A. Brezezinski. "Ritualistic Female Genital Mutilation: Current Status and Future Outlook." *Obstetrical and Gynecological Survey* 52, no. 10 (1997): 643-653.

James, Stephen A. "Reconciling International Human Rights and Cultural Relativism: The Case of Female Circumcision." *Bioethics* 8, no. 1 (1994): 1-26.

Kluge, E. W. "Female Genital Mutilation: Cultural Values and Ethics." *Journal of Obstetrics and Gynecology* 16, no. 2 (1997): 71.

Lyons, Harriet. "Anthropologists, Moralities, and Relativities: The Problem of Genital Mutilations." *Canadian Review of Sociology and Anthropology* 18 (1981): 499-578.

Van Deer Kwaak, Anke. "Female Circumcision and Gender Identity: A Questionable Alliance?" *Social Science and Medicine* 35, no. 6 (1992): 777-787.

Walker, Alice, and Pratiibha Parmar. *Warrior Marks: Female Genital Mutilation and the Sexual Blinding of Women.* New York: Harcourt Brace, 1993.

Circumcision, male

Procedure

Anatomy or system affected: Genitals, reproductive system

Specialties and related fields: General surgery, pediatrics, urology

Definition: The removal of the foreskin (prepuce) covering the head of the penis.

Key terms:

chordee: the downward curvature of the penis, most apparent on erection, caused by the shortness of the skin on the downward side of the penile shaft *glans or glans penis:* the head of the penis

necrosis: the death of one or more cells or a portion of a tissue or organ resulting from irreversible damage

phimosis: the narrowing of the opening of the skin covering the head of the penis sufficient to prevent retraction of the skin back over the glans

sepsis: an infection in the circulating blood

smegma: a pasty accumulation of shed skin cells and secretions of the sweat glands which collects in the moist areas of the foreskin-covered base of the glans

urinary tract infections: infections of the bladder, kidneys, the urethra (which connects the bladder to the opening at the end of the penis), and the ureters (which connect the bladder to the kidneys); infection may be limited to one area of these organs or spread throughout the urinary tract

INDICATIONS AND PROCEDURES

Routine circumcision of the newborn male—in which the foreskin of the penis is stretched, clamped, and cut—is becoming an increasingly controversial procedure. Famed pediatrician Benjamin Spock once contended that circumcision is a good idea, especially if most of the boys in the neighborhood are circumcised; then a boy feels "regular." Yet, many wonder if that is justification for circumcision. Allowing routine circumcision of newborns as a religious and cultural rite still leaves the debate over medical necessity. The United States is the only country in the world that circumcises a majority of newborn males without a religious reason. In fact, circumcision has been termed a "cultural surgery."

True medical indications for the surgery are seldom present at birth. Such conditions as infections of the head and/or shaft of the penis may be indications for circumcision; an inability to retract the foreskin in the newborn is not an indication. Some argue that circumcision should be delayed until the foreskin has become retractable, making an imprecise surgical procedure presumably less traumatic. In 96 percent of infant boys, however, the foreskin is not fully retractable; it is normally so tight and adherent that it cannot be pulled back and the penis cleaned. By age three, that percentage decreases to 10 percent.

There are other definite contraindications to newborn circumcision. Circumcising infants with abnormalities of the penal head or shaft makes treatment more difficult because the foreskin may later be needed for use in reconstruction. Prematurity, instability, or a bleeding problem also preclude early circumcision. The foreskin is a natural protective membrane, representing 50 to 80 percent of the skin system of the penis, having 240 feet of nerve fibers, more than 1,000 nerve endings, and 3 feet of veins, arteries, and capillaries. It keeps the sensitive head protected, facilitating intercourse, and prevents the surface of the glans from thickening and becoming desensitized. Also, within the inner surface of the foreskin are a series of tiny ridged bands that contribute significantly to stimulating the glans.

The two most persistent arguments for the operation, however, are the risks of infection and cancer in the uncircumcised. Without circumcision, smegma accumulates beneath the base of the covered head of the penis. This cheeselike material of dead skin cells and secretions of the sweat glands is thought to be a cause of cancer of the penis and prostate gland in uncircumcised men and cancer of the cervix in their female partners. Doctors who argue against circumcision, however, say that the presence of smegma in the uncircumcised is simply a sign of poor hygiene and that poor sexual hygiene, inadequate hygienic facilities, and sexually transmitted diseases cause an increased incidence of cancer in ethnic groups or populations that do not practice circumcision. Doctors who argue against circumcision also point out that complete circumcision is found as often in male partners of women without cancer of the cervix as in male partners of women who have cervical cancer. In Sweden, moreover—where newborn circumcision is not routinely practiced but where good hygiene is practiced—the rates of these cancers are essentially the same as those found in Israel, where ritualistic circumcision is practiced.

The increased incidence of urinary tract infections and sexually transmitted diseases (STDs) in uncircumcised males sufficiently argue for circumcision, say its proponents. They warn that the intact foreskin invites bacterial colonization, which leads to urethral infection ascending to the bladder that ultimately may spread upward to the kidneys and sometimes cause permanent kidney damage. On the other hand, no proof exists that uncircumcised male infants who sustain urinary tract infections will have future urologic problems. Furthermore, the operation is not a simple procedure and is not without peril. Penile amputation, life-threatening infections, and even death have been well documented.

Slightly increased rates of infection with sexually transmitted diseases in the uncircumcised argue the case for some proponents, but it is acquired immunodeficiency syndrome (AIDS) that they most fear. In Africa, where circumcision is seldom practiced, the acquisition of AIDS by heterosexual men from infected women during vaginal intercourse is the most common mode of transmission.

Proponents say that infection with human immunodeficiency virus (HIV), the virus that leads to AIDS, depends on a break or an abrasion of the skin to gain entry. The intact foreskin provides a site for transfer of infected cervical secretions. In Africa, doctors at the University of Nairobi noted a relationship of HIV infection to genital ulcers and lack of circumcision. Uncircumcised men had a history of genital ulcers more often than did the circumcised, and they were more often HIV-positive. They were also more frequently HIV-positive even if they did not have a history of genital ulcer disease.

Every evaluation of circumcision, pro or con, should reflect the confounding genetic and environmental variables, as well as the actual increased risks and benefits. Two percent is twice 1 percent, but 2 percent may not be twice as dangerous or better than 1 percent. All the pros and cons should be explained to parents before informed consent is obtained.

USES AND COMPLICATIONS

In 1989, the American Academy Pediatrics Task Force on Circumcision concluded that "newborn circumcision has potential medical benefits and advantages as well as disadvantages and risks. When circumcision is being considered, the benefits and risks should be explained to the parents and informed consent obtained." This neutral statement does not lessen the anxiety of parents who are trying to weigh the pros and cons of routine newborn circumcision, but examination of the evidence does allow parents to weigh the individual benefits and risks and see if the scale tips in either direction.

Worldwide studies of predominantly uncircumcised populations have shown a higher incidence of urinary tract infection in boys during the first few months of life, which is the reverse of what is found in older infants and children, where girls predominate. In 1986, Brooke Army Medical Center in Fort Sam Houston, Texas, took a closer look. The doctors found the incidence of urinary tract infection in circumcised infant males to be 0.11 percent but 1.12 percent in the uncircumcised. Even without proof that the uncircumcised male infants who get urinary tract infections will have future urologic problems, the proponents for the surgical procedure claim about a 1 percent advantage.

The evidence for an increase in sexually transmitted diseases (such as genital herpes, gonorrhea, and syphilis) among the uncircumcised is conflicting. Furthermore, apparent correlations between circumcision status and these diseases do not reflect confounding genetic and environmental variables. It is also difficult to factor in the risk from HIV infections. The studies from Africa do not look at any variables in the transmission of HIV except circumcision status and previous history of genital ulcers. The nutritional and economic status of the men was not examined, even though it is known that malnourishment suppresses the immune systems. Moreover, if everyone practiced "safe sex," the argument for circumcision would be moot.

Almost all the surgical complications of circumcision can be avoided if doctors performing the procedure adhere to strict asepsis, are properly trained and experienced in the procedure, remove the appropriate and correct amount of tissue, and provide adequate hemostasis. The variety of circumstances, populations, and physicians affects the incidence of complications. In the larger, teaching hospitals, often the newest physicians with the least experience or supervision perform the operation. As a result, complica-

tions may arise. Excessive bleeding is the most frequent complication. The incidence of bleeding after circumcision ranges from 0.1 percent to as high as 35 percent in some reports. Most of the episodes are minor and can be controlled by simple measures, such as compression and suturing, but some of these efforts can lead to diminished blood supply to the head and shaft of the penis with necrosis of the affected part. Chordee can result if improper technique or bad luck intervenes, and such penile deformity begets the risk of emotional distress. The urethral opening on the end of the penis can become infected or ulcerated when the glans is no longer protected by foreskin; such infection rarely occurs in the uncircumcised. Finally, any surgical procedure runs the risk of infection. These localized infections rarely spread to the blood, but death from sepsis and its sequela has been documented.

Overall, the surgical complication rate after circumcision runs around 0.19 percent, which could be lowered with strict protocols, meticulous technique, strict asepsis, and well-trained, experienced physicians. Strict protocols, it is hoped, would ensure that absolute contraindications to the procedure—such as anomalies of the penis, prematurity, instability, or a bleeding disorder—were honored.

Another human factor must be considered. Many insurance companies do not provide payment for newborn care, since it is considered preventive medicine. Moreover, newborn care has historically been underpaid, considering the time that a conscientious physician spends providing it. If charges for a circumcision are added to the charges for the lower-valued newborn care, then compensation becomes less irritating. How often this affects the rate of circumcision is unknown. It is known that, in 1997, a physician's fee for performing a circumcision ranged to approximately $400, with a nationwide average of $137. Interestingly, a growing number of circumcised men are undergoing expensive foreskin restoration procedures.

In part because of an additional cost that arises with anesthesia, the vast majority of infant circumcisions are performed without pain control. The surgery is painful, and yet some physicians claim that the minute that the operation ends, the circumcised baby no longer cries and frequently falls asleep. Continuing pain, therefore, is probably not present.

Another perspective to examine is the experience of adult males, who are circumcised by their own choice. Many complain of at least a week's discomfort after the operation. The most compelling argument against adult circumcision, however, comes from their answer to "Would you do it again?" In one study of several hundred men who were circumcised as adults, they were asked five years later if they would do it again. All said no.

PERSPECTIVE AND PROSPECTS

Routine newborn circumcision originated in the United States in the 1860's, ostensibly as prophylaxis against disease. Some medical historians, however, believe that non-religious circumcision was a deliberate surgical procedure to desensitize and debilitate the penis to prevent masturbation. During this era, and for nearly a hundred years afterward, most American physicians viewed masturbation as an inevitable cause of blindness, weak character, insanity, nervousness, tuberculosis, venereal disease, and even death. One physician maintained that a painful circumcision would have a salutary effect upon the newborn's mind, so that pain would be associated with masturbation. As late as 1928, the *American Medical Journal* published an editorial that justified male circumcision as an effective means of preventing the dire effects of masturbation. During World Wars I and II, soldiers were forcibly circumcised under threat of court martial, being told that the surgery was for reasons of hygiene and the prevention of epilepsy and other diseases.

Eventually, a general change in attitude occurred, notably in Great Britain and New Zealand, which virtually have abandoned routine circumcision. Rates of circumcision have also fallen dramatically in Canada, Australia, and even the United States. As recently as the mid-1970's, approximately 90 percent of U.S. male babies were circumcised. Not until 1971 did the American Academy of Pediatrics determine that circumcision is not medically valid. By 1995, however, the incidence of newborn circumcision had declined to 59 percent.

In 1971, the American Academy of Pediatrics' Committee on the Fetus and Newborn issued an advisory that said, "There are no valid medical indications for routine circumcision in the neonatal period." In 1978, when the American College of Obstetricians and Gynecologists affirmed this statement, the circumcision rate had already declined to an estimated 70 percent of newborn males, compared to previous rates of between 80 and 90 percent. In response to the critics who were worried about increased urinary tract infections in the uncircumcised, the 1989 American Academy of Pediatrics' Task Force on Circumcision concluded that "newborn circumcision has potential medical benefits and advantages as well as disadvantages and risks. When circumcision is being considered, the benefits and risks should be explained to the parents and informed consent obtained."

Undoubtedly, the future will bring improved surgical techniques. More emphasis will be placed on avoiding surgical complications by more rigid monitoring of the operation and who performs the procedure. It is unlikely that circumcision will disappear completely.

Organizations such as Doctors Opposing Circumcision and the National Organization to Halt the Abuse and Routine Mutilation of Males, however, are actively proposing an end to routine neonatal circumcision. Some nursing groups and concerned mothers have formed local groups to oppose circumcision in male neonates. They argue that subjecting a baby to this procedure may impair mother-infant bonding. Another question posed by some physicians and parents is the ethics involved in the unnecessary removal of a functioning body organ, particularly without the patient's consent. Others claim that the baby's rights are being violated, noting that it is the child who must live with the outcome of the decision to perform a circumcision. As a result of these efforts, the rates of circumcision will probably continue to fall.

—*Wayne R. McKinny, M.D., updated by John Alan Ross*

See also Circumcision, female, and genital mutilation; Ethics; Genital disorders, male; Neonatology; Pediatrics; Reproductive system; Urology, pediatric.

FOR FURTHER INFORMATION:

Behrman, Richard E., ed. *Nelson Textbook of Pediatrics.* 15th ed. Philadelphia: W. B. Saunders, 1996. This standard pediatric textbook briefly covers the medical risks and benefits of routine newborn circumcision fairly and without bias or excessive medical jargon. Draws no conclusions.

Berkow, Robert, and Andrew J. Fletcher, eds. *The Merck Manual of Diagnosis and Therapy.* 16th ed. Rahway, N.J.: Merck Sharp & Dohme Research Laboratories, 1992. This classic textbook does say that circumcision "is rarely indicated medically." In contrast to longer review articles, however, *The Merck Manual* states that bleeding disorders in infants should include a history of the mother's taking medication for bleeding disturbances, such as anticoagulants or aspirin.

Bigelow, Jim. *The Joy of Uncircumcising!: Exploring Circumcision—History, Myths, Psychology, Restoration, Sexual Pleasure, and Human Rights.* 2d ed. Aptos, Calif.: Hourglass, 1995. This book provides an alternative view of this controversial procedure.

King, L. R., ed. *Urologic Surgery in Neonates and Young Infants.* Philadelphia: W. B. Saunders, 1988. J. W. Duckett's contribution, "The Neonatal Circumcision Debate," is an excellent review of the controversies surrounding this operation. Although written for doctors, it will present minimal difficulty for laypersons.

Snyder, Howard M. "To Circumcise or Not." *Hospital Practice* 26 (January 15, 1991): 201-207. This widely available medical journal article examines in detail the medical evidence for and against circumcision. With a minimum of medical jargon, the author also states his own personal bias against the routine use of the procedure.

Wiswell, T. E., and D. W. Beschke. "Risks from Circumcision During the First Month of Life Compared with Those for Uncircumcised Boys." *Pediatrics* 83 (1989): 1011. Laypersons will be able to appreciate the importance of this article, which focuses on the first month of life. The authors are recognized authorities in their field and are widely published.

CIRRHOSIS

DISEASE/DISORDER

ANATOMY OR SYSTEM AFFECTED: Liver

SPECIALTIES AND RELATED FIELDS: Family practice, internal medicine, psychology

DEFINITION: The formation of scar tissue in the liver, which interferes with its normal function.

CAUSES AND SYMPTOMS

The liver is a large, spongy organ that lies in the upper-right abdomen. Regarded as primarily part of the digestive system because it manufactures bile, the liver has many other functions, including the synthesis of blood-clotting factors and the detoxification of such harmful substances as alcohol.

Cirrhosis describes the fibrous scar tissue (or nodules) that replaces the normally soft liver after repeated long-term injury by toxins such as alcohol or viruses. The liver may form small nodules (micronodular cirrhosis), large nodules (macronodular cirrhosis), or a combination of the two types (mixed nodular cirrhosis). Cirrhosis is a frequent cause of death among middle-aged men, and increasingly among women. While alcoholism is the most common cause, chronic hepatitis and other rarer diseases can also produce the irreversible liver damage that characterizes cirrhosis. The resulting organ is shrunken and hard, unable to perform its varied duties. Because of its altered structure, the cirrhotic liver causes serious problems for surrounding organs, as blood flow becomes difficult. The barrier to normal circulation leads to two serious complications: portal hypertension (the buildup of pressure in the internal veins) and ascites (fluid leakage from blood vessels into the abdominal cavity).

TREATMENT AND THERAPY

Diagnosis is usually made from a history of alcoholism; a physical examination revealing a small, firm liver; a fluid-filled abdomen (ascites); and laboratory studies that show low concentrations of the blood products that the liver manufactures. A definitive diagnosis can only be made by biopsy, although radiographic methods such as computed tomography (CT) scanning and magnetic resonance imaging (MRI) can be quite conclusive.

The mortality rate is very high, as the damage is irreversible. Deaths from internal vein rupture and hemorrhage (the results of portal hypertension) and from kidney failure are most common. Repeated hospitalizations attempt to control the variety of complications that arise with agents that stop bleeding, bypass tubes that relieve pressure, the removal of the ascitic fluid, and nutritional support for malnutrition. Eventually, kidney failure ensues or one of these control measures fails, and death rapidly follows. Cases of mild cirrhosis, where sufficient normal tissue remains, have a clearly better course. *—Connie Rizzo, M.D.*

See also Alcoholism; Hepatitis; Jaundice; Liver; Liver cancer; Liver disorders; Liver transplantation.

Cirrhosis

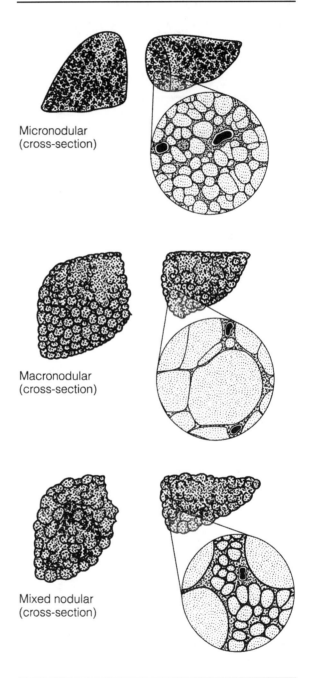

Micronodular (cross-section)

Macronodular (cross-section)

Mixed nodular (cross-section)

Cirrhosis appears in three forms, detectable under the microscope, each depending primarily on the cause of the liver damage. All, however, are characterized by the replacement of normally soft, spongy tissue with hard, fibrous scarring. Alcohol-related cirrhosis usually produces the micronodular form.

FOR FURTHER INFORMATION:

Bennett, J. Claude, et al., eds. *Cecil Textbook of Medicine.* 20th ed. Philadelphia: W. B. Saunders, 1996.

Fishman, Mark, et al. *Medicine.* 4th ed. Philadelphia: J. B. Lippincott, 1996.

Mulvihill, Mary. *Human Diseases: A Systemic Approach.* 4th ed. Norwalk, Conn.: Appleton and Lange, 1995.

CLAUDICATION

DISEASE/DISORDER

ANATOMY OR SYSTEM AFFECTED: Blood vessels, circulatory system, muscles, musculoskeletal system, nerves, nervous system

SPECIALTIES AND RELATED FIELDS: Internal medicine, neurology, vascular medicine

DEFINITION: Claudication describes a cramplike pain in one or both legs while walking, which eventually may develop into a limp. It is caused by atherosclerosis in the legs, in which the arteries become blocked or narrowed, restricting blood flow. Another, more rare form of claudication involves spinal stenosis, in which the spinal cord is constricted, putting pressure on the nerve roots going toward the legs. People suffering intermediate claudication are able to walk short distances, with rests in between to alleviate the pain.

—*Jason Georges and Tracy Irons-Georges*

See also Arteriosclerosis; Nervous system; Neuralgia, neuritis, and neuropathy; Neurology; Thrombosis and thrombus; Vascular medicine; Vascular system.

CLEFT LIP AND PALATE REPAIR

PROCEDURE

ANATOMY OR SYSTEM AFFECTED: Bones, gums, mouth, musculoskeletal system, skin

SPECIALTIES AND RELATED FIELDS: General surgery; neonatology; otorhinolaryngology; pediatrics; plastic, cosmetic, and reconstructive surgery

DEFINITION: The surgical closure of cleft lip and cleft palate, deformities of the mouth that are often described as either the failure of tissue migration to allow fusion or the failure of tissue ingrowth (filling in).

INDICATIONS AND PROCEDURES

Cleft lip is more common in males than in females. Additionally, males tend to have more severe cleft deformities than females. Cleft lip repair is classically performed according to the rule of tens: The infant should be ten weeks old, weigh at least ten pounds, and have a white blood cell count under 10,000 (no infections) and a hemoglobin count of ten grams (not anemic). Today, many surgeons prefer to perform repairs earlier in healthy, full-term newborns ranging in age from one day to fourteen days old. Cleft lip repairs typically involve making flaps around the lip area and merging the gaping sides together. The muscular layer around the mouth must be sealed into a functional unit, as must the skin.

Cleft palate is more prevalent in females than males by a 2:1 ratio. A cleft palate may involve only the soft palate, or it may involve both the hard and the soft palates. Suckling can be a greater challenge with a cleft palate than with cleft lip. Moreover, middle-ear disease and infections are a greater problem for an infant with a cleft palate, because the reflux of fluids or solids into the nasal or middle-ear regions can occur. Surgical closure of a cleft palate, usually is performed on infants between nine months and one year of age; delays can permanently retard speech and phonation development, while premature closure can stunt facial bone growth and contribute to dentition problems. Typically, if both the hard and the soft palates are open, they will be

The Repair of Cleft Lip

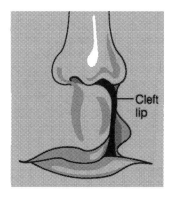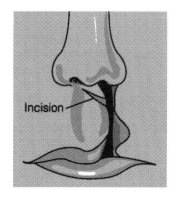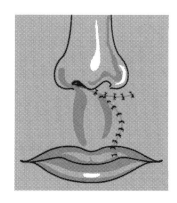

A cleft lip, a congenital deformity in which the tissues between the lip and nostril have failed to fuse, can be corrected surgically through realignment and suturing.

surgically closed at the same time. Closure of the soft palate occurs in a three-layer manner, while closure of the hard palate is done in a two-layer approach.

Cleft lip coupled with cleft palate is more common in males and tends to be left-sided more often than right-sided. Combined cleft lip and palate repair follows the same plans as described above, but there is greater concern about the well-being of an infant with the combined deformity.

—*Mary C. Fields*

See also Birth defects; Bones and the skeleton; Cleft palate; Pediatrics; Plastic, cosmetic, and reconstructive surgery; Surgery, pediatric.

CLEFT PALATE
DISEASE/DISORDER

ANATOMY OR SYSTEM AFFECTED: Bones, musculoskeletal system

SPECIALTIES AND RELATED FIELDS: Neonatology; Otorhinolaryngology; pediatrics; plastic, cosmetic, and reconstructive surgery; speech pathology

DEFINITION: A fissure in the midline of the palate so that the two sides fail to fuse during embryonic development; in some cases, the fissure may extend through both hard and soft palates into the nasal cavities.

KEY TERMS:

alveolus: the bony ridge where teeth grow

ectrodactyly: a congenital anomaly characterized by the absence of part or all of one or more of the fingers or toes

hard palate: the bony portion of the roof of the mouth, contiguous with the soft palate

Logan's bow: a metal bar placed, for protection and tension removal, on the early postoperative cleft lip

obturator: a sheet of plastic shaped like a flattened dome which fits into the cleft and closes it well enough to permit nursing

soft palate: a structure of mucous membrane, muscle fibers, and mucous glands suspended from the posterior border of the hard palate

syndactyly: a congenital anomaly characterized by the fusion of the fingers or toes

uvula: the small, cone-shaped process suspended in the mouth from the posterior of the soft palate

CAUSES AND SYMPTOMS

Cleft palate is a congenital defect characterized by a fissure along the midline of the palate. It occurs when the two sides fail to fuse during embryonic development. The gap may be complete, extending through the hard and soft palates into the nasal cavities, or may be partial or incomplete. It is often associated with cleft lip or "hare lip." About one child in eight hundred live births is affected with some degree of clefting, and clefting is the most common of the craniofacial abnormalities.

Cleft palate is not generally a genetic disorder; rather, it is a result of defective cell migration. Embryonically, in the first month, the mouth and nose form one cavity destined to be separated by the hard and soft palates. In addition, there is no upper lip. Most of the upper jaw is lacking; only the part near the ears is present. In the next weeks, the upper lip and jaw are formed from structures growing in from the sides, fusing at the midline with a third portion growing downward from the nasal region. The palates develop in much the same way. The fusion of all these structures begins with the lip and moves posteriorly toward, then includes, the soft palate. The two cavities are separated by the palates by the end of the third month of gestation.

If, as embryonic development occurs, the cells that should grow together to form the lips and palate fail to move in the correct direction, the job is left unfinished. Clefting of the palate generally occurs between the thirty-fifth and thirty-seventh days of gestation. Fortunately, it is an isolated defect not usually associated with other disabilities or with mental retardation.

If the interference in normal growth and fusion begins early and lasts throughout the fusion period, the cleft that results will affect one or both sides of the top lip and may continue back through the upper jaw, the upper gum ridge, and both palates. If the disturbance lasts only part of the time that development is occurring, only the lip may be cleft, and the palate may be unaffected. If the problem begins a little into the fusion process, the lip is normally formed, but the palate is cleft. The cleft may divide only the soft palate or both the soft and the hard palate. Even the uvula may be affected; it can be split, unusually short, or even absent.

About 80 percent of cases of cleft lip are unilateral; of these, 70 percent occur on the left side. Of cleft palate cases, 25 percent are bilateral. The mildest manifestations of congenital cleft are mild scarring and/or notching of the upper lip. Beyond this, clefting is described by degrees. The first degree is incomplete, which is a small cleft in the uvula. The second degree is also incomplete, through the soft palate and into the hard palate. Another type of "second-degree incomplete" is a horseshoe type, in which there is a bilateral cleft proceeding almost to the front. Third-degree bilateral is a cleft through both palates but bilaterally through the gums; it results in a separate area of the alveolus where the teeth will erupt, and the teeth will show up in a very small segment. When the teeth appear, they may not be normally aligned. In addition to the lip, gum, and palate deviations, abnormalities of the nose may also occur.

Cleft palate may be inherited, probably as a result of the interaction of several genes. In addition, the effect of some environmental factors that affect embryonic development may be linked to this condition. They might include mechanical disturbances such as an enlarged tongue, which prevents the fusion of the palate and lip. Other disturbances may be caused by toxins introduced by the mother (drugs such as cortisone or alcohol) and defective blood. Other associated factors include deficiencies of vitamins or minerals in the mother's diet, radiation from X rays, and infectious diseases such as German measles. No definite cause has been identified, nor does it appear that one cause alone can be implicated. It is likely that there is an interplay between mutant genes, chromosomal abnormalities, and environmental factors.

There are at least 150 syndromes involving oral and facial clefts. Four examples of cleft syndromes that illustrate these syndromes are EEC (ectrodactyly, ectodermal dysplasia, cleft lip/palate), popliteal pterygium syndrome, van der Woude's syndrome, and trisomy 13 syndrome. EEC and trisomy 13 both result in mental retardation as well as oral clefts, plus numerous other disabilities more serious than clefting. Popliteal pterygium has as its most common feature skin webbing (pterygium), along with clefts and skeletal abnormalities. Van der Woude's syndrome usually shows syndactyly as well as clefting and lower-lip pitting.

Problems begin at birth for the infant born with a cleft palate. The most immediate problem is feeding the baby. If the cleft is small and the lip unaffected, nursing may proceed fairly easily. If the cleft is too large, however, the baby cannot build up enough suction to nurse efficiently. To remedy this, the hole in the nipple of the bottle can be enlarged, or a plastic obturator can be fitted to the bottle.

Babies with cleft palate apparently are more susceptible to colds than other children. Since there is an open connection between the nose and mouth, an infection that starts in either location will easily and quickly spread to the other. Frequently, the infection will spread to the middle ear via the Eustachian tube. One end of a muscle is affixed to the Eustachian tube opening and the other end is attached to the middle of the roof of the mouth (palate). Normal contraction opens the tube so that air can travel through the tube and equalize air pressure on both sides of the eardrum. As long as the eardrum has flexibility of movement, the basics for good hearing are in place. Children with cleft palates, however, do not have good muscle reactions; therefore, air cannot travel through the tube. If the tube remains closed after swallowing, the air that is trapped is absorbed into the middle-ear tissue, resulting in a vacuum. This pulls the eardrum inward and decreases its flexibility, and hearing loss ensues. The cavity of the middle ear then fills with fluid, which often breeds bacteria, causing infection. The infection may or may not be painful; if there is no pain, the infection may go unnoticed and untreated. The accumulated fluid can cause erosion of the tiny bones, which would decrease sound transmission to the auditory nerve. This conductive hearing loss is permanent. Persistent and prolonged fluid buildup can also cause accumulation of dead matter, forming a tumorlike growth called a cholesteotoma.

Other problems associated with cleft palate are those related to dentition. In some children there may be extra teeth, while in others the cleft may prevent the formation of tooth buds so that teeth are missing. Teeth that are present may be malformed; those malformations include injury during development, fusion of teeth to form one large tooth, teeth lacking enamel, and teeth that have too little calcium in the enamel. If later in development and growth the teeth are misaligned, orthodontia may be undertaken. Another possible problem met by patients with a cleft palate is maxillary (upper-jaw) arch collapse; this condition is also remedied with orthodontic treatment.

TREATMENT AND THERAPY

One of the first questions a parent of a child with a cleft palate will pose regards surgical repair. The purpose of surgically closing the cleft is not simply to close the hole—although that goal is important. The major purpose is to achieve a functional palate. Whether this can be accomplished depends on the size and shape of the cleft, the thickness of the available tissue, and other factors. When the child is scheduled for surgery, it is a tangible sign that the condition is correctable. When the lip is successfully closed, it is positive affirmation that a professional team can help the family. The goals of both the team and the family are extremely similar: Both want the patient to look as normal as possible and to have a functional palate.

Cleft lip surgery is performed when the healthy baby weighs at least seven pounds; it is done under a general anesthetic. If the cleft is unilateral, one operation can accomplish the closure, but a bilateral cleft lip is often repaired in two steps at least a month apart. When the lip is repaired, normal lip pressure is restored, which may help in closing the cleft in the gum ridge. It may also reduce the gap in the hard palate, if one is present. Successive operations may be suggested when, even years after surgery, scars develop on the lip.

Surgery to close clefts of the hard and soft palate is typically done when the baby is at least nine months of age, unless there is a medical reason not to do so. Different surgeons prefer different times for this surgery. The surgeon attempts to accomplish three goals in the repair procedure. The surgeon will first try to ensure that the palate is long enough so that function and movement will result (this is essential for proper speech patterns). Second, the musculature around the Eustachian tube should work properly in order to cut down the incidence of ear infections. Finally, the surgery should promote the development of the facial bones and, as much as possible, normal teeth. This goal aids in eating and appearance. All this may be accomplished in one operation, if the cleft is not too severe. For a cleft that requires more procedures, the surgeries are usually spaced at least six months apart so that complete healing can occur. This schedule decreases the potential for severe scarring.

At one time, it was thought that if surgery were performed before the child began talking, speech problems would be avoided. In reality, not only did the surgery not remedy that problem but the early closure often resulted in a narrowing of the upper jaw and interference with facial growth as well. Thus the trend to put off the surgery until the child was four or five years of age developed; by this age, more than 80 percent of the lateral growth of the upper jaw has occurred. Most surgeons can perform the corrective surgery when the child is between one and two years of age without affecting facial growth.

Successful repair greatly improves speech and appearance, and the physiology of the oral and nasal cavities is also improved. Additional surgery may be necessary to improve appearance, breathing, and the function of the palate. Sometimes the palate may partially reopen, and surgery is needed to reclose it.

When the baby leaves the operating room, there are stitches in the repaired area. Sometimes a special device called a Logan's bow is taped to the baby's cheeks; this device not only protects the stitches but also relieves some of the tension on them. In addition, the baby's arms may be restrained in order to keep the baby's hands away from the affected area. (The child has been fitted for elbow restraints before surgery; the elbows are encased in tubes which prevent them from bending.) A parent of a child that has just undergone cleft palate repair should not panic at the sight of bleeding from the mouth. To curb it, gauze may be packed into the repaired area and remain about five days after surgery. As mucus and other body fluids accumulate in the area, they may be suctioned out.

During the initial recovery, the child is kept in a moist, oxygen-rich environment (an oxygen tent) until respiration is normal. The patient will be observed for signs of airway obstruction or excessive bleeding. Feeding is done by syringe, eyedropper, or special nipples. Clear liquids and juices only are allowed. The child sits in a high chair to drink, when possible. After feeding, the mouth should be rinsed well with water to help keep the stitches clean and uncrusted. Peroxide mixed with the water may help, as well as ointment. Intake and output of fluids are measured. Hospitalization may last for about a week, or however long is dictated by speed of healing. At the end of this week, stitches are removed and the suture line covered and protected by a strip of paper tape.

An alternative to surgery is the use of an artificial palate known as an obturator. It is specially constructed by a dentist to fit into the child's mouth. The appliance, or prosthesis, is carefully constructed to fit precisely and snugly, but it must be easily removable. There must be enough space at the back so the child can breathe through the nose. While speaking, the muscles move back over this opening so that speech is relatively unaffected.

Speech problems are likely the most residual of the problems in the cleft palate patient. The speech of the untreated, and sometimes the treated, cleft palate patient is very nasal. If the soft palate is too short, the closure of the palate may leave a space between the nose and the throat, allowing air to escape through the nose. There is little penetrating quality to the patient's voice, and it does not carry well. Some cleft palate speakers are difficult to understand because there are several faults in articulation. Certainly not all cleft lip or palate patients, however, will develop communication problems; modern surgical procedures help ensure that most children will develop acceptable speech and language without necessitating the help of a speech therapist.

Genetic counseling may help answer some of the family's questions about why the cleft palate occurred, whether

Forms of Cleft Palate

unilateral cleft lip

bilateral cleft lip

partial cleft palate

complete cleft palates

it will happen with future children, and whether there is any way to prevent it. There are no universal answers to these questions. The answers are dependent on the degree and type of cleft, the sex of the child, the presence of other problems, the family history, and the history of the pregnancy. Genetic counseling obtained at a hospital or medical clinic can determine whether the condition was heritable or a chance error and can establish the risk level for future pregnancies.

PERSPECTIVE AND PROSPECTS

Oral clefts, as well as other facial clefts, have been a part of historical record for thousands of years. Perhaps the earliest recorded incidence is a Neolithic shrine with a two-headed figurine dated about 6500 B.C. The origination and causative agent of such clefts remain mysterious today.

Expectant parents are rarely alerted prior to birth that their child will be born with a cleft, so it is usually in the hospital, just after birth, that parents first learn of the birth defect. Even if it is suspected that a woman is at risk for producing a child with a cleft palate, there is no way to determine if the defect is indeed present, as neither amniocentesis nor chromosomal analysis reveals the condition. When the baby is delivered, the presence of the cleft can evoke a feeling of crisis in the delivery room. Shocklike reactions may be caused by the unexpectedness of the event or can occur because the doctors and medical personnel in the room have had little exposure to the defect. The parents may feel personal failure.

The problems accompanying clefting may alter family morale and climate, increasing the complexity of the problem. A team of specialists usually work together to help the patient and the family cope with these problems. This team may include a pediatrician, a speech pathologist, a plastic surgeon, an orthodontist, a psychiatrist, a social worker, an otologist, an audiologist, and perhaps others. The formation and cooperation of a team of professionals and the emotional support that they provide for an affected family hopefully will enable that family to perceive the baby more positively, to focus on the child's potential rather than on the disability.

The cooperating team should monitor these situations: feeding problems, family and friend reactions to the baby's appearance, how parents encourage the child to talk or how they respond to poor speech, and whether the parents are realistic about the long-term outcome for their child. The grief, guilt, and shock that the parents often feel can be positively altered by how the professional team tackles the problem and by communication with the parents. Usually the team does not begin functioning in the baby's life until he or she is about a month old. Some parents have confronted their feelings, while others are still struggling with the negative feeling that the birth brought to bear. Therefore, the first visit that the parents have with the team is important, because it establishes the foundation of a support system which should last for years.

If the cleft was only a structural defect, the solution would simply be to close the hole. Yet, since there are problems concerning feeding and health, facial appearance, communication, speech, dental functioning, and hearing loss, as well as the potential for psychosocial difficulties, additional surgical, orthodontic, speech, and otolaryngological interventions may be necessary. In other words, after the closure has been made, attention is focused on aesthetic, functional, and other structural deficits.

—*Iona C. Baldridge*

See also Birth defects; Cleft lip and palate repair; Speech disorders.

FOR FURTHER INFORMATION:

Batshaw, Mark L. *Children with Disabilities*. Baltimore: Paul H. Brookes, 1997. This book first takes the reader through the basics of genetics. Based on this information, diagnoses and descriptions of birth defects are made relative to the various organ systems. Concludes by examining the emotional aspects of living with a handicapped child.

Clifford, Edward. *The Cleft Palate Experience*. Springfield, Ill.: Charles C Thomas, 1987. This author writes from the perspective of a cleft palate team participant and incorporates the value of the team in his chapters. Much space is given to the child's development of a positive self-image and the parents' role, from birth, in forming this image.

Dronamraju, Krishna R. *Cleft Lip and Palate*. Springfield, Ill.: Charles C Thomas, 1986. A compilation of research emphasizing population genetics, dental genetics, evolution, teratology, reproductive biology, and epidemiology. The purpose is to provide a basis for genetic counseling. An extensive bibliography is included.

Johnson, Wendell, and Dorothy Moeller, eds. *Speech Handicapped School Children*. 3d ed. New York: Harper & Row, 1967. Although this is a text for courses in speech pathology, the development and treatment of cleft palate are addressed. Psychological factors are considered, along with physical factors and associated problems with several speech handicaps.

Stengelhofen, Jackie, ed. *Cleft Palate*. Edinburgh: Churchill Livingstone, 1989. Explores the various communication problems met by those with a cleft palate. An appeal to the entire team of professionals treating the patient and their partnership with parents. Case histories are discussed.

Wynn, Sidney K., and Alfred L. Miller. *A Practical Guide to Cleft Lip and Palate Birth Defects*. Springfield, Ill.: Charles C Thomas, 1984. A very readable book that is actually a series of dialogues between the parents and doctors of affected children. The tone is a reassuring one, and most physical and psychological aspects are addressed forthrightly.

CLONING

PROCEDURE

ANATOMY OR SYSTEM AFFECTED: All

SPECIALTIES AND RELATED FIELDS: Biotechnology, embryology, ethics, genetics

DEFINITION: The production of new individuals who have exactly the same genes as another individual.

KEY TERMS:

cell: the basic structural unit of life; a human starts as a single cell (the fertilized egg) and develops into an adult with a trillion or more cells, almost all of which contain a nucleus with a complete set of genes

gene: a long string of chemical code letters that spell out the information needed for each feature of an individual; every human has thousands of genes, inherited from both parents, which are identical copies of those in the fertilized egg from which that individual developed

mammals: a large group of animals that share a pattern of reproduction in which offspring develop during pregnancy inside the female's body; includes many species of wild and farm animals, as well as humans

micropipette: a tiny glass tube that can be used under a microscope to manipulate and transfer cells and their parts

nucleus: a saclike structure inside each cell within which the genes are found

INDICATIONS AND PROCEDURES

A personal library of genes is responsible for all human features and is different for each person; every individual is genetically unique. The only naturally occurring exception to this rule is identical twins. This type of twinning occurs right after a fertilized egg has divided into two identical cells. For some reason, these two cells separate from each other rather than sticking together as normally happens. Each of these two separated cells then develops into a complete, normal individual. Because the two individuals are derived from the same fertilized egg, they contain identical sets of genes.

The process of natural twinning reveals much about the way in which new individuals develop. Both of the first two cells of a new individual must contain a complete library of genes. Adult cells also contain copies of all genes, or are the genes sorted out among cells as each individual develops and grows? Early experimental attempts at artificial cloning explored this question. The first breakthroughs were made by Robert Briggs and Thomas King in the 1950's. They attempted artificially to clone frogs, mainly because frogs have very large eggs that are easy to manipulate. The technique was to replace the nucleus (and therefore the genes) of a fertilized frog egg with a nucleus from a cell of a frog embryo or tadpole. If a normal frog grew from the fertilized egg, then the replacement nucleus must have contained all the genes needed to make the features of a complete frog. In some experiments, this was the result.

Many more experiments of this type were then done by John Gurdon and Donald Brown during the 1960's. They were able finally to reach the important conclusion that every adult cell (of a frog, at least) contains a complete set of genes.

In principle, it was also possible to perform the same type of procedure using the eggs and cells of mammals, to test whether artificial cloning was possible with this group of animals as well. The procedures, however, proved to be much more difficult with mammals. It was not until 1981 that Karl Ilmensee and Peter Hoppe succeeded in cloning a mammal, a mouse, for the first time. This was done by implanting a nucleus from a mouse embryo cell into a fertilized mouse egg whose own nucleus had been removed. This hybrid egg was then returned to the womb of a female mouse and went through development to a normal birth.

In 1996, Scottish investigator Ian Wilmut finally succeeded in producing a clone of an adult mammal, a sheep, by transplanting the nucleus from an adult sheep cell into a sheep's fertilized egg. This proved that adult cells of mammals also contain complete sets of genes. It now became possible artificially to clone adults of other mammals, including adult human beings.

The first step in cloning a mammal is to obtain a fertilized egg. This can be done in one of two ways. First, an egg fertilized normally can be removed from the female's womb for use in this procedure. The egg must be obtained very shortly after fertilization by the male sperm cell. This procedure is not particularly difficult but requires precise timing, and it is rarely possible to obtain more than a single egg in this way. The success rate of cloning is less than 100 percent, so it is important to start with as many eggs as possible. The second approach is more efficient: A large number of unfertilized eggs are harvested and fertilized with the male's sperm outside the female's body. By treating an egg-donating female with a fertility drug beforehand, as many as twenty fertilizable eggs can be harvested at once. These eggs are then fertilized in a dish in a warmed salt bath. The exact composition of this salt solution is critical in order to keep the eggs alive. The recipes were perfected in the 1960's by several investigators, including Ralph G. Edwards and Ruth Fowler.

The next step in cloning is to obtain a single cell from the donor to be cloned. The donor can be an embryo, youngster, or adult of the same species as the fertilized egg. As an individual matures, the nuclei become more specialized for one kind of function, and the success rate for cloning decreases. It seems, however, that no particular cell type—for example, from the liver, skin, or lung—works better than others. Tissue samples from adults can be obtained in many ways, such as biopsies of organs, skin scrapings, or from body fluids. Once a tissue specimen is obtained, the cells of the specimen (or embryo) are separated from one another by chemically digesting the connections between them. Then, a single cell is drawn into a tiny pipette. The width of the pipette is made exactly right so that the cell breaks, freeing the nucleus inside but not damaging it.

Now, the nucleus of the fertilized egg (containing its genes) must be carefully removed. This is done with a micropipette, which is inserted inside the fertilized egg. Because fertilized eggs are many times larger than adult cells, this does not harm or break the egg. The nucleus is located and gently sucked into the pipette, and the pipette is withdrawn. This nucleus is discarded, and the donor nucleus is injected into this large egg cell. At this point, then, there is a fertilized egg ready to begin development using the genetic instructions from a different cell.

It is now necessary to implant this fertilized egg into the womb of an adult female, hopefully leading to a normal pregnancy. This individual can be the female from whom the fertilized egg was originally obtained or a surrogate (replacement). The outcome should be the same in either case, since the female does not supply genetic directions during pregnancy that would influence features of the newborn.

USES AND COMPLICATIONS

Cloning research has greatly improved the understanding of how genes work to control the development of a fertilized egg into a complete and functional individual. First and most significant, cloning has shown that nearly every cell of the adult body inherits a complete set of genes from the fertilized egg. (Red blood cells and a few others are exceptions.) Of equal importance, it has shown that if the nucleus of an adult cell is returned to the inside of a fertilized egg, it becomes reprogrammed, and its genetic library responds appropriately by directing the construction of a complete new individual. This reprogramming has been studied in detail and has provided an intimate glimpse of how genes conduct development. It is these two facts of biology that make it possible to clone an individual by inserting one of its nuclei into a fertilized egg.

Cloning is now being used to make identical copies of superior farm animals. The simplest way to do this is to copy the process of natural twin formation described above, to produce artificial twins. This is done by recovering a fertilized egg after it has cleaved into a few cells. These cells are then chemically separated from each other, and each cell is reimplanted into a surrogate female to continue the pregnancy. One advantage of the procedure is that many offspring can be obtained from a single breeding between the parents. Another advantage is that the cells can be frozen and stored for later use or can be conveniently shipped to another part of the world. These procedures are particularly valuable for such purposes as breeding and distributing superior cattle and horses. It is interesting to note that these same procedures are helpful for preserving species of animals that are threatened with extinction. Many individual animals can be produced from a single success-

ful breeding, and some of the cells can be frozen and preserved for future use.

It is also possible to use the nuclear transplantation procedure to make genetically identical clones of a superior adult animal. Although much more complex and risky, this procedure is more predictable for duplicating the qualities of the cloned animal (for example, milk production or meat quality). The simpler twinning method by separating embryo cells will produce offspring whose traits are a random mix of those of the two parents, which may or may not result in a superior animal.

The methods for cloning are essentially microsurgical techniques, involving delicate operations on tiny eggs and embryos. The procedures have been steadily improved until they are almost as reliable as other small-scale surgical techniques. Inevitable risks and complications, however, must be taken into account. Cloning of mammals involves removing eggs from the female reproductive system, moving nuclei into and out of them outside the female's body, and then returning the eggs to the female's body. The cells being operated on are small and fragile, and they are easily damaged at any stage in this process. Also, the environment is quite different outside the mammalian female's body than inside the womb, and some small error—for example, with temperature or nutrients in the bathing solutions where the eggs are kept—can cause death or an abnormality in the development of the individual later on. Success rates with the nuclear transplantation procedure decline with the age of the donor of the transplanted nucleus. Thus, although the techniques are reliable, there is still a substantial risk of failure, as with any procedure involving stress on delicate cells.

PERSPECTIVE AND PROSPECTS

Studies of animal cloning have a long history, starting with simple attempts to transplant nuclei into frog eggs in the 1940's. The procedures gradually improved, and, by the 1960's, frog nuclei could be transplanted and result in normal adult frogs. These intensive studies set the stage for cloning work with mammals. The additional difficulties to be overcome to clone mammals were substantial. A critical breakthrough was the development of the precise conditions for keeping eggs alive outside the female's body. This step was a key to mammalian cloning, and it came after years of tedious research.

Since the 1980's, it has been technically possible to clone almost any animal, including humans. The limitations on human cloning now are not in the methods but in the ethical, legal, economic, and moral questions that accompany this procedure. The success rate cannot be 100 percent, so potential human beings (that is, fertilized human eggs) are being placed at risk by the procedure. If something does go wrong, it is not entirely clear whose fault it might be. The cloning procedures are also complex and expensive, and they cannot be made available to everyone.

It is important to note that a clone of an individual will

not be exactly identical to the "parent" that donated the nucleus. The clone will be younger than the donor because it must go through the complete process of development. Also, genes are not the only factor that affects development; very minor differences in the egg's environment can have major effects on the features of an individual. No one will ever be able to have a truly identical clone.

Clearly, human cloning is difficult enough that it will not be undertaken without good reasons. Less radical procedures, however, that make use of similar techniques promise to improve greatly human well-being. In particular, it is now possible to transplant copies of individual genes into the nuclei of fertilized eggs. This gene therapy can be done to correct an inherited genetic defect, such as cystic fibrosis, that is caused by abnormal copies of genes inherited from one or both parents. This kind of genetic surgery on embryos, which takes advantage of many years of hard work on cloning methods, is risky, but less so than cloning. It is a valuable tool in the field of molecular medicine.

—*Howard L. Hosick, Ph.D.*

See also Cells; Conception; Embryology; Ethics; Gene therapy; Genetic diseases; Genetic engineering; Genetics and inheritance; In vitro fertilization; Law and medicine; Multiple births; Pregnancy and gestation.

FOR FURTHER INFORMATION:

Alpern, Kenneth D., ed. *The Ethics of Reproductive Technology*. New York: Oxford University Press, 1992. A series of essays by experts on the techniques, ethical issues, and significance of various ways of influencing the development of human embryos.

Begley, Sharon, Mariana Gosnell, Timothy Nater, and Phyllis Malamud. "The Three Cloned Mice." *Newsweek*, January 19, 1981, 65-66. This well-written article clearly describes the first cloning of a mammal. It discusses both the procedure and some of its ethical implications. An excellent illustration makes clear each step in the procedure and its purpose.

Capecchi, Mario R. "Targeted Gene Replacement." *Scientific American* 270 (March, 1994): 52-59. Good coverage of how defective genes can be replaced with normal copies by inserting the genes into eggs. Recommended for those interested in this topic related to cloning.

Corea, Gena. *The Mother Machine*. New York: Harper & Row, 1985. This book presents a strong viewpoint about how cloning and other reproductive technologies can affect women. This book is representative of the literature on biotechnology from a feminist perspective.

Edwards, Ralph G., and Ruth E. Fowler. "Human Embryos in the Laboratory." *Scientific American* 201 (December, 1970): 44-54. An excellent introduction to the problems associated with keeping eggs and embryos alive outside the female's body and how those problems were solved.

Gurdon, John B. "Transplanted Nuclei and Cell Differentiation." *Scientific American* 219 (January, 1968): 24-35. A clear and well-illustrated summary of many years of work on cloning, primarily of frogs and toads. Gurdon describes the procedures beautifully.

Nossal, G. J. V., and Ross L. Coppel. *Reshaping Life: Key Issues in Genetics Engineering*. 2d ed. New York: Cambridge University Press, 1989. Includes chapters on how cells work, how genes work, and how genes can be transplanted, as well as several chapters on the implications of such techniques for human life.

CLUSTER HEADACHES
DISEASE/DISORDER
ANATOMY OR SYSTEM AFFECTED: Brain, head, nervous system, psychic-emotional system

SPECIALTIES AND RELATED FIELDS: Family medicine, internal medicine, neurology

DEFINITION: Cluster headaches are characterized by intense pain behind one eye. They are generally recurrent in nature and are of such severity that they may wake the sufferer nightly for periods of weeks or months. Some researchers have suggested that cluster headaches are one category of migraine headache. Cluster headaches may be precipitated by the injection of histamine, a vasodilator that causes a fall in blood pressure; they are sometimes termed histaminic headaches or cephalalgia.

—*Jason Georges and Tracy Irons-Georges*

See also Brain; Brain disorders; Head and neck disorders; Headaches; Migraine headaches; Stress.

COLITIS
DISEASE/DISORDER
ANATOMY OR SYSTEM AFFECTED: Abdomen, gastrointestinal system, intestines, stomach

SPECIALTIES AND RELATED FIELDS: Gastroenterology, internal medicine

DEFINITION: A potentially fatal but manageable disease of the colon which inflames and ulcerates the bowel lining, occurring in both acute and chronic forms.

KEY TERMS:

diarrhea: persistent liquid or mushy, shapeless stool

dysentery: bloody diarrhea caused by infectious agents affecting the colon

ileum: the last section of the small bowel, which passes food wastes to the colon through the ileocecal valve

inflammation: swelling caused by the accumulation of fluids and chemical agents

mucosa: the membrane of cells that lines the bowel; admits fluids and nutrients but also serves as the first-line protection against infectious agents and other materials foreign to the body

procedure: any medical treatment that entails physical manipulation or invasion of the body

stoma: an opening, formed by surgery, from the bowel to the exterior surface of the body

stool: the food wastes mixed with fluid, bacteria, mucus, and dead cells that exit the body upon defecation

ulcer: an area of the mucosa that has been abraded or dissolved by infection or chemicals, creating an open sore

CAUSES AND SYMPTOMS

The colon is the section of the lower bowel, or intestines, extending from the ileocecal valve to the rectum. It is wider in diameter than the small bowel, although shorter in length at about one meter. From behind the pelvis, the colon rises along the right side of the body (ascending colon), turns left to cross the upper abdominal cavity (transverse colon), and then turns down along the left side of the body (descending colon) until it joins the sigmoid (S-shaped) colon. The sigmoid colon empties into the rectum, a pouch that stores the waste products of digestion that are excreted through the anus. The colon absorbs most of the fluid passed to it from the small bowel, so that wastes solidify; meanwhile, bacteria in the colon break down undigested proteins and carbohydrates, creating hydrogen, carbon dioxide, and methane gases in the process.

A key structure in colonic activity is its mucosa. This thin sheet of cells lining the bowel wall permits passage of fluids and certain nutrients into the bloodstream but resists bacteria and toxins (poisonous chemical compounds). When the mucosa is torn or worn away, bacteria and toxins enter, infecting the bowel wall. The body responds to infection by rushing fluids and powerful chemicals to the endangered area to confine and kill the infecting agents. In the process, the tissues of the bowel wall swell with the fluids; this is known as inflammation. The medical suffix denoting this response is *-itis*; when it occurs in the colon, physicians call it colitis.

A variety of agents can cause colitis, which is divided into two major types depending on the duration of the disease: acute colitis and chronic ulcerative colitis. Acute colitis is a relatively brief, single episode of inflammation. It is often caused by bacteria or parasites. For example, *Giardia lamblia*, a bacterium in many American streams, is a common infectious agent in colitis, and the amoebas in polluted water supplies are responsible for the type of colitis known as amebic dysentery. Some medicines, however, especially antibiotics, can also induce colitis. Acute colitis either disappears on its own or can be cured with drugs. Untreated, however, it may be fatal.

Chronic ulcerative colitis and Crohn's disease constitute a category of serious afflictions called inflammatory bowel disease (IBD) whose primary physical effects include swelling of the bowel lining, ulcers, and bloody diarrhea. Although some medical researchers think that these afflictions may be two aspects of the same disease, ulcerative colitis affects only the colon, whereas Crohn's disease can involve the small bowel as well as the colon. Moreover, colitis chiefly involves the colonic mucosa, but Crohn's disease delves into the full thickness of the bowel wall.

Chronic ulcerative colitis is a permanent disease that manifests itself either in recurring bouts of inflammation or in continuous inflammation that cannot be cleared up with drugs. It is commonly called ulcerative colitis because ulcers, open sores in the mucosa, spread throughout the colon and rectum, where the disease usually starts. Researchers have not yet discovered the causes of chronic ulcerative colitis, although there are many theories, of which three are prominent. The first is bacterial or viral infection, and many agents have been proposed as the culprit. Because such a multitude of organisms commonly reside in or pass through the colon, researchers have enormous difficulty separating out a specific kind in order to show that it is always present during colitis attacks. Second is autoimmune reaction. Research in other diseases has shown that sometimes the body's police system, enforced by white blood cells, mistakes native, healthy tissue for a foreign agent and attacks that tissue in an attempt to destroy it. Yet no testing in chronic ulcerative colitis has yet proven the theory. Third is a combination of foreign infection and autoimmune response; it is as if the immune system overreacts to an infectious agent and continues its attack even after the agent has been neutralized. Many researchers have suspected that the disease is inherited, because certain families have higher rates of the disease than others. This genetic theory is not universally accepted, however, because it is just as likely that family members share infection rather than having passed on a genetic predisposition for the disease. Other theories propose food allergies as the cause; even toothpaste has been considered.

Regardless of the cause, there is no doubt that colitis is a painful, disabling, bewildering disease. When the bowel inflames, the tissues heat up and fever results. Cramps are common, and sufferers feel an urgent, frequently uncontrollable urge to defecate. When they reach the toilet (if they do so in time), they have soft, loose stool or diarrhea, which can seem to explode from the anus. They may have as many as ten to twenty bowel movements a day. Because ulcers often erode blood vessels, blood can appear in the stool, as well as mucus and pus from the bowel wall. Severe weight loss, anemia, lack of energy, dehydration, and anorexia often develop as the colitis persists. The symptoms may clear up on their own only to recur months or years later; attacks may come with increasing frequency thereafter. The first attack, if it worsens rapidly, is fatal in about 5 to 10 percent of patients, although the death rate can rise to 25 percent among first-time sufferers who are more than sixty years old.

Complications from colitis can be life-threatening. These include perforation of the bowel wall, strictures, hemorrhaging, and toxic megacolon (hyperinflation of the colon, an emergency medical condition). Furthermore, studies show that patients who have had ulcerative colitis for more than ten years have about a 20 percent chance of developing cancer in the colon or rectum.

Because colitis is a relapsing, embarrassing disease, patients often suffer psychological turmoil. In *Colitis* (1992), Michael P. Kelly reports the results of his study of forty-five British colitis patients. According to Kelly, they typically denied that early symptoms were the signs of serious illness, passing them off as the result of overeating or influenza. The denial continued until the continual, desperate urge to defecate made them despair of controlling their bowels without help. Often, they suffered embarrassment because they had to flee family gatherings or work in order to find a toilet or because they passed stool inadvertently in public. Many feared being beyond easy access to a toilet, shunned public places, and felt humiliated. Only then did some visit a physician, and even after chronic ulcerative colitis was diagnosed, a portion hoped they could still cope on their own. When they could not, they grew depressed, insomniac, angry at their fate, or antisocial. Even with treatment, the strain of enduring the disease can be debilitating.

Treatment and Therapy

Fortunately, medical science has several well-tested methods of controlling or curing colitis. In the case of acute colitis, patients usually resume normal bowel functions on their own and emerge as healthy as they were before the onset of symptoms. For chronic ulcerative colitis patients, however, the body is rarely the same again, and they must adjust to the effects of medication, surgery, or both—an adjustment that some authors claim is essentially a redefinition of the self.

After interviewing a patient and assessing the reported symptoms, the physician suspecting colitis orders a stool sample to check for blood, bacteria, parasites, and pus. If any of these are present, the physician directly examines the rectum and colon by inserting a fiberoptic endoscope into the rectum and up the colon. Early in the disease, the mucosa looks granular with scattered hemorrhages and tiny bleeding points. As the disease progresses, the mucosa turns spongy and has many ulcers that ooze blood and pus. An X ray often helps determine the extent of inflammation, and tissue samples taken by endoscopic biopsy can establish if it is ulcerative colitis or infection, and not Crohn's disease, that is present.

There is no easy treatment for chronic ulcerative colitis. Dietary restrictions—especially the elimination of fibrous foods such as raw fruits and vegetables or of milk products—may reduce the irritation to the inflamed colon, and symptoms then may improve if the disease is mild. Antidiarrheal drugs can firm the stool and reduce the patient's urgency to defecate, although such drugs must be used very cautiously to avoid dangerous dilation of the bowels.

Such nonspecific measures are seldom more than delaying tactics, and drugs are needed to counteract the colon's inflammation. Two types are most common. The first, sulfasalazine, is a sulfa drug developed in the 1940's. It is an anti-inflammatory agent that is most effective in mild to moderate ulcerative colitis and helps prevent recurrence of inflammation. Corticosteroids, the second type, behave like the hormones produced by the adrenal gland that suppress inflammation. The drug works well in relieving the symptoms of moderate to moderately severe attacks. Both types of drugs have serious side effects, so physicians must carefully tailor dosages for each patient and check repeatedly for reactions. In some patients, sulfasalazine induces nausea, vomiting, joint pain, headaches, rashes, dizziness, and hepatitis (liver inflammation). The effects of corticosteroids include sleeplessness, mood swings, acne, high blood pressure, diabetes, cataracts, thinning of the bones (especially the spine), and fluid retention and swelling of the face, hands, abdomen, and ankles. Women may grow facial hair; adolescents may have delayed sexual maturation. In most cases, the side effects clear up when patients stop taking the drugs.

With medication, people who suffer mild or moderate chronic ulcerative colitis can control it for years, often for the rest of their lives. Severe colitis requires surgery, and sometimes patients with milder forms choose to have surgery rather than live with the disease's unpredictable recurrence or the ever-present side effects of drugs. In any case, surgery is the one known cure for chronic ulcerative colitis, although fewer than one-third of patients undergo surgical procedures. Several types of these surgeries have high success rates.

Because ulcerative colitis eventually spreads throughout the colon, complete removal of the large bowel and rectum is the surest way to eliminate the disease. This "total proctocolectomy" takes place in three steps. The surgeon first cuts through the wall of the abdomen, the incision extending from the mid-transverse colon to the rectum, and removes the colon. Next, the end of the ileum is pulled through a hole in the abdomen to form a stoma (a procedure called an ileostomy). Finally, the rectum is removed and the anus sutured shut. Thereafter the patient defecates through the stoma. Either of two arrangements prevents stool from simply spilling out unchecked. Most patients affix plastic bags around their stomas into which stool flows without their control; when full, the bag is either emptied and reattached or thrown away and replaced. To avoid external bags, some patients prefer a "continent ileostomy," so called because it allows them to control defecation. The surgeon constructs a pouch out of a portion of the ileum and attaches it right behind the stoma, a procedure called a Kock pouch after its inventor, Nils Kock of Sweden. When this pouch is full, the patient empties it with a catheter inserted through the stoma. Some patients can choose to have an ileoanal anastomosis. In this procedure, the surgeon forms the end of the ileum into a pouch, which is attached to the anus and collects wastes in place of the rectum. The patient continues to defecate through the anus rather than through a stoma.

None of these surgical procedures is free of problems, and all require extensive recovery in the hospital and rehabilitation. Moreover, both infections and mechanical failures can occur. If healthy portions of the colon are left intact, they often flare with colitis later, and more operations become necessary. Patients with stomas are vulnerable to bacterial inflammation of the small intestine, resulting in diarrhea, vomiting, and dehydration. Stomas and pouches sometimes leak or close up, and even after successful operations patients lose some capacity to absorb zinc, bile salts, and vitamin B_{12}, although food supplements can make up for these deficiencies.

Any major surgery is an emotional trial. One that leaves a basic function of the body permanently altered, as with proctocolectomy or ileostomy, is difficult to accept afterward, even when the surgery was an emergency to save the patient's life. Patients must live with a bag of stool on their abdomen or a pouch that they must empty with a plastic straw—bags and pouches that sometimes leak stool or gas and that, even when functioning smoothly, are not pleasant to handle. They must pay close attention to body functions that they rarely had to think about before the ulcerative colitis began. The changes can severely depress patients, who then may need psychiatric help and antidepressant drugs to recover their spirits. Patients with anastomoses, who continue to defecate through their anus, also find their bowel functions changed, although not so severely. For example, it takes many months before normal stool forms, and diarrhea plagues these patients.

After their operations, patients have access to considerable help in addition to physicians and surgeons. Special nurses train patients to care for their stomas, check regularly for infection or malfunction, and generally ease them into their new lives. Formal support groups and informal networks are common, through which the afflicted can get information and reassurance. In the United States, the National Foundation for Ileitis and Colitis arranges many support groups, as well as sponsoring medical research and education programs.

PERSPECTIVE AND PROSPECTS

Acute forms of colitis, especially amebic dysentery, have long been recognized as among the endemic diseases of polluted water, and until the development of antibiotics, they regularly killed significant portions of local populations, especially the young and elderly. Chronic ulcerative colitis was first described in 1859, but no effective treatment for it existed until the 1940's. At that time, Nana Svartz of Sweden noticed that when rheumatoid arthritis patients were given sulfasalazine, the bowel condition of those who had colitis improved as well. J. Arnold Bargen, an American physician, confirmed Svartz's observation in a formal clinical trial, and sulfasalazine soon was mass-produced for distribution in the United States and later throughout the world. Since the 1940's, medications and surgical techniques for

ulcerative colitis have proliferated, although none restores a patient's original state of health.

Because the agents causing ulcerative colitis are unknown, the historical and geographical origin of the disease likewise cannot be determined. Nevertheless, three somewhat odd social facets of the disease are recognized.

Evidence suggests that ulcerative colitis is a disease of urban industrial society. Along with Crohn's disease, colitis appears to be entrenched in Scandinavia, the United States, Western Europe, Israel, and England. It rarely occurs in rural Africa, Asia, or South America, despite the poor nutrition and sanitation in some of these areas. Yet the disease does not appear to vary solely by racial type or nationality, although Jewish people tend to fall ill with it more often than any other group. For example, African Americans, whether from families long-established in the United States or recently immigrated, show an incidence of colitis as high as residents of European descent.

Furthermore, ulcerative colitis strikes the young. It most often begins between the ages of fifteen and thirty; men and women are equally likely to come down with it. This fact, taken with the high rate of inflammatory bowel disease (IBD) sufferers who have family members also with the disease (20 to 25 percent), has led some researchers to believe that a genetic factor creates a susceptibility for IBD.

Finally, IBD patients bear some social stigma, or at least believe they do. Ulcerative colitis involves bowel incontinence and often ends with surgical replacement of the anus with a stoma; in such cases, bowel movements can dominate a patient's life and become obvious to family members, coworkers, and even strangers. Because the subject of stool is taboo to many and the odor offends most people, patients can feel severe embarrassment and come to see themselves as pariahs. Even though the causes of ulcerative colitis remain obscure and the treatment is often distressing, modern medicine saves people who otherwise would die.

—*Roger Smith, Ph.D.*

See also Colon and rectal surgery; Colon cancer; Crohn's disease; Diarrhea and dysentery; Diverticulosis and diverticulitis; Gastroenterology; Gastrointestinal disorders; Gastrointestinal system; Intestinal disorders; Intestines.

FOR FURTHER INFORMATION:

Berkow, Robert, and Andrew J. Fletcher, eds. *The Merck Manual of Diagnosis and Therapy.* 16th ed. Rahway, N.J.: Merck, 1992. This is a reference work for physicians, and the nomenclature can be daunting. It is best consulted after more general introductory reading. The sections on colitis describe the physical symptoms, tests, and treatments systematically and thoroughly.

Brandt, Lawrence J., and Penny Steiner-Grossman, eds. *Treating IBD: A Patient's Guide to the Medical and Surgical Management of Inflammatory Bowel Disease.* New York: Raven, 1989. The most thorough introduction to ulcerative colitis and Crohn's disease. Writing for patients, the authors, who are all medical experts, present technical information and guidelines on symptoms, drugs, surgical procedures, nutritional management, psychotherapy, and counseling. Illustrations, tables, and very helpful glossaries accompany the text.

Kelly, Michael P. *Colitis.* New York: Routledge, 1992. Kelly begins his book with a description of symptoms and treatments, but his is primarily a sociological study. Based on interviews with forty-five patients, the work discusses typical effects that the disease had on their lives and how they coped with the treatments, especially surgical procedures. Essential reading for anyone diagnosed as having chronic ulcerative colitis.

Oppenheim, Michael. *The Complete Book of Better Digestion: A Gut-Level Guide to Gastric Relief.* Emmaus, Pa.: Rodale Press, 1990. Oppenheim's discussion of colitis is brief, but it provides a good generalized guide to symptoms and treatment. The book is most valuable as an introduction to the entire digestive tract's functions and maladies.

Plaut, Martin E. *The Doctor's Guide to You and Your Colon.* New York: Harper & Row, 1982. Although somewhat out of date, this guide is a simple and often-humorous survey of the colon and its diseases, including ulcerative colitis. Adorned with illustrations and cartoons and supplemented with recipes, it is useful as background for more specific literature about colitis.

Steiner-Grossman, Penny, Peter A. Banks, and Daniel H. Present, eds. *People . . . Not Patients: A Source Book for Living with Inflammatory Bowel Disease.* New York: National Foundation for Ileitis and Colitis, 1985. Written to help IBD patients live with their diseases, this book combines very practical information—about support groups and patients' rights, for example—with overviews of symptoms and treatments. Its main strength, however, lies in case histories of patients from different walks of life.

Thompson, W. Grant. *The Angry Gut: Coping with Colitis and Crohn's Disease.* New York: Plenum Press, 1993. The author discusses inflammatory bowel diseases. Includes bibliographic references and an index.

COLON AND RECTAL POLYP REMOVAL
PROCEDURE

ANATOMY OR SYSTEM AFFECTED: Abdomen, anus, gastrointestinal system, intestines

SPECIALTIES AND RELATED FIELDS: Gastroenterology, general surgery, proctology

DEFINITION: The surgical removal of overgrowths of the tissue lining the rectum and colon.

INDICATIONS AND PROCEDURES

Rectal and colon polyps often cause no symptoms. They are usually detected by visible blood present on feces or by routine screening for colorectal cancers. The fecal occult

blood test will detect blood that is not visible. When polyps are suspected, the physician will perform special tests such as barium enema X rays, flexible sigmoidoscopy, or colonoscopy. The latter two examinations require the passage of a small fiber-optic tube into the rectum and colon via the anus. This allows the physician to visualize the lining of the bowel.

If rectal or colon polyps are found, they are usually removed, even if they cause no symptoms, because of the possibility that these benign growths will develop into an invasive cancer. Removal is accomplished using colonoscopy to visualize the polyps and specialized forceps to detach and remove the growths. Snare forceps can be used to surround a polyp and cut it from the lining of the colon or rectum. Electrocautery forceps use heat to sever the polyp from the surrounding healthy tissue and seal off blood vessels. Special precautions must be taken, however, to remove gas from the colon so that the combustion of hydrogen or methane gas does not occur. These gases are normally produced by bacteria that inhabit the colon.

USES AND COMPLICATIONS

Since this procedure is somewhat uncomfortable for the patient, sedatives may be given. General anesthesia is usually not necessary, as rectal and colon polyp removal is typically done as an outpatient procedure.

Repeat colonoscopy should be performed so that recurrent polyps can be removed and examined for malignancy. Colorectal cancer is the second leading cause of cancer deaths in the United States, and the majority of these cancers arise from colorectal polyps.

—*Matthew Berria, Ph.D., and Douglas Reinhart, M.D.*

See also Biopsy; Cancer; Colon and rectal surgery; Colon cancer; Colonoscopy; Electrocauterization; Endoscopy; Enemas; Gastroenterology; Gastrointestinal system; Hemorrhoid banding and removal; Hemorrhoids; Intestinal disorders; Intestines; Oncology; Proctology; Screening.

COLON AND RECTAL SURGERY
PROCEDURE

ANATOMY OR SYSTEM AFFECTED: Abdomen, anus, gastrointestinal system, intestines

SPECIALTIES AND RELATED FIELDS: Gastroenterology, general surgery, proctology

DEFINITION: Surgery that is required to correct pathologies of the colon, rectum, and anus.

KEY TERMS:

abscess: a pocket of infection or inflammation

acute: referring to a short, immediate disease state

chronic: referring to an enduring disease state

ulcer: a lesion that destroys tissue

INDICATIONS AND PROCEDURES

The large intestine, or colon, is shaped like an inverted *U*. It starts at the lower right side of the pelvis, where the small intestine empties into the cecum. The colon rises from the cecum to the center of the abdomen, crosses to the left, and descends to the S-shaped sigmoid colon, the rectum, and the anus. Common disorders of the colon, rectum, and anus that require surgery are hemorrhoids, Crohn's disease, ulcerative colitis, cancer, diverticulosis, and diverticulitis.

Hemorrhoids are swollen veins in the lower part of the rectum and the anus. They protrude as nodes or lumps that can cause severe pain, itching, and inflammation. Hemorrhoids can be tied off with tiny rubber bands. After a few days, they fall off painlessly. Medications can shrink internal hemorrhoids, or hemorrhoidal tissue can be removed by photocoagulation, a process that uses electromagnetic energy to eradicate affected tissues. Sometimes, a hemorrhoidectomy is required. This procedure involves the extensive excision of hemorrhoidal tissue and can be quite painful.

Crohn's disease and ulcerative colitis are chronic inflammatory bowel diseases (IBDs) that can affect the colon. Crohn's disease usually occurs in the small intestine, although it may be limited to the colon. When Crohn's disease is severe and restricted to the colon, the surgeon may perform an ileostomy. This procedure involves removing the entire lower intestine, rectum, and anus. The anal opening is closed, and a new opening, or stoma, is made in the abdominal wall. The ileum, the lower end of the small intestine, is then attached to the opening. A removable pouch is sealed to the opening to collect fecal matter, which must be emptied manually.

Ulcerative colitis may exist with no symptoms other than an occasional flare-up, or it can be a chronic, serious, or life-threatening disease. It is characterized by a series of ulcers on the inner wall of the colon. Bloody diarrhea, abdominal pain, and painful bowel movements are symptoms. In severe cases, there is danger of perforation of the colon wall or of swelling (toxic megacolon), either of which can be life-threatening. Ulcerative colitis may also be a precursor of colon cancer. In severe cases of ulcerative colitis, surgery is required. Ileostomy is the surgical procedure usually performed, but recently a procedure was developed called ileoanal anastomosis. As in ileostomy, the surgeon removes the entire colon and rectum but leaves the anal sphincter muscles. The ileum is then attached to the anus. This procedure allows the patient to have natural bowel movements and avoids the necessity of the ileostomy pouch.

Cancers of the colon or rectum, called colorectal cancers, are major causes of morbidity and mortality. The possibility of colon cancer is often signaled by the presence of polyps on the lower intestinal wall. Symptoms such as mucus or blood in the stool may alert the physician to look for polyps and determine whether they are likely to become cancerous. Benign polyps are usually removed surgically.

When polyps are likely to become cancerous, and in the presence of actual colorectal cancer, surgery is usually performed to remove diseased tissue. This often requires excising part or all of the colon. Sometimes a colostomy is performed, an operation similar to an ileostomy. In this procedure, the diseased sections of the colon, the rectum, and the anus are removed. The anal opening is sealed, and the remaining colon is brought to an opening in the abdominal wall. This opening, or stoma, is fitted with a removable colostomy bag or pouch to collect fecal matter.

Diverticula are small, saclike pouches that develop in the colon wall, most often in the sigmoid colon. Their presence is known as diverticulosis. These sacs can collect stagnant fecal matter and become inflamed, resulting in diverticulitis. Abscesses and infection may develop. As inflammation progresses or recurs, the wall of the colon thickens, reducing the width of the passage and increasing the possibility of obstruction and distension of the colon. Perforations in the colon wall may develop and cause peritonitis (infection of the membrane that covers the abdomen).

In severe cases, it may be necessary to perform a temporary colostomy. The diseased section of colon is removed, and the rectum and anus are closed. A stoma is made in the abdominal wall and attached to the remaining colon and covered by a pouch to collect fecal matter. After the bowel has healed, the rectum and anus can be reopened and attached to the colon.

USES AND COMPLICATIONS

Patients with permanent ileostomies and colostomies are disfigured by a hole in their abdomens that is often 5 or more centimeters (2 or more inches) in diameter. Patients are required to wear removable pouches sealed to their stomas to collect fecal matter so that it can be eliminated. The apparatus is unsightly, and the entire process can be unpleasant enough to cause serious depression in the patient. Patients' spouses and other family members are often involved in changing and emptying the bags, particularly with older, infirm persons. Ileoanal anastomosis solves some of these problems because it allows natural bowel movements, but it is useful only in certain conditions.

PERSPECTIVE AND PROSPECTS

Current surgical procedures are often effective in serious colorectal conditions. The success rate of these surgeries for the treatment of cancer is quite high if the cancer is caught before it spreads to other parts of the body. Nevertheless, patients may have to endure the inconvenience of ostomy bags and paraphernalia for the rest of their lives. Ostomy equipment has been improved: Better sealing adhesives are now in use so that the bags do not slip or leak as they once did. The configuration of belts, bags, and other appliances has been altered to make them more convenient and easier to live with. New surgical procedures that could maintain normal bowel function for more patients, however, would be a major advancement. —*C. Richard Falcon*

See also Abdomen; Abdominal disorders; Biopsy; Cancer; Colitis; Colon and rectal polyp removal; Colon cancer; Colonoscopy; Crohn's disease; Diverticulitis and diverticulosis; Electrocauterization; Endoscopy; Enemas; Fistula repair; Gastroenterology; Gastrointestinal system; Hemorrhoid banding and removal; Hemorrhoids; Hernia repair; Hernias; Ileostomy and colostomy; Intestinal disorders; Intestines; Oncology; Proctology; Tumor removal; Tumors.

FOR FURTHER INFORMATION:

Larson, David E., ed. *Mayo Clinic Family Health Book.* 2d ed. New York: William Morrow, 1996.

Phillips, Robert, H. *Coping with an Ostomy.* Wayne, N.J.: Avery, 1986.

COLON CANCER

DISEASE/DISORDER

ANATOMY OR SYSTEM AFFECTED: Abdomen, anus, gastrointestinal system, intestines, lymphatic system

SPECIALTIES AND RELATED FIELDS: Gastroenterology, genetics, immunology, oncology, proctology

DEFINITION: Cancer occurring in the large intestine, which is the second deadliest type of this disease.

CAUSES AND SYMPTOMS

With an estimated 60,000 deaths per year in the United States, cancer of the colon and rectum (also called large bowel or colorectal cancer) is the second most deadly cancer, ranking only behind lung cancer. About 90 percent of colorectal cancers arise from the glandular epithelium lining the inner surface of the large bowel and are termed adenocarcinomas. The cells of this layer are constantly being replaced by new cells. This fairly rapid cell division, along with the relatively hostile environment within the bowel, promotes internal cellular errors that lead to the formation of aberrant cells. These cells can become disordered and produce abnormal growths or tumors. Often, colorectal tumors protrude into the lumen (the spaces within the bowel), forming growths called polyps. Some polyps are benign and do not spread to other parts of the body, but they may still disturb normal bowel functions. Other polyps become malignant by forming more aggressive cell types, which allows them to grow larger and spread to other organs. The cancer can grow through the layers of the colon wall and extend into the body cavity and nearby organs such as the urinary bladder. Cancer cells can also break away from the main tumor and spread (metastasize) through the blood or lymphatic vessels to other organs, such as the lungs or liver. If not controlled, the spreading cancer eventually causes death by impairment of organ and system functions.

The risk of colorectal cancer is increased by certain hereditary and environmental factors. The dietary intake of fat and fiber also influences colorectal cancer risk. Researchers believe that fiber reduces the exposure of colon cells to cancer-causing chemicals (carcinogens) by diluting them and causing them to move more rapidly through the colon. Fats may promote colorectal cancer by triggering the excess secretion of bile, which is known to be carcinogenic in animals. In addition, fat may be converted to carcinogens

by bacteria that live in the colon. Diets high in protein or low in fruit and vegetables may also elevate the risk. The tendency to develop colorectal polyps and cancer can be inherited; this genetic predisposition may be responsible for about 5 to 7 percent of all colorectal cancers. One example is an inherited disorder called familial adenomatous polyposis (FAP), in which multiple polyps develop in the colon; it often leads to colorectal cancer. Some of the defective genes that cause this and other types of colorectal cancers have been identified and are being studied to determine their role. The interplay between the various oncogenes (mutated cell division and growth genes) and tumor suppressor genes (cell division and growth inhibitor genes) has been determined. Whether inherited or caused by carcinogens, damage to these specific genetic regions disrupts the delicate balance that regulates orderly and perfectly timed cell reproduction and development, producing cancer cells. Irritable bowel syndrome (IBS) and exposure to certain occupational carcinogens are also known to increase the risk.

TREATMENT AND THERAPY

The chances for survival are greatly increased when colorectal cancer is detected and treated at an early stage. Early detection in the general population is possible with the use of three common medical tests: digital rectal examination, in which the physician checks the inner surface of the rectal wall with gloved finger for abnormal growths; fecal occult blood test, in which a stool sample is tested for hidden blood that may have emanated from a cancerous growth; and sigmoidoscopy, in which the physician examines the rectal and lower colon inner lining with a narrow tubular optical instrument inserted through the anus. If cancer is suspected, further tests will be done to arrive at a diagnosis. These tests may include a computed tomography (CT) scan, double-contrast barium enema X-ray series, and colonoscopy. The CT scan and contrast X rays reveal abnormal growths, and colonoscopy is similar to sigmoidoscopy but uses a longer, flexible tube in order to inspect the entire colon. During sigmoidoscopy and colonoscopy, the physician can remove polyps and obtain tissue samples for biopsy. Microscopic examination of the tissue samples by a pathologist can determine the stage or extent of growth of the cancer. This is important because it helps determine the type of treatment. In one type of staging, the following criteria are used: stage 0 (cancer confined to epithelium lining of the bowel), stage 1 (cancer confined to the bowel wall), stage 2 (cancer penetrating through all layers of the bowel wall and possibly invading adjacent tissues), stage 3 (cancer invading lymph nodes and/or adjacent tissues), and stage 4 (cancer spreading to distant sites, forming metastases).

Surgery is the primary treatment for colorectal cancer. Very small tumors in stage 0 can be removed surgically with the colonoscope. Tumors in more advanced stages require abdominal surgery in which the tumor is removed along with a portion of the bowel and possibly some lymph nodes. For cases in which the bowel cannot be reconnected, an opening is created through the abdominal wall (colostomy). This is usually a temporary procedure, and the hole will be closed when the bowel can be rejoined. Some advanced cancers cannot be cured by surgery alone. Adjuvant therapies—chemotherapy, radiation therapy, and biological therapy—may be used in combination with surgery. Chemotherapy drugs kill spreading cancer cells. The most common is 5-fluorouracil (5-FU), a chemical that interferes with the production of deoxyribonucleic acid (DNA) in dividing cells. 5-FU is more effective when given together with leucovorin (a compound similar to folic acid) and levamisole (an immune system stimulant). Levamisole and other treatments that reinforce the immune system are forms of biological therapy. Radiation therapy, given either before or after surgery, is helpful in killing undetected cancer cells near the site of the tumor.

PERSPECTIVE AND PROSPECTS

More than 150,000 new cases of colorectal cancer are diagnosed in the United States each year, or roughly 15 percent of all cancers. The incidence of colorectal cancer is lower among females than males and rises dramatically after the age of fifty. Colorectal cancer is more common in developed countries such as the United States and in densely populated, industrialized regions. American mortality rates from colorectal cancer are higher in the Northeast and north-central regions of the country than in the South and Southwest. Populations moving from low-risk parts of the world, such as Asia or Africa, to high-risk areas, such as the United States or Europe, take on the higher risk within a generation or two, and vice versa.

—Rodney C. Mowbray, Ph.D.
updated by Connie Rizzo, M.D.

See also Biopsy; Cancer; Chemotherapy; Colon and rectal polyp removal; Colon and rectal surgery; Colon therapy; Colonoscopy; Ileostomy and colostomy; Intestinal disorders; Intestines; Malignancy and metastasis; Oncology; Radiation therapy; Stomach, intestinal, and pancreatic cancers; Tumor removal; Tumors.

FOR FURTHER INFORMATION:

Bennett, J. Claude, et al., eds. *Cecil Textbook of Medicine.* 20th ed. Philadelphia: W. B. Saunders, 1996.

Methods of Treatment for Colon Cancer

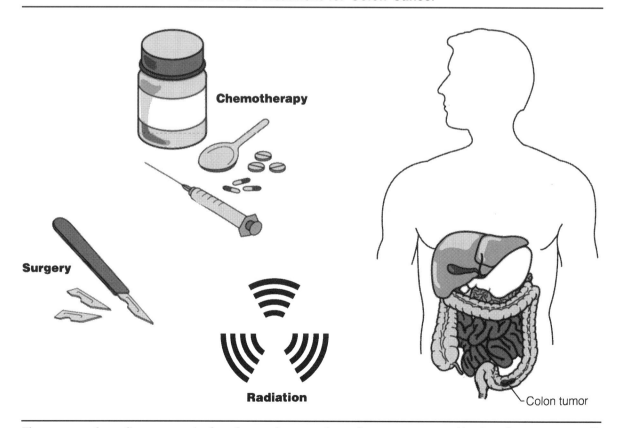

The presence of a malignant tumor in the colon requires some form of treatment or a combination of treatments, usually beginning with its surgical removal and followed by radiation therapy and/or chemotherapy (the use of anticancer drugs).

Cooper, Geoffrey M. *Elements of Human Cancer*. Boston: Jones and Bartlett, 1992.

De Vita, Vincent T., Jr., Samuel Hellman, and Steven A. Rosenberg, eds. *Cancer: Principles and Practice of Oncology*. 5th ed. Philadelphia: J. B. Lippincott, 1997.

Holleb, Arthur I., ed. *The American Cancer Society Cancer Book*. Garden City, N.Y.: Doubleday, 1986.

Murphy, G., L. Morris, and D. Lange. *Informed Decisions: The Complete Book of Cancer Diagnosis, Treatment, and Recovery*. New York: Viking Press, 1997.

U.S. Department of Health and Human Services. Public Health Service. National Institutes of Health. *Cancer of the Colon and Rectum*. Bethesda, Md.: Author, 1991.

_____. *What You Need to Know About Cancer of the Colon and Rectum*. Bethesda, Md.: Author, 1987.

COLON THERAPY

PROCEDURE

ANATOMY OR SYSTEM AFFECTED: Abdomen, anus, gastrointestinal system, intestines

SPECIALTY: Alternative medicine

DEFINITION: The irrigation of the colon, or large intestine, with water in order to detoxify it is called colon therapy. Also known as colonic irrigation and colon hydrotherapy, the procedure involves washing out the entire colon with pure water in order to dislodge any stagnating fecal material. It is believed that through poor dietary habits, lack of fluid intake, and physical or emotional stress or illness, the colon may not function properly. Such malfunction leads to a buildup of waste material, which in turn causes other body organs to overwork themselves in the detoxification process. During the forty-five-minute procedure, a tube is inserted into the anus and water is slowly pumped into the intestine. Pressure is regulated in order to avoid injury. Alternation of warm and cool water leads to contraction and relaxation of the intestinal walls, which helps to remove impacted pieces of dry feces from the walls. Feces, gas, mucus, and bacteria exit through the same tube. A cleaner internal surface of the colon provides more surface area for the absorption of nutrients and water. Side effects may include diarrhea and a loss of necessary intestinal bacteria.

—*Karen E. Kalumuck, Ph.D.*

See also Alternative medicine; Gastrointestinal system; Intestines; Preventive medicine.

COLONOSCOPY

PROCEDURE

ANATOMY OR SYSTEM AFFECTED: Abdomen, anus, gastrointestinal system, intestines

SPECIALTIES AND RELATED FIELDS: Gastroenterology, internal medicine, proctology

DEFINITION: A visual examination of the interior surface of the colon using a long, flexible tube.

INDICATIONS AND PROCEDURES

As part of the aging process, most adults develop small growths, called polyps, on the inside wall of the large intestine. Polyps generally are not a health risk unless they grow to be 1.25 centimeters (.5 inch) in diameter or larger. Blood cells are discharged from the surface of a polyp during growth. Adults over fifty are therefore encouraged to have periodic screening tests for traces of blood in the stool. If the test result is positive, an examination of the colon's interior by means of colonoscopy is indicated.

To prepare for colonoscopy, the patient must have no solid food for twelve hours, an overnight laxative, and an enema before starting the procedure.

The physician inserts a flexible cable, called an endoscope, into the patient through the anus. Optical fibers in the cable carry light into the body and return a visual image. The colon wall is examined while the cable is advanced in small steps. If polyps are found, samples of tissue can be removed through the endoscope for biopsy.

If laboratory analysis shows the tissue samples to be cancerous, abdominal surgery may be necessary to remove the diseased portion of the colon. Even if the tissue samples are benign (noncancerous), the physician may recommend removing the polyps as a preventive measure. Such surgery can be done through the endoscope cable.

USES AND COMPLICATIONS

The fiber-optic endoscope to view interior body surfaces was first developed in the 1960's. It has been enthusiastically adopted by the medical profession as a diagnostic tool, greatly reducing the need for exploratory surgery.

Biomedical engineers have designed a variety of attachments for the endoscope. For example, a wire loop with electrical connections can be inserted through the endoscope to perform surgery. The wire is slipped over the neck of a polyp and drawn tight. When electric current is applied, the hot wire slices through the connection with underlying tissue. The severed polyp then can be withdrawn.

Potential complications of colonoscopy are hemorrhage and perforation of the colon wall, but such problems are rare. The major benefit of colonoscopy is to reduce the risks of colon cancer by early detection and treatment.

—*Hans G. Graetzer, Ph.D.*

See also Colon and rectal polyp removal; Colon and rectal surgery; Colon cancer; Endoscopy; Enemas; Gastroenterology; Gastrointestinal system; Intestines; Oncology; Proctology; Tumor removal; Tumors.

COLOR BLINDNESS

DISEASE/DISORDER

ANATOMY OR SYSTEM AFFECTED: Eyes

SPECIALTIES AND RELATED FIELDS: Genetics, ophthalmology

DEFINITION: Color blindness is a genetic condition of the eye in which the patient is unable to distinguish between some colors. Common forms involve an inability to distinguish between red and green; red and green color blindness affects about 10 percent of men and is very rare in women. Total color blindness is the inability to perceive any color at all and is extremely rare. Both conditions are sex-linked disorders inherited from the mother, who carries a defective gene on one of her X chromosomes but is not affected herself.

—*Jason Georges and Tracy Irons-Georges*
See also Eyes; Genetic diseases; Visual disorders.

COLOSTOMY. *See* ILEOSTOMY AND COLOSTOMY.

COMA
DISEASE/DISORDER
ANATOMY OR SYSTEM AFFECTED: Brain, head, nervous system, psychic-emotional system
SPECIALTIES AND RELATED FIELDS: Critical care, emergency medicine
DEFINITION: A loss of consciousness from which a person cannot be aroused; a symptom signifying a variety of causes.

KEY TERMS:
alcoholic coma: coma accompanying severe alcohol intoxication
apoplectic coma: coma induced by cerebrum, cerebellar, or brain-stem hemorrhage, as well as by embolism or cerebral thrombosis
brain death: irreversible brain damage so extensive that the organ enjoys no potential for recovery and can no longer maintain the body's internal functions
coma: a loss of consciousness from which the patient cannot be aroused
conscious: having an awareness of one's existence
hepatic coma: coma accompanying cerebral damage caused by the degeneration of liver cells (especially that associated with cirrhosis of the liver)
traumatic coma: coma following a head injury
CAUSES AND SYMPTOMS
Consciousness is defined by the normal wakeful state, with its self-aware cognition of past events and future anticipation. Disease or dysfunction that impairs this state usually causes readily identifiable conditions such as coma. The self-aware. cognitive aspects of consciousness depend largely on the interconnected neural networks of the cerebral hemispheres. Normal conscious behavior depends on the continuous, effective interaction of these systems. Loss of consciousness from medical causes can be brief (a matter of minutes to an hour or so) or it can be sustained for many hours, days, or sometimes even weeks. The longer the duration of the comatose state, the more likely it is to reflect structural damage to the brain rather than a transient alteration in its function.

The word "coma" comes from the Greek *koma*, meaning to put to sleep or to fall asleep. This state of unarousable unresponsiveness results from disturbance or damage to areas of the brain involved in conscious activity or the maintenance of consciousness—particularly parts of the cerebrum (the main mass of the brain), upper parts of the brain stem, and central regions of the brain, especially the limbic system. A wide spectrum of specific conditions can injure the brain and cause coma. The damage to the brain may be the result of a head injury or of an abnormality such as a brain tumor, brain abscess, or intracerebral hemorrhage. Often there has been a buildup of poisonous substances that intoxicates brain tissues. This buildup can occur because of a drug overdose, advanced kidney or liver disease, or acute alcoholic intoxication. Encephalitis (inflammation of the brain) and meningitis (inflammation of the brain coverings) can also cause coma, as can cerebral hypoxia (lack of oxygen in the brain, possibly attributable to the impairment of the blood flow to some areas). Whatever the underlying mechanism, coma indicates brain failure, and the high degree or organization of cerebral biochemical systems has been disrupted. Coma is easily distinguishable from sleep in that the person does not respond to external stimulation (such as shouting or pinching) or to the needs of his or her body (such as a full bladder).

Comas are classified according to the event or condition that caused the comatose state. Some of the most frequently encountered types of comas are traumatic coma, alcoholic coma, apoplectic coma, deanimate coma, diabetic coma, hepatic coma, metabolic coma, vigil coma, pseudo coma, and irreversible coma. Traumatic coma follows a head injury. It enjoys a somewhat more favorable outcome than that of comas associated with medical illness. About 50 percent of patients in a coma from head injuries survive, and the recovery is closely linked to age: The younger the patient, the greater the chance for recovery. Alcoholic coma refers to the coma accompanying severe alcohol intoxication, usually more than 400 milligrams alcohol per 100 milliliters of blood. This coma is marked by rapid, light respiration, usually with tachycardia and hypotension. Apoplectic coma is induced by cerebrum, cerebellar, or brain-stem hemorrhage, as well as by embolism or cerebral thrombosis. The term "deanimate coma" refers to a deep coma with loss of all somatic and autonomic reflex activity. The maintenance of life depends wholly upon such supportive measures as assisted respiration, and cardiac arrest will quickly follow if the respirator is stopped; this may be a transient or irreversible state. Diabetic coma is the coma of severe diabetic acidosis. Hepatic coma is the coma accompanying cerebral damage resulting from degeneration of liver cells, especially that associated with cirrhosis of the liver. "Metabolic coma" is the term applied to the coma occurring in any metabolic disorder in the absence of a demonstrable macroscopic physical abnormality of the brain. Vigil coma is defined as a state of stupor in which the patient is mute and shows no verbal or motor responses to stimuli although the eyes are open and give a false impression of alertness. Pseudo coma refers to states resembling acute unconsciousness but with self-awareness preserved. Irreversible coma, or brain death, occurs when irreversible brain damage is so extensive that the organ enjoys no potential for recovery and can no longer maintain the body's internal functions.

TREATMENT AND THERAPY

Of the acute problems in clinical medicine, none is more difficult than the prompt diagnosis and effective management of the comatose patient. The difficulty exists partly because the causes of coma are so many and partly because the physician possesses only a limited time in which to make the appropriate diagnostic and therapeutic judgment.

Measurements of variations in the depth of coma are important in its assessment and treatment. Varying depths of coma are recognized. In less severe forms, the person may respond to stimulation by, for example, moving an arm. In severe cases, the person fails to respond to repeated vigorous stimuli. Yet even deeply comatose patients may show some automatic responses, as they may continue to breathe unaided, may cough, yawn, blink, and show roving eye movement. These actions indicate that the lower brain stem, which controls these responses, is still functioning.

Assessment of the patient in coma includes an evaluation of all vital signs, the level of consciousness, neuromuscular responses, and reaction of the pupils to light. In most hospitals, a printed form for neurologic assessment is used to measure and record the patient's responses to stimuli in objective terms. The Glasgow coma scale also provides a standardized tool that aids in assessing a comatose patient and eliminates the use of ambiguous and easily misinterpreted terms such as "unconscious" and "semicomatose." Additional assessment data should include evaluation of the gag and corneal reflexes. Abnormal rigidity and posturing in response to noxious stimuli indicate deep coma.

The definitive treatment of altered states of consciousness requires removing, correcting, or halting the specific process responsible for the state to whatever degree possible. Often, accurate diagnosis and specific therapy require time, and the first priority is to protect the brain from permanent damage.

General treatment measures that apply to all patients include the following: ensurance of an adequate airway passage and oxygenation; maintenance of proper circulation; intravenous administration of glucose or thiamine if the patient is undernourished; any measures necessary to stop generalized seizures; the restoration of the blood acid-base and osmolar balance; the treatment of any detected infection; the treatment and control of extreme body temperatures; the administration of specific antidotes for situations such as drug overdoses; control of agitation; and the protection of the corneas.

In the absence of the gag reflex, regurgitation and aspiration are potential problems. Tube feeding, if necessary, must be done slowly and with the head of the bed raised during the feeding and for about half an hour later. Absence of the corneal reflex can inhibit blinking and natural moistening of the eye. The cornea cannot be allowed to dry, since blindness can result; therefore, artificial tears are instilled in the eyes to keep them moist.

Once the cause leading to the comatose state has been determined, the appropriate steps should be taken to minimize or eliminate it whenever possible. For many causes of coma, rapid intervention and treatment can mean recuperation for the patient, such as in the cases of diabetes, removable hematomas, and drug overdose.

Comatose patients are predisposed to all the hazards of immobility, including impairment of skin integrity and the development of ulcers, contractures and joint disabilities, problems related to respiratory and circulatory status, and alterations in fluid and electrolyte balance. All these factors must be taken into consideration when dealing with the comatose patient.

The outcome from severe medical coma depends on its cause and, with the exception of depressant drug poisoning, on the initial severity and extent of neurologic damage. Depressant drug poisoning reflects a state of general anesthesia, and, barring severe complications, almost all patients who survive drug intoxication can recover physically unscathed.

The clinical tests most valuable for estimating the capacity for recovery after medical coma are identical to those used in making the initial diagnosis. Within a few hours or days after the onset of coma, many patients show neurologic signs that can differentiate, with a high probability, the future extremes of either no improvement or the capacity for good recovery. After a period of about six hours (except for patients on drugs), certain neurological findings begin to correlate with the potential for neurologic recovery and can predict the outcome of about one-third of patients who will do badly. By the end of the first day, tests can predict the two-thirds of the patients who will do well. With each successive day, the signs develop greater predictive power. Persistence of coma in an adult for more than four weeks is almost never associated with later complete recovery.

PERSPECTIVE AND PROSPECTS

Attempts to define *coma* must give at least brief consideration to the concepts of consciousness. Consciousness involves not only the reception of stimuli but also the emotional implications of such stimuli, as well as the construction of intricate mental images.

Since the days of the ancient Greeks, people have known that normal conscious behavior depends on intact brain function and that disorders of consciousness are a sign of cerebral insufficiency. The range of awake and intelligent behavior is so rich and variable, however, that clinical abnormalities are difficult to recognize unless there are substantial deviations from the norm. Impaired, reduced, or absent conscious behavior implies the presence of severe brain dysfunction and demands urgent attention if recovery is to be expected. The brain can tolerate only a limited amount of physical or metabolic injury without suffering irreparable harm, and the longer the failure lasts, the narrower the margin between recovery and the development of permanent neurologic invalidism.

Since such researchers as Pierre Mollaret and Maurice Goulon first examined the question in 1959, many others have tried to establish criteria that would accurately and unequivocally determine that the brain is dead, or about to die no matter what therapeutic measures one undertakes. In 1968, the Harvard Medical School Ad Hoc Committee to Examine the Definition of Brain Death established criteria for determining irreversible coma, or brain death. These criteria are often used to complement the traditional criteria for determining death. All other existing guidelines, such as the Swedish, British, and United States Collaborative Study Criteria, include nearly identical clinical points but contain some differences as to the duration of observation necessary to establish the diagnosis as well as the emphasis to be placed on laboratory procedures in diagnosis.

Techniques such as computed tomography (CT) scanning and electroencephalography (EEG) have transformed the process of diagnosis in clinical neurology, with technology sometimes replacing clinical deduction. The art of diagnosis, however, is to comprehend the whole picture—where the lesion is, what it comprises, and above all, what it is doing to the patient.

Advances in resuscitative medicine have made obsolete the traditional clinical definition of death, that is, the cessation of heartbeat. Cardiac resuscitation can salvage patients after periods of asystole lasting up to several minutes. Cardiopulmonary bypass machines permit the patient's heartbeat to cease for several hours with full clinical recovery after resuscitation. While respiratory depression formerly meant death within minutes, modern mechanical ventilators can maintain pulmonary oxygen exchange indefinitely. Such advances have permitted many patients with formerly lethal cardiac, pulmonary, and neuromuscular disease to return to relatively full and useful lives. Abundant clinical evidence, however, demonstrates that severe damage to the brain can completely destroy the organ's vital functions and capacity to recover, even when the other parts of the body still live. The result has been to switch the emphasis in defining death to a cessation of brain function. Brain death occurs when brain damage is so extensive that the organ has no potential for recovery and cannot maintain the body's internal functions. Countries worldwide have adopted the principle that death occurs when either the brain or the heart irreversibly fails in its functions. In the United States, the time of brain death has been accepted as the time of the person's death in legal terms.

The determination of whether a comatose patient is brain-dead or can possibly recuperate is extremely important. Issues such as organ transplant programs that require donation of healthy organs and the economic and emotional expense involved in the treatment and care of a comatose patient make it critical to know when to fight for life and when to diagnose death.

In carrying out the many details of the physical care and assessment of the comatose patient, health care personnel must not lose sight of the fact that the patient is a fellow human being and a member of a family. One cannot always be sure exactly how much the patients are aware of what is being said or done as care is given. Whatever the level of awareness and response, comatose patients are told what will be done to and for them, as they deserve the same respect afforded alert and aware patients.

—*Maria Pacheco, Ph.D.*

See also Concussion; Death and dying; Ethics; Euthanasia; Unconsciousness.

FOR FURTHER INFORMATION:
Bennett, J. Claude, et al., eds. *Cecil Textbook of Medicine.* 20th ed. Philadelphia: W. B. Saunders, 1996. Offers in-depth coverage of numerous medical conditions and a comprehensive presentation of the comatose state. The discussion is technical, however, and requires a good science background.

Clayman, Charles B., ed. *The American Medical Association Encyclopedia of Medicine.* New York: Random House, 1989. A concise presentation of numerous medical terms and illnesses. A very good general reference.

Fazekas, J. F., and Ralph W. Alman. *Coma: Biochemistry, Physiology, and Therapeutic Principles.* Springfield, Ill.: Charles C Thomas, 1962. A good basic reference work that presents eight different types of comas, their causes and treatment, as well as a general introduction to the subject.

Landau, Sidney I., et al., eds. *International Dictionary of Medicine and Biology.* 3 vols. Vol. 1. New York: John Wiley & Sons, 1986. Offers a brief presentation of medical and biological terms. A useful general reference work.

Miller, Benjamin Frank, and Claire B. Keane. *Encyclopedia and Dictionary of Medicine, Nursing, and Allied Health.* 5th ed. Philadelphia: W. B. Saunders, 1992. Contains a concise presentation of the topic of coma.

Plum, Fred, and J. B. Posner. *The Diagnosis of Stupor and Coma.* 3d ed. Philadelphia: F. A. Davis, 1980. An excellent book dealing in detail with the diagnosis, treatment, and management of the comatose patient. Well organized and easy to read, it also includes an excellent bibliography for individuals who are interested in more specific presentations of the topic.

COMMON COLD
DISEASE/DISORDER

ANATOMY OR SYSTEM AFFECTED: Chest, lungs, nose, respiratory system

SPECIALTIES AND RELATED FIELDS: Family medicine, internal medicine, otorhinolarnygology, public health, virology

DEFINITION: A class of viral respiratory infections that form the world's most prevalent illnesses.

KEY TERMS:

acute: referring to a disease process of sudden onset and short duration

chronic: referring to a disease process of long duration and frequent recurrence

coronavirus: a microorganism causing respiratory illness; one of the most prevalent causes of the common cold

pathogen: any disease-causing microorganism

rhinovirus: a microorganism causing respiratory illness; one of the most prevalent causes of the common cold

virus: an extremely small pathogen that can replicate only within a living cell

CAUSES AND SYMPTOMS

One of the reasons that no cure has ever been found for the common cold is that it is caused by literally hundreds of different viruses. More than two hundred distinct strains from eight genera have been identified, and no doubt more will be discovered. Infection by one of these viruses may confer immunity to it, but there will still be scores of others to which that individual is not immune. The common cold is usually restricted to the nose and surrounding areas—hence its medical name, rhinitis (*rhin-* meaning "nose" and *-itis* meaning "inflammation").

Children get the most colds, averaging six to eight per year until they are six years old. From that age, the number diminishes until, for adults, the rate is three to five colds per year. Colds and related respiratory diseases are the largest single cause of lost workdays and school days. Colds and related respiratory diseases are probably the world's most expensive illnesses. In the United States, about a million and a half person-years are lost from work each year; this figure accounts for one-half of all absences. Worldwide, the costs of lost workdays, medications, physician's visits, and the complications that may require extensive medical care are incalculable.

Among the virus types that cause the common cold are rhinovirus, coronavirus, influenza virus, parainfluenza virus, enterovirus, adenovirus, respiratory syncytial virus, and coxsackie virus. They are not all equally responsible for cold infections. Rhinoviruses and coronaviruses between them are thought to cause 25 to 60 percent of all colds. Rhinoviruses appear to be responsible for colds that occur in the peak cold seasons of late spring and early fall. Coronaviruses appear to be responsible for colds that occur when rhinovirus is less active, such as in the late fall, winter, and early spring.

A respiratory syncitial virus can cause the common cold in adults; in children it causes much more severe diseases, including pneumonia and bronchiolitis (inflammation of the bronchioles, small air passages in the lungs). Similarly, influenza and parainfluenza viruses, adenoviruses, and enteroviruses can be responsible for rhinitis and sore throat, but they are also capable of more serious illnesses such as pneumonia and influenza.

Viruses are the smallest of the invading microorganisms that cause disease, so small that they are not visible using ordinary microscopes. They can be seen, however, with an electron microscope, and their presence in the body can be detected through various laboratory tests.

Viruses vary enormously in their size and structure. Some consist of three or four proteins with a core of either deoxyribonucleic acid (DNA) or ribonucleic acid (RNA); some have more than fifty proteins and other substances. Viruses can only replicate within living cells. They invade the body and produce disease conditions in different ways. Some travel through the body to find their target host cells. A good example is the measles virus, which enters through the mucous membranes of the nose, throat, and mouth and then finds its way to target tissues throughout the body. Some, such as the viruses that cause the common cold, enter the body through the nasal passages and settle directly into nearby cells.

Rhinoviruses are members of the Picornaviridae family (*pico-*from "piccolo," meaning "very small"; *rna* from RNA, the genetic material that it contains; and *viridae* denoting a virus family). Coronaviruses are members of the Coronaviridae family, and they also contain RNA. Most viruses that are pathogenic to humans can thrive only at the temperature inside the human body, 37 degrees Celsius (98.6 degrees Fahrenheit). Rhinoviruses prefer the cooler temperatures found in the nasal passages, 33 to 34 degrees Celsius (91.4 to 93.2 degrees Fahrenheit). More than one hundred different rhinovirus types have been identified.

Exactly how a patient contracts a cold is better understood than it once was. Exposure to a cold environment—for example, getting a chill in winter weather—does not cause a cold unless the individual is exposed to the infecting virus at the same time. Fatigue or lack of sleep does not increase susceptibility to the cold virus, and even the direct exposure of nasal tissue to cold viruses does not guarantee infection.

A group in England, the Medical Research Council's Common Cold Unit, studied the disease from 1945 to 1990 and made many fundamental discoveries—even though the researchers never found a cure, or for that matter, any effective methods to prevent the spread of the disease. As part of their research, they put drops containing cold virus into the noses of volunteers. Only about one-third of the subjects thus inoculated developed cold symptoms, showing that direct exposure to the infecting agent does not necessarily bring on a cold.

What appears to be essential in the spread of the disease is bodily contact, particularly handshaking or touching. The infected individual wipes his or her nose or coughs into his or her hand, getting nasal secretions on the fingers. These infected secretions are then transferred to the hand of another person who, if susceptible, can become infected by bringing the hand up to the mouth or nose. Sneezing and coughing also spread the disease. Many viral and bacterial diseases are transmissible through nasopharyngeal (nose and throat) secretions; these include measles, mumps, rubella, pneumonia, influenza, and any number of other infections.

One or more individuals in a group become infected and bring the disease to a central place, such as a classroom, office, military base, or day care center. In the case of the common cold, transferring infected particles by touch exposes another person to the infection. In other respiratory diseases, breathing, sneezing, or coughing virus-laden particles into the air will spread the disease. The infected individual then becomes the means by which the disease is brought into the home. By far, the largest number of colds are brought into the family by children who have contracted the infection in classrooms or day care centers.

The pathogenesis of the common cold—that is, what happens when an individual is exposed to the cold virus—is not fully understood. It is believed that the virus enters the nasal passages and attaches itself to receptors on a cell of the nasal mucous membrane and then invades the cell. Viruses traveling freely in the blood or lymphatic system are subject to attack by white blood cells called phagocytes in

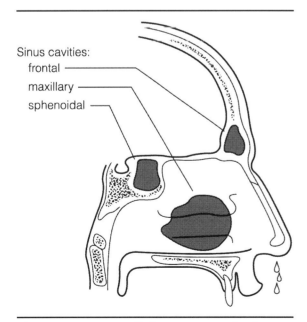

Sinus cavities:
frontal
maxillary
sphenoidal

The sinus cavities typically become congested with mucus as the body fights the virus that has caused the cold.

what is part of the body's nonspecific defense system against invading pathogens.

Once inside the host cell, the virus replicates itself by stealing elements of the protoplasm of the cell and using them to build new viruses under the direction of the RNA component. These new viruses are released by the host cell to infect other cells. This process can injure or kill the host cell, activating the body's specific immune response system and starting the chain of events that will destroy the invading virus and create immunity to further infection from it.

In response to cell death or injury, certain chemicals are released that induce inflammation in the nasal passages. Blood vessels in the nasal area enlarge, increasing blood flow to the tissues and causing swelling. The openings in capillary walls enlarge and deliver lymphocytes, white blood cells that produce antibodies to fight the virus, as well as other specialized white blood cells.

Nasal mucosa swell and secretions increase, a condition medically known as rhinorrhea (-*rrhea* meaning "flowing," denoting the runny nose of the common cold). During the first few days of infection, these secretions are thin and watery. As the disease progresses and white blood cells are drawn to the area, the secretions become thicker and more purulent, that is, filled with pus. A sore throat is common, as is laryngitis, or inflammation of the larynx or voice box. Fever is not a usual symptom of the common cold, but a cough will often develop as excess mucus or phlegm builds up in the lungs and windpipe.

As mucus accumulates and clogs nasal passages, the body attempts to expel it by sneezing. In this process, impulses from the nose travel to the brain's "sneeze reflex center," where sneezing is triggered to help clear nasal passages. Similarly, as phlegm accumulates in the windpipe and bronchial tree of the lungs, a message is sent to the "cough reflex center" of the brain, where coughing is initiated to expel the phlegm.

The common cold is self-limiting and usually resolves within five to ten days, but there can be complications in some cases. Patients who have asthma or chronic bronchitis frequently develop bronchoconstriction (narrowing of the air passages in the lungs) as a result of a common cold. If severe, purulent tracheitis and bronchitis develop, there may be a concomitant bacterial infection. In some patients, the infection may spread to other organs, such as the ears, where an infection called otitis media can develop. Sinusitis, infection of the cavities in the bone of the skull surrounding the nose, is common. If the invading organism spreads to the lungs, bronchitis or pneumonia may develop.

Other possible complications of the common cold depend on the individual virus. Rhinoviruses, usually limited to colds, may infrequently cause pneumonia in children. Coronaviruses, also usually limited to colds, infrequently cause pneumonia and bronchiolitis. A respiratory syncitial virus causes pneumonia and bronchiolitis in children, the common cold in adults, and pneumonia in the elderly. Parainfluenza virus, which causes croup and other respiratory diseases in children, can cause sore throat and the common cold in adults and, rarely, may cause tracheobronchitis in these patients. Influenza B virus, an occasional cause of the common cold, also causes influenza and, infrequently, pneumonia.

Another condition that can closely resemble the common cold, but which is not caused by a virus, is allergic rhinitis. The major form of allergic rhinitis is hay fever. It has many of the same symptoms as the common cold: sneezing, runny nose, nasal congestion, and sometimes, sore throat. In addition, the hay fever victim may suffer from itching in the eyes, nose, mouth, and throat. Hay fever is an allergic reaction to certain pollens. Because the pollens that cause hay fever are abundant at certain times of the year, it may be prevalent at the same times as some colds. Spring is a peak season for the common cold and also for hay fever, because of the many tree pollens that are carried in the air. In the fall, weed pollens, such as ragweed, affect hay fever sufferers during another peak period for colds. Colds occur less frequently in summer, but summer is another peak season for hay fever.

TREATMENT AND THERAPY

The nose is the first barrier of defense against the bacteria and viruses that cause upper respiratory infections. The nasal cavity is lined with a thin coating of mucus, a thick liquid that is constantly replenished by the mucous glands. Inner nasal surfaces are filled with tiny hairs, or cilia. Dust, bacteria, and other foreign matter are trapped by the mucus and moved by the cilia toward the nasopharynx to be expectorated or swallowed.

The blood vessels in the nasopharyngeal bed respond automatically to stimulation from the brain. Certain stimuli cause the vessels to constrict, widening air passages and at the same time reducing the flow of mucus. Other stimuli, such as those that are sent in response to a viral infection, allergen, or other irritant, cause blood vessels to dilate and increase the flow of mucus. Nasal passages become swollen, and airways are blocked.

The mucus-covered lining of the nasal passages contains various substances that help ward off infection and irritation by allergens. Lysozyme (lyso- meaning "dissolution" and -zyme from "enzyme," a catalyst that promotes an activity) attacks the cell walls of certain bacteria, killing them. It also attacks pollen granules. Mucus also contains glycoproteins that temporarily inhibit the activity of viruses. Mucus has small amounts of the antibodies immunoglobulin IgA and IgC that also may inhibit the activity of invading viruses.

Bed rest is usually the first element of treatment. Limiting physical stress may help keep the cold from worsening and may avoid secondary infections. The medications used to treat the common cold are directed at relieving individual symptoms: There is nothing available that will kill the viruses that cause it. Most cases of the common cold are treated at home with over-the-counter cold preparations. Children's colds and the complications that may arise from colds, such as bacterial and viral superinfection, may require the services of a physician.

Many medications for the common cold contain antihistamines. Histamine is a naturally occurring chemical in the body that is released in response to an allergen or an infection. It is a significant cause of the inflammation, swelling, and runny nose of hay fever. When these symptoms are seen with the common cold, however, they are probably caused by the body's inflammatory defense system rather than by histamine.

When antihistamines were first discovered, it was thought that they could inhibit the inflammatory defense against a cold. Patients were advised to take antihistamines at the first sign of a cold, in the hope of avoiding a full infection. Current thinking is that antihistamines have little value in the treatment of the common cold. They may have a minor effect on a runny nose, but there are better agents for this purpose. Antihistamines are usually highly sedative—most over-the-counter sleeping pills are antihistamines—so they may cause drowsiness. Patients taking many antihistamines are cautioned to avoid driving or operating machinery that could be dangerous.

The mainstays of therapy for the common cold are the decongestants that are applied topically (that is, directly to the mucous membranes in the nose) or taken orally. They are also called sympathomimetic agents because they mimic the effects of certain natural body chemicals that regulate many body processes. A group of these, called adrenergic stimulants, regulate vasoconstriction and vasodilation—in other words, they can narrow or widen blood vessels, respectively. Their vasoconstrictive capability is useful in managing the common cold, because it reduces the size of the blood vessels in the nose, reduces swelling and congestion, and inhibits excess secretion.

Topical decongestants are available as nasal sprays or drops. The sprays are squirted up into each nostril. The patient is usually advised to wait three to five minutes and then blow his or her nose to remove the mucus. If there is still congestion, the patient is advised to take another dose, allowing the medication to reach further into the nasal cavity. Nose drops are taken by tilting the head back and squeezing the medication into the nostrils through the nose-dropper supplied with the medication. Clearance of nasal congestion is prompt, and the patient can breathe more easily. Nasal irritation is reduced, so there is less sneezing. Some nasal sprays and drops last longer than others, but none works around-the-clock, so applications must be repeated throughout the day.

Patients who use nasal sprays and drops are advised to follow the manufacturer's directions exactly. Applied too often or in too great a quantity, these preparations can cause unwanted problems, such as rhinitis medicamentosa, or nasal inflammation caused by a medication (also called rebound congestion). As the vasoconstrictive effect of the drugs wears down, the blood vessels dilate, the area becomes swollen, and secretions increase. This reaction may be attributable to the fact that the drug's vasoconstrictive effect has deprived the area of blood, and thus excited an increased inflammatory state, or it may simply be attributable to irritation by the drug. Use of sprays or drops should be limited to three or four days.

Oral decongestants are also effective in reducing swelling and relieving a runny nose, although they do not have as great a vasoconstrictive effect concentrated in the nasal area as sprays or drops. Because they circulate throughout the body, their vasoconstrictive effects may be seen in other vascular beds. There are many patients who are warned not to use oral decongestants unless they are under the care of a physician. These people include patients with high blood pressure, diabetics, heart patients, and patients taking certain drugs such as monoamine oxidase (MAO) inhibitors, guanethidine, bethanidine, or debrisoquin sulfate.

Three kinds of coughs may accompany colds: coughs that produce phlegm or mucus; hyperactive nagging coughs, which result from overstimulation of the cough reflex; and dry, unproductive coughs. If the phlegm or mucus collecting in the lungs is easily removed by occasional coughing, a soothing syrup, cough drop, or lozenge may be all that the patient requires. If the cough reflex center of the brain is overstimulated, there may be hyperactive or uncontrollable coughing and a cough suppressant, such as dextromethorphan, may be needed. Dextromethorphan works in the brain to raise the level of stimulus that is required to trigger the cough reflex. Some antihistamines, such as diphenhydramine hydrochloride, are effective cough suppressants. If coughing is unproductive—that is, if the mucus has thickened and dried and is not easily removed—an expectorant should be taken. Currently, the only expectorant used in over-the-counter drugs is guaifenesin. It helps soften and liquefy mucus deposits, so that coughs become productive. When a cough of a cold is serious enough for a physician to be consulted, prescription drugs may have to be used, such as codeine to stop hyperactive coughing and potassium iodide for unproductive coughs.

For allergic rhinitis or hay fever, avoidance of allergens is recommended but is not always possible. For hay fever outbreaks, antihistamines are the mainstays of therapy, with other agents added to relieve specific symptoms. For example, topical and oral decongestants may be required to relieve a runny nose.

PERSPECTIVE AND PROSPECTS

Viruses are among the most intriguing and baffling challenges to medical science. Great progress has been made in preventing some virus diseases, such as by immunization against smallpox and hepatitis B. There has been only limited success, however, in finding agents to cure virus diseases, and so far nothing has been found to prevent or cure the common cold. Vaccines have been developed against certain rhinoviruses, and no doubt many more could be developed. Yet because the common cold is caused by so many different types of virus—more than two hundred—and vaccines against one virus are not necessarily effective against others, it is questionable whether such vaccines would ever be useful. A helpful vaccine would be one that could immunize against an entire family of viruses such as rhinoviruses or coronaviruses, the two leading causes of the common cold.

The search goes on for agents to cure the common cold. Substances, such as interferons, have been found that are effective against a wide range of viruses. One of the interferons was used by the British Medical Research Council's Common Cold Unit. They reported that interferon applied as an intranasal spray was highly effective in protecting subjects from cold infection. After some years, however, experimentation with interferon in the common cold was abandoned because the agent had significant side effects, nasal congestion among them.

The science of virology only began in the 1930's, so it is not surprising that viruses continue to hide their mysteries. Nevertheless, many fundamental discoveries have been made and one can predict increasing success. As scientists unravel the intricacies of viral infections, they find clues that help them devise ways of interfering with virus life processes. In some cases, effective drugs have been developed, such as the interferons, acyclovir for herpes simplex, and amantadine for the influenza virus. It is likely that the cure for the common cold will continue to be elusive, unless a broad-spectrum antiviral agent could be developed that works against multiple viral infections in the way that broad-spectrum antibiotics work against multiple bacterial infections.
                                                    —*C. Richard Falcon*

See also Allergies; Bronchitis; Coughing; Fever; Influenza; Nasopharyngeal disorders; Nausea and vomiting; Otorhinolarnygology; Pneumonia; Rhinitis; Sinusitis; Sore throat; Viral infections.

FOR FURTHER INFORMATION:

American Pharmaceutical Association. *Handbook of Nonprescription Drugs*. 9th ed. Washington, D.C.: Author, 1990. The section on drugs for colds, coughs, and allergies contains a thorough background discussion of these conditions. All major over-the-counter medications are listed.

Gallo, Robert. *Virus Hunting*. New York: Basic Books, 1991. Gallo gives a good general account of viruses—how they live and how modern medical science is trying to combat them.

Larson, David E., ed. *Mayo Clinic Family Health Book*. 2d ed. New York: William Morrow, 1996. One of the most thorough and accessible medical texts for the layperson.

Scott, Andrew. *Pirates of the Cell*. Oxford, England: Basil Blackwell, 1985. A superior text on viruses for the layperson, this book is particularly successful in clarifying the enormous range of pathogenic viruses, describing the infective process, and outlining the state of antiviral vaccines, medications, and procedures.

Young, Stuart H., Bruce S. Dobozin, and Margaret Miner. *Allergies*. Yonkers, N.Y.: Consumer Reports Books, 1992. A useful book that covers the treatment of allergic coldlike conditions, such as hay fever, and gives advice on how to manage them.

COMPUTED TOMOGRAPHY (CT) SCANNING

PROCEDURE

ANATOMY OR SYSTEM AFFECTED: Abdomen, brain, head, nervous system

SPECIALTIES AND RELATED FIELDS: Biotechnology, emergency medicine, gastroenterology, radiology

DEFINITION: The combination of X rays and computer technology to provide detailed cross-sectional images of tissue.

KEY TERMS:

CAT (computer axial tomography) scan: an older term for the result of a CT procedure

cathode-ray tube: a vacuum tube which focuses an electron beam on a screen, producing the image from the CT scan

metastasis: the spread of cancer from its site of origin

INDICATIONS AND PROCEDURES

Computed tomography (CT) scanning, formerly referred to as a computed axial tomography (CAT) scan, describes a procedure which combines an X ray of tissue with a computer, providing a detailed cross-sectional image of the area of the body under analysis. The major advantage of this procedure is that it is noninvasive, providing a relatively easy and safe analysis of internal organs or structures.

The CT scan is applicable for the analysis of most internal organs. Most commonly, it is used in the analysis of brain disorders (brain CT scan) or for problems elsewhere in the body (body CT scan). The quality of images seen on the screen allows the detection of minute differences within both soft tissue (brain or other organs) and harder structures such as bone.

Often, the symptoms described by a patient to a physician can be interpreted many ways, some of which are minor and some of which may be life-threatening. For example, the patient may describe vague symptoms such as headache or dizziness. The problem may be as simple as a migraine or tension headache or as serious as a stroke or brain tumor. Prior to the development of the CT scan, proper diagnosis of the cause of such symptoms required complicated, sometimes dangerous procedures; standard X-ray analysis was often not sensitive enough to detect small abnormalities. Among the advantages of the CT scan is its ability to detect such small changes.

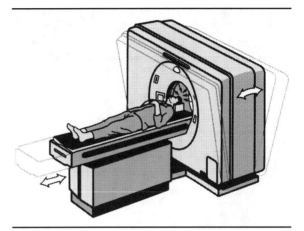

In the imaging technique called computed tomography (CT) scanning (formerly known as a CAT scan), multiple X-ray pictures are taken as the scanner tilts and rotates around the patient. These images are then assembled by a computer to create a three-dimensional view of a body part, such as the head.

Diagnosis of the underlying problem that is causing headaches, for example, may warrant the use of the brain CT scan. The patient lies horizontally on a table, with the head placed within a large scanner or box. If warranted, as in the analysis of small abnormalities, a contrast material may first be injected. Contrast dyes are not always used.

The scanner produces a narrow beam of X rays as it moves in a 360-degree circular motion around the head of the patient; the X rays are monitored by a series of detectors placed around the body. Each slice, or photograph, is produced in only several seconds; between ten and thirty photographs are taken. The total amount of radiation emitted is less than that encountered during a dental X ray.

Associated with the monitors is a computer which produces a cross-sectional image of the brain, creating a composite picture which appears on a cathode-ray tube. The picture can then be stored or printed. The total procedure usually can be carried out in less than one hour. The results can then be reviewed by a radiologist or other physician. In an analogous manner, other areas of the body may be scanned when symptoms warrant it. Brain tumors or tumors that have metastasized from other sites stand out as abnormalities against the normal background.

USES AND COMPLICATIONS

CT scanning can be used to detect small changes or abnormalities within most organs of the body. It is particularly useful in the analysis of the brain or abdominal regions, especially if symptoms suggest the presence of a tumor. Likewise, tumor metastasis can be observed. Small growths that might ordinarily require surgery for their detection can be monitored with the scan, and the extent of metastasis from the primary site can be followed.

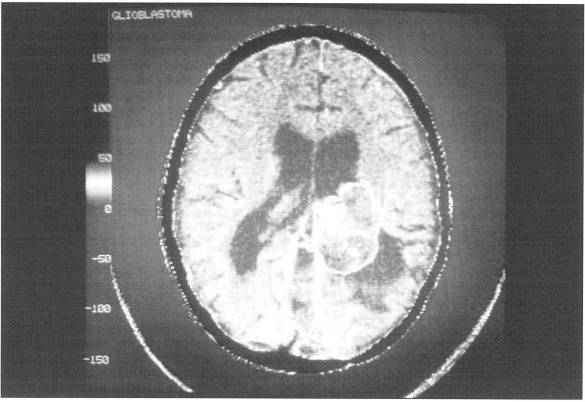

Brain tumors can be visualized used computed tomography (CT) scanning. This scan shows a large glioblastoma in the middle of the brain. (Dan McCoy/Rainbow)

The procedure is not used solely in the detection of cancer or tumor metastasis. It has been applied to the analysis of brain damage resulting from strokes or of dementia from any cause. In the case of strokes, damaged areas of the brain may appear darker than normal, standing out by their contrast. The procedure can also be applied in the analysis of bone damage resulting from a break. The cross-sectional image of the bone can allow for more sensitive observation of the extent of the damage than can be obtained with conventional X rays. Indeed, the CT scan has been reported to be one hundred times as sensitive as normal X rays.

Preparation for the procedure can be mildly discomforting but generally presents no danger. When a body scan is to be carried out, the person cannot eat for several hours prior to the procedure; an enema may also be administered. Occasionally, the patient may have an allergy to the contrast dye, in which case either an alternative must be used or the allergic response must be dampened with medication. During the procedure, the patient must lie still, sometimes with difficulty, for an hour. A sedative may be administered. Since for a brain CT scan the patient's head is surrounded by a scanner, it is also possible that the patient may feel claustrophobic.

PERSPECTIVE AND PROSPECTS

The CT scan was developed in the early 1970's to provide a convenient, noninvasive method of internal analysis. Previously, analysis of symptoms associated with tumors, headaches, or strokes required either surgery or uncomfortable tests such as angiography, the intravascular injection of a radiopaque solution to allow X-ray analysis of the organ, the resulting image being limited in detail. Some procedures such as pneumoencephalography, the replacement of portions of cerebrospinal fluid with gas to delineate the brain, are also inherently dangerous. The CT scan can be carried out on an outpatient basis, is much faster than some alternative techniques, and is relatively inexpensive when compared to most hospital procedures.

During the 1980's, CT scanning was combined with the procedure of stereotaxic surgery to add another dimension to diagnostic and clinical medicine. In this procedure, an electrode or probe is inserted into the brain while the organ is monitored with the CT scanner. The combination of techniques allows for pinpoint accuracy with the stereotaxic apparatus.

—*Richard Adler, Ph.D.*

See also Brain; Brain disorders; Headaches; Imaging and radiology; Magnetic resonance imaging (MRI); Non-invasive tests; Nuclear medicine; Positron emission tomography (PET) scanning; Strokes and TIAs; Tumors; Ultrasonography.

FOR FURTHER INFORMATION:
Altman, Roberta, and Michael Sarg. *The Cancer Dictionary*. New York: Facts on File, 1992.
Dollinger, Malin, et al. *Everyone's Guide to Cancer Therapy*. Kansas City, Mo.: Andrews & McMeel, 1994.
Moskowitz, Mark, and Michael Osband. *The Complete Book of Medical Tests*. New York: W. W. Norton, 1984.
Romans, Lois E. *Introduction to Computed Tomography*. Baltimore: Williams & Wilkins, 1995.
Sobel, David, and Tom Ferguson. *The People's Book of Medical Tests*. New York: Summit Books, 1985.

CONCEPTION

BIOLOGY

ANATOMY OR SYSTEM AFFECTED: Cells, reproductive system, uterus

SPECIALTIES AND RELATED FIELDS: Embryology, gynecology, obstetrics

DEFINITION: The process of creating new life, encompassing all the events from deposition of sperm into the female to the first cell divisions of the fertilized ovum.

KEY TERMS:

cervix: the lowest part of the uterus in contact with the vagina; contains an opening filled with mucus through which sperm can pass

ejaculation: the reflex activated by sexual stimulation that results in sperm mixed with fluid being expelled from the male's body

fertilization: the union of the sperm and the ovum, which usually occurs in the female's oviduct

menstruation: the process of shedding the lining of the uterus that occurs about once a month

oviduct: the thin tube that leads from near the ovary to the upper part of the uterus; also called the Fallopian tube

ovulation: the process by which the mature ovum is expelled from the ovary

ovum: the round cell produced by the female that carries her genetic material; also called the egg

sperm: the motile cells produced within the male that carry his genetic material

uterus: the organ above the vagina through which the sperm must pass on their way to the ovum; also called the womb

vagina: the stretchy, tube-shaped structure into which the male's penis is inserted during intercourse; the site of sperm deposition

PROCESS AND EFFECTS

The process of conception begins with the act of intercourse. When the male's penis is inserted into the female's vagina, the stimulation of the penis by movement within the vagina triggers a reflex resulting in the ejaculation of sperm. During ejaculation, involuntary muscles in many of the male reproductive organs contract, causing semen, a mixture of sperm and fluid, to move from its sites of storage out through the urethra within the penis.

The average volume of semen in a typical human ejaculation is only 3.5 milliliters, but this small volume normally contains 200 million to 400 million sperm. Other constituents of semen include prostaglandins, which cause contractions of involuntary muscles in both the male and the female; the sugar fructose, which provides energy to the sperm; chemicals that adjust the activity of the semen; and a number of enzymes and other chemicals.

In a typical act of intercourse, the semen is deposited high up in the woman's vagina. Within a minute after ejaculation, the semen begins to coagulate, or form a clot, because of the activation of chemicals within the semen. Sperm are not able to leave the vagina until the semen becomes liquid again, which occurs spontaneously fifteen to twenty minutes after ejaculation.

Once the semen liquefies, sperm begin moving through the female system. The path to the ovum (if one is present) lies through the cervix, then through the hollow cavity of the uterus, and up through the oviduct, where fertilization normally occurs. The sperm are propelled through the fluid within these organs by the swimming movements of their tails, as well as by female organ contractions that are stimulated by the act of intercourse and by prostaglandins contained in the semen. It is not necessary for the woman to experience orgasm, a pleasurable climax, in order for these contractions to occur. The contractions allow sperm to reach the oviduct within five minutes after leav-

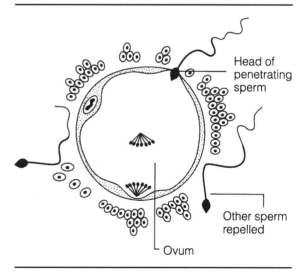

Head of penetrating sperm

Other sperm repelled

Ovum

Male sperm cells propel themselves toward the ovum (female egg) by the swimming movements of their tails; fertilization occurs when a sperm cell penetrates the layers surrounding the ovum and fuses its membrane with the membrane of the ovum.

ing the vagina, a rate of movement that far exceeds their own swimming abilities.

Although some sperm can reach the oviduct quite rapidly, others never enter the oviduct at all. Of the two hundred million to four hundred million sperm deposited in the vagina, it is estimated that only one hundred to one thousand enter the oviducts. Some of the other millions of sperm may be defective, lacking the proper swimming ability. Other apparently normal sperm may become lost within the female's organs, possibly trapped in clefts between cells in the organ linings. The damaged and lost sperm will eventually be destroyed by white blood cells produced by the female.

Sperm movement through the female system is enhanced around the time of ovulation. For example, at the time of ovulation, the hormones associated with ovulation cause changes in the cervical mucus that aid sperm transport. The mucus at that time is extremely liquid and contains fibers that align themselves into channels, which are thought to be used by the sperm to ease their passage through the cervix. The hormones present at the time of ovulation also increase the contractions produced by the uterus and oviduct, and thus sperm transport through the structures is enhanced as well.

During transport through the female, sperm undergo a number of important chemical changes, collectively called capacitation, that enable them to fertilize the ovum successfully. Freshly ejaculated sperm are not capable of penetrating the layers surrounding the ovum, a fact that was uncovered when scientists first began to experiment with in vitro fertilization (the joining of sperm and ovum outside the body). Capacitation apparently occurs during transport of the sperm through the uterus and possibly the oviduct, and it is presumably triggered by some secretion of the female. With in vitro fertilization, capacitation is achieved by adding female blood serum to the dish that contains the sperm and ovum. Capacitation is not instantaneous; it has been estimated that this process requires an hour or more in humans. Thus, even though the first sperm may arrive in the vicinity of the ovum within twenty minutes after ejaculation, fertilization cannot take place until capacitation is completed.

The site where ovum and sperm typically come together is within the oviduct. At the time of ovulation, an ovum is released from the surface of the ovary and drawn into the upper end of the oviduct. Once within the oviduct, the ovum is propelled by contractions of the oviduct and possibly by wavelike motions of cilia, hairlike projections that line the inner surface of the oviduct. It takes about three days for the ovum to travel the entire length of the oviduct to the uterus, and since the ovum only remains fertilizable for twelve to twenty-four hours, successful fertilization must occur in the oviduct.

Upon reaching the ovum, the sperm must first penetrate two layers surrounding it. The outermost layer, called the corona radiata, consists of cells that break away from the ovary with the ovum during ovulation; the innermost layer, the zona pellucida, is a clear, jellylike substance that lies just outside the ovum cell membrane. Penetration of these two layers is accomplished by the release of enzymes carried by the sperm. Once through the zona pellucida, the sperm are ready to fertilize the ovum.

Fertilization occurs when a sperm fuses its membrane with the membrane of the ovum. This act triggers a protective change in the zona pellucida that prevents any additional sperm from reaching the ovum and providing it with extra chromosomes. Following fusion of the fertilizing sperm and ovum, the chromosomes of each become mingled; the resulting one-celled zygote contains a complete set of chromosomes, half contributed by the mother and half by the father.

It is at the moment of fertilization that the sex of the new child is decided. Genetic sex is determined by a pair of chromosomes denoted X and Y. Female body cells contain two X's, and each ovum produced contains only one X. Male body cells contain an X and a Y chromosome, but each sperm contains either an X or a Y chromosome. Men usually produce equal numbers of X- and Y-type sperm. The sex of the new individual is determined by which type of sperm fertilizes the ovum: If it is a Y-bearing sperm, the new individual will be male, and if it is an X-bearing sperm, the new individual will be female. Since entry of more than one sperm is prohibited, the first sperm to reach the ovum is the one that will fertilize it.

Following fertilization, the zygote or early embryo begins a series of cell divisions while it travels down the oviduct. When it arrives at the uterus about three days after ovulation, the zygote will be in the form of a hollow ball of cells. Initially, this ball of cells floats in the fluid-filled cavity of the uterus, but two or three days after its arrival in the uterus (five to six days after ovulation), it will attach to the uterine lining. Over the next nine months, the body of the embryo will take on a human form and develop the ability to live independently outside the uterus.

COMPLICATIONS AND DISORDERS

Three factors limit the time frame in which conception is possible: the fertilizable lifetime of the ovulated ovum, estimated to be between twelve and twenty-four hours; the fertilizable lifetime of ejaculated sperm in the female tract, usually assumed to be about forty-eight hours; and the time required for sperm capacitation, which is one hour or more. The combination of these factors determines the length of the fertile period, the time during which intercourse must occur if conception is to be achieved. Taking the three factors into account, the fertile period is said to extend from forty-eight hours prior to ovulation until perhaps twenty-four hours after ovulation. For example, if intercourse occurs forty-eight hours before ovulation, the sperm will be capacitated in the first few hours and will still be within their fertilizable lifetime when ovulation occurs. On the other hand, if intercourse occurs twenty-four hours after ovulation, the sperm will still require time for capacitation, but the ovum will be near the end of its viable period. Thus the later limit of the fertile period is equal to the fertilizable lifetime of the ovum, minus the time required for capacitation.

Obviously, a critical factor in conception is the timing of ovulation. In a typical twenty-eight-day menstrual cycle, ovulation occurs about halfway through the cycle, or fourteen days after the first day of menstrual bleeding. In actuality, cycle length varies widely, both among individual women and in a single woman from month to month. It appears that generally the first half of the cycle is more variable in length, with the second half more stable. Thus, no matter how long the entire menstrual cycle is, ovulation usually occurs fourteen days prior to the first day of the next episode of menstrual bleeding. Therefore, it is relatively easy to determine when ovulation occurred by counting backward, but difficult to predict the time of ovulation in advance.

Assessment of ovulation time in women is notoriously difficult. There is no easily observable outward sign of ovulation. Some women do detect slight abdominal pain about the time of ovulation; this is referred to as *Mittelschmerz*, which means, literally, pain in the middle of the cycle. This slight pain may be localized on either side of the abdomen and is thought to be caused by irritation of the abdominal organs by fluid released from the ovary during ovulation. Other signs of ovulation are an increased volume and stretchiness of the cervical mucus and a characteristic fern-like pattern of the mucus when it is dried on a glass slide. There is also a slight rise in body temperature after ovulation, which again makes it easier to determine the time of ovulation after the fact rather than in advance. It is also possible to measure the amount of luteinizing hormone (LH) in urine or blood; this hormone shows a marked increase about sixteen hours prior to ovulation. Home test kits to detect LH levels are available for urine samples. There are additional signs of the time of ovulation, such as a slight opening of the cervix and a change in the cells lining the vagina, that can be used by physicians to determine the timing and occurrence of ovulation.

Since ovulation time is so difficult to detect in most women on an ongoing basis, most physicians would counsel that, to achieve a pregnancy, couples should plan on having intercourse every two days. This frequency will ensure that sperm capable of fertilization are always present, so that the exact time of ovulation becomes unimportant. A greater frequency of intercourse is not advised, since sperm numbers may be reduced when ejaculation occurs often. Approximately 85 to 90 percent of couples will achieve pregnancy within a year when intercourse occurs about three times a week.

Couples often wonder if it is possible to predetermine the sex of their child by some action taken in conjunction with intercourse. Scientists have found no consistent effect of parental diet, position assumed during intercourse, timing of intercourse within the menstrual cycle, or liquids that are introduced into the vagina to kill one type of sperm selectively. In the laboratory, it is possible to achieve partial separation of sperm in a semen sample by subjecting the semen to an electric current or other procedure. The separated sperm can then be used for artificial insemination (the introduction of semen through a tube into the uterus). This method is not 100 percent successful in producing offspring of the desired sex and so is available only on an experimental basis.

Some couples have difficulty in conceiving a child, in a few cases as a result of some problem associated with intercourse. For example, the male may have difficulty in achieving erection or ejaculation. The vast majority of these cases are caused by psychological factors such as stress and tension rather than any biological problem. Fortunately, therapists can teach couples how to overcome these psychological problems.

About 15 percent of couples in the United States suffer from some type of biological infertility—that is, infertility that persists when intercourse occurs successfully. In 10 percent of the cases of infertility, doctors are unable to establish a cause. In another 20 percent of couples, both partners are infertile. In the remaining 70 percent of cases, about half the problems are in the male and half in the female.

In men, the most commonly diagnosed cause of infertility is low sperm count. Sometimes low sperm count is caused by a treatable imbalance of hormones. If not treatable, this problem can sometimes be circumvented by the use of pooled semen samples in artificial insemination or through in vitro fertilization. In vitro fertilization may also be a solution for men who produce normal numbers of sperm but whose sperm lack swimming ability. Another cause of male infertility is blockage of the tubes that carry the semen from the body, which may be caused by a previous infection. Surgery is sometimes successful in removing such a blockage.

In women, a common cause of infertility is a hormonal problem that interferes with ovulation. Treatment with one of a number of so-called fertility drugs may be successful in promoting ovulation. Fertility drugs, however, have some disadvantages: They have a tendency to cause ovulation of more than one ovum, thus raising the possibility of multiple pregnancy, which is considered risky; and they may alter the environment of the uterus, making implantation of a resulting embryo less likely.

Another common cause of female infertility is blockage of the oviducts resulting from scar tissue formation in the aftermath of some type of infection. Because surgery is not always successful in opening the oviducts, this condition may require the use of in vitro fertilization or the new technique of surgically introducing ova and sperm directly into the oviduct at a point below the blockage.

Finally, some cases of infertility result from biological incompatibility between the man and the woman. It may be that the sperm are unable to penetrate the cervical mucus, or perhaps that the woman's body treats the sperm cells as invaders, destroying them before they can reach the ovum. Techniques such as artificial insemination and in vitro fertilization offer hope for couples experiencing these problems.

PERSPECTIVE AND PROSPECTS

For most of history, the events surrounding conception were poorly understood. For example, microscopic identification of sperm did not occur until 1677, and the ovum was not identified until 1827 (although the follicle in which the ovum develops was recognized in the 1600's). Prior to these discoveries, people held the belief espoused by early writers such as Aristotle and Galen that conception resulted from the mixing of male and female fluids during intercourse.

There was also confusion about the timing of the fertile period. Some early doctors thought that menstrual blood was involved in conception and therefore believed that the fertile period coincided with menstruation. Others recognized that menstrual bleeding was a sign that pregnancy had not occurred; they assumed that the most likely time for conception to result was immediately after the menstrual flow ceased. It was not until the 1930's that the first scientific studies on the timing of ovulation were completed.

Since there was little scientific understanding of the processes involved in conception, medical practice for most of human history was little different from magic, revolving around the use of rituals and herbal treatments to aid or prevent conception. Gradually, people rejected these practices, often because of religious teachings. By the 1900's, conception had been established as an area of intense privacy, thought by physicians and the general public to be unsuitable for medical intervention.

In the early part of the twentieth century, the role of physicians in aiding conception was mostly limited to educating and advising couples finding difficulty in conceiving. There were few techniques, other than artificial insemination and fertility drug treatment, available to assist in conception at that time.

The situation changed with the first successful in vitro fertilization in 1978. This event ushered in an era of intense medical and public interest in assisting conception. Other methods to aid conception were soon introduced, including embryo transfer, frozen storage of embryos, and surgical placement of ova and sperm directly into the oviduct.

Paralleling the development of these techniques has been demand on the part of society for medicine to apply them.

Infertility rates in the United States have been gradually increasing. One reason for increased infertility has been the increasing age at which couples decide to start a family, since the fertility of women appears to undergo a decline past the age of thirty. Another factor affecting fertility rates of both men and women has been an increased incidence of various sexually transmitted diseases, which can result in chronic inflammation of the reproductive organs and infertility caused by scar tissue formation.

People's attitudes toward medical intervention in conception have also changed. The earlier religious taboos against interference in conception have been somewhat relaxed, although some churches still do not approve of certain methods of fertility management. Although there remain ethical issues to be resolved, the general public seems to have accepted the idea that medicine should provide assistance to those who wish to, but cannot, conceive children.

—Marcia Watson-Whitmyre, Ph.D.

See also Childbirth; Cloning; Contraception; Gynecology; In vitro fertilization; Infertility in females; Infertility in males; Menstruation; Multiple births; Obstetrics; Pregnancy and gestation; Reproductive system.

FOR FURTHER INFORMATION:

Birke, Lynda, Susan Himmelweit, and Gail Vines. *Tomorrow's Child: Reproductive Technologies in the Nineties.* London: Virago Press, 1990. Written for the general reader, this book is unique in its multifaceted coverage of medically assisted conception. Provides accurate information on the procedures involved and also covers ethical issues.

Hafez, E. S. E., ed. *Human Reproduction: Conception and Contraception.* Hagerstown, Md.: Harper & Row, 1980. Written by expert scientists, this text provides complete coverage of human conception. The first two sections cover male and female anatomy and physiology.

Harkness, Carol. *The Infertility Book.* San Francisco: Volcano Press, 1987. Presents a comprehensive guide to problems of infertility and combines both a medical and an emotional perspective. Contains anecdotal accounts in the patients' own words.

Jones, Richard E. *Human Reproductive Biology.* 2d ed. San Diego: Academic Press, 1997. This college-level textbook provides comprehensive coverage of all biological aspects of human reproduction. There is a separate chapter on fertilization, and information on the timing of ovulation, contraception, and infertility treatment is also presented.

Liebman-Smith, Joan. *In Pursuit of Pregnancy.* New York: Newmarket Press, 1987. This well-written book presents the stories of three couples as they discover and cope with their infertility. Contains good descriptions of diagnostic and treatment procedures.

Silber, Sherman J. *How to Get Pregnant.* New York: Charles Scribner's Sons, 1980. Written by a physician, this text is as straightforward as its title implies. Accurate, comprehensive, and easy to read.

Weschler, Toni. *Taking Charge of Your Infertility*. New York: HarperPerennial, 1995. This book encourages women to become responsible for their own reproductive health. Includes excellent discussions of infertility, natural birth control, and achieving pregnancy.

Wisot, Arthur, and David Meldrum. *Conceptions and Misconceptions*. Vancouver: Harley and Marks, 1997. Written by two leading fertility experts, this book is an excellent guide through the maze of in vitro fertilization and other assisted reproductive techniques. Includes an excellent discussion of the basic physiology of conception and reproduction.

CONCUSSION
DISEASE/DISORDER
ANATOMY OR SYSTEM AFFECTED: Brain, head, nervous system, psychic-emotional system

SPECIALTIES AND RELATED FIELDS: Emergency medicine, neurology

DEFINITION: The most common injury to the head is the concussion. When the head is struck by a hard blow or shaken violently, the brain is jostled, striking the inside of the skull. The result is temporary neural dysfunction, which may cause confusion, dizziness, nausea, headache, lethargy, changes in character, and amnesia concerning the time just before or after the injury. These symptoms are normal for a concussion and are not usually serious; some may last for weeks. Any worsening of these symptoms following the injury, however, may require further medical care and could indicate more severe damage to the brain, such as a cerebral contusion.

—*Jason Georges and Tracy Irons-Georges*
See also Amnesia; Bleeding; Brain; Brain disorders; Coma; Dizziness and fainting; Head and neck disorders; Nausea and vomiting; Nervous system; Neurology; Sports medicine; Unconsciousness.

CONGENITAL HEART DISEASE
DISEASE/DISORDER
ANATOMY OR SYSTEM AFFECTED: Chest, circulatory system, heart

SPECIALTIES AND RELATED FIELDS: Cardiology, neonatology, pediatrics, vascular medicine

DEFINITION: Conditions resulting from malformations of the heart that occur during embryonic and fetal development, accounting for about 25 percent of all congenital defects.

KEY TERMS:
atrium: one of two heart chambers that receive blood, the left from the lungs and the right from the body

great arteries and veins: large vessels channeling blood into and out of the heart, including the aorta (to the body),

the pulmonary artery (to the lungs), the vena cava (from the body), and the pulmonary veins (from the lungs)

heart failure: the inability of the heart to pump adequate amounts of blood to maintain the organs and tissues of the body; often results in tissue fluid retention and congestion

murmur: a sound made by the heart other than the normal two-step beat; murmurs are caused by the turbulent movement of blood and may indicate a heart defect

septum: a membrane which serves as a wall of separation; in the heart, the interatrial septum divides the two atria and the interventricular septum divides the two ventricles

ventricles: heart chambers that pump blood, the left to the body and the right to the lungs

CAUSES AND SYMPTOMS
Congenital heart disease collectively includes various structural and functional defects of the heart and blood vessels resulting from errors that occur during embryonic development. The defects may cause heart murmurs, high or low blood pressure, congestive heart failure, cyanosis (blue skin), abnormal heart rhythms and rates, and incidences of low oxygen (hypoxia). Congenital heart disease is detected in about 0.7 percent of live births and 2.7 percent of stillbirths. Babies born with congenital heart disease have the most difficulty during the first few weeks of life. Some problems, however, are not easily detected at the time of birth and are discovered at various stages of life. Heart defects may be inherited from parents, induced by environmental agents such as drugs, or caused by an interaction of genetic and environmental factors. Defects are more common in children with genetic disorders such as Down syndrome. With intensive treatment, including surgery, many forms of congenital heart disease can be corrected, allowing those affected to lead normal lives.

Knowledge of normal heart development will help in understanding how congenital heart disease occurs and will provide a means for categorizing these defects. Near the end of the third week of embryonic development, the heart begins to form from two cords of tissue that hollow out and fuse to form a primitive heart tube. This tube undergoes some constrictions and dilations to form the early divisions of the heart, including a receiving chamber, the atrium, and a pumping chamber, the ventricle, which exits into a muscular tube called the truncus arteriosus. At about twenty-two days, the heart begins to contract and pump blood. A day later, it bends or loops upon itself to form an S shape, with the atrium on one side, the truncus arteriosus on the other side, and the ventricle in the middle. If it bends to the left instead of to the right, a rare heart defect called dextrocardia results. The heart will be displaced to the right side of the body and may have some accompanying abnormalities.

During the fourth and fifth week of development, the heart begins to divide into four chambers by first forming a septum (dividing membrane) in the canal between the atrium and the ventricle. This septum is formed by heart tissue called the endocardial cushions. Failure of this septum to form properly causes atrioventricular canal defects. These are often associated with Down syndrome. During the fifth week of development, a spiral septum forms in the truncus arteriosus which divides it into two vessels: the pulmonary artery, which connects to the right ventricle, and the aorta, which connects to the left ventricle. The formation of this septum and the ventricular connections are subject to error and may result in a group of anomalies called conotruncal defects.

As these large arteries are forming, a shunt (bypass) develops between them called the ductus arteriosus. This short vessel allows the blood to be diverted away from the nonfunctional fetal lungs into the aorta and on to the placenta, where it will receive oxygen and nutrients. Persistence of this shunt after birth is responsible for a defect called patent ductus. A septum dividing the atrium into right and left halves also forms during the fourth and fifth weeks of development; however, blood is allowed to pass from the right atrium to the left atrium through a small hole in this septum called the foramen ovale. This hole normally closes after birth but is necessary during fetal life to shunt blood away from the fetal lungs and toward the placenta in a manner similar to that of the ductus arteriosus. At about the same time, a septum forms from the floor of the ventricle and divides it into right and left halves. Failure of the atrial and ventricular septa to form properly and to close at the time of birth results in septal defects.

After the appearance of the four chambers, two pairs of valves form in the heart to prevent the back flow of blood and to ensure greater efficiency in pumping. The semilunar valves (also called the pulmonary and aortic valves) form between the ventricles and their respective outlet arteries (pulmonary artery and aorta), and the atrioventricular valves (bicuspid or mitral on the left and tricuspid on the right) form between the atria and the ventricles. Improperly formed valves can lead to flow defects. During development, the heart also makes connections with veins returning from the general circulation and the lungs. Errors in these connections and other structural errors cause several other less common congenital heart defects.

The most common congenital heart defects are the septal defects and patent ductus, which together account for about 37 percent of all heart defects. After birth, because the pressure becomes higher in the left side of the heart, blood moves from left to right through the openings in the heart that come with such defects, causing too much to flow to the lungs and a mixing of systemic and pulmonary blood. The child's lungs will be congested, causing difficulty in breathing and eventually heart failure.

About 29 percent of congenital heart defects are categorized as right-heart and left-heart flow defects. These defects impede the flow of blood from either the right or the left side of the heart to its normal destination. Right-heart flow defects include bicuspid pulmonary valve (a valve with two cusps instead of three), pulmonary valve stenosis (a narrowing of the valve), dysplastic pulmonary valve (a malformed valve), peripheral pulmonary stenosis (a narrowing of the walls of the pulmonary artery), infundibular pulmonary stenosis (a narrowing below the valve), and hypoplastic right ventricle (incomplete formation of the valve). These defects impede blood flow to the lungs, which results in poor oxygenation of the blood (cyanosis). Left-heart flow defects include bicuspid aortic valve, aortic valve stenosis, coarctation of the aorta (narrowing), aortic atresia (a blocked aorta), and hypoplastic left ventricle. These defects impede blood flow to the body and often result in altered blood pressure, hypoxia of body tissues, and congestive heart failure.

The principal conotruncal defects, which account for about 17 percent of heart defects, are tetralogy of Fallot and transposition of the great arteries. Tetralogy of Fallot includes a group of four defects which results in cyanosis; they are pulmonary stenosis, a ventricular septal defect, an overriding or displaced aorta, and hypertrophy or enlargement of the right ventricle. With transposition of the great arteries, the aorta connects to the right ventricle and the pulmonary artery to the left ventricle, the opposite of the normal formation. The blood is not properly oxygenated, and survival is not possible without medical intervention or a

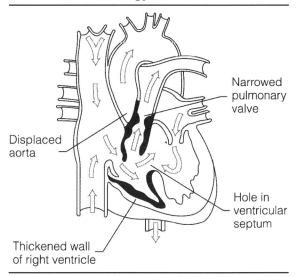

Tetralogy of Fallot

Narrowed pulmonary valve

Displaced aorta

Hole in ventricular septum

Thickened wall of right ventricle

A relatively common congenital heart defect, tetralogy of Fallot comprises four defects: an overriding or displaced aorta, pulmonary stenosis (a narrowed pulmonary valve), a ventricular septal defect (a hole in the ventricular septum), and a thickened, or enlarged, right ventricle. These together result in cyanosis: poor blood oxygenation.

natural shunt such as patent ductus. Other rare conotruncal defects include double outlet right ventricle (the aorta and the pulmonary artery attached to right ventricle), truncus arteriosus (failure of the truncus to separate into the aorta and the pulmonary artery), and aortopulmonary window (an opening between the aorta and the pulmonary artery).

Defects resulting from improper fusion of the endocardial cushions and surrounding tissues cause atrioventricular defects, which affect about 9 percent of patients with congenital heart disease. Complete atrioventricular canal defect occurs in about 20 percent of Down syndrome cases, but it is rare outside this group. The defect produces a large open space in the center of the heart, allowing blood to intermix freely between the right and left sides of the heart. The defect is sometimes accompanied by hypoplastic ventricle. If the condition is not treated, the heart will fail. Patent foramen primum or ostium primum is a milder form of atrioventricular canal defect in which the atrial septum fails to fuse with the endocardial cushions, resulting in a problem similar to atria septal defect. In addition, the mitral valve is usually deformed.

Other less common defects include looping defects such as dextrocardia, in which the apex of the heart points to the right instead of to the left. This change in symmetry normally does not affect heart function, but some looping defects are associated with other problems such as transposition of the great arteries. Another less common defect is anomalous venous return, in which the veins returning blood to the heart from the lungs attach to the right atrium or return to the right atrium by attaching to other large veins rather than to the left atrium. Errors in the coronary artery connections may also occur, causing poor circulation of blood to the heart muscles. Very rarely, the heart may protrude through the chest wall at birth, causing a difficult-to-treat problem called ectopia cordis.

TREATMENT AND THERAPY

Congenital heart disease can often be diagnosed shortly after birth, especially if the baby experiences certain symptoms such as cyanosis, shortness of breath, fatigue and sweating while eating, and inability to gain weight. A physical examination by a physician will include checking the heart and breathing rates for abnormalities and listening to the heart for possible murmurs. Heart murmurs are whooshing sounds caused by turbulent movement of blood that may indicate faulty valves, patent ductus, and other heart defects. A cardiologist will make the definitive diagnosis by administering such tests as the electrocardiogram, the Doppler-echocardiogram, and the cardiac catheterization. The electrocardiogram measures the rhythmic electrical signal that passes through the heart with each beat. An abnormal signal will often indicate problems with a particular region of the heart and is especially useful in identifying rhythm disorders. The echocardiogram produces visual images of the heart by sending out ultrasound waves that bounce off and return to a receiving device. Most structural heart defects can be detected with this technique, and many are discovered prenatally with routine fetal ultrasound monitoring. At the same time, a second receiving device (the Doppler) analyzes ultrasound signals from blood moving through the heart and is able to provide information about the speed and direction of blood flow within the heart. This helps detect abnormal functions such as reverse blood flow. The Doppler-echocardiogram has revolutionized congenital heart disease diagnosis and in most cases provides enough information to define the patient's problem accurately.

If the cardiologist believes that it is necessary, further tests can be done. A chest X ray may be taken to determine if there is any lung involvement in the disorder. Cardiac catheterization can add information about the internal heart blood pressures and blood oxygen levels and can help visualize some defects better with the administration of contrast dyes in combination with X-ray analysis. Special monitors can be used to record the electrocardiogram for one or two days to check for intermittent rhythm irregularities, and older children can be monitored while exercising to see how the heart performs under stress. These and other tests allow physicians to assess the seriousness of the problem and to recommend timely and appropriate treatment.

Serious heart malformations need to be treated immediately upon diagnosis. Often these include defects that cause cyanosis, including transposition of the great arteries, left-heart flow defects such as coarctation of the aorta, and defects that cause heart failure such as truncus arteriosus. Immediate emergency surgery may be needed to save the life of the newborn infant. Additional follow-up surgeries may also be required to correct the defect completely. For example, one way of correcting transposition of the great arteries is by performing an atrial switch operation in which systemic blood returning from the body is diverted to the left side of the heart (so it can be pumped to the lungs) and pulmonary blood from the lungs is diverted to the right side of the heart (so it can be pumped to the body). This is accomplished by first enlarging the foramen ovale with a balloon catheter, a procedure called Rashkind balloon atrial septostomy, followed by a second operation several months later to enlarge the opening between the two atria further and to install a flap to enhance the cross flow of blood, which is known as a Mustard or Senning atrial switch operation. A more recently developed procedure for correcting this defect requires only one operation. The misplaced aorta and pulmonary artery are both cut and then reattached to the correct heart chamber; this is called a Jatene arterial switch operation. At the same time, the coronary arteries are moved to the new aorta.

Some defects require no surgery but can be treated with drugs and other less traumatic procedures, such as the balloon catheter. Drugs are also used to help improve heart performance before and after surgery. When fluid accumulates in the lungs or other body tissues, the heart has problems pumping all the blood that returns to it because of the congestion. The overworked heart suffers under this stress, and thus the condition is called congestive heart failure. Diuretics such as Lasix (furosemide) improve the kidneys' ability to remove the excess fluid and relieve the congestion. Another drug, digitalis, can be helpful in treating congestive heart failure by slowing the heart rate and causing it to beat more forcefully. An open ductus is beneficial to children born with cyanotic heart defects because it allows a more even distribution of oxygenated blood. Treatment with prostaglandin E1 helps keep the ductus open until corrective surgery can be performed. Indomethacin has the opposite effect and is often used to promote closing of a patent ductus in premature babies. As in adults, drugs such as digitalis, beta-blockers, and calcium channel blockers can be used to treat abnormal heart rhythms (arrhythmia) in children with congenital heart disease. The balloon catheter is a nonsurgical technique that is used to enlarge narrow vessels and passages and has been used successfully to treat pulmonary and aortic valve stenosis in a technique called balloon valvuloplasty.

Types of surgery done later in infancy or childhood include closed heart operations such as repair of a patent ductus and partial treatment of some types of cyanosis with a Blalock-Taussig shunt (connecting the subclavian artery to the pulmonary artery to bring more blood to the lungs). Open heart surgery is used to repair defects inside the heart such as septal defects. A heart-lung machine is used to bypass the heart and lungs while the operation is underway, and the body is cooled so that the brain and other tissues require less oxygen. Children with very serious heart defects such as hypoplastic right or left ventricles may require a series of corrective surgical operations, and for some the only hope is a heart transplant. For example, children with hypoplastic right ventricle are given a Blalock-Taussig shunt shortly after birth to improve blood flow to their lungs and then are later given the Fontan operation, which involves closing off the Blalock-Taussig shunt and connecting the pulmonary artery to the right atrium so that blood returning from the body will flow directly to the lungs, completely bypassing the defective right ventricle.

Some heart defects require no treatment. For example, most small septal defects close on their own during the first one or two years of life. Also, mild disorders such as benign valve defects usually require no treatment, and many children with heart murmurs have no detectable problems.

PERSPECTIVE AND PROSPECTS

In the late nineteenth and early twentieth centuries, physicians were beginning to understand that certain congenital heart defects such as patent ductus could be diagnosed by listening to the heart. Treatment, however, was not possible at that time. The *Atlas of Congenital Cardiac Disease* was published in 1936 by Maude Abbot of McGill University.

This work greatly assisted other physicians in recognizing and diagnosing congenital heart disease. In 1939, Robert Gross of Boston repaired a patent ductus, and in 1944, Alfred Blalock and Helen Taussig developed and performed their famous shunt operation in order to treat children with tetralogy of Fallot. Open heart surgery had to wait until the mid-1950's, when the heart-lung machine was perfected. Even then, open heart surgery could only be performed on older children. These operations were pioneered by Walton Lillehei of the University of Minnesota and John Kirlin of the Mayo Clinic. Open heart surgery on newborn infants was developed in the 1970's by Brian Barratt-Boyes of New Zealand.

During the period while heart surgery was being developed, cardiac catheterization was also advancing. It was used primarily for diagnosis, but in 1966, William Rashkind of Philadelphia began to use the balloon catheter to enlarge openings in the atrial septum in order to treat transposition of the great arteries. Microsurgical catheters are currently being developed to repair patent ductus and other heart defects without the need for major surgery. The echocardiogram was pioneered by Inge Edler in the 1950's, and the Doppler-echocardiogram came into widespread use as a diagnostic tool in the 1980's. This instrument has greatly reduced the need for other diagnostic tests that were used in the past.

The modern strategy for treatment of congenital heart defects is to perform the corrective surgery as early in infancy as possible. This eliminates the need for numerous hospitalizations and diagnostic tests and reduces the need for extensive drug treatment. Children with multiple defects will still need more than one surgery. Modern treatment also emphasizes the roles of the child, the family, and health care personnel in fostering an understanding of the condition, treatment, and outcome. Even children who have been successfully treated will sometimes have physical limitations. These children need to be encouraged and supported by their families and allowed to pursue their goals to the fullest extent possible. Overcoming congenital heart disease is now possible for the vast majority of those who are afflicted.   —*Rodney C. Mowbray, Ph.D.*

See also Arrhythmias; Birth defects; Bypass surgery; Cardiology; Cardiology, pediatric; Genetic diseases; Heart; Heart disease; Heart failure; Heart transplantation; Mitral insufficiency; Neonatology; Shunts.

FOR FURTHER INFORMATION:

Berkow, Robert, and Andrew J. Fletcher, eds. *The Merck Manual of Diagnosis and Therapy.* 16th ed. Rahway, N.J.: Merck Sharp & Dohme Research Laboratories, 1992. Chapter 25, "Disease of the Heart and Pericardium: Congenital Heart Disease," contains complete medical descriptions of the common congenital heart defects and appropriate methods of diagnosis and treatment. This reference work is found in most libraries.

Johnson, Robert Arnold, Edgar Haber, and W. Gerald Austen, eds. *The Practice of Cardiology*. Boston: Little, Brown, 1980. A thorough discussion of congenital heart disease is provided in two chapters: chapter 29, "Heart Disease in the Infant and Young Child," and chapter 30, "Congenital Heart Disease in the Child, Adolescent, and Adult Patient." Written for physicians, but much information can be gleaned by the layperson.

McGoon, M. *The Mayo Clinic's Heart Book*. New York: William Morrow, 1993. The most respected text for laypeople on heart disease. Covers all aspects of anatomy, physiology, diagnosis, treatment, and prevention.

Mackintosh, Alan. *The Heart Disease Reference Book*. London: Harper & Row, 1984. A comprehensive reference book of heart problems, including congenital heart disease, written for the nonphysician seeking more in-depth information than provided by books written for the general public. Contains excellent line diagrams and descriptions of congenital heart defects.

Moore, Keith L., and T. V. N. Persaud. *The Developing Human*. 5th ed. Philadelphia: W. B. Saunders, 1993. An outstanding textbook on human embryonic development. Chapter 14 deals with the development of the circulatory system. The diagrams and descriptions allow the reader to compare normal and abnormal development and to see exactly how errors in development result in congenital heart defects.

Neill, Catherine A., Edward B. Clark, and Carleen Clark. *The Heart of a Child*. Baltimore: The Johns Hopkins University Press, 1992. A comprehensive, up-to-date work on heart disease affecting children written for the layperson by medical professionals. The authors give a thorough description of all congenital heart defects and explain their developmental basis. In addition to diagnosis, treatment, and rehabilitation, the book deals with the special problems of children with heart disease. The best reference for the general reader.

Roberts, William C., ed. *Adult Congenital Heart Disease*. Philadelphia: F. A. Davis, 1987. A medical text that focuses on adults with congenital heart defects. This book will be of interest to those that have survived congenital heart disease and now need follow-up medical care as adults.

CONGESTIVE HEART FAILURE. *See* HEART FAILURE.

CONJUNCTIVITIS
DISEASE/DISORDER
ANATOMY OR SYSTEM AFFECTED: Eyes
SPECIALTIES AND RELATED FIELDS: Ophthalmology
DEFINITION: One of the most common eye disorders, conjunctivitis is an inflammation of the white part of the eye, the conjunctiva. In addition to the redness caused

by the presence of excess blood, symptoms often include pain and discharge; the patient's vision remains unaffected. Conjunctivitis is highly contagious and is usually spread from one eye to the other by the patient. The condition has many possible causes, ranging from bacterial infections to viral infections, from allergies to the sexually transmitted disease chlamydia. Acute bacterial conjunctivitis, commonly known as pinkeye, generally lasts two weeks and is characterized by itching and burning as well. —*Jason Georges and Tracy Irons-Georges*
See also Bacterial infections; Chlamydia; Eyes.

CONSTIPATION
DISEASE/DISORDER
ANATOMY OR SYSTEM AFFECTED: Abdomen, gastrointestinal system, intestines
SPECIALTIES AND RELATED FIELDS: Family practice, gastroenterology, internal medicine
DEFINITION: The slow passage of feces through the bowels or the presence of hard feces.

CAUSES AND SYMPTOMS
People of every age group, from infants to the elderly, can experience the unpleasant symptoms of constipation, which is characterized primarily by discomfort. Certain disease states such as diabetes mellitus, paralysis of the legs, colon cancer, and hypothyroidism predispose a person to constipation. Possible causes of constipation are medications, iron supplements, toilet training procedures, pregnancy, lack of adequate fluids, a low-fiber diet, and lack of physical activity.

TREATMENT AND THERAPY
Most cases of constipation can be treated by the patient at home. Drinking adequate fluids makes it easier for fecal material to pass through the large intestine. Without adequate hydration, a person may experience small, pelletlike stools. Eight to ten glasses of liquids per day are recommended, including water, milk, cocoa, fruit juice, herbal tea, and soup. Once adequate hydration is achieved, a high-fiber diet can gradually be started. Without enough fluids, a high-fiber diet can worsen the problems of constipation. A high-fiber diet adds bulk to the bowel movement (increasing stool volume, decreasing pressure within the colon, and decreasing the intestinal transit time of foods) and thus can lead to more regular bowel habits and partial relief of the symptoms. One can increase fiber in the diet by eating prunes, high-fiber breakfast cereals, beans or legumes, raw fruits and vegetables, and whole-grain breads. In order to minimize gastrointestinal discomforts such as increased flatulence (gas), it is recommended to increase one's fiber consumption gradually.

In addition to adequate liquids and a high-fiber diet, exercise is important in treating constipation. Any sort of physical activity, such as walking, running, tennis, or swimming, can help to stimulate the activity of the large intestine.

Laxatives and enemas should not be used until after a discussion with a physician. Mineral oil should also not be used because many essential fat-soluble vitamins (such as vitamins A, D, E, and K) may be excreted as well. Persistent constipation should be evaluated by a physician.

—*Martha M. Henze, R.D.*

See also Diarrhea and dysentery; Enemas; Gastroenterology; Gastroenterology, pediatric; Gastrointestinal disorders; Gastrointestinal system; Hemorrhoid banding and removal; Hemorrhoids; Indigestion; Intestinal disorders; Intestines; Obstruction.

CONTRACEPTION

PROCEDURE

ANATOMY OR SYSTEM AFFECTED: Endocrine system, genitals, glands, reproductive system, uterus

SPECIALTIES AND RELATED FIELDS: Family practice, gynecology

DEFINITION: The use of techniques to prevent pregnancy, which may interfere with ovulation, sperm transport, or the implantation of the embryo.

KEY TERMS:

barrier method: a contraceptive that physically prevents sperm from meeting the ovum; includes the male condom, female condom, diaphragm, cervical cap, and vaginal sponge

cervix: the entrance to the uterus from the vagina; it secretes mucus, which appears as vaginal discharge

ejaculation: the release of sperm from the male's body during sexual activity

failure rate: the percentage of women who become pregnant while using a given contraceptive method for one year; used to describe numerically how well a contraceptive works

hormone: a chemical signal carried in the blood that allows distant body parts to coordinate their actions; synthetic hormones mimic natural ones

implantation: the process in which the embryo attaches to the uterine lining

ovulation: the monthly release of a mature ovum (egg) from the ovary; ovulation must occur for pregnancy to be possible

spermicide: a chemical that kills sperm after they are ejaculated

uterus: the organ that supports the embryo during its development

vagina: the tube-shaped cavity of the female into which the male's penis is inserted during intercourse; the diaphragm, cervical cap, vaginal sponge, or spermicide can be inserted into the vagina as contraceptives

TYPES OF CONTRACEPTION

Theoretically, pregnancy can be prevented by interfering with the process of conception at any number of sites in the male or female anatomy. In practice, it has proven much easier to interfere with events that occur in women: ovulation, sperm transport through the female system, or implantation of the newly fertilized ovum. Only one nonsurgical method for male contraception has proven useful: the condom, which prevents sperm from being deposited in the female at the time of ejaculation.

Oral contraceptives, commonly referred to as "the pill," are one of the most widely used forms of female contraception. Oral contraceptives contain synthetic estrogen and progesterone, which are similar to the hormones normally produced by the woman's ovaries. All the different formulas of oral contraceptives work by the same mechanism: The hormones in the pills prevent ovulation. In a woman not taking birth control pills, ovulation occurs once a month, triggered by a particular set of hormonal changes. These hormonal changes do not occur in women who take oral contraceptives; these women do not ovulate. Menstruation, which is normally caused by a reduction in progesterone, does occur in women who take oral contraceptives because the pills mimic this hormonal event.

A similar mechanism of contraception occurs with long-acting hormones given by injection. Depo-Provera is a synthetic progesterone that is injected once every three months; during this time, the hormone persists in the body and prevents ovulation. In addition, the uterine lining does not undergo the normal periodic thickening necessary to prepare it for supporting an embryo. Menstruation is often absent or irregular in women who use Depo-Provera, because of the lack of development of the uterine lining and because progesterone levels remain fairly high.

A third hormonal method of contraception for the female is the Norplant system, which employs silicon capsules containing a synthetic progesterone. The capsules are implanted under the skin, typically on the arm, and release the hormone constantly as long as they remain in place. One set of capsules can provide continuous contraceptive protection for up to five years, but they can be removed earlier if the woman wishes. Like oral contraceptives and Depo-Provera, Norplant works in part by preventing ovulation. Even if ovulation does occur, women using Norplant do not become pregnant because the hormone has other effects, including inhibition of sperm transport in the female and changes in the uterus. Lack of menstrual bleeding or irregular bleeding may occur with Norplant.

An intrauterine device (IUD), a small piece of plastic or metal inserted into the uterus, appears to prevent pregnancy by interfering with implantation of the early embryo. Women who use IUDs continue to ovulate and menstruate, but they do not become pregnant because of changes in the uterine lining that make the uterus unable to support an embryo.

Another contraceptive technique is to introduce a spermicide (sperm-killing chemical) into the vagina prior to intercourse. The most commonly used spermicide is

Types of Contraceptive Devices

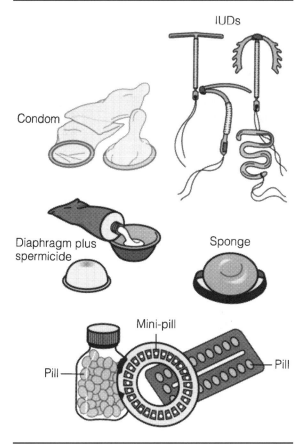

Many different kinds of devices have been designed to prevent pregnancy, from barrier methods such as condoms and diaphragms to hormonal methods such as birth control pills. Each method has its own advantages, disadvantages, and failure rates.

nonoxynol-9, which is supplied in the form of foams, creams, gels, or suppositories. The spermicide is placed in the vagina before intercourse and will kill sperm that are deposited there during ejaculation.

Spermicides can be used alone or in combination with barrier contraceptives, devices that mechanically block the passage of sperm through the female system. Barrier contraceptives include the male condom, female condom, diaphragm, and cervical cap. Another barrier method, the vaginal sponge, was taken off the market in 1995. Condoms are sheaths made of latex rubber, polyurethane, or animal intestine (called "skin" or "natural" condoms). Condoms are worn on the erect penis during intercourse and collect sperm during ejaculation. The female condom is a polyurethane sheath placed into the vagina prior to intercourse; it is held in place by a flexible ring and, like the male con-

dom, collects sperm to prevent them from moving through the female system. Diaphragms and cervical caps are dome-shaped or thimble-shaped rubber devices that cover the woman's cervix. Filled with spermicide and placed into the woman's vagina prior to intercourse, they prevent sperm passage through the female system.

Possibly the simplest method of contraception, at least in theory, is the avoidance of intercourse around the time of ovulation, known as periodic abstinence, the rhythm method, or natural family planning. In actual practice, the method is complicated by the fact that detection of ovulation is difficult in humans. The woman attempts to determine her time of ovulation by keeping careful calendar records of her menstrual cycles, by charting monthly changes in her body temperature, or by noting monthly changes in her cervical mucus, which appears as a vaginal discharge. The number of days that the woman may safely engage in intercourse may be few, depending on the length and reliability of her menstrual cycles.

A method of contraception found widely in developing countries, but not recommended because of low effectiveness, is the use of a postcoital spermicidal douche, that is, a liquid introduced into the vagina after intercourse with the intention of killing sperm and/or washing sperm out of the vagina. Studies have shown, however, that a postcoital douche can aid sperm movement into the woman's uterus and thus may actually increase the chance of pregnancy. Douches may also cause vaginal or uterine infections.

Some couples use coitus interruptus (interrupted intercourse) as a contraceptive method. In coitus interruptus, the man withdraws the penis from the woman's vagina prior to ejaculation. In practice, the method has a high failure rate, because some sperm may be deposited in the female along with secretions from the penis prior to ejaculation, and also because it may be difficult for the man to predict when ejaculation will occur and to withdraw successfully before that time.

Another contraceptive tactic is to prevent implantation of the fertilized ovum if unprotected intercourse, rape, or a contraceptive failure has occurred around the time of ovulation. Emergency contraceptive pills, sometimes called "the morning-after pill," may be given in a high-dose regimen. This treatment is most effective if started within the first twelve to twenty-four hours and is not likely to be effective if begun more than seventy-two hours after the unprotected event. Danazol or progestin-only pills may also be used for this purpose. For some women, insertion of a copper IUD within five to seven days of the event may be appropriate. Diethylstilbestrol (DES) was formerly approved for emergency contraception, but it is no longer recommended as a result of severe side effects.

In some countries, mifepristone (RU-486) is available as a postcoital contraceptive, and it is under study for this use in the United States. RU-486, which is sometimes called the French abortion pill, blocks the action of progesterone, thinning the lining of the uterus and making it unsuitable for implantation of the embryo. This progesterone blockade also causes the cervix (the opening of the uterus) to soften and open and the uterus to be more sensitive to prostaglandins. Research has shown that a single dose taken within seventy-two hours of unprotected intercourse is highly effective in preventing pregnancy and has a low incidence of unpleasant side effects, so RU-486 may become the preferred morning-after pill. If the woman has an established pregnancy, RU-486 may be used as an alternative to surgical abortion. It is followed by treatment with misoprostol, a prostaglandin, to cause the uterus to contract strongly and expel its contents.

Another drug called methotrexate, which is available in the United States, stops cell division in the products of conception (the embryo and other tissues). If misoprostol is inserted into the vagina or taken orally one week after administration of methotrexate to stimulate uterine contractions, the effectiveness is 90 to 96 percent.

Because both of these methods are most effective early in pregnancy, their use is usually not an option after seven weeks from the first day of the last menstrual period. Medical abortions take anywhere from three days to four weeks for completion and require repeated visits to a health care provider. If the medical method is not successful, the woman must then undergo a surgical abortion.

PROCEDURES AND RATES OF EFFECTIVENESS

The choice of a contraceptive should be made after a couple weighs the effectiveness and ease of use against the possible health risk factors and disadvantages of a particular method.

The easiest method to use is Norplant: Once the capsules have been inserted, the woman does not need to do anything else until the capsules are replaced at the end of five years. Insertion is performed under local anesthesia in a medical office or clinic. The most common problem is menstrual irregularity. Norplant is considered to be safe for most women and has a failure rate of less than 1 percent.

Depo-Provera is almost as easy to use as Norplant: The woman simply goes to a health care provider for an injection once every three months. No serious health problems have been reported, and the failure rate is less than 1 percent.

An IUD is another method that is easy to use. The IUD is inserted in a health care provider's office or clinic; thereafter, the woman will be continually protected from pregnancy. The woman should have the IUD replaced every two years, and once a month should check that it is still in place by feeling for the threads that trail from the IUD into the vagina. The pregnancy rate in IUD users is 5 percent or less. The most common complaint is of increased bleeding and painful cramping during menstruation, especially during the first year of IUD use. IUD users are more likely than other women to develop pelvic infections, including

those caused by sexually transmitted diseases. More seriously, the IUD may become imbedded in the wall of the uterus or cause a tear in the uterus, but these complications are unlikely with the devices now available.

Oral contraceptives are widely used because they have low failure rates (4 percent to 9 percent) and the protection from pregnancy is continuous, not requiring any additional act at the time of intercourse (such as putting on a condom). The possibility of pregnancy increases if the woman forgets to take her pills every day, or if she does not take them at approximately the same time every day. Oral contraceptives are available only by prescription because they carry some health risks, primarily for women with a history of diabetes, liver disease, blood-clotting disorders, heart disease, or high blood pressure or for those who smoke. There is also concern about increased risk of certain cancers and liver tumors. Minor side effects may include headache, abnormal menstrual bleeding, nausea, or depression.

Vaginal spermicide used alone has a failure rate ranging from 22 percent to 26 percent. Failure rates as low as 5 percent, however, have been observed when couples use both vaginal spermicide and a condom, whereas the condom alone has a failure rate of 10 percent to 19 percent. The only health problem associated with spermicide or condom use is an occasional allergic reaction. It is important that directions for use be followed: The spermicide must be inserted into the vagina, or the condom put on the penis, before intercourse starts. The condom should cover the entire penis and must be worn throughout the act of intercourse. The condom should be held at the base of the penis as the man withdraws from the vagina. Latex condoms are more reliable than "skin" condoms, and no condom should ever be reused. Polyurethane condoms are available for those with latex allergies. A petroleum-based lubricant, such as petroleum jelly, should not be used because it may weaken the condom. Both spermicide and condoms are sold without a prescription.

The diaphragm and cervical cap have failure rates ranging from 12 percent to 39 percent, with the large variation attributable to the fact that not everyone who uses these methods follows the instructions. These barriers should be used every time the woman has intercourse. The diaphragm should be filled with a cream or jelly-type spermicide prior to insertion, no sooner than six hours before intercourse. The diaphragm should also be left in place for at least six hours after intercourse, in order to allow the spermicide time to kill any sperm that may have gotten past the barrier. If the couple wishes to repeat intercourse within this six-hour period, more spermicide should be added directly to the vagina, without removing the diaphragm. The diaphragm should not be left in place for longer than twenty-four hours total, since the possibility of infection is increased by prolonged use. The diaphragm must be cleaned well and dried after each use and should be examined for tears or holes. Diaphragms should be replaced every two years, or more often if necessary. They must be fitted by a physician, since they come in different sizes. If the woman has a weight change of ten pounds or more, or has been pregnant, she should be fitted for a new diaphragm. The only health problems associated with the diaphragm are allergies and increased risk of bladder infections.

Use of a cervical cap is similar to that of the diaphragm, except that the cap can be left in place for up to forty-eight hours. Additional spermicide need not be added for repeated acts of intercourse. Many women find that the cervical cap is more difficult to place and remove, since it fits the cervix snugly.

The female condom is filled with spermicide prior to insertion into the vagina. Like other barriers, it should be in place before intercourse begins and be worn throughout the sexual act. The main advantage of the female condom over the male condom is not in pregnancy prevention, but in decreasing disease transmission, since the female condom covers most of the external female genital region, thus reducing skin-to-skin contact between the couple.

The failure rate of periodic abstinence varies from 14 percent to 19 percent. Couples with high motivation and self-control have better success with this method, as do women with regular, predictable menstrual periods. Ovulation prediction may be made by the calendar method, in which it is assumed that the woman will ovulate twelve to sixteen days before the start of her next expected menstrual period. In addition, the woman may monitor changes in her body temperature and cervical mucus: Body temperature increases around the time of ovulation, and the cervical mucus becomes wet, thick, and stretchy, like uncooked egg white, at about the same time. It is considered safe to have intercourse three days after the increased body temperature occurs, or four days after the peak in wetness of the cervical mucus. Periodic abstinence carries no health risks, because no foreign substance or hormone is introduced to the body, however the method cannot be used if the woman is breast-feeding a baby, because menstrual cycles are absent or irregular at that time, even though the woman can still become pregnant.

PERSPECTIVE AND PROSPECTS

Possibly the oldest form of contraception is coitus interruptus, mentioned in the Bible in the story of Onan, who used this practice to avoid impregnating his brother's widow. Other early accounts of contraceptive attempts refer to various potions or magical practices on which people relied in a superstitious manner.

Some present-day contraceptives developed from previous, less effective methods. Early people experimented widely with barrier-type contraceptives. Balls, natural sea sponges, or wads of leaves placed in the vagina prior to intercourse have been used throughout history and in dif-

ferent parts of the world as barrier contraceptives. Condoms made of animal intestines or of fine linen were first described in writings and drawings of ancient Rome and Egypt. Condoms were originally used, however, solely for the prevention of disease transmission; their contraceptive properties were apparently not recognized until the seventeenth or eighteenth century.

IUDs became popular in the 1950's, but the first ones designed expressly to achieve contraception date back to the early part of the twentieth century. Prior to this time, doctors sometimes fitted women with a "stem pessary," an object with a stem protruding into the uterus from a base in the vagina, with the aim of actually promoting pregnancy. The contraceptive action of these stem pessaries was gradually recognized, and by the late 1800's wealthy women resorted to them to avoid pregnancy.

The hormonal methods of contraception are the newest developments, with oral contraceptives first tested in the 1950's and introduced to the market in the 1960's. Injection and implant methods of delivering contraceptive hormones were also developed and tested starting in the 1960's and were soon adopted for use in most countries. The United States, however, did not approve the use of these methods until the early 1990's.

A number of new contraceptive methods are under study in the United States and other countries, with emphasis on female-controlled methods that both prevent pregnancy and protect against sexually transmitted disease. Researchers are also attempting improvements on existing methods, including biodegradable hormone implants and frameless IUDs. Hormonal methods to suppress sperm production in men (the "male pill") tested in the late 1990's included injectable synthetic testosterone and implants with testosterone derivatives. These and contraceptive vaccines for men or for women were not expected to be available before the end of the decade.

With so many methods of contraception available today, it is difficult to realize that not so long ago, it was illegal in many countries to distribute contraceptives or information about contraception. In the United States, information about the "prevention of conception" was explicitly listed in the Comstock Act of 1873, which outlawed the mailing of obscene material. The driving force behind the law, lobbyist Anthony Comstock, believed that any attempt to prevent conception was immoral. Punishment for breaking the law included heavy monetary fines and imprisonment. In the United States, federal enforcement of this law continued until the mid-1900's, but in 1971 contraceptive information was finally removed from the list of materials banned by the Comstock Act.

Although contraceptives are now legal and widely available in the United States, they are still not used as widely as they could be. Studies have shown that more than half of the pregnancies in the United States each year are unintended. A little more than half of these unintended pregnancies occur in women who are not using any contraceptive method; the others result from contraceptive failure, including cases of human error or misuse.

Aside from the personal reasons for choosing to avoid pregnancy, there are also global concerns about population growth. Based on the growth rates in the early 1990's, the world population was expected to double in the next forty years. Scientists fear that Earth's ability to sustain a sizable human population may have already been surpassed.

—Marcia Watson-Whitmyre, Ph.D.,
updated by Rebecca Lovell Scott, Ph.D.

See also Abortion; Conception; Ethics; Gynecology; Hormones; Hysterectomy; Menstruation; Pregnancy and gestation; Reproductive system; Sterilization; Tubal ligation; Vasectomy.

FOR FURTHER INFORMATION:

Covington, Timothy R., and J. Frank McClendon. *Sex Care: The Complete Guide to Safe and Healthy Sex.* New York: Pocket Books, 1987. Detailed information on how to use contraceptives. Sexually transmitted diseases and other reproductive health problems are also covered.

Fathalla, Mahmoud F., Allan Rosenfield, and Cynthia Indriso, eds. *Family Planning.* Vol. 2 in *The FIGO Manual of Human Reproduction,* edited by Fathalla and Rosenfield. 2d ed. Park Ridge, N.J.: Parthenon, 1990. Sponsored by the World Health Organization and the International Federation of Gynecology and Obstetrics and written by an array of international experts, this volume contains accurate, well-explained information on contraception, with informative figures.

Fathalla, Mahmoud F., Allan Rosenfield, Cynthia Indriso, Dilup K. Sen, and Shan S. Ratnam, eds. *Reproductive Health: Global Issues.* Vol. 3 in *Reproduction,* edited by Fathalla and Rosenfield. 2d ed. Park Ridge, N.J.: Parthenon, 1990. Another volume in the same series as the preceding book. Readers may be interested in the chapters that cover social issues in reproduction, population growth, and contraceptive safety.

Green, Shirley. *The Curious History of Contraception.* London: Ebury Press, 1971. A lighthearted account of contraceptive history, this book makes entertaining reading, with ample coverage of some of the more outlandish methods of contraception that people have used.

Harlap, Susan, Kathryn Kost, and Jacqueline Darroch Forrest. *Preventing Pregnancy, Protecting Health: A New Look at Birth Control Choices in the United States.* New York: Alan Guttmacher Institute, 1991. This well-researched book presents information on the health impact of different forms of contraception, such as sexually transmitted diseases, cancer, and later infertility. Highly recommended.

Hatcher, Robert A., et al. *Contraceptive Technology.* 16th ed. New York: Irvington, 1994. This frequently revised book offers a thorough and readable discussion of most aspects of contraception.

Lader, Lawrence. *RU 486: The Pill That Could End the Abortion Wars and Why American Women Don't Have It.* Reading, Mass.: Addison-Wesley, 1991. The title adequately explains the subject matter of the book. The author is a longtime campaigner for abortion rights and was prominently cited by the Supreme Court in the landmark *Roe v. Wade* decision that legalized abortion in the United States.

Rodman, Hyman, Susan H. Lewis, and Saralyn B. Griffith. *The Sexual Rights of Adolescents.* New York: Columbia University Press, 1984. This text examines the legal rights of teenagers in various areas of sexuality, including the right to obtain contraception and abortion. Well written and easy to read.

Sitruck-Ware, Régine, and C. Wayne Bardin, eds. *Contraception: Newer Pharmacological Agents, Devices, and Delivery Systems.* New York: Marcel Dekker, 1992. With chapters written by various researchers in the field of contraception, this text covers both contemporary methods and a number of methods still in the development phases.

Weschler, Toni. *Taking Charge of Your Infertility.* New York: HarperPerennial, 1995. This book encourages women to become responsible consumers of their own reproductive health. Includes excellent discussions of infertility, natural birth control, and achieving pregnancy.

CORNEAL TRANSPLANTATION

PROCEDURE

ANATOMY OR SYSTEM AFFECTED: Eyes

SPECIALTIES AND RELATED FIELDS: General surgery, ophthalmology

DEFINITION: A delicate surgical operation involving the removal and replacement of the cornea, the transparent outer covering of the eye.

KEY TERMS:

endothelium: the inner surface of the cornea, which is separated from the rest of the eye by an essential layer of transparent fluid

lamellar keratoplasty: the partial removal or transplantation of a portion of the cornea; usually possible in younger patients or those with less advanced disorders

penetrating keratoplasty: the surgical transplantation of the entire thickness of the cornea, which is made up of four distinct layers of tissue

trephine: a specialized surgical instrument which is used to cut a perfectly vertical incision to remove corneas from both the donor and the recipient

INDICATIONS AND PROCEDURES

The cornea, which has four distinct layers, is the transparent outer coating of the eye. It serves both to protect the eye and to provide the main refracting surface as light reaches the eye and is transmitted to the lens and retina. Its total thickness is approximately .52 millimeter. The layers of specialized tissue pass from the epithelium through the stroma and Descemet's membrane to the endothelium, or inner surface of the cornea.

Several types of corneal disorders may lead to a decision to perform partial or total keratoplasty. Most of these fall under the general term "corneal dystrophy." The most common, or classical, cases of corneal dystrophy involve the deposit of abnormal material in the cornea, resulting in irritation and eventually damage. Frequently, such disorders stem from genetic factors, making it possible to diagnose the dystrophy during the patient's childhood and perform a lamellar keratoplasty. Other dystrophies include granular dystrophy and macular dystrophy. The former involves lesions in the center of the cornea, which may multiply and coalesce. At that stage, they may extend into the deeper layers of the stroma, the second layer of the cornea. Macular dystrophy actually begins in the stroma, causing all layers to become opaque.

Entirely different types of disorders that may call for corneal transplantation are interstitial keratitis (a type of inflammation) and trachoma. The latter condition can reach near epidemic levels in underdeveloped areas of the world, where low levels of hygiene allow the implantation and rapid multiplication of bacteria in the cornea. The effect is a breakdown of tissue accompanied by the discharge of mucus.

Whether the cornea has been affected by disease or injury, the goal of corneal transplantation is to eliminate any opacity that can hamper vision. The graft operation itself may be described in only a few stages, each marked by the need for a high degree of technical skill to increase the likelihood of success. First, the surgeon must calculate the exact size of the graft in question. This is done through the use of a special tool called a trephine, which will make the cuts to remove both the donor and the host eye corneas. Some trephines are equipped with transparent lenses to give the surgeon maximum levels of accuracy. When the two vital incisions are made, great care is taken to obtain a perfectly vertical cut.

Beginning with this initial stage, the surgeon may add a bubble of air through the incision to protect the endothelium and reduce the likelihood of an immune system reaction once the donor cornea has been transplanted. As the transfer occurs, another air bubble is introduced. After suturing, this bubble will be replaced by a balanced salt solution called acetylcholine.

This suturing, which must be very precise, almost always begins with four sutures at the cardinal points to ensure even tension. The last stage of the operation involves checking the wound for leakage of acetylcholine. This step is necessary not only to avoid infection but also to guard against rejection of the cornea by the host organ.

USES AND COMPLICATIONS

Significant differences in the healing process following corneal transplantation occur according to the method of suturing. A choice is made between a continuing or an interrupted series of sutures around the circumference of the cornea. Interrupted sutures may be preferred if there is a chance of uneven healing of the wound, something the physician may judge following examination of the degree of vascularization in particular corneal graft beds. In some cases, surgeons may opt for double suturing.

The chief complication that can follow corneal transplantation is rejection by the immune system. Surgeons try to obviate this risk by close study of the factors that can affect the receptivity of the eye to a new cornea. Earlier literature on corneal transplantation tended to assume that there was a lack of antigenicity—the production of disease-fighting antigenes, or antibodies, as a defense system against viruses, bacteria, or foreign tissues—in the cornea. As ophthalmologists developed a fuller understanding of the immunological role of blood vessels and the lymphatic system, however, the need to give considerable attention to the degree of vascularization of the graft bed zone became more obvious. One method that surgeons can use to reduce antigene activity and enhance host acceptance is part of the transplantation operation itself: constant maintenance of a liquid layer between the host tissue and the new cornea tissue being transplanted.

Although the period for healing and suture removal varies from patient to patient, the surgeon looks for the normal development of a gray-tinged scar tissue in the incision area as a sign of success. Failure, if discovered in time, may lead to a second transplantation attempt.

PERSPECTIVE AND PROSPECTS

The first attempts to perform corneal transplantation—all unsuccessful—date from the nineteenth century. In the 1820's, German doctor F. Reisinger experimented with corneal grafts using rabbits and chickens. In the 1830's, Samuel Bigger of Ireland and R. S. Kissam of the United States tried to pioneer surgical grafts on humans, but both made the error of trying to replace human corneas with animal corneas. Success with living tissue (as opposed to the application of a glass product) finally came in 1905 when Moravian doctor Edward Zirm transplanted a child donor's cornea to the eye of a chemical burn victim. Zirm's success was based on cumulative medical knowledge of antiseptics, anesthesia, and technical aids such as the ophthalmoscope and the trephine. After a long period without major changes, in 1935 a Russian scientist named Filatov experimented with two innovations that were copied in other countries: the use of egg membrane to enhance a firm fix and the insertion of a delicate spatula between the cornea and lens to protect the intraocular tissues.

The greatest advances were made soon after antibiotics and steroids were introduced in the 1940's. By the 1950's, the use of extremely delicate surgical needles helped reduce postsurgical rejection rates. Major contributions to the development of delicate surgical instruments were made by the Spanish ophthalmologist Ramón Castroviejo, who performed many operations in the United States. By the 1980's, Castroviejo was urging others to follow the example of Townley Paton, who founded New York's first eye bank some two decades earlier.

The prospects for increasingly higher success rates in the field of corneal transplantation are linked to technical progress in donor organ conservation and the level of precision that can be achieved in carrying out transplantation operations.   —*Byron D. Cannon, Ph.D.*

See also Eye surgery; Eyes; Grafts and grafting; Ophthalmology; Transplantation; Visual disorders.

FOR FURTHER INFORMATION:

Brightbill, Frederick S., ed. *Corneal Surgery.* 2d ed. St. Louis: C. V. Mosby, 1993. This rather technical text is divided into sections in which the authors discuss their specific areas of expertise.

Casey, T. A., and D. J. Mayer. *Corneal Grafting.* Philadelphia: W. B. Saunders, 1984. Less technical than some texts, but a bit dated, reflecting an earlier state of medical science and the techniques of corneal surgery.

Leibowitz, Howard, ed. *Corneal Disorders.* Philadelphia: W. B. Saunders, 1984. This text concentrates on the diagnosis of inflammations and infections, as well as the effects of trauma, that may require corneal surgery, including corneal transplantation.

Smolin, Gilbert, and Richard A. Throft, eds. *The Cornea.* Boston: Little, Brown, 1994. This covers some cornea-related topics that either are absent from standard texts (for example, congenital anomalies) or reflect recent surgical advances (for example, corneal surgery to make refractive corrections to reduce or remove myopia).

Spaeth, George L., ed. *Ophthalmic Surgery.* 2d ed. Philadelphia: W. B. Saunders, 1990. The subsections of this text deal with all aspects of eye surgery, including corneal surgery and operations to correct glaucoma, cataracts, and retinal displacement.

COSMETIC SURGERY. *See* PLASTIC, COSMETIC, AND RECONSTRUCTIVE SURGERY.

COUGHING

DISEASE/DISORDER

ANATOMY OR SYSTEM AFFECTED: Chest, lungs, respiratory system

SPECIALTIES AND RELATED FIELDS: Family practice, internal medicine, pulmonary medicine

DEFINITION: A cough is produced when air is suddenly forced through the glottis, the vocal apparatus of the larynx; this response is triggered by irritation of the tra-

chea or the bronchi in the lungs. Such irritation can be caused by environmental factors, such as smoke or dust, or by infections or disease of the throat or the lungs themselves. Coughing is commonly seen with the common cold, bronchitis, pneumonia, croup, influenza, lung cancer, and tuberculosis. The nature of a cough may provide information for diagnosing a condition, such as the barking cough of croup, and coughing is often beneficial in removing secretions from the lungs, as with cystic fibrosis.   —*Jason Georges and Tracy Irons-Georges*

See also Bronchitis; Choking; Common cold; Cystic fibrosis; Diphtheria; Influenza; Lung cancer; Lungs; Otorhinolaryngology; Pertussis; Pneumonia; Pulmonary diseases; Pulmonary medicine; Pulmonary medicine, pediatric; Respiration; Sore throat; Tuberculosis.

CRANIOTOMY

PROCEDURE

ANATOMY OR SYSTEM AFFECTED: Bones, brain, head, nervous system

SPECIALTIES AND RELATED FIELDS: General surgery, neurology

DEFINITION: Craniotomy is the opening of or surgical entry into the skull. Brain tumors, blood clots, and other factors that cause pressure on the brain must be corrected to prevent brain damage and consequent physical and/or mental impairment. Craniotomy allows physicians to enter the brain and correct such potentially serious problems. The growth or area of pressure is localized with computer tomography (CT) scanning and magnetic resonance imaging (MRI). A felt pen is used to outline the surgical incisions on the patient's shaved skull. The skin is cut to the skull bone and small bleeding arteries are sealed with electric current. After the skin is pulled back, three holes, called Burr holes, are drilled into the skull, and a fine-wire Gigli's saw is used to connect the holes in the skull. The skull piece is hinged opened, and the dura mater, a tough membrane covering the brain, is dissected away. After the required procedure on the brain is completed, the dura mater is stitched together, the bone flap is replaced and secured with soft wire, and the scalp incision is closed. Recovery is usually quick, and any pain is managed with drug therapy.

—*Karen E. Kalumuck, Ph.D.*

See also Bones and the skeleton; Brain; Brain disorders; Neurology; Neurology, pediatric; Neurosurgery.

CREUTZFELDT-JAKOB DISEASE AND MAD COW DISEASE

DISEASE/DISORDER

ANATOMY OR SYSTEM AFFECTED: Brain, muscles, nervous system

SPECIALTIES AND RELATED FIELDS: Environmental health, microbiology, neurology, public health, virology

DEFINITION: Creutzfeldt-Jakob disease (CJD) is a central nervous system disorder of humans that is characterized by a progressive dementia, myoclonus, and distinctive electroencephalographic and neuropathologic findings. Although uncommon, it is the most prevalent of the human subacute spongiform encephalopathies, fatal diseases caused by transmissible pathogens of uncertain type. Mad cow disease is a spongiform encephalopathy that affects cattle but can be transmitted to humans.

KEY TERMS:

dementia: a progressive, organic mental disorder characterized by chronic personality disintegration, confusion, disorientation, stupor, deterioration of intellectual capacity and function, and impairment of control of memory, judgment, and impulses

encephalopathy: any abnormal condition of the structure or function of the tissues of the brain

myoclonus: a spasm of a single muscle or a group of muscles

spongiform: shaped like or resembling a sponge

subacute: pertaining to a disease or other abnormal condition present in a person who appears to be clinically well

CAUSES AND SYMPTOMS

Several animal diseases are caused by chemical agents that replicate slowly and have long latent intervals in their hosts. Experts have termed these agents proteinaceous infectious particles; they are resistant to most procedures that modify nucleic acids. Increasingly, these diseases are being referred to as prions.

Five major slow virus diseases of humans have been identified and are thought to be caused by prions. Kuru is characterized by cerebellar ataxia, tremors, dysarthria and emotional lability. Subacute sclerosing panencephalitis is a slowly progressive disorder that is typically a disease of children. Progressive multifocal leukoencephalopathy is a disorder that progressively demyelinates central nervous system tissue. Creutzfeldt-Jakob disease and the recently recognized bovine spongiform encephalopathy, or "mad cow disease," round out this group.

Creutzfeldt-Jakob disease (CJD) belongs to a group of diseases called spongiform encephalopathies. This term refers to the appearance of characteristic tissue in the central nervous systems of victims on examination. CJD usually occurs sporadically in middle-aged adults without known exposure. A family history is evident in 5 percent of victims, suggesting common exposure or a genetic susceptibility. Human-to-human transmission has been reported. Incubation periods are between four and twenty-one years, emphasizing the astonishingly long incubation times of the spongiform encephalopathies. Most victims are between sixty and eighty years old. Some cases have been documented in people as young as thirty. Men and women are equally affected.

The pathologic findings in CJD are limited to the central nervous system, although the transmissible agent can be detected in many organs. Vague psychiatric or behavioral symptoms suggesting a personality change often precede the onset of CJD. Within a few weeks or months, a relentlessly progressive dementia becomes evident. Myoclonus is usually present at some time during the course. Deterioration is usually rapid, and 90 percent of victims die within one year. CJD patients do not have fevers, and their blood and cerebrospinal fluid are normal.

Mad cow disease is a spongiform encephalopathy that affects cattle. It can be transmitted to other animals by eating the brains of infected animals. In this manner, mad cow disease has been transmitted to livestock given feed to which contaminated animal tissue has been added. It has also been transmitted to humans, primarily in Great Britain. The symptoms of mad cow disease in humans resemble those of CJD.

TREATMENT AND THERAPY

The CJD, kuru, and animal spongiform encephalopathy agents are unlike any known virus or other well-characterized transmissible agent. These pathogens provoke no inflammatory response or specific antibody production. They are resistant to chemical and physical treatments that inactivate most viruses. Such treatments include heat, formaldehyde, nuclease digestion, and ultraviolet and ionizing radiation. The agents can be inactivated by procedures that denature proteins.

No effective treatment is available for Creutzfeldt-Jakob disease; it appears to be uniformly fatal. Although CJD can be transmitted, the risk to health care workers and others having contact with patients is no higher than to the general population. Isolation of patients is not suggested, but reasonable care should be exercised. No organs, tissues, or tissue products from patients with CJD or with any ill-defined neurologic disease should be used for transplantation or replacement therapy.

There is no treatment for mad cow disease; it too is thought to be 100 percent fatal. The most effective prevention is the destruction of animals suspected of being exposed to the disease.

PERSPECTIVE AND PROSPECTS

Creutzfeldt-Jakob disease is closely related to kuru and scrapie. Scrapie is a spongiform encephalopathy of sheep that is experimentally transmissible to other animal species. The scrapie agent is not known to cause disease in humans. Kuru is a disease previously endemic among the Fore people inhabiting an area in the eastern highlands of Papua New Guinea. Cerebellar dysfunction, dementia, and progression to death within two years were typical symptoms. Women and children were affected much more frequently than were men. Evidence indicates that the kuru agent was transmitted through the ritual handling and consumption of affected tissues, especially brains, from deceased relatives. These cultural practices were discontinued, and the incidence of kuru has decreased dramatically since 1959.

Brain tissues from patients dying of kuru were inoculated

into the brains of chimpanzees that, after a prolonged incubation period, developed a similar disease. Subsequently, the pathology of kuru and CJD were noted to be similar, and experimental transmission studies using CJD-affected brain were undertaken. These experiments also were positive, and CJD has been transmitted to a wide range of laboratory animals.

Clinically, Creutzfeldt-Jakob disease can be mistaken for other disorders that cause dementia, especially Alzheimer's disease. CJD, however, usually has a shorter clinical course with myoclonus. The recent development of scrapie antibodies that cross-react with CJD-specific proteins allows rapid immunologic confirmation of the diagnosis by brain biopsy or postmortem examination of specimens.

On a worldwide basis, the incidence of Creutzfeldt-Jakob disease is one case per million people. Higher rates of CJD have been noted in Israel among Libyan-born Jews and in some areas of the Czech Republic and Chile. Approximately 250 deaths occur in the United States each year. Some individuals receiving growth hormone extracts from human pituitary glands developed Creutzfeldt-Jakob disease. This practice was discontinued in the United States in 1985, but additional cases may develop. Mad cow disease has not been a problem in the United States, primarily as a result of strict quarantines and the testing of imported beef. —*L. Fleming Fallon, Jr., M.D., M.P.H.*

See also Brain; Brain disorders; Dementia; Food poisoning; Prion diseases; Viral infections; Zoonoses.

FOR FURTHER INFORMATION:

Johnson, R. T. "Prion Disease." *New England Journal of Medicine* 326 (1992): 486-490. This review article organizes most known information about proteinaceous infections particles. It is well written.

Prusiner, Stanley B., and Michael McKinley, eds. *Prions: Novel Infectious Pathogens Causing Scrapie and Creutzfeldt-Jakob Disease.* New York: Academic Press, 1988. This text is somewhat dated but still contains a wealth of information. Experts contributed the many chapters.

Ramton, Sheldon, and John C. Stauber. *Mad Cow U.S.A.: Could the Nightmare Happen Here?* New York: Common Courage Press, 1997. The authors argue that the U.S. and British governments colluded with beef producers to suppress important facts about interspecies transmission of mad cow disease, facts that might have prevented several painful deaths. They fear grave consequences for public health and make a strong case against these laws and, inadvertently, for vegetarianism.

CRITICAL CARE
SPECIALTY
ANATOMY OR SYSTEM AFFECTED: All
SPECIALTIES AND RELATED FIELDS: Anesthesiology, cardiology, emergency medicine, gastroenterology, geriat-

rics and gerontology, neurology, nursing, obstetrics, pharmacology, pulmonary medicine, radiology, sports medicine, toxicology
DEFINITION: The care of patients who are experiencing severe health crises—short-lived or prolonged, accidental or anticipated—which require continuous monitoring.
KEY TERMS:
asphyxia: an impaired exchange of oxygen and carbon dioxide in the lungs; if prolonged, this condition leads to death

aspirate: to suck in fluid or a foreign body into an airway of the lungs, which frequently leads to aspiration pneumonia

debridement: the excision of bruised, injured, or otherwise devitalized tissue from a wound site

electrocardiogram (EKG or ECG): a graphic record of the electrical activity of the heart, obtained with an electrocardiograph and displayed on a computer screen or paper strip

emphysema: an increase in the size of air spaces at the terminal ends of bronchioles in the lungs; this damage reduces the ability of the lungs to exchange oxygen and carbon dioxide

esophagus: the portion of the digestive system connecting the mouth and stomach; it is muscular, propelling food during the act of swallowing

hypothermia: a subnormal body temperature; clinically, it is a sustained cooling of the body to lower-than-normal temperatures

resuscitation: the restoration to life after apparent death; the methods used to restore normal organ functioning, primarily referring to the heart

sternum: the breastbone; found in the midline of the chest cavity and lying over the heart

trauma: an injury caused by rough contact with a physical object; it can be accidental or induced

SCIENCE AND PROFESSION

Critical care is the branch of medicine that provides immediate services, usually on an emergency basis. It also encompasses some forms of ongoing care provided in a hospital setting for patients who are so sick that they are medically unstable and must be monitored constantly. Such patients are at an ongoing high risk for disastrous complications.

Critical care personnel must be specially trained, and standards for training and evaluation in this field have been prepared for physicians, nurses, and other hospital personnel. Some critical care facilities are available in the United States. Ninety percent of hospitals with fewer than two hundred beds have a single critical care unit, usually called an intensive care unit (ICU). Only 9 percent of these hospitals have a second intensive care facility, typically dedicated solely to the care of heart attack victims. In total, 7 to 8 percent of all hospital beds in the United States are used for intensive care. Because ICU facilities are at a premium and are expensive to operate, patients are transferred to a regular hospital bed as quickly as possible, given their specific medical condition. Of the physicians who are certified in critical care, most are anesthesiologists, followed by internists. A shortage of trained critical care physicians has existed in the United States for many years.

Critical care facilities are available in several varieties, providing specialized care to particular patients. The most common type of ICU is for individuals who require care for medical crises. These patients frequently have a short-term condition or disease that can be treated successfully. Others are admitted to a medical ICU for multiple organ system failure. These people are often very sick with conditions that overwhelm even the best available care and equipment. Heart attack victims are often admitted to a coronary ICU, which has specialized equipment for support and resuscitation if needed. Once medically stable, coronary ICU patients are transferred to a regular hospital bed.

Larger hospitals may have an ICU for surgical patients. Typically, these individuals are admitted to the surgical ICU from the operating room after a procedure. In the ICU, they are stabilized while the effects of anesthesia wear off. They, too, are transferred to a normal hospital room as soon as is medically safe. Neonatal ICUs exist in some larger hospitals to provide care for premature and very sick infants. Such infants may stay in neonatal ICUs for extended periods of time (weeks to months) depending on their specific condition. There may also be a pediatric ICU specially designed for very sick children.

DIAGNOSTIC AND TREATMENT TECHNIQUES

Critical care is synonymous with immediate care: Swift action is required on an emergency basis to sustain or save a life. The most immediate of critical care needs are to establish and maintain a patent airway for ventilation and to maintain sufficient cardiac functioning to provide minimal perfusion or blood supply to critical organs of the body.

Resuscitation is the support of life by external means when the body is unable to maintain itself. Basic life support is for emergency situations and consists of delivering oxygen to the lungs, maintaining an airway, inflating the lungs if necessary, and assisting with circulation. These methods are collectively known as cardiopulmonary resuscitation (CPR). Oxygen can be transferred from one mouth to another by forceful breathing or by the means of pumps

An Intensive Care Unit

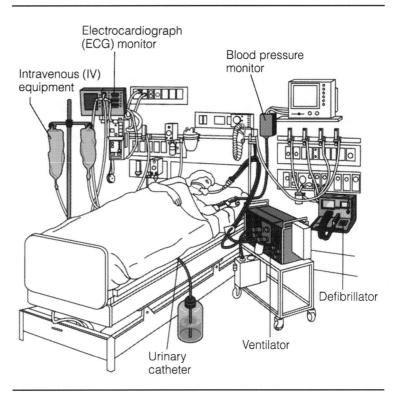

Critical care involves the constant monitoring of patients with life-threatening conditions. This care is usually provided in an intensive care unit (ICU).

and pure oxygen from a container. The airway is commonly maintained by positioning the head and neck so as to extend the chin and open the trachea. It is also possible to make an incision in the trachea, insert a tube, and provide oxygen through the tube. The lungs may be inflated by using the force of exhaled air from one person breathing into another's mouth or by utilizing a machine that inflates the lungs to a precise level and delivers oxygen in accurate, predetermined amounts. When a victim's heart is not working, the circulation of blood is provided by external compression of the chest. This action squeezes the heart between the sternum and the spine, forcing blood into the circulatory system.

Advanced life support includes attempts to restart a nonfunctioning heart. This goal is commonly accomplished by electrical means (defibrillation). The heart is given a brief shock which is sufficient to start it beating on its own. Drugs can also be used to restore spontaneous circulation in cardiac arrest. Epinephrine (adrenaline) is the most commonly used drug, although sodium bicarbonate is used for some conditions. A heart can be restarted by manual compression. This technique requires direct access to the heart and is limited to situations in which the heart stops beating during a surgical procedure involving the thorax, when the heart is directly accessible.

Prolonged life support is administered after the heart has been restarted and is concerned chiefly with the brain and other organs such as the kidneys that are sensitive to oxygen levels in the blood. Drugs and mechanical ventilation are used to supply oxygen to the lungs. Prolonged life support uses sophisticated technology to deliver oxygenated blood to the organs continuously. The body can be maintained in this manner for long periods of time. Once begun, prolonged life support is continued until the patient regains consciousness or until brain death has been certified by a physician. A patient's state of underlying disease may be determined to be so severe that continuing prolonged life support becomes senseless. The factors entering into a decision to terminate life support are complex and involve a patient's family, physician, and other pro--fessionals.

Individuals who are critically ill must be closely monitored. Many of the advancements in the care of these patients have been attributable to improvements in monitoring. While physiologic measurements cannot replace the clinical impressions of trained professionals, monitoring data often provide objective information that reinforces clinical opinions. More people die from the failure of vital organs than from the direct effects of injury or disease. The most commonly monitored events are vital signs: heart rate, blood pressure, breathing rate, and temperature. These are frequently augmented by electrocardiograms (ECGs or EKGs). Other, more sophisticated electronic methods are available for individuals in intensive care units.

Vital signs are still frequently assessed manually, although machinery is available to accomplish the task. Modern intensive care units are able to store large amounts of data that can be analyzed by computer programs. Data can be transmitted to distant consoles, thus enabling a small number of individuals to monitor several patients simultaneously. Monitoring data can also be displayed on computer screens, allowing more rapid evaluation. Automatic alarms can be used to indicate when bodily functions exceed predetermined parameters, thus rapidly alerting staff to critical or emergency situations.

Breathing—or, more correctly, ventilation—can be monitored extensively. The volume of inspired air can be adjusted to accommodate different conditions. The amount of oxygen can be changed to compensate for emphysema or other loss of oxygen exchange capacity. The rate of breathing can also be regulated to work in concert with the heart in order to provide maximum benefit to the patient. The effectiveness of pulmonary monitoring is itself monitored by measuring the amount of oxygen in arterial blood. This, too, can be accomplished automatically and adjustments made by instruments.

Common situations that require critical care are chok-

ing, drowning, poisoning, physical trauma, psychological trauma, and environmental disasters.

Choking. Difficulty in either breathing or swallowing is termed choking. The source of the obstruction may be either internal or external: Internal obstructions can result from a foreign body becoming stuck in the mouth (pharynx), throat (esophagus or trachea), or lungs (bronchi). The blockage may be partial or total. A foreign body that is caught in the esophagus will create difficulty in swallowing; one that is caught in the trachea will obstruct breathing. Any foreign body may become lodged and create a blockage. Objects that commonly cause obstructions include teeth (both natural and false), food (especially meat and bones from fish), and liquids such as water and blood.

Obstructions can occur externally. Examples of external causes of choking include compression of the larynx or trachea that are the result of blunt trauma (a physical blow or other injury sustained in an accident), a penetrating projectile such as a bullet or stick, and toys or small items of food that are swallowed accidentally. Foods such as nuts or candy are frequently aspirated as the result of trying to catch one in the mouth after tossing it in the air. An object that becomes stuck in the lungs frequently does not cause an acute shortage of breath, but this situation can lead to aspiration pneumonia, which is extremely difficult to treat.

The symptoms of choking are well known: gagging, coughing, and difficulty in breathing. Pain may or may not be present. Frequently, there is a short episode of difficulty in breathing followed by a period when no symptoms are experienced. The foreign body may be moved aside or pushed deeper into the body by the victim's initial frantic movements. A foreign body lodged in the esophagus will not interfere with breathing but may cause food or liquids to spill into the trachea and become aspirated; as with an object in the lungs, this usually leads to pneumonia or other serious respiratory conditions.

Drowning. Drowning is defined as the outcome (usually death) of unanticipated immersion into a liquid (usually water). Consciousness is an important determinant of how an individual reacts to immersion in water. A person who is conscious will attempt to escape from the fluid environment, which involves attempts to regain orientation and not to aspirate additional liquids. An unconscious person has none of these defenses and usually dies when the lungs fill rapidly with water. Normal persons can hold their breath for thirty seconds or more. Frequently, this is sufficient time for a victim to escape from immersion in a fluid environment. When a victim exhales just prior to entering water, this time period is not available; indeed, panic frequently develops, and the victim aspirates water.

Most but not all victims of drowning die from aspirating water. Approximately 10 percent of drowning victims die from asphyxia while underwater, possibly because they hold their breath or because the larynx goes into spasms. The brain of the average person can survive without oxygen for about four minutes. After that time, irreversible damage starts to occur; death follows in a matter of minutes. After four minutes, survival is possible but unlikely to be without the permanent impairment of mental functions.

The physical condition of the victim exerts a profound influence on the outcome of a drowning situation. Physically fit persons have a far greater chance of escaping from a drowning environment. Individuals who are in poor condition, who are very weak, or who have handicaps must overcome these conditions when attempting to escape from a drowning situation; frequently, they are unable to remove themselves and die in the process.

Another physical condition such as exhaustion or a heart attack may also be present. An exhausted person is weak and may not have the physical strength or endurance to escape. A person who experiences a heart attack at the moment of immersion is at a severe disadvantage. If the heart is unable to deliver blood and nutrients to muscles, even a physically fit person is weakened and may be less likely to escape a drowning situation.

The temperature of the water is critical. Immersing the face in cold water (below 20 degrees Celsius or 56 degrees Fahrenheit) initiates a reflex that slows the person's heart rate and shunts blood to the heart and brain, thus delaying irreversible cerebral damage. Immersion in water even colder leads to hypothermia (subnormal body temperature). In the short term, hypothermia reduces the body's consumption of oxygen and allows submersion in water for slightly longer periods of time. There have been reports of survival after immersion of ten minutes in warm water and forty minutes in extremely cold water. Age is also a factor: Younger persons are more likely to tolerate such conditions than older persons.

Poisoning. Whether intentional or accidental, poisoning demands immediate medical care. Intoxication can also initiate a crisis that requires critical care. Alcohol is the most common intoxicant, but a wide range of other substances are accidentally ingested. Accidental poisoning is the most common cause of death in young children. When an individual is poisoned, the toxic substance must be removed from the body. This removal may be accomplished in a variety of ways and is usually done in a hospital. Supportive care may be needed during the period of acute crisis. The brain, liver, and kidneys are usually at great risk during a toxic crisis; steps must be taken to protect these organs.

Physical trauma. In the United States, more than 1.5 million persons are hospitalized each year as a result of trauma; some 100,000 of these patients die. Trauma is the leading cause of death in persons under the age of forty and, overall, is the third most common cause of death. Approximately three million people have died as a result of motor vehicle accidents alone in the United States; the first such

death occurred in 1899. Trauma is commonly characterized as either blunt or penetrating.

Blunt trauma occurs when an external force is applied to tissue, causing compression or crushing injuries as well as fractures. This force can be applied directly from being hit with an object or indirectly through the shear forces generated by sudden deceleration. In the latter event, relatively mobile organs or structures continue moving until stopped by adjacent, relatively fixed organs or structures. Any of these injuries can result in extensive internal bleeding. Damage may also cause fluids to be lost from tissues and lead to shock, circulatory collapse, and ultimately death.

The most frequent sources for penetrating wounds are knives and firearms. A knife blade produces a smaller wound; fewer organs are likely to be involved, and adjacent structures are less likely to sustain damage. In contrast, gunshot wounds are more likely to involve multiple tissues and to damage adjacent structures. More energy is released by a bullet than by a knife. This energy is sufficient to fracture a bone and usually leads to a greater amount of tissue damage.

The wound must be repaired, typically through surgical exploration and suturing. Extensively damaged tissue is removed in a process called debridement. Any visible sources of secondary contamination must also be removed. With both knife and firearm wounds often comes contamination by dirt, clothing, and other debris; this contamination presents a serious threat of infection to the victim and is also a problem for critical care workers. The wound is then covered appropriately, and the victim is given antibiotics to counteract bacteria that may have been introduced with the primary injury.

Psychological trauma. Critical care is often required in situations that lead to psychological stress. Individuals taking drug overdoses require critical supportive care until the drug has been metabolized by or removed from the body. Respiratory support is needed when the drug depresses the portion of the brain that controls breathing. Some drugs cause extreme agitation, which must be controlled by sedation.

Severe trauma to a loved one can initiate a psychological crisis. Psychological support must be provided to the victim; frequently, this is done in a hospital setting. An entire family may require critical care support for brief periods of time in the aftermath of a catastrophe. Severe trauma, disease, or the death of a child may require support by outsiders. Most hospitals have professionals who are trained to provide such support. In addition, people with psychiatric problems sometimes fail to take the medications that control mental illness. Critical care support in a hospital is often needed until these people are restabilized on their medications.

Environmental disasters. The need for psychological support, as well as urgent medical care, is magnified with natural or environmental disasters such as earthquakes, hurricanes, floods, or tornadoes. Environmental disasters seriously disrupt lives and normal services; they arise with little or no warning. The key to providing critical care in a disaster situation is adequate prior planning.

Responses to disasters occur at three levels: institutional (hospital), local (police, fire, and rescue), and regional (county and state). The plan must be simple and evolve from normal operations; individuals respond best when they are asked to perform tasks with which they are familiar and for which they are trained. The response must integrate all existing sources of emergency medical and supportive services. Those who assume responsibilities for overall management must be well trained and able to adapt to different conditions that may be encountered. Because no two disasters are ever alike, such flexibility is essential. Summaries of individual duties and responsibilities should be available for all involved individuals. Finally, the disaster plan should be practiced and rehearsed using specific scenarios. Experience is the single best method to ensure competency when a disaster strikes.

Environmental disasters such as earthquakes, hurricanes, floods, or tornadoes cause loss of life and extensive loss of property. Essential services such as water, gas, electricity, and telephone communication are often lost. Victims must be provided food, shelter, and medical care on an immediate basis. Critical care is usually required at the time of the disaster, and the need for support may continue long after the immediate effects of the disaster have been resolved.

PERSPECTIVE AND PROSPECTS

One of the most important issues with regard to critical care is sometimes controversial: when to discontinue life support. Life-support equipment is usually withdrawn as soon as patients are able to function independent of the machinery. These patients continue to recover, are discharged from the hospital, and complete their recovery at home. For some, however, the outcome is not as positive. Machines may be used to assist breathing. For a patient who does not improve, or who deteriorates, there comes a point in time when a decision to stop life support must be made. This is not an easy decision, nor should it be made by a single individual.

The patient's own wishes must be paramount. These wishes, however, must have been clearly communicated while the individual was in good health and with unimpaired thought processes. A patient's family is entitled to provide input in the decision to terminate care, but others are also entitled to provide input: the patient's physician, representatives of the hospital or institution, a representative of the patient's religious faith, and the state.

Medical science has developed criteria for death. The application of these criteria, however, is not uniform. The final decision to terminate life support is frequently a consensus of all the parties mentioned above. When there is a dispute, the courts are often asked to intervene. Extensive disagreements exist concerning the ethics of terminating critical care. It is beyond the scope of this discussion to provide definitive guidelines. This logical extension of critical care may not have a uniform resolution; the values and beliefs of each individual determine the outcome of each situation.

—*L. Fleming Fallon, Jr., M.D., M.P.H.*

See also Aging, extended care for the; Choking; Coma; Critical care, pediatric; Death and dying; Disease; Electrocardiography (ECG or EKG); Electroencephalography (EEG); Emergency medicine; Ethics; Euthanasia; Hospitals; Nursing; Paramedics; Poisoning; Psychiatric disorders; Respiration; Resuscitation; Surgery, general; Terminally ill, extended care for the; Tracheostomy; Unconsciousness; Wounds.

FOR FURTHER INFORMATION:

Ayres, Stephen M., et al., eds. *Textbook of Critical Care.* 3d ed. Philadelphia: W. B. Saunders, 1995. This medical text, written by experts in the field, represents the views of the Society of Critical Care Medicine. The general reader will find it interesting but may elect to skip some sections containing highly technical details.

Foster, Harold D., ed. *Disaster Planning.* New York: Springer-Verlag, 1980. This text provides extensive information on preparing for disasters. The section authors are experts in their own fields. A well-written excellent reference.

Heimlich, H. J. "A Life-Saving Maneuver to Prevent Food-Choking." *Journal of the American Medical Association* 234 (October 27, 1975): 398-401. A classic article written by the originator of the Heimlich maneuver. Describes a way to dislodge foreign bodies trapped in the throats of choking victims who are conscious but who cannot speak.

Safar, Peter. *Cardiopulmonary Cerebral Resuscitation.* Stavanger, Norway: Asmund S. Laerdal, 1981. A text that completely describes the process of cardiopulmonary resuscitation (CPR). The general reader can learn much from it but is cautioned to take a training course taught by the Red Cross or American Heart Association before attempting to use CPR.

Walt, Alexander J., and Robert F. Wilson. *Management of Trauma: Pitfalls and Practice.* Philadelphia: Lea & Febiger, 1975. The reader seeking further information about trauma is referred to this book. The text is written for critical care professionals; the serious reader will find a wealth of material.

CRITICAL CARE, PEDIATRIC
SPECIALTY

ANATOMY OR SYSTEM AFFECTED: All

SPECIALTIES AND RELATED FIELDS: Anesthesiology, cardiology, emergency medicine, gastroenterology, neonatology, neurology, nursing, pediatrics, pharmacology, pulmonary medicine, radiology, toxicology

DEFINITION: The hospital care of seriously ill or injured infants and children.

KEY TERMS:

computed tomography (CT) scanning: a radiographic technique using computer-enhanced X-ray images to show the anatomy of cross sections of the body

magnetic resonance imaging (MRI): a technique using strong electromagnets to show the anatomy of cross sections of the body in great detail

SCIENCE AND PROFESSION

When a serious illness or injury occurs to children, they cannot simply be treated as small adults. The serious illnesses from which they suffer are different from those of adults. Children's bodies respond differently to illness and injuries and require different types of resuscitative fluids and medications. The critical care pediatrician is specially trained to provide this special care.

A critical care pediatrician has undergone, in addition to four years of medical school, three years of pediatric residency and three years of fellowship training in the care of critically ill or injured children. Critical care pediatricians usually practice in large referral hospitals or children's hospitals.

The care of a seriously ill or injured child requires many skills, including the resuscitation and stabilization of the patient's condition, consultation with other specialists, and the establishment and execution of a plan of action. The plan is often complicated, especially if more than one organ system is involved. The critical care pediatrician coordinates the work of the patient's health team.

Resuscitation usually begins in the emergency room and is directed by the emergency room physician. The critical care pediatrician may take over care in the emergency room or when the patient is moved from there or from the operating room to the intensive care unit (ICU).

On the patient's arrival at the hospital, the team first ensures that the patient is able to breathe adequately, and, if not, begins to ventilate the patient's lungs. The patient's cardiac output is quickly evaluated, and chest compression is begun if it is inadequate. The degree of shock is evaluated next and is treated with intravenous fluid. As this resuscitation is being carried out, the critical care pediatrician obtains a history of the illness or injury and conducts a thorough examination of the patient. Based on this information, the physician orders appropriate laboratory and radiographic tests and calls on other specialists, as needed, for help and advice.

Once the patient arrives in the ICU, the critical care pediatrician must continue to treat the initial problem as well as any complications and difficulties added by surgery or other therapies. The physician must be able to relate these problems to his or her knowledge of anatomy and physiology. A quick and accurate assessment of a large number of factors is required as is the ability to gain an overview of all the conditions faced in the care of the patient.

The critical care pediatrician's day is largely spent in a hospital emergency room and its intensive care areas. This type of specialist does not usually practice in a clinic except for occasional follow-up examinations of patients who have been discharged from the hospital.

DIAGNOSTIC AND TREATMENT TECHNIQUES

The critical care pediatrician utilizes a wide variety of diagnostic techniques. Complete blood counts, blood chemistry tests, and cultures of blood, urine, and cerebrospinal fluid are initially helpful, especially in looking for bacterial infections. These tests must be performed periodically to assess the patient's progress. Depending on the patient's problem, more specific tests may be necessary. Imaging studies, such as X rays, ultrasonography, and computed tomography (CT) and magnetic resonance imaging (MRI) scans, are often critical to this evaluation.

Besides closely monitoring the patient's condition, the critical care pediatrician must be able to perform a number of procedures. One is the management of ventilators, machines that can breathe for a child who is too ill or injured to breathe adequately on his or her own. The critical care physician is also expert at inserting a number of intravascular devices, such as central intravenous catheters for intravenous (IV) fluids and for monitoring the function of the heart and intra-arterial catheters for monitoring blood pressure and drawing blood gas tests, which are used to evaluate the function of the lungs.

A complicated form of cardiopulmonary support for some critically ill children is called extracorporeal membrane oxygenation (ECMO). It is the circulation of the child's blood through an artificial lung machine using large intravenous tubes, generally inserted in the neck. This machine adds oxygen to and removes carbon dioxide from the child's circulation. ECMO requires a team of highly trained technicians. Its use is overseen by the critical care pediatrician when the patient is older than a newborn. ECMO is available only in the largest referral hospitals.

The care of critically ill children requires much emotional maturity on the part of the physician. The child's family is frightened and anxious, and the child is under great emotional stress. The team of caregivers feels the stress of working with these children as well. The critical care pediatrician must be able to provide empathetic support to all people involved in the health crisis. Despite its share of tragedies, critical care pediatrics is a richly rewarding field. The outcome for critically ill children is better than that for equally ill adults.

PERSPECTIVE AND PROSPECTS

While there have always been pediatricians with an interest in critical pediatric care, fellowships in the specialty were first developed in the last quarter of the twentieth century. Critical care was recognized as a subspecialty of pediatrics in 1987. By 1994, there were only sixty-five pediatricians who had been accepted as fellows of the American College of Critical Care Medicine. By then, there was a rapidly increasing demand for these specialists, with four to six positions being advertised for pediatric critical care doctors for every one adult position.

—*Thomas C. Jefferson, M.D.*

See also Choking; Coma; Critical care; Death and dying; Disease; Electrocardiography (ECG or EKG); Electroencephalography (EEG); Emergency medicine; Ethics; Euthanasia; Hospitals; Nursing; Paramedics; Pediatrics; Poisoning; Psychiatric disorders; Respiration; Resuscitation; Surgery, pediatric; Terminally ill, extended care for the; Tracheostomy; Unconsciousness; Wounds.

FOR FURTHER INFORMATION:

The Pediatric Clinics of North America 41, no. 6 (December, 1994).

Todres, I. David, and John H. Fugate, eds. *Critical Care of Infants and Children*. Boston: Little, Brown, 1996.

CROHN'S DISEASE

DISEASE/DISORDER

ANATOMY OR SYSTEM AFFECTED: Abdomen, gastrointestinal system, intestines, stomach

SPECIALTIES AND RELATED FIELDS: Gastroenterology, internal medicine

DEFINITION: A serious, chronic inflammatory disease of the gastrointestinal tract.

CAUSES AND SYMPTOMS

Crohn's disease, one of the two inflammatory bowel diseases (IBDs), can cause inflammation and ulceration within any region of the digestive tract. Though a break in the mucous membrane of the digestive tract can occur anywhere from the mouth to the anus, in this disease the inflammation occurs primarily in the ileum, the section of the small intestine that meets the large intestine. (Ulcerative colitis, the other IBD, occurs only in the colon or rectum.) Because of the patchy, nonuniform distribution of the inflamed areas in the small intestine, Crohn's disease is also known as regional enteritis.

Crohn's disease affects not only the mucosa or surface layer of the digestive tract but also often progresses so that all three layers of the intestinal wall become inflamed. Frequently, fistulas (connections) between the digestive tract and other body structures develop, causing further physical complications. Mechanical obstructions and stricture formation, in which the bowel abnormally narrows, can also occur.

The common symptoms of Crohn's disease are diarrhea, abdominal pain, nausea, and vomiting. These symptoms can lead to systemic complications of weight loss, dehydration, anemia, and fever. Malnutrition often also occurs because of the inability of the small intestine to absorb nutrients properly.

TREATMENT AND THERAPY

Since no medical cure exists for Crohn's disease, the goal of treatment is to decrease the inflammation of the diseased intestinal segment. This can be done by rest, nutritional

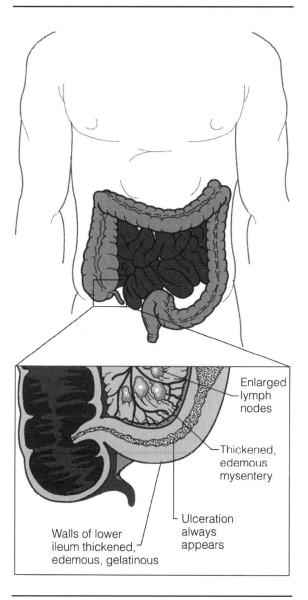

Crohn's Disease

Enlarged lymph nodes

Thickened, edemous mysentery

Ulceration always appears

Walls of lower ileum thickened, edemous, gelatinous

Crohn's disease can cause inflammation and ulceration within any region of the digestive tract, but most often in the ileum.

therapy, and medication. In severe cases, surgical resection may be done; however, this procedure is not recommended because of the high rate of recurrence of Crohn's disease. The disease is characterized by periods of exacerbations and remissions. For acute flare-ups, bed rest is recommended and oral feeding may be stopped. Though nutritional management of Crohn's disease needs to be individualized, often a diet low in fiber and fat and high in protein and carbohydrates is tolerated best. Immunosuppressive and anti-inflammatory medications are the most commonly prescribed drugs for treatment. —*Martha M. Henze, R.D.*

See also Colitis; Colon and rectal surgery; Colon cancer; Diarrhea and dysentery; Diverticulosis and diverticulitis; Fistula repair; Gastroenterology; Gastroenterology, pediatric; Gastrointestinal disorders; Gastrointestinal system; Intestinal disorders; Intestines.

FOR FURTHER INFORMATION:

Steiner-Grossman, Penny, Peter A. Banks, and Daniel H. Present, eds. *People . . . Not Patients: A Source Book for Living with Inflammatory Bowel Disease*. New York: National Foundation for Ileitis and Colitis, 1985.

Thompson, W. Grant. *The Angry Gut: Coping with Colitis and Crohn's Disease*. New York: Plenum Press, 1993.

CRYOTHERAPY AND CRYOSURGERY

PROCEDURE

ANATOMY OR SYSTEM AFFECTED: All

SPECIALTIES AND RELATED FIELDS: Dermatology, family practice, general surgery, oncology

DEFINITION: Cryotherapy is the use of exceptionally cold temperatures to achieve several therapeutic purposes, including relief of pain and reduction of inflammation; cryosurgery is a form of cryotherapy employing special devices to freeze and destroy diseased tissue.

KEY TERMS:

cryogenic agent: one of various mediums used to achieve the low temperatures needed to produce therapeutic effects

cryoprobe: an instrument used by physicians to apply cryogenic agents to diseased tissue; cryoprobes have differently shaped tips which affect the size and depth of the freezing

INDICATIONS AND PROCEDURES

Cryosurgery can be used by family physicians or dermatologists to treat a variety of skin lesions in the office setting. Abscesses, actinic keratoses, basal cell carcinomas, freckles, granulation tissue, keloids, papular nevi, and some warts are examples of skin lesions that are treated by use of cryosurgery.

The hand of the physician touching the patient is used to brace the cryoprobe and position it just above the lesion to be treated. The probe is turned on and quickly lowered onto the lesion. An ice ball forms around the probe within a few seconds, and the physician keeps the probe on the lesion until adequate freezing occurs. Freeze times for skin lesions vary from about thirty seconds to a cycle of freezing, thawing, and refreezing lasting less than two minutes.

When treating skin lesions, the physician uses the size of the ice ball which forms around the tip of the cryoprobe to judge the depth and extent of the freezing process. The shape of the tip and the pressure applied to the skin lesion determine the depth of the freeze zone.

Many factors come into play to set the resistance of the lesion to freezing; lesions with keratin coverings greatly resist freezing and require debriding well in advance of treatment.

The simple equipment of cryosurgery can be used to treat easily accessible cancers, such as tumors of the skin, ears, eyes, eyelids, lip, tongue, anus, rectum, and cervix. (More complex equipment and combined approaches are needed to treat other cancers.) For example, physicians have learned that use of cryosurgery to treat tumors of the maxillary sinus is effective and achieves even better results when combined with radiation and chemotherapy.

In the simplest form of cryosurgery used to treat cancer, the cooling agent is applied through a specialized tool to the cancerous tissue, which is killed by freezing and allowed to slough. The tissue is rapidly frozen, allowed to thaw slowly, then refrozen and rethawed. This method avoids surgical excision, minimizes blood loss, and reduces operative pain. After the treatment is completed, the resulting wound is monitored carefully to ensure that no cancer survives. Most sites require only one treatment to effect a cure, but some large tumors may require repeated treatments. Soft tissue heals normally and with little scarring. Treated bones heal more slowly. Liquid nitrogen is the only cryogenic agent used to treat invasive cancer, while liquid nitrous oxide is used when treatment involves only a thin layer of tissue.

USES AND COMPLICATIONS

The use of cryosurgery to treat lesions on the eyelids can cause them to swell shut for a prolonged period. Treating lesions near nerves, especially those with sensory function, can cause temporary impairment. The skin of infants and elderly people are more susceptible to blistering and sloughing. Skin treated with cryosurgery can lose its pigment, sweat glands, and hair follicles.

After cryosurgery, the wound requires only simple care, and the patient can even bathe and swim while it heals. The wound generally heals with little or no scarring, although complete healing may take as long as eight weeks. Some patients report that they feel a burning sensation during the procedure, which becomes more intense as the area thaws. Infection of the wound is rare. Family physicians generally use liquid nitrous oxide in a cryogun or liquid nitrogen in a spray apparatus to freeze skin tissue. The nitrous oxide lowers the tip temperature to −89 degrees Celsius, a far higher temperature than liquid nitrogen; therefore, use of liquid nitrous oxide may be more limited in its applications and requires longer freezing times.

PERSPECTIVE AND PROSPECTS

The use of cryotherapy in treating cancer dates from 1850, when English physicians used iced salt water to treat cancers found in the breast and uterus. The physicians reported that cryotherapy relieved pain, reduced tumor size, and stemmed bleeding and discharge. These benefits are still cited today, even through cryotherapy equipment and techniques have improved. By 1900, scientists were able to liquefy commonly occurring gases, and medical investigators began to use liquid air to freeze and kill skin cancer. The conducting of further studies and the introduction of improved equipment in the 1950's and 1960's were key factors in the development of modern cryosurgery. The use of liquid nitrogen, capable of reaching temperatures of –196 degrees Celsius, was introduced into clinical practice.

Cryosurgery has become the standard method of treating skin cancer. It is an accepted form of treatment for many other cancers as well, such as those found in the oral cavity, prostate gland, and liver. This technique can be employed in conjunction with other forms of therapy or as an alternative when other methods fail. Moreover, in areas of the world where technology is not advanced, facilities are less satisfactory, and the number of patients is high, cryosurgery is considered an important and effective tool in the treatment of cancer.   —*Russell Williams, M.S.W.*

See also Abscess drainage; Abscesses; Cancer; Cervical procedures; Dermatology; Electrocauterization; Malignant melanoma removal; Skin; Skin cancer; Skin disorders; Skin lesion removal; Tumor removal; Tumors.

FOR FURTHER INFORMATION:

Bolton, Ruth. "Nongenital Warts: Classification and Treatment Options." *American Family Physician* 43, no. 6 (June, 1991): 2049-2056.

Gage, Andrew. "Cryosurgery in the Treatment of Cancer." *Surgery, Gynecology, and Obstetrics* 174, no. 1 (January, 1992): 73-92.

Harper, Diane. "Pain and Cramping Associated with Cryosurgery." *The Journal of Family Practice* 39, no. 6 (December, 1994): 551-557.

Hocutt, John, Jr. "Skin Cryosurgery for the Family Physician." *American Family Physician* 48, no. 3 (September, 1993): 445-452; 455-456.

Winburn, Ginger, et al. "Current Role of Cryoamputation." *The American Journal of Surgery* 162, no. 6 (December, 1991): 647-651.

CT SCANNING. *See* COMPUTED TOMOGRAPHY (CT) SCANNING.

CULDOCENTESIS
PROCEDURE
ANATOMY OR SYSTEM AFFECTED: Genitals, reproductive system, uterus
SPECIALTIES AND RELATED FIELDS: Gynecology
DEFINITION: The removal of fluid from the space immediately behind the vagina is termed culdocentesis. Under some circumstances, the cavity behind the vagina may fill with fluid, which must be removed. During a pelvic exam, the physician may notice pressure and/or fluid in this space, which will be confirmed by ultrasound analy-

sis. This fluid accumulation may be the result of a ruptured ectopic pregnancy or from untreated pelvic inflammatory disease (PID). To remove the fluid, culdocentesis is performed in the doctor's office without anesthesia. The cervix is grasped and pulled up, and a thin needle is inserted through the vagina to the cavity. The fluid is analyzed: If it is blood, the patient will be immediately transported to surgery to determine and fix the cause of bleeding. The procedure takes approximately one hour and is somewhat painful. Spotting may occur for a day after culdocentesis.   —*Karen E. Kalumuck, Ph.D.*

See also Abscess drainage; Abscesses; Ectopic pregnancy; Gynecology; Pelvic inflammatory disease (PID).

CUSHING'S SYNDROME
DISEASE/DISORDER
ANATOMY OR SYSTEM AFFECTED: All
SPECIALTIES AND RELATED FIELDS: Endocrinology
DEFINITION: Cushing's syndrome is an endocrine disorder that consists of a group of abnormalities; it usually strikes

---

Cushing's Syndrome

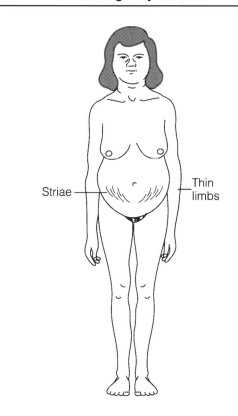

Striae   Thin limbs

An adrenal disorder, Cushing's syndrome causes symptomatic fatty deposits, striae, and thin limbs and may be associated with a variety of mild to serious conditions.

women. The result of excessive levels of adrenocortical hormones in the body, the syndrome causes characteristic fatty deposits in the face, neck, and trunk. Various other disorders may result, including diabetes mellitus, muscle wasting, bone fractures, peptic ulcers, insomnia, hypertension, a compromised immune system, as well as amenorrhea (cessation of menstruation), acne, and hirsutism (excessive hairiness) in women. Treatment of the syndrome may include radiation, drug therapy, or surgery, depending on the source of the hormone secretions, such as a tumor.

—*Jason Georges and Tracy Irons-Georges*
See also Addison's disease; Endocrine disorders; Endocrinology; Hormones.

CYST REMOVAL
PROCEDURE
ANATOMY OR SYSTEM AFFECTED: Breasts, genitals, glands, joints, reproductive system, skin
SPECIALTIES AND RELATED FIELDS: Dermatology; general surgery; gynecology; plastic, cosmetic, and reconstructive surgery
DEFINITION: A surgical procedure to remove a fluid or solid nodule performed in a physician's office or a hospital, depending on the type and location of the cyst.
KEY TERMS:
aspirate: to remove a substance using suction; a cyst can be aspirated using a needle and syringe to withdraw its contents
cyst: a sac containing a fluid, semifluid, or solid substance
incision: a cut made with a scalpel during a surgical procedure
laparoscope: a small surgical tube which can be inserted through a small incision into the abdominal cavity to view and perform surgery on abdominal organs

INDICATIONS AND PROCEDURES

Many different types of cysts may require surgical removal. Baker's, Bartholin's, ovarian, sebaceous, thyroglossal, and breast cysts are among the most common.

Baker's cysts are small lumps that form behind the knee. Fluid-filled sacs found around joints, known as bursa, normally protect the moving joint from causing damage to overlying skin, tendons, and muscles. When the bursas behind the knee accumulate excess fluid, they can expand and form a Baker's cyst. This fluid accumulation often occurs if the knee is arthritic. Physicians usually apply pressure bandages to reduce the bursal swelling. If this does not work, the cyst must be surgically removed.

Bartholin's cysts are formed when the Bartholin's glands found in the female genital area become swollen with fluid. These glands normally secrete a lubricating fluid during sexual excitation and aid in intercourse by reducing friction around the entrance of the vagina. Infections occasionally occur in the ducts of these glands, which may cause scar-

ring and obstruction. Cysts that develop in these glands do not usually cause pain. They may repeatedly become infected, however, and must be removed if antibiotic therapy does not eradicate the bacteria.

Ovarian cysts typically cause vague symptoms and may disappear without treatment. When symptoms occur, they may include abdominal discomfort, pain during intercourse, and painful or irregular menses. Ovarian cysts are formed when a follicle which houses an egg accumulates excess fluid. They may also arise from the corpus luteum that forms after an egg has been released during ovulation. If an ovarian cyst is suspected, the physician will perform a pelvic exam, an ultrasound exam, or a laparoscopic exam. The latter procedure requires the patient to undergo an operation in which a viewing tube (laparoscope) is inserted into the pelvic cavity and the ovaries are visualized. If these cysts are thought to be cancerous (95 percent are benign), interfere with reproductive function, or cause severe symptoms, they are surgically removed. In most cases, only the cyst need be removed. If the cysts are large or tend to recur, however, then the entire ovary may be removed.

Removal of the ovarian cyst or of the ovary (oophorectomy) requires general anesthesia and an abdominal incision. The surgeon must ligate (tie off) the blood vessels to the ovary before removal to prevent excessive blood loss. Once the cystic ovary is removed, the abdomen is sutured and the patient is allowed to recover. She can usually return to normal activities within about six weeks.

A sebaceous cyst may develop when a duct from a sebaceous gland in the skin becomes blocked and the oily fluid is unable to escape. These glands, which are associated with hair follicles, secrete sebum to lubricate the hair and skin. If the sebaceous cyst is very large or infected with bacteria, surgical removal is usually indicated. This operation can be done in a physician's office under local anesthesia. A small incision is made in the skin, and the entire cyst is removed or drained. If the complete wall of the cyst is not removed, it may recur. A few sutures are needed to close the wound.

Thyroglossal cysts usually arise because of a congenital defect in which the duct that connects the base of the tongue to the thyroid gland fails to disappear. If a cyst develops in this area, a noticeable swelling will occur above the thyroid cartilage (Adam's apple). This cyst nearly always becomes infected and thus should be surgically removed. This procedure involves an incision just above the thyroid cartilage and gland. The surgeon then separates surrounding tissue up to the base of the tongue to gain access to the cyst. The cyst can then be removed and the skin sutured.

Fibrocystic breast disease, usually detected as a breast lump, is usually a benign condition. Nevertheless, all breast masses should be examined by a physician. Most of these fluid-filled cysts can be drained in a physician's office if they are causing discomfort. A long, sterile needle attached to a syringe is inserted into the lump, and the fluid is aspirated.

USES AND COMPLICATIONS

The most common complication of ovarian cysts occurs in the pregnant patient. These cysts can rupture or displace the reproductive organs so that delivery becomes difficult. If the cyst is large, the physician may perform a laparotomy, which involves an operation to open the abdominal cavity to remove the cyst. If possible, the surgery is done before the fourth month of gestation in order to reduce the risks to the fetus.

Thyroglossal cyst removal has the potential complication of damaging the thyroid gland, which can lead to thyroid hormone deficiency. Such a surgical error may leave the patient with a relatively low metabolic rate. This complication can be treated with the appropriate use of thyroid hormone drugs.

—*Matthew Berria, Ph.D., and Douglas Reinhart, M.D.*

See also Abscess drainage; Abscesses; Biopsy; Breast biopsy; Breast disorders; Breasts, female; Colon and rectal polyp removal; Colon and rectal surgery; Cysts and ganglions; Dermatology; Endometrial biopsy; Ganglion removal; Glands; Gynecology; Hydrocelectomy; Laparoscopy; Myomectomy; Nasal polyp removal; Skin; Skin disorders; Skin lesion removal.

FOR FURTHER INFORMATION:

Clayman, Charles B., ed. *The American Medical Association Encyclopedia of Medicine.* New York: Random House, 1989.

Cunningham, F. Gary, et al., eds. *Williams Obstetrics.* 20th ed. Stamford, Conn.: Appleton and Lange, 1997.

Hellmann, David B. "Arthritis and Musculoskeletal Disorders." In *Current Medical Diagnosis and Treatment,* edited by Lawrence M. Tierney, Jr., et. al. 37th ed. Norwalk, Conn.: Appleton and Lange, 1998.

CYSTECTOMY

PROCEDURE

ANATOMY OR SYSTEM AFFECTED: Abdomen, bladder, urinary system

SPECIALTIES AND RELATED FIELDS: General surgery, gynecology, proctology, urology

DEFINITION: The surgical removal of the bladder and accompanying structures or organs.

INDICATIONS AND PROCEDURES

Cystectomy is often the treatment of choice in cases of bladder cancer, which may be treated with chemotherapy or radiation in combination with surgery. The procedure, usually performed under general anesthesia, is carried out by making an incision in the abdomen, after which the ducts that carry urine from the bladder, called ureters, are cut and tied. The affected bladder is removed and, in men, the prostate gland is also excised. In women, the uterus, Fal-

Cystectomy

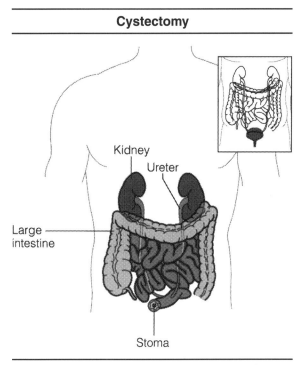

Kidney
Ureter
Large intestine
Stoma

The removal of the bladder, usually as a result of cancer, necessitates the creation of a stoma, in which the ureters are connected to a section of small intestine, through which urine is voided from the body.

lopian tubes, and ovaries are removed along with the diseased bladder.

At this point, a permanent opening is made in the abdomen. The two ureters are joined to a tiny section of small intestine that has been removed from the rest of the intestines, formed into a loop, and inserted through the abdominal wall. Urine is excreted through this opening, called a stoma.

USES AND COMPLICATIONS

A cystectomy has serious consequences. In men, the result is usually impotence because the nerve tracts that permit penile erections are usually damaged severely by the surgery. In women, the outcome is infertility as a result of the combination of cystectomy and hysterectomy. Because most women who undergo the procedure have already experienced the menopause, however, this consequence usually does not affect them adversely.

In addition to the complications from infection and systemic shock that can accompany any major surgery, cystectomy poses another problem: Following surgery and for the remainder of a patient's life, urine is passed outside the body and must be collected in a pouch that is worn externally. It takes some patients considerable time to adapt to this inevitable complication. Enterostomy therapists teach patients how to care for the stoma; patients are usually referred to these specialists following a cystectomy.

Some patients also experience problems with proper intestinal function in the days immediately following a cystectomy. This difficulty is overcome through the regular administration of a solution of saline fluids and glucose intravenously beginning soon after the surgery.

—*R. Baird Shuman, Ph.D.*

See also Cancer; Cystoscopy; Hysterectomy; Oncology; Prostate gland removal; Urinalysis: Urinary system; Urology.

CYSTIC FIBROSIS

DISEASE/DISORDER

ANATOMY OR SYSTEM AFFECTED: Chest, lungs, respiratory system, most bodily systems

SPECIALTIES AND RELATED FIELDS: Genetics, neonatology, pediatrics, pulmonary medicine

DEFINITION: A disease that affects the exocrine glands and, secondarily, most physical systems, resulting in death usually between the ages of sixteen and thirty.

KEY TERMS:

chloride transport: the movement of one of the ions found in ordinary salt across a membrane from the inside of a cell to the outside; this transport is common in human cells and is critical for many important metabolic functions

cystic fibrosis transmembrane-conductance regulator (CFTR): the protein product of the cystic fibrosis gene and a chloride transport channel

meconium ileus: the puttylike plug found in the intestines of some cystic fibrosis babies when they are born

mutation: an alteration in the deoxyribonucleic acid (DNA) sequence of a gene, which usually leads to the production of a nonfunctional enzyme or protein and thus a lack of a normal metabolic function

recessive genetic disease: a disease caused by mutated genes that must be inherited from both parents in order for that individual to show its symptoms

secretory epithelium: tissues or groups of cells that have the ability to move substances, such as chloride ions, from the inside of cells to a duct or tube

CAUSES AND SYMPTOMS

Genetic diseases are inherited, rather than caused by any specific injury or infectious agent. Thus, unlike many other types of diseases, genetic diseases rage throughout a person's entire lifetime and often begin to exert their debilitating effects prior to birth. Since in many cases the primary defect or underlying cause of the disease is unknown, treatment is difficult or impossible and is usually restricted to treating the symptoms of the disease. Genetic diseases include sickle-cell anemia; thalassemia; Tay-Sachs disease; some forms of muscular dystrophy, diabetes, and hemophilia; and cystic fibrosis.

In each disease, a specific normal function is missing because of a defect in the individual's genes. Genes are sequences of deoxyribonucleic acid (DNA) contained on the chromosomes of an individual that are passed to the next generation via ova and sperm. Usually, the primary defect in a genetic disease is the inability to produce a normal enzyme, the class of proteins used to speed up, or catalyze, the chemical reactions that are necessary for cells to function. A defective gene, also called a mutation, may not allow the production of a necessary enzyme; therefore, some element of metabolism is missing from an individual with such a mutation. This lack of function leads to the symptoms associated with a genetic disease, such as the

Cystic Fibrosis

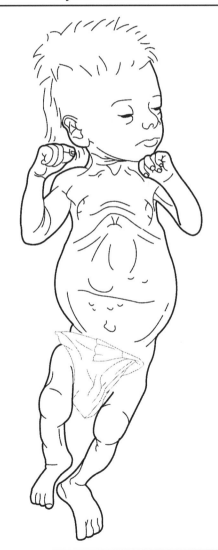

Approximately 10% of newborns with cystic fibrosis have a puttylike plug of undigested material in their intestines called the meconium ileus, which results in emaciation with a distended abdomen.

lack of insulin production in juvenile diabetes or the inability of the blood to clot in hemophilia. In the 1940's and 1950's, when the understanding of basic cellular metabolism made clear the relationship between genes, enzymes, mutant genes, and lack of enzyme function, the modern definition of genetic disease came into routine medical use.

Cystic fibrosis, one such genetic disease, has several major effects on an individual. These effects begin before birth, extend into early childhood, and become progressively more serious as the affected individual grows. The primary diagnosis for the disease is a very simple test which looks for excessive saltiness in perspiration. Although the higher-than-normal level of salt in the perspiration is, of itself, not life-threatening, the associated symptoms are. Because these other symptoms may vary from one individual to the next, the perspiration test is a very useful early diagnostic tool.

Major symptoms of cystic fibrosis include the blockage of several important internal ducts. This blockage occurs because the cystic fibrosis mutation has a critical effect on the ability of certain internal tissues called secretory epithelia to transport normal amounts of salt and water across their surfaces. These epithelia are often found in the ducts that contribute to the digestive and reproductive systems.

The blockage of ducts resulting from the production and export of overly viscous secretions reduces the delivery of digestive enzymes from the pancreas to the intestine; thus proteins in the intestine are only partly digested. Fat-emulsifying compounds, called bile salts, are often blocked as well on their route from the pancreas to the intestine, so the digestion of fats is often incomplete. These two conditions often occur prior to birth. Approximately 10 percent of newborns with cystic fibrosis have a puttylike plug of undigested material in their intestines called the meconium ileus. This plug prevents the normal movement of foods through the digestive system and can be very serious.

Because of their overall inefficiency of digestion, young children with cystic fibrosis can seem to be eating quite normally yet remain severely undernourished. They often produce bulky, foul-smelling stools as a result of the high proportion of undigested material. This symptom serves as an indicator of the progress of the disease, as such digestive problems often increase as the affected child ages.

As individuals with cystic fibrosis grow older, their respiratory problems increase because of the secretion of a thick mucus on the inner lining of the lungs. This viscous material traps white blood cells that release their contents when they rupture, which makes the mucus all the more thick and viscous. The affected individuals constantly cough in an attempt to remove this material. Of greater importance is that the mucus forms an ideal breeding ground for many types of pathogenic bacteria, and the affected individual suffers from continual respiratory infections. Male patients are almost always infertile as a result

of the blockage of the ducts of the reproductive system, while female fertility is sometimes reduced as well.

Traditional treatments for cystic fibrosis have improved an individual's chance of survival and have dramatically affected the quality of life. In the 1950's, a child afflicted with cystic fibrosis usually lived only a year or two. Thus, cystic fibrosis was originally described as a children's disease and was intensively studied only by pediatricians. Today, aggressive medical intervention has changed survival rates dramatically. Affected individuals are treated by a package of therapies designed to alleviate the most severe symptoms of the disease, and taken together, they had extended the median age of survival of cystic fibrosis patients to twenty-nine years by the early 1990's. In fact, since this figure contains many individuals who were born before many of the effective treatments were developed and so did not benefit from them throughout their entire lifetimes, the true average life expectancy may be as high as forty years.

The available treatments, however, do not constitute a cure for the disease. The major roadblock to developing a cure was that the primary genetic defect remained unknown. All that was clear until the mid-1980's was that many of the secretory epithelia had a salt and water transport problem. By the late 1980's, the defect was further restricted to a problem in the transport of chloride ions, one of the two constituents of ordinary salt and a critical chemical in many important cellular processes. Because individuals who had severe forms of cystic fibrosis could still live, however, this function was deemed important but not absolutely essential for survival. Furthermore, only certain tissues and organs in the body seemed to show abnormal functions in a cystic fibrosis patient, while other organs—the heart, brain, and nerves—seemed to function normally. Thus, the defect was not uniform.

The pattern of inheritance of cystic fibrosis was relatively easy to determine. The disease acts as a recessive trait. Humans, like most animals, have two copies of each gene: one that is inherited on a chromosome from the egg, and the other on a similar chromosome from the sperm. There is a gene in all humans that controls some normal cellular function related to the transport of chloride from the inside of a cell to the outside. If this function is missing or impaired, the individual shows the symptoms of cystic fibrosis.

A recessive trait is one that must be inherited from both the mother and the father in order to take effect. Inheriting only a single copy of the mutation from one parent does not have a deleterious effect on an individual, who would not demonstrate any of the disease symptoms. Such a person, however, is a carrier of the disease and can still pass that mutation on to his or her own children. Thus genetic diseases caused by recessive mutations, such as cystic fibrosis, can remain hidden in a family for many generations. Only when two carriers of the disease marry are some of their children at risk. The rules of genetics, as first described by Gregor Mendel in the nineteenth century, predict that in such a marriage, approximately one in four children will have cystic fibrosis. Another one-fourth will be normal, and the remaining half will be carriers of the disease like their parents. Because the production of eggs and sperm involves a random shuffling of genes and chromosomes, however, the occurrence of normal individuals, carriers, and affected individuals cannot be predicted; only average probabilities can be discussed.

TREATMENT AND THERAPY

The traditional treatments for cystic fibrosis usually include dietary supplements which contain the digestive enzymes and bile salts that cannot pass through the blocked ducts; this is a daily requirement. Individuals with cystic fibrosis are also placed on special balanced diets to ensure proper nutrition despite their difficulties in digesting fats and proteins. One characteristic of cystic fibrosis treatment is the long daily ritual of backslapping, which is designed to help break up the thick mucus in the lungs. Aggressive antibiotic therapy can keep infections of the lungs from forming or spreading. In the 1990's, an additional therapy was begun using a special enzyme which when inhaled can break down DNA in the lung mucus. Many white blood cells rupture while trapped in the thick mucus lining of the lungs, and the release of their DNA adds to the high viscosity of the mucus. Genetically engineered deoxyribonuclease (DNase), an enzyme produced from bacteria, has been found to be helpful in degrading this extra DNA, thus making it easier to break up and cough out the mucus found in the lungs of affected patients.

Another treatment approach for cystic fibrosis focused on determining the nature of the primary genetic defect. The ultimate goal was to determine which of the thousands of human genes was the one that, when defective, led to cystic fibrosis. Once accomplished, the next step would be to determine the normal function of this gene so that therapies designed to replace this function could be developed.

The classic approach to studying any genetic phenomenon involves mapping the gene. First, it must be determined which of a human's twenty-three chromosomes contains the DNA that makes up the gene. By studying the inheritance of the disease, along with other human traits, the gene was located on chromosome number 7. To localize the gene more precisely, however, modern molecular techniques had to be applied. Success came when two independent groups announced that they had identified the location of the gene in 1989. The groups were led by Lap-Chee Tsui of the Hospital for Sick Children in Toronto, Canada, and Francis Collins of the University of Michigan in Ann Arbor. The groups not only located the exact chromosomal location of the gene but also purified the gene from the vast amount of DNA in a human cell so that it could be studied in isolation. Then the structure of the normal form of the gene

was compared to the DNA structure found in individuals with the disease.

DNA from more than thirty thousand individuals with cystic fibrosis was analyzed, and to the surprise of most, more than 230 differences between these defective cystic fibrosis genes and normal genes were found. Although about 70 percent of the affected individuals did have a single type of DNA difference or mutation, the other 30 percent had a tremendous variety of differences. Thus unlike sickle-cell anemia, which seems to be attributable to the same defect in every affected individual, cystic fibrosis is a widely varying group of differences, which accounts for the range in severity of its symptoms. More important, this enormous diversity of defects makes developing a single, simple DNA-based screening procedure difficult. The only thing that all these individuals had in common was that, in each case, the same gene and gene product were affected.

Tsui's and Collins' groups, as well as several others, tried to determine the normal function of the protein that was coded by the cystic fibrosis gene. This protein was called cystic fibrosis transmembrane-conductance regulator (CFTR) because it was soon shown to create a channel or passage by which cells move chloride ions across their membranes. In an individual afflicted with cystic fibrosis, this channel does not work properly; both the salt and the water balance of the affected cell, and ultimately of the whole tissue, is disturbed. The thick mucus buildup in the lungs is a direct consequence of this disturbance, as is the higher-than-normal salt concentration in the patient's perspiration.

Remarkably, CFTR is an enormous protein that is embedded in the membrane of cells found in the lungs, pancreas, and the reproductive tracts. CFTR contains 1,480 amino acids linked end to end. The CFTR found in 70 percent of individuals with cystic fibrosis contains the same amino acids as normal genes, with one exception: The 508th amino acid found in a normal individual is missing. Thus, the extensive debilitating symptoms of this disease result from the mere omission of one amino acid from a long chain containing 1,479 identical ones. The other mutations affect different parts of this protein and, in all cases, reduce the ability of the CFTR protein to carry out its normal function.

In the cases of several other genetic diseases, screening programs have been developed to help patients make informed choices about having children. For Tay-Sachs disease, a fatal neurological disease found in 1 in 3,600 Ashkenazi Jews, a screening program coupled with a strong educational program has combined to reduce the incidence of the disease from approximately 100 births a year in the 1970's to an average of 13 by the early 1980's. Similar screening programs have been developed for a rare genetic disease called phenylketonuria (PKU). A screening program for cystic fibrosis, however, would be much more difficult for several reasons.

First, the population at risk for cystic fibrosis is much larger; hence the costs and scope of the program would be enormous. Second, since there are many different mutations that can affect the gene responsible for causing cystic fibrosis, it may not be easy to develop a simple test which could detect this enormous variation accurately without missing affected individuals or falsely concluding that some normal individuals are affected. Finally, the symptoms shown by individuals affected with cystic fibrosis range from quite severe to nearly normal, thus making it even more difficult to provide definitive genetic counseling. For such counseling to be truly effective, large numbers of individuals from groups known to be at risk for the disease would have to undergo screening and counseling. Furthermore, a prenatal diagnostic test would need to be available to allow couples at risk to ascertain with some degree of certainty whether any particular child is going to be born with the disease. Developing these tests and coupling them with widely available, low-cost counseling remain major challenges to the medical community.

Therapies for cystic fibrosis, like those of any genetic disease, once consisted solely of ways to treat the symptoms. Since every cell in the affected individual lacked a particular metabolic function as a result of the disease, there was no easy way to replace these functions. For cystic fibrosis, this problem was exacerbated by the lack of understanding of the primary defect. The work of Tsui's and Collins' teams allowed a more direct assault on the actual defect. Gene therapy involves either replacing a defective gene with a normal one in affected cells, or adding an additional copy or copies of the normal gene to affected cells, in an attempt to restore the same functional enzymes and thus reestablish a normal metabolic process. In the case of cystic fibrosis, animal studies have shown that it is possible to produce normal lung function when either genes or genetically engineered viruses containing normal genes are sprayed into the lungs of affected animals. Yet since there is no similar direct route for getting engineered viruses or purified genes to the pancreas or reproductive system, because of their location deep within the body, other procedures will need to be developed. In the case of the lung cells, only those cells that actually receive the purified gene change, becoming normal. Since the cells lining the lung are continuously being replenished, lung gene therapy would need to be an ongoing process.

PERSPECTIVE AND PROSPECTS

Patients with the symptoms of cystic fibrosis were first described in medical records dating back to the eighteenth century. The disease was initially called mucoviscidosis and later cystic fibrosis of the pancreas. It was not clear that these symptoms were related to a single specific disease, however, until the work of Dorothy Anderson of Columbia University in the late 1930's. Anderson studied a large number of cases of persons who died with similar lung and pancreas problems. She noticed that siblings were sometimes affected and thus suspected that the disease had a genetic cause. Anderson was responsible for naming the disease on the basis of the fibrous cysts on the pancreas that she often saw in autopsies performed on affected individuals.

In the United States, cystic fibrosis is the most prevalent lethal genetic disease among Caucasians. Estimates vary, but most are in the range of 1 affected child in every 2,000 births. In the early 1990's, there were approximately 25,000 affected Americans and more than 50,000 affected people worldwide. The incidence of cystic fibrosis among Asian American or African American populations is considerably lower, ranging from 1 in 17,000 births for African Americans and less than 1 in 80,000 births for certain Asian American groups. What is particularly striking about this disease is that approximately 1 in 25 Caucasians is a carrier. Such individuals do not show disease symptoms but can have affected children if they marry another carrier.

Since this rate is so high, a premium has been placed on the development of inexpensive and accurate diagnostic procedures, which along with good genetic counseling, could greatly reduce the incidence of cystic fibrosis in the population. Yet, since carriers are perfectly normal and often do not realize that they are indeed carrying the gene, conventional genetic counseling cannot easily reduce the incidence of the mutation in human populations at risk. Only the widespread use of a DNA-based diagnostic procedure could serve to identify the large population of carriers, but even then, since three-fourths of the children of a marriage between two carriers would be normal, counseling would be fraught with severe ethical problems. Why such a deleterious gene remains in such high frequencies in the population remains a mystery. —*Joseph G. Pelliccia, Ph.D.*

See also Birth defects; Coughing; Genetic counseling; Genetic diseases; Lungs; Respiration.

FOR FURTHER INFORMATION:

Boat, T. F., M. J. Welsh, and A. L. Beaudet. "Cystic Fibrosis." In *The Metabolic Basis of Inherited Disease.* 6th ed. New York: McGraw-Hill, 1989. Offers a full description of how the primary defect in chloride ion transport leads to the various symptoms associated with cystic fibrosis.

Garber, Edward B., ed. *Genetic Perspectives in Biology and Medicine.* Chicago: University of Chicago Press, 1985. Clearly written essays that cover some of the basic issues of human genetics, genetic disease, birth defects, and the molecular diagnosis of genetic disease.

Harris, Ann, and Maurice Super. *Cystic Fibrosis: The Facts.* 2d ed. Oxford, England: Oxford University Press, 1991. An excellent overview of the disease, its symptoms, and its treatment in a readable text.

Pierce, Benjamin A. *The Family Genetic Sourcebook.* New York: John Wiley & Sons, 1990. Contains good background reading on genetics and genetic diseases. Cystic fibrosis is not the main focus of the text, but it is discussed.

Tsui, Lap-Chee. "Cystic Fibrosis, Molecular Genetics." In *The Encyclopedia of Human Biology*, edited by Renato Dulbecco. Vol. 2. New York: Academic Press, 1991. The pursuit of the cystic fibrosis gene is documented, along with some discussion of the function of the CFTR. Readable by someone with a strong high school science background.

U.S. Congress. Office of Technology Assessment. *Cystic Fibrosis and DNA Tests: Implications of Carrier Screening*. OTA-BA-532. Washington, D.C.: Government Printing Office, 1992. An excellent overview of the scientific, ethical, social, economic, and political issues involved with screening for cystic fibrosis or for any genetic disease.

_____. *Genetic Counseling and Cystic Fibrosis Carrier Screening: Results of a Survey-Background Paper*. OTA-BP-BA-97. Washington, D.C.: Government Printing Office, 1992. A survey that looks at issues related to genetic screening for cystic fibrosis.

CYSTITIS

DISEASE/DISORDER

ANATOMY OR SYSTEM AFFECTED: Bladder, urinary system

SPECIALTIES AND RELATED FIELDS: Bacteriology, gynecology, urology

DEFINITION: An inflammation of the bladder, primarily caused by bacteria and resulting in pain, a sense of urgency to urinate, and sometimes hematuria (blood in the urine).

KEY TERMS:

cytoscopy: a minor operation performed so that the urologist can examine the bladder

dysuria: painful urination, usually as a result of infection or an obstruction; the patient complains of a burning sensation when voiding

Escherichia coli: bacteria found in the intestines that may cause disease elsewhere

hematuria: the abnormal presence of blood in the urine

perineum: the short bridge of flesh between the anus and vagina in women and the anus and base of the penis in men

ureters: the two tubes that carry urine from the kidneys to the bladder

urethra: the tube carrying urine from the bladder to outside the body

CAUSES AND SYMPTOMS

The term "cystitis" is a combination of two Greek words: *kistis*, meaning hollow pouch, sac, or bladder, and *itis* meaning inflammation. Cystitis is often used generically to refer to any nonspecific inflammation of the lower urinary tract. Specifically, however, it should be used to refer to

inflammation and infection of the bladder. Three true symptoms denote cystitis: dysuria, frequent urination, and hematuria. In a given year, about two million people are afflicted with cystitis; most of them are women. Fifteen percent of those affected will be struck again.

The symptoms of cystitis may appear abruptly and, often, painfully. One of the trademark symptoms signaling an onset is dysuria (burning or stinging during urination). It may precede or coincide with an overwhelming urge to urinate, and very frequently, although the amount passed may be extremely small. In addition some sufferers may experience nocturia (sleep disturbance because of a need to urinate). In many cases there may be pus in the urine. Origination of hematuria (blood in the urine), which often occurs with cystitis, may be within the bladder wall, in the urethra, or even in the upper urinary tract. These painful symptoms should be enough to spur one to seek medical attention; if left untreated, the bacteria may progress up the ureters to the kidneys, where a much more serious infection may develop. Pyelonephritis can cause scarring of the kidney tissue and even life-threatening kidney failure. Usually kidney infections are accompanied by chills, high fever, nausea and/or vomiting, and back pain that may radiate downward.

Acute cystitis can be divided into two groups. One is when infection occurs with irregularity and with no recent history of antibiotic treatments. This type is commonly caused by the bacteria *Escherichia coli*. Types of bacteria other than *E. coli* that can cause cystitis are *Proteus*,

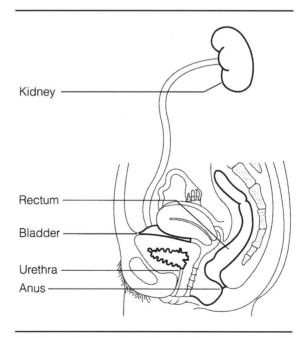

Cystitis, an inflammation of the bladder, may progress to the kidneys if left untreated.

Klebsiella, *Pseudomonas*, *Streptococcus*, *Enterobacter*, and, rarely, *Staphylococcus*. The second group of sufferers have undergone antibiotic treatment; those bacteria not affected by the antibiotics can cause infection. Most urinary tract infections are precipitated by the patient's own rectal flora. Once bacteria enter the bladder, whether they will cause infection depends on how many bacteria invade the bladder, how well the bacteria can adhere to the bladder wall, and how strongly the bladder can defend itself. The bladder's inherent defense system is the most important of the factors.

One of the natural defense mechanisms employed by the bladder is the flushing provided by regular urination at frequent intervals. If fluid intake is sufficient—most urologists consider this amount to be eight 8-ounce glasses daily—there will be regular and efficient emptying of the bladder, which can wash away the bacteria that have entered. This large volume of fluid also helps dilute the urine, thereby decreasing bacterial concentration. Another defense mechanism is the low pH of the bladder, which also helps control bacterial multiplication. It may be, too, that the bladder lining employs some means to repel bacteria and to inhibit their adherence to the wall. Others theorize that genetic, hormonal, and immune factors may help determine the defensive capability of the bladder.

Many women experience their first episode of cystitis as they become sexually active. So-called honeymoon cystitis, that related to sexual activity, comes about because intercourse may massage bacteria into the bladder, as can repeated thrusts of the penis, penetration of the vagina by fingers or other objects, or manual stimulation of the clitoris. Bacteria are boosted into and forced upward through the urethra. Also, a change in position—from back to front but not from front to back—may precede an attack of cystitis. When intercourse from the rear occurs, the penis may be contaminated with bacteria from the anal region, which then are transferred to the urethra. From the urethra, it is a short trip to the bladder for the bacteria. Unless they are voided upon conclusion of intercourse, they may multiply, causing inflammation and infection. Sex late in the day may be particularly hazardous if the perineal area has not been thoroughly cleansed after a bowel movement. Bathing after intercourse is too late to prevent the *E. coli* from being pushed into the urethral opening. Some instances of cystitis may be reduced if there is adequate vaginal lubrication prior to intercourse and avoidance of vaginal sprays and douches.

Women who use a diaphragm as birth control are more than twice as likely to develop urinary tract infections than other sexually active women. The reason for this increased likelihood may be linked to the more alkaline vaginal environment in diaphragm users, or perhaps to the spring in the rim of the diaphragm that exerts pressure on the tissue around the urethra. Urine flow may be restricted, and the stagnant urine is a good harbor for bacterial growth.

When urine remains in the bladder for an extended period of time, its stagnation may allow for the rapid growth of bacteria, thereby leading to cystitis. Besides the use of a diaphragm, urine flow may be restricted by an enlarged prostate or pregnancy. Diabetes mellitus may also lead to cystitis, as the body's resistance to infection is lowered. Infrequent voiding for whatever reason is associated with a greater likelihood of cystitis.

Less frequently, cases have been linked to vaginitis as a result of *Monilia* or *Trichomonas*. Yeasts such as these change the pH of the vaginal fluid, which will allow and even encourage bacterial growth in the perineal region. Sometimes, it is an endless cycle: A patient takes antibiotics for cystitis, which kills her protective bacteria and allows the overgrowth of yeasts. The yeasts cause vaginitis, which may promote another case of cystitis, and the cycle continues. In fact, recurrent cystitis may be a result of an inappropriate course of antibiotic treatment; the antibiotic is not specific to the bacteria. More rarely, recurrent cases may be a result of constant seeding by the kidneys or a bowel fistula. The most common cause of recurrent cystitis, however, is new organisms from the rectal area that invade the perineal area. This new pool may be inadvertently changed by antibiotic treatment.

A less common but often more severe kind of cystitis is interstitial cystitis, an inflammation of the bladder caused by nonbacterial causes, such as an autoimmune or allergic response. With this type of cystitis, there may be inflammation and/or ulceration of the bladder, which may result in scarring. These problems usually cause frequent and painful urination and possible hematuria. What separates interstitial cystitis from acute cystitis is that it primarily strikes women in their early to mid-forties and that, while urine output is normal, soon after urination, the urge to void again is overwhelming. Delaying urination may cause a pink tinge to appear in the urine. This minimal bleeding is most often a result of an overly small bladder being stretched so that minute tears in the bladder wall bleed into the urine. This form is often hard to diagnose, as the symptoms may be mild or severe and may appear and disappear or be constant.

Treatment and Therapy

Medical students are typically underprepared to deal with the numerous cases of cystitis. The student is told to test urine for the presence of bacteria, prescribe a ten-day course of antibiotics, sometimes take a kidney X ray and/or perform a cytoscopy, and then perhaps prescribe more antibiotics. If the patient continues to complain, perhaps a painful dilation of the urethra or cauterizing (burning away) of the inflamed skin is performed. None of these procedures guarantees a cure.

Diagnosis of cystitis should be relatively easy; however, in a number of cases it is misdiagnosed because the doctor has failed to identify the type of bacteria, the patient's history of past cases, and possible links between cystitis and life factors (sexual activity, contraceptive method, and diet, for example). A more appropriate antibiotic given at this point might lower the risks of frequent recurrences. Diagnosis of urinary tract infection takes into account the medical history, a physical examination of the patient, and performance of special tests. The history begins with the immediate complaints of the patient and is completed with a look back at the same type of infections that the patient has had from childhood to the present. The physician should conduct urinalysis but be cognizant that, if the urine is not examined at the right time, the bacteria may not have survived and thus a false-negative reading may occur.

One special test, a cytoscopy, is used to diagnose some of the special characteristics of cystitis. These include redness of the bladder cells, enlarged capillaries with numerous small hemorrhages, and in cases of severe cystitis, swelling of bladder tissues. Swelling may be so pronounced that it partially blocks the urethral opening, making incomplete emptying of the bladder likely to occur. Pus pockets may be visible.

In a woman who first experiences cystitis when she becomes sexually active, the doctor usually instructs the patient to be alert to several details. She should wash or shower before intercourse and be warned that contraceptive method and position during intercourse may increase her chances of becoming infected. To decrease the chance of introducing the contamination of bowel flora to the urethra, wiping after urination and defecation from front to back is advised.

Children are not immune to attacks of cystitis; in fact, education at an early age may aid children in lowering their chances of developing cystitis. Some of the following may be culprits in causing cystitis and maintaining a hospitable environment for bacteria to grow: soap or detergent that is too strong, too much fruit juice, overuse of creams and ointments, any noncotton underwear, shampoo in the bath water, bubble bath, chlorine from swimming pools, and too little fluid intake. Once children reach the teenage years, many of the above remain causes. Added to them are failure to change underwear daily, irregular periods, use of tampons, and the use of toiletries and deodorants. Careful monitoring of these conditions can greatly reduce the risk of recurrent infections.

The symptoms of cystitis are often urgent and painful enough to alert a sufferer to visit a physician as quickly as possible. Such a visit not only makes the patient feel better but also decreases the chances that the bacteria will travel toward and even into the kidney, causing pyelonephritis. Antibiotic therapy is the typical mode of treating acute or bacterial cystitis. The antibiotics chosen should reach a high concentration in the urine, should not cause the proliferation of drug-resistant bacteria, and should not kill helpful bacteria. Some antibiotics used to treat first-time sufferers of cystitis with a high success rate (80 to 100 percent) are

TMP-SMX, sulfisoxazole, amoxycillin, and ampicillin. Typically, a three-day course of therapy not only will see the patient through the few days of symptoms but, also will not change bowel flora significantly. When *E. coli* cause acute cystitis, there is a greater than 80 percent chance that one dose of an antibiotic such as penicillin will effectively end the bout, and again, the bowel flora will not be upset. Such antibiotics, when chosen carefully by the physician to match the bacteria, are useful in treating cystitis because they act very quickly to kill the bacteria. Sometimes, enough bacteria can be killed in one hour that the symptoms begin to abate immediately.

Yet antibiotics are not without their drawbacks: They may cause nausea, loss of appetite, dizziness, diarrhea, and fatigue and may increase the likelihood of yeast infections. The most common problem is the one posed by antibiotics that destroy all bacteria of the body. When the body's normal bacteria are gone, yeasts may proliferate in the body's warm, moist places. In one of the areas, the vagina, vaginitis causes a discharge which can seep into the urethra. The symptoms of cystitis may begin all over again.

For those suffering from recurrent cystitis, the treatment usually is a seven- to ten-day course of antibiotic treatment that will clear the urine of pus, indicating that the condition should be cured. If another bout recurs fairly soon, it is probably an indication that treatment was ended too quickly, as the infective bacteria were still present. To ensure that treatment has been effective, the urine must be checked and declared sterile.

Because cystitis is so common, and because many are frustrated by the inadequacies of treatment, self-treatment has become very popular. Self-treatment does not cure the infection but certainly makes the patient more comfortable while the doctor cultures a urine specimen, determines the type of bacteria causing the infection, and prescribes the appropriate antibiotic. Monitoring the first signs that a cystitis attack is imminent can save a victim from days of intense pain.

Those advocating home treatment do not all agree, however, on the means and methods that reduce suffering. All agree that once those first sensations are felt, the sufferer should start to drink water or water-based liquids; there is some disagreement on whether this intake should include fruit juice, especially cranberry juice. Some believe that the high acidic content of the juice may act to kill some of the bacteria, while others believe that the acid will only decrease the pH of the urine, causing more intense burnings as the acidic urine passes through the inflamed urethra. Through an increased fluid intake, more copious amounts of urine are produced. The excess urine acts to leach the bacteria from the bladder and, by diluting the urine, decreases its normal acidity. More dilute urine will relieve much of the burning discomfort during voiding. If a small amount of sodium bicarbonate is added to the water, it will aid in alkalinizing the urine. The best self-treatment is to drink one cup of water every twenty minutes for three hours; after this period, the amount can be decreased. A teaspoonful of bicarbonate every hour for three or four hours is safe (unless the person suffers from blood pressure problems or a heart condition). Additionally, the patient may wish to take a painkiller, such as acetaminophen. If lifestyle permits, resting will enhance the cure, especially if a heating pad is used to soothe the back or stomach. After the frequent visits to the toilet, cleaning the perineal area carefully can reduce continued contamination.

Diagnosis of interstitial cystitis can only be made using a cytoscope. Since the cause is not bacterial, antibiotics are not effective in treating this type of cystitis. To enhance the healing process of an inflamed or ulcerated bladder as a result of interstitial cystitis, the bladder may be distended and the ulcers cauterized; both procedures are done under anesthesia. Corticosteroids may be prescribed to help control the inflammation.

PERSPECTIVE AND PROSPECTS

Writings throughout history indicate that people have always suffered from bladder problems, including cystitis, although the prevalence probably was not as high. The first urologists likely were the Hindus of the Vedic era, about 1500 B.C. They were considered experts in removing bladder stones and relieving obstructions of the urinary tract.

The recorded incidence of cystitis was possibly lower because the topic would have been taboo; women in particular would not have mentioned the problem. Couples of generations past would not have participated in intercourse as frequently; both sexes wore so many clothes and had so many children underfoot or servants around that daytime sexual activity would have been rare. Without contraception, intercourse was often for procreation; once there were several children, the couple might choose to inhabit separate bedrooms. Life spans were clearly shorter; women frequently died in childbirth. Thus, the primary causes of cystitis were not common until the twentieth century.

Those forebears did not have antibiotics, but apparently those who suffered from cystitis recovered. The treatment they did use, though, has some merit. They drank copious amounts of herb teas—chamomile, mint, and parsley. They probably added some belladonna for pain relief. All this fluid would have served to help quench the "fire." It would also have had the benefit of helping flush the bacteria from the bladder.

Infection in males is far less frequent than in females; in fact, cystitis occurs ten times more often in females than in males, and it affects about 30 percent of women at some time in their lives. Unfortunately, most urologists are versed in male problems. Female specialists, gynecologists, treat the reproductive system but may not have studied female urinary dysfunction. If a male suffers from urinary dysfunction, he should seek the services of a urologist. A woman who has interstitial cystitis should also see a urologist, specifically one who knows about this form of cystitis. If a female is experiencing recurrent cystitis, she is probably already seeing a gynecologist or an internist; however, if she is not getting relief, she should avail herself of a urologist, especially one specializing in female urology, if possible.

A strong social stigma is associated with bladder dysfunction, which may create an obstacle when treatment is necessary. From the time of infancy, some children are taught that anything to do with bladder or bowel function is shameful or dirty. Therefore, when dysfunction occurs, self-esteem may be decreased. As a result, the sufferer may fail to ask for help. Such a reaction must be overcome if there is to be significant progress in treating and conquering cystitis.   —*Iona C. Baldridge*

See also Antibiotics; Bacterial infections; Urethritis; Urinalysis; Urinary disorders; Urinary system; Urology; Urology, pediatric.

FOR FURTHER INFORMATION:

Chalker, Rebecca, and Kristene E. Whitmore. *Overcoming Bladder Disorders*. New York: HarperCollins, 1990. This book was written to inform the general public about bladder disorders. It is meant to aid in diagnosis and in the selection of the right physician. Diagrams and a glossary help make this work easy to read.

Dalton, John R., and Erick J. Bergquist. *Urinary Tract Infections*. London: Croom Helm, 1987. One of a series written to update clinicians' and epidemiologists' knowledge of urinary infections. Included are clinical, epidemiological, and bacteriological aspects of infection that can be used for diagnosis and treatment. To understand this text, some knowledge of the subject is helpful.

Gillespie, Larrian, with Sandra Blakeslee. *You Don't Have to Live with Cystitis*. Rev. and updated ed. New York: Avon Books, 1996. A popular work on cystitis and women's health.

Kilmartin, Angela. *Cystitis*. New York: Warner Books, 1980. A layperson's view of coping with cystitis. This easy-to-read book takes the reader through the steps that can help assuage and control recurring attacks of cystitis. Many case histories are quoted, and the seeking of knowledgeable medical help is strongly advised.

Memmler, Ruth Lundeen, Barbara J. Cohen, and Dena L. Wood. *The Human Body in Health and Disease*. 7th ed. Philadelphia: J. B. Lippincott, 1992. This textbook offers a clear presentation of how human systems maintain homeostasis through their interactions. Integral to the discussion of each system is a detailed list of the conditions that produce disease.

Yalla, Subbarao V., Edward J. McGuire, Ahmed Elbadawi, and Jerry G. Blaivas, eds. *Neurourology and Urodynamics*. New York: Macmillan, 1988. A complicated volume compiled to answer specific questions regarding urodynamics. The sections are designed to lead one from physiology through diagnostic tools and treatment. Not for the general reader.

CYSTOSCOPY
PROCEDURE

ANATOMY OR SYSTEM AFFECTED: Bladder, urinary system

SPECIALTIES AND RELATED FIELDS: Urology

DEFINITION: The internal examination of the bladder with a long, thin optical instrument is called cystoscopy. Chronic bladder infections, interstitial cystitis, bladder stones, polyps, and suspected cancer are all conditions that may necessitate an internal examination of the bladder by cystoscopy. In this procedure, the lubricated cystoscope, a thin, straight instrument with a viewing camera at its tip, is passed through the urethra into the bladder. Sterile water is run through the instrument to fill the bladder. The entire membranous lining of the organ is visible to the surgeon through manipulation of the cystoscope within the bladder. Local diagnosis of the problem can be made, and the presence of the cystoscope allows additional procedures to be conducted, such as the crushing of bladder stones by forceps that have been inserted through the cystoscope and the taking of tissue for microscopic analysis. Cystoscopy is usually conducted under local anesthesia.

—Karen E. Kalumuck, Ph.D.

See also Cystectomy; Cystitis; Endoscopy; Pediatrics; Stone removal; Stones; Urinalysis; Urinary system; Urology; Urology, pediatric.

CYSTS AND GANGLIONS
DISEASE/DISORDER

ANATOMY OR SYSTEM AFFECTED: Breasts, glands, joints, kidneys, muscles, musculoskeletal system, nerves, nervous system, reproductive system, skin, urinary system, uterus

SPECIALTIES AND RELATED FIELDS: dermatology, gastroenterology, gynecology, nephrology, neurology

DEFINITION: A cyst is a swelling or nodule containing fluid or soft material that results from a blocked duct from a gland or abnormal growth in tissue that produces fluid. Cysts can occur in any tissue of the body. When surrounding a tendon, usually in the wrists, fingers, or feet, they are called ganglions. Cysts in the skin form when sebaceous glands become blocked. Ganglions and sebaceous cysts are benign but may be removed surgically if they become painful or unsightly. Such swellings occurring in body organs, where fluid cannot escape, may be more serious. For example, polycystic ovaries are enlarged from the presence of hundreds of tiny cysts, which can rupture and cause considerable pain. Polycystic kidney disease is a fatal condition.

—Jason Georges and Tracy Irons-Georges

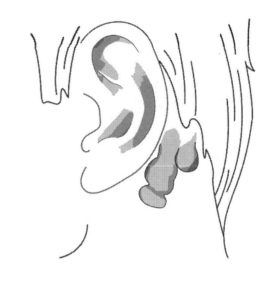

Cysts can occur in any tissue of the body; common sebaceous cysts may appear, among other places, behind the ears and at the base of the neck.

See also Abscess removal; Abscesses; Acne; Ganglion removal; Kidney disorders; Kidneys; Ovarian cysts; Pimples; Reproductive system; Skin; Skin disorders; Tendon disorders.

CYTOLOGY
SPECIALTY

ANATOMY OR SYSTEM AFFECTED: Cells, immune system

SPECIALTIES AND RELATED FIELDS: Bacteriology, hematology, histology, immunology, oncology, pathology, serology

DEFINITION: The study of the appearance of cells, usually with the aid of a microscope, in order to diagnose diseases.

KEY TERMS:

cell: a tiny baglike structure within which the basic functions of the body are carried out

chromosomes: rodlike cell parts made up of the genes that are the blueprints for every feature of the body; located in the nucleus of almost all cells

electron: a tiny particle with an electronic charge; a component of an atom

enzyme: a protein that is able to speed up a particular chemical reaction in the body

membranes: sheetlike structures that enclose each cell and separate the various organelles from one another

nucleus: the "control center" of plant and animal cells; a large spherical mass occupying up to one-third of the volume of a typical cell

organelles: specialized parts of cells

pathologist: a physician who is specially trained to use cytology and related methods to diagnose disease

protein: an abundant kind of molecule found in cells; proteins have many functions, from acting as enzymes to forming mechanical structures such as tendons and hair

SCIENCE AND PROFESSION

Cytology is the study of the appearance of cells, the fundamental units that make up all living organisms. Cells are complex structures constructed from many different subcomponents that must work together in a precisely regulated fashion. Each cell must also cooperate with neighboring cells within the organism. A cell is like a complex automobile: many separate components must be synchronized, and the cell (or car) must follow a strict order of function in order to coordinate successfully with its neighbors. Because illness results from the malfunction of cells, physicians must be able to measure key cell functions accurately. The normal and abnormal function of cells can be evaluated in many different ways; cytology is the study of cells using microscopes. A sophisticated collection of cytological techniques is available to pathologists, with which a precise diagnosis of cellular malfunction is possible.

All cells share several basic features. They are surrounded by a membrane, a flexible, sheetlike structure which encloses the fluid contents of the cell but allows required materials to move into the cell and waste products to move out of it. The complex salty fluid contained by the membrane is the cytoplasm; the other subcomponents of the cell, called organelles, are suspended in this substance. Each cell contains a set of genes, located on chromosomes, which function as blueprints for all other structures of the cell; the genes are inherited from one's parents. In plant and animal cells, the chromosomes are contained in a prominent organelle called the nucleus, which is surrounded by its own membrane inside the cell. Cells must also have a collection of enzymes used to convert food into energy in order to power the cell. In the cells of animals and plants, these enzymes are packaged into organelles called mitochondria. Membranes, the nucleus, and the mitochondria are the most prominent parts of a cell that are visible in the microscope, but cells also contain a variety of other specialized parts that are required for them to function properly. In addition, cells can also export (secrete) a variety of materials. For example, secreted materials make up bone, cartilage, tendons, mucus, sweat, and saliva.

Despite these basic features, the different types of cells have very distinct appearances. The cells of bacteria, plants, and animals are easily distinguishable from one another in the microscope. Bacterial cells are simplified, lacking organized nuclei and mitochondria. Different kinds of bacteria can be precisely distinguished in the microscope; for example, strep throat is caused by spherical bacteria that form chains, like beads of a necklace. Some dangerous bacteria can be colored with dyes that do not stain harmless bacteria. Because so many human diseases are caused by bacteria, highly accurate procedures have been developed for their identification.

The adult human body is made up of several trillion individual cells. Although much larger than bacteria, all of these are far too small to be seen with the naked eye (typically about 20 microns in diameter). Each organ of the body—the brain, liver, kidney, skin, and so on—is made up of several kinds of cells, specialized for particular functions. They must cooperate closely: Mistakes in the activities of any of these many cells can cause disease. A pathologist is able to recognize small changes in the appearance of each of many different cell types.

A few of the characteristic cell types in the human body include nerve, muscle, secretory, and epithelial cells. Nerve cells are designed to pass information throughout the nervous system. The nerve cells function much like electrical wires, so they have slender wirelike extensions that can be several feet long. Defects in the wiring circuits, for example in patients with Alzheimer's disease, can be readily detected. Muscle cells are easily identified because they are elongated cylinders packed with special fibers that cause muscular contraction. Secretory cells produce and release such substances as digestive enzymes. Such cells are often filled with membrane-bound packets of their specialized product, ready to be released from the cell. The skin and the surfaces of various internal organs are encased in a cell type called epithelium. Epithelial cells are tilelike and are often fastened tightly to neighboring epithelial cells by special kinds of connectors. Numerous other specialized cell types are found in the body as well, but these four types represent the most common cell designs.

Cells are sophisticated and delicate structures that carry out specific functions efficiently. The structure and function of normal cells are stable and predictable. If significant numbers of cells are somehow damaged, disease is the result. Such defective cells change in their appearance in characteristic ways. Therefore, cytology is an important element in the diagnosis of many diseases and for monitoring the cellular response to therapy.

Many different types of stress can cause cell damage. One of the most common stresses is oxygen deprivation, known as hypoxia. Even a brief interruption of oxygen can cause irreversible damage to cells because it is needed for energy production. Since oxygen is transported in the blood, the most common cause of hypoxia is loss of blood supply, which can occur with blockage by blood clots or narrowed blood vessels and with several kinds of lung or heart problems. Carbon monoxide poisoning results from interference with the blood's ability to absorb and carry oxygen, while the poison cyanide interferes with a cell's ability to make use of oxygen.

Poisons such as cyanide can damage cells in many other

ways, as can drugs. Prolonged use of barbiturates or alcohol can damage liver cells. These cells are also sensitive to common chemicals such as carbon tetrachloride, one used widely as a household cleaning agent. The liver is where foreign chemicals are changed to harmless forms, which explains why the liver cells are often damaged. Even useful chemicals, however, can cause harm to cells in some circumstances. Constant high levels of glucose, a sugar used by all cells, may overwork certain cells of the pancreas to the point where they become defective. Some foods (especially fats) and certain food additives, if they are eaten in excess, can interfere with how cells work.

Physical damage to cells—caused, for example, by blows to the body—can dislocate parts of cells, preventing their proper coordination. Extreme cold can interfere with the blood supply, causing hypoxia; extreme heat can cause cells to speed up their rate of metabolism, again exceeding the oxygen-carrying capacity of the circulatory system. The "bends," the affliction suffered by surfacing deep-sea divers, results from tiny bubbles of nitrogen that block capillaries. Various kinds of radiant energy, such as radioactivity or ultraviolet light, can damage specific chemicals of cells, causing them to malfunction. Electrical energy generates extreme local heat within the body, which can damage cells directly.

Many small living organisms can interfere with cellular function as well. Viruses are effective parasites of cells, using cells for their own survival. This relationship can result in cell death, as in poliomyelitis; in depressed cell function, as in viral hepatitis; or in abnormal cell growth, as in some cancers. Bacteria can also live as parasites, releasing toxins that interfere with cellular function in a variety of ways. Malaria is caused by a single-celled animal that damages blood cells, athlete's foot is caused by a fungus, and tiny worms called nematodes can invade cells and cause them to work improperly.

All cell types are not equally sensitive to damage by each agent. Liver cells are particularly sensitive to damage by toxic chemicals. Nerve and muscle cells are the first to be injured by hypoxia. Kidney cells are also easily damaged by loss of blood supply. Lung cells are affected by anything that is inhaled.

DIAGNOSTIC AND TREATMENT TECHNIQUES

Before cells can be successfully observed, they must be prepared through several steps. First, it is necessary to select a relatively small sample of a particular organ for closer scrutiny. Such a sample is called a biopsy when it is collected by a physician who wishes to test for a disease. The biopsy must then be preserved, or fixed, so that its parts will not deteriorate. Next, the specimen must be encased within a solid substance so that it can be handled without damage. Most often, the fixed specimen is soaked in melted paraffin, which then is allowed to solidify in a mold. For some kinds of microscopes, harder plastic materials are

used. Next, the specimen must be thinly sliced so that the internal details can be seen. The delicate slices are mounted on a support, typically a thin glass slide for light microscopy. Finally, the parts of the cell must be colored, or stained. Without this coloring, the cell parts would be transparent and thus unobservable.

The basic tool of the cytologist is the light microscope. It can magnify up to about seven hundred times. Numerous sophisticated methods are used with light microscopy. Specific stains have been developed for distinguishing the different molecules that make up cells. For example, Alcian blue is a dye that stains a type of complex sugar that accumulates outside certain abnormal cells, making it easier to identify these cells. Also, specially prepared antibodies can recognize particular proteins within cells. Disease-causing proteins, including the proteins of dangerous viruses and bacteria, can be precisely identified in this way.

A major advance in cytology is the electron microscope. It forms images in essentially the same way as a light microscope does, but using electrons rather than visible light. Because of the properties of electrons, this type of microscope can magnify tens of thousands of times beyond life size. A wide range of new cell features has been revealed with the electron microscope. The details of how genes work, how materials enter and leave cells, how energy is produced, and how molecules are synthesized have been made clearer. The steps for preparing specimens for electron microscopy are delicate, time-consuming, and demanding. Furthermore, the electron microscope itself is complex and expensive. Considerable skill is required to use it effectively. For these reasons, electron microscopy is not commonly used for routine medical diagnoses.

Cell injury causes predictable changes in cells that can be interpreted by a pathologist to suggest the underlying cause of the damage and how best to treat it. Almost all forms of reversible injury cause changes in the size and shape of cells. Cellular swelling is an obvious symptom that almost always reflects a serious underlying problem. Such cells also have a characteristic cloudy appearance. Swelling and cloudiness indicate loss of energy reserves and abnormal uptake of water into the cell through improperly functioning cell-surface membranes. An indication of serious damage is the accumulation within the cell of vacuoles—small, fluid-filled sacs that have a characteristic clear appearance when viewed through a microscope. More severe injury can cause the formation of vacuoles that contain fat, giving the cells a foamy appearance. Such damage is most often seen in cells of the heart, kidneys, and lungs. These changes appear to reflect both membrane abnormalities and the defective metabolism of fats.

Cells that are damaged beyond the point of repair will die, a process called necrosis. The two key processes in necrosis are the breakdown and mopping up of cellular contents, and large changes in structure of cellular proteins in ways that can be identified under the microscope. The most conspicuous and reliable indicators of necrosis are changes in the appearance of the nucleus, which can shrink or even break into pieces and which eventually disappears completely. Ultimately, the entire cell disappears.

Cancer provides a good illustration of how cytology is employed in the diagnosis of a specific disease. A skilled cytologist can detect cells at an early stage of cancer development and, with accuracy, can gauge how dangerous a cancer cell is or is likely to become. Cancer is a disease of abnormal growth. Cancer cells may have few abnormal features other than their improper growth; tumors made up of such cells are generally not dangerous and so are labeled benign. Malignant tumor cells, on the other hand, are highly

abnormal. They can damage and invade other parts of the body, making these cells much more dangerous.

The cells of benign tumors may have nearly the same appearance as the cells of the normal tissue from which they arose. Benign cancers of skin, bone, muscle, and nerve keep the obvious structures that allow these highly specialized cell types to carry out their normal functions. Ironically, however, continued normal function can itself become a problem, because there are too many cells producing specialized products. For example, tumors in tissues that produce hormones can result in massive excesses of such hormones, causing severe imbalances in the function of the body's organs. Malignant tumor cells, on the other hand, have lost some or all of the functional and cytological fea-

The Methods of Cytology

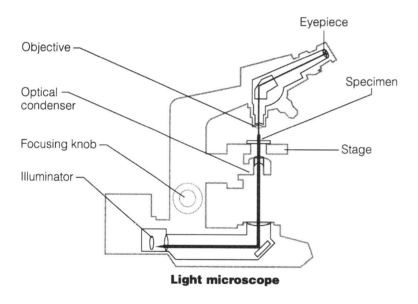

Light microscope

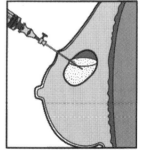

Needle aspiration

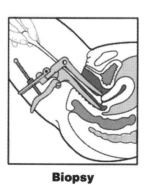

Biopsy

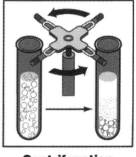

Centrifugation

Cytologists study cells in both normal and abnormal states. Cells and fluid to be examined may be obtained through biopsy, separated by centrifugation, and studied under a light microscope.

tures of their parent normal cells. They have a simpler and more primitive appearance, termed anaplasia by pathologists. The degree of anaplasia is one of the most reliable hallmarks of how malignant a cell has become.

Almost any part of the cell can become anaplastic. A common change is in the chromosomes of a cancer cell. The number, size, and shape of chromosomes change, and detailed analysis of these changes is often important in diagnosis, as in leukemia. Many malignant tumor cells secrete enzymes that attack surrounding connective tissue, changing its appearance in characteristic ways. Membrane systems of anaplastic cells are also abnormal, with serious consequences. The movement of materials in and out of cells becomes defective, and energy production mechanisms are upset, causing the characteristic changes in appearance described above. A general feature of tumors made up of anaplastic cells is the variability among individual cells. Some cells can appear virtually normal, while other tumor cells nearby can appear highly abnormal in several ways.

The cells of benign tumors remain where they arose. The cells of malignant tumors, however, have the ability to spread through the body (metastasize), penetrating and damaging other organs in the process. These abilities, to invade and metastasize, have serious effects on the rest of the body. Invading cells often can be identified easily with a microscope. Extensions of the tumor cells may reach into surrounding normal organ parts. Tumor cells can be observed penetrating into blood and lymph vessels and other body cavities, such as the abdominal cavity and air pockets in the lung. Small clusters of tumor cells can be found in blood and identified in distant organs. These cells can begin the process of invasion all over again, producing so-called secondary tumors in other organs. How malignant cancer cells can cause so much harm becomes clear.

PERSPECTIVE AND PROSPECTS

Of the diagnostic procedures that are available to physicians, cytologic techniques are among the most popular. Because the cells being examined are so tiny, the microscopes used must be able to magnify the cells enough to allow observation of their characteristics. Historically, the use of cytology in medical practice has closely paralleled the development of adequate microscopes and methods for preparing specimens.

Magnifying lenses by themselves lack the power required for observing cells. A microscope of adequate power must use several such lenses stacked together. The first crude microscopes with this design appeared late in the sixteenth century. During the next several hundred years, microscopes were mostly used to observe cells of plant material because the woody parts of plants can be thinly sliced and then observed directly, without the need for further preparation. The word "cell" was first employed by Robert Hooke (1635-1703) in a paper published in 1665. He observed small chambers in pieces of cork, which were where cells had been

located in the living cork tree. These chambers reminded Hooke of monks' cells in a monastery, hence the name.

The great anatomist Marcello Malpighi (1628-1694) may have been the first to observe mammalian cells, within capillaries. The real giant of this era, however, was the Dutch microscopist Antoni van Leeuwenhoek (1632-1723), who greatly improved the quality of microscopes and then used them to observe single-celled animals, bacteria, sperm, and the nuclei within certain blood cells. Although most progress continued to be made with plants, numerous observations accumulated during the seventeenth and eighteenth centuries which suggested that animals are made up of tiny saclike units, and Hooke's word "cell" was applied to describe them. This concept was clearly stated in 1839 by Theodor Schwann (1810-1882); his idea that all animals are composed of cells and cellular products quickly gained acceptance. At this time, however, there was essentially no comprehension of how cells work. Without an understanding of normal cell function, cytology was still of little use in identifying and understanding disease.

During the late nineteenth and early twentieth centuries, the appearance of different cell types was carefully described. The main organelles of cells were identified, and such fundamental processes as cell division were observed and understood. At last it was possible to utilize cytology for medical purposes. The principles of medical cytology were established by the great pathologist Rudolf Virchow (1821-1902), who suggested for the first time that diseases originate from changes in specific cells of the body.

Rapid progress in cytology was made in the 1940's and 1950's, for two reasons. First, improved microscopes were developed, allowing greater accuracy in observing cell structure. The second reason—rapid progress in genetics and biochemistry—greatly increased the knowledge of how cells function and of the significance of specific changes in their appearance. Because cells are the basic units of life, scientists will continue to study them in detail, and the medical world will benefit directly from further, improved understanding in this field.   —*Howard L. Hosick, Ph.D.*

See also Bacterial infections; Bacteriology; Biopsy; Blood and blood components; Blood testing; Cancer; Cells; Cytopathology; Gram staining; Hematology; Hematology, pediatric; Histology; Laboratory tests; Malignancy and metastasis; Microbiology; Microscopy; Oncology; Pathology; Serology; Urinalysis; Viral infections.

FOR FURTHER INFORMATION:

Berns, Michael W. *Cells.* 2d ed. Philadelphia: Saunders College Publishing, 1983. This small book is among the most easily read of a number of introductory surveys designed for beginning college students. Contains considerable solid information on cytology that should be understandable to the interested nonstudent. Overviews of cells and of microscopy are followed by more detailed discussions of each cell component. Well illustrated.

Cairns, John. *Cancer: Science and Society.* San Francisco: W. H. Freeman, 1978. Cancer is a common disease, and cytology is particularly important for its proper diagnosis. For the reader interested in the medical importance of cancer cytology, this eloquent but nontechnical overview should be particularly useful.

Cohn, Norman S. *Elements of Cytology.* 2d ed. New York: Harcourt, Brace and World, 1969. The classic beginning textbook in cytology. Offers a good section on various cytological methods (microscopy, fixation, staining, and others). Many useful illustrations and good photographs are included. More detailed than most readers will require, but selective reading of the straightforward text will be helpful.

Robbins, Stanley L., Ramzi S. Cotran, and Vinay Kumar, eds. *Basic Pathology.* 6th ed. Philadelphia: W. B. Saunders, 1997. Presents a reasonably concise overview of the entire field of pathology, but the emphasis is on cytology. The chapter on disease at the cellular level is excellent and readable. The authors are unusually adept at explaining the facts in a simple and interesting way. Should be of use to the reader who wishes to find more information on how cytology is used to diagnose a particular disease.

Taylor, Ron. *Through the Microscope.* Vol. 22 in *The World of Science.* New York: Facts on File, 1986. A fine introduction to the wonders of microscopy, recommended for all readers. In a large format with more than one hundred beautiful photographs. The clear, simple, and brief text explains how microscopes work and what is being seen. The section "Microscopes, Health, and Disease" is particularly relevant, explaining cytological detective work. Contains a useful glossary of cytological terms.

Wolfe, Stephen L. *Cell Ultrastructure.* Belmont, Calif.: Wadsworth, 1985. This book consists mostly of electron microscope photographs of the important structures of viruses, bacteria, and plant and animal cells. Included for most structures are three-dimensional drawings that are particularly useful for visualizing how cells are put together. The text is brief, and most of it should be understandable to the general reader.

Cytomegalovirus (CMV)

Disease/disorder

Anatomy or system affected: Blood, brain, cells, ears, eyes, gastrointestinal system, immune system, liver, lungs

Specialties and related fields: Family practice, gastroenterology, hematology, immunology, obstetrics, pediatrics, virology

Definition: A viral disease normally producing mild symptoms in healthy individuals but severe infections in the immunocompromised. Congenital infection may lead to malformations or fetal death.

Key terms:

hepatitis: inflammation of the liver; usually caused by viral infections, toxic substances, or immunological disturbances

hepatosplenomegaly: enlargement of the liver and spleen such that they may be felt below the rib margins

heterophil antibodies: antibodies that are detected using antigens other than the antigens that induced them

jaundice: yellow staining of the skin, eyes, and other tissues and excretions with excess bile pigments in the blood

latency: following an acute infection by a virus, a period of dormancy from which the virus may be reactivated during times of stress or immunocompromise

microcephaly: a congenital condition involving an abnormally small head associated with an incompletely developed brain

Causes and Symptoms

Cytomegalovirus (CMV) is a member of the herpesvirus group that includes such viruses as the Epstein-Barr virus, which causes infectious mononucleosis, and the varicella-zoster virus, which causes chickenpox. CMV is a ubiquitous virus that is transmitted in a number of different ways. A newly infected woman may transmit the virus across the placenta to her unborn child. Infection may also occur in the birth canal or via mother's milk. Young children commonly transmit CMV by means of saliva. Sexual transmission is common in adults. Blood transfusions and organ transplants may also transmit cytomegalovirus to recipients. More than 80 percent of adults worldwide have antibodies indicating exposure to cytomegalovirus.

Congenital cytomegaloviral infection is universally common and especially prevalent in developing nations. Approximately 1 percent of live births in the United States are infected. Most congenitally infected infants exhibit no symptoms. Normal development may follow, but some infants suffer problems such as deafness, visual impairment, and/or mental retardation. Approximately 10 to 20 percent exhibit clinically obvious evidence of cytomegalic inclusion disease: hepatosplenomegaly, jaundice, microcephaly, deafness, seizures, cerebral palsy, and blood disorders such as thrombocytopenia (a decrease in platelets) and hemolytic anemia (in which red blood cells are destroyed). Giant cells having nuclei containing large inclusions are found in affected organs. Cytomegalovirus is a leading cause of mental retardation and responsible for about 10 percent of cases of microcephaly.

In immunocompetent adults and older children, cytomegalovirus can cause heterophil-negative mononucleosis, an infectious mononucleosis in which no heterophil antibodies are formed. Such antibodies are found in infectious mononucleosis caused by the Epstein-Barr virus. Heterophil-negative mononucleosis is characterized by fever, hepatitis, lethargy, and abnormal lymphocytes in blood.

Severe systemic cytomegalovirus infections are frequently seen in the immunocompromised. Transplant patients are intentionally immunosuppressed to reduce the likelihood of graft rejection, making them vulnerable to infection by cytomegalovirus either by reactivation or by acquisition of the virus from the donor organ. Resulting systemic infections are manifested in diseases such as pneumonia, hepatitis, and retinitis. In addition to these CMV diseases, acquired immunodeficiency syndrome (AIDS) patients suffer from infections of the central nervous system and gastrointestinal tract. Their blood cells may also be affected, resulting in disorders such as thrombocytopenia. AIDS patients frequently have intestinal CMV infections leading to chronic diarrhea. Cytomegalovirus retinitis in AIDS patients is particularly serious and may lead to retinal detachment and blindness. This is the most common sight-damaging opportunistic eye infection found in AIDS patients.

TREATMENT AND THERAPY

Two antiviral drugs, ganciclovir and foscarnet, have been found to be moderately efficacious in the treatment of cytomegaloviral infection in the immunocompromised. Toxic properties, however, can limit their long-term administration. Ganciclovir exhibits hematopoietic toxicity; that is, it has an adverse affect on blood cells that may result in neutropenia, a decrease in the number of neutrophils in the blood. Foscarnet has more side effects than ganciclovir. It is a nephrotoxic substance, which means that it may damage the kidneys and thus cannot be used in patients with renal failure.

Both ganciclovir and foscarnet have been found to be beneficial when used as prophylaxis in transplants. Each of these drugs successfully decreases the incidence of post-transplant cytomegaloviral infection in patients receiving solid organ or bone marrow transplants. Another material employed as a prophylaxis for bone marrow and renal transplant recipients is intravenous cytomegalovirus immune globulin.

Therapy for cytomegalovirus retinitis involves intravenous treatment with either ganciclovir or foscarnet. Both drugs stop the progression of retinitis in 90 percent of cases, but if therapy is then discontinued, progressive deterioration occurs in most AIDS patients. Thus, therapy must be continued indefinitely. Further complicating treatment is the emergence of resistant strains, possibly requiring increased dosage and/or a combined dosage of both drugs.

Retinal detachment is another complication arising from cytomegalovirus retinitis. It may occur even in those undergoing successful antiviral treatment. Surgical intervention is required to restore functional vision in these cases.

PERSPECTIVE AND PROSPECTS

The term "cytomegalia" was first used in 1921 to describe the condition of an infant with intranuclear inclusions in the lungs, kidney, and liver. This condition in an adult was first attributed to a virus of the herpes group in 1925. Twenty-five

cases of apparent cytomegalic inclusion disease had been described by 1932. Cytomegalovirus was pursued and isolated in the mid-1950's by Margaret Smith in St. Louis. Around the same time, independently and serendipitously, groups in Boston and in Bethesda also isolated the virus.

Antiviral drugs such as interferon and acyclovir have been found to be ineffective in the treatment of cytomegalovirus infections. An analogue of acyclovir, ganciclovir, was shown in 1982 to be much more effective against CMV than acyclovir. Since then, foscarnet, a pyrophosphate analogue, has also proved effective in the treatment of CMV diseases in immunocompromised patients.

—Nancy Handshaw Clark, Ph.D.

See also Acquired immunodeficiency syndrome (AIDS); Birth defects; Eye surgery; Eyes; Hepatitis; Herpes; Immune system; Immunodeficiency disorders; Immunology; Mental retardation; Mononucleosis; Pregnancy and gestation; Stillbirth; Transplantation; Viral infections; Visual disorders.

FOR FURTHER INFORMATION:

Bellenir, Karen, and Peter D. Dresser, eds. *Contagious and Non-Contagious Infectious Diseases Sourcebook*. Detroit: Omnigraphics, 1996.

Roizman, Bernard, ed. *Infectious Diseases in an Age of Change*. Washington, D.C.: National Academy Press, 1995.

Roizman, Bernard, Richard J. Whitley, and Carlos Lopez, eds. *The Human Herpesviruses*. New York: Raven Press, 1993.

CYTOPATHOLOGY

SPECIALTY

ANATOMY OR SYSTEM AFFECTED: Cells, immune system

SPECIALTIES AND RELATED FIELDS: Bacteriology, cytology, forensic pathology, hematology, histology, oncology, pathology, serology

DEFINITION: The medical field that deals with changes in cell structure or physiology as a result of injuries, infectious agents, or toxic substances.

SCIENCE AND PROFESSION

The profession of cytopathology deals with the search for lesions or abnormalities within individual cells or groups of cells. Generally speaking, a pathologist is a physician trained in pathology, the study of the nature of diseases. Observations of tissue or cell lesions are utilized in the diagnosis of disease or other agents associated with damage to cells.

Cell damage may result from endogenous phenomena, including the aging process, or from exogenous agents such as biological organisms (viruses or bacteria), chemical agents (bacterial toxins or other poisons), and physical agents (heat, cold, or electricity). For example, particular biological agents produce recognizable lesions that may be useful in the diagnosis of disease, such as the crystalline structures characteristic of certain viral infections.

The type of necrosis, or cell death, encountered is useful in diagnosing the problem. For example, certain types of enzymatic dissolution of cells, which result in areas of liquefaction, are the result of bacterial infection. Gangrenous necrosis often follows the restriction of the blood supply, because of either infection or a blood clot.

Pathologic changes within the cell can also help pinpoint the time of death. Organelles degenerate at a rate dependent on their use of oxygen. For example, mitochondria, which utilize significant amounts of oxygen, are among the first organelles to degenerate.

DIAGNOSTIC AND TREATMENT TECHNIQUES

The diagnosis and treatment of cancer are prime examples of the use of cytopathology. The extent of pleomorphism in cell size and shape, irregularity of the nucleus, and presence (or absence) of organelles all provide the basis for the choice of treatment and help determine the ultimate prognosis. Specific organelles are stained with characteristic histochemicals, followed by microscopic observation. A preponderance of large, irregularly shaped cells provides for a poorer prognosis than if cells appeared more normally differentiated. The nuclei in highly malignant tumors show a greater variation in size and chromatin pattern, as compared with those of cells from benign growths. Such differences lead directly to decisions on the choice of treatment: surgical removal, chemotherapy, or radiation.

—*Richard Adler, Ph.D.*

See also Bacteriology; Biopsy; Blood and blood components; Blood testing; Cancer; Cells; Cytology; Gram staining; Hematology; Hematology, pediatric; Histology; Laboratory tests; Malignancy and metastasis; Microbiology; Microscopy; Oncology; Pathology; Serology; Toxicology; Tumors; Urinalysis.

DEATH AND DYING

DISEASE/DISORDER

ANATOMY OR SYSTEM AFFECTED: Psychic-emotional system, all bodily systems

SPECIALTIES AND RELATED FIELDS: Family practice, geriatrics and gerontology, psychology

KEY TERMS:

anticipatory depression: a depressive reaction to the awaited death of either oneself or a significant other; also called anticipatory grieving, preparatory grieving, or preparatory depression

bereavement: the general, overall process of mourning and grieving; considered to have progressive stages which include anticipation, grieving, mourning, postmourning, depression, loneliness, and reentry into society

depression: a general term covering mild states (sadness, inhibition, unhappiness, discouragement) to severe states (hopelessness, despair); typically part of normal, healthy grieving; considered the fourth stage of death and dying, between bargaining and acceptance

grief: the emotional and psychological response to loss; always painful, grieving is a type of psychological work and requires some significant duration of time

mourning: the acute phase of grief; characterized by distress, hopelessness, fear, acute loss, crying, insomnia, loss of appetite, anxiety, guilt, and restlessness

reactive depression: depression occurring as a result of overt events that have already taken place; it universally occurs in the bereaved

uncomplicated bereavement: a technical psychiatric label describing normal, average, and expectant grieving; despite an experience of great psychological pain, it is considered normal and healthy unless it continues much beyond one year

thanatology: the study and investigation of life-threatening actions, terminal illness, suicide, homicide, death, dying, grief, and bereavement

CAUSES AND SYMPTOMS

Medicine determines that death has occurred by assessing bodily functions in either of two areas. Persons with irreversible cessation of respiration and circulation are dead; persons with irreversible cessation of ascertainable brain functions are also dead. There are standard procedures used to diagnose death, including simple observation, brain-stem reflex studies, and the use of confirmatory testing such as electrocardiography (ECG or EKG), electroencephalography (EEG), and arterial blood gas analysis (ABG). The particular circumstances—anticipated or unanticipated, observed or unobserved, the patient's age, drug or metabolic intoxication, or suspicion of hypothermia—will favor some procedures over others, but in all cases both cessation of functions and their irreversibility are required before death can be declared.

Between 60 and 75 percent of all people die from chronic terminal conditions. Therefore, except in sudden death (as in a fatal accident) or when there is no evidence of consciousness (as in a head injury which destroys cerebral, thinking functions while leaving brain-stem, reflexive functions intact), dying is both a physical and a psychological process. In most cases, dying takes time, and the time allows patients to react to the reality of their own passing. Often, they react by becoming vigilant about bodily symptoms and any changes in them. They also anticipate changes that have yet to occur. For example, long before the terminal stages of illness become manifest, dying patients commonly fear physical pain, shortness of breath, invasive procedures, loneliness, becoming a burden to loved ones, losing decision-making authority, and facing the unknown of death itself.

As physical deterioration proceeds, all people cope by resorting to what has worked for them before: the unique means and mechanisms which have helped maintain a sense of self and personal stability. People seem to go through the process of dying much as they have gone through the process of living—with the more salient features of their personalities, whether good or bad, becoming sharper and more prominent. People seem to face death much as they have faced life.

Medicine has come to acknowledge that physicians should understand what it means to die. Indeed, while all persons should understand what their own deaths will mean, physicians must additionally understand how their dying patients find this meaning. Physicians who see death as the final calamity coming at the end of life, and thus primarily as something that only geriatric medicine has to face, are mistaken. Independent of beliefs about "life after life," the life process on this planet inexorably comes to an end for everyone, whether as a result of accident, injury, or progressive deterioration.

In 1969, psychiatrist Elisabeth Kübler-Ross published the landmark *On Death and Dying*, based on her work with two hundred terminally ill patients. Technologically driven, Western medicine had come to define its role as primarily dealing with extending life and thwarting death by defeating specific diseases. Too few physicians saw a role for themselves once the prognosis turned grave. In the decades that followed *On Death and Dying*, the profession has reaccepted that death and dying are part of life and that, while treating the dying may not mean extending the length of life, it can and should mean extending its quality.

Kübler-Ross provided a framework which explained how people cope with and adapt to the profound and terrible news that their illness is going to kill them. Although other physicians, psychologists, and thanatologists have shortened, expanded, and adapted her five stages of the dying process, neither the actual number of stages nor what they are specifically called is as important as the information and insight that any stage theory of dying yields. As with any human process, dying is complex, multifaceted, multi-dimensional, and polymorphic.

Well-intentioned, but misguided, professionals and family members may try to help move dying patients through each of the stages only to encounter active resentment or passive withdrawal. Patients, even dying patients, cannot be psychologically moved to where they are not ready to be. Rather than making the terminally ill die the "right" way, it is more respectful and helpful to understand any stage as a description of normal reactions to serious loss, and that these reactions normally vary among different individuals and also within the same individual over time. The reactions appear, disappear, and reappear in any order and in any combination. What the living must do is respect the unfolding of an adaptational schema which is the dying person's own. No one should presume to know how someone else should die.

COMPLICATIONS AND DISORDERS

Denial is Kübler-Ross' first stage, but it is also linked to shock and isolation. Whether the news is told outright or gradual self-realization occurs, most people react to the knowledge of their impending death with existential shock: Their whole selves recoil at the idea, and they say, in some fashion, "This cannot be happening to me. I must be dreaming." Broadly considered, denial is a complex cognitive-emotional capacity which enables temporary postponement of active, acute, but in some way detrimental, recognition of reality. In the dying process, this putting off of the truth prevents a person from being overwhelmed while promoting psychological survival. Denial plays an important stabilizing role, holding back more than could be otherwise managed while allowing the individual to marshall psychological resources and reserves. It enables patients to consider the possibility, even the inevitability, of death and then to put the consideration away so that they can pursue life in the ways that are still available. In this way, denial is truly a mechanism of defense.

Many other researchers, along with Kübler-Ross, report anger as the second stage of dying. The stage is also linked to rage, fury, envy, resentment, and loathing. When "This cannot be happening to me," becomes, "This is happening to me. There was no mistake," patients are beginning to replace denial with attempts to understand what is happening to and inside them. When they do, they often ask, "Why me?" Though logically an unanswerable question, the logic of the question is clear. People, to remain human, must try to make intelligible their experiences and reality. The asking of this question is an important feature of the way in which all dying persons adapt to and cope with the reality of death.

People react with anger when they lose something of value; they react with greater anger when something of value is taken away from them by someone or something. Rage and fury, in fact, are often more accurate descriptions of people's reactions to the loss of their own life than anger.

Anger is a difficult stage for professionals and loved ones, more so when the anger and rage are displaced and projected randomly into any corner and crevice of the patient's world. An unfortunate result is that caretakers often experience the anger as personal, and the caretakers' own feelings of guilt, shame, grief, and rejection can contribute to lessening contact with the dying person, which increases his or her sense of isolation.

Bargaining is Kübler-Ross' third stage, but it is also the one about which she wrote the least and the one that other thanatologists are most likely to leave unrepresented in their own models and stages of how people cope with dying. Nevertheless, it is a common phenomenon wherein dying people fall back on their faith, belief systems, or sense of the transcendent and the spiritual and try to make a deal—with God, life, fate, a higher power, or the composite of all the randomly colliding atoms in the universe. They ask for more time to help family members reconcile or to achieve something of importance. They may ask if they can simply attend their child's wedding or graduation or if they can see their first grandchild born. Then they will be ready to die; they will go willingly. Often, they mean that they will die without fighting death, if death can only be delayed or will delay itself. Some get what they want; others do not.

At some point, when terminally ill individuals are faced with decisions about more procedures, tests, surgeries, or medications or when their thinness, weakness, or deterioration becomes impossible to ignore, the anger, rage, numbness, stoicism, and even humor will likely give way to depression, Kübler-Ross' fourth stage and the one reaction that all thanatologists include in their models of how people cope with dying.

The depression can take many forms, for indeed there are always many losses, and each loss individually or several losses collectively might need to be experienced and worked through. For example, dying parents might ask themselves who will take care of the children, get them through school, walk them down the aisle, or guide them through life. Children, even adult children who are parents themselves, may ask whether they can cope without their own parents. They wonder who will support and anchor them in times of distress, who will (or could) love, nurture, and nourish them the way that their parents did. Depression accompanies the realization that each role, each function, will never be performed again. Both the dying and those who love them mourn.

Much of the depression takes the form of anticipatory grieving, which often occurs both in the dying and in those who will be affected most by their death. It is a part of the dying process experienced by the living, both terminal and nonterminal. Patients, family, and friends can psychologically anticipate what it will be like when the death does occur and what life will, and will not, be like afterward. The grieving begins while there is still life left to live.

Bereavement specialists generally agree that anticipatory grieving, when it occurs, seems to help people cope with what is a terrible and frightening loss. It is an adaptive psychological mechanism wherein emotional, mental, and existential stability is painfully maintained. When depression develops, not only in reaction to death but also in preparation for it, it seems to be a necessary part of how those who are left behind cope in order to survive the loss themselves. Those who advocate or advise cheering up or looking on the bright side are either unrealistic or unable to tolerate the sadness in themselves or others. The dying are in the process of losing everything and everyone they love. Cheering up does not help them; the advice to "be strong" only helps the "helpers" deny the truth of the dying experience.

Both preparatory and reactive depression are often accompanied by unrealistic self-recrimination, shame, and guilt in the dying person. Those who are dying may judge themselves harshly and criticize themselves for the wrongs that they committed and for the good that they did not accomplish. They may judge themselves to be unattractive, unappealing, and repulsive because of how the illness and its treatment have made them appear. These feelings and states of minds, which have nothing to do with the reality of the situation, are often amenable to the interventions of understanding and caring people. Disfigured breasts do not make a woman less a woman; the removal of the testes does not make a man less a man. Financial and other obligations can be restructured and reassigned. Being forgiven and forgiving can help finish what was left undone.

Kübler-Ross' fifth stage, acceptance, is an intellectual and emotional coming to terms with death's reality, permanence, and inevitability. Ironically, it is manifested by diminished emotionality and interests and increased fatigue and inner (many would say spiritual) self-focus. It is a time without depression or anger. Envy of the healthy, the fear of losing all, and bargaining for another day or week are also absent. This final stage is often misunderstood. Some see it either as resignation and giving up or as achieving a happy serenity. Some think that acceptance is the goal of dying well and that all people are supposed to go through this stage. None of these viewpoints is accurate. Acceptance, when it does occur, comes from within the dying person. It is marked more by an emotional void and psychological detachment from people and things once held important and necessary and by an interest in some transcendental value (for the atheist) or his or her God (for the theist). It has little to do with what others believe is important or "should" be done. It is when dying people become more intimate with themselves and appreciate their separateness from others more than at any other time.

PERSPECTIVE AND PROSPECTS

All patients die—a fact that the actual practice of clinical Western medicine has too often discounted. Dealing with death is difficult in life, and it is difficult in medicine. As the ultimate outcome of all medical interventions, however, it is unavoidable. Dealing with the dying and those who care about them is also difficult. Patients ask questions that cannot be answered; families in despair and anger seek to find cause and sometimes lay blame. It takes courage to be with individuals as they face their deaths, struggling to find meaning in the time that they have left. It takes special courage simply to witness this struggle in a profession which prides itself on how well it intervenes. Working with death also reminds professionals of their own inevitable death. Facing that fact inwardly, spiritually, and existentially also requires courage.

Cure and treatment become care and management in the dying. They should live relatively pain-free, be supported in accomplishing their goals, be respected, be involved in decision making as appropriate, be encouraged to function as fully as their illness allows, and be provided with others to whom control can comfortably and confidently be passed. The lack of a cure and the certainty of the end can intimidate health care providers, family members, and close friends. They may dread genuine encounters with those whose days are knowingly numbered. Yet the dying have the same rights to be helped as any of the living, and how a society assists them bears directly on the meaning that its members are willing to attach to their own lives.

Today, largely in response to what dying patients have told researchers, medicine recognizes its role to assist these patients in working toward an appropriate death. Caretakers must determine the optimum treatments, interventions, and conditions which will enable such a death to occur. For each terminally ill person, these should be unique and specific. Caretakers should respond to the patient's needs and priorities, at the patient's own pace and as much as possible following the patient's lead. For some dying patients, the goal is to remain as pain-free as is feasible and to feel as well as possible. For others, finishing whatever unfinished business remains becomes the priority. Making amends, forgiving and being forgiven, resolving old conflicts, and reconciling with self and others may be the most therapeutic and healing of interventions. Those who are to be bereaved fear the death of those they love. The dying fear the separation from all they know and love, but they fear as well the loss of autonomy, letting family and friends down, the pain and invasion of further treatment, disfigurement, dementia, loneliness, the unknown, becoming a burden, and the loss of dignity.

The English writer C. S. Lewis said that bereavement is the universal and integral part of the experience of loss. It requires effort, authenticity, mental and emotional work, a willingness to be afraid, and an openness to what is happening and what is going to happen. It requires an attitude which accepts, tolerates suffering, takes respite from the reality, reinvests in whatever life remains, and moves on.

The only way to cope with dying or witnessing the dying of loved ones is by grieving through the pain, fear, loneliness, and loss of meaning. This process, which researcher Stephen Levine has likened to opening the heart in hell, is a viscous morass for most, and all people need to learn their own way through it and to have that learning respected. Healing begins with the first halting, unsteady, and frightening steps of genuine grief, which sometimes occur years before the "time of death" can be recorded as an historical event and which may never completely end.

—*Paul Moglia, Ph.D.*

See also Acquired immunodeficiency syndrome (AIDS); Aging; Depression; Ethics; Euthanasia; Grief and guilt; Midlife crisis; Phobias; Psychiatry; Psychiatry, child and adolescent; Psychiatry, geriatric; Stress; Sudden infant death syndrome (SIDS); Suicide; Terminally ill, extended care for the.

FOR FURTHER INFORMATION:

Becker, Ernest. *The Denial of Death.* New York: Free Press, 1997. Written by an anthropologist and philosopher, this is an erudite and insightful analysis and synthesis of the role that the fear of death plays in motivating human activity, society, and individual actions. A profound work.

Bluebond-Langer, Myra. *The Private Worlds of Dying Children.* Princeton, N.J.: Princeton University Press, 1978. Based on research that she conducted with hospitalized leukemic children, the anthropologist-author describes how children deal with their impending deaths in ways that give meaning and instruction to those who deal with the terminally ill. Filled with transcribed dialogue; at times a moving work.

Cook, Alicia Skinner, and Daniel S. Dworkin. *Helping the Bereaved: Therapeutic Interventions for Children, Adolescents, and Adults.* New York: BasicBooks, 1992. Although not a self-help book, this work is useful to professionals and nonprofessionals alike as a review of the state of the art in grief therapy. Practical and readable. Of special interest for those becoming involved in grief counseling.

Corr, Charles A., Clyde M. Nabe, and Donna M. Corr. *Death and Dying, Life and Living.* 2d ed. Pacific Grove, Calif.: Brooks/Cole, 1997. This book provides perspective on common issues associated with death and dying for family members and others affected by life-threatening circumstances.

Feifel, Herman, ed. *The Meaning of Death.* New York: McGraw-Hill, 1959. A classic of thanatological thinking before thanatology became a recognized specialty. Brings together systematized knowledge about death from multiple disciplines. An excellent resource of information fostering reflection.

Kübler-Ross, Elisabeth, ed. *Death: The Final Stage of Growth.* Englewood Cliffs, N.J.: Prentice Hall, 1975. A psychiatrist by training, Kübler-Ross brings together other researchers' views of how death provides the key to how human beings make meaning in their own personal worlds. The author, who is regarded as the pioneer in death and dying studies, addresses practical concerns over how people express grief and accept the death of those close to them, and how they might prepare for their own inevitable ends.

_____, ed. *Living with Death and Dying.* New York: Macmillan, 1981. Written in response to the concerns and questions of professionals and parents in dealing with dying generally and with children's understanding of death in particular, this is a conversational work based on the experience and insights of Kübler-Ross and two of her colleagues. Moving and genuine.

Kushner, Harold. *When Bad Things Happen to Good People.* New York: Summit, 1985. The first of Rabbi Kushner's works on finding meaning in one's life, it was originally his personal response to make intelligible the death of his own child. It has become a highly regarded reference for those who struggle with the meaning of pain, suffering, and death in their lives. Highly recommended.

Levine, Stephen. *Meetings at the Edge: Dialogues with the Grieving and the Dying, the Healing and the Healed.* Garden City, N.Y.: Anchor Press, 1984. An encouraging, realistic, and reassuring work by a nonphysician who addresses the suffering and pain of the dying and the bereaved. Advocates opening oneself to grief as a means of healing oneself with it. Although nonsectarian, this work has an Eastern, even Buddhist, slant. Clearly written with much practical application.

Linn, Matthew, Dennis Linn, and Sheila Fabricant. *Healing the Greatest Hurt.* New York: Paulist Press, 1985. A wonderful, reflective, and practical work written within the Christian tradition that would be of benefit to believers in other traditions as well. Grapples with the great unknown of what lies after death through the eschatological metaphor known as "the communion of saints."

DEMENTIA

DISEASE/DISORDER

ANATOMY OR SYSTEM AFFECTED: Brain, nervous system, psychic-emotional system

SPECIALTIES AND RELATED FIELDS: Geriatrics and gerontology, neurology, psychiatry

DEFINITION: A generally irreversible decline in intellectual ability resulting from a variety of causes; differs from mental retardation, in which the affected person never reaches an expected level of mental growth.

KEY TERMS:

basal ganglia: a collection of nerve cells deep inside the brain, below the cortex, that controls muscle tone and automatic actions such as walking

cortical dementia: dementia resulting from damage to the brain cortex, the outer layer of the brain that contains the bodies of the nerve cells

delirium: an acute condition characterized by confusion, a fluctuating level of consciousness, and visual, auditory, and even tactile hallucinations; often caused by acute disease, such as infection or intoxication

hydrocephalus: a condition resulting from the accumulation of fluid inside the brain in cavities known as ventricles; as fluid accumulates, it exerts pressure on the neighboring brain cells, which may be destroyed

subcortical dementia: dementia resulting from damage to the area of the brain below the cortex; this area contains nerve fibers that connect various parts of the brain with one another and with the basal ganglia

vascular dementia: dementia caused by repeated strokes, resulting in interference with the blood supply to parts of the brain

CAUSES AND SYMPTOMS

Dementia affects about four million people in the United States and is a major cause of disability in old age. Its prevalence increases with age. Dementia is characterized by a permanent memory deficit affecting recent memory in particular and of sufficient severity to interfere with the patient's ability to take part in professional and social activities. Although the aging process is associated with a gradual loss of brain cells, dementia is not part of the aging process. It also is not synonymous with benign senescent forgetfulness, which is very common in old age and affects recent memory. Although the latter is a source of frustration, it does not significantly interfere with the individual's professional and social activities because it tends to affect only trivial matters (or what the individual considers trivial). Furthermore, patients with benign forgetfulness usually can remember what was forgotten by utilizing a number of subterfuges, such as writing lists or notes to themselves and leaving them in conspicuous places. Individuals with benign forgetfulness also are acutely aware of their memory deficit, while those with dementia—except for in the early stages of the disease—have no insight into their memory deficit and often blame others for their problems.

In addition to the memory deficit interfering with the patient's daily activities, patients with dementia have evidence of impaired abstract thinking, impaired judgment, or other disturbances of higher cortical functions such as aphasia (the inability to use or comprehend language), apraxia (the inability to execute complex, coordinated movements), or agnosia (the inability to recognize familiar objects).

Dementia may result from damage to the cerebral cortex (the outer layer of the brain), as in Alzheimer's disease, or from damage to the subcortical structures (the structures below the cortex), such as white matter, the thalamus, or the basal ganglia. Although memory is impaired in both cortical and subcortical dementias, the associated features are different. In cortical dementias, for example, cognitive functions such as the ability to understand speech and to talk and the ability to perform mathematical calculations are severely impaired. In subcortical dementias, on the other hand, there is evidence of disturbances of arousal, motivation, and mood, in addition to a significant slowing of cognition and of information processing.

Alzheimer's disease, the most common cause of presenile dementia, is characterized by progressive disorientation, memory loss, speech disturbances, and personality disorders. Pick's disease is another cortical dementia, but unlike Alzheimer's disease, it is rare, tends to affect younger patients, and is more common in women. In the early stages of Pick's disease, changes in personality, disinhibition, inappropriate social and sexual conduct, and lack of foresight may be evident—features that are not common in Alzheimer's disease. Patients also may become euphoric or apathetic. Poverty of speech is often present and gradually progresses to mutism, although speech comprehension is usually spared. Pick's disease is characterized by cortical atrophy localized to the frontal and temporal lobes.

Vascular dementia is the second most common cause of dementia in patients over the age of sixty-five and is responsible for 8 percent to 20 percent of all dementia cases. It is caused by interference with the blood flow to the brain. Although the overall prevalence of vascular dementia is decreasing, there are some geographical variations, with the prevalence being higher in countries with a high incidence of cardiovascular and cerebrovascular diseases, such as Finland and Japan. About 20 percent of patients with dementia have both Alzheimer's disease and vascular dementia. Several types of vascular dementia have been identified.

Multiple infarct dementia (MID) is the most common type of vascular dementia. As its name implies, it is the result of multiple, discrete cerebral infarcts (strokes) that have destroyed enough brain tissue to interfere with the patient's higher mental functions. The onset of MID is usually sudden and is associated with neurological deficit, such as the paralysis or weakness of an arm or leg or the inability to speak. The disease characteristically progresses in steps: With each stroke experienced, the patient's condition suddenly deteriorates and then stabilizes or even improves slightly until another stroke occurs. In about 20 percent of patients with MID, however, the disease displays an insidious onset and causes gradual deterioration. Most patients also show evidence of arteriosclerosis and other factors predisposing them to the development of strokes, such as hypertension, cigarette smoking, high blood cholesterol, diabetes mellitus, narrowing of one or both carotid arteries, or cardiac disorders, especially atrial fibrillation (an irregular heartbeat). Somatic complaints, mood changes, depression, and nocturnal confusion tend to be more common in vascular dementias, although there is relative preservation of the patient's personality. In such cases, magnetic resonance imaging (MRI) or a computed tomography (CT) scan of the brain often shows evidence of multiple strokes.

Strokes are not always associated with clinical evidence of neurological deficits, since the stroke may affect a "silent" area of the brain or may be so small that its immediate impact is not noticeable. Nevertheless, when several of these small strokes have occurred, the resulting loss of brain tissue may interfere with the patient's cognitive functions. This is, in fact, the basis of the lacunar dementias. The infarcted tissue is absorbed into the rest of the brain, leaving a small cavity or lacuna. Brain-imaging techniques and especially MRI are useful in detecting these lacunae.

A number of neurological disorders are associated with dementia. The combination of dementia, urinary incontinence, and muscle rigidity causing difficulties in walking should raise the suspicion of hydrocephalus. In this condition, fluid accumulates inside the ventricles (cavities within the brain) and results in increased pressure on the brain cells. A CT scan demonstrates enlargement of the ventricles. Although some patients may respond well to surgical shunting of the cerebrospinal fluid, it is often difficult to identify those who will benefit from surgery. Postoperative complications are significant and include strokes and subdural hematomas.

Dementia has been linked to Parkinson's disease, a chronic, progressive neurological disorder that usually manifests itself in middle or late life. It has an insidious onset and a very slow progression rate. Although intellectual deterioration is not part of the classical features of Parkinson's disease, dementia is being recognized as a late manifestation of the disease, with as many as one-third of the patients eventually being afflicted. The dementing process also has an insidious onset and slow progression rate. Some of the medication used to treat Parkinson's disease also may induce confusion, particularly in older patients.

Subdural hematomas (collections of blood inside the brain) may lead to mental impairment and are usually precipitated by trauma to the head. Usually, the trauma is slight and the patient neither loses consciousness nor experiences any immediate significant effects. A few days or even weeks later, however, the patient may develop evidence of mental impairment. By that time, the patient and caregivers may have forgotten about the slight trauma that the patient had experienced. A subdural hematoma should be suspected in the presence of a fairly sudden onset and progressing course. Headaches are common. A CT scan can reveal the presence of a hematoma. The surgical removal of the hematoma is usually associated with a good prognosis if the surgery is done in a timely manner, before irreversible brain damage occurs.

Brain tumors may lead to dementia, particularly if they are slow growing. Most tumors of this type can be diagnosed by CT scanning or MRI. Occasionally, cancer may induce dementia through an inflammation of the brain.

Many chronic infections affecting the brain can lead to dementia; they include conditions that, when treated, may reverse or prevent the progression of dementia, such as syphilis, tuberculosis, slow viruses, and some fungal and protozoal infections. Human immunodeficiency virus (HIV) infection is also a cause of dementia, and it may be suspected if the rate of progress is rapid and the patient has risk factors for the development of HIV infection. Although the dementia is part of the acquired immunodeficiency syndrome (AIDS) complex, it may occasionally be the first manifestation of the disease.

It is often difficult to differentiate depression from dementia. Nevertheless, sudden onset—especially if preceded by an emotional event, the presence of sleep disturbances, and a history of previous psychiatric illness—is suggestive of depression. The level of mental functioning of patients with depression is often inconsistent. They may, for example, be able to give clear accounts of topics that are of personal interest to them but be very vague about, and at times may not even attempt to answer, questions on topics that are of no interest to them. Variability in performance during testing is suggestive of depression, especially if it improves with positive reinforcement.

TREATMENT AND THERAPY

It is estimated that dementia affects about 0.4 percent of the population aged sixty to sixty-four years and 0.9, 1.8, 3.6, 10.5, and 23.8 percent of the population aged sixty-five to sixty-nine, seventy to seventy-four, seventy-five to seventy-nine, eighty to eighty-four, and eighty-five to ninety-three years, respectively. Different surveys may yield different results, depending on the criteria used to define dementia.

For physicians, an important aspect of diagnosing patients with dementia is detecting potentially reversible causes which may be responsible for the impaired mental functions. A detailed history followed by a meticulous and thorough clinical examination and a few selected laboratory tests are usually sufficient to reach a diagnosis. Various investigators have estimated that reversible causes of dementia can be identified in 10 percent to 20 percent of patients with dementia. Recommended investigations include brain imaging (CT scanning or MRI), a complete blood count, and tests of erythrocyte sedimentation rate, blood glucose, serum electrolytes, serum calcium, liver function, thyroid function, and serum B_{12} and folate. Some investigators also recommend routine testing for syphilis. Other tests, such as those for the detection of HIV infection, cerebrospinal fluid examination, neuropsychological testing, drug and toxin screen, serum copper and ceruloplasmin analysis, carotid and cerebral angiography, and electroencephalography, are performed when appropriate.

It is of paramount importance for health care providers to adopt a positive attitude when managing patients with dementia. Although at present little can be done to treat and reverse dementia, it is important to identify the cause of the dementia. In some cases, it may be possible to prevent the disease from progressing. For example, if the dementia is the result of hypertension, adequate control of this condition may prevent further brain damage. Moreover, the prevalence of vascular dementia is decreasing in countries where efforts to reduce cardiovascular and cerebrovascular diseases have been successful. Similarly, if the dementia is the result of repeated emboli (blood clots reaching the brain) complicating atrial fibrillation, then anticoagulants or aspirin may be recommended.

Even after a diagnosis of dementia is made, it is important for the physician to detect the presence of other conditions that may worsen the patient's mental functions, such as the inadvertent intake of medications that may induce confusion and mental impairment. Medications with this potential are numerous and include not only those that act on the brain, such as sedatives and hypnotics, but also hypotensive agents (especially if given in large doses), diuretics, and antibiotics. Whenever the condition of a patient with dementia deteriorates, the physician meticulously reviews all the medications that the patient is taking, both medical prescriptions and medications that may have been purchased over the counter. Even if innocuous, some over-the-counter preparations may interact with other medications that the patient is taking and lead to a worsening of mental functions. Inquiries are also made into the patient's alcohol intake. The brain of an older person is much more sensitive to the effects of alcohol than that of a younger person, and some medications may interact with the alcohol to impair the patient's cognitive functions further.

Many other disease states also may worsen the patient's mental functions. For example, patients with diabetes mellitus are susceptible to developing a variety of metabolic abnormalities including a low or high blood glucose level, both of which may be associated with confusional states. Similarly, dehydration and acid-base or electrolyte disorders, which may result from prolonged vomiting or diarrhea, may also precipitate confusional states. Infections, particularly respiratory and urinary tract infections, often worsen the patient's cognitive deficit. Finally, patients with dementia may experience myocardial infarctions (heart attacks) that are not associated with any chest pain but that may manifest themselves with confusion.

The casual observer of the dementing process is often overwhelmed with concern for the patient, but it is the family that truly suffers. The patients themselves experience no physical pain or distress, and except for in the very early stages of the disease, they are oblivious to their plight as a result of their loss of insight. Health care professionals therefore are alert to the stress imposed on the caregivers by dealing with loved ones with dementia. Adequate support from agencies available in the community is essential.

When a diagnosis of dementia is made, the physician discusses a number of ethical, financial, and legal issues with the family, and also the patient if it is believed that he or she can understand the implications of this discussion. Families are encouraged to make a list of all the patient's assets, including insurance policies, and to discuss this information with an attorney in order to protect the patient's and the family's assets. If the patient is still competent, it is recommended that he or she select a trusted person to have durable power of attorney. Unlike the regular power of attorney, the former does not become invalidated when the patient becomes mentally incompetent and continues to be in effect regardless of the degree of mental impairment of the person who executed it. Because durable power of attorney cannot be easily reversed once the person is incompetent, great care should be taken when selecting a person and the specific powers granted should be clearly specified. It is also important for the patient to make his or her desires known concerning advance directives and the use of life support systems.

Courts may appoint a guardian or conservator to have charge and custody of the patient's property (including real estate and money) when no responsible family members or friends are willing or available to serve as guardian. Courts supervise the actions of the guardian, who is expected to report all the patient's income and expenditures to the court once a year. The court may also charge the guardian to ensure that the patient is adequately housed, fed, and clothed and receiving appropriate medical care.

PERSPECTIVE AND PROSPECTS

Dementia is a very serious and common condition, especially among the older population. Dementia permanently robs patients of their minds and prevents them from functioning adequately in their environment by impairing memory and interfering with the ability to make rational decisions. It therefore deprives patients of their dignity and independence.

Because dementia is mostly irreversible, cannot be adequately treated at present, and is associated with a fairly long survival period, it has a significant impact not only on the patient's life but also on the patient's family and caregivers and on society in general. The expense of long-term care for patients with dementia, whether at home or in institutions, is staggering. Every effort, therefore, is made to reach an accurate diagnosis and especially to detect any other condition that may worsen the patient's underlying dementia. Finally, health care professionals do not treat the patient in isolation but also concern themselves with the impact of the illness on the patient's caregivers and family.

Much progress has been made in defining dementia and determining its cause. Terms such as "senile dementia" are no longer in use, and even the use of the term "dementia" to diagnose a patient's condition is frowned upon because there are so many types of dementia. The recognition of the type of dementia affecting a particular patient is important because of its practical implications, both for the patient and for research into the prevention, management, and treatment of dementia. The prevalence of vascular dementia, for example, is decreasing in many countries where the prevention of cardiovascular diseases such as hypertension and arteriosclerosis has been successful.

Unfortunately, there is little that can be done to cure dementia and no effective means to regenerate nerve cells. Researchers, however, are feverishly trying to identify factors that control the growth and regeneration of nerve cells. Although no single medication is expected to be of benefit to all types of dementia, it is hoped that effective therapy for many dementias will be developed.

—*Ronald C. Hamdy, M.D., Louis A. Cancellaro, M.D., and Larry Hudgins, M.D.*

See also Aging; Aging, extended care for the; Alzheimer's disease; Amnesia; Brain; Brain disorders; Hallucinations; Memory loss; Parkinson's disease; Psychiatric disorders; Psychiatry; Psychiatry, geriatric; Strokes and TIAs.

FOR FURTHER INFORMATION:

Coons, Dorothy H., ed. *Specialized Dementia Care Units.* Baltimore: The Johns Hopkins University Press, 1991. A collection of articles reviewing the benefits and disadvantages of caring for patients with dementia in specialized care units. Several problems encountered when running such units are addressed.

Hamdy, Ronald C., J. M. Turnbull, L. D. Norman, and M. M. Lancaster, eds. *Alzheimer's Disease: A Handbook for Caregivers.* 2d ed. St. Louis: Mosby Year Book, 1994. A comprehensive discussion of the symptoms and characteristic features of Alzheimer's disease and other dementias. Abnormal brain structure and function in these patients are discussed, and the normal effects of aging are reviewed. Gives caregivers practical advice concerning the encouragement of patients with dementia.

Howe, M. L., M. J. Stones, and C. J. Brainerd, eds. *Cognitive and Behavioral Performance Factors in Atypical Aging.* New York: Springer-Verlag, 1990. A review of the factors controlling behavior, test performance, and brain function in both young and older patients.

Kovach, Christine, ed. *Late Stage Dementia Care: A Basic Guide.* Washington, D.C.: Taylor & Francis, 1997. Provides information on assessment and treatment management for individuals experiencing dementia. A valuable source for caregivers and family members of those affected.

Terry, Robert D., ed. *Aging and the Brain.* New York: Raven Press, 1988. A review of the application of concepts in neurobiology and technology in the study of brain structure and function in normal elderly people and those with different types of dementia.

U.S. Congress. Office of Technology Assessment. *Confused Minds, Burdened Families: Finding Help for People with Alzheimer's and Other Dementias.* Washington, D.C.: Government Printing Office, 1990. A report from the Office of Technology Assessment analyzing the problems of locating and arranging services for people with dementia in the United States. Also presents a framework for an effective system to provide appropriate services and discusses congressional policy options for establishing such a system.

_____. *Losing a Million Minds: Confronting the Tragedy of Alzheimer's Disease and Other Dementias.* Washington, D.C.: Government Printing Office, 1987. A comprehensive report from the Office of Technology Assessment reviewing the nature and psychological, sociological, and economic implications of dementia in the United States. The various programs and services available are reviewed, and recommendations concerning future policies are made. The issues of personnel training and quality assurance are also addressed.

West, Robin L., and Jan D. Sinnott, eds. *Everyday Memory and Aging.* New York: Springer-Verlag, 1992. A review of issues relating to memory research and methodology, especially as they apply to aging.

DENTAL DISEASES
DISEASE/DISORDER

ANATOMY OR SYSTEM AFFECTED: Gums, mouth, teeth
SPECIALTIES AND RELATED FIELDS: Dentistry
DEFINITION: Diseases that affect the teeth, such as dental caries, and the gums, such as gingivitis, pyorrhea, or cancer.

KEY TERMS:

dental caries: tooth decay
dentin: a hard, bonelike tissue lying beneath the tooth enamel
enamel: the hard surface covering of teeth
gingivae: the soft tissue surrounding the teeth; the gums
gingivitis: an inflammation of the gums
periodontal diseases: diseases characterized by inflammation of the gingivae
pyorrhea: the second stage of gingivitis
tooth pulp: the tissue at the center of teeth, surrounded by dentin
Vincent's infection: a bacterial infection of the gingivae, also known as trench mouth

CAUSES AND SYMPTOMS

Dental diseases fall into four major categories: dental caries, or tooth decay; periodontal disease, including gingivitis and pyorrhea; Vincent's infection, or trench mouth; and oral cancer. The first of these diseases was the largest contributor to tooth loss among people under thirty-five in the United States before the widespread fluoridation of drinking water was begun; it remains a major cause of tooth loss in much of the world. Periodontal disease in its two stages, gingivitis and pyorrhea, is the most widespread dental problem for people over thirty-five. Most people who suffer the loss of all of their teeth are victims of this condition. Vincent's infection, which shares many characteristics with gingivitis, is a bacterial infection. The infection flares up, is treated, and disappears, whereas gingivitis is more often a continuing condition that requires both persistent home treatment and specialized treatment. The most serious but least frequently occurring dental disease is oral cancer. It is the only dental disease commonly considered life-threatening, and there is a risk that it may spread to other parts of the body.

Dental caries occur because the food that one eats becomes trapped in the irregularities of the teeth, creating lactic acids that penetrate the enamel through holes (often microscopic) in it. Once lodged between the teeth or below the gum line, carbohydrates and starches combine with saliva to form acids that, over time, can penetrate a tooth's enamel, enter the dentin directly below it, and progressively destroy the dentin while spreading toward the tooth's center, the pulp.

This process often is not confined to a single tooth. As decay spreads, adjoining teeth may be affected. Some people have much harder tooth enamel than others. Therefore, some individuals may experience little or no decay, whereas others who follow similar diets and practice similar methods of dental hygiene may develop substantial decay.

Toothache occurs when decay eats through the dentin and enters the nerve-filled dental pulp, causing inflammation, infection, and pain. A dull, continuous ache, either mild or severe and often pulsating, may indicate that the infection has entered the jawbone beneath the tooth. An aching or sensitivity in the back teeth during chewing is sometimes a side effect of sinusitis.

Periodontal disease. One of dentistry's nagging problems is periodontal disease, which results from a buildup of cal-

Dental Plaque

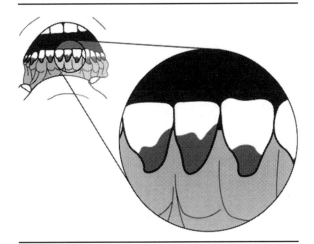

Plaque—a buildup of bacteria, mucus, and food debris—leads to dental caries (tooth decay) if not regularly removed by brushing, flossing, and professional tooth cleaning.

culus, or tartar, formed by hardened plaque. Plaque is formed when food, particularly carbohydrates and starches, interact with the saliva that coats the teeth, creating a yellowish film. If this film is not removed, it inevitably lodges between the gums and the teeth, where, within twenty-four hours, it hardens into calculus. Dental hygienists can remove most of this calculus mechanically. If it is allowed to build up over extended periods, however, the calculus will irritate the gums, causing the soreness, swelling, and bleeding that signal gum infection. Eventually, this infection becomes entrenched and difficult to treat.

Periodontists can control but not cure most periodontal disease. In its early manifestations, periodontal disease results in gingivitis, marked by inflammation and bleeding. Untreated, it progresses to pyorrhea, which is characterized by gums that recede from the teeth and form pockets in which infections flourish. As pyorrhea advances, the bone that underlies the teeth and holds them in place is compromised and ultimately destroyed, causing looseness and eventual tooth loss.

Vincent's infection (trench mouth) is communicable through kissing or sharing eating utensils. Although it is sometimes mistaken for gingivitis, Vincent's infection has one distinguishing characteristic that gingivitis does not have: It is accompanied by a fever stemming from sustained bacterial infection, which also causes extremely foul breath. Vincent's infection is curable through proper treatment. It is unlikely to recur unless one is again exposed to the infection.

Oral cancer is the most serious of oral diseases. It often spreads quickly, destroying the tissues of the mouth during its ravaging advance. It not only threatens its original site but also can spread to other areas of the body and to vital organs. Fortunately, oral cancer is uncommon. Nevertheless, dentists look vigilantly for signs of it when they perform mouth examinations because early detection is vital to successful treatment, containment, and cure. People who have persistent mouth sores that do not heal may be experiencing the early manifestations of oral cancer and should see their dentists or physicians immediately.

Other conditions. Two other dental conditions afflict many people: malocclusion and toothache. Malocclusion occurs when, for a variety of reasons, the teeth are out of alignment. People with malocclusion are prime candidates for dental caries and periodontal disease, largely because their teeth are difficult to reach and hard to clean. Malocclusion may also cause one or more teeth to strike the teeth above or below them, causing injury to teeth and possibly fracturing them.

TREATMENT AND THERAPY

Modern dentistry has succeeded in controlling most dental diseases. In the United States, dental caries have been almost eliminated in the young, for example, by the addition of fluoride to most water systems. Used over time, fluoride strengthens the teeth by increasing the hardness of the enamel, making it resistant to the acids that form in the mouth and cause decay.

Since the 1950's, many American children have been reared on fluoridated water. Those whose water supply is not fluoridated have usually had their teeth treated with fluoride by their dentists. Many have brushed their teeth regularly with fluoridated toothpaste, which offers considerable protection from dental caries. From the 1950's to the 1990's, fluoride reduced dental decay in Americans under the age of twenty-one by more than 70 percent.

Current research into ways of preventing dental decay centers on several projects of the National Institute of Dental Research. Researchers for this organization discovered in the mid-1960's that a substance found in the mouth's streptococcal bacteria creates dextran. Dextran enables bacteria to cling to the surface of the teeth and invade them with the lactic acid that they generate. Researchers ultimately discovered dextrase, an enzyme effective in dissolving dextran. Strides are being made to use dextrase in toothpaste or mouthwash in order to reduce or eliminate the effects of dextran.

Some people's teeth seem to be impervious to tooth decay. It has been determined that such people have a common substance in their blood that protects their teeth from dental caries. Attempts are being made to identify and isolate this substance and to make it generally available to the public and to dentists in an applicable form. Some dentists coat the teeth with a durable plastic substance to make them resistant to penetration by the acids that cause dental decay, creating a hard protective coating above the enamel and making it difficult for food to lodge between the teeth or in irregularities in the teeth.

Because malocclusion can lead to tooth decay, dentists have become increasingly aware of the need to replace lost teeth so that the alignment of the remaining teeth will not be disturbed. Tooth implantation, a process by which a tooth, either artificial or natural, is anchored directly and permanently in the gum, solves many dental problems that in the past were addressed by attaching artificial teeth to existing ones beside them. In situations where malocclusion is caused by malformations, the use of orthodontic braces results in a more regular alignment.

Nutrition has come to the forefront of recent research in dental health. A lack of calciferol, a form of vitamin D₂, may result in dental abnormalities, including malocclusion. Among substantial numbers of hospital patients who suffer from nutritional problems, the earliest symptoms occur in the soft tissue of the mouth.

Brushing the teeth after meals and before bed controls plaque, as does regular flossing. Such daily attention must be supplemented by twice-yearly cleaning, performed by a dentist or dental hygienist, and by annual or biennial whole-mouth X rays to reveal incipient decay. Various mouthwashes also contain substances that control decay.

People who cannot brush after every meal should use a mouthwash or rinse the mouth out with water after eating, then brush as soon as they can. Special attention must be given to the back surfaces of the lower front teeth because the salivary glands are located there. This area is a breeding ground for the bacteria that cause the formation of lactic acid. Routine home care of this kind, particularly daily flossing, will help prevent both tooth decay and periodontal disease, and can also reverse some of the inroads that periodontal disease has made. When gingivitis advances to pyorrhea, however, dental surgery may be indicated.

The major villain in both gingivitis and pyorrhea is tartar, or calculus, which is produced when plaque hardens. When tartar accumulates beneath the gums, it causes an irritation that can lead to infection. Sometimes, this infection moves to other parts of the body, causing joint problems and other difficulties.

People can control plaque by practicing daily dental hygiene at home. They must also have accumulated tartar regularly scraped away or removed by ultrasound in the dentist's office. Malocclusions and defects in the production of saliva can be corrected by dentists and can greatly reduce the progress of periodontal disease.

When gum surgery is advised for the removal of the deep gum pockets that occur with pyorrhea, further surgery can usually be avoided by regular home care. Meanwhile, researchers are trying to develop a vaccine to immunize its recipients against the bacteria that cause tooth decay. Other decay-inhibiting agents are being studied closely with the expectation that they may in time be added to common foods and beverages.

Vincent's infection is successfully treated with antibiotics, accompanied by a prescribed course of dental hygiene that is begun in the dentist's office and continues at home on a daily basis. Some patients have found a peroxide mouthwash helpful in treating this disease.

Oral cancer, when it is discovered by a dentist, is usually referred immediately to the patient's family physician, who then refers the case to an oncologist. Laser treatment and radiation are used in controlling this sort of cancer, as are chemotherapy and surgery. The most important element in cancer treatment is time. It is essential, therefore, that specialized treatment be initiated as soon as oral cancer is discovered or suspected. In cases of oral cancer, a delay of even days can affect outcomes negatively.

The most immediate treatments for toothache range from the application of cold compresses to the taking of aspirin or some other analgesic every few hours. If the decayed part of the tooth is visible and reachable, sometimes applying a mixture of oil of cloves and benzocaine to the decayed area on a small swab soothes the pain. These treatments, however, offer only temporary relief.

Dentists resist treating toothache by removing the tooth,

although removal offers an immediate solution to the problem. In some cases, dentists can drill out the decay and fill the tooth with silver amalgam, gold, or plastic. Quite often, by the time a tooth begins to ache, the pulp and dentin have been ravaged by decay and the best solution is endodontistry, or root canal, which will preserve the tooth but may necessitate the attachment of a crown.

PERSPECTIVE AND PROSPECTS

Great strides have been made in the United States in preventing and treating dental disease as researchers have reached deeper understandings of the root causes of such disease. Dentistry has become increasingly less painful through the use of anesthetics and high-speed, water-cooled drills. The public at large has grown aware of the close relationship between dental health and general health. People are unwilling to accept tooth loss as a natural consequence of aging. They have also begun to realize that orthodontistry is more than a cosmetic procedure. Rather, it is a necessary procedure for correcting misalignments of the teeth that can result in difficulty if uncorrected.

National attention has been given to preventing tooth decay through the fluoridation of water supplies and, although some groups still fight fluoridation, it is for most Americans an accepted fact of modern life. Fluoridation more than any other factor has changed the emphasis in dentistry from preventing and treating dental caries to more sophisticated pursuits such as orthodontistry, endodontistry, and periodontistry. The establishment of the National Institute for Dental Research by Congress in 1948 has, more than any other single factor, stimulated dental research in the United States.

Advances in preventing and treating dental disease are constantly being made. Through genetic engineering, it is almost inevitable that substances will soon be available to increase an individual's resistance to tooth decay. Nevertheless, controlling the buildup of calculus, the major factor in periodontal disease, will probably remain the responsibility of individuals through daily home care and twice yearly visits to their dentists.   —*R. Baird Shuman, Ph.D.*

See also Caries, dental; Dentistry; Endodontic disease; Fracture repair; Gingivitis; Jaw wiring; Orthodontics; Periodontal surgery; Periodontitis; Root canal treatment; Teeth; Tooth extraction; Toothache.

FOR FURTHER INFORMATION:

Anderson, Pauline C., and Martha R. Burkard. *The Dental Assistant*. 5th ed. Albany, N.Y.: Delmar, 1987. Designed as a textbook for dental hygienists, this popular volume is particularly clear in its discussion of periodontal disease and dental caries. Although it is not directed specifically to laypersons, the book is easily accessible to nonspecialized readers.

Foster, Malcolm S. *Protecting Our Children's Teeth: A Guide to Quality Dental Care from Infancy Through Age Twelve*. New York: Insight Books, 1992. This book, meant for parents, is clear and easy to understand. The illustrations are useful. A good starting point.

McGuire, Thomas. *The Tooth Trip: An Oral Experience*. New York: Random House, 1972. Although somewhat dated, this book provides accurate information about dental diseases. Its pen-and-ink drawings clarify some of the technical information that McGuire provides. Aimed at laypersons.

Renner, Robert. *An Introduction to Dental Anatomy and Esthetics*. Chicago: Quintessence, 1985. This standard work in the field is thorough and accurate. Presents extensive information about dental disease, its prevention and treatment. A fundamental resource.

Ring, Malvin E. *Dentistry: An Illustrated History*. New York: Harry N. Abrams, 1985. Ring's coverage of dentistry is broad and accurate. The illustrations are particularly useful in helping readers understand dental diseases. An excellent starting point for those unfamiliar with the topic.

Ward, Brian R. *Dental Care*. New York: Franklin Watts, 1986. Ward emphasizes the daily care of the teeth and the prevention of dental disease. Presents this information lucidly and directly, using selective illustrations appropriately and well.

Woodall, Irene R., ed. *Comprehensive Dental Hygiene Care*. 4th ed. St. Louis: C. V. Mosby, 1993. This illustrated text addresses topics in dental hygiene and prophylaxis.

DENTISTRY

SPECIALTY

ANATOMY OR SYSTEM AFFECTED: Gums, mouth, teeth

SPECIALTIES AND RELATED FIELDS: Anesthesiology, orthodontics

DEFINITION: The field of health involving the diagnosis and treatment of diseases of the teeth and related tissues in the oral cavity.

KEY TERMS:

dental caries: the scientific term for tooth decay

dentist: a doctor with specialized training to diagnose and treat diseases of the teeth and oral tissues

endodontics: the dental specialty that treats diseases of infected pulp tissue

oral surgery: the dental specialty that surgically removes diseased teeth and oral tissues and treats fractures of the jawbone

orthodontics: the dental specialty that treats malocclusions or improperly aligned teeth by straightening the teeth in the jaws

pedodontics: the dental specialty that treats children

periodontics: the dental specialty that treats the diseases of the supporting tissues of the teeth

prosthodontics: the dental specialty that restores missing teeth with fixed or removable dentures

SCIENCE AND PROFESSION

The practice of dentistry is a highly specialized area of medicine that treats the diseases of the teeth and their surrounding tissues in the oral cavity. Dental education normally takes four years to complete, with predental training preceding it. Prior to entering a dental school, students are usually required to have a bachelor's degree from a college or university. This degree should have major emphasis in biology or chemistry. Predental courses are concentrated in both inorganic and organic chemistry. The biology courses can cover such subjects as comparative anatomy, histology, physiology, and microbiology. Other courses that can help students to prepare for both dental school and the future practice of dentistry are English, speech skills, economics, physics, computer technology, and subjects such as sculpture that teach spatial relationships. Upon entering dental school, students are faced with two distinct parts of their education: didactics and techniques.

The didactic courses offered in dental schools are required to achieve knowledge of the human body, most particularly the head and neck. Some of the courses required are human anatomy (including dissection of a human cadaver), physiology, biochemistry, microbiology, general and oral histology and pathology, dental anatomy, pharmacology, anesthesiology, and radiology. One course specific to dental school is occlusion, which emphasizes the structure of the temporomandibular joint and its accompanying neurology and musculature.

In addition, students must know the properties of the materials used in the practice of dentistry. The physical properties of metals, acrylic plastics, gypsum plasters, impression materials, porcelains, glass ionomers, dental composites, sealant resins, and other substances must be thoroughly understood to determine the proper restorations for diseased tissues in the mouth. Knowledge of resistance to wear by chewing forces, thermal conductivity, and corrosion and staining by mouth fluids and foods is important. Information concerning the materials used in dental treatment in terms of resistance to recurrent decay, possible toxicity, or irritation to the hard and soft tissues of the oral cavity is also necessary.

The technical phase of dental education addresses the practical use of this didactic knowledge in treating diseases of the mouth. Students are trained to operate on diseased teeth and to prepare the teeth to receive restorations that will function as biomechanical prostheses in, or adjacent to, living tissue. An understanding of anatomy, physiology, and pathology is necessary for successful restoration of the teeth. During this course of study, students are required to construct fillings, cast-gold crowns and inlays, fixed and removable dentures, porcelain crowns and inlays, and other restorations on mannequins, plastic models, or extracted teeth. These activities are undertaken prior to working on patients. Through practice and repetition of these techniques, dental students soon become aware of the importance of mastering this phase of the education prior to their application in a clinical environment.

The clinical phase of dental education integrates the didactic and technical instruction that has taken place throughout the first years of professional study. Students learn to treat patients under the close supervision of their instructors. The treatment of patients in all the specialties of dentistry is required of students before they receive the degree for general dentistry. Some students may opt for extra training in one of several specialties. In order to become a specialist, postgraduate education is required. This

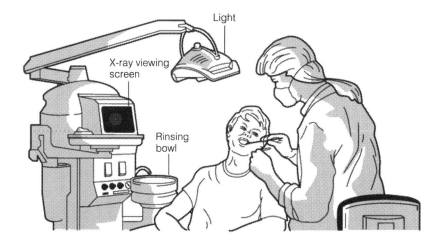

A dentist's office is equipped with specialized instruments for the cleaning and repair of teeth.

education commonly encompasses two years of study but is sometimes longer.

Upon graduation, students receive their professional degrees. Before they can legally practice dentistry in the United States, however, they must successfully pass an examination offered by the board of dental examiners in their chosen state. National exams in didactics are offered during dental school, and most states accept them as part of their state examination. The technical portion of the exam may only be taken after the student has received a doctorate. The emphasis regarding techniques may vary from state to state. Many states allow reciprocity, which means that a student who has passed the examination in one state may become licensed to practice in another. In states that do not

Some Conditions Treated in Dentistry

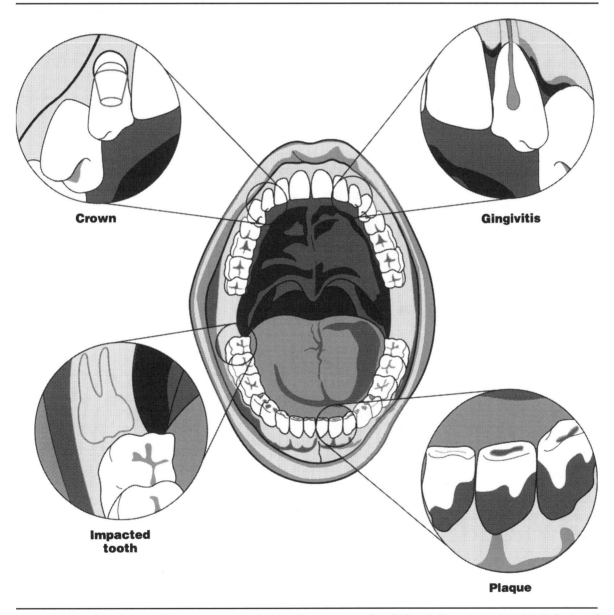

Care of the teeth and supporting structures may involve the treatment of such dental diseases as gingivitis (infection of the gums), the removal of dental plaque (hard deposits on the teeth), the surgical excision of impacted molars (teeth trapped beneath the gums), and the fitting of a crown (an artificial covering for a tooth) following root canal treatment.

accept reciprocity, the student must pass the practical examination of that state prior to obtaining a license. There have been attempts to make reciprocity universal among all states, but several states insist on governing the quality of their dental health care.

Dental education can be quite expensive. After a dentist receives a license to practice, the cost of equipping an office must also be borne. A dental office must have dental chairs, office and reception room furniture, a dental laboratory, a sterilizing room, X-ray units, instruments, and various supplies. Because of these expenses, new dentists often initially practice as an associate or partner of an established dentist, as an employee of a dental clinic, in the military or Public Health Service, or in state institutions. Some dentists enjoy the academic atmosphere of dental schools and return to become part-time or full-time educators.

DIAGNOSTIC AND TREATMENT TECHNIQUES

The practice of dentistry is quite different in modern times compared to the past. While some techniques and materials are still in use, there have been improvements in materials and instruments because of expanded knowledge in many scientific fields. This knowledge has increased to such an extent that dentistry has divided into several specialties. While the general dentist uses all disciplines of dentistry to treat patients, complex problems often require referral and the expertise of a specialist.

The general dentist is involved primarily in the treatment of caries or tooth decay and the replacement of missing teeth. Bacterial acids that dissolve the enamel and dentin of teeth cause caries. A diseased or damaged tooth must be prepared mechanically by the removal of the decayed material using a dental drill and tough, sharp bits called burs. The amount of damage and the position of the tooth in the mouth determine the type of restoration. In the posterior or back teeth, initial cavities may be restored with silver amalgam or bonded composite resins. In addition to removing the decayed tooth structure, the dentist must take into consideration the closeness of the dental pulp, the chewing forces of the opposing teeth, and the aesthetics of the finished restoration. In the anterior or front teeth, aesthetic restorative materials are used to fill small cavities. In this case also, the size and position of the defect determine the choice of restorative material.

When the amount of tooth destruction caused by decay becomes too large for conservative filling materials, the remaining tooth structure must be reinforced by the use of cast metal or porcelain restorations. The tooth is prepared for the specific restoration, and accurate impressions are taken of the prepared teeth. The crown or inlay is fabricated on hard plaster models reproduced from the impressions and then cemented into place on the tooth. This process is also used for fixed partial dentures, or bridges, which are used to replace one or more missing teeth. Two or more teeth are prepared on either end of the space of missing

teeth to support the span. The bridge is constructed with metal and porcelain as a single unit. It is then cemented on the prepared abutment teeth.

The health of the supporting tissues of the teeth, the periodontium, is necessary for the long-term retention of any mechanical restoration. When teeth become loose in the jaws because of periodontal disease, or pyorrhea, the restoration of these teeth often depends on the treatment by a periodontist, the specialist in this field. Periodontists treat the diseased tissues by scraping off harmful deposits on the roots of the teeth and by removing the diseased soft tissue and bone through curettage, surgery, or both techniques. At present, there is no means to regenerate or regrow bone lost by periodontal disease. Some newer techniques of grafting the patient's bone with sterile freeze-dried bone, implanting stainless steel pins or using other artificial materials, show great promise.

If the tooth decay reaches the dental pulp and infects it, there are two choices of treatment: removal of the tooth or endodontic therapy, commonly known as root canal treatment. If the tooth is well supported by a healthy periodontium, it is better to save the tooth by endodontics. The basic procedure of a root canal is to enter the tooth through the chewing surface on teeth toward the rear of the mouth or the inside surface or lingual aspect of teeth in the front of the mouth. Files, reamers, and broaches to the tip of the root remove diseased or decaying (necrotic) material of the dental pulp. The now-empty canal is filled by cementing a point that fits into it. Although the tooth is now nonvital, meaning that it has lost its blood supply and nerve, it can remain in the mouth for many years and provide good service.

The maintenance of the health of the primary dentition, or baby teeth, is very important. These deciduous teeth, although lost during childhood and adolescence, are important not only to the dental health of the child but to the permanent teeth as well. The deciduous teeth act as guides and spacers for the correct placement of adult teeth when they erupt. A pediodontist, who specializes in the practice of dentistry for children, must have a good knowledge of the specific mechanics of children's mouths in treating primary teeth. This specialist must also have a thorough foundation in the treatment of congenital diseases. The pediodontist prepares the way for dental treatment by an adult dentist and often assists an orthodontist by doing some preliminary straightening of teeth.

An orthodontist treats malocclusions, or ill-fitting teeth (so-called bad bites) with mechanical appliances that reposition the teeth into an occlusion that is closer to ideal. These appliances, known commonly as braces, move the teeth through the bone of the jaws until the opposing teeth occlude in a balanced bite. The side benefit of this treatment is that the teeth become properly positioned for an attractive smile.

Sometimes the teeth or their supporting tissues become so diseased that there is no alternative but to remove them.

A general dentist often does routine extractions of these diseased teeth. If the patient has complications beyond the training of a general dentist or is medically compromised by systemic illness, an oral surgeon, with specialized training, is typically consulted. This specialist not only removes teeth under difficult conditions but also is trained to remove tumors of the oral cavity, treat fractures of the jaws, and perform the surgical placement of dental implants.

Although the total loss of teeth is becoming rarer, there are still many patients who are without teeth. Often, they have been wearing complete, removable dentures that, over a period of time, have caused the loss or resorption of underlying bone. Prosthodontists are specialists trained to construct fixed and removable dentures for difficult cases. The increased success of titanium implants in the jaws and the appliances connected to them have aided prosthodontists in treating the complex cases. They also construct appliances to replace tissues and structures lost from cancer surgery of the oral cavity and congenital deformities such as cleft palate.

PERSPECTIVE AND PROSPECTS

In the past, dentistry only treated pain caused by a diseased tooth; the usual mode of treatment was extraction. Today, the prevention of disease, the retention of teeth, and the restoration of the dentition are the treatment goals of dentists.

The development of composite resins has successfully addressed many aesthetic problems associated with restorations. Although metal fillings of silver amalgam (actually a mixture of silver, lead, and a small amount of mercury) and cast-gold restorations are often the treatments of choice, the display of metal is offensive to some patients. Plastic composite materials that are chemically bonded to the enamel and dentin of teeth are more aesthetically pleasing than metals. They have also shown great promise for longevity. There is still some concern about the resistance of these materials to chewing forces and leakage of the bonding to the tooth, but the techniques and materials are improving.

Dental porcelains improved greatly in the last half of the twentieth century. Although porcelain fused to metal crowns is often the material of choice, in certain cases crowns, inlays, and fixed bridges of a newer type of porcelain are being used. Thin veneers of porcelain are also used to restore front teeth that are congenitally or chemically stained. The result is cosmetically more appealing. Through a similar bonding process of composites, these veneers on the front surfaces of the teeth offer maximum aesthetics with minimum destruction of tooth structure.

While implantation of metals into the jawbones to support dentures and other prosthetic appliances is not new, the recent use of titanium implants and precision techniques promises long-term retention. Special drills are used to prepare the implant site, and titanium cylinders are either threaded into the bone or pushed into the jaw. The implant is covered by the gum tissue and allowed to heal for six to eight months, so that the process of osseointegration (joining of bone and metal) can occur. The bone will actually fuse to the pure metal, anchoring the implant for an eventual prosthetic appliance.

Laser technology is an exciting field that may have some applications in dentistry. Lasers have been used in gum surgery. Some theorists believe that if the enamel surface of the teeth were to be fused, it would be highly resistant to decay. The heat generated by lasers is a concern, but steps are being taken to control this problem. One of the most promising uses of lasers is in the specialty of endodontics. A thin laser fiberoptic probe advanced down the root canal, preparing and sterilizing the canal prior to filling, vaporizes diseased or degenerating pulp.

Computer science is also being integrated into the treatment phase of dentistry. For example, after scanning a patient's mouth, projected results of treatment can be displayed on a computer screen. In addition, restorations can be developed using the concept of computer-aided design/computer-aided manufacturing (CAD/CAM). A computer scans a prepared tooth for a crown or inlay. The restoration is then designed for a three-dimensional model on the screen. After the model restoration has been chosen, the computer transfers the data to a computer-activated milling machine in the dental laboratory, and a restoration is reproduced in a ceramic or composite resin material in the designed image. The restoration is then cemented into the prepared tooth.

Such improvements in techniques and materials have advanced dentistry into a new era in providing treatment for patients. The basic fundamentals of treatment of the teeth and their surrounding tissues must be maintained, however, in view of the peculiar anatomy and physiology of the teeth.

The above discussion reflects the state of dentistry in North America and Western Europe. In other parts of the world, resources are not available for such advanced techniques. In these countries, teeth are still more likely to be extracted than restored. Prosthetic devices are less common, and many chemical treatments are simply not available. The underlying reason is lack of money.

—*William D. Stark, D.D.S.*
updated by L. Fleming Fallon, Jr., M.D., M.P.H.

See also Anesthesia; Anesthesiology; Caries, dental; Dental diseases; Endodontic disease; Fracture repair; Gastrointestinal system; Gingivitis; Halitosis; Head and neck disorders; Jaw wiring; Orthodontics; Periodontal surgery; Periodontitis; Root canal treatment; Teeth; Temporomandibular joint (TMJ) syndrome; Tooth extraction; Toothache.

FOR FURTHER INFORMATION:

Foster, Malcolm S. *Protecting Our Children's Teeth: A Guide to Quality Dental Care from Infancy Through Age*

Twelve. Ann Arbor, Mich.: Insights Books, 1992. This book is written for parents and other interested readers. It gives insights and suggestions for promoting general dental health.

Kendall, Bonnie L. *Opportunities in Dental Care Careers*. Lincolnwood, Ill.: VGM Career Horizons, 1991. This text provides guidance for students interested in the field of dentistry. It provides information about careers in all allied dentistry fields. Admission requirements for different careers and the names of professional schools that can supply the training are listed.

Moss, Stephen J. *Growing Up Cavity Free: A Parent's Guide to Prevention*. New York: Edition Q, 1994. This rather brief book is written in easy-to-understand language. There are standard suggestions for preventing dental problems.

Smith, Rebecca W. *The Columbia University School of Dental and Oral Surgery's Guide to Family Dental Care*. New York: W. W. Norton, 1997. This classic text provides easy-to-understand explanations of all common dental problems and procedures and many less common procedures. The text is written for the general reader.

Woodforde, John. *The Strange Story of False Teeth*. New York: Universe Books, 1983. This interesting book covers the development of prosthetic appliances to replace missing teeth. There is much dental history described in the text, and the illustrations demonstrate some of the more bizarre attempts to construct appliances to restore dentition. The book is most likely to be found in a library.

DEPRESSION

DISEASE/DISORDER

ANATOMY OR SYSTEM AFFECTED: Brain, heart, musculoskeletal system, psychic-emotional system

SPECIALTIES AND RELATED FIELDS: Family practice, geriatrics and gerontology, psychiatry, psychology

DEFINITION: The single most common psychiatric disorder, caused by biological and/or psychological factors; approximately 15 percent of cases result in suicide.

KEY TERMS:

bipolar disorder: a mood disorder characterized by one or more manic and major depressive episodes occurring simultaneously or in cycles

cyclothymia: a mood disorder characterized as a less intense form of bipolar disorder

dysthymia: a mood disorder characterized as a less intense form of depressive disorder

electroconvulsive therapy: the use of electric shocks to induce seizure in depressed patients as a form of treatment

major depressive disorder: a pattern of major depressive episodes that form an identified psychiatric disorder

major depressive episode: a syndrome of symptoms characterized by depressed mood; required for the diagnosis of some mood disorders

manic episode: a syndrome of symptoms characterized by elevated, expansive, or irritable mood; required for the diagnosis of some mood disorders

psychopharmacology: the drug treatment of psychiatric disorders

psychosurgery: the surgical removal or destruction of part of the brain of depressed patients as a form of treatment

psychotherapy: the "talk" therapies that target the emotional and social contributors and consequences of depression

seasonal affective disorder: a mood disorder associated with the winter season, when the amount of daylight hours is reduced

CAUSES AND SYMPTOMS

The term "depression" is used to describe a fleeting mood, an outward physical appearance of sadness, or a diagnosable clinical disorder. It is estimated that 13 million Americans suffer from a clinically diagnosed depression, a mood disorder that often affects personal, vocational, social, and health functioning. The *Diagnostic and Statistical Manual of Mental Disorders* (4th ed., 1994, DSM-IV) of the American Psychiatric Association delineates a number of mood disorders that subsume the various types of clinical depression.

A major depressive episode is a syndrome of symptoms, present during a two-week period and representing a change from previous functioning. The symptoms include at least five of the following: depressed or irritable mood, diminished interest in previously pleasurable activities, significant weight loss or weight gain, insomnia or hypersomnia, physical excitation or slowness, loss of energy, feelings of worthlessness or guilt, indecisiveness or a diminished ability to concentrate, and recurrent thoughts of death. The clinical depression cannot be initiated or maintained by another illness or condition, and it cannot be a normal reaction to the death of a loved one (some symptoms of depression are a normal part of the grief reaction).

In major depressive disorder, the patient experiences a major depressive episode and does not have a history of mania or hypomania. Major depressive disorder is often first recognized in the patient's late twenties, while a major depressive episode can occur at any age, including infancy. Women are twice as likely to suffer from the disorder than are men.

There are several potential causes of major depressive disorder. Genetic studies suggest a familial link with higher rates of clinical depression in first-degree relatives. There also appears to be a relationship between clinical depression and levels of the brain's neurochemicals, specifically serotonin and norepinephrine. It is important to keep in mind, however, that 20 to 30 percent of adults will experience depression in their lifetime. Common causes of clinical depression include psychosocial stressors, such as the death of a loved one or the loss of a job, or any of a number of personal stressors; it is unclear why some people respond to a specific psychosocial stressor with a clinical depression and others do not. Finally, certain prescription medications have been noted to cause clinical depression. These drugs include muscle relaxants, heart medications, hypertensive medications, ulcer medications, oral contraceptives, and steroids. Thus there are many causes of clinical depression, and no single cause is sufficient to explain all clinical depressions.

Another category of depressive disorder are bipolar disorders, which affect approximately 1 to 2 percent of the population. Bipolar I disorder is characterized by one or more manic episodes along with persisting symptoms of depression. A manic episode is defined as a distinct period of abnormally and persistently elevated, expansive, or irritable mood. Three of the following symptoms must occur during the period of mood disturbance: inflated self-esteem, decreased need for sleep, unusual talkativeness or pressure to keep talking, racing thoughts, distractibility, excessive goal-oriented activities (especially in work, school, or social areas), and reckless activities with a high potential for negative consequences (such as buying sprees or risky business ventures). For a diagnosis of bipolar disorder, the symptoms must be sufficiently severe to cause impairment in functioning and/or concern regarding the person's danger to himself/herself or to others, must not be superimposed on another psychotic disorder, and must not be initiated or maintained by another illness or condition. Bipolar II disorder is characterized by a history of a major depressive episode and current symptoms of mania.

Patients with bipolar disorder will display cycles in which they experience a manic episode followed by a short episode of a major depressive episode, or vice versa. These cycles are often separated by a period of normal mood. Occasionally, two or more cycles can occur in a year without a period of remission between them, in what is referred to as rapid cycling. The two mood disorders can also occur simultaneously in a single episode. Bipolar disorder is often first recognized in adolescence or in the patient's early twenties; it is not unusual, however, for the initial recognition to occur later in life. Bipolar disorder is equally common in both males and females.

Genetic patterns are strongly involved in bipolar disorder. Brain chemicals (particularly dopamine, acetylcholine, GABA, and serotonin), hormones, drug reactions, and life stressors have all been linked to its development. Of particular interest are findings which suggest that, for some patients with bipolar disorder, changes in the seasons affect the frequency and severity of the disorder. These meteorological effects, while not well understood, have been observed in relation to other disorders of mood.

Cyclothymia is another cyclic mood disorder related to depression; it has a reported lifetime prevalence of approximately 1 to 2 percent. This chronic mood disorder is characterized by manic symptoms without marked social or occupational impairment ("hypomanic" episodes) and symptoms of major depressive episode that do not meet the clinical criteria (less than five of the nine symptoms described above). These symptoms must be present for at least two years, and if the patient has periods without symptoms, these periods cannot be longer than two months. Cyclothymia cannot be superimposed on another psychotic disorder and cannot be initiated or maintained by another illness or condition. This mood disorder has its onset in adolescence and early adulthood and is equally common in men and women. It is a particularly persistent and chronic disorder with an identified familial pattern.

Dysthymia is another chronic mood disorder affecting approximately 2 to 4 percent of the population. Dysthymia is characterized by at least a two-year history of depressed mood and at least two of the following symptoms: poor appetite, insomnia or hypersomnia, low energy or fatigue, low self-esteem, poor concentration or decision making, or feelings of hopelessness. There cannot be evidence of a major depressive episode during the first two years of the dysthymia or a history of manic episodes or hypomanic episodes. The patient cannot be without the symptoms for more than two months at a time, the disorder cannot be superimposed on another psychotic disorder, and it cannot be initiated or maintained by another illness or condition. Dysthymia appears to begin at an earlier age, as young as childhood, with symptoms typically evident by young adulthood. Dysthymia is more common in adult females, equally common in both sexes of children, and with a greater prevalence in families. The causes of dysthymia are believed to be similar to those listed for major depressive disorder.

TREATMENT AND THERAPY

Crucial to the choice of treatment for clinical depression is determining the variant of depression being experienced. Each of the diagnostic categories has associated treatment approaches that are more effective for a particular diagnosis. Multiple assessment techniques are available to the health care professional to determine the type of clinical depression. The most valid and reliable is the clinical interview. The health care provider may conduct either an informal interview or a structured, formal clinical interview assessing the symptoms that would confirm the diagnosis of clinical depression. If the patient meets the criteria set forth in the DSM-IV, then the patient is considered for depression treatments. Patients who meet many but not all diagnostic criteria are sometimes diagnosed with a "subclinical" depression. These patients might also be considered appropriate for the treatment of depression, at the discretion of their health care providers.

Another assessment technique is the "paper-and-pencil" measure, or depression questionnaire. A variety of questionnaires have proven useful in confirming the diagnosis of clinical depression. Questionnaires such as the Beck Depression Inventory, Hamilton Depression Rating Scale, Zung Self-Rating Depression Scale, and the Center for Epidemiologic Studies Depression Scale are used to identify persons with clinical depression and to document changes with treatment. This technique is often used as an adjunct to the clinical interview and rarely stands alone as the definitive assessment approach to diagnosing clinical depression.

Laboratory tests, most notably the dexamethasone suppression test, have also been used in the diagnosis of depression. The dexamethasone suppression test involves injecting a steroid (dexamethasone) into the patient and measuring the production levels of another steroid (cortisol) in response. Studies have demonstrated, however, that certain severely depressed patients do not reveal the suppression of cortisol production that would be expected following the administration of dexamethasone. The test has also failed to identify some patients who were depressed and has mistakenly identified others as depressed. Research continues to determine the efficacy of other laboratory measures of brain activity to include computed tomography (CT) scanning, positron emission tomography (PET) scanning, and magnetic resonance imaging (MRI). At this time, laboratory tests are not a reliable diagnostic strategy for depression.

Once a clinical depression (or a subclinical depression) is identified, there are at least four general classes of treatment options available. These options are dependent on the subtype and severity of the depression and include psychopharmacology (drug therapy), individual and group psychotherapy, light therapy, family therapy, electroconvulsive therapy (ECT), and other less traditional treatments. These treatment options can be provided to the patient as part of an outpatient program or, in certain severe cases of clinical depression in which the person is a danger to himself/herself or others, as part of a hospitalization.

Clinical depression often affects the patient physically, emotionally, and socially. Therefore, prior to beginning any treatment with a clinically depressed individual, the health care provider will attempt to develop an open and communicative relationship with the patient. This relationship will allow the health care provider to provide patient education on the illness and to solicit the collaboration of the patient in treatment. Supportiveness, understanding, and collaboration are all necessary components of any treatment approach.

Three primary types of medications are used in the treatment of clinical depression: cyclic antidepressants, monoamine oxidase inhibitors (MAOIs), and lithium salts. These medications are considered equally effective in decreasing the symptoms of depression, which begin to resolve in three to four weeks after initiating treatment. The health care professional will select an antidepressant based on side effects, dosing convenience (once daily versus three times a day), and cost.

The cyclic antidepressants are the largest class of antidepressant medications. As the name implies, the chemical makeup of the medication contains chemical rings, or "cycles." There are unicyclic (buproprion and fluoxetine, or Prozac), bicyclic (sertraline and trazodone), tricyclic (amitriptyline, desipramine, and nortriptyline), and tetracyclic (maprotiline) antidepressants. These antidepressants function to either block the reuptake of neurotransmitters by the neurons, allowing more of the neurotransmitter to be available at a receptor site, or increase the amount of neurotransmitter produced. The side effects associated with the cyclic antidepressants—dry mouth, blurred vision, constipation, urinary difficulties, palpitations, and sleep disturbance—vary and can be quite problematic. Some of these antidepressants have deadly toxic effects at high levels, so they are not prescribed to patients who are at risk of suicide.

Monoamine oxidase inhibitors (isocarboxazid, phenelzine, and tranylcypromine) are the second class of antidepressants. They function by slowing the production of the enzyme monoamine oxidase. This enzyme is responsible for breaking down the neurotransmitters norepinephrine and serotonin, which are believed to be responsible for depression. By slowing the decomposition of these transmitters, more of them are available to the receptors for a longer period of time. Restlessness, dizziness, weight gain, insomnia, and sexual dysfunction are common side effects of the MAOIs. MAOIs are most notable because of the dangerous adverse reaction (severely high blood pressure) that can occur if the patient consumes large quantities of foods high in tyramine (such as aged cheeses, fermented sausages, red wine, foods with a heavy yeast content, and pickled fish). Because of this potentially dangerous reaction, MAOIs are not usually the first choice of medication and are more commonly reserved for depressed patients who do not respond to the cyclic antidepressants.

A third class of medication used in the treatment of depressive disorders consists of the mood stabilizers, the most notable being lithium carbonate, which is used primarily for bipolar disorder. Lithium is a chemical salt that is believed to effect mood stabilization by influencing the production, storage, release, and reuptake of certain neurotransmitters. It is particularly useful in stabilizing and preventing manic episodes and preventing depressive episodes in patients with bipolar disorder.

Another drug occasionally used in the treatment of depression is alprazolam, a muscle relaxant benzodiazepine commonly used in the treatment of anxiety. Alprazolam is believed to affect the nervous system by decreasing the sensitivity of neuronal receptors believed to be involved in depression. While this may in fact occur, the more likely explanation for its positive effect for some patients is that it reduces the anxiety or irritability often coexisting with depression in certain patients.

Psychotherapy refers to a number of different treatment

techniques used to deal with the psychosocial contributors and consequences of clinical depression. Psychotherapy is a common supplement to drug therapy. In psychotherapy, the patients develop knowledge and insight into the causes and treatment for their clinical depression. In cognitive psychotherapy, cure comes from assisting patients in modifying maladaptive, irrational, or automatic beliefs that can lead to clinical depression. In behavioral psychotherapy, patients modify their environment such that social or personal rewards are more forthcoming. This process might involve being more assertive, reducing isolation by becoming more socially active, increasing physical activities or exercise, or learning relaxation techniques. Research on the effectiveness of these and other psychotherapy techniques indicates that psychotherapy is as effective as certain antidepressants for many patients and, in combination with certain medications, is more effective than either treatment alone.

Electroconvulsive (or "shock") therapy is the single most effective treatment for severe and persistent depression. If the clinically depressed patient fails to respond to medications or psychotherapy and the depression is life-threatening, electroconvulsive therapy is considered. It is also considered if the patient cannot physically tolerate antidepressants, as with elders who have other medical conditions. This therapy involves inducing a seizure in the patient by administering an electrical current to specific parts of the brain. The therapy is quite sophisticated and safe, involving little risk to the patient. Patients undergo six to twelve treatments over a two-day to five-day period. Some temporary memory impairment is a common side effect of this treatment.

A variant of clinical depression is known as seasonal affective disorder. Patients with this illness demonstrate a pattern of clinical depression during the winter, when there is a reduction in the amount of daylight hours. For these patients, phototherapy has proven effective. Phototherapy, or light therapy, involves exposing patients to bright light (greater than or equal to 2,500 lux) for two hours daily during the depression episode. The manner in which this treatment approach modifies the depression is unclear and awaits further research.

Psychosurgery, the final treatment option, is quite rare. It refers to surgical removal or destruction of certain portions of the brain believed to be responsible for causing severe depression. Psychosurgery is used only after all treatment options have failed and the clinical depression is life-threatening. Approximately 50 percent of patients who undergo psychosurgery benefit from the procedure.

PERSPECTIVE AND PROSPECTS

Depression, or the more historical term "melancholy," has had a history predating modern medicine. Writings from the time of the ancient Greek physician Hippocrates refer to patients with a symptom complex similar to the present-day definition of clinical depression.

Major depressive episodes and the various subtypes of depression are the leading psychiatric diagnoses treated by health care professionals. Prevalence rates from large-scale studies of depression suggest that approximately 1 in 20 adults will meet the criteria for a major depressive episode at some point in their lives; 1 in 100 for bipolar disorder; 1 in 33 for dysthymia; and 1 in 100 for cyclothymia.

The rates of clinical depression have increased since the early twentieth century, while the age of onset of clinical depression has decreased. Women appear to be at least twice as likely as men to suffer from clinical depression, and people who are happily married have a lower risk for clinical depression than those who are separated, divorced, or dissatisfied in their marital relationship. These data, along with recurrence rates of 50 to 70 percent, indicate the importance of this psychiatric disorder.

While most psychiatric disorders are nonfatal, clinical depression can lead to death. Of the approximately 30,000 suicide deaths per year in the United States, 40 to 80 percent are believed to be related to depression. Approximately 15 percent of patients with major depressive disorder will die by suicide. There are, however, other costs of clinical depression. In the United States, billions of dollars are spent on clinical depression, divided among the following areas: treatment, suicide, and absenteeism (the largest). Clinical depression obviously has a significant economic impact on a society.

The future of clinical depression lies in early identification and treatment. Identification will involve two areas. The first is improving the social awareness of mental health issues to include clinical depression. By eliminating the negative social stigma associated with mental illness and mental health treatment, there will be an increased level of the reporting of depression symptoms and thereby an improved opportunity for early intervention, preventing the progression of the disorder to the point of suicide. The second approach to identification involves the development of reliable assessment strategies for clinical depression. Data suggest that the majority of those who commit suicide see a physician within thirty days of the suicide. The field will continue to strive to identify biological markers and other methods to predict and/or identify clinical depression more accurately. Treatment advances will focus on further development of pharmacological strategies and drugs with more specific actions and fewer side effects. Adjuncts to traditional drug therapies need continued development and refinement to maximize the success of integrated treatments.
—*Oliver Oyama, Ph.D.*
updated by Nancy A. Piotrowski, Ph.D.

See also Anxiety; Brain; Death and dying; Dementia; Eating disorders; Electroconvulsive therapy; Emotions, biochemical causes and effects of; Geriatrics and gerontology; Grief and guilt; Hypochondriasis; Light therapy; Manic-depressive disorder; Midlife crisis; Neurology; Neurology, pediatric; Neurosis; Neurosurgery; Obsessive-compulsive disorder; Panic attacks; Paranoia; Pharmacology; Phobias; Postpartum depression; Psychiatric disorders; Psychiatry; Psychiatry, child and adolescent; Psychiatry, geriatric; Psychoanalysis; Psychosomatic disorders; Stress; Suicide.

FOR FURTHER INFORMATION:

American Psychiatric Association. *Diagnostic and Statistical Manual of Mental Disorders.* 4th ed. Washington, D.C.: Author, 1994. This reference book lists the clinical criteria for psychiatric disorders, including the mood disorders that incorporate the depressions.

Beckham, E. Edward, and William R. Leber, eds. *Handbook of Depression: Treatment, Assessment, and Research.* Homewood, Ill.: Dorsey Press, 1985. This text reviews the field of depression from a scientific perspective. The twenty-seven chapters provide a thoroughly comprehensive review of depression assessment, treatment, and research.

Burns, David D. *Feeling Good: The New Mood Therapy.* New York: William Morrow, 1980. This well-written book is nontechnical and is designed for a general audience. The author describes depression—its assessment and treatment—from a self-help perspective. He introduces the principle of cognitive therapy, which focuses on treating depression by changing the way that people think.

DePaulo, J. Raymond, Jr., and Keith R. Ablow. *How to Cope with Depression: A Complete Guide for You and Your Family.* New York: McGraw-Hill, 1989. Written for patients diagnosed with depression and for their families and friends. The authors use case histories of patients seen at The Johns Hopkins University Hospital to highlight their clinical information. Includes a nice section on bipolar (manic-depressive) disorder.

Greist, John H., and James W. Jefferson. *Depression and Its Treatment.* Rev. ed. Washington, D.C.: American Psychiatric Press, 1992. A patient's guide to depression. The authors describe mood disorders and the identification of depression, and they review the various treatments that are available. The appendices offer a listing of national organizations concerned with depression and an excellent reading list.

Matson, Johnny L. *Treating Depression in Children and Adolescents.* New York: Pergamon Press, 1989. This book, written by one of the leaders in the scientific study of depression, presents a guide to the evaluation and treatment of depression in children and adolescents. The author describes the assessment and treatment approaches that are unique for this nonadult population.

Roesch, Roberta. *The Encyclopedia of Depression.* New York: Facts on File, 1991. This volume was written for both a lay and a professional audience. Covers all aspects of depression, including bereavement, grief, and mourning. The appendices include references, self-help groups, national associations, and institutes.

DERMATITIS

DISEASE/DISORDER

ANATOMY OR SYSTEM AFFECTED: Hair, skin

SPECIALTIES AND RELATED FIELDS: Dermatology

DEFINITION: A wide range of skin disorders, some the result of allergy, some caused by contact with a skin irritant, and some attributable to other causes.

KEY TERMS:

allergen: a substance that excites an immunologic response; also called an antigen

crusting: the appearance of slightly elevated skin lesions made up of dried serum, blood, or pus; they can be brown, red, black, tan, or yellowish

immunoglobulin E (IgE): ordinarily, a relatively rare antibody; in patients with atopic dermatitis, levels can be significantly higher than in the general population

lesion: any pathologic change in tissue

scaling: a buildup of hard, horny skin cells

secondary infection: a bacterial, viral, or other infection that results from or follows another disease

wheal: a small swelling in the skin

CAUSES AND SYMPTOMS

The term "dermatitis" does not refer to a single skin disease, but rather to a wide range of disorders. "Dermatitis" is often used interchangeably with "eczema." The two most common dermatitides are atopic (allergic) dermatitis, in which the individual appears to inherit a predilection for the disease, and contact dermatitis, in which the individual's skin reacts immediately on contact with a substance, or develops sensitivity to it.

Atopic dermatitis often occurs in individuals with a personal or family history of allergy, such as hay fever or asthma. Thirty to 50 percent of children with atopic dermatitis develop asthma or hay fever, a rate that is three to five times higher than for the general population. These people often have high serum levels of a certain antibody, immunoglobulin E (IgE), which may be associated with their skin's tendency to break out, although a specific antigen-antibody reaction has not been demonstrated.

There are many distinct characteristics of atopic dermatitis, some of which depend on the age of the patient. The disease usually starts early in childhood. It is often first discovered in infants in the first months of life when redness and weeping, crusted lesions appear mostly on the face, although the scalp, arms, and legs may also be affected. There is intense itching. Papules (pimples), vesicles (small, blisterlike lesions filled with fluid), edema (swelling), serous exudation (discharge of fluid), and scaly crusts may be seen. At one year of age, oval, scaly lesions appear on the arms, legs, face, and torso. In older children and adults, the lesions are usually localized in the crook of the elbow and the back of the knees, and the face and neck may be involved. The course of the disease is variable. It usually subsides by the third or fourth year of life, but periodic outbreaks may occur throughout childhood, adolescence, and adulthood. In 75 percent of cases, atopic dermatitis improves between the ages of ten and fourteen. Cases persisting past the patient's middle twenties, or beginning then, are the most difficult to treat.

Dryness and itching are always present in atopic dermatitis. People with atopic dermatitis seem to lose skin moisture more readily than average people: Rather than soft, pliable skin, they develop dry, rough, sensitive skin that is particularly prone to chapping and splitting. The skin becomes itchy, and the individual's tendency to scratch significantly aggravates the condition in what is called the "itch-scratch-itch" cycle or the "scratch-rash-itch" cycle: The individual scratches to relieve the itching, which causes a rash, which in turn causes increased itching, which invites increased scratching and increased irritation. After years of itching and scratching, the skin of older children and adults with atopic dermatitis develops red, lichenified (rough, thickened) patches in the crook of the arm and behind the knees, as well as on the eyelids, neck, and wrists.

Constant chafing of the affected area invites bacterial infection and lymphadenitis (inflammation of lymph nodes). Furthermore, patients with atopic dermatitis seem to have altered immune systems. They appear to be more susceptible than others to skin infections, warts, and contagious skin diseases. *Staphylococcus aureus* and certain streptococci are common infecting bacteria in these patients. Pyoderma is often seen as a result of bacterial infection in atopic dermatitis. This condition features redness, oozing, scaling, and crusting, as well as the formation of small pustules (pus-filled pimples).

Patients with atopic dermatitis are also particularly sensitive to herpes simplex and vaccinia viruses. Exposure to either could cause a severe skin disease called Kaposi's varicelliform eruption. Vaccinia virus (the agent that causes cowpox) is used in the preparation of smallpox vaccine. Therefore, patients with atopic dermatitis must not be vaccinated against smallpox. Furthermore, they must be isolated from patients with active herpes simplex and those recently vaccinated against smallpox.

Patients with atopic dermatitis may also develop contact dermatitis, which can greatly exacerbate their condition. They are also sensitive to a wide range of allergens, which can bring on outbreaks, as well as to low humidity (such as in centrally heated houses in winter), which would contribute to dry skin. They may not be able to tolerate woolen clothing.

A condition called keratosis pilaris often develops in the presence of atopic dermatitis. It is not seen in young infants, but it does appear in childhood. Hair follicles on the torso, buttocks, arms, and legs become plugged with horny matter and protrude above the skin, giving the appearance of goose bumps or "chicken skin." The palms of the hands of patients with atopic dermatitis have significantly more fine

lines than those of average people. In many patients, there is a tiny "pleat" under the eyes. They are often prone to cold hands and may have pallor, seen as a blanching of the skin around the nose, mouth, and ears.

When ordinary skin is lightly rubbed with a pointed object, almost immediately there is a red line, followed by a red flare, and finally, a wheal or slight elevation of the skin along the line. In patients with atopic dermatitis, however, there is a completely different reaction: The red line appears, but almost instantly it becomes white. The flare and the wheal do not appear.

About 4 to 12 percent of patients with atopic dermatitis develop cataracts at an early age. Normally, cataracts do not appear until the fifties and sixties; those with atopic dermatitis may develop them in their twenties. These cataracts usually affect both eyes simultaneously and develop quickly.

Psychologically, children with atopic dermatitis often show distinct personality characteristics. They are reported to be bright, aggressive, energetic, and prone to fits of anger. Children with severe, unmanageable cases of atopic dermatitis may become selfish and domineering, and some go on to develop significant personality disorders.

It is not known exactly what happens to cause the itching and dry skin that are the fundamental signs of atopic dermatitis and the root of many of its complications. Various theories suggest various origins. It is by definition an allergic disorder, but the allergens that are specifically involved and how they produce the signs of atopic dermatitis are unknown. One of the most interesting theories involves the antibody IgE. Theoretically, the union of IgE with an antigen causes certain cells to release pharmacologic mediators, such as histamine, bradykinin, and slow-reacting substance (SRS-A), that cause itching and thus begin the cycle of scratching and irritation characteristic of atopic dermatitis. The fact that patients with atopic dermatitis have

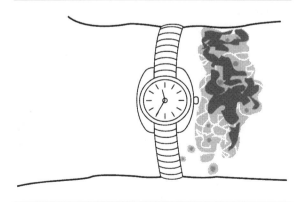

A person can be sensitive to a particular material, such as a nickel watch strap, and contract the itchy, blistering rash of contact dermatitis.

higher than normal levels of IgE, and that there is a relationship between IgE levels and the severity of atopic dermatitis, seems to lend support to this theory.

Contact dermatitis could resemble atopic dermatitis at certain stages, but the dry skin of atopic dermatitis may not be seen. Contact dermatitis is usually characterized by a rash consisting of small bumps, itchiness, blisters, and general swelling. It occurs when the skin has been exposed to a substance to which the body is sensitive or allergic. If the contact dermatitis is caused by direct irritation by a caustic substance, it is called irritant contact dermatitis. The causative agents are primary irritants that cause inflammation at first contact. Some obvious irritants are acids, alkalis, and other harsh chemicals or substances. An example is fiberglass dermatitis, in which fine glass particles from fiberglass fabrics or insulation enter the skin and cause redness and inflammation.

If the dermatitis is caused by allergic sensitivity to a substance, it is called allergic contact dermatitis. In this case, it may take hours, days, weeks, or years for the patient to develop sensitivity to the point where exposure to these substances causes allergic contact dermatitis. These agents include soaps, acetone, skin creams, cosmetics, poison ivy, and poison sumac.

Allergic contact dermatitis comprises the largest variety of contact dermatitides, many of them named for the allergens that cause them. Hence, there is pollen dermatitis; plant and flower dermatitis, such as poison ivy or poison oak; clothing dermatitis; shoe, and even sandal strap, dermatitis; metal and metal salt dermatitis; cosmetic dermatitis; and adhesive tape dermatitis, among others. They all have one thing in common: The skin is exposed to an allergen from any of these sources and becomes so sensitive to it that further exposure causes a rash, itching, and blistering.

The development of sensitivity to an allergen is an immunological response to exposure to that substance. With many allergens, the first contact elicits no immediate immunological reaction. Sensitivity develops after the allergen has been presented to the T lymphocytes that mediate the immune response.

Because it often takes a long time to develop sensitivity, patients are surprised to discover that they have become allergic to substances that they have been using for years. For example, a patient who has been applying a topical medication to treat a skin condition may one day find that the medication causes an outbreak of dermatitis. Ironically, some of the ingredients in medications commonly used to treat skin conditions are among the major allergens that cause allergic contact dermatitis. These include antibiotics, antihistamines, topical anesthetics, antiseptics, as well as the inactive ingredients used in formulating the medication, such as stabilizers.

Other substances to which the patient may develop sensitivity include the chemicals used in making fabric for clothing, tanning chemicals used in making leather, dyes, and ingredients in cosmetics. Many patients develop sensitivity to allergens found in the workplace. The list of potential allergens in the industrial setting is virtually endless. It includes solvents, petroleum products, chemicals commonly used in manufacturing processes, and coal tar derivatives.

In some cases, the allergen requires sunlight or other forms of light to precipitate an outbreak of contact dermatitis. This is called photoallergic contact dermatitis, and it may be caused by such agents as aftershave lotions, sunscreens, topical sulfonamides, and other preparations applied to the skin. Another light reaction, termed phototoxic contact dermatitis, can be caused by exposure to sunlight after exposure to perfumes, coal tar, certain medications, and various chemicals.

A different form of dermatitis involves the sebaceous glands, which secrete sebum, a fatty substance that lubricates the skin and helps retain moisture. Sebaceous dermatitis is usually seen in areas of the body with high concentrations of sebaceous glands, such as on the scalp or face, behind the ears, on the chest, and in areas where skin rubs against skin, such as the buttocks and the groin. It is seen most often in infants and adolescents, although it may persist into adulthood or start at that time.

In infants, sebaceous dermatitis can begin within the first month of life and appears as a thick, yellow, crusted lesion on the scalp called cradle cap. There can be yellow scaling behind the ears and red pimples on the face. Diaper rash may be persistent in these infants. In older children, the lesion may appear as thick, yellow plaques in the scalp. When sebaceous dermatitis begins in adulthood, it starts slowly, and usually its only manifestation is scaling on the scalp (dandruff). In severe cases, yellowish-red scaling pimples develop along the hairline and on the face and chest. Its cause is unknown, but a yeast commonly found in the hair follicles, *Pityrosporum ovale*, may be involved.

There are many other kinds of dermatitis. Diaper dermatitis, or diaper rash, is a complex skin disorder that involves irritation of the skin by urine and feces, irritation by constant rubbing, and secondary infection by *Candida albicans*. Nummular dermatitis (from *nummus*, meaning coin) is characterized by crusting, scaly, disc-shaped papules and vesicles filled with fluid and often pus. Pityriasis alba is a common dermatitis with pale, scaly patches. In lichen simplex chronicus, there is intense itching, with lesions caused by, and perpetuated by, scratching and rubbing. Stasis dermatitis occurs at the ankles; brown discoloration, swelling, scaling, and varicose veins are common. Hyperimmunoglobulin E (Hyper IgE) syndrome is characterized by extremely high IgE levels, ten to one hundred times higher than normal, and a family history of allergy; the patient has frequent skin infections, suppurative (pus-forming) lymphadenitis, pustules, plaques, and abscesses. Pompholyx occurs on the hands and soles of the feet; there is excessive sweating, with eruptions of deep vesicles accompanied by burning or itching.

Friction can also cause dermatitis. In intertrigo, the friction of skin rubbing against skin causes inflammation that can become infected. In frictional lichenoid dermatitis, or sandbox dermatitis, it is thought that the abrasive action of sand or other gritty material on the skin causes the characteristic lesions. Winter eczema seems to be caused by the skin-drying effects of low humidity as well as by harsh soaps and overfrequent bathing; dry skin and itching are common. The acrodermatitis diseases (from *acro*, meaning the extremities) may be limited to the hands and feet, or, like acrodermatitis enteropathica, may erupt in other parts of the body, such as around the mouth and on the buttocks. In fixed-drug eruption, lesions appear in direct response to the administration of a drug; the lesions are generally in the same parts of the body, but they may spread. Swimmer's itch is a parasitic infection from an organism that lives in fresh water lakes and ponds, while seabather's eruption seems to be caused by a similar saltwater organism.

TREATMENT AND THERAPY

Many dermatitides resemble one another, and it is important for a physician to identify the patient's complaint precisely in order to treat it effectively. Therefore, the physician will confirm the identity of the condition through a process known as differential diagnosis. This method allows him or her to rule out all similar conditions, pinpoint the exact nature of the patient's problem, and develop a therapeutic regimen to treat it.

In treating atopic dermatitis, one of the first goals is to relieve dryness and itching. The patient is cautioned not to bathe excessively because this dries the skin. Lotions are used to lubricate the skin and retain moisture. The patient is advised not to scratch, because this could break the skin and invite infection. The patient is advised to avoid any known offending agents and not to apply any medication to the skin without the doctor's knowledge.

Wet compresses can bring relief to patients with atopic dermatitis. Topical corticosteroids are used to help resolve acute flare-ups, but only for short-term therapy, because their prolonged use might produce undesirable side effects. Oral antihistamines are often given to relieve itching and to help the patient sleep. Diet may play a role in atopic dermatitis in infants: Some pediatric dermatologists and other physicians recommend elimination of milk, eggs, tomatoes, citrus fruits, wheat products, chocolate, spices, fish, and nuts from the diets of these patients. Soft cotton clothing is recommended, as is the avoidance of pets or fuzzy toys that might be allergenic. For secondary infections that arise from atopic dermatitis, the physician prescribes appropriate antibiotic therapy.

In primary irritant contact dermatitis, the offending agent is eliminated or avoided. In allergic contact dermatitis, one of the main goals is to discover the offending agent so that the patient can avoid contact with it. Sometimes this information can be elicited from the patient interview, and sometimes it is necessary to conduct a series of patch tests. In this procedure, known allergens are applied to the skin of the patient to find those that cause irritation. Avoidance of the offending agent can cause the patient some difficulty if the agent happens to be something that is found everywhere. An example is the metal nickel, which is in coins, jewelry, and hundreds of other objects. Patients who insist on wearing nickel-plated jewelry are advised to paint it with clear nail polish periodically to avoid contact of the metal with the skin. Similarly, many other allergens are in common use. Patients are advised to read cosmetic labels and food and medical ingredients lists in order to avoid contact with agents to which they are sensitive.

Because there is such a wide range of allergic contact dermatitides, treatment of the flare-ups varies considerably. Topical and oral steroids are used, as well as antihistamines. Sometimes the physician finds it necessary to drain large blisters and apply drying agents to weeping lesions. Sometimes the condition calls for wet compresses to relieve itching and soothe the patient. Specialized lotions, soaps, and shampoos are also used, some to treat dryness and others, as in the case of sebaceous dermatitis, to remove scales and to relieve oiliness.

Other treatments depend on the type of dermatitis from which the patient suffers. Patients with photoallergic or phototoxic dermatitis are advised to avoid light. Acrodermatitis enteropathica is caused by a zinc deficiency; in addition to palliative therapy to relieve the symptoms, these patients are given zinc sulfate, which results in complete remission of the disease. As with atopic dermatitis, bacterial infections occurring as a result of a flare-up of allergic contact dermatitis are treated with appropriate antibiotic therapy.

PERSPECTIVE AND PROSPECTS

The skin is the largest organ of the human body, and it is subject to an extraordinary range and number of diseases, with atopic dermatitis and contact dermatitis among the most common. They may afflict patients of all ages, but they are particularly prevalent in children. Many of the dermatitides start in the first weeks of life and continue through childhood. In many cases, the disease is resolved by the time that the child reaches adolescence, but in some it continues into adulthood.

In spite of the fact that disorders of the skin are readily apparent, an understanding of them has been imperfect throughout history. For example, the allergic nature of many of the dermatitides was not explained until the twentieth century. In addition, because their symptoms are similar to one another and to diseases that are not properly classified as dermatitides, there has been much confusion in identifying them. It has been suggested that many of the biblical lepers were in fact suffering only from a form of dermatitis.

With prolonged exposure, however, they probably became lepers in time.

The dermatitides are often highly complex diseases, involving genetic, allergic, metabolic, and immune and infective factors, among many others. They are not usually life-threatening, but they take an enormous toll in pain, discomfort, and disfigurement, with an equal toll in psychological distress that can be suffered by patients.

Understanding of these disorders improves constantly, and with understanding comes new methods of treating them. Nevertheless, progress will probably be limited. There is the possibility that patients can be desensitized to allow them to tolerate the allergens that bring about their eruptions, as many hay fever sufferers have been desensitized against the pollens and dusts that trigger their allergy. It is unlikely, however, that there will ever be vaccines to immunize against this group of diseases, nor can many of them be cured, except in the sense that the discomfort that they bring can be treated and the agents that cause them can be avoided.   —*C. Richard Falcon*

See also Acne; Allergies; Dermatology; Dermatopathology; Eczema; Itching; Pimples; Poisonous plants; Psoriasis; Rashes; Rosacea; Scabies; Skin disorders.

For Further Information:

Alexander, Dale. *Dry Skin and Common Sense*. West Hartford, Conn.: Witkower Press, 1978. Dry skin is a feature of atopic dermatitis. This book provides treatment tips for the layperson and suggests that dietary habits may improve the condition.

Dvorine, William. *A Dermatologist's Guide to Home Skin Treatment*. New York: Charles Scribner's Sons, 1983. This text features easy-to-understand descriptions of various skin diseases, including the dermatitides. Dvorine offers his recommendations on how to treat them at home.

Handbook of Nonprescription Drugs. 9th ed. Washington, D.C.: American Pharmaceutical Association, 1990. This drug reference work contains excellent background sections on the diseases treated by the thousands of drugs listed. It is well illustrated and particularly suited to teaching the layperson about various disease conditions and how they can be treated. The section on skin diseases is clear, with excellent illustrations.

Larson, David E., ed. *Mayo Clinic Family Health Book*. 2d ed. New York: William Morrow, 1996. An excellent general reference for the layperson, with good coverage of the dermatological diseases.

Walzer, Richard A. *Skintelligence*. New York: Appleton-Century-Crofts, 1981. This dermatologist offers advice on "how to be smart about your skin."

Dermatology

Specialty

Anatomy or system affected: Hair, immune system, nails, skin

Specialties and related fields: Cytology, histology, immunology, oncology, public health

Definition: The study of a variety of irritations or lesions affecting one of several layers of the skin.

Key terms:

allergens: foreign substances in the surrounding environment that may cause an allergic response, such as a skin reaction

dermatitis: a general term for nonspecific skin irritations that may be caused by bacteria, viruses, or fungi

keratin: a fibrous molecule essential to the tissue structure of hair, nails, or the skin

melanin: a polymer made up of several compounds (including the amino acid tyrosine) that causes pigmentation in the skin, hair, and eyes

Science and Profession

Dermatology is the subfield of medicine that deals with diseases of the skin. Some disorders affecting the hair and fingernails may also fall under this category.

Dermatological study requires attention to three distinct layers of the skin, each of which can be affected differently by different disorders. The deepest layer is the subcutaneous tissue where fat is formed and stored. It is also here that the deeper hair follicles and sweat glands originate. Blood vessels and nerves pass from this layer to the dermis. The dermis is mainly connective tissue that contains the oil-producing, or sebaceous, glands and shorter hair follicles. On the surface of the skin is the epidermis, which is itself multilayered. The innermost basal layer is made up of specialized keratin-and melanin-forming cells, whereas the outermost, horny cell layer consists of keratinized dead cells.

The diagnosis of apparent skin disease requires dermatologists to determine whether symptomatic sores, or lesions, are primary (the original symptoms of suspected disease) or secondary (such as infection or irritation caused by scratching which may overshadow the original disorder). Dermatologists are trained to recognize categories of lesions and to determine whether they represent actual diseases or relatively common disorders characteristic of age, or even genetic predispositions. The most common categories of lesions include vesicles, bullae, and crusts; scaling; keratosis; lichenification; pustules; atrophy; and tumors.

Vesicles and bullae are bubblelike eruptions filled with clear serous fluid. As primary lesions, they are often the symptoms of diseases such as chicken pox and herpes zoster. Crusts are formed by tissue fluid that remains in a dried form after the rupture of microscopic vesicles.

Scaling is noticeably different than crusting. These flakes on the surface of the skin may represent a subsiding stage of earlier inflammation. Scaling may be a secondary lesion associated with psoriasis. Keratoses are rough lesions with strongly adherent, not loose, flaking. Lichenification involves a thickening of the epidermis, with a more pronounced visibility of lined patterns on the skin surface. Pustules are lesions filled with pus, which serves as a growth medium for microorganisms. Atrophy always involves shrinkage of skin tissues, creating in some cases visible depressions in the area of the lesion. The last category of primary lesions, tumors, may be found either on the surface of or underneath the skin. Tumorous growths can signal a condition as benign as seborrheic keratosis (the appearance of thick scales in isolated spots, particularly as age advances) or as serious as one of several forms of skin cancer.

Secondary lesions appear as the primary, or causal, skin disorder progresses, creating different symptoms in the secondary stage. Examples of secondary lesions include scales (dandruff and psoriasis), crusts (impetigo), ulcers (advanced syphilis), and scarring, the growth of connective tissue that actually replaces damaged tissues following burns or other traumatic injuries.

In addition to these general categories of lesions associated with dermatological diseases, a number of localized problems in blood flow—called vascular nevoid lesions, or birthmarks—may be visible at or soon after birth. Dermatologists assume that some of these lesions may be caused by genetic factors. The most common vascular nevi categories are nevus flammeus (port-wine stain), a purple discoloring of the skin resulting from dilated dermal vessels, and capillary hemangioma (strawberry mark), which begins as a bruiselike lesion but soon grows into a protruding mass. Unlike port-wine stains, which remain throughout the individual's lifetime unless they are removed through laser surgery, strawberry marks will usually subside and disappear on their own, leaving at most visible puckering of the skin. Unless there are complications (such as ulceration), treatment is usually simple, consisting of the application of elastic bandages to maintain constant pressure, thus reducing the distortion caused by the rapid expansion of skin tissue in a localized area.

Probably the most commonly recognized dermatological disorder, acne, usually occurs among adolescents and young adults. Although this problem is likely to occur as part of the normal process of maturation, lack of proper care of acne may cause complications and lifelong scarring. Acne, as with equally common cases of seborrheic dermatitis (or dandruff, a subcategory of psoriasis), afflicts those areas of the body where oil gland secretions are plentiful and where many forms of bacteria are present on the skin (mainly the face, neck, and upper trunk). The points of lesion for acne are always specific: the hair follicles that are so numerous in these areas of the body. Two phenomena, so-called blackheads and the pimples associated with acne, occur when the normal draining of follicle secretions is blocked in a sac called a comedo. Blackheads occur when the residue trapped in the comedo—keratin, sebum, and various microorganisms—becomes chemically oxidized. When conditions associated with acne appear, an increase in bacterial growth within the comedones produces characteristic pimples which, if traumatized by scratching or picking, may burst, leading to the possibility of further infection. There is no way to prevent acne from appearing, but dermatological therapy to soothe the effects of advanced cases may be recommended.

Another relatively benign but persistently insoluble dermatological problem, the appearance of warts, occurs most often among the middle-aged or older segment of the adult population. Modern dermatological research dating from the 1960's has determined that warts are associated with particular viral strains (Papillomaviruses). At least four subtypes have been associated with the appearance of warts on the human body. Warts may vary greatly in appearance—from plantar warts, which grow well below the skin surface and exhibit a drier consistency, to plane warts, which are even with the skin surface, to a very visible brownish and moist lump, which is often found on the face or hands. All warts are localized viral infections that destroy the normal skin tissue in the area of infection. Despite their common occurrence—dermatologists experience a high rate of patient demand for their removal—warts have always carried a certain social stigma. As viruses, they may be transferred to others through contact, particularly if the lesion is an open one.

The term "seborrheic dermatitis" can refer to the recurrent and common problem of dandruff (redness and scaling mainly in skin areas where body hair is present). Like acne, seborrheic dermatitis is more a condition resulting from secretion imbalances and chemical reactions affecting the skin than an actual disease. Dermatological complications arise when excessive scratching of sensitive areas cause secondary lesions to form.

Beyond these categories of common skin disorders are far more serious diseases that require professional dermatological treatment. For example, psoriasis, although varying in possible locations all over the body (including the hands and feet), seems to share symptoms with seborrheic dermatitis, specifically the flaking away of dry skin. What begins as limited patches of flaking, usually on elbows or in the armpits, however, may spread rapidly and have traumatic effects. Dermatologists usually associate psoriasis with stress and anxiety. When irritations are limited in scope, treatment through topical medications—most containing coal tar, sulfur, salicylic acid, or ammoniated mercury solutions—may be successful. Advanced cases may demand systemic treatment with more sophisticated drugs.

Herpes simplex is another common viral infection which leads directly to surface lesions that may be communicable, in this case cold sores. As with warts, folk knowledge has it that improper hygienic practices lead to the much more virulent eruptions associated with herpes simplex. Medical observations have shown, however, that various factors may unleash a dermatological reaction from latent viral sources in an individual. A herpes simplex reaction to increased levels of exposure to sunlight is a good example. On the other hand, many cases of herpes simplex occur in both the male and female genital areas. Although these eruptions are not necessarily connected with much more serious sexually transmitted diseases, their communicability is clearly associated with levels of hygiene in intimate sexual contact. Whatever the cause of herpes simplex, its highly contagious nature may demand dermatological attention to avoid more serious complications. Any occurrence of herpes simplex inflammation near a vital organ, for example, must be treated immediately to prevent the spread of viral infection, particularly in the area surrounding the eyes.

Herpes zoster, commonly referred to as shingles, is thought to be a recurrence in the adult years of a common viral infection that most people experience at an earlier age: chickenpox. The persistence of the symptoms of shingles among adults, however, is not comparable to the mild effect of the virus during childhood. The appearance of painful lesions, usually but not always in the trunk area, may come after a short period of tingling. Although inflammation may pass, many elderly patients, especially those suffering from systemic diseases such as diabetes mellitus, are plagued by continuous long-term discomfort. In addition to discomfort, there may be (as in herpes simplex) a danger of complications if the area of inflammation is close to vulnerable tissues or key organs, such as the eyes or ears. In cases where lesions may affect the eyes, dermatologists must go beyond topical treatment to enhance the healing process. Additional emergency therapy may include systemic steroid treatment, the intravenous administration of corticotropin, or oral doses of prednisone.

DIAGNOSTIC AND TREATMENT TECHNIQUES

The diagnosis of specific dermatoses, or potentially serious skin diseases, may or may not require cutaneous biopsies; because their symptoms are not shared by other diseases, a diagnosis can often be made by observation alone. Less easily recognized problems include lichen planus, an uncommon chronic pruritic disease; such potentially dangerous bullous diseases as pemphigus vulgaris, which is characterized by flat-topped papules on the wrists and legs that resemble poison ivy reactions; and skin cancer. Such conditions usually require biopsy to ensure that a mistaken diagnosis does not lead to the wrong treatment. Several methods of biopsy are employed, according to the nature of the lesion under examination. For example, the cutaneous punch technique, which utilizes a special surgical tool that penetrates to about 4 millimeters, may not be appropriate if the lesion is close to the surface. In this case, either curettage (scraping) or shave biopsy (cutting a layer corresponding to the thickness of the lesion) may be used in combination with the cutaneous punch method.

The total number of dermatoses that can be diagnosed is far too great for review here. The conditions that are most commonly treated, however, range from mildly seri-

ous but clearly irritating lesions such as acne or warts to much more serious phenomena such as psoriasis and lupus erythematosus. Several early and potentially dangerous conditions, especially basal cell carcinoma, may deteriorate into fatal skin cancers.

Dermatologists classify serious skin diseases under several key divisions. Pruritic dermatoses are characterized by itching. Vascular dermatoses, including several categories of urticaria, are all characterized by sudden outbreaks of papules—some temporary in their irritation and therefore merely disorders, as with hives as a reaction to poison ivy or medicines such as penicillin, and others more serious, such as swelling of the glottis, which may accompany angioneurotic edema. Papulosquamous dermatoses include psoriasis and lichen planus, both localized irritations that involve redness and flaking. In addition to these categories of dermatoses, a wide variety of common dermatologic viruses demand special medical attention because they are socially communicable. These include herpes simplex and herpes zoster. Other serious viruses affecting the skin, such as smallpox and measles, have been controlled by preventive vaccinations. Impetigo, once common during childhood in certain environments, is a bacterial infection, not a viral one. One formerly lethal sexually transmitted disease is syphilis, a form of spirochetal infection. Although far from eradicated, syphilis has been treatable through the use of benzathine penicillin since the mid-twentieth century.

The most serious challenge to dermatologists is the early diagnosis and treatment of skin cancer. The most common forms of skin cancer are basal cell epithilioma, which originates in the epidermis, often as a result of excessive exposure to the sun, and squamous cell carcinoma, which may affect the epidermis or mucosal surfaces (the inside of the mouth or throat). Early diagnosis of both types is essential to prevent metastasis (spreading). The most dangerous skin cancer is malignant melanoma, which may reveal itself through changes in size or color of a body mark such as a mole. This cancer can metastasize very rapidly and endanger the life of the patient.

Possible treatments for different types of skin disease vary considerably. Surgical operations, although certainly not unknown, tend to be associated with more extreme disorders, most notably skin cancer. In such cases, it is usually not the dermatologist but a specialized surgeon who performs the procedure.

The most common treatments used by dermatologists involve the application of various pharmaceutical preparations directly to the surface of the skin. For the treatment of common skin disorders, dermatologists may choose between a variety of medications.

The effect of antipruritic agents (menthol, phenol, camphor, or coal tar solutions) is to reduce itching. Keratoplastic agents (salicylic acid) and keratolytic agents (stronger doses of salicylic acid, resorcinol, or sulfur) affect the relative thickness or softness of the horny layer of the skin. They are associated with the treatment of diseases or disorders characterized by flaking.

Antieczematous agents, including coal tar solutions and hydrocortisone, halt oozing from vesicular lesions. By far the most commonly used drugs in dermatology are antiseptics which, according to their classification, control or kill bacteria, fungi, and viruses. Antibacterial agents that have been widely used for many years include iodochlorhydroxyquin and ammoniated mercury. Ointments to combat viral infections are much less common on the pharmaceutical market, but the recently developed drug acyclovir has been marketed under the name Zovirax.

These and many other topical applications may be only the first steps, however, in soothing the irritating side effects of more serious or chronically persistent dermatological diseases. Doctors may turn to more active therapies to treat specific ailments, beginning with the general category of electrosurgery, of which there are five specialized subtreatments: electrodesiccation, or the drying of tissues; electrocoagulation, which involves more intense heat; electrocautery, the actual burning of tissues; electolysis, which produces the cauterization of lesions by chemical reaction; and electrosection, or the removal of tissues by cutting, achieved by the focus of electrical currents produced by various forms of vacuum tubes. By the 1990's, rapid progress in laser beam technology—particularly the carbon dioxide laser, which is a beam of infrared electromagnetic energy with an almost infinitesimal wavelength of 10,600 nanometers—began to replace some of these time-tested methods in cases in which electrosurgery had been commonplace for almost half a century.

Other modes of treatment that penetrate the subsurface layers of the skin include radiation therapy and cryosurgery, which is the immediate freezing of tissues by application of agents such as solid carbon dioxide (−78.5 degrees Celsius) or liquid nitrogen (−195.8 degrees Celsius). These methods are used to treat conditions ranging from psoriasis and pruritic dermatoses to skin cancer.

Perspective and Prospects

One common feature—visible body surface symptoms—means that the medical identification and attempted treatment of human skin diseases can be traced to almost all cultures in all historical periods. An outstanding example of ancient peoples' concerns for eruptions on the skin can be found in the Old Testament or Talmud in Leviticus. In the Scripture, however, as well as in many medieval texts, one sees that a variety of skin diseases tended to be classified as leprosy. The physical location of skin lesions often determined the results of very general attempts at diagnosis.

It was not until the last quarter of the eighteenth century that Viennese physicians ushered in what could be called the first phase of scientific study of the skin and its disorders, or dermatology. This early Viennese school insisted on the study of the morphological nature of the lesions. Until this time, physicians had grouped skin diseases according to their appearance in different places on the body. By the mid-nineteenth century another Austrian, Ferdinand von Hebra, made considerable progress in classifying skin diseases.

Because so many lesions of the skin could potentially lead to diagnoses of sexually transmitted diseases, early generations of dermatologists concentrated most of their emphasis in this area. Discovery of a treatment for syphilis in the early twentieth century freed researchers to diversify their physiological investigations, opening the field to broader applications of biochemistry for treatment of different skin conditions, a field developed by the American doctor Stephen Rothman in the 1930's. Some categories, such as fungal diseases, were brought under control by treatments that were developed fairly quickly. By the second half of the century, dermatologists could alleviate most of the complications caused by psoriasis. Then, during the last quarter of the twentieth century, impressive advances in the discovery and patenting of sophisticated drugs brought most of the major dermatological diseases, including those caused in large part by nervous stress, under general control.

Although the treatment of life-threatening diseases, particularly skin cancers, continues to fall short of guaranteed cures, early recognition of their symptoms has steadily increased patients' chances for survival.

—*Byron D. Cannon, Ph.D.*

See also Abscess drainage; Abscesses; Acne; Albinism; Athlete's foot; Biopsy; Burns and scalds; Cancer; Carcinoma; Chickenpox; Cryotherapy and cryosurgery; Cyst removal; Cysts and ganglions; Dermatitis; Dermatopathology; Eczema; Electrocauterization; Fungal infections; Glands; Grafts and grafting; Hair loss and baldness; Hair transplantation; Healing; Histology; Itching; Keratoses; Lice, mites, and ticks; Lupus erythematosus; Malignant melanoma removal; Nail removal; Neurofibromatosis; Pigmentation; Pimples; Plastic, cosmetic, and reconstructive surgery; Poisonous plants; Psoriasis; Rashes; Rosacea; Scabies; Sense organs; Skin; Skin cancer; Skin disorders; Skin lesion removal; Tattoo removal; Touch; Warts.

For Further Information:

Braverman, Irwin M. *Skin Signs of Systemic Disease*. Philadelphia: W. B. Saunders, 1998. This book deals with the side effects of chronic diseases such as lymphomas and leukemia that may, at certain stages, be diagnosed through dermatological analysis.

Monk, B. E., et al., eds. *Skin Disorders in the Elderly*. Oxford, England: Blackwell Scientific Publications, 1988. As the title suggests, this collection of studies deals with typical skin problems among the elderly, many of which stem from infections elsewhere in the body.

Pillsbury, Donald M. *A Manual of Dermatology*. Philadelphia: W. B. Saunders, 1971. A somewhat dated but well-organized treatment of the main clinical facets of dermatology, including indicated therapies.

Roenigk, Henry H., ed. *Office Dermatology*. Baltimore: Williams & Wilkins, 1981. Less technical than most medical texts, this general work addresses the most common skin diseases in concise terms.

Sauer, Gordon C. *Manual of Skin Diseases*. 6th ed. Philadelphia: J. B. Lippincott, 1991. This very detailed and frequently updated text is among the most widely used in medical schools. Part of its organization consists of "reminder boxes" to emphasize salient points for diagnosis and therapy.

DERMATOPATHOLOGY

SPECIALTY

ANATOMY OR SYSTEM AFFECTED: Immune system, skin

SPECIALTIES AND RELATED FIELDS: Cytology, dermatology, forensic medicine, histology, immunology, oncology, pathology

DEFINITION: The study of the causes and characteristics of diseases or changes involving the skin.

KEY TERMS:

basal cells: cells at the base of the epidermis that migrate upward and become the principal source of epidermal tissue

dermatoses: disorders of the skin

dermis: the layer of skin just below the surface, in which is found blood and lymphatic vessels, sebaceous (oil) glands, and nerves; also called the corium

epidermis: the outer layer of the skin, consisting of a dead superficial layer and an underlying cellular section

SCIENCE AND PROFESSION

Dermatopathology is the medical specialty that utilizes external clinical features of the body's surface, as well as histological changes that are observed microscopically, to define diseases of the skin. The dermatopathologist is a physician who has specialized in pathology, the clinical study of disease, and/or in histology, the microscopic study of cells and tissues. Although the specific clinical field of this specialty involves the skin, the practitioner has also received broader training in pathology.

The skin is the tough, cutaneous layer that covers the entire surface of the body. In addition to the epidermal tissue of the surface, the skin contains an extensive network of underlying structures, including lymphatic vessels, nerves and nerve endings, and hair follicles. The dead cells on the surface of the epidermis continually slough off, to be replaced by dividing cells from the underlying basal layers. As these cells proceed to the surface, they mature and die, forming the outer layer of the skin.

When a disease or condition of the skin is being diagnosed, the initial observations are often carried out by a general practitioner or dermatologist. This person will make a gross observation; if warranted, biopsies or samples of the lesion may then be provided to the dermatopathologist for examination. The most common forms of skin lesions are those associated with allergies, such as contact dermatitis associated with exposure to plant oils (poison ivy) or chemicals (antibiotics). More serious dermatologic diseases may also require diagnosis. Specific types of disease are often represented by specific kinds of lesions; these may include a variety of forms of skin cancers, lesions associated with bacterial or viral infections (such as impetigo or herpes simplex), and autoimmune disorders (such as lupus). The dermatopathologist may also be concerned with diseases of underlying tissue, such as lymphoid cancers or lesions penetrating into mucous membranes.

The dermatopathologist is involved in the diagnosis of the problem but generally is not involved with specific forms of treatment. Nevertheless, his or her recommendations may certainly influence any decisions. The major role of the dermatopathologist is observation; this may then be followed by an interpretation of results, including a possible prognosis or outcome.

DIAGNOSTIC AND TREATMENT TECHNIQUES

The clinical examination of skin lesions initially falls within the realm of the dermatologist. If the gross observations are insufficient to warrant diagnosis, however, a sample of the lesion can be sent to the dermatopathologist for further examination. In addition to the tissue sample, information on the age, sex, and skin color of the patient should be included, along with any history of the suspected condition.

If the lesion is superficial, as in dermatoses such as warts or even certain types of cancer, a superficial shave biopsy is sufficient for examination. If the lesion involves an infiltrating tumor, inflammation, or possible metabolic problems, a deeper section of tissue is necessary. The specimen is immediately placed in a fixative solution such as formalin, in order to prevent deterioration.

The dermatopathologist initially embeds the sample in paraffin, which can be sectioned into thin slices after hardening. The tissue is stained, most commonly with hematoxylin and eosin (H & E), and observed microscopically.

Anything about the cells that is out of the ordinary may be helpful in the diagnosis of the problem. For example, in the case of basal cell carcinoma, the cells may be abnormally shaped, with enlarged nuclei. They may also be observed infiltrating other layers of tissue. With contact dermatitis, the lesion is characterized by infiltration of large numbers of white blood cells, particularly lymphocytes, with their easily observed large nuclei. Edema, the abnormal accumulation of fluid, is also common with these types of lesions.

The presence of bacteria, as with boils or impetigo, warrants the use of antibiotics, unlike other inflammatory lesions. In this matter, the dermatopathology of the sample can determine the appropriate form of treatment.

While dermatopathology is primarily observational, recommendations regarding treatment may be made by its practitioners. For example, the study of a sample for the type and extent of cancer may lead to a recommendation concerning how extensive the surgical removal of the tumor should be.

PERSPECTIVE AND PROSPECTS

The use of the physical appearance of the skin as a means of diagnosis represents one of the earliest attempts to understand disease. With the microscopic examination of tissue, first performed during the nineteenth century, it became possible to match the presence of histological lesions to specific diseases and to differentiate these diseases from one another.

The field of dermatopathology was greatly refined during the twentieth century. The development of differential and immunological staining methods allowed for a greater understanding of the roles played by the wide variety of cells in the body. For example, the dendritic cells of the skin were found to have a critical function in the immune responses which begin at that level.

In many Western countries, there was a significant shift during the twentieth century in the types of skin disease most commonly seen, mostly reflecting changes in lifestyle. The prevalence of malignant melanomas and basal cell carcinomas became much higher as a result of increased exposure to sun during leisure hours. The recognition of such problems has become an important aspect of the training of clinicians less specialized than dermatopathologists, such as family physicians. —*Richard Adler, Ph.D.*

See also Autoimmune disorders; Bacterial infections; Biopsy; Cancer; Carcinoma; Cytopathology; Dermatitis; Dermatology; Edema; Electrocauterization; Grafts and grafting; Herpes; Histology; Lupus erythematosus; Malignant melanoma removal; Microscopy; Oncology; Pathology; Pigmentation; Plastic, cosmetic, and reconstructive surgery; Skin; Skin cancer; Skin disorders; Skin lesion removal; Viral infections; Warts.

FOR FURTHER INFORMATION:

McKee, Phillip. *A Concise Atlas of Dermatopathology.* New York: Gower Medical, 1993.

Mehregan, Amir. *Pinkus' Guide to Dermatohistopathology.* 6th ed. Norwalk, Conn.: Appleton-Century-Crofts, 1995.

Tierney, Lawrence M., Jr., et al., eds. *Current Medical Diagnosis and Treatment.* 37th ed. Norwalk, Conn.: Appleton and Lange, 1998.

Vasarinsh, P. *Clinical Dermatology: Diagnosis and Therapy of Common Skin Diseases.* Boston: Butterworth, 1982.

DIABETES MELLITUS

DISEASE/DISORDER

ANATOMY OR SYSTEM AFFECTED: Abdomen, blood vessels, circulatory system, endocrine system, eyes, gastrointestinal system, glands, nervous system, pancreas

SPECIALTIES AND RELATED FIELDS: Endocrinology, family practice, genetics, internal medicine, pediatrics, vascular medicine

DEFINITION: A hormonal disorder in which the pancreas is not able to produce sufficient insulin to process and maintain proper blood sugar levels; if left untreated, it leads to secondary complications such as blindness, dementia, and eventually death.

KEY TERMS:

beta cells: the insulin-producing cells located at the core of the islets of Langerhans in the pancreas; the alpha, or glucagon-producing, cells form an outer coat

cross-linking: a chemical reaction, triggered by the binding of glucose to tissue proteins, that results in the attachment of one protein to another and the loss of elasticity in aging tissues

glucosuria: a condition in which the concentration of blood glucose exceeds the ability of the kidney to reabsorb it; as a result, glucose spills into the urine, taking with it body water and electrolytes

insulin-dependent diabetes mellitus (IDDM): type 1 diabetes, a state of absolute insulin deficiency in which the body does not produce sufficient insulin to move glucose into the cells

insulin resistance: a lack of insulin action; a reduction in the effectiveness of insulin to lower blood glucose concentrations; characteristic of type 2 diabetes

insulitis: the selective destruction of the insulin-producing beta cells in type 1 diabetes

islets of Langerhans: clusters of cells scattered throughout the pancreas; they produce three hormones involved in sugar metabolism: insulin, glucagon, and somatostatin

non-insulin-dependent diabetes mellitus (NIDDM): type 2 diabetes, which is the state of a relative insulin deficiency; although insulin is released, its target cells do not adequately respond to it by taking up blood glucose

CAUSES AND SYMPTOMS

Diabetes mellitus is by far the most common of all endocrine (hormonal) disorders. The word "diabetes" is derived from the Greek word for "siphon" or "running through," a reference to the potentially large urine volume that can accompany the condition. *Mellitus*, the Latin word for "honey," was added when physicians began to make the diagnosis of diabetes mellitus based on the sweet taste of the patient's urine. The disease has been depicted as a state of starvation in the midst of plenty. Although there is plenty of sugar in the blood, without insulin it does not reach the cells that need it for energy. Glucose, the simplest form of sugar, is the primary source of energy for many vital functions. Deprived of glucose, cells starve and tissues begin to degenerate. The unused glucose builds up in the bloodstream, which leads to a series of secondary complications.

The acute symptoms of diabetes mellitus are all attributable to inadequate insulin action. The immediate conse-

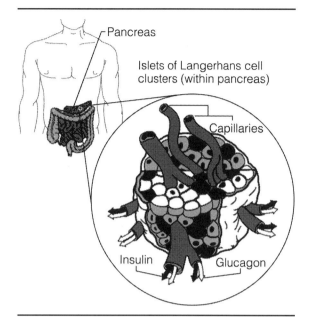

Location of the pancreas, with a section showing the specialized cells (islets of Langerhans) that produce the sugar-metabolizing hormones.

quence of an insulin insufficiency is a marked decrease in the ability of both muscle and adipose (fat) tissue to remove glucose from the blood. In the presence of inadequate insulin action, a second problem manifests itself. People with diabetes continue to make the hormone glucagon. Glucagon, which raises the level of blood sugar, can be considered insulin's biological opposite. Like insulin, glucagon is released from the pancreatic islets. The release of glucagon is normally inhibited by insulin; therefore, in the absence of insulin, glucagon action elevates concentrations of glucose. For this reason, diabetes may be considered a "two-hormone disease." With a reduction in the conversion of glucose into its storage forms of glycogen in liver and muscle and lipids in adipose cells, concentrations of glucose in the blood steadily increase (hyperglycemia). When the amount of glucose in the blood exceeds the capacity of the kidney to reabsorb this nutrient, glucose begins to spill into the urine (glucosuria). Glucose in the urine then drags additional body water along with it so that the volume of urine dramatically increases. In the absence of adequate fluid intake, the loss of body water and accompanying electrolytes (sodium) leads to dehydration and, ultimately, death caused by the failure of the peripheral circulatory system.

Insulin deficiency also results in a decrease in the synthesis of triglycerides (storage forms of fatty acids) and stimulates the breakdown of fats in adipose tissue. Although glucose cannot enter the cells and be used as an energy source, the body can use its supply of lipids from the fat cells as an alternate source of energy. Fatty acids increase in the blood, causing hyperlipidemia. With large amounts of circulating free fatty acids available for processing by the liver, the production and release of ketone bodies (breakdown products of fatty acids) into the circulation are accelerated, causing both ketonemia and an increase in the acidity of the blood. Since the ketone levels soon also exceed the capacity of the kidney to reabsorb them, ketone bodies soon appear in the urine (ketonuria).

Insulin deficiency and glucagon excess also cause pronounced effects on protein metabolism and result in an overall increase in the breakdown of proteins and a reduction in the uptake of amino acid precursors into muscle protein. This leads to the wasting and weakening of skeletal muscles and, in children who are diabetics, results in a reduction in overall growth. Unfortunately, the increased level of amino acids in the blood provides an additional source of material for glucose production (gluconeogenesis) by the liver. All these acute metabolic changes in carbohydrates, lipids, and protein metabolism can be prevented or reversed by the administration of insulin.

There are two distinct types of diabetes mellitus. Type I, or insulin-dependent diabetes mellitus (IDDM), is an absolute deficiency of insulin that accounts for approximately 10 percent of all cases of diabetes. Until the discovery of insulin, people stricken with Type I diabetes faced certain death within about a year of diagnosis. In Type II or non-insulin-dependent diabetes mellitus (NIDDM), insulin secretion may be normal or even increased, but the target cells for insulin are less responsive than normal (insulin resistance); therefore, insulin is not as effective in lowering blood glucose concentrations. Although either type can be manifested at any age, Type I diabetes has a greater prevalence in children, whereas the incidence of Type II diabetes increases markedly after the age of forty and is the most common type of diabetes. Genetic and environmental factors are important in the expression of both types of diabetes mellitus.

Type I diabetes is an autoimmune process that involves the selective destruction of the insulin-producing beta cells in the islets of Langerhans (insulitis). The triggering event that initiates this process in genetically susceptible persons may be a virus or, more likely, the presence of toxins in the diet. The body's own T lymphocytes progressively attack the beta cells but leave the other hormone-producing cell types intact. T lymphocytes are white blood cells that normally attack virus-invaded cells and cancer cells. For up to ten years, there remains a sufficient number of insulin-producing cells to respond effectively to a glucose load, but when approximately 80 percent of the beta cells are destroyed, there is insufficient insulin release in response to a meal and the deadly spiral of the consequences of diabetes mellitus is triggered. Insulin injection can halt this lethal process and prevent it from recurring but cannot mimic the normal pattern of insulin release from the pancreas. It is interesting that not everyone who has insulitis actually progresses to experience overt symptoms of the disease, although it is known that the incidence of Type I diabetes around the world is on the increase.

Type II diabetes is normally associated with obesity and lack of exercise as well as with genetic predisposition. Family studies have shown that as many as 25 to 35 percent of persons with Type II diabetes have a sibling or parent with the disease. The risk of diabetes doubles if both parents are affected. Because there is a reduction in the sensitivity of the target cells to insulin, people with Type II diabetes must secrete more insulin to maintain blood glucose at normal levels. Because insulin is a storage, or anabolic, hormone, this increased secretion further contributes to obesity. In response to the elevated insulin concentrations, the number of insulin receptors on the target cell gradually decreases, which triggers an even greater secretion of insulin. In this way, the excess glucose is stored despite the decreased availability of insulin binding sites on the cell. Over time, the demands for insulin eventually exceed even the reserve capacity of the "genetically weakened" beta cells, and symptoms of insulin deficiency develop as the plasma glucose concentrations remain high for increasingly larger periods of time. Because the symptoms of Type II diabetes are usually less severe than those of Type I diabetes, many persons have the disease but remain unaware of it. Unfor-

tunately, once the diagnosis of diabetes is made in these individuals, they also exhibit symptoms of long-term complications that include atherosclerosis and nerve damage. Hence, Type II diabetes has been called the "silent killer."

TREATMENT AND THERAPY

Insulin is the only treatment available for Type I diabetes, and in many cases it is used to treat individuals with Type II diabetes. Insulin is available in many formulations, which differ in respect to the time of onset of action, activity, and duration of action. Insulin preparations are classified as fast-acting, intermediate-acting, and long-acting; the effects of fast-acting insulin last for thirty minutes to twenty-four hours, while those of long-acting preparations last from four to thirty-six hours. Some of the factors that affect the rate of insulin absorption include the site of injection, the patient's age and health status, and the patient's level of physical activity. For a person with diabetes, however, insulin is a reprieve, not a cure.

Because of the complications that arise from chronic exposure to glucose, it is recommended that glucose concentrations in the blood be maintained as close to physiologically normal levels as possible. For this reason, it is preferable to administer multiple doses of insulin during the day. By monitoring plasma glucose concentrations, the diabetic person can adjust the dosage of insulin administered and thus mimic normal concentrations of glucose rela-

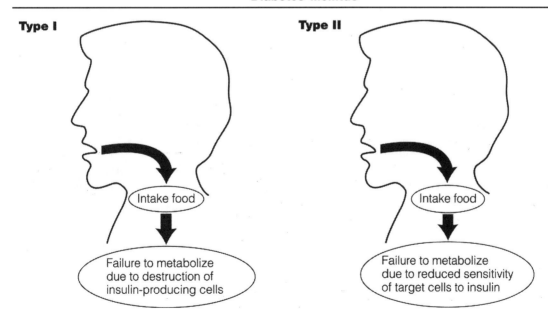

Diabetes Mellitus

Type I

Intake food

Failure to metabolize due to destruction of insulin-producing cells

Type II

Intake food

Failure to metabolize due to reduced sensitivity of target cells to insulin

Diabetes mellitus results from the body's failure to metabolize sugar properly. Type I diabetes is an autoimmune process that destroys insulin-producing cells and is often found in children. Type II diabetes results from the reduced sensitivity of target cells to insulin, requiring increased secretion of insulin to maintain blood sugar levels; this type generally affects adults and is often caused by poor eating habits and lack of exercise over years.

tively closely. Basal concentrations of plasma insulin can also be maintained throughout the day by means of electromechanical insulin delivery systems. Whether internal or external, such insulin pumps can be programmed to deliver a constant infusion of insulin at a rate designed to meet minimum requirements. The infusion can then be supplemented by a bolus injection prior to a meal. Increasingly sophisticated systems automatically monitor blood glucose concentrations and adjust the delivery rate of insulin accordingly. These alternative delivery systems are intended to prevent the development of long-term tissue complications.

There are a number of chronic complications that account for the shorter life expectancy of diabetic persons. These include atherosclerotic changes throughout the entire vascular system. The thickening of basement membranes that surround the capillaries can affect their ability to exchange nutrients. Cardiovascular lesions are the most common cause of premature death in diabetic persons. Kidney disease, which is commonly found in longtime diabetics, can ultimately lead to kidney failure. For these persons, expensive medical care, including dialysis and the possibility of a kidney transplant, overshadows their lives. Diabetes is the leading cause of new blindness in the United States. In addition, diabetes leads to a gradual decline in the ability of nerves to conduct sensory information to the brain. For example, the feet of some diabetics feel more like stumps of wood than living tissue. Consequently, weight is not distributed properly; in concert with the reduction in blood flow, this problem can lead to pressure ulcers. If not properly cared for, areas of the foot can develop gangrene, which may then lead to amputation of the foot. Finally, in male patients, there are problems with reproductive function that generally result in impotence.

The mechanism responsible for the development of these long-term complications of diabetes is genetic in origin and dependent on the amount of time the tissues are exposed to the elevated plasma glucose concentrations. What, then, is the link between glucose concentrations and diabetic complications?

As an animal ages, most of its cells become less efficient in replacing damaged material, while its tissues lose their elasticity and gradually stiffen. For example, the lungs and heart muscle expand less successfully, blood vessels become increasingly rigid, and ligaments tighten. These apparently diverse age-related changes are accelerated in diabetes, and the causative agent is glucose. Glucose becomes chemically attached to proteins and deoxyribonucleic acid (DNA) in the body without the aid of enzymes to speed the reaction along. What is important is the duration of exposure to the elevated glucose concentrations. Once glucose is bound to tissue proteins, a series of chemical reactions is triggered that, over the passage of months and years, can result in the formation and eventual accumulation of

cross-links between adjacent proteins. The higher glucose concentrations in diabetics accelerate this process, and the effects become evident in specific tissues throughout the body.

Understanding the chemical basis of protein cross-linking in diabetes has permitted the development and study of compounds that can intervene in this process. Certain compounds, when added to the diet, can limit the glucose-induced cross-linking of proteins by preventing their formation. One of the best-studied compounds, aminoguanidine, can help prevent the cross-linking of collagen; this fact is shown in a decrease in the accumulation of trapped lipoproteins on artery walls. Aminoguanidine also prevents thickening of the capillary basement membrane in the kidney. Aminoguanidine acts by blocking glucose's ability to react with neighboring proteins. Vitamins C and B_6 are also effective in reducing cross-linking. All these substances may be considered antiaging compounds.

Alternatively, transplantation of the entire pancreas is an effective means of achieving an insulin-independent state in persons with Type I diabetes mellitus. Both the technical problems of pancreas transplantation and the possible rejection of the foreign tissue, however, have limited this procedure as a treatment for diabetes. Diabetes is usually manageable; therefore, a pancreas transplant is not necessarily lifesaving. Some limited success in treating diabetes has been achieved by transplanting only the insulin-producing islet cells from the pancreas or grafts from fetal pancreas tissue. It may one day be possible to use genetic engineering to permit cells of the liver to self-regulate glucose concentrations by synthesizing and releasing their own insulin into the blood.

Some of the less severe forms of Type II diabetes mellitus can be controlled by the use of oral hypoglycemic agents that bring about a reduction in blood glucose. These drugs can be taken orally to drive the beta cells to release even more insulin than usual. These drugs also increase the ability of insulin to act on the target cells, which ultimately reduces the insulin requirement. The use of these agents remains controversial, because they overwork the already strained beta cells. If a diabetic person is reliant on these drugs for extended periods of time, the insulin cells could "burn out" and completely lose their ability to synthesize insulin. In this situation, the previously non-insulin-dependent person would have to be placed on insulin therapy for life.

If obesity is a factor in the expression of Type II diabetes, as it is in most cases, the best therapy is a combination of a reduction of calorie intake and an increase in activity. More than any other disease, Type II diabetes is related to lifestyle. It is often the case that people prefer having an injection or taking a pill to improving their quality of life by changing their diet and level of activity. Attention to diet and exercise results in a dramatic decrease in the need for drug therapy in nine out of ten diabetics. In some cases, the loss of only a small percentage of body weight results in an increased sensitivity to insulin. Exercise is particularly helpful in the management of both types of diabetes, because working muscle does not require insulin to metabolize glucose. Thus, exercising muscles take up and use some of the excess glucose in the blood, which reduces the overall need for insulin. Permanent weight reduction and exercise also help to prevent long-term complications and permit a healthier and more active lifestyle.

PERSPECTIVE AND PROSPECTS

Diabetes mellitus is a disease of ancient origin. The first written reference to diabetes, which was discovered in the tomb of Thebes in Egypt (1500 B.C.), described an illness associated with the passage of vast quantities of sweet urine and an excessive thirst.

The study of diabetes owes much to the Franco-Prussian War. In 1870, during the siege of Paris, it was noted by French physicians that the widespread famine in the besieged city had a curative influence on diabetic patients. Their glycosuria decreased or disappeared. These observations supported the view of clinicians at the time who had previously prescribed periods of fasting and increased muscular work for the treatment of the overweight diabetic individual.

It was Oscar Minkowski of Germany who, in 1889, accidentally traced the origin of diabetes to the pancreas. Following the complete removal of the pancreas from a dog, Minkowski's technician noted the animal's subsequent copious urine production. Acting on the basis of a hunch, Minkowski tested the urine and determined that its sugar content was greater than 10 percent.

In 1921, Frederick Banting and Charles Best, at the University of Toronto, successfully extracted the antidiabetic substance "insulin" using a cold alcohol-hydrochloric acid mixture to inactivate the harsh digestive enzymes of the pancreas. Using this substance, they first controlled the disease in a depancreatized dog and then, a few months later, successfully treated the first human diabetic patient. The clinical application of a discovery normally takes a long time, but in this case a mere twenty weeks had passed between the first injection of insulin into the diabetic dog and the first trial with a diabetic human. Three years later, in 1923, Banting and Best were awarded the Nobel Prize in Physiology or Medicine for their remarkable achievement.

Although insulin, when combined with an appropriate diet and exercise, alleviates the symptoms of diabetes to such an extent that a diabetic can lead an essentially normal life, insulin therapy is not a cure. The complications that arise in diabetics are typical of those found in the general population except that they happen much earlier in the diabetic. With regard to these glucose-induced complications, it was first postulated in 1908 that sugars could react with proteins. In 1912, Louis Camille Maillard further characterized this reaction at the Sorbonne and realized that the

consequences of this reaction were relevant to diabetics. Maillard suggested that sugars were destroying the body's amino acids, which then led to increased excretion in diabetics. It was not until the mid-1970's, however, that Anthony Cerami in New York introduced the concept of the nonenzymatic attachment of glucose to protein and recognized its potential role in diabetic complications. A decade later, this development led to the discovery of aminoguanidine, the first compound to limit the cross-linking of tissue proteins and thus delay the development of certain diabetic complications.

In 1974, Josiah Brown published the first report showing that diabetes could be reversed by transplanting fetal pancreatic tissue. By the mid-1980's, procedures had been devised for the isolation of massive numbers of human islets that could then be transplanted into diabetics. For persons with diabetes, both procedures represent more than a treatment; they may offer a cure for the disease.

—Hillar Klandorf, Ph.D.

See also Endocrine disorders; Endocrinology; Endocrinology, pediatric; Gangrene; Gastroenterology; Gastroenterology, pediatric; Gastrointestinal system; Glands; Hormones; Hypoglycemia; Internal medicine; Obesity; Pancreas; Pancreatitis.

FOR FURTHER INFORMATION:

Biermann, June, and Barbara Toohey. *The Diabetic's Book.* 3d ed. New York: G. P. Putnam's Sons, 1994. This extremely helpful book deals with both Type I and Type II diabetes. It is filled with useful information to help patients live a more healthful and satisfying life and contains answers to 130 frequently asked questions about the disease, including lifestyle, diet, and therapy.

_____. *The Peripatetic Diabetic.* Los Angeles: Jeremy P. Tarcher, 1984. Written for the diabetic patient and parents of the diabetic child, the book uses sound medical information and practical advice to help find solutions to problems in the real world. A popular and sometimes humorous book for people with diabetes.

Bliss, Michael. *The Discovery of Insulin.* Edinburgh: Paul Harris, 1987. An excellent historical perspective on the events leading to the discovery of insulin. The complete dedication of those individuals in their pursuit of what was hoped to be the "cure" for diabetes is well documented.

Cerami, Anthony, Helen Vlassara, and Michael Browlee. "Glucose and Aging." *Scientific American* 256 (May, 1987): 90-96. A pioneering article written by experts in the field of diabetic complications. This important work clearly explains the development of cross-linking in the tissues and challenges the reader with new approaches to treating a very old problem. Contains excellent figures and diagrams of the processes involved.

Jovanovic-Peterson, Lois, Charles M. Peterson, and Morton B. Stori. *A Touch of Diabetes.* Minneapolis: Chronimed, 1995. A straightforward guide for people with Type II diabetes. Provides useful information on the disease and suggestions of how to change eating habits and monitor one's lifestyle.

Krall, Leo P., and Richard S. Beaser. *Joslin Diabetes Manual.* 12th ed. Philadelphia: Lea & Febiger, 1989. First published in 1918, this book serves as a guide for people with diabetes. Its intent is to help diabetics understand the disease and permit them to take control of their lives.

Powers, Margaret A., ed. *Handbook of Diabetes Medical Nutrition Therapy.* Rev. ed. Gaithersburg, Md.: Aspen, 1996. A comprehensive book written by dietitians for persons interested in the nutritional treatment of diabetes; blends new scientific knowledge and thought with recent advances in clinical practice.

DIALYSIS

PROCEDURE

ANATOMY OR SYSTEM AFFECTED: Abdomen, blood, circulatory system, kidneys, urinary system

SPECIALTIES AND RELATED FIELDS: Biotechnology, hematology, internal medicine, nephrology, serology, urology

DEFINITION: The artificial replacement of renal (kidney) function, which involves the removal of toxins in the blood by selective diffusion through a semipermeable membrane.

KEY TERMS:

hemodialysis: the removal of toxins from blood through the process of dialysis

osmosis: the diffusion of molecules through a semipermeable membrane until there is an equal concentration on either side of the membrane

peritoneal dialysis: the removal of toxins from blood by dialysis in the peritoneal cavity

peritoneum: the membrane lining the walls of the abdominal cavity and enclosing the viscera

INDICATIONS AND PROCEDURES

The two major functions of the kidneys are to produce urine, thereby excreting toxic substances and maintaining an optimal concentration of solutes in the blood, and to produce and secrete hormones that regulate blood flow, blood production, calcium and bone metabolism, and vascular tone. These functions can be impaired or even completely halted by kidney failure that may or may not be related to diseases such as hepatitis and diabetes. The kidney is the only human organ with a function—that is, the excretion of toxic substances from the blood—that can be artificially replaced on a reliable and chronic basis. Although dialysis cannot duplicate the intricate processes of normal renal function, it is possible to provide patients with a tolerable level of life.

If a solute is added to a container of water, it will be distributed at uniform concentration through the water. This process is called diffusion and results from random movement of the solute molecules in the solvent; it can be seen as a chemical mixing of the solution. The mixing will ensure an even distribution of solute molecules throughout the solution. The time required for complete mixing depends on factors such as the nature of the solute, its molecular size, the temperature of the solution, and the size of the container. The process of dialysis is based on the diffusion of solute molecules (urea and other substances) from the blood or fluids of a patient to a sterile solution called dialysate. The artificial kidney or dialysis system is designed to provide controllable osmosis, or the transfer of solutes and water across a semipermeable membrane separating streams of blood (contaminated as a result of renal failure) and dialysate (a sterile solution). For solutes such as urea, the outflowing blood concentration is high, while the concentration in the inflowing dialysate is usually zero. The result is a concentration gradient that guarantees osmosis of urea molecules from the blood to the dialysate solution. The same process will take place for other toxins present in the blood but absent from the dialysate solution.

There are two types of clinical dialysis, hemodialysis and peritoneal dialysis. In hemodialysis, the device utilized is called a dialyzer. The three basic structural elements of all dialyzers are the blood compartment, the membrane, and the dialysate compartment. In a perfect dialyzer, diffusion equilibrium would result in the blood and dialysate streams during passage through the device, and virtually all the urea and toxins contained in the inflowing blood stream would be transferred to the dialysate stream. This level of efficiency is not achieved, however, and for maximum efficiency, dialysate flow rate should be from two to two and one-half times the actual blood flow rate.

Several fundamental material and design requirements must be met in the construction of efficient dialyzers suitable for clinical use. First, the surfaces in contact with blood and the flow geometry must not induce the formation of blood clots. The materials used must be nontoxic and free of leachable toxic substances. The ratio of membrane surface area to contained volume must be high to ensure maximum transference of substances, and the resistance to blood flow must be low and predictable.

There are three basic designs for a dialyzer: the coil, parallel plate, and hollow fiber configurations. The coil dialyzer was the earliest design. In it, the blood compartment consisted of one or two membrane tubes placed between support screens and then wound with the screens around a plastic core. This resulted in a coiled tubular membrane laminated between support screens, which was then enclosed in a rigid cylindrical case. This design had serious performance limitations, such as a high hydraulic resistance to blood flow and an increase in contained blood volume as blood flow through the device was increased.

The coil design has all but been replaced by more efficient devices. In the parallel plate dialyzer, sheets of membrane are mounted on a plastic support screen and then stacked in multiple layers, allowing for multiple parallel blood and dialysate flow channels. The original design had problems with membrane stretching and nonuniform channel performance. In order to minimize these problems, smaller plates and better membrane supports have been developed. The hollow fiber dialyzer is the most effective design for providing low volume and high efficiency together with modest resistance to flow. Developed in the 1970's, the membrane is composed of tiny cellulose or synthetic hollow fibers about the size of a human hair. Between seven thousand and twenty-five thousand of those fibers are enclosed in a cylindrical jacket, with the blood inlet and outlet at the top and bottom of the cylinder and the dialysate inlet and outlet being simply expanded sections of the jacket itself. This is the most commonly used geometry for hemodialysis. Extreme care must be taken to ensure that all the extra fluids that might have entered the blood during dialysis are removed. Ultrafiltration refers to the removal of water from the blood after dialysis and is a critical component of the dialysis process.

The delivery system of a dialyzer provides on-line proportioning of water with dialysate concentrate and monitors the dialysate for temperature, composition, and blood leaks. It also controls the ultrafiltration rate and regulates the dialysate flow. Normally included in the system are a blood pump, blood pressure and air monitors, and an anticoagulant pump.

The composition of the dialysate is designed to approximate the normal electrolyte concentration found in plasma and extracellular water; it contains calcium, magnesium, sodium and potassium chloride, sodium acetate, sodium carbonate, and lactic acid, kept at a pH of 7.4. The water used in this preparation is purified, heated to between 35 and 37 degrees Celsius and deaerated to prevent air embolism. An anticoagulant must be added in the process to prevent the formation of blood clots. Heparin is the most commonly used anticoagulant, mainly because its effect is immediate, is easily measured, and can be almost immediately terminated by adding protamine. In addition, because of its high molecular weight and substantial protein binding, it is not dialyzable and will not be lost from the blood in the process.

Several types of polymers are commonly employed for the manufacture of the membranes utilized in hemodialysis.

The Administration of Hemodialysis

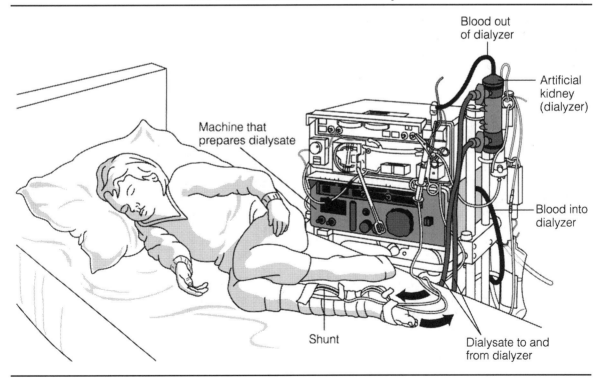

Dialysis is a method of removing wastes from the blood when the kidneys have failed to do so. Hemodialysis, which employs a machine that acts as an artificial kidney, is performed in a hospital in a session lasting two to six hours in which the blood is filtered to eliminate wastes, toxins, and excess fluid.

Cellulosic membranes, or membranes generated from the plant product cellulose, are the most commonly used polymers. (Cellophane was originally used, and later cuprophan and hemophan were introduced.) Noncellulosic artificial membranes made from synthetic polymers such as polycarbonate and polyamide are also used.

The development of efficient and more permeable synthetic membranes and ultrafiltration control delivery systems have reduced treatment time to two or three hours. Dialysis remains a potentially lethal procedure, and careful monitoring of equipment and solutions is necessary. For example, the dialysate must be monitored for hypertonic or hypotonic conditions that can result in hemolysis and death, and the flow from the dialyzer outlet back to the patient must have, among other things, an air bubble detector and filters to remove clots.

Peritoneal dialysis involves the transfer of solutes and water from the peritoneal capillary blood to the dialysate in the peritoneal cavity and the absorption of glucose and other solutes from the peritoneal fluid into the blood. The physiology of this process is less understood than that of hemodialysis. The process involves the introduction in the peritoneal cavity of a certain volume of dialysate and its removal after the dialysis process is complete. The main type of procedure is chronic intermittent peritoneal dialysis (CIPD). This process is performed three to seven times per week and takes from eight to twelve hours. It is mostly done overnight, when a pump introduces the dialysate to the peritoneal cavity and gravity removes it. Two systems are commonly used for this purpose: One is the reverse osmosis machine, which provides continuous flow through the night in a fast manner, while the other system utilizes a cycler for the cycling of the dialysate during the night. Cyclers are semiautomated systems with simple operation and a low initial expense that provide basically trouble-free performance but are expensive in the long run because they use premixed dialysates and many disposable components. Chronic ambulatory peritoneal dialysis (CAPD) is the most versatile and manageable of the techniques. In this case, the inflow and outflow of dialysate is done manually by gravity. With about 2 liters of dialysate used per exchange, it normally takes ten minutes for inflow and fifteen to twenty minutes for outflow. There are an average of four exchanges per day and one overnight. This is an easy, safe, and effective method of dialysis. A variation of CAPD is continuous cycling peritoneal dialysis (CCPD), introduced in 1980. It basically reverses the CAPD cycle: Cyclers are used during the night to achieve three to four exchanges, and there is a long period without exchange during the day. This minimizes the inconvenience of scheduling exchanges during the day, and many patients can alternate between the two methods without experiencing problems.

For peritoneal dialysis, the dialysate includes dextrose, lactate, sodium, calcium, and magnesium salts. An antico-agulant such as heparin can be added when needed, such as if blood is seen in the peritoneal fluid. Other substances—such as insulin for both diabetic and nondiabetic patients, antibiotics if there is peritonitis, and bicarbonate to prevent abdominal discomfort—can also be added without major complications.

Peritoneal dialysis may be a better choice than hemodialysis for certain patients when factors such as coronary artery disease, diabetes mellitus, age, or severe hemodialysis-related symptoms are present. It is also the choice for patients whose residence is remote from a dialysis center, who wish to travel frequently, or who live alone.

USES AND COMPLICATIONS

Hemodialysis is used in acute and chronic renal failure patients. Some individuals, however, do not tolerate hemodialysis well, such as children, infants, geriatric patients, diabetics, and victims of traumatic injuries. Therefore, the selection of patients for this procedure must be closely monitored. The process can be also used for treatment of drug overdose (since drugs can be removed from the blood during the dialysis procedure) and hypercalcemia, an excess of calcium.

For many years, peritoneal dialysis was reserved for the treatment of acute renal failure (ARF) or for those patients awaiting transplantation or the availability of hemodialysis. Although it is used principally for the treatment of patients with end-stage renal disease, it remains a valuable tool in the management of ARF because of its simplicity and widespread availability. Essentially, it can be provided in any hospital by most internists or surgeons without the need for specially trained nephrology personnel. It also avoids the need for systematic anticoagulation, making it a good choice for patients in the immediate postoperative period with severe trauma, intracerebral hemorrhage, or hypocoagulable states. It is most suitable for the treatment of patients with an unstable cardiovascular system and for pediatric or elderly patients. It could be impossible to use, however, in postsurgical patients with many abdominal drains, with hernias, or with severe gastroesophageal reflux.

For many years, peritoneal dialysis was not used for patients with CRF (chronic renal failure) because of the problems involved in the maintenance of permanent peritoneal access, the inconvenience of manual dialysate exchanges, the high rate of peritonitis observed in these patients, and the rapid progress made in hemodialysis in the early 1960's. The advent of a safe, permanent peritoneal catheter in the late 1960's and the simultaneous development of automated reverse osmosis peritoneal delivery systems created new interest in the technique and resulted in safer, more effective systems. Peritoneal dialysis can also be used or is recommended in the following cases: for diabetic patients, since it provides a continuous source of insulin and also has the advantage of providing blood pressure control; for edema patients, since the process is useful in the treatment of intractable edema states such as congestive heart failure; and for pancreatitis patients or individuals who suffer from the release of pancreatic enzymes into the abdominal cavity and their subsequent absorption into the circulation. For the latter, the removal of the enzymes through peritoneal dialysis may prevent the necrotic process. Individuals exhibiting hypothermia as a consequence of accidental exposure, cold water immersion, central nervous system disorders, intoxication, or burns can be treated by performing peritoneal dialysis with dialysate solutions between 40 and 45 degrees Celsius. This will bring the body back to 34 degrees Celsius (a stable temperature) in a few hours, and, if the cause of the hypothermia is intoxication, the drugs causing the condition can be removed at the same time.

PERSPECTIVE AND PROSPECTS

As early as the 1600's, the relationship between blood and various diseases was known. At that time, however, great difficulties existed in the transport and study of blood. By the 1800's, the techniques for entering the blood vessels had been refined. The dangers of air embolization (air entering the patient) and clotting were well recognized. Prior to 1850, there was no treatment for patients with renal failure, but crude methods such as applying heat, immersing in warm baths, bloodletting, or administering diaphoretic (perspiration-inducing) mixtures of nitric acid in alcohol and wine were commonly used. (In fact, diaphoretic mixtures and bloodletting for renal failure were used as late as the 1950's.)

In 1854, Thomas Graham, a Scottish chemist, presented a paper on osmotic force, which was the first reference to the process of separating a substance using a semipermeable membrane. His definitions and experimental proofs of the laws of diffusion and osmosis form the foundation upon which dialysis is based. Between 1872 and 1900, the control of membrane manufacture and the dialysis of animal blood were critical developments. One of the key turning points in the development of dialysis occurred in 1913, when John Jacob Abel, using anticoagulants, created the fist extracorporeal device that could be used to diffuse a substance from blood and developed methods to quantify this diffusion. World War I brought the development of the first plate dialyzer, by Heinrich Necheles, a German-born physician. It included an air bubble trap, continuous blood flow, and an entry port for a saline solution to be used as dialysate; it was only used for animals. George Haas must be credited as the first to perform dialysis on a uremic human, in October, 1924. He used heparin, an anticoagulant discovered by William H. Howell and Luther E. Holt, two Americans. Haas had all the pieces together: a dialyzer with a large surface area, a workable membrane, a blood pump, and an anticoagulant.

The emergence of manufactured membranes in the 1930's (such as cellophane, which allows small molecules to pass through it) was crucial in the development of the technique. The lifesaving potential of an artificial kidney was shown by Willem Kolff, a physician from The Netherlands, who saved a patient from coma. His classic work *New Ways of Treating Uraemia*, published in 1947, laid out the principles that are still used and was the first manual for the treatment of patients undergoing hemodialysis. In the United States, the first clinical dialysis was performed on January 26, 1948, at Mt. Sinai Hospital in New York City, by physicians Irving Kroop and Alfred Fishman. The number of groups developing artificial kidney devices and programs between 1945 and 1950 was large. The first complete artificial kidney system commercially available came into existence in 1956, and the first home patient was treated in 1964 by Belding Scribner, from the University of Washington.

Soon the dialyzing fluid delivery systems became smaller and easier to use, the designs were simplified and made more compact, and a better understanding of the physiology of the patient was obtained. Calcium depletion, bone disease, neuropathy, dietary management, and anemia were being looked at closely in order to determine better how much dialysis was required for effective treatment. The late 1960's brought the miniaturization of the systems, in-home care, and lower prices. In fact, in 1973, legislation was enacted in the United States that provided payment through the Social Security system for the care of dialysis patients.

In the latter part of the 1970's, a shift to totally automated systems and an emphasis on negative-pressure dialysis had major impacts, resulting in a move from coil to hollow-fiber dialyzers. Some patients, however, such as diabetics, children, and older patients, did not tolerate hemodialysis well. Therefore, a closer look was taken at peritoneal and automated peritoneal dialysis delivery systems. The earliest reference to peritoneal diffusion was in 1876, and in 1895 it was formally presented as an alternative to remove toxins from the bloodstream. Nevertheless, peritoneal dialysis lay dormant until the 1940's. The basic procedure of using solutions and instilling them into the peritoneal cavity in order to reduce the toxin levels in the blood was first used in 1945 by a group of physicians in Beth Israel Hospital in Boston. The full implications of its use came in the late 1970's, with the development of reverse osmosis technology and the introduction of continuous ambulatory peritoneal dialysis. In the 1980's, the introduction of continuous intermittent peritoneal dialysis gave patients yet another treatment option.

One of the main goals of the medical community and industry is to provide the quality of care that will minimize the burden of those afflicted with renal disease. The main goal, however, remains to obtain the necessary knowledge to understand the causes of progressive renal failure and then prevent, control, or eliminate the consequences of renal disease.   —*Maria Pacheco, Ph.D.*

See also Blood and blood components; Circulation; Diabetes mellitus; Edema; Heart failure; Hematology; Hematology, pediatric; Hepatitis; Hyperthermia and hypothermia; Kidney disorders; Kidney transplantation; Kidneys; Nephrectomy; Nephritis; Nephrology; Nephrology, pediatric; Pancreatitis; Renal failure.

FOR FURTHER INFORMATION:

Cogan, Martin G. and Patricia Schoenfeld, eds. *Introduction to Dialysis.* 2d ed. New York: Churchill Livingstone, 1991. An excellent and thorough presentation of the topic. Somewhat technical, however, since it includes derivations for the equations governing the different parts of the process. A good reference work for those interested in the theoretical and practical aspects of the dialysis process.

Fine, Leonard, and Herbert Beall. *Chemistry for Engineering and Scientists.* Philadelphia: W. B. Saunders, 1990. A good chemistry book that explains the chemical and physical bases of diffusion and dialysis in a nontechnical presentation.

Nissenson, Allen R., and Richard N. Fine, eds. *Dialysis Therapy.* 2d ed. Philadelphia: Hanley and Belfus, 1993. A compilation of works dealing with the theory, applications, advantages, and complications of dialysis. The reader will need some background in the area to make the best use of the book.

Nissenson, Allen R., Richard N. Fine, and Dominik E. Gentile, eds. *Clinical Dialysis.* 2d ed. Norwalk, Conn.: Appleton and Lange, 1990. A compilation of works by various authorities in the field of dialysis. Contains an excellent presentation of the development of the technique and of its many aspects and applications. Because of the heavy use of medical terminology, this work is better suited to individuals with some background in the area.

Voet, Donald, and Judith G. Voet. *Biochemistry.* New York: John Wiley & Sons, 1990. A good book to use for the description and explanation of the chemical processes taking place in the kidney and other areas of the body.

DIARRHEA AND DYSENTERY

DISEASE/DISORDER

ANATOMY OR SYSTEM AFFECTED: Abdomen, gastrointestinal system, intestines

SPECIALTIES AND RELATED FIELDS: Family practice, gastroenterology, internal medicine, pediatrics, public health

DEFINITION: Intestinal disorders that may indicate minor emotional distress or a variety of diseases, some serious; diarrhea is loose, watery, copious bowel movements, whereas dysentery is an intestinal infection characterized by severe diarrhea.

KEY TERMS:

electrolytes: inorganic ions dissolved in body water, including sodium, potassium, calcium, magnesium, chloride, phosphate, bicarbonate, and sulphate

functional disease: a derangement in the way that normal anatomy operates

gastroenterology: the medical subspecialty devoted to care of the digestive tract and related organs

intestines: the tube connecting the stomach and anus in which nutrients are absorbed from food; divided into the small intestine and the colon, or large intestine

mucosa: the semipermeable layers of cells lining the gut, through which fluid and nutrients are absorbed

organic disease: disease resulting from an identifiable cause, such as an enzyme deficiency, growth, hole, or organism

pathogen: an organism that causes disease

peristalsis: the wavelike muscular contractions that move food and waste products through the intestines; problems with peristalsis are called motility disorders

stool: the waste products expelled from the anus during defecation

CAUSES AND SYMPTOMS

A symptom of various diseases rather than a disease in itself, diarrhea is so difficult to define and can result from so many disparate causes that it is sometimes called the gastroenterologist's nightmare. Dysentery (bloody diarrhea), a more threatening symptom, presents even further complexity.

Uncontrolled, some forms of diarrhea result in dehydration, weakness, and malnutrition and quickly turn deadly. Diarrhea is implicated in more infant deaths worldwide than any other affliction. Even in mild forms, it produces so much distress in victims and has inspired so many remedies that its psychological and economic toll is monumental. During the 1980's, diarrhea accounted for an estimated $23 billion annually in medical expenses and lost productivity in the United States alone, a figure that surpassed the government budgets of many states.

Common medical definitions of diarrhea seek to bring diagnostic precision to a nebulous complaint and to distinguish between acute and chronic forms and between organic and functional causes. For example, *The Merck Manual* (15th ed., 1987), a widely respected reference for physicians, associates diarrhea with increased amount and fluidity of fecal matter and frequent defecation relative to a person's usual pattern, emphasizing the importance of volume (more than three hundred grams of stool daily, of which 60 to 90 percent is water) in the definition. The key phrase here is "relative to a usual pattern": Because quantity, frequency, and firmness of bowel movements vary greatly among healthy people, a more precise generalization is difficult to make. Yet some specialists demand greater specificity from the definition. For example, W. Grant Thompson, a professor of medicine and popular author on the digestive tract, proposes the operational definition of "loose or watery stools more than 75 percent of the time" in *Gut Reactions* (1989). Acute diarrhea seldom lasts more than five days, although acute dysentery may continue up to ten days; most causes are infections, that is, resulting from the presence of microorganisms (viruses, bacteria, or parasites). Physicians differ over how long the symptoms must persist before a condition is identified as chronic diarrhea, proposing from two weeks to three months; impaired functioning of the intestinal tract (functional diarrhea) is usually responsible, although persistent malfunctions may originate from pathogens that in most cases provoke only acute diarrhea.

In a single day, water intake, saliva, gastric juice, bile, pancreatic juices, and electrolyte secretions in the upper small intestine produce about nine to ten liters of fluid in the average person. One to two liters of this amount empty into the colon, and 100 to 150 milligrams are excreted in the stool; the rest is absorbed through the intestinal mucosa. If for any reason more fluid enters the colon than it can absorb, diarrhea results. Schemes classifying diarrhea according to the biochemical mechanisms causing it vary considerably, although all authorities agree on three broad types of malfunction.

The first is secretory diarrhea. The intestines, especially the small intestine, normally add water and electrolytes—principally sodium, potassium, chloride, and bicarbonate—into the nutrient load during the biochemical reactions of digestion. In a healthy person, more fluid is absorbed than is secreted. Many agents and conditions can reverse this ratio and stimulate the mucosa to exude more water than can be absorbed: toxin-producing bacteria; various organic chemicals, including caffeine and some laxatives; acids; hormones; some cancers; and inflammatory diseases of the bowel. Large stool volume (more than one liter a day), with little or no decrease during fasting and with normal sodium and potassium content in the body fluid, characterizes secretory diarrhea.

Second, the nutrient load in the gut may include substances that exert osmotic force but cannot be absorbed, causing osmotic diarrhea. Some laxatives (especially those containing magnesium), an inability to absorb the lactose in dairy products or the artificial sweeteners in diet foods, and enzyme deficiencies are the principal causes. Stool volume tends to be less than one liter a day and decreases during fasting; the sodium and potassium content of stool water is low.

Third, motility disorders occur when peristalsis, the natural wavelike contractions of the bowel wall that move waste matter toward the rectum for defecation, becomes deranged. Some drugs, irritable bowel syndrome (IBS), hyperthyroidism, and gut nerve damage (as from diabetes mellitus) may have this effect. Fluid passes through the intestines too quickly or in an uncoordinated fashion, and too little is removed from the waste matter.

These mechanisms do not conform exactly with popular names for diarrhea. For example, travelers' diarrhea, the most infamous, comprises a diverse group of microorganism infections that come from drinking polluted water or eating tainted foods. When a person is not a native to an area, and so has little or no resistance to locally abundant pathogens, these pathogens can radically alter the balance of intestinal flora or attack the mucosa, increasing secretion and disrupting absorption and motility. Similarly, terms such as "Montezuma's revenge," "the backdoor trots," and "beaver fever" can refer to a variety of organic diseases, although the last commonly refers to *Giardia lamblia* infection.

Dysentery occurs with infectious diarrhea, most commonly from bacteria and amoebas, such as shigella, salmonella, and *Escherichia coli* (*E. coli*), and with inflammatory diseases of the bowel, such as colitis and Crohn's disease. Any pathogen that injures and inflames the bowel wall, ulcerating the mucosa, may cause blood and pus to ooze into the feces. To the greatest threat from diarrhea—dehydration—dysentery often adds fever, chills, cramping, blood loss, and nausea, and in extreme cases delirium, convulsions, and coma.

Although most diarrheas result from physiological mechanisms, one relatively rare form of chronic diarrhea ultimately has a psychological origin: laxative abuse. Physicians consider this curious phenomenon a specialized manifestation of Münchausen's syndrome, named after the German soldier Baron Münchausen (1720-1797) who was famous for his wild tales of military exploits and injuries in battles. In order to be admitted to hospitals, patients mutilate themselves in such a way that the injuries mimic acute, dramatic, and convincing symptoms of serious physiological diseases. Laxative abusers secretly dose themselves with nonprescription laxatives and suffer continual diarrhea, weight loss, and weakness. When they present themselves to physicians, they lie about taking laxatives, which makes a correct diagnosis extremely difficult; even when confronted with irrefutable evidence of the abuse, they deny it and persist in taking the laxatives.

TREATMENT AND THERAPY

Almost everyone, at one time or another, produces stools that seem somehow unusual; if the bowel movement comes swiftly and is preceded by intestinal cramps and if the stool has anything from a watery to an oatmeal-like consistency, victims are likely to believe that they have diarrhea. Such episodes seldom indicate anything except perhaps a dietary excess or a temporary motility disturbance. Normal bowel movement returns on its own, and no medical treatment is called for. When loose feces are uncontrollable, even explosive, however, and other symptoms coexist, such as nausea, bleeding, fever, bloating, and persistent intestinal pain, the distress may indicate serious illness.

Because so many organic and functional diseases can lead to diarrhea, physicians follow carefully designed algorithms when treating patients. Essentially, such an algorithm seeks to eliminate possibilities systematically. Step by step, physicians interview patients, conduct physical examinations, and, when called for, perform tests that gradually narrow the range of possible causes until one seems most likely. Only then can the physician decide upon an effective therapy. This painstaking approach is necessary because treatments for some mechanisms of diarrhea prove useless against or worsen other mechanisms. If the underlying disease is complex or uncommon, the process can be long and frustrating.

One treatment, however, always precedes a complete investigation. Because dehydration is the most immediately serious effect of diarrhea, the physician first tries to prevent or reduce dehydration in a patient through oral rehydration; that is, the patient is given fluids with electrolytes to drink. Often, mineral water or fruit juice with soda crackers is sufficient to restore fluid balance.

If the diarrhea lasts fewer than three days and no other serious symptoms accompany it, the physician is unlikely to recommend treatment other than oral rehydration because whatever caused the upset is already resolving itself. If the diarrhea is persistent, however, the physician queries the patient about his or her recent experience, which is called "taking a history." Fever, tenesmus (the urgent need to defe-

cate without the ability to do so satisfactorily), blood in the stool, and abdominal pain will suggest that a pathogen has infected the patient. If the patient has recently eaten seafood, traveled abroad, suffered an immune system disorder, or engaged in sexual activity without the protection of condoms, the physician has reason to suspect that viruses, bacteria, or parasites are responsible.

At that point, a stool sample is taken. If few or no white cells turn up in the stool, then the diarrhea has not caused inflammation. Several common bacteria and parasites, usually contracted during travel, induce diarrhea without inflammation, most notably some types of *E. coli*, cryptosporidium, rotavirus, Norwalk virus, and *Giardia lamblia*. Further tests, such as the culturing and staining of stool samples and electron microscopy of stool or bowel wall tissue, will distinguish between bacterial and parasite infection. Most noninflammatory bacterial diarrheas are allowed to run their course without drug therapy; only the effects of the diarrhea (especially dehydration) are treated. If the agent responsible is a parasite, the patient is given specific antiparasite medications.

The presence of white cells in the stool is evidence of inflammatory diarrhea, and the physician considers a completely separate group of microorganisms, especially

Cycle of Amebic Dysentery

Encysted in food
(four amoebas in cyst)

Ingestion

Cyst digested; amoebas
set free in large intestine

New amoebic cysts form
and are passed in feces

shigella, salmonella, amoebas, and various forms of *E. coli*. Because the inflammation may cause bleeding and pockets of pus, which in turn can lead to anemia and fever, inflammatory diarrhea often requires aggressive treatment. Cell cultures help identify the specific microorganism involved, and that identification enables the physician to select the proper antibiotic to kill the infecting agents.

If cell cultures, microscopic examination of stool samples, biopsies, or staining fails to identify a microorganism (and some, like the parasite *Giardia lamblia*, are difficult to spot), the physician suspects that the diarrhea derives from a source other than an infectious agent. Irritable bowel syndrome (IBS), a chronic and relapsing disorder, may be making its first appearance. Overuse of antibiotics, antacids, or laxatives is frequently the cause, in which case the cure is simple: Elimination of the drugs clears up the symptom.

When neither drugs nor IBS is responsible, the physician looks for other diseases, organic or functional; these can range from the readily identifiable to the obscure, and they are often chronic. Chemical tests, for example, can show that a patient has enzyme deficiencies that produce intolerance to types of food, such as dairy products, or conditions resulting from malfunctioning organs, such as hyperthyroidism and pancreatic insufficiency. Looking through an endoscope, a long flexible fiberoptic tube, the physician can locate diarrhea-causing tumors or the abrasions and inflammation typical of colitis and Crohn's disease. Yet neither tests nor direct examination may pin down the dysfunction. For example, diarrhea figures prominently among a group of symptoms, probably derived from assorted dysfunctions, that characterize IBS; this mild functional disease is estimated to afflict between 10 and 20 percent of Americans.

Cancers, Crohn's disease, and some forms of colitis can be alleviated with surgery, although in the case of Crohn's disease the relief from diarrhea may be only temporary. The surgery itself, however, may impair bowel function, worsening diarrhea rather than stopping it. Food intolerances are managed by removing the offending food from the patient's diet; similarly, some types of colitis and IBS sometimes improve after the physician and patient experiment with altering the patient's diet. Medications are available that supplement or counteract the biochemical imbalances created by malfunctioning organs, such as treatment for hyperthyroidism. Yet, in many cases, the disease must simply be endured and the diarrhea can only be palliated with bulking agents, which often contain aluminum and bismuth, or opiates, such as morphine and codeine, which slow peristalsis.

The surest protection from diarrhea of all types is a balanced, moderate, pathogen-free diet, although diet alone seldom prevents organic diseases. When dietary control is difficult, such as when a person travels and especially when the itinerary includes underdeveloped countries, other measures may help. Bacterial infection accounts for 80 percent of cases of travelers' diarrhea, so some physicians recommend regular doses of antibiotics or a bismuth subsalicylate preparation (such as Pepto Bismol) to kill off the pathogens before they can cause trouble. Such prophylactic treatment is controversial because the drugs, taken over long periods, can have serious side effects, including rashes, tinnitus (ringing in the ear), sensitivity to sunlight, and shock. Also, preventive doses of drugs may give travelers a false sense of security so that they fail to exercise caution in eating foreign foods. Also, widespread use of antibiotics for this purpose fosters the emergence of bacteria that are resistant to them, ultimately making the treatment of disease more difficult.

Perspective and Prospects

In effect, diarrhea is an urgent message from the body that something is wrong. Although it is often difficult for a physician to interpret, persistent diarrhea sends a signal that cannot be ignored without endangering the patient. Similarly, when significant numbers of people in an area suffer diarrhea, the disease is an urgent social and political message to local governments: Public health is endangered and steps must be taken to improve living conditions.

Although some endemic diarrheal diseases do exist in wealthy industrialized countries such as the United States, most severe, long-lasting plagues of diarrhea occur in impoverished nations that have inadequate sanitation systems and poor standards for food handling. Most viral, bacterial, and parasitic diarrheas are transmitted by food and water. Any food can harbor bacteria after being grown in or washed with infected water. Meat is especially vulnerable during slaughtering, but refrigerating, drying, salting, fermenting, freezing, or irradiating it prevents the bacteria from proliferating to numbers that cause illness. If the food is stored in a warm place, as is often the case in countries lacking the resources for refrigeration or other safe storage techniques, the diarrhea-causing organisms can spoil the food in hours. Spoiled food becomes a particular nuisance when served at restaurants or by street vendors, because great numbers and varieties of people are infected.

Organisms that cause many forms of diarrhea travel in human excrement. When an infected person defecates, the organism-rich stool enters the sewer system, and if that system is not well designed, the infected excrement may leak into the local water supply, spreading the infection when the water is drunk or used to wash food. Furthermore, infected persons, if they fail to wash themselves well, may have traces of excrement on their hands, and when they touch food during its preparation or touch other people directly, the organism can find a new host.

In 1989, the World Health Organization (WHO) issued ten rules for safe food preparation in an attempt to improve food handling practices worldwide and combat diarrheal diseases. The effort, it was hoped, would reduce infant mortality in developing countries, since diarrheal dehydration kills children younger than two years of age at rates disproportionate to other age groups. WHO advises food handlers to choose foods that are already processed, to cook foods thoroughly, to serve cooked foods immediately, to store foods carefully, to reheat foods thoroughly, to prevent raw and cooked foods from touching, to wash their hands repeatedly, to clean all kitchen surfaces meticulously, to protect foods from insects and rodents, and to use pure water.

Eliminating endemic infectious diarrheal diseases would improve general health significantly throughout the world, since diarrhea is one of the most incapacitating of afflictions even in its mild forms. International travel would also become safer; of the estimated 300 million people who cross national borders yearly, 20 to 50 percent contract diarrheal illnesses. Noninfectious diarrhea from chronic functional diseases will remain a knotty problem, but it is rare in comparison to acute infectious diarrhea, cannot be transmitted, and so has little or no effect on public health.

—Roger Smith, Ph.D.

See also Abdominal disorders; Bacterial infections; Colitis; Colon cancer; Crohn's disease; Digestion; *E. coli* infection; Food poisoning; Gastroenterology; Gastroenterology, pediatric; Gastrointestinal disorders; Gastrointestinal system; Incontinence; Indigestion; Intestinal disorders; Intestines; Lactose intolerance.

FOR FURTHER INFORMATION:

DuPont, Herbert L., and Charles D. Ericsson. "Drug Therapy: Prevention and Treatment of Traveler's Diarrhea." *The New England Journal of Medicine* 328 (June 24, 1993): 1821-1826. This article, one of the Center for Infectious Diseases' periodic updates on the subject, is a review of existing knowledge. It should be basic reading for international travelers, or anyone who wants an accurate overview of travelers' diarrhea.

Gracey, Michael, ed. *Diarrhea*. Boca Raton, La.: CRC Press, 1991. The fourteen essays in this collection cover major types of acute and chronic diarrhea in depth. Although written by academic physicians, the essays are accessible to readers with a basic knowledge of physiology, and the clarity and wealth of information make the book a valuable resource. Extensive bibliographies are included.

Greenberger, Norton J. *Gastrointestinal Disorders: A Pathophysiologic Approach*. 4th ed. Chicago: Year Book Medical Publishers, 1989. A medical text that requires college-level preparation in biochemistry and physiology to appreciate fully, yet its discussion of diseases is lucid and orderly. A solid introduction into the mechanisms involved in diarrhea and dysentery.

Janowitz, Henry D. *Your Gut Feelings: A Complete Guide to Living Better with Intestinal Problems*. New York: Oxford University Press, 1987. An eminent gastroenterologist and popular writer on intestinal subjects, Janowitz writes plainly and offers much helpful advice. His section on travelers' diarrhea is particularly valuable.

Sachar, David B., Jerome D. Waye, and Blair S. Lewis, eds. *Gastroenterology for the House Officer*. Baltimore: Williams & Wilkins, 1989. This handbook has two virtues:

Incidence of Amebic Dysentery

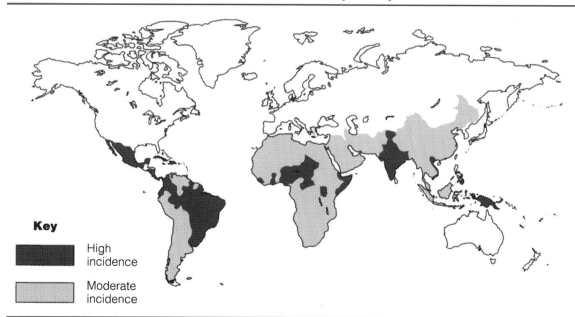

Key

High incidence

Moderate incidence

first, crisp definitions of disease types and mechanisms and, second, an easy-to-reference outline format. Readers must know medical and pharmaceutical terminology, however, to derive the full benefit of the text.

Scarpignato, Carmelo, and P. Rampal. *Traveler's Diarrhea: Recent Advances.* New York: S. Karger, 1995. The authors discuss the latest methods in the prevention, control, and treatment of diarrhea.

Thompson, W. Grant. *Gut Reactions: Understanding Symptoms of the Digestive Tract.* New York: Plenum Press, 1989. With much charm, Grant writes for the general reader, laying out the essential information that patients need in order to comprehend most gastrointestinal ailments. His chapter on diarrhea addresses only the functional diseases, and the book is perhaps best read as a thorough introduction to the gut and the medical specialties that care for it.

DIET. *See* NUTRITION.

DIETARY DEFICIENCIES. *See* MALNUTRITION; NUTRITION; VITAMINS AND MINERALS.

DIGESTION
BIOLOGY

ANATOMY OR SYSTEM AFFECTED: Abdomen, gastrointestinal system, intestines, pancreas, stomach

SPECIALTIES AND RELATED FIELDS: Biochemistry, family practice, gastroenterology, internal medicine, nutrition, pharmacology

DEFINITION: The chemical breakdown of food materials in the stomach and small intestine and the absorption into the bloodstream of essential nutrients through the intestinal walls.

KEY TERMS:

amino acids: the product of proteins broken down by digestive enzymes; essential for the building of tissue throughout the body

cecum: the dividing passageway between the small intestine and the large intestine, or colon

chyme: partially broken down food materials that pass from the stomach into the small intestine

dyspepsia: a general term applied to several forms of indigestion

villi: fingerlike projections on the intestinal lining that absorb essential body nutrients after enzymes break down chyme

STRUCTURE AND FUNCTIONS

In the most general terms, digestion is a multiple-stage process that begins by breaking down foodstuffs taken in by an organism. Some specialists consider that the actual process of digestion occurs after this breaking-down stage, when essential nutritional elements are absorbed into the

body. Even after division of the digestive process into two main functions, there remains a third, by-product stage: disposal by the body of waste material in the form of urine and feces.

Several different vital organs, all contained in the abdominal cavity, contribute either directly or indirectly to the digestive process at each successive stage. Certain imbalances in the functioning of any one, or a combination of, these organs can lead to what is commonly called indigestion. Chronic imbalances in the functioning of any of the key digestive organs—the stomach, small intestine, large intestine (or colon), liver, gallbladder, and pancreas—may indicate symptoms of diseases that are far more serious than mere indigestion.

In a very broad sense, the process of digestion begins even before food that has been chewed and swallowed passes into the stomach. In fact, while chewing is underway, a first stage of glandular activity—the release of saliva by the salivary glands into the food being chewed (a process referred to as intraluminal digestion)—provides a natural lubricant to help propel masticated material down the esophagus. Although the esophagus does not perform a digestive function, its muscular contractions, which are necessary for swallowing, are like a preliminary stage to the muscular operation that begins in the stomach.

The human stomach has two main sections: the baglike upper portion, or fundus, and the lower part, which is twice as large as the fundus, called the antrum. The function of the fundus is essentially to receive and hold foods that reach the stomach via the esophagus, allowing intermittent delivery into the antrum. Here two dynamic elements of the breaking-down process occur, one physical, the other chemical. The muscular tissue surrounding the antrum acts to churn the partially liquefied food in the lower stomach, while a series of what are commonly called gastric juices flow into the mixture held by the stomach.

The most active element that is secreted from special parietal cells in the mucous membranes lining the stomach is hydrochloric acid. The possibility of damage to the stomach lining is minimized (but not removed entirely) first by the fact of chemical reaction between the acid and the mildly alkaline chewed food and second by the presence of other gastric juices that are present in the antrum. Primary among these is the enzyme pepsin, which is secreted by a different set of specialized cells in the gastric lining. Secretions of both hydrochloric acid and pepsin become mixed and interact chemically with food materials, while the antrum itself moves in rhythmic pulses caused by muscular contractions (peristalsis). One of the key functions of pepsin during this stage is to break down protein molecules into shorter molecular strings of less complicated amino acids, which eventually serve as building material for many body tissues.

At a certain point, food materials are sufficiently reduced

to pass beyond the antrum into the duodenum, the first section of the small intestine, where a different stage in the digestive process takes place. At this juncture, the partially broken-down food material is referred to as chyme. The transfer of food from one digestive organ to another is actually monitored by a special autonomic nerve, called the vagus nerve, which originates in the medulla at the head of the spinal cord. Although the vagus nerve innervates a number of vital zones in the abdominal cavity, its function here is quite specific: It adjusts the intensity of muscular movement in the stomach wall and thus limits the amount of food passing into the small intestine.

The exact amount of food that is allowed to enter the intestinal tract represents only part of the essential question of balance between agents contributing to the digestive process. The presence of a now slightly acidic food-gastric juice mixture in the duodenum sparks what is called an enterogastric reflex. Two hormones, secretin and cholecystokinin, begin to flow from the mucous membranes of the duodenum. These hormones serve to limit the acidic strength of stomach secretions and trigger reactions in the liver, gallbladder, and pancreas—other key organs that contribute to digestion as the chyme passes through the intestines.

While in the compact, coiled mass of the small intestine (compared to the thicker, but much shorter colon, or large intestine), food materials, especially proteins, are broken down into one of twenty possible amino acid components by the chemical action of two pancreatic enzymes, trypsinogen and chymotrypsinogen, and two enzymes produced in the intestinal walls themselves, aminopeptidase and dipeptidase. It is interesting to note that the body, which is itself in large part constructed of protein material, has its own mechanism to prevent protein-splitting enzymes from devouring the very organs that produce them. Thus, when they leave the pancreas, both trypsinogen and chymotrypsinogen are inactive compounds. They become active "protein-breakers" only when joined by another enzyme—enterokinase—which is secreted from cells in the wall of the small intestine itself.

Other nutritional components contained in chyme interact chemically with other specialized enzymes that are secreted into the small intestine. Carbohydrate molecules, especially starch, begin to break down when exposed to the enzyme amylase in saliva. This process is intensified greatly when pancreatic amylase flows into the small intestine and mixes with the chyme. The products created when carbohydrates break down are simple sugars, including disaccharides and monosaccharides, especially maltose. As these sugars are all broken down into monosaccharides, a final process that occurs in the wall of the small intestine itself (which contains more specialized enzymes such as maltase, sucrase, and lactase), they become the most rapidly assimilated body nutrients.

The process needed to break down fats is more complicated, since fats are water insoluble and enter the intestine in the form of enzyme-resistant globules. Before the fat-splitting enzyme lipase can be chemically active, bile, a fluid produced by the liver and stored in the gallbladder, must be present. Bile serves to dissolve fat globules into tiny droplets that can be broken down for absorption, like all other nutritive elements, into the body via the epithelial lining of the intestinal wall. Such absorption is locally specialized. Iron and calcium pass through the epithelial lining of the duodenum. Protein, fat, sugars, and vitamins pass through the lining of the jejunum, or middle small intestine. Finally, salt, vitamin B_{12}, and bile salts pass through the lining of the lower small intestine, or ileum.

It is this stage that many scientists consider to be the true process of digestion. Absorption occurs through enterocytes, which are specialized cells located on the surface of the epithelium. The surface of the epithelium is increased substantially by the existence of fingerlike projections called villi. These tiny protrusions are surrounded by the fluid elements of chemically altered food. Specialized enterocyte cells selectively absorb these elements into the capillaries that are inside each of the hundreds of thousands of villi. From the capillaries, the nutrients enter the blood and are carried by the portal vein to the liver. This organ carries out the essential chemical processes that prepare fats, carbohydrates, and proteins for their eventual delivery, through the main bloodstream, to various parts of the body.

Elements that are left after the enzymes in the small intestine have done their work are essentially waste material, or feces. These pass from the small intestine to the large intestine, or colon, through a dividing passageway called the cecum. The disposal of waste materials may or may not be considered to be technically part of the main digestive process.

After essential amounts of water and certain salts are absorbed into the body through the walls of the colon, the remaining waste material is expulsed from the bowels through the rectum and anus. If any prior stage in the digestive process is incomplete or if chemical imbalances have occurred, the first symptoms of indigestion may manifest themselves as bowel movement irregularities.

DISORDERS AND DISEASES

Malfunctions in any of the delicate processes that make up digestion can produce symptoms that range from what is commonly called simple indigestion to potentially serious diseases of the gastrointestinal tract. Functional indigestion, or dyspepsia, is one of the most common sources of physical discomfort experienced not only by human beings but by most animals as well. Generally speaking, dyspepsias are not the result of organic disease, but rather of a temporary imbalance in one of the functions described above. There are many possible causes of such an imbalance, including nervous stress and changes in the nature and content of foods eaten.

The most common causes of dyspepsia and their symptoms, although serious enough in chronic cases to require expert medical attention, are far less dangerous than diseases afflicting one of the digestive organs. Such diseases include gallstones, pancreatitis, peptic ulcers (in which excessive acid causes lesions in the stomach wall), and, most serious of all, cancers afflicting any of the abdominal organs.

Dyspepsia may stem from either physical or chemical causes. On the physical side, it is clear that an important part of the digestive process depends on muscular or nerve-related impulses that move partially digested food through the gastrointestinal tract. When, for reasons that are not yet fully understood, the organism fails to coordinate such physical reactions, spasms may occur at several points from the esophagus through to the colon. If extensive, such muscular contractions can create abdominal pains that are symptomatic of at least one category of functional indigestion.

Problems of motility, or physical movement of food materials through the digestive tract, may also cause one common discomfort associated with indigestion: heartburn. This condition occurs when the system fails to move adequate quantities of the mixture of food and gastric juices, including hydrochloric acid, from the stomach into the duodenum. The resultant backup of food forces part of the acidic liquid mass into the esophagus, causing an instant discomfort.

Insufficient motility may also cause delays in the movement of feces through the colon, resulting in constipation. Just as the vagus nerve monitors the muscular movements that are necessary to move food from the stomach to the small intestine, an essential gastrocolic reflex, tied to the organism's nervous system, is needed to ensure a constant rhythm in the movement of feces into the rectum for elimination. If this function is delayed (as a result of nervous stress in some individuals, or because of the dilated physical state of the colon in aged persons) food residues become too tightly compressed in the bowels. As the colon continues to carry out its normal last-stage digestive function of reabsorbing essential water from waste material before it is eliminated, the feces become drier and even more compacted, making defecation difficult and sometimes painful.

Most other imbalances in digestive functions are chemical in nature. Highly spiced or unfamiliar foods frequently upset the balance in the body's chemical digestion. Symptoms may appear either in the abdomen itself (in particular, a bloated stomach accompanied by what is commonly called gas, a symptom of chemical disharmony in the digestive process) or in the stool. If the chemical breakdown of chyme is incomplete because of an imbalance in the proportion (either excessive or inadequate) of enzymes secreted into the stomach or intestines, the normal process of absorption will not take place, creating one of a number of symptoms of indigestion.

The most common symptom of indigestion is diarrhea, which can result from a variety of causes. Because movement in the bowels is affected by different nerve signals, some diarrhea attacks may be linked to nonchemical reactions, such as extreme nervousness. Relaxation of the sphincter, however, as well as the rise in the contractile pressure of the lower colon that precedes defecation (the gastroileal reflex), are also affected by the presence of gastrointestinal hormones, particularly gastrin itself. An imbalance in the amount of concentration of such components in the gastrointestinal tract (attributable to incomplete digestive chemistry) tends to relax the bowels to such a degree that elimination cannot be prevented except through determined mental resistance. It is important to note that if diarrhea continues for an extended time, its effect on the body is not simply the loss of essential body nutrients that pass through the bowels without being fully digested; the inability of the colon to reabsorb into the body an adequate proportion of the water content from the feces can lead to dehydration of the organism, especially in infants.

In most areas of the world, there is widespread consensus that treatment of indigestion is a matter of taking over-the-counter drugs whose function is to right the imbalance in some of the chemical processes described above. In theory as well as in practice, such treatments do work since the basic chemical imbalance, if it is has not extended beyond the point of indigestion (in the case of peptic ulcers, for example), is fairly easily diagnosed, even by pharmacists. Increasingly, however, the public is becoming aware that digestion can be aided, and indigestion avoided, by paying closer attention to dietary habits, particularly the importance of increasing fiber intake to facilitate the digestive process. Critical advances are also being made in knowledge of the potentially harmful effects on digestion of the chemical additives to processed foods.

PERSPECTIVE AND PROSPECTS

Historical traces of the medical observation of indigestion, as well as the prescription of remedies, can be found as far back as ancient Egypt. A famous medical text from about 1600 B.C. known as the Ebers Papyrus contains suggested remedies (mainly herbal drugs) for digestive ailments, as well as instructions for the use of suppositories to loosen the lower bowel. For centuries, however, such practical advice for treating indigestion were never accompanied by an adequate theoretical conception of the digestion function itself.

In the medieval Western world, many erroneous guidelines for understanding the digestive process were handed down from the works of Galen of Pergamum (129-c.199). Galen taught that food material passed from the intestines to the liver, where it was transformed into blood. At this point, a vital life-giving spirit, or "pneuma," gave the blood power to drive the body. Similar misconceptions would continue until, following the work of William Harvey (1578-1657), medical science gained more accurate knowledge of the circulatory function of the bloodstream. By the eighteenth century, rapid advances had been made in studies of the function of the stomach and intestines, notably by the French naturalist René de Réaumur (1683-1757), who demonstrated that food is broken down by gastric juices in the stomach, and by the Italian physiologist Lazzaro Spallanzani (1729-1799), who discovered that the stomach itself is the source of gastric juices.

It was an American army surgeon, William Beaumont (1785-1853), who wrote what became, until well into the twentieth century, the most complete medical guide to digestive functions. Beaumont carried out direct clinical observations of the actions of gastric juices in humans. He also observed the way in which the anticipation of eating can spark not only the secretion of such fluids but also the muscular stimuli that promote motility in the digestive process. Soon after Beaumont's findings were published, the German physiologist Theodor Schwann (1810-1882) first isolated pepsin. Others would show that a variety of enzymes in the gastrointestinal tract are secreted by different organs in the abdomen, notably the pancreas.

—Byron D. Cannon, Ph.D.

See also Acid-base chemistry; Constipation; Diarrhea and dysentery; Enzymes; Food biochemistry; Food poisoning; Gastroenterology; Gastroenterology, pediatric; Gastrointestinal disorders; Gastrointestinal system; Heartburn; Indigestion; Intestines; Metabolism; Nutrition; Peristalsis; Ulcer surgery; Ulcers; Vagotomy.

FOR FURTHER INFORMATION:

Brooks, Frank P. *Control of Gastrointestinal Function.* New York: Macmillan, 1970. A short and readable guide to the more detailed topics contained in formal medical texts.

Jackson, Gordon, and Philip Whitfield. *Digestion: Fueling the System.* New York: Torstar Books, 1984. This compact and excellently illustrated volume is designed for the informed layperson.

Janowitz, Henry D. *Indigestion.* New York: Oxford University Press, 1992. Deals with common problems of indigestion and includes medical approaches to the treatment of chronic cases.

Johnson, Leonard R., ed. *Gastrointestinal Physiology.* 5th ed. St. Louis: C. V. Mosby, 1997. This book contains a variety of different "self-contained" specialized topics dealt with by experts. Offers the excellent chapters "Gastric Motility" and "Pancreatic Secretion."

Magee, Donal F., and Arthur F. Dalley. *Digestion and the Structure and Function of the Gut.* Basel, Switzerland: S. Karger, 1986. This textbook is part of a continuing education publication series. Although it covers all topics with full technical detail, it is easily understood by a well-informed reader.

DIPHTHERIA

DISEASE/DISORDER

ANATOMY OR SYSTEM AFFECTED: Lungs, nervous system, respiratory system

SPECIALTIES AND RELATED FIELDS: Bacteriology, emergency medicine, public health

DEFINITION: A major cause of death in children until effective immunization was developed, diphtheria is a highly contagious bacterial infection that usually affects the respiratory system. When the bacteria, spread through the air or physical contact, cause a thick, grayish green membrane to form over the larynx, tonsils, pharynx, and sinus cavities, the result is hoarseness, a raspy cough, a sore throat, and a fever. Serious complications in the heart, kidneys, and nervous systems may occur when the bacteria release a dangerous toxin into the bloodstream. Treatment consists of the use of antitoxins and penicillin, which can destroy the diphtheria organisms. Although it has become rare in developed countries, diphtheria still has a mortality rate of 10 percent.

—Jason Georges and Tracy Irons-Georges

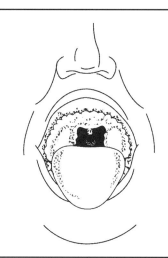

Diphtheria causes a thick, grayish green membrane to form over the larynx, tonsils, pharynx, and sinus cavities.

See also Antibiotics; Bacterial infections; Bacteriology; Childhood infectious diseases; Pulmonary diseases; Respiration.

DISEASE

DISEASE/DISORDER

ANATOMY OR SYSTEM AFFECTED: All

SPECIALTIES AND RELATED FIELDS: All

DEFINITION: A morbid (pathological) process with a characteristic set of symptoms that may affect the entire body or any of its parts; the cause, pathology, and course of a disease may be known or unknown.

KEY TERMS:

diagnosis: the art of distinguishing one disease from another

lesion: any pathologic or traumatic discontinuity of tissue or loss of function of a body part

pathology: the study of the essential nature of disease, especially as it relates to the structural and functional changes that are caused by that disease

prognosis: a forecast regarding the probable cause and result of an attack of disease

syndrome: a congregation of a set of signs and symptoms that characterize a particular disease process, but without a specific etiology or a constant lesion

TYPES OF DISEASE

It is difficult to answer the question "What is disease?" To the patient, disease means discomfort and disharmony with the environment. To the treating physician or surgeon, it means a set of signs and symptoms. To the pathologist, it means one or more structural changes in body tissues, called lesions, which may be viewed with or without the aid of magnifying lenses.

The study of lesions, which are the essential expression of disease, forms part of the modern science of pathology. Pathology had its beginnings in the morgue and the autopsy room, where investigations into the cause of death lead to the appreciation of "morbid anatomy"—at first by gross (naked-eye) examination and later microscopically. Much later, the investigation of disease moved from the cold autopsy room to the patient's bedside, from the dead body to the living body, on which laboratory tests and biopsies are performed for the purpose of establishing a diagnosis and addressing proper treatment.

Diagnosis is the art of determining not only the character of the lesion but its etiology, or cause. Because so much of this diagnostic work is done in the laboratories, the term "laboratory medicine" has gained in popularity. The explosion in high technology has expanded the field of laboratory medicine tremendously. The diagnostic laboratory today is highly automated and sophisticated, containing a team of laboratory technologists and scientific researchers rather than a single pathologist.

The lesions laid bare by the pathologist usually bear an obvious relation to the symptoms, as in the gross lesions of acute appendicitis, the microscopic lesions in poliomyelitis, or even the chromosomal lesions in genetically inherited conditions such as Down syndrome. Yet there may be lesions without symptoms, as in early cancer or "silent" diseases such as tuberculosis. There may also be symptoms without obvious lesions, as in the so-called psychosomatic disease, functional disorders, and psychiatric illnesses. It is likely that future research will reveal the presence of "biochemical lesions" in these cases. The presence of lesions distinguishes organic disease, in which there are gross or microscopic pathologic changes in an organ, from functional disease, in which there is a disturbance of function without a corresponding obvious organic lesion. Although most diagnoses consist largely of naming the lesion (such as cancer of the lung or a tooth abscess), diseases should truly be considered in the light of disordered function rather than altered structure. Scientists are searching beyond the presence of obvious lesions in tissues and cells to the submicroscopic, molecular, and biochemical alterations affecting the chemistry of cells.

Not all diseases have a specific etiology. A syndrome is a complex of signs and symptoms with no specific etiology or constant lesion. It results from interference at some point with a chain of body processes, causing impairment of body function in one or more systems. With a syndrome, a specific biochemical molecular derangement caused by yet undiscovered agents is usually found. An example is acquired immunodeficiency syndrome (AIDS), for which a specific human immunodeficiency virus (HIV) agent is now accepted as its etiologic agent.

Some diseases have an acute (sudden) onset and run a relatively short course, as with acute tonsillitis (strep throat) or the common cold. Others run a long, protracted course, as with tuberculosis and rheumatoid arthritis; these are called chronic illnesses. The healthy body is in a natural state of readiness to combat disease, and thus there is a natural tendency to recover from disease. This is especially true in acute illness, in which inflammation tends to heal with full resolution of structure and function. Sometimes, however, healing does not occur and the disease overwhelms the body and leads to death. Therefore, a patient with acute pneumonia may have a full recovery, with complete healing and resolution of structure and function, or may die. The outcome of disease can vary between the extremes of full recovery or death and can run a chronic, protracted course eventually leading to severe loss of function. This outcome is the prognosis, a forecast of what may be expected to happen. The accurate diagnosis of disease is essential for its treatment and prognosis.

There are four aspects to the study of disease. The first is etiology or cause; for example, the common cold virus causes the common cold. The second is pathogenesis, or course; it refers to the sequence of events in the body that occurs in response to injury and the method of the lesion's production and development. The relation of an etiologic agent to disease, of cause to effect, is not always as simple a matter as it is in most acute illnesses; for example, a herpesvirus causes the development of fever blisters. In many illnesses, indeed in most chronic illnesses, the concept of one agent causing one disease is an oversimplification. In tuberculosis, for example, the causative agent is a characteristic slender microbe called tubercle bacillus (*Mycobacterium tuberculosis*). Many people may be exposed to and inhale the tuberculosis bacteria, but only a few will get the disease; also, the bacteria may lurk in the body for years and only become clinically active as a result of an unrelated, stressful situation that alters the body's immunity, such as prolonged strain, malnutrition, or another infection. In investigating the causation and pathogenesis of disease, several factors—such as heredity, sex, environment, nutrition, immunity, and age—must be considered. That is why there is no simple answer to the questions, "Does cigarette smoking cause cancer?" or "Does a cholesterol-rich diet cause hardening of the blood vessels (atherosclerosis)?" The third aspect to the study of disease relates to morphologic and structural changes associated with the functional alterations in cells and tissues that are characteristic of the disease. These are the gross and microscopic findings that allow the pathologist to establish a diagnosis. The fourth aspect to disease study is the evaluation of functional abnormalities and their clinical significance; the nature of the morphologic changes and their distribution in different organs or tissues influence normal function and determine the clinical features, signs and symptoms, and course and outcome (prognosis) of disease.

All forms of tissue injury start with molecular and structural changes in cells. Cells are the smallest living units of tissues and organs. Along with their substructural components, they are the seat of disease. Cellular pathology is the study of disease as it relates to the origins, molecular mechanisms, and structural changes of cell injury.

The normal cell is similar to a factory. It is confined to a fairly narrow range of function and structure, dictated by its genetic code, the constraints of neighboring cells, the availability of and access to nutrition, and the disposal of its waste products. It is said to be in a "steady state," able to handle normal physiologic demands and to respond by adapting to other excessive or strenuous demands (such as the muscle enlargement seen in bodybuilders) to achieve a new equilibrium with a sustained workload. This type of adaptive response is called hypertrophy. Conversely, atrophy is an adaptive response to decreased demand, with a resulting diminished size and function.

If the limits of these adaptive responses are exceeded, or if no adaptive response is possible, a sequence of events follows which results in cell injury. Cell injury is reversible up to a certain point, but if the stimulus persists or is severe, then the cell suffers irreversible injury and eventual death. For example, if the blood supply to the heart muscle is cut off for only a few minutes and then restored, the heart muscle cells will experience injury but can recover and function normally. If the blood flow is not restored until one hour later, however, the cells will die.

Whether specific types of stress induce an adaptive response, a reversible injury, or cell death depends on the nature and severity of the stress and on other inherent, variable qualities of the cell itself. The causes of cell injury are many and range from obvious physical trauma, as in automobile accidents, to a subtle, genetic lack of enzymes or

hormones, as in diabetes mellitus. Broadly speaking, the causes of cell injury and death can be grouped into the following categories: hypoxia, or a decrease in the delivery of available oxygen; physical agents, as with mechanical and thermal injuries; chemical poisons, such as carbon monoxide, alcohol, tobacco, and other addictive drugs; infectious agents, such as viruses and bacteria; immunological and allergic reactions, as in patients with certain sensitivities; genetic defects, as with sickle-cell anemia; and nutritional imbalances, such as severe malnutrition and vitamin deficiencies or nutritional excesses predisposing a patient to heart disease and atherosclerosis.

CAUSES OF DISEASE

By far the most common cause of disease is infection, especially by bacteria. Certain lowly forms of animal life known as animal parasites may also live in the body and produce disease; parasitic diseases are common in poor societies and countries. Finally, there are viruses, forms of living matter so minute that they cannot be seen with the most powerful light microscope; they are visible, however, with the electron microscope. Viruses, as agents of disease, have attracted much attention for their role in many diseases, including cancer.

Bacteria, or germs, can be divided into three morphologic groups: cocci, which are round; bacilli, which are rod-shaped; and spirilla or spirochetes, which are spiral-shaped, like a corkscrew. Bacteria produce disease either by their presence in tissues or by their production of toxins (poisons). They cause inflammation and either act on surrounding tissues, as in an abscess, or are carried by the bloodstream to other distant organs. Strep throat is an example of a local infection by cocci—in this case, streptococci. Some dysenteries and travelers' diarrheas are caused by coliform bacilli. Syphilis is an example of disease caused by a spirochete. The great epidemics of history, such as bubonic plague and cholera, are caused by bacteria, as are tuberculosis, leprosy, typhoid, gas gangrene, and many others. Bacterial infections are treatable with antibiotics, such as penicillin.

Viruses, on the other hand, are not affected by antibiotics; they infect the cell itself and live within it, and are therefore protected. Viruses cause a wide variety of diseases. Some are short-lived and run a few days' course, such as many childhood diseases, the measles, and the common cold. Others can cause serious body impairment, such as poliomyelitis and AIDS. Still others are probably involved in causing cancer and such diseases as multiple sclerosis.

Of the many physical agents causing injury, trauma is the most obvious; others relate to external temperatures, ones that are either too high or too low. A high temperature may produce local injury, such as a burn, or general disease, as in heat stroke. Heat stroke results from prolonged direct exposure to the sun (sunstroke) or from very high temperatures, so that the heat-regulating mechanism of the body becomes paralyzed. The internal, body temperature shoots up to alarming heights; collapse, coma, and even death may result. Low temperatures can cause local frostbite or general hypothermia, which can also lead to death.

Other forms of physical agents causing injury are radiation and atmospheric pressure. Increased atmospheric pressure is best illustrated by the "bends," a decompression sickness which can affect deep sea divers. The pressure of the water causes inert gases, such as nitrogen, to be dissolved in the blood plasma. If the diver passes too rapidly from a high to a normal atmospheric pressure, the excessive nitrogen is released, forming gas bubbles in the blood. These tiny bubbles can cause the blockage of small vessels of the brain and result in brain damage. The same problem can occur in high-altitude aviators unless the airplane is pressurized.

The study of chemical poisoning, or toxicology, as a cause of disease is a large and specialized field. Poisons may be introduced into the body by accident (especially in young children), because of suicide or homicide, and most important as industrial pollution. Lead poisoning is a danger because of its use in paints and soldering. Acids and carbon monoxide are emitted into the atmosphere by industry, and various chemicals are dumped into the ground and water. Such environmental damage will eventually affect plants, livestock, and humans.

Hypoxia (lack of oxygen) is probably the most common cause of cell injury, and it may also be the ultimate mechanism of cell death by a wide variety of physical, biological, and chemical agents. Loss of adequate blood and oxygen supply to a body part, such as a leg, is called ischemia. (This is a local loss of blood, in contrast to anemia, which is a general condition of poor oxygen-carrying capacity affecting the entire body.) If the blood loss is very severe, the result is hypoxia, or anoxia. This condition may also result from narrowing of the blood vessels, called atherosclerosis. If this narrowing occurs in the artery of the leg, as may be seen in patients with advanced diabetes, then the tissues of the foot will eventually die, a condition known as gangrene. An even more critical example of ischemia is blockage of the coronary arteries of the heart, resulting in a myocardial infarction (heart attack), with damage to the heart muscle. Similarly, severe blockage of arteries to the brain can cause a stroke.

Nutritional diseases can be caused either by an excessive intake and storage of foodstuffs, as in extreme obesity, or by a deficiency. Obesity is a complex condition, often associated with hereditary tendencies and hormonal imbalances. The deficiency conditions are many. Starvation and malnutrition can occur because of intestinal illnesses that prevent the delivery of food to the blood (malabsorption) or because of debilitating diseases such as advanced cancer. Even more important than general malnutrition as a cause of disease is a deficiency of essential nutrients such as min-

erals, vitamins, and other trace elements. Iron deficiency causes anemia, and calcium deficiency causes osteoporosis (bone fragility). Vitamin deficiencies are also numerous, and deficiency of the trace element iodine causes a thyroid condition called goiter.

Genetic defects as a cause of cellular injury and disease are of major interest to many biologists. The genetic injury may be as gross as the congenital malformations seen in patients with Down syndrome or as subtle as molecular alterations in the coding of the hemoglobin molecule that causes sickle-cell anemia.

Cellular injuries and diseases can be induced by immune mechanisms. The anaphylactic reaction to a foreign protein, such as a bee sting or drug, can actually cause death. In the so-called autoimmune diseases, such as lupus erythematosus, the immune system turns against the cellular components of the very body that it is supposed to protect.

Finally, neoplastic diseases, or cancer, are presently of unknown etiology. Some are innocuous growths, while others are highly lethal. Diagnosing cancer and determining its precise nature can be an elaborate, and elusive, process. The methods involve clinical observations and laboratory tests; a biopsy of the involved organ may be taken and analyzed.

PERSPECTIVE AND PROSPECTS

It is sometimes said that the nature of disease is changing, that one hears more often of people dying of heart failure and cancer than was once the case. This does not mean that these diseases have actually become more common, although more people do die from them. This increase is attributable to a longer life span and vastly improved diagnostic methods.

For primitive humans, there were no diseases, only patients stricken by evil; therefore, magic was the plausible recourse. Magic entails recognition of the principle of causality—that, given the same predisposing conditions, the same results will follow. In a profound sense, magic is early science. In ancient Egypt, the priests assumed the role of healers. Unlike magic, however, religion springs from a different source. Here the system is based on the achievement of results against, or in spite of, a regular sequence. Religion heals with miracles and antinaturals that require the violation of causality. The purely religious concept of disease, as an expression of the wrath of gods, became embodied in many religious traditions.

The ancient Greeks are credited with attempts at introducing reason to the study of disease by asking questions about the nature of things and considering the notion of health as a harmony, as the adjustment of such opposites as high and low, hot and cold, dry and moist. Disease, therefore, was a disharmony of the four elements that make up life: earth, air, fire, and water. This concept was refined by Galen in the second century and became dogma throughout the Dark Ages until the Renaissance, when the seat of disease was finally assigned to organs within the body itself through autopsy studies. Much later, in the nineteenth century, the principles espoused by French physiologist Claude Bernard were introduced, whereby disease was considered not a thing but a process that distorts normal physiologic and anatomic features. The nineteenth century German pathologist Rudolf Virchow emphasized the same principle—that disease is an alteration of life's processes—by championing the concept of cellular pathology, identifying the cell as the smallest unit of life and as the seat of disease.

As new diseases are discovered and old medical mysteries are deciphered, as promising new medicinal drugs and vaccines are tested and public health programs implemented, the age-old goal of medicine as a healing art seems to be closer at hand. —*Victor H. Nassar, M.D.*

See also Arthropod-borne diseases; Childhood infectious diseases; Dental diseases; Environmental diseases; Gallbladder diseases; Genetic diseases; Infection; Motor neuron diseases; Parasitic diseases; Pathology; Prion diseases; Protozoan diseases; Pulmonary diseases; Sexually transmitted diseases; Zoonoses; *specific diseases.*

FOR FURTHER INFORMATION:

Boyd, William. *Boyd's Introduction to the Study of Disease.* 11th ed. Philadelphia: Lea & Febiger, 1992. A textbook for students in the medical and allied health sciences. The text and illustrations emphasize the view of disease as a disturbed functional alteration.

Grist, Norman R., et al. *Diseases of Infection: An Illustrated Textbook.* 2d ed. Oxford, England: Oxford University Press, 1992. An informative survey of communicable diseases. Contains copious illustrations.

Jones, Kenneth L., Louis W. Shainberg, and Curtis O. Byer. *Disease.* 2d ed. San Francisco: Canfield Press, 1975. A popular work designed to educate the general reader about both communicable and noncommunicable diseases. Examines the causes of these diseases, as well as general theories of causation.

Perez-Tamayo, Ruy. *Mechanisms of Disease: An Introduction to Pathology.* 2d ed. Chicago: Yearbook Medical Publishers, 1985. A fascinating examination of the nature and mechanism of disease. Written for the advanced student.

Robbins, Stanley L., Ramzi S. Cotran, and Vinay Kumar. *Robbins' Pathologic Basis of Disease.* 5th ed. Philadelphia: W. B. Saunders, 1994. The standard textbook on disease for medical students.

Shaw, Michael, ed. *Everything You Need to Know About Diseases.* Springhouse, Pa.: Springhouse Press, 1996. This well-illustrated consumer reference, compiled by more than one hundred doctors and medical experts, describes five hundred illnesses and conditions, their causes, symptoms, diagnosis, treatment, and prevention. A valuable reference book for everyone interested in health and disease.

DISK REMOVAL

PROCEDURE

ANATOMY OR SYSTEM AFFECTED: Back, bones, nervous system, spine

SPECIALTIES AND RELATED FIELDS: General surgery, neurology, orthopedics, physical therapy

DEFINITION: A surgical procedure used to remove intervertebral disks that are compressing on nerves that enter and exit the spinal cord.

KEY TERMS:

cervical vertebrae: the first seven bones of the spinal column, located in the neck

disk prolapse: the protrusion (herniation) of intervertebral disk material, which may press on spinal nerves

intervertebral disks: flattened disks of fibrocartilage that separate the vertebrae and allow cushioned flexibility of the spinal column

lumbar vertebrae: the five bones of the spinal column in the lower back, which experience the greatest stress in the spine

spinal cord: a column of nervous tissue housed in the vertebral column which carries messages to and from the brain

INDICATIONS AND PROCEDURES

A relatively common disorder which causes lower back and sometimes leg pain is the herniation or prolapse of an intervertebral disk in the lower back. These disks are made of cartilage and serve to separate the bones that make up the vertebral column. The spinal cord is located within the bony structure of the vertebrae and has nerves which enter and exit between these bones. These sensory and motor nerves must pass alongside the intervertebral disks. When a disk's jellylike center bulges out through a weakened area of the firmer outer core, the disk is said to be herniated or prolapsed. This may compress the spinal cord or the nerve roots and yield such symptoms as interference with muscle strength or pain and numbness of the lower back and leg.

More than 90 percent of disk prolapses occur in the lumbar region of the back, but they may also occur in the cervical vertebrae. Occasionally, disk herniation is caused by improper lifting of heavy objects, sudden twisting of the spinal column, or trauma to the back or neck. More typically, however, a prolapsed disk develops gradually as the patient ages and the intervertebral disks degenerate.

In order to diagnosis a prolapsed disk, a physician will likely want to visualize the vertebrae and spinal cord using X rays, computed tomography (CT) scans, or magnetic resonance imaging (MRI). Once diagnosed, most cases can be treated with analgesics, muscle relaxants (such as cyclobenzaprine and methocarbamol), and physical therapy. If the symptoms recur, however, it may be necessary to have the protruding portion of the disk or the whole disk surgically removed. This procedure usually requires that the patient have general anesthesia and remain hospitalized for several days.

For a lumbar procedure, the patient is anesthetized and placed on the operating room table in a modified kneeling position, with the abdomen suspended and the legs placed over the end of the table. The lower back is then prepared for a sterile procedure, and the surgeon makes an incision in the middle of the back along the spine. The surrounding tissues are retracted, and the vertebrae are exposed. At this time, the surgeon must make a careful dissection of the tissues in order to identify the affected nerves and intervertebral disk. Once the prolapsed disk is found, the physician will cut away the fragment of the disk impinging on the nerve. It is important that all free fragments be removed, as these could cause symptoms at a later time. Often, the surgeon must remove some of the vertebrae to gain access to the disk. This is known as a laminectomy.

USES AND COMPLICATIONS

Because the vertebral column houses the spinal cord, any surgical manipulation of this area must be approached with extreme caution. Very large arteries (the aorta) and veins (the vena cava) lie adjacent to the spinal column and, if accidentally cut, can lead to rapid blood loss. The spinal cord is surrounded by a covering called the meninges, which helps to protect the cord and which contains the cerebral spinal fluid. Trauma to the meninges may cause the fluid to leak out or lead to meningitis (inflammation of the meninges). One surgical approach to reduce the adverse affects of a lesion to the meninges is to use some of the patient's fat to pack the leak and help prevent scarring. Patients with operative trauma to the meninges may complain of headache, which usually decreases in severity as the lesion heals.

Other complications that may arise include infections in approximately 3 percent of patients, thromboembolism in less than 1 percent, and death in about one patient per 1,000. One study reports an overall complication rate of 4 percent. Unfortunately, one of the major long-term complications reported in the study involved a worsening of symptoms after surgery.

PERSPECTIVE AND PROSPECTS

Even with some potential complications, disk removal typically has a favorable outcome, although this varies somewhat depending on the patient, the treatment method, and what the patient and physician consider "a good result." Typically favorable outcomes range from 50 to 95 percent. The number of patients who need a second operation ranges from 4 to 25 percent.

Health care professionals are beginning to emphasize the importance of prevention of back pain. Educating patients on proper lifting techniques, such as bending the legs rather than the back and avoiding twisting, will reduce the potential for damage to the intervertebral disks. Individuals who are overweight are also at risk for developing lower back pain because of the added stress to the lumbar spine, as well as because of their relatively weak abdominal muscles. The abdominal muscles are important in stabilizing and supporting the lower back. Exercises which help strengthen these muscles are recommended for a weight-reducing exercise and diet program. Patients who must sit for long periods of time are also at risk for lower back pain. These people should take several quick breaks to stand and stretch, which reduces the constant stress on the lumbar spine.

—*Matthew Berria, Ph.D., and Douglas Reinhart, M.D.*

See also Bone disorders; Bones and the skeleton; Laminectomy and spinal fusion; Meningitis; Orthopedic surgery; Orthopedics; Slipped disk; Spinal disorders; Spine, vertebrae, and disks.

FOR FURTHER INFORMATION:

Aminoff, Michael J. "Nervous System." In *Current Medical Diagnosis and Treatment*, edited by Lawrence M. Tierney, Jr., et. al. 37th ed. Norwalk, Conn.: Appleton and Lange, 1998.

Bradford, David S., ed. *The Spine*. Philadelphia: Lippincott-Raven, 1997.

Clayman, Charles B., ed. *The American Medical Association Encyclopedia of Medicine*. New York: Random House, 1989.

Stutzman, Ray E., and Patrick C. Walsh. "The Spine: Lower Back Pain and Disorders of Intervertebral Disc." In *Campbell's Operative Orthopaedics*, edited by A. H. Crenshaw. 8th ed. 5 vols. St. Louis: Mosby Year Book, 1992.

DISLOCATION. *See* FRACTURE AND DISLOCATION.

DIVERTICULITIS AND DIVERTICULOSIS
DISEASE/DISORDER

ANATOMY OR SYSTEM AFFECTED: Abdomen, gastrointestinal system, intestines

SPECIALTIES AND RELATED FIELDS: Gastroenterology, internal medicine, proctology

DEFINITION: Diverticulosis is a disease involving multiple outpouchings, or diverticuli, of the wall of the colon; these diverticuli may become inflamed, leading to the painful condition called diverticulitis.

KEY TERMS:

colon: the portion of the large intestine excluding the cecum and rectum; it includes the ascending, transverse, descending, and sigmoid colon

dietary fiber: indigestible plant substances that humans eat; fiber may be soluble, meaning that it dissolves in water, or insoluble, meaning that it does not dissolve in water

hernia: the bulging out of part or all of an organ through the wall of the cavity that usually contains it

infection: multiplication of disease-causing microorganisms in the body; the body normally also contains microorganisms that do not cause disease *inflammation:* a tissue response to injury involving local reactions that attempt to destroy the injurious material and begin healing

lumen: the channel within a hollow or tubular organ

mucosa: the inner lining of the digestive tract; in the colon, the major function of the mucosal cells is to reabsorb liquid from feces, creating a semisolid material

perforation: an abnormal opening, such as a hole in the wall of the colon

peritoneal cavity: the cavity in the abdomen and pelvis that contains the internal organs

prevalence: the frequency of disease cases in a population, often expressed as a fraction (such as cases per 100,000)

CAUSES AND SYMPTOMS

Diverticulosis is an acquired condition of the colon that involves a few to hundreds of blueberry-sized outpouchings of its wall called diverticuli. Diverticular disease is usually manifested by the presence of multiple diverticuli that are at risk of causing abdominal pain, inflammation, or bleeding.

Although the wall of the colon is thin, microscopically it has four layers. The innermost layer is called the mucosa. Its main function is to absorb fluids from the substance entering the colon, turning it into a semisolid material called feces. Outside the mucosa is the submucosa, a layer which contains blood vessels as well as nerve cells that control the functions of mucosal cells. Outside the submucosa is the muscularis, which contains muscle cells that are able to contract, pushing feces along the colon and eventually out through the rectum. Outside the muscularis is the serosa, which forms a wrap around the colon and helps prevent infections in this organ from spreading beyond its walls.

The definition of a diverticulum, taken from *Stedman's Medical Dictionary* (25th ed., 1990), is "a pouch or sac opening from a tubular or saccular organ, such as the gut or bladder." The diverticuli that form in the colon are not true diverticuli, in that the entire wall is not present in the outpouching. If examined microscopically, only the mucosal and submucosal layers pouch out through weakened areas in the muscularis layer. If examined by the naked eye, however, it appears as if the entire wall of the colon is involved in the tiny outpouching. The mucosa bulges out in the part of the colonic wall that is weakened: This is where arteries penetrate through clefts in the muscularis.

The large intestine begins with the cecum, which is connected to the small intestine. The cecum is a pouch leading to the colon, whose components are the ascending, transverse, descending, and sigmoid colon. The sigmoid colon leads to the rectum, which is connected to the outside of the body by the anal canal. Although diverticuli can appear at a variety of locations in the gastrointestinal (GI) tract, they are usually located in the colon, most commonly in the sigmoid colon.

The most common form of diverticulosis is called spastic colon diverticulosis, which is a condition involving diverticuli in the sigmoid colon whose lumen is abnormally narrowed. Since the circumference of the colon normally alternately narrows and widens along its length, muscle contractions may result in local occlusions of the lumen at the narrowed sections. Occlusion may cause the lumen of the colon to become multiple, separate chambers. When this happens, the pressure within the chambers can increase to the point where the mucosa herniates out through small clefts in the muscularis, creating diverticuli.

Most people with diverticulosis never notice it. When abdominal pain related to painful diverticular disease develops, it is felt in the lower abdomen and may last for hours or days. Eating usually makes it worse, whereas passing gas or having a bowel movement may relieve it.

Besides causing abdominal pain, diverticuli may cause rectal bleeding, which may vary from mild to life-threatening. Usually, there is a sudden urge to defecate followed by passage of red blood, clots, or maroon-colored

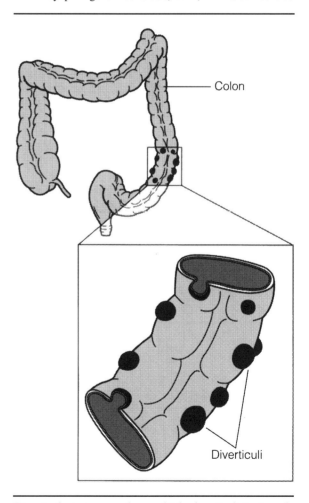

Diverticulosis occurs when multiple diverticuli (outpouchings) appear on the colon wall.

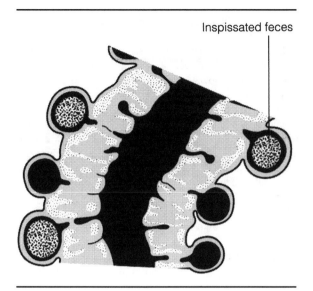

Inspissated feces

Diverticulitis begins when fecal material invades diverticuli and thickens (inspissated feces); when a diverticulum perforates, bacteria travel outside the colon into other regions and cause serious symptoms, including lower abdominal pain, fever, chills, and abscesses.

stool. If the stool is black, the bleeding is probably from the upper GI tract.

Since the colon may be studded with multiple diverticuli, and the bleeding may stop by the time of evaluation, it is often difficult to tell which one bled. Diverticulosis is most common in elderly people, who may have other conditions of the colon that are associated with bleeding. Therefore, it is often impossible to confirm that the cause of bleeding was from diverticular disease—even if the colon is lined with hundreds of diverticuli.

What is most important is to establish what part of the GI tract is bleeding. To find out if the bleeding could have come from the upper GI tract, a tube is passed through the nose into the stomach and the contents are aspirated. If blood is not present, this suggests lower GI bleeding. In addition, the esophagus, stomach, and upper small intestine can be visualized with a flexible, snakelike instrument called an endoscope to exclude a source such as a bleeding ulcer.

It is more difficult to examine the lower GI tract. The simplest procedure is anoscopy, by which the physician can examine the inside of the anal canal for hemorrhoids. Proctosigmoidoscopy, a procedure similar to endoscopy, offers a view of the rectum and part of the sigmoid colon. It may reveal diverticuli or other lesions such as a bleeding growth called a polyp.

Angiography is a test done in the radiology department; it involves injecting dye into the vessels that lead to the colon. If there is active bleeding, it can help localize the source. Even if the bleeding has stopped, this procedure

can sometimes identify abnormal blood vessel formations suggestive of cancer or a blood vessel abnormality called angiodysplasia. Colonoscopy is most easily performed after bleeding has stopped. It requires cleaning out the contents of the colon and then inserting a long, flexible instrument called a colonoscope all the way to the cecum. The entire lining of the colon can be visualized while withdrawing the colonoscope.

About 15 percent of people with diverticulosis suffer from one or more episodes of diverticulitis, which is an inflammatory condition that may progress to an infection. Initially, feces may become trapped and inspissated (thickened) in a diverticulum, irritating it and leading to inflammation. Inflammation is a tissue response to injury which involves local reactions that attempt to destroy the injurious material and begin the healing process. It is usually the first step in the body's attempt to prevent infection and involves the migration of white blood cells out of blood vessels and into tissues, where they begin to fight off bacteria. The white blood cells release enzymes that cause tissue destruction. Because it is thin, the wall of the diverticulum may develop a tiny perforation.

Feces are made up of waste material and bacteria that normally do not cause problems when confined within the lumen of the colon. When a diverticulum perforates, however, they travel outside the colon and into other regions such as the peritoneal cavity, causing an infection. This infection along the outside of the colon is often limited, because many adjacent structures are able to wall off the bacteria, limiting their ability to extend through the peritoneal cavity. Although they become sealed off, they often form a pus-filled lesion called an abscess.

Fever and abdominal pain are the most common symptoms of diverticulitis. The fever may be high and associated with shaking chills. The pain is often sudden in onset, continuous, and may radiate from the left lower abdomen to the back. Laboratory findings usually include an elevated white blood cell count, a nonspecific finding that occurs with a variety of infections.

Radiographic studies are helpful for diagnosing and assessing the severity of diverticulitis. For example, a computed tomography (CT) scan can detect diverticuli or a thickening of the bowel wall associated with diverticulitis and can help assess whether abscesses are present.

TREATMENT AND THERAPY

There are two treatment goals in treating uncomplicated, painful diverticular disease: prevention of further development of diverticuli and pain relief. It is important to understand that the pressure that is able to develop inside the lumen of the colon is inversely related to the radius of the lumen. Therefore, if the lumen's radius can be increased, the pressures within the lumen will lessen, theoretically decreasing the chance of diverticuli formation. One key to increasing the radius of the lumen of the colon is to increase the bulk of the stool by the addition of dietary fiber.

A Western diet tends to be high in fiber-free animal foods and to lose much of its fiber during processing. This low-fiber diet may contribute to the cause of diverticulosis, which is prevalent in countries that have low-fiber diets. The typical American diet contains an average of 12 grams of fiber per day, whereas diets from Africa and India contain from 40 to 150 grams of fiber per day. A high-fiber diet can increase stool bulk by 40 to 100 percent. Fiber adds bulk to the stool because it acts like a sponge, retaining water that would normally be reabsorbed by the colonic mucosa. Fiber also increases stool bulk because 50 to 70 percent of the fiber is degraded by the bacteria in the colon and the products of degradation attract water by a process called osmosis.

The main fibers that increase stool bulk are the water-insoluble fibers, such as cellulose, hemicellulose, and lignin; they are derived from plants such as vegetables and whole grain cereals. Diets high in these fibers have been shown to decrease the intraluminal pressure in the sigmoid colon, as well as to relieve the pain associated with uncomplicated diverticular disease. The best results have been with the addition of 10 to 25 grams per day of coarse, unprocessed wheat bran to various liquid and semisolid foods. The sudden addition of large amounts of bran to one's diet, however, may cause bloating. Commercial preparations such as methylcellulose may be better tolerated during the first few weeks of therapy; their use may then be tapered off as bran is added to the diet. There are also various antispasmodic drugs available for inhibiting the muscle spasms of the colon, but many of those used in the United States are not very effective for decreasing symptoms.

For diverticular bleeding, the most effective therapy is patience. Most episodes stop on their own, and conservative treatments such as maintaining the patient's blood volume with intravenous fluids and possibly performing blood transfusions are all that is necessary. In those patients with continued active bleeding and in whom the source of the bleeding can be identified with angiography, a drug called vasopressin may be administered into the artery over several hours. This causes constriction of the vessel and stops bleeding most of the time. Once the vasopressin is stopped, however, patients may resume bleeding.

If vasopressin fails, surgery may be necessary. Surgery is most often successful if the bleeding site has been well localized before the operation. In that case, only the involved segment of the colon needs to be removed. If the bleeding site cannot be identified, it may be necessary to remove a majority of the colon; this procedure is associated with a higher rate of postoperative complications.

Diverticulitis that warrants hospitalization is initially treated with intravenous antibiotics for seven to ten days. Antibiotics help prevent 70 to 85 percent of patients from needing surgery. Most of those who respond to antibiotics will not have future attacks severe enough to warrant hospitalization.

Other measures may be necessary for the care of someone with diverticulitis, because the inflammation around the colon may be associated with problems such as narrowing of the bowel lumen to the point where it causes a partial or complete colonic obstruction. In this case, nothing should be given by mouth, and a tube should be passed through the nose into the stomach in order to suck out air and the stomach contents. This suction helps to reduce the amount of material that can pass through the colon and worsen the dilation of the colon that occurs proximal to the obstruction.

If the fever persists for more than a few days, the diverticulitis may be associated with complications. One complication is the formation of a large abscess outside the colon, which may be detected by a CT scan. An abscess has a rim around it that makes it difficult for antibiotics to penetrate the liquid center. If it does not go away despite antibiotic therapy, surgery may be necessary. If the abscess is small, it is possible to remove the involved segment of bowel and reattach the two free ends. If the abscess is very large, it may be necessary first to drain the abscess and then to cut across the colon proximal to the diseased segment, attaching the free end of the proximal segment to the abdominal wall, a procedure called a diverting colostomy. Later, the diseased segment of colon can be removed, and the remaining two free ends of colon can be joined. Another option is to drain the abscess with the aid of visual guidance by the CT scan and then operate on the colon. Draining the abscess in this manner helps get the infection under control before surgery is performed. Other indications for surgery in diverticulitis include complications such as a persistent bowel obstruction. In this case, it is often necessary to use a two-stage approach rather than to cure the problem in one operation.

Another complication of diverticulitis is a generalized infection of the peritoneal cavity, called peritonitis. Surgery for peritonitis involves removing the leaking segment of bowel and attaching the remaining two free ends of the colon to the abdominal wall. In addition, the peritoneal cavity is rinsed with a sterile solution in an attempt to clean out the contaminating materials.

Diverticulitis may also be complicated by the presence of a perforation of a diverticulum leading to a fistula, an abnormally existing channel connecting two hollow organs. When there is a fistula between the colon and the bladder, stool can travel into the bladder. The bacteria in the stool can cause severe, recurrent urinary tract infections. Another symptom is that bowel gas gets into the bladder; when the patient urinates, there is an intermittent stream because of colonic gas being passed along with the urine. When a fistula exists, it is necessary to remove the diseased segment of colon, the fistula tract, and a small portion of the bladder where the tract entered it.

Even if a patient with diverticulitis seems to improve and is able to return home from the hospital without needing surgery, there is still a chance that surgery will be necessary in the future. Surgery may be needed if the patient continues to have repeated, severe attacks of diverticulitis, or when a fistula between the colon and bladder causes recurring urinary tract infections. Another reason for surgery is when there is persistent partial colonic obstruction and it is impossible to inspect the narrowed region of colon to exclude a constricting cancerous lesion as the cause of the obstruction.

PERSPECTIVE AND PROSPECTS

Diverticuli are quite common in the United States and other developed countries that tend to eat processed, low-fiber foods. In the United States, for example, diverticulosis is uncommon before the age of forty but is seen in 30 to 50 percent of elderly people at autopsy. Of those with diverticuli, only about one-fifth suffer any symptoms. Although members of ethnic groups who live in underdeveloped countries and eat a high-fiber diet tend to have a low prevalence of diverticulosis, their risk of developing this disease increases within ten years of moving to more developed countries.

Before 1900, the presence of colonic diverticuli in the United States was considered a curiosity, whereas now it is found in one-third to one-half of all autopsies of people over the age of sixty. There are a few possible explanations for why this increasing prevalence is seen.

First, the change in the American diet probably plays a large part in the pathogenesis of diverticular disease. Fiber consumption may have fallen off by as much as 30 percent during the twentieth century. Many people in the United States eat foods such as quick-cooking rice, highly processed cereals, and processed flour, all which contains less fiber than their unprocessed counterparts. In addition, the population tends to eat more fats and proteins and less carbohydrates. Many fibers are from food sources rich in carbohydrates and are carbohydrates themselves.

The increasing prevalence of diverticular disease may also be attributable to the changing survival pattern. In 1900, the average life expectancy in the United States was forty-nine; in 1983, it was seventy-one years for men and seventy-eight years for women. The proportion of people over sixty-five has risen: It was 4.1 percent in 1900 and increased to 11.6 percent in 1986. Thus, the American population is not only growing but also getting older. Since diverticulosis is seen in increasing frequencies with aging, it is understandable that more of it was seen in the late twentieth century than during the early 1900's.

Most poor people in the world live largely on plant foods rich in fiber, being largely dependent on cereal grains such as wheat, rice, and corn for both their calorie and their protein sources. Although one can look at the amount of fiber in the diet of rural Africans and compare it to that in the United States, there may be other differences in lifestyles that contribute to the higher prevalence of diverticular disease in the United States. Living in rural Africa, without traffic jams and the fast pace of developed countries, may cause people to have less stressful lives, and the lower stress is associated with fewer muscle spasms in the colon. Since it has been documented that stress can increase colonic contractions, and stress may worsen another disorder of the colon involving muscle spasm called irritable bowel syndrome (IBS), one might postulate that the stress of Western society contributes to the spasms in the sigmoid colon that may lead to diverticular disease.

Another reason for the increase in the prevalence of diverticular disease could be improvements in detection. Now it is detected not only at autopsy but also by barium enema, during sigmoidoscopy, and during surgery. Thus, there are more opportunities for discovering diverticulosis.

—Marc H. Walters, M.D.

See also Colon and rectal polyp removal; Colon and rectal surgery; Colon cancer; Colon therapy; Colonoscopy; Constipation; Digestion; Gastroenterology; Gastroenterology, pediatric; Gastrointestinal disorders; Gastrointestinal system; Intestinal disorders; Intestines; Nutrition; Peritonitis.

FOR FURTHER INFORMATION:

Achkar, Edgar, et al. *Clinical Gastroenterology*. 2d ed. Philadelphia: Lea & Febiger, 1992. This book is written by gastroenterologists from the Cleveland Clinic. Contains excellent chapters on abdominal pain, gastrointestinal bleeding, and diverticular disease. Less detailed but more readable than Marvin Sleisenger and John Fordtran's textbook (below).

Ganong, William F. *Review of Medical Physiology*. 18th ed. Stamford, Conn.: Appleton and Lange, 1997. This classic book has a nice section emphasizing normal gastrointestinal physiology which would provide a solid background for understanding diverticulosis.

Hackford, Alan W., and Malcolm C. Veidenheimer. "Diverticular Disease of the Colon: Current Concepts and Management." *Surgical Clinics of North America* 65 (April, 1985): 347-363. This article emphasizes the medical and surgical options for treating diverticulitis.

Kumar, Vinay, Ramzi S. Cotran, and Stanley L. Robbins. *Basic Pathology*. 6th ed. Philadelphia: W. B. Saunders, 1997. An introductory pathology textbook. Less detailed than texts used by physicians, but still contains useful information on diverticular disease.

Segal, I. A. Solomon, and J. A. Hunt. "Emergence of Diverticular Disease in the Urban South African Black." *Gastroenterology* 72 (February, 1977): 215-219. This article discusses the emergence of diverticulosis in urban South African blacks, coincident with decreasing dietary fiber intake.

Sleisenger, Marvin H., and John S. Fordtran, eds. *Sleisenger* and Fordtran's Gastrointestinal and Liver Disease: Pathophysiology, Diagnosis, Management. 6th ed. 2 vols. Philadelphia: W. B. Saunders, 1998. This text is the best comprehensive textbook of gastrointestinal diseases and physiology. Contains excellent information on diverticular disease.

Tortora, Gerard J., and Sandra R. Grabowski. *Principles of Anatomy and Physiology.* 8th ed. New York: HarperCollins, 1996. An outstanding textbook of human anatomy and physiology, and a good first text to consult before reading more advanced gastroenterology and journal articles. Many supplements are available, including an anatomy and physiology laserdisc.

DIZZINESS AND FAINTING
DISEASE/DISORDER

ANATOMY OR SYSTEM AFFECTED: Blood vessels, brain, circulatory system, head, nervous system, psychic-emotional system

SPECIALTIES AND RELATED FIELDS: Cardiology, emergency medicine, family practice, internal medicine, neurology

DEFINITION: Dizziness is a feeling of light-headedness and unsteadiness, sometimes accompanied by a feeling of spinning or other spatial motion; fainting is a loss of consciousness as a result of insufficient amounts of blood reaching the brain. Both are symptoms of many conditions, which may be harmless or serious.

KEY TERMS:

cardiac output: the amount of blood that the heart can pump per unit time (usually per minute); if the brain does not receive enough of the cardiac output, the person becomes dizzy and may faint

dizziness: a sensation of whirling with difficulty balancing

fainting: a weak feeling followed by a loss of consciousness, usually due to a lack of blood flow to the brain; also called syncope

hypertension: a condition in which the patient's blood pressure is higher than what the body demands

hypotension: decrease in blood pressure to the point that insufficient blood flow causes symptoms

vasoconstriction: a reduction in the diameter of arteries, which increases the amount of work required for the heart to move blood

vasodilation: an increase in the diameter of arteries, which decreases the amount of work required for the heart to move blood

venous return: the amount of blood returning to the heart; one factor that determines the amount of blood the heart can pump out

vertigo: a sensation of moving in space or having objects move about when the patient is stationary, the most common symptom of which is dizziness; vertigo results from a disturbance in the organs of equilibrium

CAUSES AND SYMPTOMS

Humans have evolved several mechanisms by which adequate blood flow to organs is maintained. Without a constant blood supply, the body's tissues would die from a lack of essential nutrients and oxygen. In particular, the brain and heart are very sensitive to changes in their blood supply as they, more than any other organs, must receive oxygen and nutrients at all times. If they do not, their cells will die and cannot be replaced.

While the heart supplies most of the force needed to propel the blood throughout the body, tissues rely on changes in the size of arteries to redirect blood flow to where it is needed most. For example, after a large meal the blood vessels that lead to the gastrointestinal tract enlarge (vasodilate) so that more blood can be present to collect the nutrients from the meal. At the same time, the blood vessels that supply muscles decrease in diameter (vasoconstrict) and effectively shunt the blood toward the stomach and intestines. On the other hand, during exercise, the blood vessels that supply the muscles dilate and the ones leading to the intestinal tract vasoconstrict. This mechanism allows the cardiovascular system to supply the most blood to the most active tissues.

The brain is somewhat special in that the body tries to maintain a nearly constant blood flow to it. Located in the walls of the carotid arteries, which carry blood to the brain, are specialized sensory cells that have the ability to detect changes in blood pressure. These cells are known as baroreceptors. If the blood pressure going to the brain is too low, the baroreceptors send an impulse to the brain which in turn speeds up the heart rate and causes a generalized vasoconstriction. This reflex response raises the body's blood pressure, reestablishing adequate blood flow to the brain. If the baroreceptors detect too high a blood pressure, they send a signal to the brain which in turn slows the heart rate and causes the arteries of the body to dilate. These reflexes prevent large fluctuations in blood flow to the brain and other tissues.

Most people have experienced a dizzy feeling or maybe even a fainting response when they have stood up too quickly from a prone position. The ability of the baroreceptors to maintain relatively constant arterial pressure is extremely important when a person stands after having been lying down. Immediate upon standing, the pressure in the carotid arteries falls and a reduction of this pressure can cause dizziness or even fainting. Fortunately, the falling pressure at the baroreceptors elicits an immediate reflex, resulting in a more rapid heart rate and vasoconstriction and minimizing the decrease in blood flow to the brain.

Blood pressure is not the only factor that is essential in maintaining tissue viability. The accumulation of waste products and a lack of essential nutrients and gases can also have a profound effect on how much blood flows through a particular tissue and how quickly. In a region of the carotid arteries near the baroreceptors are chemoreceptors. Chemoreceptors detect the concentration of the essential gas, oxygen, and the concentration of the gaseous waste product, carbon dioxide. When carbon dioxide concentrations increase and oxygen concentrations decrease, the chemoreceptors stimulate regions in the brain to increase the heart rate and blood pressure in an attempt to supply the tissues with more oxygen and flush away the excess carbon dioxide. If the chemoreceptors detect high levels of oxygen and low levels of carbon dioxide, an impulse is transmitted to the brain which in turn slows the heart rate and decreases the blood pressure.

Normally, most of the control of blood flow to the brain is accomplished by the baroreceptor and chemoreceptor reflexes. However, the brain has a backup system. If blood flow decreases enough to cause a deficiency of nutrients and oxygen and an accumulation of waste products, special nerve cells respond directly to the lack of adequate energy sources and become strongly excited. When this occurs, the heart is stimulated and blood pressure rises.

Dizziness is a sensation of light-headedness often accompanied by a sensation of spinning (vertigo). Occasionally, a person experiencing dizziness will feel nauseous and may even vomit. Most attacks of dizziness are harmless, resulting from a brief reduction in blood flow to the brain. There are several causes of dizziness, and each alters blood flow to the brain for a slightly different reason.

A person rising rapidly from a sitting or lying position may become dizzy. This is known as postural hypotension, which is caused by a relatively slow reflexive response to the reduced blood pressure in the arteries providing blood to the brain. Rising requires increased blood pressure to supply the brain with adequate amounts of blood. Postural hypotension is more common in the elderly and in individuals prescribed antihypertensive medicines (drugs used to lower high blood pressure).

If the patient experiences vertigo with dizziness, the condition is usually caused by a disorder of the inner ear equilibrium system. Two disorders of the inner ear that can cause dizziness are labyrinthitis and Ménière's disease. Labyrinthitis, inflammation of the fluid-filled canals of the inner ear, is usually caused by a virus. Since these canals are involved in maintaining equilibrium, when they become infected and inflamed one experiences the symptom of dizziness. Ménière's disease is a degenerative disorder of the ear in which the patient experiences not only dizziness but also progressive hearing loss.

Some brain-stem disorders also cause dizziness. The brain stem houses the vestibulocochlear nerve, which transmits messages from the ear to several other parts of the nervous system. Any disorder that alters the functions of this nerve will result in dizziness and vertigo. Meningitis (inflammation of the coverings of the brain and spinal cord), brain tumors, and blood-flow deficiency disorders such as atherosclerosis may affect the function of the vestibulocochlear nerve.

Syncope (fainting) is often preceded by dizziness. Syncope is the temporary loss of consciousness as a result of an inadequate blood flow to the brain. In addition to losing consciousness, the patient may be pale and sweaty. The most common cause of syncope is a vasovasal attack, in which an overstimulation of the vagus nerve slows the heart down. Often vasovagal syncope results from severe pain, stress, or fear. For example, people may faint when hearing bad news or at the sight of blood. More commonly, individuals who have received a painful injury will faint. Rarely, vasovagal syncope may be caused by prolonged coughing, straining to defecate or urinate, pregnancy, or forcing expiration. Standing still for long periods of time or standing up rapidly after lying or sitting can cause fainting. With the exception of vasovagal syncope, all the other causes of syncope are attributable to inadequate blood returning to the heart. If blood pools in the lower extremities, there is a reduced amount available for the heart to pump to the brain. In vasovagal syncope and some disorders of heart rhythm such as Adams-Stokes syndrome, it is the heart itself that does not force enough blood toward the brain.

TREATMENT AND THERAPY

Short periods of dizziness usually subside after a few minutes. Deep breathing and rest will usually help relieve the symptom. Prolonged episodes of dizziness and vertigo should be brought to the attention of a physician.

Recovery from fainting likewise will occur when adequate blood flow to the brain is reestablished. This happens within minutes because falling to the ground places the head at the same level as the heart and helps return the blood from the legs. If a person does not regain consciousness within a few minutes, a physician or emergency medical team should be notified.

The most common cause of syncope is decreased cerebral blood flow resulting from limitation of cardiac output. When the heart rate falls below its normal seventy-five beats per minute to approximately thirty-five beats per minute, the patient usually becomes dizzy and faints. Although slow heart rates can occur in any age group, it is most often found in elderly people who have other heart conditions. Drug-induced syncope can also occur. Drugs for congestive heart failure (digoxin) or antihypertensive medications that slow the heart rate (propranolol, metoprolol) may reduce blood flow to the brain sufficiently to cause dizziness and fainting.

Exertional syncope occurs when individuals perform some physical activity to which they are not accustomed. These physical efforts demand more work from the cardiovascular system, and in patients with some obstruction of the arteries which leave the heart, the cardiovascular system is overstressed. This defect, combined with the vasodilation in the blood vessels that provide blood to the working muscles, reduces the amount of blood available for use by the brain. If the person also hyperventilates during exercise, he or she will effectively reduce the amount of carbon dioxide in the blood and rid the cardiovascular system of this normal stimulus for increasing heart rate and blood flow to the brain. Some persons also hold their breath during periods of high exertion. For example, people attempting to lift something very heavy often take a deep breath just prior to exerting and then hold their breath when they lift the object. This practice, known as the Valsalva maneuver, increases the pressure within the chest cavity, which in turn reduces the amount of blood returning to the heart. A decrease in blood returning to the heart (venous return) causes a decrease in the availability of blood to be pumped out of the heart and reduces cardiac output. The reduction in cardiac output decreases the amount of blood flowing to the brain and initiates a fainting response. It is interesting to note that humans also use the Valsalva maneuver when defecating or urinating, particularly when they strain. These acts can also lead to exertional syncope.

In order for a physician to diagnose and treat dizziness and fainting accurately, he or she must take an accurate medical history, paying particular attention to cardiovascular and neurological problems. In addition to experiencing episodes of dizziness and fainting, patients often have a weak pulse, low blood pressure (hypotension), sweating, and shallow breathing. Heart rate and blood pressure are monitored while the patient assumes different positions. The clinician also listens to the heart and carotid arteries to determine whether there are any problems with these tissues, such as a heart valve problem or atherosclerosis of the carotid arteries. An electrocardiogram (ECG or EKG) can detect abnormal heart rates and rhythms that may reduce cardiac output. Laboratory tests are used to determine whether the patient has low blood sugar (hypoglycemia), too little blood volume (hypovolemia), too few red blood cells (anemia), or abnormal blood gases suggesting a lung disorder. Finally, if the physician suspects a neurological problem such as a seizure disorder, he or she may run an electroencephalogram (EEG) to record brain activity.

Treatment for any of these underlying disorders may cure the dizziness and fainting episodes. In patients with postural hypotension, merely being aware of the condition will allow them to change their behavior to lessen the chances of becoming dizzy and fainting. These patients should not make any sudden changes in posture that could precipitate an attack. Often, this means simply slowing down their movements and learning to assume a horizontal position if they feel dizzy. Patients also can learn to contract their leg muscles and not hold their breath when rising. This increases the amount of blood available for the heart to pump toward the brain. If these techniques do not provide an adequate solution for postural hypotension, then a physician can prescribe drugs such as ephedrine, which increase blood pressure.

Heart rhythm disturbances that cause an abnormally fast or slow heart rate can be corrected with drug therapy such as quinidine or disopyramide (if the rate is too rapid) or a pacemaker (if the rate is too slow). It is interesting to note that even too fast a heart rate can cause dizziness and fainting. In patients with this type of arrhythmia, the heart beats at such a rapid rate that it cannot efficiently fill with blood before the next contraction. Therefore, less blood is pumped with each beat.

Other treatments for dizziness and fainting may include correcting the levels of certain blood elements. Patients with hypoglycemia often feel dizzy. The brain and spinal cord require glucose as their energy source. In fact, the brain and spinal cord have a very limited ability to utilize other substrates such as fat or protein for energy. Because of this, patients often feel light-headed when there are inadequate levels of glucose in the blood. Patients can correct this condition by eating more frequent meals, and if necessary, physicians can administer drugs such as epinephrine or glucagon. These agents liberate glucose from storage sites in the liver.

Individuals with a low blood volume are often dehydrated and upon becoming rehydrated no longer have dizziness or fainting episodes. If dehydration is not corrected and becomes worse, the patient can go into shock, a state of inadequate blood flow to tissues that will result in death if left untreated. In addition to being dizzy or fainting, the patient is often cold to the touch and has a rapid heart rate, low blood pressure, bluish skin, and rapid breathing. These patients are treated by emergency medical personnel, who keep the individual warm, elevate the legs, and infuse fluid into a vein. Drugs may be used to help bring blood pressure back to normal. The cause of the shock should be identified and corrected.

PERSPECTIVE AND PROSPECTS

As humans evolved, they assumed an upright posture. This was advantageous because it allows for the use of the front limbs for other things besides locomotion. Unlike most four-legged animals, however, humans have their brains above their hearts and must continually force blood uphill to reach this vital tissue. This adaptation to the upright posture is a continuing physiological problem because the cardiovascular system must counteract the forces of gravity to provide the brain with blood. If this does not occur, the individual becomes dizzy and faints.

Another significant problem that humans face is adaptation to brain blood flow during exercise. The amount of blood flowing to a tissue is usually proportional to the metabolic demand of the tissue. At rest, various organs throughout the body receive a certain amount of the cardiac output. For example, blood flow to abdominal organs such as the spleen and the kidneys requires about 43 percent of the total blood volume. The total flow to the brain is estimated to be only 13 percent, and the skin and skeletal muscles require 21 percent and 9 percent, respectively. Other areas such as the gastrointestinal tract and heart receive the remaining 14 percent. During exercise, the skeletal muscles may receive up to 80 percent of the cardiac output while the rest of the organs are perfused at a much-reduced rate.

Most data indicate that the brain receives only 3 percent of the total cardiac output during heavy exercise. Even though there is a large change in the redistribution of cardiac output, physiologists do not know the absolute amount of blood reaching the brain or the mechanism for the change in the perfusion rate.

With strenuous aerobic exercise such as jogging, there is an increase in cardiac output. During strenuous anaerobic exercise such as weight lifting, however, there may be a decrease in cardiac output attributable to the Valsalva maneuver. Therefore, it has been difficult to predict accurately, using available techniques, the volume of blood reaching this critical tissue. —*Matthew Berria, Ph.D.*

See also Anxiety; Brain; Brain disorders; Ear infections and disorders; Ears; Exercise physiology; Headaches; Ménière's disease; Meningitis; Migraine headaches; Narcolepsy; Nausea and vomiting; Nervous system; Neuralgia, neuritis, and neuropathy; Neurology; Neurology, pediatric; Palpitations; Unconsciousness.

FOR FURTHER INFORMATION:

Astrand, Per-Olof, and Kaare Rodahl. *Textbook of Work Physiology: Physiological Bases of Exercise*. 3d ed. New York: McGraw-Hill, 1986. This text can be used by individuals who want a basic understanding of how the cardiovascular system responds to physical stresses. It can also be used by readers with an extensive background in physiology. For these professionals, some of the text includes highly detailed explanations of physiological adaptations to exercise.

Babakian, Viken K., and Lawrence R. Wechsler, eds. *Transcranial Doppler Ultrasonography*. St. Louis: Mosby Year Book, 1993. Describes a noninvasive way to measure blood flow to the brain using ultrasound techniques. The authors provide information on how drugs such as anesthetics alter blood flow to the brain. They also discuss the importance of monitoring cerebral blood flow during surgeries.

Clayman, Charles B., ed. *The American Medical Association Encyclopedia of Medicine*. New York: Random House, 1989. This encyclopedia lists in alphabetical order medical terms, diseases, and medical procedures. It does an excellent job of explaining rather complex medical subjects for the nonprofessional audience. In the sections on dizziness and fainting, flow charts detail the appropriate first aid treatments.

Geelen, G., and J. E. Greenleaf. "Orthostasis: Exercise and Exercise Training." *Exercise and Sport Sciences Re-* views 21 (1993): 201-230. Provides an excellent, complete discussion of the relationship between exercise and dizziness and fainting. These authors describe the current theories on blood flow regulation to the brain in athletes.

Guyton, Arthur C. *Human Physiology and Mechanisms of Disease*. 6th ed. Philadelphia: W. B. Saunders, 1997. This textbook introduces human physiology and basic pathology for individuals without an extensive background in medicine. Guyton offers several chapters on blood pressure regulation in humans and gives brief explanations as to what happens when blood pressure is not adequately regulated.

DNA AND RNA

BIOLOGY

ANATOMY OR SYSTEM AFFECTED: Cells

SPECIALTIES AND RELATED FIELDS: Genetics

DEFINITION: Molecules that store coded genetic information and express this information as functional proteins; deoxyribonucleic acid (DNA) is a long, thin, double-stranded fibrous molecule which holds coded information that determines the type, amount, and timing of protein production, while ribonucleic acid (RNA) is a long, single-stranded molecule that amplifies, transports, and expresses this coded information.

KEY TERMS:

genetic disease: a disease state that exists because of a decrease in or the absence of normal protein activity as the result of an alteration in the information carried in the DNA

mutation: an alteration in the information stored in DNA that may lead to an alteration in the structure of proteins produced from this information

replication: the process by which the DNA of a cell is duplicated so that the information stored there can be passed on to new cells after cell division

transcription: the process by which the information stored in DNA is copied into the structure of RNA for transport to the cytoplasm

translation: the process by which the copied information in RNA is utilized in the production of a protein

STRUCTURE AND FUNCTIONS

With the exception of a few sets of identical twins, each human being is a biologically unique individual. That uniqueness has its basis in one's cellular makeup. Appearance derives from the arrangement of cells during fetal development, size depends on the cells' ability to grow and divide, and the function of organs depends on the biochemical function of the individual cells that constitute each organ. The functions of cells depend on the types and amounts of the different proteins that they synthesize. The substance that holds the information that determines the structure of proteins, when they should be produced, and in what amounts is deoxyribonucleic acid (DNA).

DNA is the molecule of heredity, and as a child receives half of its DNA from each parent, each individual is the product of a mixture of information. Therefore, while children resemble their parents, they are unique. Each cell in an individual's body has a complete set of genetic information contained in the chromosomes of the cell's nucleus. Human cells have forty-six chromosomes (twenty-three pairs). Each chromosome is a single piece of DNA associated with many types of proteins. The major function of DNA is to store, in a stable manner, the information that is the "blueprint" for all physiological aspects of an individual. Stability is one of the key attributes of DNA. An information storage molecule is of little use if it can be altered or damaged easily. Another key characteristic of DNA is its ability to be replicated. When a cell divides, the information in the DNA must be replicated so that each of the two new cells can have a complete set.

Stability, the ability to be replicated, and the ability to store vast amounts of coded information have their basis in the structure of DNA. DNA is a long, incredibly thin fiber. The chromosomes in some cells would be as long as a foot or more if they were fully extended. The shape of the DNA molecule can be imagined as a long ladder whose rails are chains of two alternating molecules: deoxyribose (a sugar) and phosphate (an acid containing phosphorus and oxygen). The steps of the ladder are made of pairs of organic bases, of which there are four types: adenine (A), guanine (G), thymine (T), and cytosine (C). Adenine always pairs up with thymine to form a step in the ladder (A-T), and guanine always pairs with cytosine (C-G). This complementarity of base-pairing is the basis for DNA replication and for transferring information from DNA out of the nucleus and into the cytoplasm. Finally, the whole DNA molecule is twisted into a stable right-handed spiral, or helix. Because there is no restriction on the sequence in which the base pairs appear along the molecule, the bases have the potential to be used as a four-letter alphabet that can encode information into "words" of varying lengths, called genes. Each information sequence, or gene, holds the information needed to synthesize a linear chain of amino acids, which are the building blocks of proteins. The information encoded in the base sequences of DNA determines the quantities and composition of all proteins made in the cell.

Under certain conditions, DNA can be separated lengthwise into two halves, or denatured, by breaking the base pairs so that one of each pair remains attached to one sugar-phosphate chain and the other base remains attached to the other sugar-phosphate chain. Because this forms two strands of DNA, whole DNA is usually referred to as being double-stranded. Such separation rarely happens by accident because of the extreme length of DNA. If any area becomes denatured, the rest of the base pairs hold the mole-cule together. In addition, an area of denaturation will automatically try to renature, since complementary bases have a natural attraction for each other. As stable as these traits make it, DNA must be capable of being duplicated so that newly divided cells each have a complete copy of the stored information. DNA is replicated by breaking the base pairs, separating the DNA into two halves, and building a new half onto each of the old halves. This is possible because the complementarity rule (A pairs with T, and C pairs with G) allows each half of a denatured DNA molecule to hold the information needed to construct a new second half. This is accomplished by special sets of proteins that separate the old DNA as they move along the molecule and build new DNA in their wake.

All the information needed to produce proteins is located in the DNA within the nucleus of the cell, but all protein synthesis occurs outside the nucleus in the cytoplasm. An information transfer molecule is required to copy or transcribe information from the genes of the DNA and carry it to the cytoplasm, where large globular protein complexes called ribosomes take the information and translate it into the amino acid structure of specific proteins. This information transfer molecule is ribonucleic acid (RNA). Many RNA copies can be made for any single piece of information on the DNA and used as a template to synthesize many proteins. In this way, the information in DNA is also amplified by RNA. RNA also participates in the synthesis of proteins from the genetic information. RNA resembles one half of a DNA molecule and is usually referred to as being single-stranded. It consists of a single chain of alternating sugars and phosphates with a single organic base attached to each sugar. The sugar in this case is ribose, similar to deoxyribose, and the bases are identical to those in DNA with the exception of thymine, which is replaced by a very similar base called uracil (U).

There are three major types of RNA. Messenger RNA (mRNA), is responsible for the transfer of information from the DNA sequences in the nucleus to the ribosomes in the cytoplasm. Ribosomal RNA (rRNA) interacts with dozens of proteins to form the ribosome. It aids in the interaction between mRNA and the ribosome. Transfer RNA (tRNA) is a group of small RNAs that helps translate the information coded in the mRNA into the structure of specific proteins. They carry the amino acids to the ribosome and match the correct amino acid to its corresponding sequence of bases in the mRNA.

The first step in producing a specific protein is the accurate copying or transcription of information in a gene into information on a piece of mRNA. There are specific sets of proteins that separate the double-stranded DNA in the immediate vicinity of a gene into two single-stranded portions and then, using the DNA as a template, build a piece of mRNA that is a complementary copy of the information in the gene. This is possible because RNA also uses organic bases in its structure. The A, C, G, and T of the single-stranded portion of DNA form base pairs with the U, G, C, and A of the mRNA, respectively. The complementary copy of mRNA, when complete, falls away from the DNA and moves to the cytoplasm of the cell.

In the cytoplasm, the mRNA binds to a ribosome. As the ribosome moves down the length of the mRNA, the tRNAs interact with both the ribosome and the mRNA in order to

The Structure of DNA

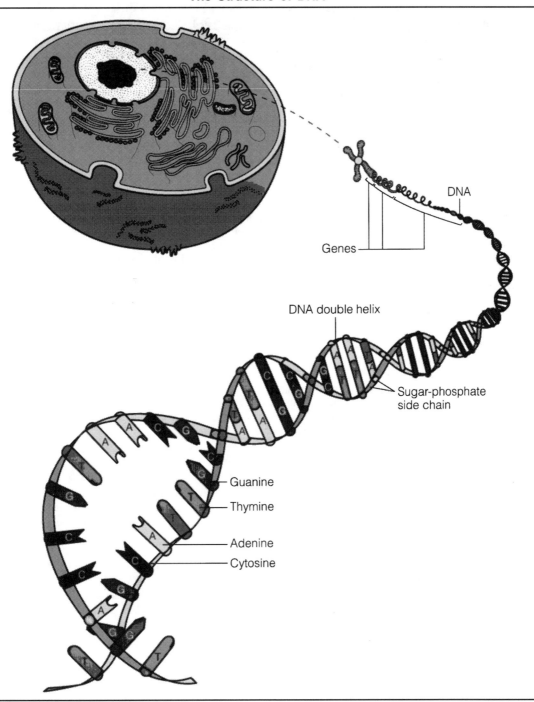

Genes

DNA

DNA double helix

Sugar-phosphate side chain

Guanine

Thymine

Adenine

Cytosine

match the proper amino acid (carried by the tRNAs) to the proper sequence of bases in the mRNA. The order of amino acids in the protein is thus determined by the order of bases in the DNA. Achieving the correct order of amino acids is critical for the correct functioning of the protein. The order of amino acids in the chain determines the way in which it interacts with itself and folds into a three-dimensional structure. The function of all proteins depends on their assuming the correct shape for interaction with other molecules. Therefore, the sequence of bases in the DNA ultimately determines the shape and function of proteins.

DISORDERS AND DISEASES

When the normal structure of DNA is altered (a process called a mutation), the amount of proteins produced and/or the functions of proteins may be affected. At the one extreme, a mutation may cause no problem at all to the person involved. At the other extreme, it may cause devastating damage to the person and result in genetic disease or cancer.

Mutations are changes in the normal sequence of bases in the DNA that carry the information to build a protein or that regulate the amount of protein to be produced. There are different types of mutations, such as the alteration of one base into another, the deletion of one or many bases, or the insertion of bases that were not in the sequence previously. Mutations can have many different causes, such as ultraviolet rays, X rays, mutagenic chemicals, invading viruses, or even heat. Sometimes mutations are caused by mistakes made during the process of DNA replication or cell division. Cells have several systems that constantly repair mutations, but occasionally some of these alterations slip by and become permanent.

Mutations may affect protein structure in several ways. The protein may be too short or too long, with amino acids missing or new ones added. It might have new amino acids substituting for the correct ones. Sometimes as small a change as one amino acid can have noticeable effects. In any of these cases, changes in the amino acid sequence of a protein may drastically affect the way the protein interacts with itself and folds itself into a three-dimensional structure. If a protein does not assume the correct three-dimensional structure, its function may be impaired. It is important to note that how severely a protein's function is affected by a mutation depends on which amino acids are involved. Some amino acids are more important than others in maintaining a protein's shape and function. A change in amino acid sequence may have virtually no effect on a protein or it may destroy that protein's ability to function.

If a mutation occurs that affects the regulation of a particular protein, that gene may be perfectly normal and the protein may be fully functional, but it may exist in the cell in an improper amount—too much, too little, or even none at all. It is important to note that the overproduction of a protein, as well as its underproduction or absence, can be harmful to the cell or to the person in general. The genetic

disease known as Down syndrome is the result of the overproduction of many proteins at the same time.

The term "genetic disease" is used for a heritable disease that can be passed from parent to child. The mutation responsible for the disease is contributed by the parents to the affected child via the sperm or the egg or (as is usually the case) both. The parents are, for the most part, quite unaffected. Because all creatures more complex than bacteria have at least two copies of all their genes, a person may carry a mutated gene and be perfectly healthy because the other normal gene compensates by producing adequate amounts of normal protein. If two individuals carrying the same mutated gene produce a child, that child has a chance of obtaining two mutant genes—one from each parent. Every cell in that child's body carries the error with no normal genes to compensate, and every cell that would normally use that gene must produce an abnormal protein or abnormal amounts of that protein. The medical consequences vary, depending on which gene is affected and which protein is altered. The following are two specific examples of genetic diseases in which the connection between specific mutations and the disease states are well documented.

Sickle-cell anemia is a genetic disease that results from an error in the gene that carries the information for the protein beta globin. Beta globin is one of the building blocks of hemoglobin, the molecule that binds to and carries oxygen in the red blood cells. The error or mutation is a surprisingly small one and serves to illustrate the fact that the replacement of even a single amino acid can change the chemical nature and function of a protein. Normal beta globin has a glutamic acid as the sixth amino acid in the protein chain. The mutation of a single base in the DNA changes the coded information such that the amino acid valine replaces glutamic acid as the sixth position in the protein chain. This single alteration causes the hemoglobin in the red blood cell to crystallize under conditions of low oxygen concentration. As the crystals grow, they twist and deform the normally flexible and disk-shaped red blood cells into rigid sickle shapes. These affected cells lose their capacity to bind and hold oxygen, thereby causing anemia, and their new structure can cause blockages in small capillaries of the circulatory system, causing pain and widespread organ damage. There is no safe and effective treatment or cure for this condition.

Phenylketonuria (PKU) is caused by a mutation in the gene that controls the synthesis of the protein phenylalanine hydroxylase (PAH). There are several mutations of the PAH gene that can lead to a drastic decrease in PAH activity (by greater than 1 percent of normal activity). Some are changes in one base that lead to the replacement of a single amino acid for another. For example, one of the most common mutations in the PAH gene is the alteration of a C to a T that results in amino acid number 408 changing from an

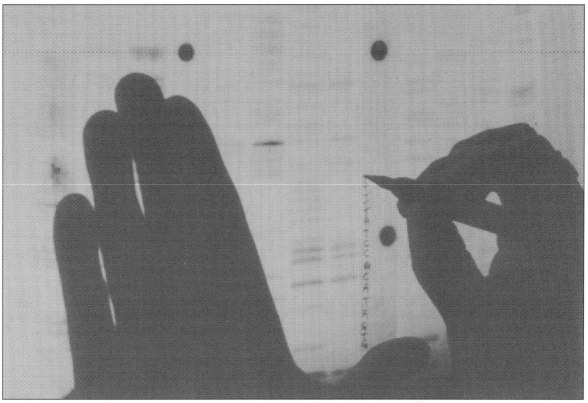

A researcher labels proteins on a radiograph of DNA. (Dan McCoy/Rainbow)

arginine to a tryptophan. Some mutations are deletions of whole sequences of bases in the gene. One such deletion removes the tail end of the gene. In any case, the amino acid structure of PAH is altered significantly enough to remove its ability to function. Without this protein, the amino acid phenylalanine cannot be converted into tyrosine, another useful amino acid. The problem is not a shortage of tyrosine, since there is plenty in most foods, but rather an accumulation of undesirable products that form as the unused phenylalanine begins to break down. Since developing brain cells are particularly sensitive to these products, the condition can cause mental retardation unless treated immediately after birth. While there is no cure, the disease is easily diagnosed and treatment is simple. The patient must stay on a diet in which phenylalanine is restricted. Food products that contain the artificial sweetener aspartame (NutraSweet) must have warnings to PKU patients printed on them since phenylalanine is a major component of aspartame.

PERSPECTIVE AND PROSPECTS

Genetics is a young science whose starting point is traditionally considered to be 1866, the year in which Gregor Mendel published his work on hereditary patterns in pea plants. While he knew nothing of DNA or its structure, Mendel showed mathematically that discrete units of inheritance, which are now called genes, existed as pairs in an organism and that different combinations of these units determined that organism's characteristics. Unfortunately, Mendel's work was ahead of its time and thus ignored until rediscovered by several researchers simultaneously in 1900.

DNA itself was discovered in 1869 by Friedrich Miescher, who extracted it from cell nuclei but did not realize its importance as the carrier of hereditary information. Chromosomes were first seen in the 1870's as threadlike structures in the nucleus, and because of the precise way they are replicated and equally parcelled out to newly divided cells, August Weismann and Theodor Boveri, in the 1880's, postulated that chromosomes were the carriers of inheritance.

In 1900, Hugo de Vries, Karl Correns, and Erich Tschermak von Seysenegg—all plant biologists who were working on patterns of inheritance—independently rediscovered Mendel's work. De Vries had in the meantime discovered mutation around 1890 as a source of hereditary variation, but he did not postulate a mechanism. Mendel's theories and the then-current knowledge of chromosomes merged perfectly. Mendel's units of inheritance were thought somehow to be carried on the chromosomes. Pairs of chromosomes would carry Mendel's pairs of hereditary units which, in 1909, were dubbed "genes."

At this point, genes were still a theoretical concept and has not been proved to be carried on the chromosomes. In 1909, Thomas Hunt Morgan began the work that would provide that proof and allow the mapping of specific genes to specific areas of a chromosome. The nature of a gene, or how it expressed itself, was still a mystery. In 1941, George Beadle and Edward Tatum proved that genes regulated the production of proteins, but the nature of genes was still in debate. There were two candidates for the chemical substance of genes; one was protein and the other was the deceptively simple DNA. In 1944, Oswald Avery proved in experiments with pure DNA that DNA was indeed the molecule of inheritance. In 1953, James D. Watson and Francis Crick elucidated the chemical structure of the double helix, and soon after, Matthew Meselson and Franklin Stahl proved that DNA replicated itself. By the end of the 1950's, RNA was being implicated in protein synthesis, and much of the mechanism of translation was postulated by Marshall Nirenberg and Johann Matthaei in 1961.

The concept of heritable genetic disease is also a relatively recent one. The first direct evidence that a mutation can result in the production of an altered protein came in 1949 with studies on sickle-cell anemia. Since then, thousands of genetic diseases have been characterized. The advent of recombinant DNA technology in the 1970's, which allows the direct manipulation of DNA, has increased the knowledge of these diseases manyfold, as well as demonstrating the genetic influences in maladies such as cancer and behavioral disorders. This technology has led to vastly improved diagnostic methods and therapies while pointing the way toward potential cures. —*Robert D. Meyer, Ph.D.*

See also Cells; Gene therapy; Genetic counseling; Genetic diseases; Genetic engineering; Genetics and inheritance; Mutation.

FOR FURTHER INFORMATION:

Campbell, Neil A. *Biology*. 4th ed. Redwood City, Calif.: Benjamin/Cummings, 1997. This classic introductory textbook provides an excellent discussion of essential biological structures and mechanisms. Its extensive and detailed illustrations help to make even difficult concepts accessible to the nonspecialist. Of particular interest are the chapters comprising the unit entitled "The Gene."

Drlica, Karl. *Understanding DNA and Gene Cloning: A Guide for the Curious*. 3d ed. New York: John Wiley & Sons, 1997. This book for the uninitiated explains the basic principles of genetic mechanisms without requiring knowledge of chemistry. The first third is especially good on the fundamentals, but the remainder may be too deep for some readers.

Edey, Maitland A., and Donald C. Johanson. *Blueprints: Solving the Mystery of Evolution*. Boston: Little, Brown, 1989. Although the thrust of this excellently written book is the history of evolutionary theory, it necessarily covers the history of genetic theory as well. A fascinating look at the steps leading to contemporary knowledge of DNA and genes.

Frank-Kamenetskii, Maxim D. *Unraveling DNA—The Most Important Molecule of Life*. Rev. ed. Reading, Mass.: Addison-Wesley, 1997. This very readable book provides an excellent history of the discovery of DNA. Also describes the nature of DNA and discusses genetic engineering and the ethical questions that surround its use.

Gonick, Larry, and Mark Wheelis. *The Cartoon Guide to Genetics*. Rev. ed. HarperPerennial, 1991. An effective mixture of humor and fact makes this book a nonthreatening reference on genetics for nonscientists. Presented using historical context, it covers DNA and RNA structure and function and much more.

Gribbin, John. *In Search of the Double Helix*. New York: Bantam Books, 1985. Gribbin is a renowned science writer who is capable of explaining complex subjects in a way that anyone can understand. In this book, he goes from Charles Darwin's theories to quantum mechanics in his rendition of the history of the discovery of DNA. Very readable.

Hofstadter, Douglas R. "The Genetic Code: Arbitrary?" In *Metamagical Themas: Questing for the Essence of Mind and Pattern*. New York: Basic Books, 1985. While only a thirty-page chapter in a large book, this piece by Hofstadter is an excellent and thought-provoking explanation of transcription and translation written for the nonscientist.

Nicholl, Desmond. *Introduction to Genetic Engineering*. Cambridge, England: Cambridge University Press, 1994. A valuable textbook for the nonspecialist and anyone interested in genetic engineering. It provides an excellent foundation in molecular biology and builds on that foundation to show how organisms can be genetically engineered. Particularly useful is the glossary of terms.

Watson, James D. *The Double Helix*. New York: Signet Books, 1968. This classic of science literature covers the events leading up to the discovery of the structure of DNA. It is highly readable, and because the structure of DNA is a critical part of the narrative, the reader is left with a clear understanding of that structure.

DOMESTIC VIOLENCE
DISEASE/DISORDER

ANATOMY OR SYSTEM AFFECTED: Psychic-emotional system, all bodily systems

SPECIALTIES AND RELATED FIELDS: Emergency medicine, family practice, geriatrics and gerontology, internal medicine, pediatrics, psychiatry, psychology, public health

DEFINITION: Assaultive behavior intended to punish, dominate, or control another in an intimate family relationship; physicians are often best able to identify situations of domestic violence and assist victims to implement preventive interventions.

KEY TERMS:

cycle of violence: a repeating pattern of violence characterized by increasing tension, culminating in violent action, and followed by remorse

family violence: violence against an intimate partner, typically to assert domination, control actions, or punish, which occurs as a pattern of behavior, not as a single, isolated act; also called battering, marital violence, domestic violence, relationship violence, child abuse, or elder abuse

funneling: an interviewing technique for assessing violence in a patient's relationship, beginning with broad questions of relationship conflict and gradually narrowing to focus on specific violent actions

hands-off violence: indirect attacks meant to terrorize or control a victim; may include property or pet destruction, threats, intimidating behavior, verbal abuse, stalking, and monitoring

hands-on violence: direct attacks upon the victim's body, including physical and sexual violence; comprises a continuum of acts ranging from seemingly minor to obviously severe

lethality: the potential, given the particular dynamics of violence in a relationship, for one or both partners to be killed

safety planning: the development of a specific set of actions and strategies to enable a victim either to avoid violence altogether or, once violence has begun, to escape and minimize damage and injury

CAUSES AND SYMPTOMS

Domestic or family violence is the intentional use of violence against an intimate partner. The purpose of the violence is to assert domination, to control the victim's actions, or to punish the victim for some actions. Family violence generally occurs as a pattern of behavior over time rather than as a single, isolated act.

Forms of family violence include child physical abuse, child sexual abuse, spousal or partner abuse, and elder abuse. These forms of violence are related, in that they occur within the context of the family unit. Therefore, the victims and perpetrators know one another, are related to one another, may live together, and may love one another. These various forms of violence also differ insofar as victims may be children, adults, or frail, elderly adults. The needs of victims differ with age and independence, but there are also many similarities between the different types of violence. One such similarity is the relationship between the offender and the victim. Specifically, victims of abuse are always less powerful than abusers. Power includes the ability to exert physical and psychological control over situations. For example, a child abuser has the ability to lock a child in a bathroom or to abandon him or her in a remote area in order to control access to authorities. A spouse abuser has the ability to physically injure a spouse, discon-

nect the phone, and keep the victim from leaving for help. An elder abuser can exert similar control. Such differences in power between victims and offenders are seen as a primary cause of abuse; that is, people batter others because they can.

Families that are violent are often isolated. The members usually keep to themselves and have few or no friends or relatives with whom they are involved, even if they live in a city. This social isolation prevents victims from seeking help from others and allows the abuser to establish rules for the relationship without answering to anyone for these actions. Abuse continues and worsens because the violence occurs in private, with few consequences for the abuser.

Victims of all forms of family violence share common experiences. In addition to physical violence, victims are also attacked psychologically, being told they are worthless and responsible for the abuse that they receive. Because they are socially isolated, victims do not have an opportunity to take social roles where they can experience success, recognition, or love. As a result, victims often have low self-esteem and truly believe that they cause the violence. Without the experience of being worthwhile, victims often become severely depressed and anxious, and they experience more stress-related illnesses such as headaches, fatigue, or gastrointestinal problems.

Child and partner abuse are linked in several ways. About half of the men who batter their wives also batter their children. Further, women who are battered are more likely to abuse their children than are nonbattered women. Even if a child of a spouse-abusing father is not battered, living in a violent home and observing the father's violence has negative effects. Such children often experience low self-esteem, aggression toward other children, and school problems. Moreover, abused children are more likely to commit violent offenses as adults. Children, especially males, who have observed violence between parents are at increased risk of assaulting their partners as adults. Adult sexual offenders have an increased likelihood of having been sexually abused as children. Yet, while these and other problems are reported more frequently by adults who were abused as children than by adults who were not, many former victims do not become violent. The most common outcomes of childhood abuse in adults are emotional problems. Although much less is known about the relationship between child abuse and future elder abuse, many elder abusers did suffer abuse as children. While most people who have been abused do not themselves become abusers, this intergenerational effect remains a cause for concern.

In its various forms, family violence is a public health epidemic in the United States. Once thought to be rare, family violence occurs with high frequency in the general population. Although exact figures are lacking and domestic violence tends to be underreported, it is estimated that each year 1.9 million children are physically abused; 250,000 children are sexually molested; 1.6 million women are assaulted by their male partners; and between 500,000 and 2.5 million elders are abused. Rates of violence directed toward unmarried heterosexual women, married heterosexual women, and members of homosexual male and female couples tend to be similar. No one is immune: Victims come from all social classes, races, and religions. Partner violence directed toward heterosexual men, however, is rare and usually occurs in relationships in which the male hits first.

Because family violence is so pervasive, physicians encounter many victims. One out of every three to five women visiting emergency rooms is seeking medical care for injuries related to partner violence. In primary care clinics, including family medicine, internal medicine, and obstetrics and gynecology, one out of every four female patients reports violence in the past year, and two out of five report violence at some time in their lives. It is therefore reasonable to expect all physicians and other health care professionals working in primary care and emergency rooms to provide services for victims of family violence.

Family violence typically consists of a pattern of behavior occurring over time and involving both hands-on and hands-off violence. Hands-on violence consists of direct attacks against the victim's body. Such acts range from pushing, shoving, and restraining to slapping, punching, kicking, clubbing, choking, burning, stabbing, or shooting. Hands-on violence also includes sexual assault, ranging from forced fondling of breasts, buttocks, and genitals; to forced touching of the abuser; to forced intercourse with the abuser or with other people.

Hands-off violence includes physical violence that is not directed at the victim's body but is intended to display destructive power and assert domination and control. Examples include breaking through windows or locked doors, punching holes through walls, smashing objects, destroying personal property, and harming or killing pet animals. The victim is often blamed for this destruction and forced to clean up the mess. Hands-off violence also includes psychological control, coercion, and terror. This includes name calling, threats of violence or abandonment, gestures suggesting the possibility of violence, monitoring of the victim's whereabouts, controlling of resources (such as money, transportation, and property), forced viewing of pornography, sexual exposure, or threatening to contest child custody. These psychological tactics may occur simultaneously with physical assaults or may occur separately. Whatever the pattern of psychological and physical tactics, abusers exert extreme control over their partners.

Neglect—the failure of one person to provide for the basic needs of another dependent person—is another form of hands-off abuse. Neglect may involve failure to provide food, clothing, health care, and shelter. Children, older

adults, and developmentally delayed or physically handicapped people are particularly vulnerable to neglect.

Family violence differs in two respects from violence directed at strangers. First, the offender and victim are related and may love each other, live together, share property, have children, and share friends and relatives. Hence, unlike victims of stranger violence, victims of family violence cannot quickly or easily sever ties with or avoid seeing their assailants. Second, family violence often increases slowly in intensity, progressing until victims feel immobilized, unworthy, and responsible for the violence that is directed toward them. Victims may also feel substantial and well-grounded fear about leaving their abusers or seeking legal help, because they have been threatened or assaulted in the past and may encounter significant difficulty obtaining help to escape. In the case of children, the frail and elderly, or people with disabilities, dependency upon the caregiver and cognitive limitations make escape from an abuser difficult. Remaining in the relationship increases the risk of continued victimization. Understanding this unique context of the violent family can help physicians and other health care providers understand why battered victims often have difficulty admitting abuse or leaving the abuser.

Family violence follows a characteristic cycle. This cycle of violence begins with escalating tension and anger in the abuser. Victims describe a feeling of "walking on eggs." Next comes an outburst of violence. Outbursts of violence sometimes coincide with episodes of alcohol and drug abuse. Following the outburst, the abuser may feel remorse and expect forgiveness. The abuser often demands reconciliation, including sexual interaction. After a period of calm, the abuser again becomes increasingly tense and angry. This cycle generally repeats, with violence becoming increasingly severe. In partner abuse, victims are at greatest risk when there is a transition in the relationship such as pregnancy, divorce, or separation. In the case of elder abuse, risk increases as the elder becomes increasingly dependent on the primary caregiver, who may be inexperienced or unwilling to provide needed assistance. Without active intervention, the abuser rarely stops spontaneously and often becomes more violent.

TREATMENT AND THERAPY

Physicians play an important role in stopping family violence by first identifying people who are victims of violence, then taking steps to intervene and help. Physicians use different techniques with each age group because children, adults, and older adults each have special needs and varying abilities to help themselves. This section will first consider the physician's role with children and then will examine the physician's role with adults and older adults.

Because children do not usually tell a physician directly if they are being abused physically or sexually, physicians use several strategies to identify child and adolescent victims. Physicians screen for abuse during regular checkups by asking children if anyone has hurt them, touched them in private places, or scared them. To accomplish this screening with five-year-old patients having a routine checkup, physicians may teach their young patients about private areas of the body; let them know that they can tell a parent, teacher, or doctor if anyone ever touches them in private places; and ask the patients if anyone has ever touched them in a way that they did not like. For fifteen-year-old patients, physicians may screen potential victims by providing information on sexual abuse and date rape, then ask the patients if they have ever experienced either.

A second strategy that physicians use to identify children who are victims of family violence is to remain alert for general signs of distress that may indicate a child or youth lives in a violent situation. General signs of distress in children, which may be caused by family violence or by other stressors, include depression, anxiety, low self-esteem, hyperactivity, disruptive behaviors, aggressiveness toward other children, and lack of friends.

In addition to general signs of distress, there are certain specific signs and symptoms of physical and sexual abuse in children which indicate that the child has probably been exposed to violence. For example, bruises that look like a handprint, belt mark, or rope burn would indicate abuse. X rays can show a history of broken bones that are suspicious. Intentional burns from hot water, fire, or cigarettes often have a characteristic pattern. Sexually transmitted diseases in the genital, anal, or oral cavity of a child who is aged fourteen or under would suggest sexual abuse.

A physician observing specific signs of abuse or violence in a child, or even suspecting physical or sexual abuse, has an ethical and legal obligation to provide this information to state child protective services. Every state has laws that require physicians to report suspected child abuse. Physicians do not need to find proof of abuse before filing a report. In fact, the physician should never attempt to prove abuse or interview the child in detail because this can interfere with interviews conducted by experts in law, psychology, and the medicine of child abuse. When children are in immediate danger, they may be hospitalized so that they may receive a thorough medical and psychological evaluation while also being removed from the dangerous situation. In addition to filing a report, the physician records all observations in the child's medical chart. This record includes anything that the child or parents said, drawings or photographs of the injury, the physician's professional opinion regarding exposure to violence, and a description of the child abuse report.

The physician's final step is to offer support to the child's family. Families of child victims often have multiple problems, including violence between adults, drug and alcohol abuse, economic problems, and social isolation. Appropriate interventions for promoting safety include foster care for children, court-ordered counseling for one or both parents, and in-home education in parenting skills. The physician's goal, however, is to maintain a nonjudgmental manner while encouraging parental involvement.

Physicians also play a key role in helping victims of partner violence. Like children and adolescents, adult victims will usually not disclose violence. Therefore physicians should screen for partner violence and ask about partner violence whenever they notice specific signs of abuse or general signs of distress. Physicians screen for current and past violence during routine patient visits, such as during initial appointments; school, athletic, and work physicals; premarital exams; obstetrical visits; and regular checkups. General signs of distress include depression, anxiety disorders, low self-esteem, suicidal ideation, drug and alcohol abuse, stress illnesses (headache, stomach problems, chronic pain), or patient comments about a partner being jealous, angry, controlling, or irritable. Specific signs of violence include physical injury consistent with assault, including those requiring emergency treatment.

When a victim reports partner violence, there are five steps that a physician can take to help. Communicating belief and support is the first step. Sometimes abuse is extreme and patient reports may seem incredible. The physician validates the victim's experience by expressing belief in the story and exonerating the patient of blame. The physician can begin this process by making eye contact and telling the victim, "You have a right to be safe and respected" and "No one should be treated this way."

The second step is helping the patient assess danger. This is done by asking about types and severity of violent acts, duration and frequency of violence, and injuries received. Specific factors that seem to increase the risk of death in violent relationships include the abuser's use of drugs and alcohol, threats to kill the victim, and the victim's suicidal ideation or attempts. Finally, the physician should ask if the victim feels safe returning home. With this information, the physician can help the patient assess lethal potential and begin to make appropriate safety plans.

The third step is helping the patient identify resources and make a safety plan. The physician begins this process by simply expressing concern for the victim's safety and providing information about local resources such as mandatory arrest laws, legal advocacy services, and shelters. For patients planning to return to an abusive relationship, the physician should encourage a detailed safety plan by helping the patient identify safe havens with family members, friends, or a shelter; assess escape routes from the residence; make specific plans for dangerous situations or when violence recurs; and gather copies of important papers, money, and extra clothing in a safe place in or out of the home in the event of a quick exit. Before the patient leaves, the physician should give the patient a follow-up appointment within two weeks. This provides the victim with a specific, known resource. Follow-up visits should continue until the victim has developed other supportive resources.

The physician's final step is documentation in the patient's medical chart. This written note includes the victim's report of violence, the physician's own observations of injuries and behavior, assessment of danger, safety planning, and follow-up. This record can be helpful in the event of criminal or civil action taken by the victim against the offender. The medical chart, and all communications with the patient, is kept strictly confidential. Confronting the offender about the abuse can place the victim at risk of further, more severe violence. Improper disclosure can also result in loss of the patient's trust, precluding further opportunities for help.

There are several things that a physician should never do when working with a patient-victim. The physician should not encourage a patient to leave a violent relationship as a first or primary choice. Leaving an abuser is the most dangerous time for victims and should be attempted only with adequate planning and resources. The physician should not recommend couples counseling. Couples counseling endangers victims by raising the victim's expectation that issues can be discussed safely. The abuser often batters the victim after disclosure of sensitive information. Finally, the physician should not overlook violence if the violence appears to be "minor." Seemingly minor acts of aggression can be highly injurious.

Physicians also play an important role in helping adults who are older, developmentally delayed, or physically disabled. People in all three groups experience a high rate of family violence. Each group presents unique challenges for the physician. One common element among all three groups is that the victims may be somewhat dependent upon other adults to meet their basic needs. Because of this dependence, abuse may sometimes take the form of failing to provide basic needs such as adequate food or medical care. In many states, adults who are developmentally delayed are covered by mandatory child abuse reporting laws.

The signs and symptoms of the abuse of elders are similar to the other forms of family violence. These include physical injuries consistent with assault, signs of distress, and neglect, including self-neglect. Elder abuse victims are often reluctant to reveal abuse because of fear of retaliation, abandonment, or institutionalization. Therefore, a key to intervention is coordinating with appropriate social service and allied health agencies to support an elder adequately, either at home or in a care center. Such agencies include aging councils, visiting nurses, home health aids, and respite or adult day care centers. Counseling and assistance for caregivers is also an important part of intervention.

Many states require physicians to report suspected elder abuse. Because many elder abuse victims are mentally competent, however, it is important that they be made part of the decision-making and reporting process. Such collaboration puts needed control in the elder's hands and therefore facilitates healing. Many other aspects of intervention described for partner abuse apply to working with elders, including providing emotional support, assessing danger, safety planning, and documentation.

In addition to helping the victims of acute, ongoing family violence, physicians have an important role to play in helping survivors of past family violence. People who have survived family violence may continue to experience negative effects similar to those experienced by acute victims. Physicians can identify survivors of family violence by screening for past violence during routine exams. A careful history can determine whether the patient has been suffering medical or psychological problems related to the violence. Finally, the physician should identify local resources for the patient, including a mutual help group and a therapist.

Physicians can also help prevent family violence. One avenue of prevention is through education of patients by discussing partner violence with patients at key life transitions, such as during adolescence when youths begin dating, prior to marriage, during pregnancy, and during divorce or separation. A second avenue of prevention is making medical clinic waiting rooms and examination rooms into education centers by displaying educational posters and providing pamphlets.

PERSPECTIVE AND PROSPECTS

Despite its frequency, family violence has not always been viewed as a problem. In the 1800's, it was legal in the United States for a man to beat his wife, or for parents to use brutal physical punishment with children. Although the formation of the New York Society for the Prevention of Cruelty to Children in 1874 signaled rising concern about child maltreatment, the extent of the problem was underestimated. As recently as 1960, family violence was viewed as a rare, aberrant phenomenon and women who were victims of violence were often seen as partially responsible because of "masochistic tendencies." Several factors combined to turn the tide during the next thirty years. Medical research published in the early 1960's began documenting the severity of the problem of child abuse. By 1968, every state in the United States had passed a law requiring that physicians report suspected child abuse, and many states established child protective services to investigate and protect vulnerable children.

Progress in the battle against partner violence was slower. The battered women's movement brought new attention and a feminist understanding to the widespread and serious nature of partner violence. This growing awareness provided the impetus, during the 1970's and 1980's, for reform in the criminal justice system, scientific research, continued growth of women's shelters, and the development of treatment programs for offenders.

The medical profession's response to partner abuse followed these changes. In 1986, Surgeon General C. Everett Koop declared family violence to be a public health problem and called upon physicians to learn to identify and intervene with victims. In 1992, the American Medical Association (AMA) echoed the Surgeon General and stated that physicians have an ethical obligation to identify and assist victims of partner violence, and it established standards and protocols for identifying and helping victims of family violence. Because partner and elder abuse have been recognized only recently by the medical community, many physicians are just beginning to learn about their essential role.

Family violence has at various times been considered as a social problem, a legal problem, a political problem, and a medical problem. Because of this shifting understanding and because of the grassroots political origins of the child and partner violence movements, some may question why physicians should be involved. There are three compelling reasons.

First, there is a medical need: Family violence is one of the most common causes of injury, illness, and death for women and children. Victims seeking treatment for acute injuries make up a sizable portion of emergency room visits. Even in outpatient clinics, women report high rates of recent and ongoing violence and injury from partners. In addition to physical injuries, many victims experience stress-related medical problems for which they seek medical care. Among obstetrical patients who are battered, there is a risk of injury to both the woman and her unborn child. Hence, physicians working in clinics and emergency rooms will see many people who are victims.

Second, physicians have a stake in breaking the cycle of violence because they are interested in injury prevention and health promotion. When a physician treats a child or adult victim for physical or psychological injury but does not identify root causes, the victim will return to a dangerous situation. Prevention of future injury requires proper diagnosis of root causes, rather than mere treatment of symptoms.

Third, physicians have a stake in treatment of partner violence because it is a professional and ethical obligation. Two principles of medical ethics apply. First, a physician's actions should benefit the patient. Physicians can benefit patients who are suffering the effects of family violence only if they correctly recognize the root cause and intervene in a sensitive and professional manner. Physicians should also "do no harm." A physician who fails to recognize and treat partner violence will harm the patient by providing inappropriate advice and treatment.

—*L. Kevin Hamberger, Ph.D., and Bruce Ambuel, Ph.D.*

See also Addiction; Alcoholism; Depression; Ethics; Intoxication; Manic-depressive disorder; Paranoia; Psychiatric disorders; Psychiatry; Psychiatry, child and adolescent; Psychiatry, geriatric; Psychoanalysis; Psychosis; Schizophrenia; Stress.

FOR FURTHER INFORMATION:

Barnett, Ola W., Cindy-Lou Miller-Perrin, and Robert D. Perrin. *Family Violence Across the Lifespan: An Introduction.* Thousand Oaks, Calif.: Sage Publications, 1997. Provides information about the different ways that domestic violence, and the warning signs associated with it, may be recognized at various stages in the life spans of individuals and families.

Bass, Ellen, and Laura Davis. *The Courage to Heal: A Guide for Women Survivors of Child Sexual Abuse.* 3d rev. and updated ed. New York: HarperPerennial, 1994. A practical guide to understanding child sexual abuse for female survivors. Informative, but not intended as a substitute for professional therapy.

Island, David, and Patrick Letellier. *Men Who Beat the Men Who Love Them.* New York: Haworth Press, 1991. The first published book that tackles the issue of gay male partner violence. The authors write in a lively, straightforward manner that is easy to understand. Proposes novel ways of thinking about partner violence.

Jones, Ann, and Susan Schechter. *When Love Goes Wrong: What to Do When You Can't Do Anything Right.* New York: HarperCollins, 1992. Contains practical and useful information for women caught in controlling and abusive relationships, such as how to leave an abusive relationship.

Levine, Murray, and Adeline Levine. *Helping Children: A Social History.* New York: Oxford University Press, 1992. The Levines provide an excellent history of child maltreatment in the United States, as well as the various legal, social, and medical strategies that have been used to help abused children.

Pagelow, Mildred. *Family Violence.* New York: Praeger, 1984. One of the most comprehensive texts on family violence available. Though an academic text, it is easy to read and provides a balanced discussion of the major definitions, issues, and controversies in the field of family violence.

Straus, Murray A., Richard J. Gelles, and Suzanne K. Steinmetz. *Behind Closed Doors: Violence in the American Family.* Garden City, N.Y.: Anchor Press/Doubleday, 1980. A report of the first national survey on violence in the American family. Though many statistics are presented, they are explained in layperson's terms.

Wolfe, David A., Christine Wekerle, and Katreena Scott. *Alternatives to Violence: Empowering Youth to Develop Healthy Relationships.* Thousand Oaks, Calif.: Sage Publications, 1997. Offers information about how to recognize problems related to the development of violence in relationships, as well as strategies to help adolescents develop healthy relationship habits.

DOWN SYNDROME

DISEASE/DISORDER

ANATOMY OR SYSTEM AFFECTED: Brain, nervous system, psychic-emotional system

SPECIALTIES AND RELATED FIELDS: Embryology, genetics, obstetrics, pediatrics

DEFINITION: A congenital abnormality characterized by moderate to severe mental retardation and a distinctive physical appearance caused by a chromosomal aberration, the result of either an error during embryonic cell division or the inheritance of defective chromosomal material.

KEY TERMS:

chromosomes: small, threadlike bodies containing the genes that are microscopically visible during cell division

gametes: the egg and sperm cells that unite to form the fertilized egg (zygote) in reproduction

gene: a segment of the DNA strand containing instructions for the production of a protein

homologous chromosomes: chromosome pairs of the same size and centromere position that possess genes for the same traits; one homologous chromosome is inherited from the father and the other from the mother

meiosis: the type of cell division that produces the cells of reproduction, which contain one-half of the chromosome number found in the original cell before division

mitosis: the type of cell division that occurs in nonsex cells, which conserves chromosome number by equal allocation to each of the newly formed cells

translocation: an aberration in chromosome structure resulting from the attachment of chromosomal material to a nonhomologous chromosome

CAUSES AND SYMPTOMS

Down syndrome is an example of a genetic disorder, that is, a disorder arising from an abnormality in an individual's genetic material. Down syndrome results from an incorrect transfer of genetic material in the formation of cells. Genetic information is contained in large "library" molecules of deoxyribonucleic acid (DNA). DNA molecules are formed by joining together units called nucleotides which come in four different varieties: adenosine, thymine, cytosine, and guanine (identified by their initials A, T, C, and G). These nucleotides store hereditary information by forming "words" with this four-letter alphabet. In a gene, a section of DNA which contains the chemical message controlling an inherited trait, three consecutive nucleotides combine to specify a particular amino acid. This word order forms the "sentences" of a recipe telling cells how to construct proteins, such as those coloring the hair and eyes, from amino acids.

In living systems, tissue growth occurs through cell division processes in which an original cell divides to form two cells containing duplicate genetic material. Just before a cell divides, the DNA organizes itself into distinct, com-

pact bundles called chromosomes. Normal human cells, diploid cells, contain twenty-three pairs (or a total of forty-six) of these chromosomes. Each pair is a set of homologues containing genes for the same traits. These chromosomes are composed of two DNA strands, chromatids, joined at a constricted region known as the centromere. The bundle is similar in shape to the letter *X*. The arms are the parts above and below the constriction, which may be centered or offset toward one end (giving arms of equal or different lengths, respectively). During mitosis, the division of nonsex cells, the chromatids separate at the centromere, forming two sets of single-stranded chromosomes, which migrate to opposite ends of the cell. The cell then splits into two genetically equivalent cells, each containing twenty-three single-stranded chromosomes that will duplicate to form the original number of forty-six chromosomes.

In sexual reproduction, haploid egg and sperm cells, each containing twenty-three single-stranded chromosomes, unite in fertilization to produce a zygote cell with forty-six chromosomes. Haploid cells are created through a different, two-step cell division process termed meiosis. Meiosis begins when the homologues in a diploid cell pair up at the equator of the cell. The attractions between the members of each pair then break, allowing the homologues to migrate to opposite ends of the cell, each twin to a different pole, without splitting at the centromere. The parent cell then divides once to give two cells containing twenty-three double-stranded chromosomes, and then divides again through the process of mitosis to form cells that contain only twenty-three single-stranded chromosomes. Thus, each cell contains half of the original chromosomes.

Although cell division is normally a precise process, occasionally an error called nondisjunction occurs when a chromosome either fails to separate or fails to migrate to the proper pole. In meiosis, the failure to move to the proper pole results in the formation of one gamete having twenty-four chromosomes and one having twenty-two chromosomes. Upon fertilization, zygotes of forty-seven or forty-five chromosomes are produced, and the developing embryo must function with either extra or missing genes. Since every chromosome contains a multitude of genes, problems result from the absence or excess of proteins produced. In fact, the embryos formed from most nondisjunctional fertilizations die at an early stage in development and are spontaneously aborted. Occasionally, nondisjunction occurs in mitosis, when a chromosome migrates before the chromatids separate, yielding one cell with an extra copy of the chromosome and no copy in the other cell.

Down syndrome is also termed trisomy 21 because it most commonly results from the presence of an extra copy of the smallest human chromosome, chromosome 21. Actually, it is not the entire extra chromosome 21 that is responsible, but rather a small segment of the long arm of this chromosome. Only two other trisomies occur with any significant frequency: trisomy 13 (Patau's syndrome) and trisomy 18 (Edwards' syndrome). Both of these disorders are accompanied by multiple severe malformations, resulting in death within a few months of birth. Most incidences of Down syndrome are a consequence of a nondisjunction during meiosis. In about 75 percent of these cases, the extra chromosome is present in the egg. About 1 percent of Down syndrome cases occur after the fertilization of normal gametes from a mitosis nondisjunction, producing a mosaic in which some of the embryo's cells are normal and some exhibit trisomy. The degree of mosaicism and its location will determine the physiological consequences of the nondisjunction. Although mosaic individuals range from apparent normality to completely affected, typically the disorder is less severe.

In about 4 percent of all Down syndrome cases, the individual possesses not an entire third copy of chromosome 21 but rather extra chromosome 21 material, which has been incorporated via a translocation into a nonhomologous chromosome. In translocation, pieces of arms are swapped between two nonrelated chromosomes, forming "hybrid" chromosomes. The most common translocation associated with Down syndrome is that between the long arm (Down gene area) of chromosome 21 and an end of chromosome 14. The individual in whom the translocation has occurred shows no evidence of the aberration, since the normal complement of genetic material is still present, only at different chromosomal locations. The difficulty arises when this individual forms gametes. A mother who possesses the 21/14 translocation, for example, has one normal 21, one normal 14, and the hybrid chromosomes. She is a genetic carrier for the disorder, because she can pass it on to her offspring even though she is clinically normal. This mother could produce three types of viable gametes: one containing the normal 14 and 21; one containing both translocations, which would result in clinical normality; and one containing the normal 21 and the translocated 14 having the long arm of 21. If each gamete were fertilized by normal sperm, two apparently normal embryos and one partial trisomy 21 Down syndrome embryo would result. Down syndrome that results from the passing on of translocations is termed familial Down syndrome and is an inherited disorder.

The presence of an extra copy of the long arm of chromosome 21 causes defects in many tissues and organs. One major effect of Down syndrome is mental retardation. The intelligence quotients (IQs) of affected individuals are typically in the range of 40-50. The IQ varies with age, being higher in childhood than in adolescence or adult life. The disorder is often accompanied by physical traits such as short stature, stubby fingers and toes, protruding tongue, and an unusual pattern of hand creases. Perhaps the most recognized physical feature is the distinctive slanting of the eyes, caused by a vertical fold (epicanthal fold) of skin near

the nasal bridge which pulls and tilts the eyes slightly toward the nostrils. For normal Caucasians, the eye runs parallel to the skin fold below the eyebrow; for Asians, this skin fold covers a major portion of the upper eyelid. In contrast, the epicanthal fold in trisomy 21 does not cover a major part of the upper eyelid.

It should be noted that not all defects associated with Down syndrome are found in every affected individual. About 40 percent of Down syndrome patients have congenital heart defects, while about 10 percent have intestinal blockages. Affected individuals are prone to respiratory infections and contract leukemia at a rate twenty times that of the general population. Although Down syndrome children develop the same types of leukemia in the same proportions as other children, the survival rate of the two groups is markedly different. While the survival rate for non-Down syndrome patients after ten years is about 30 percent, survival beyond five years is negligible in Down syndrome patients. It appears that the extra copy of chromosome 21 not only increases the risk of contracting the cancer but also exerts a decisive influence on the disease's outcome. Reproductively, males are sterile while some females are fertile. Although many Down syndrome infants die in the first year of life, the mean life expectancy is about thirty years. This reduced life expectancy results from defects in the immune system, causing a high susceptibility to infectious disease. Most older Down syndrome individuals develop an Alzheimer's-like condition, and less than 3 percent live beyond fifty years of age.

TREATMENT AND THERAPY

Trisomy 21 is one of the most common human chromosomal aberrations, occurring in about 0.5 percent of all conceptions and in one out of every seven hundred to eight hundred live births. About 15 percent of the patients institutionalized for mental deficiency suffer from Down syndrome.

Even before the chromosomal basis for the disorder was determined, the frequency of Down syndrome births was correlated with increased maternal age. For mothers at age twenty, the incidence of Down syndrome is about 0.05 percent, which increases to 0.9 percent by age thirty-five and 3 percent for age forty-five. Studies comparing the chromosomes of the affected offspring with both parents have shown that the nondisjunction event is maternal about 75 percent of the time. This maternal age effect is thought to result from the different manner in which the male and female gametes are produced. Gamete production in the male is a continual, lifelong process, while it is a one-time event in females. Formation of the female's gametes begins early in embryonic life, somewhere between the eighth and twentieth weeks. During this time, cells in the developing ovary divide rapidly by mitosis, forming cells called primary oocytes. These cells then begin meiosis by pairing up the homologues. The process is interrupted at this point,

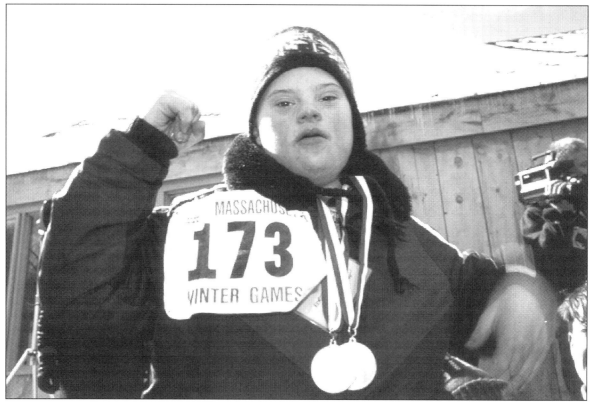

A young person with Down syndrome taking part in the Special Olympics. (William McCoy/Rainbow)

and the cells are held in a state of suspended animation until needed in reproduction, when they are triggered to complete their division and form eggs. It appears that the frequency of nondisjunction events increases with the length of the storage period. Studies have demonstrated that cells in a state of meiosis are particularly sensitive to environmental influences such as viruses, X rays, and cytotoxic chemicals. It is possible that environmental influences may play a role in nondisjunction events. Up to age thirty-two, males contribute an extra chromosome 21 as often as do females. Beyond this age, there is a rapid increase in nondisjunctional eggs, while the number of nondisjunctional sperm remains constant. Where the maternal age effect is minimal, mosaicism may be an important source of the trisomy. An apparently normal mother who possesses undetected mosaicism can produce trisomy offspring if gametes with an extra chromosome are produced. In some instances, characteristics such as abnormal fingerprint patterns have been observed in the mothers and their Down syndrome offspring.

Techniques such as amniocentesis, chorionic villus sampling, and alpha-fetoprotein screening are available for prenatal diagnosis of Down syndrome in fetuses. Amniocentesis, the most widely used technique for prenatal diagnosis, is generally performed between the fourteenth and sixteenth weeks of pregnancy. In this technique, about one ounce of fluid is removed from the amniotic cavity surrounding the fetus by a needle inserted through the mother's abdomen. Although some testing can be done directly on the fluid (such as the assay for spina bifida), more information is obtained from the cells shed from the fetus that accompany the fluid. The mixture obtained in the amniocentesis is spun in a centrifuge to separate the fluid from the fetal cells. Unfortunately, the chromosome analysis for Down syndrome cannot be conducted directly on the amount of cellular material obtained. Although the majority of the cells collected are nonviable, some will grow in culture. These cells are allowed to grow and multiply in culture for two to four weeks, and then the chromosomes undergo karyotyping, which will detect both trisomy 21 and translocational aberration.

In karyotyping, the chromosomes are spread on a microscope slide, stained, and photographed. Each type of chromosome gives a unique, observable banding pattern when stained which allows it to be identified. The chromosomes are then cut out of the photograph and arranged in homologous pairs, in numerical order. Trisomy 21 is easily observed, since three copies of chromosome 21 are present, while the translocation shows up as an abnormal banding pattern. Termination of the pregnancy in the wake of an unfavorable amniocentesis diagnosis is complicated, because the fetus at this point is usually about eighteen to twenty weeks old, and elective abortions are normally performed between the sixth and twelfth weeks of pregnancy. Earlier sampling of the amniotic fluid is not possible because of the small amount of fluid present.

An alternate testing procedure called chorionic villus sampling became available in the mid-1980's. In this procedure, a chromosomal analysis is conducted on a piece of placental tissue that is obtained either vaginally or through the abdomen during the eighth to eleventh week of pregnancy. The advantages of this procedure are that it can be done much earlier in the pregnancy and that enough tissue can be collected to conduct the chromosome analysis immediately, without the cell culture step. Consequently, diagnosis can be completed during the first trimester of the pregnancy, making therapeutic abortion an option for the parents. Chorionic villus sampling does have some negative aspects. One disadvantage is the slightly higher incidence of test-induced miscarriage as compared to amniocentesis—around 1 percent (versus less than 0.5 percent). Also, because tissue of both the mother and the fetus are obtained in the sampling process, they must be carefully separated, complicating the analysis. Occasionally, chromosomal abnormalities are observed in the tested tissue that are not present in the fetus itself.

Prenatal maternal alpha-fetoprotein testing has also been used to diagnose Down syndrome. Abnormal levels of a substance called maternal alpha-fetoprotein are often associated with chromosomal disorders. Several research studies have described a high correlation between low levels of maternal alpha-fetoprotein and the occurrence of trisomy 21 in the fetus. By correlating alpha-fetoprotein levels, the age of the mother, and specific female hormone levels, between 60 percent and 80 percent of fetuses with Down syndrome can be detected. Although techniques allow Down syndrome to be detected readily in a fetus, there is no effective intrauterine therapy available to correct the abnormality.

The care of a Down syndrome child presents many challenges for the family unit. Until the 1970's, most of these children spent their lives in institutions. With the increased support services available, however, it is now common for such children to remain in the family environment. Although many Down syndrome children have happy dispositions, a significant number have behavioral problems that can consume the energies of the parents, to the detriment of the other children. Rearing a Down syndrome child often places a large financial burden on the family: Such children are, for example, susceptible to illness; they also have special educational needs. Since Down syndrome children are often conceived late in the parents' reproductive period, the parents may not be able to continue to care for these children throughout their offspring's adult years. This is prob-

lematic because many Down syndrome individuals do not possess sufficient mental skills to earn a living or to manage their affairs without supervision.

All women in their mid-thirties have an increased risk of producing a Down syndrome infant. Since the resultant trisomy 21 is not of a hereditary nature, the abnormality can be detected only by the prenatal screening, which is recommended for all pregnancies of women older than age thirty-four.

For parents who have produced a Down syndrome child, genetic counseling can be beneficial in determining their risk factor for future pregnancies. The genetic counselor determines the specific chromosomal aberration that occurred utilizing chromosome studies of the parents and affected child, along with additional information provided by the family history. If the cause was nondisjunction and the mother is young, the recurrence risk is much less than 1 percent; for mothers over the age of thirty-four, it is about 5 percent. If the cause was translocational, the Down syndrome is hereditary and risk is much greater—statistically, a one-in-three chance. In addition, there is a one-in-three chance that clinically normal offspring will be carriers of the syndrome, producing it in the next generation. For couples who come from families having a history of spontaneous abortions, which often result from lethal chromosomal aberrations and/or incidence of Down syndrome, it is suggested that they undergo chromosomal screening to detect the presence of a Down syndrome translocation.

PERSPECTIVE AND PROSPECTS

English physician John L. H. Down is credited with the first clinical description of Down syndrome, in 1886. Since the distinctive epicanthic fold gave Down children an appearance that John Down associated with Asians, he termed the condition "mongolism"—an unfortunate term showing a certain racism on Down's part, since it implies that those affected with the condition are throwbacks to a more "primitive" racial group. Today, the inappropriate term has been replaced with the term "Down syndrome."

A French physician, Jérôme Lejeune, suspected that Down syndrome had a genetic basis and began to study the condition in 1953. A comparison of the fingerprints and palm prints of affected individuals with those of unaffected individuals showed a high frequency of abnormalities in the prints of those with Down syndrome. These prints are developed very early in development and serve as a record of events that take place early in embryogenesis. The extent of the changes in print patterns led Lejeune to the conclusion that the condition was not a result of the action of one or two genes but rather of many genes or even an entire chromosome. Upon microscopic examination, he observed that Down syndrome children possess forty-seven chromosomes instead of the forty-six chromosomes found in normal children. In 1959, Lejeune published his findings, showing that Down syndrome is caused by the presence of an extra chromosome which was later identified as an extra copy of chromosome 21. This first observation of a human chromosomal abnormality marked a turning point in the study of human genetics. It demonstrated that genetic defects not only were caused by mutations of single genes but also could be associated with changes in chromosome number. Although the presence of an extra chromosome allows varying degrees of development to occur, most of these abnormalities result in fetal death, with only a few resulting in live birth. Down syndrome is unusual in that the affected individual often survives into adulthood.

—*Arlene R. Courtney, Ph.D.*

See also Amniocentesis; Birth defects; Chorionic villus sampling; DNA and RNA; Genetic diseases; Genetics and inheritance; Leukemia; Mental retardation; Mutation.

FOR FURTHER INFORMATION:

Blatt, Robin J. R. *Prenatal Tests.* New York: Vintage Books, 1988. Discusses tests available for prenatal screening, their benefits, the risk factors of the tests, and how to decide whether to have prenatal testing.

Holtzman, Neil A. *Proceed with Caution: Predicting Genetic Risks in the Recombinant DNA Era.* Baltimore: The Johns Hopkins University Press, 1989. Discusses genetic counseling, how genetic disorders are diagnosed, and social implications.

Nyhan, William L. *The Heredity Factor: Genes, Chromosomes, and You.* New York: Grosset & Dunlap, 1976. Provides a good introduction to the field of medical genetics. Discusses chromosomal disease and how chromosomes are analyzed.

Pueschel, Siegfried. *A Parent's Guide to Down Syndrome.* Baltimore: Paul H. Brookes, 1990. An informative guide highlighting the important developmental stages in the life of a child with Down syndrome.

Rondal, Jean A., et al., eds. *Down's Syndrome: Psychological, Psychobiological, and Socioeducational Perspectives.* San Diego: Singular, 1996. An academic text on issues surrounding Down syndrome. Includes references and an index.

Shaw, Michael, ed. *Everything You Need to Know About Diseases.* Springhouse, Pa.: Springhouse Press, 1996. This well-illustrated consumer reference, compiled by more than one hundred doctors and medical experts, describes five hundred illnesses and conditions, their causes, symptoms, diagnosis, treatment, and prevention. A valuable reference book for everyone interested in health and disease. Of particular interest is chapter 21, "Genetic Disorders."

Tingey, Carol, ed. *Down Syndrome: A Resource Handbook.* Boston: Little, Brown, 1988. A practical resource for rearing a Down syndrome child, including guidelines on daily life, developmental expectations, and health and medical needs.

DRUG ADDICTION. *See* ADDICTION.

DRUG RESISTANCE
DISEASE/DISORDER
ANATOMY OR SYSTEM AFFECTED: All

SPECIALTIES AND RELATED FIELDS: Bacteriology, microbiology, pharmacology, public health, virology

DEFINITION: The ability of a pathogen, formerly susceptible to a particular medication, to change in such a way that it is no longer affected by it.

KEY TERMS:

antibiotic: a substance that kills or prevents the growth of bacteria

bacteria: microscopic single-celled organisms

bacteriophage: a virus that attaches itself to bacteria

chromosomes: rod-shaped cell components that contain deoxyribonucleic acid (DNA)

conjugation: the direct exchange of genetic material between bacteria

pathogen: a living organism that causes disease

plasmids: circular pieces of DNA within bacteria

transduction: the transfer of genetic material between bacteria by a bacteriophage

transposons: pieces of DNA which can be transferred between plasmids and chromosomes

virus: a microscopic organism consisting of DNA or ribonucleic acid (RNA) within a protein coating

CAUSES AND SYMPTOMS

Drug resistance occurs whenever pathogens—microscopic organisms such as bacteria, viruses, and fungi, or larger organisms such as parasites—that have been successfully eradicated with a certain agent develop the ability to resist that agent. The most common and most important form of drug resistance is the ability of bacteria to develop resistance to antibiotics.

An antibiotic attacks a bacterial cell by binding to the cell wall and penetrating it to reach the interior of the cell, where it interferes with a vital biochemical process. Bacteria can develop resistance to an antibiotic in several ways. The bacterial cell may develop the ability to produce a substance that inactivates the antibiotic. The structure of the cell wall may be altered so that the antibiotic can no longer bind to or penetrate it. The cell may increase the activity of the biochemical process being attacked, or it may develop a new process to replace the old one.

Resistance to a particular antibiotic arises in a bacterial cell by random genetic mutation. Because this cell survives antibiotic treatment that destroys other bacteria of the same kind, it is able to reproduce, resulting in numerous offspring that are also resistant. The bacteria that were formerly susceptible to the antibiotic are now resistant.

Even if an antibiotic is completely successful at eradicating a particular type of bacteria, problems with drug resistance can arise. The human body contains billions of bacteria of many different kinds. When one or more of these kinds of bacteria are eliminated by an antibiotic, those kinds that happen to be resistant will multiply in greater numbers. Even if these resistant bacteria are harmless, they often have the ability to transfer antibiotic resistance to harmful bacteria.

Use of multiple antibiotics or antibiotics that attack many kinds of bacteria, known as broad-spectrum antibiotics, can cause other problems. By eliminating a large number of the bacteria normally present, powerful antibiotics encourage the growth of fungi such as *Candida albicans*. Fungal infections are resistant to antibiotics and require special antifungal drugs.

The ability to resist a particular antibiotic is encoded as genetic information on deoxyribonucleic acid (DNA) molecules. DNA is located in chromosomes, which are found in all living cells, or in plasmids, which are found only in bacteria. Plasmids are of particular importance because they allow antibiotic resistance to be transferred from one kind of bacteria to another.

Two bacterial cells may exchange plasmids by direct contact in a process known as conjugation. Not all plasmids can be exchanged in this way, but the genetic information that encodes for resistance may be transferred from a plasmid that cannot be exchanged to one that can. This occurs when a small piece of DNA known as a transposon breaks away from one plasmid and attaches itself to another. A transposon may also break away from a chromosome and attach itself to another chromosome or to a plasmid.

Antibiotic resistance can also be transferred between bacteria by a bacteriophage. A bacteriophage is a virus that attaches itself to a bacterial cell. It then incorporates DNA from the bacterial cell into its own DNA. The virus may then transfer this DNA to the next bacterial cell to which it attaches itself. In this way, it can transfer drug resistance between bacteria that are unable to undergo conjugation.

The various ways in which genetic information is exchanged between bacteria may result in organisms with multiple drug resistance. Some bacteria are known to be resistant to at least ten different antibiotics.

An important factor in the emergence of antibiotic resistance is the misuse of antibiotics. For example, antibiotics have no effect on viruses but are often used on viral illnesses. A study published in 1997 revealed that at least half of all patients in the United States who visited doctors' offices with colds, upper respiratory tract infections, and bronchitis received antibiotics, even though 90 percent of these illnesses are caused by viruses. The same study showed that almost a third of all antibiotic prescriptions written in doctors' offices were used for these kinds of illnesses. Similar problems are also seen in hospitals. A 1997 study of the misuse of the antibiotic vancomycin in U.S. hospitals revealed that 63 percent of vancomycin orders violated guidelines set up by the Centers for Disease Control.

Several public health concerns have arisen as a result of drug resistance. One of the earliest serious problems to arise was an outbreak of dysentery caused by bacteria resistant to four antibiotics in Japan in 1955. From the 1950's to the 1990's, multiple antibiotic resistance emerged in bacteria that caused pneumonia, gonorrhea, meningitis, and other serious illnesses.

A case documented in Nashville, Tennessee, from 1973 to 1974 demonstrates the severity of the problem. A patient with a history of being treated with broad-spectrum antibiotics was exposed to bacteria known as *Serratia* while in the hospital. The *Serratia*, normally susceptible to many antibiotics, picked up the genetic information encoding for multiple antibiotic resistance from otherwise harmless bacteria in the patient's body. The newly resistant *Serratia* spread to other patients in the hospital and to patients in other nearby hospitals. Meanwhile, the *Serratia* transferred resistance to bacteria known as *Klebsiella*. By the end of 1974, more than four hundred patients in four hospitals were infected with multiply resistant *Serratia* or *Klebsiella*. Seventeen of these patients died.

In the 1980's, drug-resistant tuberculosis emerged as a public health concern. In New York City in 1991, for example, 33 percent of all tuberculosis infections were resistant to at least one drug, and 19 percent were resistant to both of the two most effective drugs used to treat the disease. Because of resistance, many tuberculosis patients require treatment with four drugs for several months. Because of public health concerns and the difficulty of taking so many drugs properly for such an extended period of time, some patients are required to be directly observed by a health care worker every time that they take a dose of medication. The use of multiple drugs and the need for increased numbers of health care workers greatly increase the cost of treating tuberculosis.

A new challenge appeared in 1997, when patients in Japan and the United States developed infections caused by bacteria known as *Staphylococcus aureus* that were partially resistant to the drug vancomycin. These patients required multiple antibiotics for extended periods of time. *Staphylococcus aureus* is an organism normally found on human skin that can cause potentially fatal infections when it enters the blood. Many of these bacteria are resistant to multiple antibiotics, leaving vancomycin as the only effective treatment. Medical researchers fear that if *Staphylococcus aureus* with full resistance to vancomycin appears in the near future, it could cause infections that would be nearly impossible to treat.

TREATMENT AND THERAPY

Several different strategies have been suggested for dealing with the problem of antibiotic resistance. In general, these strategies involve educating the public and health care workers, monitoring antibiotic use, and promoting research into methods to deal with resistant bacteria.

The general public should be aware of the proper use of antibiotics. Many patients expect to be given antibiotics for illnesses that do not respond to them, such as viral infections. They may pressure physicians into prescribing antibiotics even when physicians are aware that they are useless. Some patients may use another person's antibiotics or may use old supplies of antibiotics that they have saved from previous illnesses. Even when antibiotics are properly prescribed, patients who begin to feel better may fail to take the entire amount prescribed, leading to an increased risk of drug resistance without completely eliminating the original infection. Public education is even more critical in those nations where many antibiotics can be purchased without a prescription.

All health care workers should be aware of the importance of avoiding the spread of resistant pathogens from one patient to another. In the late 1990's, about two million Americans per year acquired new infections while in hospitals. These infections, known as nosocomial infections, were responsible for about eighty thousand deaths per year. The most important factor in reducing the rate of nosocomial infections is frequent, thorough hand-washing with effective disinfectants.

Physicians need to be aware of the proper ways to use antibiotics. Experts have suggested better education in antibiotic use in medical schools, more continuing education in the subject for practicing physicians, and the development of computer programs to aid physicians in selecting antibiotics. Some have suggested that all physicians prescribing antibiotics in hospitals be required to consult with physicians who specialize in infectious diseases. Standardized order forms that include guidelines for proper use of each antibiotic have also been proposed.

Pharmacists need to be aware of appropriate antibiotic use. They must be able to tell patients how to use antibiotics properly and to use them only under the direction of a physician. Some hospitals have given pharmacists the authority to make changes in antibiotic therapy when appropriate.

Experts agree that monitoring antibiotic use is critical to fighting drug resistance. A study published in 1997 demonstrated the effectiveness of education and monitoring in reducing resistance. Physicians in Finland were educated in the proper use of the antibiotic erythromycin, and use of the drug was monitored. In 1992, 16.5 percent of bacteria known as group A streptococci were resistant to erythromycin. In 1996, only 8.6 percent were resistant. Some experts have proposed using computers to share information about antibiotic use and resistance among as many health care facilities as possible.

Faster development of new antibiotics for use on multiply resistant bacteria has been proposed. Experts stress, however, that these new antibiotics must be used only when necessary in order to avoid promoting resistance to them.

Increased use of vaccines and the development of new vaccines would reduce the need for antibiotics by preventing certain types of bacterial infections. The vaccine that provides protection against pneumonia caused by bacteria known as pneumococci, for example, is recommended for use by all elderly persons in the United States. Despite this suggestion, in 1985 less than 15 percent of older Americans had received the vaccine.

Research into less familiar ways of fighting infections has also been suggested. These methods include developing drugs that strengthen the human immune system. Drugs may also be developed to attack the bacterial genes that encode for drug resistance or to attack the genes that cause certain bacteria to be pathogens. By the late 1990's, these methods remained mostly speculative.

Other methods have been proposed for minimizing antibiotic resistance. Because patients often expect or demand prescriptions when they visit physicians, some experts have suggested that the physician write a "lifestyle" prescription when drug use is not appropriate. Such a prescription would explain why antibiotics should not be used in a particular situation and would give the patient specific instructions on how to treat the illness without them.

Organized action to deal with the problem may be helpful. Physicians and others are encouraged to join the Alliance for Prudent Use of Antibiotics, founded in 1981. This organization educates health care professionals and the general public on proper use of antibiotics and draws attention to cases of improper use worldwide.

Political action has been suggested to encourage governments to deal with antibiotic resistance. Many developing countries have little or no control over antibiotics, many of which are sold without medical supervision for illnesses that do not respond to antibiotics. In the United States, a two-day House of Representatives Subcommittee Hearing on Antibiotic Resistance held in December, 1984, led to no government action. Many experts believe that more should be done.

A more controversial suggestion is eliminating the routine use of antibiotics in farm animals. These animals are often given small amounts of antibiotics to promote growth. Experts disagree about whether evidence exists to link antibiotic use in animals with drug resistance in bacteria that cause human illnesses. In 1970, the United Kingdom banned the use of antibiotics for growth promotion in animals except for substances prescribed by veterinarians and not used in humans. Similar restrictions were later adopted in several European nations and in Canada. A similar ban was proposed in the United States in 1977 but was not approved by Congress. Since then, many American farmers have voluntarily chosen to replace antibiotics with other growth-promoting substances.

PERSPECTIVE AND PROSPECTS

Drug resistance was first noted in the early twentieth century by the German researcher Paul Ehrlich (1854-1915). He discovered that the pathogen which causes syphilis could become resistant to Salvarsan, the substance that he had recently developed to treat the disease. The discovery of antibiotics such as sulfas and penicillins in the first half of the twentieth century led to their extensive use in the 1940's. Almost immediately, antibiotic resistance was seen in several organisms.

Multiply resistant bacteria were first noted in the 1950's. The problem of drug resistance continued to increase in the late twentieth century and was expected to become a major public health concern in the twenty-first century unless steps were taken to educate health care professionals and the public in the proper use of antibiotics. —*Rose Secrest*

See also Antibiotics; Bacterial infections; Bacteriology; Epidemiology; Fungal infections; Hospitals; Iatrogenic disorders; Infection; Microbiology; Mutation; Pharmacology; Pharmacy; Viral infections.

FOR FURTHER INFORMATION:

Fisher, Jeffrey A. *The Plague Makers: How We Are Creating Catastrophic New Epidemics—and What We Must Do to Avert Them.* New York: Simon & Schuster, 1994. A discussion of antibiotic resistance and steps that can be taken to prevent it. Includes controversial chapters on AIDS and on antibiotic use in animals.

Lappe, Marc. *Germs That Won't Die: Medical Consequences of the Misuse of Antibiotics.* New York: Anchor Press, 1982. A clear and concise description of the mechanisms by which antibiotic resistance arises in bacteria.

Levy, Stuart B. *The Antibiotic Paradox: How Miracle Drugs Are Destroying the Miracle.* New York: Plenum Press, 1992. A wide-ranging, in-depth study of the problem of antibiotic resistance by the founder of the Alliance for Prudent Use of Antibiotics. Includes clear diagrams explaining the methods by which resistance transfers between bacteria.

Murray, Barbara E. "Can Antibiotic Resistance Be Controlled?" *New England Journal of Medicine* 330, no. 17 (April 28, 1994): 1229-1230. An editorial that outlines the future consequences of increasing drug resistance and offers several suggestions for fighting it.

Smaglik, Paul. "Proliferation of Pills." *Science News* 151, no. 20 (May 17, 1997): 310-311. An account of the frequent misuse of antibiotics, with opinions from several experts.

DRUG THERAPY. *See* ANTIBIOTICS; NARCOTICS.

DWARFISM
DISEASE/DISORDER
ANATOMY OR SYSTEM AFFECTED: Back, bones, brain, endocrine system, glands, hips, legs, musculoskeletal system, nervous system

SPECIALTIES AND RELATED FIELDS: Endocrinology, genetics, orthopedics, pediatrics

DEFINITION: Underdevelopment of the body, most often caused by a variety of genetic or endocrinological dysfunctions and resulting in either proportionate or disproportionate development, sometimes accompanied by other physical abnormalities and/or mental deficiencies.

KEY TERMS:
amino acid: the building blocks of protein
autosomal: refers to all chromosomes except the X and Y chromosomes (sex chromosomes) that determine body traits
cleft palate: a gap in the roof of the mouth, sometimes present at birth and frequently combined with harelip
collagen: protein material of which the white fibers of the connective tissue of the body are composed
hypoglycemia: low blood sugar
laminae: arches of the vertebral bones
spondylosis: a condition characterized by restriction of movement of the vertebral bones; occurs naturally as a child grows
stenosis: any narrowing of a passage or orifice of the body

CAUSES AND SYMPTOMS
A person of unusually small stature is generally termed a "dwarf." Dwarfism in humans may be caused by a number of conditions that occur either before birth or in early childhood. When short stature is the only observable feature, growth—though abnormal relative to height—is proportionate. Short stature is nearly always blamed on endocrinological dysfunction, but few cases are actually the result of endocrinopathy. If shortness is caused by endocrinopathy, it is often attributable to a deficiency in one or two glands: the pituitary gland (which produces growth hormone) and the thyroid gland. Those who are unusually short but have no other obvious disease are divided into two categories: those who were afflicted prenatally and those who were afflicted postnatally. Many of those born "growth-retarded" are actually the result of chromosomal aberrations and skeletal abnormalities; other events that may cause prenatal growth retardation might include magnesium deficiency (which would prohibit ribosome synthesis and, in turn, halt protein synthesis) or a uterus that is too small. Postnatal growth retardation may be caused by heredity if both parents are short; there is no skeletal abnormality at fault. Other short-statured children may simply mature at a much slower rate, yet grow normally. Typically, one of the parents may have had a late onset of puberty; such children may reach normal height in their late teens.

Unusually short-statured males are those who are shorter than five feet tall; in females, fifty-eight inches and below is short-statured. Children are classified as dwarfs if their height is below the third percentile for their age. When this is the case, doctors will look primarily to four major causes of dwarfism: an underactive or inactive pituitary gland, achondroplasia (failure of normal development in cartilage), emotional or nutritional deprivation, or Turner's syndrome

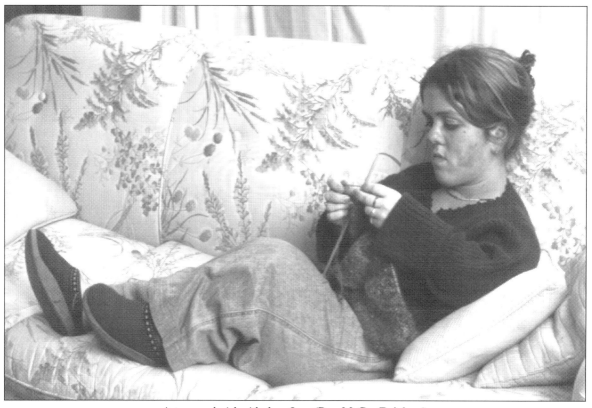

A teenaged girl with dwarfism. (Dan McCoy/Rainbow)

(the possession of a single, X chromosome). If the answer is not found in one of these alternatives, then it may be found in rarer causes, either genetically based or disease-induced.

Growth hormone, also called somatotropin, determines a person's height. Growth hormone does not affect brain growth but may influence the brain's functions. In addition, it may enhance the growth of nerves radiating from the brain so that they can reach their targets. Growth hormone elevates the appetite, increases metabolic rate, maintains the immune system, and works in coordination with other hormones to regulate carbohydrate, protein, lipid, nucleic acid, water, and electrolyte metabolism. Target areas for growth hormone include cell membranes, as well as other cell organelles, in bone, cartilage, bone marrow, adipose tissue, and the liver, kidney, heart, pancreas, mammary glands, ovaries, testes, thymus gland, and hypothalamus. Fetuses not producing growth hormone still grow normally until birth; they may even weigh more than average at birth. These babies may thrive at first, but if no growth hormone is administered, they will be "miniature" adults with a maximum height of two and one-half feet. Other telltale physical attributes include higher-than-average body fat, a high forehead, wrinkled skin, and a high-pitched voice. During childhood, there may be episodic hypoglycemia at-

tacks. If the endocrine system is functioning properly, puberty may be delayed but still will occur. Complete reproductive maturity will be reached, and there is great likelihood that the afflicted person will develop his or her complete intellectual potential. When it is inherited, growth hormone deficiency occurs as an autosomal recessive trait. Yet the genetic basis for growth hormone deficiency may not simply be caused by a gene. The condition could, in theory, be the result of a structural defect in the pituitary gland or the hypothalamus, or in the secretory mechanisms of growth hormone itself.

Prenatal thyroid dysfunction that goes untreated results in cretinism. Cretins do not undergo nervous, skeletal, or reproductive maturation; they may not grow over thirty inches tall. Before two months of age, treatment can cause a complete reversal of symptoms. Delayed treatment, however, cannot reverse brain damage, although growth and reproductive organs can be dramatically affected.

Achondroplasia is inherited as an autosomal dominant form of short-limb dwarfism. Only when one dominant gene is inherited is achondroplasia expressed; when an offspring inherits the dominant gene from both parents, the condition is lethal. Incidence of achondroplasia increases with parental age and is more closely related to the father's age. Mutations may account for a majority of cases of achondroplasia, since in only 15 to 20 percent of cases is there an afflicted parent. Achondroplasia results from abnormal embryonic development that affects bone growth; metaphyseal development is prevented, which means that cartilaginous bone growth is impaired. This impairment is accompanied by unusually small laminae of the spine, resulting in spinal stenosis. The spinal cord may become compressed during the normal process of spondylosis. These individuals may experience slowly progressing spastic weakness of the legs as a result of the spinal cord compression. The torso may be normal, but the head will be disproportionately large and the limbs may be dwarfed and curved. In addition, there will be a prominent forehead and a depressed nasal bridge. A shallow thoracic cage and pelvic tilt may cause a protuberant abdomen. Bowlegs are caused by overly long fibulae. Many infants so affected are stillborn. Those surviving to adulthood are typically three feet to five feet tall and have unusual muscular strength; reproductive and mental development are not affected, and neither is longevity.

Marasmus, severe emaciation resulting form malnutrition prenatally or in early infancy, may be considered a form of dwarfism. It is caused by extremely low caloric and protein intake, which causes a wasting of body tissues. Usually marasmus is found in babies either weaned very early or never breastfed. All growth is retarded, including head circumference. If the area housing the brain fails to grow, then it cannot house a normal-sized brain, and some degree of retardation will occur. Not only is growth stunted, but such infants will be apathetic and hyperirritable as well. As they lie in bed, they are completely unresponsive to their environment and are irritable when moved or handled. Although the symptoms are treatable and may disappear, the growth failure is permanent.

Occasionally, dwarfism may be induced by emotional starvation. This type of child abuse causes extreme growth retardation, inhibition of skeletal growth, and delayed psychomotor development. Fortunately, it can be reversed by social and dietary changes. These children are extremely small but perfectly proportioned; however, they have a distended abdomen.

The height achieved in females with Turner's syndrome is typically between four and one-half and five feet. Turner's syndrome results when an egg has no X chromosome and is fertilized by an X-bearing sperm. The offspring are females with only one X; their ovaries never develop and are unable to function. These individuals cannot undergo puberty; physical manifestations of Turner's syndrome include short stature, stocky build, and a webbed neck.

Another cause of short stature may be as a consequence of chronic disease. Children suffering from chronic renal (kidney) failure nearly always experience growth retardation because of hormonal, metabolic, and nutritional abnormalities, effects seen in 35 to 65 percent of children with renal failure. The failure to grow occurs more often in children with congenital renal disease than in those with acquired renal disease.

With congenital heart disease, several factors may prohibit growth. Growth failure may be a direct result of the disease or an indirect result of other problems associated with heart disease. These babies experience stress, with periods of cardiac failure, and either caloric or protein deficiency. These inadequacies grossly slow the multiplication of cells and hence growth. If surgery corrects the condition, some catching up can be expected, but normal growth is dependent on how much time has elapsed without treatment.

TREATMENT AND THERAPY

In the United States population in 1992, there were roughly five million people of short stature, with 40 percent of this number under the age of twenty-one. The more a child is below the average stature, the greater is the likelihood of determining the cause. A child who is short-statured should be evaluated so that, if an endocrine disorder is the root, the child can be treated. Time is an important consideration with hypothyroidism especially, since the longer it goes untreated, the more likely it is that mental development will be arrested.

Children born with congenital growth-hormone deficiency are sometimes small for their gestational age; however, the majority of growth hormone-deficient children acquire the disorder after birth. The first year or two, the children grow normally; then growth dramatically decreases. Diagnosis of growth-hormone deficiency requires numerous tests and sampling. If bone age appears the same as the child's age, then growth-hormone deficiency can be eliminated. A test for normal growth hormone secretion is done by measuring a blood sample for growth hormone twenty minutes after exercise in a fasting child. If this test shows a hormone deficiency, then growth-hormone therapy may help the child overcome the obstacles of being labeled "short."

At first, growth hormone was harvested from human pituitary glands after a person's death. This process was so expensive, however, that few children with hormone deficiency could be treated. Even worse, some of those who did get this treatment were inadvertently infected with a slow-acting virus that proved fatal. In the mid-1980's, it was found that some men who had received human growth hormone died at an early age of a neurological disorder called Creutzfeldt-Jakob disease (CJD). These men were found to have been given the disease via a growth hormone that had been obtained from pituitary glands during autopsies. Once the relationship was determined, more victims were traced. CJD is a nervous disorder caused by a slow-acting, viruslike particle. Its symptoms include difficulty in balance while walking, loss of muscular control, slurred speech, impairment of vision, and other muscular disorders including spasticity and rigidity. Behavioral changes and mental incapacities may also occur (memory loss, confusion, dementia). The symptoms appear, progress rapidly over the next months, and usually cause death in less than a year. There is no treatment or cure.

These unfortunate circumstances led to the development of a synthetic growth hormone. It is made by encoding bacterial deoxyribonucleic acid (DNA) with the sequence of human growth hormone; the bacteria used are those that grow normally in the human intestinal tract. The bacteria synthesize human growth hormone using the preprogrammed human sequence of DNA; it is then purified so that no bacteria remain in the hormone that is used for treatment. The Food and Drug Administration (FDA) approved the biosynthetic hormone in 1985. The sole difference in the synthetic and the naturally produced growth hormone was one amino acid; in 1987, a new synthetic form without the extra amino acid became available. This synthetic hormone works exactly as natural growth hormone does. Moreover, it does not carry the danger of contamination attributed to human growth hormone. In most cases, the patient's immune system fails to interfere with the synthetic growth hormone's effectiveness. In fact, no major health-threatening side effects have surfaced in using artificial growth hormone. In 1992, there were more than 150,000 growth hormone-deficient children in the United States receiving growth-hormone therapy.

Those children suffering from various forms of chondrodystrophies (cartilage disorders), such as achondroplasia, are diagnosed by using skeletal measurements, clinical manifestations, X rays, laboratory study and analysis of cartilage, and observed abnormalities of the body's proteins, such as collagen and cell membranes. In chondrodystrophies, skeletal growth is disproportionate, with shortened limbs more common than a shortened trunk. If visual examination is not confirmation enough, the diagnosis may be assured through X rays. Although histological studies do not necessarily enhance diagnosis, making an analysis of the patient's cartilage may lead to a better understanding of the disease. Biochemical studies of abnormal proteins in chondrodystrophies actually have little diagnostic value, but they too may lead to better understanding. Because achondroplasia is genetically inherited, prevention of the affliction involves genetic counseling before conception.

A child so affected may be treated symptomatically; surgery on the fibulae to correct bowlegs may be desirable, either for cosmetic reasons or for functional reasons. Laminectomies or skull surgery may be indicated for neurological problems. If hearing loss occurs because of recurrent ear infections, then corrective surgery may be necessary. Achondroplasiacs generally enjoy a normal life span, barring complications to symptoms.

Other chondrodystrophies that cause dwarfism may have more severe symptoms than achondroplasia. Cockayne syndrome, a type of progeria, is the sudden onset of premature old age in extremely young children. It is the result of in-

heritance of an autosomal recessive gene. Physical signs of the disease begin after a normal first year of life. In the second year, growth begins to falter, and psychomotor development becomes abnormal. As time passes, dwarfism, and sometimes mental retardation, becomes evident. Other observable characteristics that develop are a shrunken face with sunken eyes and a thin nose, optic degeneration, cavities of the teeth, a photosensitive skin rash that produces scarring, disproportionately long limbs with large hands and feet, and hair loss. The life span for children with this disease is very short.

Another chondrodystrophy inherited through autosomal recessive genes is thanotophoric dwarfism. All known cases have died during the first four weeks of life as a result of respiratory distress; most are stillborn. Postnatal death occurs as a result of an extremely small thoracic cage with only eleven pairs of ribs present. Other physical characteristics of the disease are that the infant has a large skull relative to its face, which is often elongated with a prominent forehead. The eyes are widely spaced, and there is a broad, flat nasal bridge. Frequently, cleft palate is present. The ears are low-set and poorly formed, and the neck is short and fleshy. The limbs, particularly the legs, are bowed; clubfoot is common, as are dislocated hip joints.

A small percentage of short-statured individuals may be unusually short because of social and psychological factors. This condition is called psychosocial dwarfism. This type of nongrowth is secondary to emotional deprivation and is representative of a type of child abuse. The behavior of such children is characterized by apathy and inadequate interpersonal relationships, with retarded motor and language development. They generally do not gain weight in spite of their extraordinary appetite and excessive thirst; they may steal and hoard food yet have the distended abdomen of a starving child. Diagnosis generally identifies a growth-hormone deficiency, and when these children are moved to stimulating and accepting environments, their behavior becomes more normal. Their caloric intake decreases as their growth hormone secretion becomes normal and their growth undergoes a dramatic catch-up.

Perspective and Prospects

Dwarfism is certainly not a new phenomenon. Two well-known Egyptian deities, Bes and Ptah, are represented as dwarfs. At one time, short-statured individuals were an attraction in the royal courts. Jeffery Hudson, a favorite of Charles I of England, is said to have been only eighteen inches high at the age of thirty; and Bébé, the celebrated dwarf in the court of Stanisław I of Poland, was thirty-three inches tall. More recently, perfectly proportioned dwarfs have made a living by working in circuses and sideshows. It is likely that the best known of these individuals was P. T. Barnum's General Tom Thumb (Charles Stratton), who at twenty-five was thirty-one inches tall.

Today, because of the negative consequences afforded the

short-statured, counseling should begin early if treatment is not feasible. Counseling would begin with a physical examination to determine the nature of the affliction. If it is ascertained that the short stature cannot be treated, both patient and parents should be informed of the nature of the disease. The patient should be assured that intelligence will not be affected, even if the head is somewhat large. Ear infections are common, and the child should be closely watched to avoid hearing loss. Normal fertility is the rule, but giving birth will necessitate a cesarean section. These characteristics of a majority of dwarfism cases should assure families that, as the child matures, he or she will not be limited physically or mentally. The problems that the patients may face usually deal with social and emotional consequences. Short-statured children will usually be thought younger than their age; finding appropriate clothes and shoes may be difficult. Children are often cruel, and as afflicted individuals are highly noticeable, they may be the butt of jokes and teasing and will experience discrimination on many fronts. Seeking affiliation with support groups may aid in coping with the difficulties that a short-statured person will undoubtedly meet.

The rate at which those diagnosed with dwarfism develop psychologically is directly related to two components: if their parents treat them according to their age rather than their size, and if they can cope with the notoriety that their size brings them. It is common for such children to lag in development; personality traits often exhibited with delayed maturation are withdrawal, inhibition, dissociation, and learning problems. There have been no observed tendencies toward aggression or acting out. Inhibition and withdrawal are likely if affected children are appalled by their notoriety; if they use it to measure popularity, they may act the clown to minimize their size difference.   —*Iona C. Baldridge*

See also Congenital heart disease; Endocrine disorders; Endocrinology; Endocrinology, pediatric; Gigantism; Growth; Hormones.

FOR FURTHER INFORMATION:

Bergsma, Daniel, ed. *Birth Defects: Atlas and Compendium*. Baltimore: Williams & Wilkins, 1973. This large volume includes a section of photographs of birth defects, followed by alphabetical descriptions of hundreds of such defects. Such important information as genetic likelihood, complications, treatment, and prognosis is included by Bergsma, an authority on types of dwarfism.

Cheek, Donald B. *Human Growth*. Philadelphia: Lea & Febiger, 1968. Every aspect of growth, including physiology, biochemistry, and psychology, is covered in this volume. More information is accorded growth-retarded children than those undergoing normal growth or overgrowth. Each chapter ends with an extensive bibliography.

Juul, Anders, and Jens O. L. Jorgensen, eds. *Growth Hormone in Adults: Physiological and Clinical Aspects*. New York: Cambridge University Press, 1996. This book

examines the use of somatotropin on adults to treat dwarfism.

Kelly, Thaddeus E. *Clinical Genetics and Genetic Counseling*. 2d ed. Chicago: Year Book Medical Publishers, 1986. This text of genetic disorders and their treatment was written to aid medical students and physicians. Aside from the sometimes difficult medical terminology, the case illustrations and discussions of genetic counseling are interesting.

Martin, Constance R. *Endocrine Physiology*. New York: Oxford University Press, 1985. This textbook covers virtually every aspect of endocrinology, gland by gland. Human physiology is emphasized, and the topics should be comprehensible to students with a basic background in animal physiology. Some knowledge in biochemistry is useful.

Morgan, Brian L. G., and Roberta Morgan. *Hormones*. Los Angeles: Body Press, 1989. A book written for use by the general reader as a resource for hormones and their roles in the human body. Very readable, it also contains sections about hormonal diseases and includes a bibliography.

Shaw, Michael, ed. *Everything You Need to Know About Diseases*. Springhouse, Pa.: Springhouse Press, 1996. This well-illustrated consumer reference, compiled by more than one hundred doctors and medical experts, describes five hundred illnesses and conditions, their causes, symptoms, diagnosis, treatment, and prevention. A valuable reference book for everyone interested in health and disease. Of particular interest is chapter 21, "Genetic Disorders."

DYSENTERY. *See* DIARRHEA AND DYSENTERY.

DYSLEXIA

DISEASE/DISORDER

ANATOMY OR SYSTEM AFFECTED: Brain, ears, eyes, nervous system, psychic-emotional system

SPECIALTIES AND RELATED FIELDS: Audiology, neurology, psychology, speech pathology

DEFINITION: Severe reading disability in children with average to above-average intelligence.

KEY TERMS:

auditory dyslexia: the inability to perceive individual sounds that are associated with written language

cognitive: relating to the mental process by which knowledge is acquired

computed tomography (CT) scan: a detailed X-ray picture that identifies abnormalities of fine tissue structure

dysgraphia: illegible handwriting resulting from impaired hand-eye coordination

electroencephalogram: a graphic record of the brain's electrical activity

imprinting: training that overcomes reading problems by use of repeated, exaggerated language drills

kinesthetic: related to sensation of body position, presence, or movement, resulting mostly from the stimulation of sensory nerves in muscles, tendons, and joints

phonetics: the science of speech sounds; also called phonology

visual dyslexia: the inability to translate observed written or printed language into meaningful terms

CAUSES AND SYMPTOMS

Nearly 25 percent of the individuals in the United States and of many other industrialized societies who otherwise possess at least average intelligence cannot read well. Many such people are viewed as suffering from a neurological disorder called dyslexia. This term was first introduced by the German ophthalmologist Rudolf Berlin in the nineteenth century. Berlin defined it as designating all those individuals who possessed average or above-average intelligence quotients (IQs) but who could not read adequately because of their inability to process language symbols. At the same time as Berlin and later, others reported on dyslexic children. These children saw everything perfectly well but acted as if they were blind to all written language. For example, they could see a bird flying but were unable to identify the written word "bird" seen in a sentence.

The problem involved in dyslexia has been defined and redefined many times, since its introduction. The modern definition of the disorder, which is close to Berlin's definition, is based on long-term, extensive studies of dyslexic children. These studies have identified dyslexia as a complex syndrome composed of a large number of associated behavioral dysfunctions that are related to visual-motor brain immaturity and/or brain dysfunction. These problems include a poor memory for details, easy distractibility, poor motor skills, visual letter and word reversal, and the inability to distinguish between important elements of the spoken language.

Understanding dyslexia in order to correct this reading disability is crucial and difficult. To learn to read well, an individual must acquire many basic cognitive and linguistic skills. First, it is necessary to pay close attention, to concentrate, to follow directions, and to understand the language spoken in daily life. Next, one must develop an auditory and visual memory, strong sequencing ability, solid word decoding skills, the ability to carry out structural-contextual language analysis, the capability to interpret the written language, a solid vocabulary which expands as quickly as is needed, and speed in scanning and interpreting written language. These skills are taught in good developmental reading programs, but some or all are found to be deficient in dyslexic individuals.

Two basic explanations have evolved for dyslexia. Many physicians propose that it is caused by brain damage or brain dysfunction. Evolution of the problem is attributed to accident, disease, and/or hereditary faults in body biochemistry. Here, the diagnosis of dyslexia is made by the use of electroencephalograms (EEGs), computed tomography (CT) scans, and related neurological technology. After such evaluation is complete, medication is often used to diminish hyperactivity and nervousness, and a group of physical training procedures called patterning is used to counter the neurological defects in the dyslexic individual.

In contrast, many special educators and other researchers believe that the problem of dyslexia is one of dormant, immature, or undeveloped learning centers in the brain. Many proponents of this concept strongly encourage the correction of dyslexic problems by the teaching of specific reading skills. While such experts agree that the use of medication can be of great value, they attempt to cure dyslexia mostly through a process called imprinting. This technique essentially trains dyslexic individuals and corrects their problems via the use of exaggerated, repeated language drills.

Another interesting point of view, expressed by some experts, is the idea that dyslexia may be the fault of the written languages of the Western world. For example, Rudolf F. Wagner notes that Japanese children exhibit an incidence of dyslexia that is less than 1 percent. The explanation for this, say Wagner and others, is that unlike Japanese, the languages of Western countries require both reading from left to right and phonetic word attack. These characteristics—absent in Japanese—may make the Western languages either much harder to learn or much less suitable for learning.

A number of experts propose three types of dyslexia. The most common type and the one most often identified as dyslexia is called visual dyslexia, the lack of ability to

b d

p q

on no

Dyslexia may make it difficult to distinguish letters and words that are mirror images of each other, thus making it difficult for an otherwise intelligent child to learn to read.

translate the observed written or printed language into meaningful terms. The major difficulty is that afflicted people see certain words or letters backward or upside down. The resultant problem is that—to the visual dyslexic—any written sentence is a jumble of many letters whose accurate translation may require five or more times as much effort as is needed by an unafflicted person. The other two problems viewed as dyslexia are auditory dyslexia and dysgraphia. Auditory dyslexia is the inability to perceive individual sounds of spoken language. Despite having normal hearing, auditory dyslexics are deaf to the differences between certain vowel and/or consonant sounds, and what they cannot hear they cannot write. Dysgraphia is the inability to write legibly. The basis for this problem is a lack of the hand-eye coordination that is required to write clearly.

Many children who suffer from visual dyslexia also exhibit elements of auditory dyslexia. This complicates the issue of teaching many dyslexic students because only one type of dyslexic symptom can be treated at a time. Also, dyslexia appears to be a sex-linked disorder, being much more common in boys than in girls. Estimates vary between three and seven times as many boys having dyslexia as girls.

TREATMENT AND THERAPY

The early diagnosis and treatment of dyslexia is essential to its eventual correction. Many experts agree that if a treatment begins before the third grade, there is an 80 percent probability that the dyslexia can be corrected. If the disorder remains undetected until the fifth grade, however, success at treating dyslexia is cut in half. If treatment does not begin until the seventh grade, the probability of successful treatment drops below 5 percent.

The preliminary identification of a dyslexic child can be made from symptoms that include poor written schoolwork, easy distractibility, clumsiness, poor coordination, poor spatial orientation, confused writing and/or spelling, and poor left-right orientation. Because numerous nondyslexic children also show many of these symptoms, a second step is required for such identification: the use of written tests designed to identify dyslexics. These tests include the Peabody Individual Achievement Test, the Halstead-Reitan Neuropsychological Test Battery, and the SOYBAR Criterion Tests.

Electroencephalograms and CT scans are often performed in the hope of pinning down concrete brain abnormalities in dyslexic patients. There is considerable disagreement, however, over the value of these techniques, beyond finding evidence of tumors or severe brain damage—both of which may indicate that the condition observed is not dyslexia. Most researchers agree that children who seem to be dyslexic but who lack tumors or damage are no more likely to have EEG or CT scan abnormalities than nondyslexics. An interesting adjunct to EEG use is a technique

called brain electrical activity mapping (BEAM). BEAM converts an EEG into a brain map. Viewed by some workers in the area as a valuable technique, BEAM is contested by many others.

Once conclusive identification of a dyslexic child has been made, it becomes possible to begin corrective treatment. Such treatment is usually the preserve of special education programs. These programs are carried out by the special education teacher in school resource rooms. They also involve special classes limited to children with reading disabilities and schools that specialize in treating learning disabilities.

An often-cited method used is that of Grace Fernald, which utilizes kinesthetic imprinting, based on combined language experience and tactile stimulation. In this popular method or adaptations of it, a dyslexic child learns to read in the following way. First, the child tells a spontaneous story to the teacher, who transcribes it. Next, each word that is unknown to the child is written down by the teacher, and the child traces its letters repeatedly until he or she can write the word without using the model. Each word learned becomes part of the child's word file. A large number of stories are handled this way. Though the method is quite slow, many reports praise its results. Nevertheless, no formal studies of its effectiveness have been made.

A second common teaching technique that is utilized by special educators is the Orton-Gillingham-Stillman method, which was developed in a collaboration between two teachers and a pediatric neurologist, Samuel T. Orton. The method evolved from Orton's conceptualization of language as developing from a sequence of processes in the nervous system that ends in its unilateral control by the left cerebral hemisphere. He proposed that dyslexia arises from conflicts between this cerebral hemisphere and the right cerebral hemisphere, which is usually involved in the handling of nonverbal, pictorial, and spatial stimuli.

Consequently, the corrective method that is used is a multisensory and kinesthetic approach, like that of Fernald. It begins, however, with the teaching of individual letters and phonemes. Then, it progresses to dealing with syllables, words, and sentences. Children taught by this method are drilled systematically, to imprint them with a mastery of phonics and the sounding out of unknown written words. They are encouraged to learn how the elements of written language look, how they sound, how it feels to pronounce them, and how it feels to write them down. Although the Orton-Gillingham-Stillman method is as laborious as that of Fernald, it is widely used and appears to be successful.

Another treatment aspect that merits discussion is the use of therapeutic drugs in the handling of dyslexia. Most physicians and educators propose the use of these drugs as a useful adjunct to the special education training of those dyslexic children who are restless and easily distracted and who have low morale because of continued embarrassment in school in front of their peers. The drugs that are utilized most often are amphetamine, Dexedrine, and methylphenidate (Ritalin).

These stimulants, given at appropriate dose levels, will lengthen the time period during which certain dyslexic children function well in the classroom and can also produce feelings of self-confidence. Side effects of their overuse, however, include loss of appetite, nausea, nervousness, and sleeplessness. Furthermore, there is also the potential problem of drug abuse. When they are administered carefully and under close medical supervision, however, the benefits of these drugs far outweigh any possible risks.

A proponent of an entirely medical treatment of dyslexia is psychiatrist Harold N. Levinson. He proposes that the root of dyslexia is in inner ear dysfunction and that it can be treated with the judicious application of proper medications. Levinson's treatment includes amphetamines, antihistamines, drugs used against motion sickness, vitamins, health food components, and nutrients mixed in the proper combination for each patient. He asserts that he has cured more than ten thousand dyslexics and documents many cases. Critics of Levinson's work pose several questions, including whether the studies reported were well controlled and whether the patients treated were actually dyslexics. A major basis for the latter criticism is Levinson's statement that many of his cured patients were described to him as outstanding students. The contention is that dyslexic students are never outstanding students and cannot work at expected age levels.

An important aspect of dyslexia treatment is parental support of these children. Such emotional support helps dyslexics to cope with their problems and with the judgment of their peers. Useful aspects of this support include a positive attitude toward an afflicted child, appropriate home help that complements efforts at school, encouragement and praise for achievements, lack of recrimination when repeated mistakes are made, and positive interaction with special education teachers.

Perspective and Prospects

The identification of dyslexia by German physician Rudolf Berlin and England's W. A. Morgan began the efforts to solve this unfortunate disorder. In 1917, Scottish eye surgeon James Hinshelwood published a book on dyslexia, which he viewed as being a hereditary problem, and the phenomenon became much better known to many physicians.

Attempts at educating dyslexics were highly individualized until the endeavors of Orton and his coworkers and of Fernald led to more standardized and widely used methods. These procedures, their adaptations, and several others not mentioned here became the standard treatments for dyslexia by the late twentieth century.

Interestingly, many famous people—including Hans Christian Andersen, Winston Churchill, Albert Einstein,

General George Patton, and Woodrow Wilson—had symptoms of dyslexia, which they subsequently overcame. This was fortunate for them, because adults who remain dyslexic are very often at a great disadvantage. In many cases in modern society, such people are among the functionally illiterate and the poor. Job opportunities open to dyslexics of otherwise adequate intelligence are quite limited.

Furthermore, with the development of a more complete understanding of the brain and its many functions, better counseling facilities, and the conceptualization and actualization of both parent-child and parent-counselor interactions, the probability of successful dyslexic training has improved greatly. Moreover, while environmental and socioeconomic factors contribute relatively little to the occurrence of dyslexia, they strongly affect the outcome of its treatment.

The endeavors of special education have so far made the greatest inroads in the treatment of dyslexia. It is hoped that many more advances in the area will be made as the science of the mind grows and diversifies, and the contributions of psychologists, physicians, physiologists, and special educators mesh even more effectively. Perhaps BEAM or the therapeutic methodology suggested by Levinson may provide or contribute to definitive understanding of and treatment of dyslexia.　　　　—Sanford S. Singer, Ph.D.

See also Learning disabilities.

For Further Information:

Huston, Anne Marshall. *Understanding Dyslexia: A Practical Approach for Parents and Teachers.* Rev. ed. Lanham, Md.: Madison Books, 1992. Explains dyslexia, describes its three main types, identifies causes and treatments, and covers useful teaching techniques. A bibliography, a useful glossary, appendices, and teaching materials are valuable additions.

Jordan, Dale R. *Dyslexia in the Classroom.* 2d ed. Columbus, Ohio: Charles E. Merrill, 1977. Seeks to provide information to "grass-roots" professionals who work with group problems seen as comprising dyslexia. Included are definitions of the three types of dyslexia, their classroom characteristics, correction methods, methods for distinguishing dyslexia from other learning disabilities, and useful screening tests.

Klasen, Edith. *The Syndrome of Specific Dyslexia: With Special Consideration of Its Physiological, Psychological, Testpsychological, and Social Correlates.* Baltimore: University Park Press, 1972. A study of five hundred dyslexics that provides much useful information on aspects of dyslexia origin, speech disorders, organic-sensory and neuropsychological symptoms, psychopathology, therapy, psychologic test results, socioeconomic and family background, and parental attitudes.

Levinson, Harold N. *Smart but Feeling Dumb.* New York: Warner Books, 1984. Based on "thousands of cases cured," this book explains the basis and treatment of dyslexia as inner ear dysfunction that can be cured with judicious application of the correct medications. Included are an overview, case studies, a summary, useful appendices, and a bibliography.

Routh, Donald K. "Disorders of Learning." In *The Practical Assessment and Management of Children with Disorders of Development and Learning*, edited by Mark L. Wolraich. Chicago: Year Book Medical Publishers, 1987. This succinct article summarizes salient facts about learning disorders, including etiology, assessment, management, and outcome. Interested readers will also find many useful references.

Snowling, Margaret. *Dyslexia: A Cognitive Developmental Perspective*. New York: Basil Blackwell, 1989. Covers aspects of dyslexia, including its identification, associated cognitive defects, the basis for language skill development, and the importance of phonetics. Also contains many references.

Valett, Robert E. *Dyslexia: A Neuropsychological Approach to Educating Children with Severe Reading Disorders*. Belmont, Calif.: David S. Lake, 1980. This text, containing hundreds of references, is of interest to readers wishing detailed information on dyslexia and on educating dyslexics. Its two main sections are the neuropsychological foundations of reading (including neuropsychological factors, language acquisition, and diagnosis) and a wide variety of special education topics.

Wagner, Rudolf F. *Dyslexia and Your Child: A Guide for Teachers and Parents*. Rev. ed. New York: Harper & Row, 1979. This clear, useful book is "for teachers and parents concerned with children referred to as dyslexic." Includes a careful exposition of dyslexic symptoms, commentary on the problem, ways to treat dyslexia and associated problems, recommended reading, and a glossary.

DYSMENORRHEA
DISEASE/DISORDER
ANATOMY OR SYSTEM AFFECTED: Reproductive system, uterus
SPECIALTIES AND RELATED FIELDS: Gynecology
DEFINITION: Dysmenorrhea is cramplike abdominal pain generally occurring just before or during a menstrual period. Primary dysmenorrhea, which is not related to an identifiable cause, has been linked to excessive levels of prostaglandin, the hormone that triggers uterine contractions; it may be treated with mild painkillers, heat, and prostaglandin inhibitors, and it usually occurs in teenage girls and young women. The source of painful menstruation in women who are over twenty-five or who have given birth is usually secondary dysmenorrhea, which is attributable to an underlying condition such as endometriosis, pelvic inflammatory disease, or tumors; treatment consists of addressing this condition, perhaps with surgery. —*Jason Georges and Tracy Irons-Georges*
See also Endometriosis; Gynecology; Hormones; Menstruation; Pelvic inflammatory disease (PID); Premenstrual syndrome (PMS); Reproductive system.

DYSPHASIA. *See* APHASIA AND DYSPHASIA.

DYSTROPHY
DISEASE/DISORDER
ANATOMY OR SYSTEM AFFECTED: All
SPECIALTIES AND RELATED FIELDS: Neurology, ophthalmology
DEFINITION: Dystrophy is a progressive condition that occurs when required nutrients do not reach tissues or organs, causing an inability of these structures to carry out their proper functions; such defective nutrition can result from poor circulation or nerve damage, and many dystrophies are inherited. Muscular dystrophies, in which the muscles degenerate, are the most common example. Dystrophy can also occur in the eyes, resulting in blindness, and in the nerve fibers of the brain, causing severe neurological problems.

—*Jason Georges and Tracy Irons-Georges*
See also Blindness; Muscle sprains, spasms, and disorders; Muscles; Muscular dystrophy; Nervous system; Neuralgia, neuritis, and neuropathy; Neurology; Neurology, pediatric.

E. COLI INFECTION

DISEASE/DISORDER

ANATOMY OR SYSTEM AFFECTED: Blood, cells, gastrointestinal system, immune system, intestines, nervous system, urinary system

SPECIALTIES AND RELATED FIELDS: Bacteriology, cytology, epidemiology, gastroenterology, internal medicine, microbiology, neonatology, nephrology, public health, urology

DEFINITION: Infection with a rod-shaped, anaerobic, self-propelling bacterium of the family Enterobacteriaceae. It normally inhabits mammal intestines without ill effect, but some strains can cause life-threatening illness.

KEY TERMS:

intestines: The bowel, a two-part tube (the small intestine and the large intestine, or colon) connecting the stomach and anus; it absorbs nutrients from food

mucosa: a mucus-secreting membrane lining the bowel wall

strain: a subgroup in a species

toxin: a substance, usually a protein made by a cell, that causes injury

CAUSES AND SYMPTOMS

Escherichia coli (*E. coli*), the organism most often used for experiments in microbiology, is the best understood type of cell. These bacteria dwell in large numbers in the colons of mammals and constitute a major part of normal feces. More than 250 strains of *E. coli* are known, nearly all harmless to humans, although some may sicken other mammals. Scientists classify those strains that are toxic to humans according to the manner in which they cause disease (pathogenesis). People infected with the bacteria do not always develop symptoms.

Enterotoxigenic *E. coli* (ETEC) strains are the most common source of "travelers' diarrhea" in the United States and Europe. They colonize the small intestine and make it secrete fluid rather than absorb fluid. The result may be watery diarrhea. The afflicted person does not have a fever or inflammation of the bowel wall, which is not damaged by the bacteria.

Enteropathogenic *E. coli* (EPEC) strains attack the lower section of the small intestine, the ileum. Binding tightly to the mucosa cells, they damage the bowel wall. The infected person may feel cramps and have bloody diarrhea (dysentery).

Enterohemorrhagic *E. coli* (EHEC) strains can inflame the colon, damaging the mucosa and causing bleeding and severe cramps, a condition known as hemorrhagic colitis. In some cases, toxins absorbed through the bowel wall enter the bloodstream and travel to the kidneys. There, the glomeruli are attacked and red blood are cells destroyed, a condition called hemolytic-uremic syndrome (HUS). The infected person will have difficulty urinating, and the urine will contain blood products such as hemoglobin. Fever may ensue, and the kidneys may fail, potentially a fatal condition. A related condition, thrombotic thrombocytopenic purpura, in which platelets and red blood cells are destroyed, produces high fever, vomiting, cramps, and damage to one or more organs. Untreated, it is almost always fatal.

Enteroinvasive *E. coli* (EIEC) strains penetrate the mucosa of the colon. The result is intense inflammation and moderate dysentery. A related set of strains afflict infants less than six months of age; the diarrhea may persist for weeks, and the resulting malnutrition and dehydration can be fatal. These strains are rare in the United States.

E. coli strains that enter the bloodstream can cause inflammation when they lodge and multiply in a localized part of the body: meningitis in the spine, prostatitis in the prostate gland, or cystitis in the bladder. After infection, people with depressed immune systems, such as those with acquired immunodeficiency syndrome (AIDS), may develop septicemia—blood poisoning throughout the body that can harm organs and cause sudden fevers, vomiting, skin eruptions, diarrhea, and, if persistent, death.

TREATMENT AND THERAPY

There is no specific treatment for *E. coli* infection. Medical research recommends managing the symptoms and providing supportive therapy while waiting for the body's immune system to clear the disease on its own. Thus, doctors seek to reduce fever, stop diarrhea, and ensure that the patient gets nourishment and enough fluid to prevent dehydration. Bed rest is often necessary in moderate and severe cases.

If the infection leads to a secondary disease, such as HUS, then doctors treat symptoms vigorously. Dialysis can support patients during kidney failure. Infusions of plasma can amend anemia from blood loss. A variety of medications can be taken to reduce the inflammation in such disorders as meningitis and prostatitis.

Most studies do not recommend antibiotics for killing *E. coli* bacteria. Clinical trials have not shown that such treatments help the patient. On the contrary, antibacterial medications appear to increase the patient's chance of developing a secondary condition, particularly HUS. Use of antidiarrheal drugs may also foster HUS.

PERSPECTIVES AND PROSPECTS

German biochemist Theodor Escherich (1857-1911) first isolated *Escherichia coli* in 1884; the species is named after him. The bacteria were best known as the "laboratory rats" of microbiologists until several outbreaks of the O157:H7 EHEC strain attracted public attention in the 1990's. *E. coli* bacteria spread most often from food or beverages contaminated by feces of cattle and humans. Hamburger was the usual culprit, although deer jerky, unpasteurized apple juice, milk, and bean sprouts have also been linked to outbreaks. Many secondary infections arose in people who had contact with those infected from foods. Dozens died, nearly all of them children or the elderly.

Proper food handling is the best defense against *E. coli*:

Making sure that foods and liquids do not touch feces prevents the bacteria from spreading. If they do spread, the bacteria are relatively easy to kill. Pasteurization cleanses liquids; thorough cooking purifies meats and vegetables.

Studies in the mid-1990's found, unexpectedly, that some strains of *E. coli*—O157:H7, for example—mutate at an extremely high rate. Most mutations are harmless, but the chance of a new toxic variety is appreciable. Additionally, some types of *E. coli* have shown increasing resistance to antibiotics; however, epidemiologists deny that an *E. coli* strain such as O157:H7 could be an epidemic-causing "superbug." *E. coli* of all types cause less sickness in the United States than *Campylobacter*, *Salmonella*, and *Shigella* bacteria.   —*Roger Smith, Ph.D.*

See also Antibiotics; Bacterial infections; Bacteriology; Colitis; Diarrhea and dysentery; Drug resistance; Food poisoning; Gastroenterology; Gastroenterology, pediatric; Gastrointestinal disorders; Gastrointestinal system; Infection; Intestinal disorders; Intestines; Meningitis; Microbiology; Mutation; Renal failure.

FOR FURTHER INFORMATION:

Dixon, Bernard. *Power Unseen: How Microbes Rule the World*. Oxford, England: W. H. Freeman, 1994.

Lederberg, Joshua, ed. *Encyclopedia of Microbiology*. San Diego: Academic Press, 1992.

Su, Chinyu, and Lawrence J. Brandt. "*Escherichia coli* O157:H7 Infection in Humans." *Annals of Internal Medicine* 123 (November 1, 1995): 698-714.

Sussman, Max, ed. *The Virulence of* Escherichia coli. London: Academic Press, 1985.

EAR INFECTIONS AND DISORDERS

DISEASE/DISORDER

ANATOMY OR SYSTEM AFFECTED: Ears

SPECIALTIES AND RELATED FIELDS: Audiology, neurology, otorhinolaryngology

DEFINITION: Infections or disorders of the outer, middle, or inner ear, which may result in hearing impairment or loss.

KEY TERMS:

conductive loss: a hearing loss caused by an outer-ear or middle-ear problem which results in reduced transmission of sound

frequency: the number of vibrations per second of a source of sound, measured in hertz; correlates with perceived pitch

intensity of sound: the physical phenomenon that correlates approximately with perceived loudness; measured in decibels

otitis: any inflammation of the outer or middle ear

sensory-neural loss: a hearing loss caused by a problem in the inner ear; this impairment is caused by a hair cell or nerve problem and is usually not amenable to surgical correction

CAUSES AND SYMPTOMS

The hearing mechanism, one of the most intricate and delicate structures of the human body, consists of three sections: the outer ear, the middle ear, and the inner ear. The outer ear converts sound waves into the mechanical motion of the eardrum (tympanic membrane), and the middle ear transmits this mechanical motion to the inner ear, where it is transformed into nerve impulses sent to the brain.

The outer ear consists of the visible portion, the ear canal, and the eardrum. The middle ear is a small chamber containing three tiny bones—the auditory ossicles, termed malleus (hammer), incus (anvil), and stapes (stirrup)—which transmit the vibrations of the eardrum (attached to the hammer) into the inner ear. The chamber is connected to the back of the throat by the Eustachian tube, which allows equalization with the external air pressure. The inner ear, or cochlea, is a fluid-filled cavity containing the complex structure necessary to convert the mechanical vibrations of the cochlear fluid into nerve pulses. The cochlea, shaped something like a snail's shell, is divided lengthwise by a slightly flexible partition into upper and lower chambers. The upper chamber begins at the oval window, to which the stirrup is attached. When the oval window is pushed or pulled by the stirrup, vibrations of the eardrum are transformed into cochlear fluid vibrations.

The lower surface of the cochlear partition, the basilar membrane, is set into vibration by the pressure difference between the fluids of the upper and lower ducts. Lying on the basilar membrane is the organ of Corti, containing tens of thousands of hair cells attached to the nerve transmission lines leading to the brain. When the basilar membrane vibrates, the cilia of these cells are bent, stimulating them to produce electrochemical impulses. These impulses travel along the auditory nerve to the brain, where they are interpreted as sound.

Although well protected against normal environmental exposure, the ear, because of its delicate nature, is subject to various infections and disorders. These disorders, which usually lead to some hearing loss, can occur in any of the three parts of the ear.

The ear canal can be blocked by a buildup of waxy secretions or by infection. Although earwax serves the useful purpose of trapping foreign particles that might otherwise be deposited on the eardrum, if the canal becomes clogged with an excess of wax, less sound will reach the eardrum and hearing will be impaired.

Swimmers' ear, or otitis externa, is an inflammation caused by contaminated water which has not been completely drained from the ear canal. A moist condition in a region with little light favors fungal growth. Symptoms of swimmers' ear include an itchy and tender ear canal and a small amount of foul-smelling drainage. If the canal is allowed to become clogged by the concomitant swelling, hearing will be noticeably impaired.

Otitis Externa

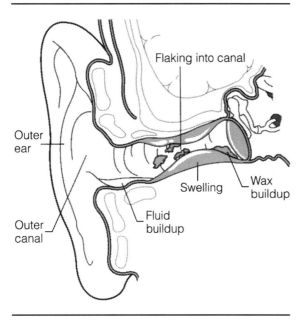

Otitis externa (swimmers' ear) results when the outer ear is inflamed by contaminated water that has not been completely drained from the ear canal.

A perforated eardrum may result from a sharp blow to the side of the head, an infection, the insertion of objects into the ear, or a sudden change in air pressure (such as a nearby explosion). Small perforations are usually self-healing, but larger tears require medical treatment.

Inflammation of the middle ear, acute otitis media, is one of the most common ear infections, especially among children. Infection usually spreads from the throat to the middle ear through the Eustachian tube. Children are particularly susceptible to this problem because their short Eustachian tubes afford bacteria in the throat easy access to the middle ear. When the middle ear becomes infected, pus begins to accumulate, forcing the eardrum outward. This pressure stretches the auditory ossicles to their limit and tenses the ligaments so that vibration conduction is severely impaired. Untreated, this condition may eventually rupture the eardrum or permanently damage the ossicular chain. Furthermore, the pus from the infection may invade nearby structures, including the facial nerve, mastoid bones, the inner ear, or even the brain. The most common symptom of otitis is a sudden severe pain and an impairment of hearing resulting from the reduced mobility of the eardrum and the ossicles.

Secretory otitis media is caused by occlusion of the Eustachian tube as a result of conditions such as a head cold, diseased tonsils and adenoids, sinusitis, improper blowing of the nose, or riding in unpressurized airplanes.

People with allergic nasal blockage are particularly prone to this condition. The blocked Eustachian tube causes the middle-ear cavity to fill with a pale yellow, noninfected discharge which exerts pressure on the eardrum, causing pain and impairment of hearing. Eventually, the middle-ear cavity is completely filled with fluid instead of air, impeding the movement of the ossicles and causing hearing impairment.

A mild, temporary hearing impairment resulting from airplane flights is termed aero-otitis media. This disorder results when a head cold or allergic reaction does not permit the Eustachian tube to equalize the air pressure in the middle ear with atmospheric pressure when a rapid change in altitude occurs. As the pressure outside the eardrum becomes greater than the pressure within, the membrane is forced inward, while the opening of the tube into the upper part of the throat is closed by the increased pressure. Symptoms are a severe sense of pressure in the ear, pain, and hearing impairment. Although the pressure difference may cause the eardrum to rupture, more often the pain continues until the middle ear fills with fluid or the tube opens to equalize pressure.

Chronic otitis media may result from inadequate drainage of pus during the acute form of this disease or from a permanent eardrum perforation that allows dust, water, and bacteria easy access to the middle-ear cavity. The main symptoms of this disease are fluids discharging from the outer ear and hearing loss. Perforations of the eardrum result in hearing loss because of the reduced vibrating surface and a buildup of fibrous tissue which further induces conductive losses. In some cases, an infection may heal but still cause hearing loss by immobilizing the ossicles. There are two distinct types of chronic otitis, one relatively harmless and the other quite dangerous. An odorless, stringy discharge from the mucous membrane lining the middle ear characterizes the harmless type. The dangerous type is characterized by a foul-smelling discharge coming from a bone-invading process beneath the mucous lining. If neglected, this process can lead to serious complications, such as meningitis, paralysis of the facial nerve, or complete sensory-neural deafness.

The ossicles may be disrupted by infection or by a jarring blow to the head. Most often, a separation of the linkage occurs at the weakest point, where the anvil joins the stirrup. A partial separation results in a mild hearing loss, while complete separation causes severe hearing impairment.

Disablement of the mechanical linkage of the middle ear may also occur if the stirrup becomes calcified, a condition termed otosclerosis. The normal bone is resorbed and replaced by very irregular, often richly vascularized bone. The increased stiffness of the stirrup produces conductive hearing loss. In extreme cases, the stirrup becomes completely immobile and must be surgically removed. Although the exact cause of this disease is unknown, it seems to be hereditary. About half of the cases occur in families in which one or more relatives have the same condition, and it occurs more frequently in females than in males. There is also some evidence that the condition may be triggered by a lack of fluoride in drinking water and that increasing the intake of fluoride may retard the calcification process.

Tinnitus is characterized by ringing, hissing, or clicking noises in the ear that seem to come and go spontaneously without any sound stimulus. While technically tinnitus is not a disease of the ear, it is a common symptom of various ear problems. Possible causes of tinnitus are earwax lodged against the eardrum, a perforated or inflamed eardrum, otosclerosis, high aspirin dosage, or excessive use of the telephone. Tinnitus is most serious when caused by an inner-ear problem or by exposure to very intense sounds, and it often accompanies hearing loss at high frequencies.

Ménière's disease is caused by an excess production of cochlear fluid which increases the pressure in the cochlea. This condition may be precipitated by allergy, infection, kidney disease, or any number of other causes, including severe stress. The increased pressure is exerted on the walls of the semicircular canals, as well as on the cochlear partition. The excess pressure in the semicircular canals (the organs of balance) is interpreted by the brain as a rapid spinning motion, and the victim experiences abrupt attacks of vertigo and nausea. The excess pressure in the cochlear

Otitis Media

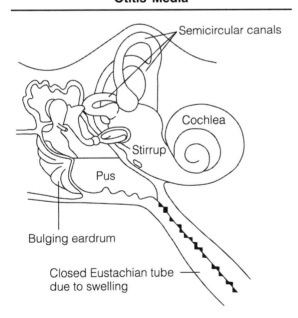

Otitis media occurs when infection spreads from the throat to the middle ear via the Eustachian tube; it is a serious condition which, left untreated, may lead to permanent ear damage and even infection of the brain.

partition has the same effect as a very loud sound and rapidly destroys hair cells. A single attack causes a noticeable hearing loss and could result in total deafness without prompt treatment.

Of all ear diseases, damage to the hair cells in the cochlea causes the most serious impairment. Cilia may be destroyed by high fevers or from a sudden or prolonged exposure to intensely loud sounds. Problems include destroyed or missing hair cells, hair cells which fire spontaneously, and damaged hair cells that require unusually strong stimuli to excite them. At the present time, there is no means of repairing damaged cilia or of replacing those which have been lost.

Viral nerve deafness is a result of a viral infection in one or both ears. The mumps virus is one of the most common causes of severe nerve damage, with the measles and influenza viruses as secondary causes.

Ototoxic (ear-poisoning) drugs can cause temporary or permanent hearing impairment by damaging auditory nerve tissues, although susceptibility is highly individualistic. A temporary decrease of hearing (in addition to tinnitus) accompanies the ingestion of large quantities of aspirin or quinine. Certain antibiotics, such as those of the mycin family, may also create permanent damage to the auditory nerves.

Repeated exposure to loud noise (in excess of 90 decibels) will cause a gradual deterioration of hearing by destroying cilia. The extent of damage, however, depends on the loudness and the duration of the sound. Rock bands often exceed 110 decibels; farm machinery averages 100 decibels.

Presbycusis (hearing loss with age) is the inability to hear high-frequency sounds because of the increasing deterioration of the hair cells. By age thirty, a perceptible high-frequency hearing loss is present. This deterioration progresses into old age, often resulting in severe impairment. The problem is accelerated by frequent unprotected exposure to noisy environments. The extent of damage depends on the frequency, intensity, and duration of exposure, as well as on the individual's predisposition to hearing loss.

TREATMENT AND THERAPY

The simplest ear problems to treat are a buildup of earwax, swimmers' ear, and a perforated eardrum. A large accumulation of wax in the ear canal is best removed by having a medical professional flush the ear with a warm solution under pressure. One should never attempt to remove wax plugs with a sharp instrument. A small accumulation of earwax may be softened by a few drops of baby oil left in the ear overnight, then washed out with warm water and a soft rubber ear syringe. Swimmers' ear can usually be prevented by thoroughly draining the ears after swimming. The disease can be treated by an application of antibiotic eardrops after the ear canal has been thoroughly cleaned. A small perforation of the eardrum will usually heal itself. Larger tears, however, require an operation, tympanoplasty, that grafts a piece of skin over the perforation.

Fortunately, the bacteria that usually cause acute otitis respond quickly to antibiotics. Although antibiotics may relieve the symptoms, complications can arise unless the pus is thoroughly drained. The two-part treatment—draining the fluid from the middle ear and antibiotic therapy—resolves the acute otitis infection within a week. Secretory otitis is cured by finding and removing the cause of the occluded Eustachian tube. The serous fluid is then removed by means of an aspirating needle or by an incision in the eardrum so as to inflate the tube by forcing air through it. In some cases, a tiny polyethylene tube is inserted through the eardrum to aid in reestablishing normal ventilation. If the Eustachian tube remains inadequate, a small plastic grommet may be inserted. The improvement in hearing is often immediate and dramatic. The pain and hearing loss of aero-otitis is usually temporary and disappears of its own accord. If, during or immediately after flight, yawning or swallowing does not allow the Eustachian tube to open and equalize the pressure, medicine or surgical puncture of the eardrum may be required. The harmless form of chronic otitis is treated with applied medications to kill the bacteria and to dry the chronic drainage. The eardrum perforation may then be closed to restore the functioning of the ear and to recover hearing. The more dangerous chronic form of this disease does not respond well to antibacterial agents, but careful X-ray examination allows diagnosis and surgical removal of the bone-eroding cyst.

Ossicular interruption can be surgically treated to restore the conductive link by repositioning the separated bones. This relatively simple operation has a very high success rate. Otosclerosis is treated by operating on the stirrup in one of several ways. The stirrup can be mechanically freed by fracturing the calcified foot plate, or by fracturing the foot plate and one of the arms. Although this operation is usually successful, recalcification often occurs. Alternatively, the stirrup can be completely removed and replaced by a prosthesis of wire or silicon, yielding excellent and permanent results.

Since tinnitus has many possible, and often not readily identifiable, causes, only about 10 percent of the cases are treated successfully. The tinnitus masker has been invented to help sufferers live with this annoyance. The masker, a noise generator similar in appearance to a hearing aid, produces a constant, gentle humming sound which masks the tinnitus.

Ménière's disease, usually treated by drugs and a restricted diet, may also require surgical correction to relieve the excess pressure in severe cases. If this procedure is unsuccessful, the nerves of the inner ear may be cut. In drastic cases, the entire inner ear may be removed.

Presently there is no cure for damaged hair cells; the only treatment is to use a hearing aid. It is more advanta-

geous to take preventive measures, such as reducing noise at the source, replacing noisy equipment with quieter models, or using ear protection devices. Recreational exposure to loud music should be severely curtailed, if not completely eliminated.

PERSPECTIVE AND PROSPECTS

For many centuries, treatment of the ear was associated with that of the eye. In the nineteenth century, the development of the laryngoscope (to examine the larynx) and the otoscope (to examine the ears) enabled doctors to examine and treat disorders such as croup, sore throat, and draining ears, which eventually led to the control of these diseases. As an offshoot of the medical advances made possible by these technological devices, the connection between the ear and throat became known, and otologists became associated with laryngologists.

The study of ear diseases did not develop scientifically until the early nineteenth century, when Jean-Marc-Gaspard Itard and Prosper Ménière made systematic investigations of ear physiology and disease. In 1853, William R. Wilde of Dublin published the first scientific treatise on ear diseases and treatments, setting the field on a firm scientific foundation. Meanwhile, the scientific investigation of the diseased larynx was aided by the laryngoscope, invented in 1855 by Manuel Garcia, a Spanish singing teacher who used his invention as a teaching aid. During the late nineteenth century, this instrument was adopted for detailed studies of larynx pathology by Ludwig Türck and Jan Czermak, who also adapted this instrument to investigate the nasal cavity, which established the link between laryngology and rhinology. Friedrich Voltolini, one of Czermak's assistants, further modified the instrument so that it could be used in conjunction with the otoscope. In 1921, Carl Nylen pioneered the use of a high-powered binocular microscope to perform ear surgery. The operating microscope opened the way for delicate operations on the tiny bones of the middle ear. With the founding of the American Board of Otology in 1924, otology (later otolaryngology) became the second medical specialty to be formally established in North America.

Prior to World War II, the leading cause of deafness was the various forms of ear infection. Advances in technology and medicine have now brought ear infections under control. Today the leading type of hearing loss in industrialized countries is conductive loss, which occurs in those who are genetically predisposed to such loss and who have had lifetime exposure to noise and excessively loud sounds. In the future, ear protection devices and reasonable precautions against extensive exposure to loud sounds should reduce the incidence of hearing loss to even lower levels.

—*George R. Plitnik, Ph.D.*

See also Altitude sickness; Audiology; Ear surgery; Ears; Hearing loss; Ménière's disease; Motion sickness; Nasopharyngeal disorders; Neurology; Neurology, pediatric;

Otorhinolaryngology; Sense organs; Sinusitis; Speech disorders; Tonsillitis.

FOR FURTHER INFORMATION:

Davis, Hallowell, and S. R. Silverman. *Hearing and Deafness.* 4th ed. New York: Holt, Rinehart and Winston, 1978. Although somewhat technical, this text is written for the nonspecialist.

Jerger, James, ed. *Hearing Disorders in Adults: Current Trends.* San Diego: College-Hill Press, 1984. A reliable and readable introductory treatise on common hearing disorders.

Lutman, M. E., and M. P. Haggard, eds. *Hearing Science and Hearing Disorders.* New York: Academic Press, 1983. A monograph on acoustic perception and impairments.

Pender, Daniel J. *Practical Otology.* Philadelphia: J. B. Lippincott, 1992. A well-illustrated text on diseases of the ear and their surgical correction.

Roland, Peter S., Bradley F. Marple, and William L. Meyerhoff, eds. *Hearing Loss.* New York: Thieme, 1997. Provides information on hearing disorders and discusses the anatomy and physiology of the ear.

Strong, W. J., and G. R. Plitnik. *Music, Speech, Audio.* Provo, Utah: Soundprint, 1992. Comprehensive treatment for the layperson covering many aspects of hearing, including chapters on the ear, hearing impairments, noise, and controlling environmental sound.

EAR, NOSE, AND THROAT MEDICINE. *See* OTORHINOLARYNGOLOGY.

EAR SURGERY

PROCEDURE

ANATOMY OR SYSTEM AFFECTED: Bones, ears, musculoskeletal system, nervous system

SPECIALTIES AND RELATED FIELDS: Audiology, general surgery, otorhinolaryngology, speech pathology

DEFINITION: An invasive procedure to correct structural problems of the ear that produce some degree of hearing loss.

KEY TERMS:

cochlea: a structure in the inner ear that receives sound vibrations from the ossicles and transmits them to the auditory nerve

myringotomy: incision of the tympanic membrane used to drain fluid and reduce middle-ear pressure

ossicles: tiny bones located between the eardrum and the cochlea

otosclerosis: a condition in which the stapes becomes progressively more rigid and hearing loss results

stapedectomy: a surgical procedure in which the stapes is replaced with an artificial substitute

stapes: the ossicle that makes contact with the cochlea

tympanic membrane: the eardrum, which separates the external ear canal from the middle ear and ossicles and which transmits sound vibration to the ossicles

tympanoplasty: a surgical procedure to repair the tympanic membrane

INDICATIONS AND PROCEDURES

Humans are able to detect sound because of the interaction between the ears and the brain. When sound waves strike the tympanic membrane (eardrum), it vibrates. The movement of the tympanic membrane then causes the movement of the ossicles, the three tiny bones within the middle ear (malleus, incus, and stapes). These moving bones transfer the vibrations to the cochlea of the inner ear, which stimulates the auditory nerve and eventually the brain.

Hearing problems may result when any part of the ear is damaged. Hearing difficulties can be categorized into two main areas: conductive and sensorineural hearing loss. In conductive hearing loss, the ear loses its ability to transmit sound from the external ear to the cochlea. Common causes include earwax buildup in the outer ear canal; otosclerosis, in which the stapes loses mobility and cannot stimulate the cochlea effectively; and otitis media, in which the middle ear becomes infected and a sticky fluid is produced which causes the ossicles to become inflexible. Otitis media is the most common cause of conductive hearing loss and typically occurs in children. If antibiotics such as amoxicillin or ampicillin fail to cure the ear of infection, surgery may be required. Sensorineural hearing loss results from damage to the cochlea or auditory nerve. Common causes include loud noises, rubella (a type of viral infection) during embryonic development, and certain drugs such as gentamicin and streptomycin. Occasionally, a tumor (neuroma) of the auditory nerve may cause sensorineural hearing loss.

Myringotomy is a surgical procedure in which an incision is made in the tympanic membrane to allow drainage of fluid (effusion) from the middle ear to the external ear canal. The surgeon usually performs this operation to treat recurrent otitis media, a condition in which pressure builds in the middle ear and pushes outward on the tympanic membrane. The patient, usually a child, is given general anesthesia. An incision is made in the eardrum so that a small tube can be inserted to allow continuous drainage of the pus. The tube usually falls out in a few months, and the tympanic membrane heals rapidly.

Otosclerosis, the overgrowth of bone that impedes the movement of the stapes, can be treated by stapedectomy (surgical removal of the stapes). General anesthesia is used to prevent pain or movement when an incision is made in the ear canal and the tympanic membrane is folded to access the ossicles. The stapes can then be removed and a metal or plastic prosthesis inserted in its place. The eardrum is then repaired.

Tympanoplasty is an operation to repair the tympanic membrane or ossicles. Sudden pressure changes in an airplane or during deep-sea diving may perforate the tympanic membrane (barotrauma) and require tympanoplasty. The procedure is similar to stapedectomy. With the patient under general anesthesia, an incision is made next to the eardrum to provide access to the tympanic membrane and ossicles. The tympanic membrane may need to be repaired if the perforated eardrum does not heal on its own. An operating microscope is employed for optimal visualization of the middle ear. If the tympanoplasty involves the ossicles, microsurgical instruments are used to reposition, repair, or replace the damaged bones. They are then reset in their natural positions, and the eardrum is repaired.

Auditory neuromas are benign tumors of the supporting cells surrounding the auditory nerve. Although rare, these tumors can cause deafness. Once neuromas are confirmed by computed tomography (CT) scanning, surgical removal is necessary. With the patient under general anesthesia, the surgeon must make a hole in the skull and attempt to remove the tumor carefully without damaging the auditory nerve or adjacent nerves.

Uses and Complications

More than 90 percent of the patients undergoing stapedectomy experience improved hearing. Approximately 1 percent, however, show deterioration of hearing or total hearing loss postoperatively. For this reason, most surgeons perform stapedectomy on one ear at a time.

Occasionally, the surgical removal of auditory neuromas causes total deafness because of damage to the auditory nerve itself. In rare cases, damage to nearby nerves may cause weakness and/or numbness in that part of the face. Depending on the extent of nerve damage, the symptoms may or may not lessen with time.

Perspective and Prospects

Improvements in technology promise new methods of treating hearing loss. For example, cochlear implants have been developed for the treatment of total sensorineural hearing loss. These implants are surgically inserted into the inner ear. Electrodes in the cochlea receive sound signals transmitted to them from a miniature receiver implanted behind the skin of the ear. Directly over the implant, the patient wears an external transmitter which is connected to a sound processor and microphone. As the microphone picks up sound, the sound is eventually conducted to the electrodes within the cochlea.

—*Matthew Berria, Ph.D., and Douglas Reinhart, M.D.*

See also Audiology; Ear infections and disorders; Ears; Hearing loss; Ménière's disease; Neurology; Neurology, pediatric; Otorhinolaryngology; Plastic, cosmetic, and reconstructive surgery; Sense organs.

For Further Information:

Clayman, Charles B., ed. *The American Medical Association Encyclopedia of Medicine.* New York: Random House, 1989.
Jackler, Robert, and Michael Kaplan. "Ear, Nose, and Throat." In *Current Medical Diagnosis and Treatment,* edited by Lawrence M. Tierney, Jr., et. al. 37th ed. Norwalk, Conn.: Appleton and Lange, 1998.
Schwartz, Seymour I., ed. *Principles of Surgery.* 6th ed. New York: McGraw-Hill, 1994.

Ears

Anatomy

Anatomy or system affected: Bones, musculoskeletal system, nervous system

Specialties and related fields: Audiology, neurology, otorhinolaryngology, speech pathology

Definition: The organs responsible for both hearing and balance.

Key terms:

auditory nerve: the nerve that conducts impulses originating in hair cells of cochlea to the brain for processing as the sensation of sound

cochlea: the fluid-filled coil of the inner ear containing hair cells that change vibrations in the fluid into nerve impulses

eardrum: the membrane separating the outer ear canal from the middle ear that changes sound waves into movements of the ossicles; also called the tympanic membrane

Eustachian tube: the tube connecting the middle ear to the back of the throat; air exchange through this tube equalizes air pressure in the middle ear with the outside air pressure

inner ear: an organ that includes the cochlea (for detection of sound) and the labyrinth (for detection of movement)

labyrinth: a structure consisting of three fluid-filled, semicircular canals at right angles to one another in the inner ear; they monitor the position and movement of the head

middle ear: the air-filled cavity in which vibrations are transmitted from the eardrum to the inner ear via the ossicles

ossicles: three small bones in the middle ear that transmit vibrations from the eardrum to the fluid of the inner ear

otoscope: an instrument for viewing the ear canal and the eardrum

outer ear: the visible, fleshy part of the ear and the ear canal; transmits sound waves to the eardrum

tympanic membrane: another term for the eardrum

Structure and Functions

The ear is composed of three parts: the outer ear, the middle ear, and the inner ear. All three parts are involved in hearing, while only the inner ear is involved in balance.

Sound can be thought of as pressure waves that travel through the air. These waves are collected by the fleshy part of the outer ear and are funneled down the ear canal to the eardrum. The eardrum, being a thin membrane, vibrates as it is hit by the sound waves. Attached to the eardrum is the first of the ossicles (the hammer or malleus), which moves when the eardrum moves. The second ossicle (the anvil or incus) is attached to the first, and the third to second. Therefore, as the first bone moves, the others move also. The base of the third bone (the stirrup or stapes) is in contact with the oval window at the beginning of the inner ear. Movement of the oval window sets up vibrations in the fluid of the cochlea. These vibrations are detected by hair cells. Depending on their position in the cochlea, the hair cells are sensitive to being moved by vibrations of different frequency. When the hair of a hair cell is bent by the fluid, an impulse is generated. The impulses are transmitted to the brain via the auditory nerve. The nerve impulses are processed in the brain, and the result is the sensation of sound, in particular the sense of pitch. Thus the three parts of the ear turn sound waves into "sound" by changing air vibrations into eardrum vibrations, then ossicle movement, then fluid vibrations, and finally nerve impulses.

DISORDERS AND DISEASES

Each of the three parts of the ear can be affected by diseases that can lead to temporary or, in some cases, permanent hearing loss. Damage to the eardrum, ossicles, or any part of the ear before the cochlea results in conductive hearing loss, as these structures conduct the sound or vibrations. Damage to the hair cells or to the auditory nerve results in sensorineural hearing loss. Sound may be conducted normally but cannot be detected by the hair cells or transmitted as nerve impulses to the brain.

Disorders of the outer ear include cauliflower ear, blockage by earwax, otitis externa, and tumors. Cauliflower ear is a severe hematoma (bruise) to the outer ear. In some cases, the blood trapped beneath the skin does not resorb and instead turns into fibrous tissue that may become cartilaginous or even bonelike.

Earwax is secreted by the cells in the lining of the ear canal. Its function is to protect the eardrum from dust and dirt, and it normally works its way to the outer opening of the ear. The amount secreted varies from person to person. In some people, or in people who are continually exposed to dusty environments, excessive amounts of wax may be secreted and may block the ear canal sufficiently to interfere with its transmission of sound waves to the eardrum.

Otitis externa can take two forms, either localized or generalized. The localized form, a boil or abscess, is a bacterial infection that results from breaks in the lining of the ear canal and is often caused by attempts to scratch an itch in the ear or to remove wax. The generalized form can be a bacterial or fungal infection, known as otomycosis. Generalized otitis externa is also called swimmers' ear because it often results from swimming in polluted wa-

The Anatomy of the Human Ear

ters or from chronic moisture in the ear canal.

Tumors of the ear can be benign (noncancerous) or malignant (cancerous) growths of either the soft tissues or the underlying bone. Bony growths, or osteomas, can cause sufficient blockage, by themselves or by leading to the buildup of earwax, that hearing loss can result.

The middle ear consists of the eardrum, three small bones called the ossicles, and the Eustachian tube. The bones of the middle ear move in an air-filled cavity. Air pressure within this cavity is normally the same as the outside air pressure because air is exchanged between the middle ear and the outside world via the Eustachian tube. When this tube swells and closes, as it often does with a head cold, one experiences a stuffy feeling, decreased hearing, mild pain, and sometimes ringing in the ears (tinnitus) or dizziness. The middle ear is susceptible to infection, such as otitis media, because bacteria and viruses can sometimes enter via the Eustachian tube. Young children are especially prone to middle-ear infections because a child's Eustachian tubes are shorter and more directly in line with the back of the throat than those of adults. Untreated ear infections can sometimes spread into the surrounding bone (mastoiditis) or into the brain (meningitis).

Fluid in the middle ear during an ear infection interferes with the free movement of the ossicles, causing hearing loss that, although significant while it lasts, is temporary. In other instances, there is the prolonged presence of clear fluid in the middle ear, resulting from a combination of infection or allergy and Eustachian tube dysfunction, which itself can result from swelling caused by allergy. This condition, known as "glue ear" or persistent middle-ear effusion, can last long enough to cause detrimental effects on speech, particularly in young children. Middle-ear infections can sometimes become chronic, as in chronic otitis media; permanent damage to the hearing can result from the ossicles being dissolved away by the pus from these chronic infections.

During a middle-ear infection, fluid can build up and increase pressure within the middle-ear cavity sufficiently to rupture (perforate) the eardrum. Very loud noises are another form of increased pressure, in this case from the outside. If a loud noise is very sudden, such as an explosion or gunshot, then pressure cannot be equalized fast enough and the eardrum can rupture. Scuba diving without clearing one's ears (that is, getting the Eustachian tube to open and allow airflow) can also result in ruptured eardrums. Other causes of ruptured eardrums include puncture by a sharp object inserted into the ear canal to remove wax or relieve itching, a blow to the ear, or a fractured skull. Some hearing is lost when the eardrum is ruptured, but if the damage is not too severe the eardrum heals itself and hearing returns.

The middle ear does not always fill with fluid if the Eustachian tube is blocked. In some instances, the middle-ear cavity remains filled with trapped air. This trapped air is taken up by the cells lining the middle-ear cavity, decreasing the air pressure inside the middle ear and allowing the eardrum to push inward. Cells that are constantly shed from the eardrum collect in this pocket and form a ball that can become infected. This infected ball, or cholesteatoma, produces pus, which can erode the ossicles. If left untreated, the erosion can continue through the roof of the middle-ear cavity (causing brain abscesses or meningitis) or through the walls (causing abscesses behind the ear). The symptoms of a cholesteatoma go beyond the symptoms of an earache to include headache, dizziness, and weakness of the facial muscles.

Permanent conductive hearing loss can also result from calcification of the ossicles, a condition called osteosclerosis. Abnormal spongy bone can form at the base of the stirrup bone, interfering with its normal movement against the oval window. Hearing loss caused by osteosclerosis occurs gradually over ten to fifteen years, although it may be accelerated in women by pregnancy. There is a hereditary component.

The inner ear begins at the oval window, which separates the air-filled cavity at the middle ear from the fluid-filled cavities of the inner ear. The inner ear consists of the cochlea, which is involved in hearing, and the labyrinth, which maintains balance.

Disorders of the cochlea result in permanent sensorineural hearing loss. Hair cells can be damaged by the high fever accompanying some diseases such as meningitis. They may also be damaged by some drugs. The largest, and most preventable, sources of damage to the hair cells are occupational and recreational exposure to loud sounds, particularly if they are prolonged. In some occupations, the hearing loss from working without ear protection may be confined to certain frequencies of sounds, while other occupations lead to general loss at all sound frequencies. Prolonged exposure to overamplified music will likewise cause permanent hearing loss at all frequencies. This is more severe and has much earlier onset than presbycusis—the progressive loss of hearing, particularly in the high frequencies, that occurs with normal aging.

The labyrinth is the part of the ear that maintains one's balance; therefore the major system of disorders of the labyrinth is vertigo (dizziness). Labyrinthitis is an infection, generally viral, of the labyrinth. The vertigo can be severe but is temporary.

With Ménière's disease, there is an increase in the volume of fluid in the labyrinth and a corresponding increase in internal pressure, which distorts or ruptures the membrane lining. The symptoms, which include vertigo, noises in the ear, and muffled or distorted hearing especially of low tones, flare up in attacks that may last from a few hours to several days. The frequency of these attacks varies from one individual to another, with some people having episodes every few weeks and others having them every few years. This condition, which may be accompanied by migraine headaches, usually clears spontaneously but in some people may result in deafness.

DIAGNOSTIC AND TREATMENT TECHNIQUES

Diagnosis of the most common ear disorders, outer-ear or middle-ear infections, is done visually with the use of an otoscope. This handheld instrument is a very bright light with a removable tip. Tips of different sizes can be attached so that the doctor can look into ear canals of various sizes. Infections or obstructions in the outer ear are readily visible. Middle-ear infections can often be discerned by the appearance of the eardrum, which may appear red and inflamed. Fluid in the middle ear can sometimes be seen through the eardrum, or its presence can be surmised if the eardrum is bulging toward the ear canal. In other cases, the eardrum will be seen to be retracted or bulging inward toward the middle-ear cavity. Holes in the eardrum can also be seen, as can scars from previous ruptures that have since healed.

Impedance testing may be used in addition to the otoscope for diagnosis of middle-ear problems. Impedance testing is based on the fact that, when sound waves hit the eardrum, some of the energy is transmitted as vibrations of the drum, while some of the energy is reflected. If the eardrum is stretched tight by fluid pushing against it or by being retracted, it will be less mobile and will reflect more sound waves than a normal eardrum. In the simplest form, the mobility of the eardrum is tested with a small air tube and bulb attached to an otoscope. The doctor gently squeezes a puff of air into the ear canal while watching through the otoscope to see how well the eardrum moves.

A far more quantitative version of impedance testing can be done in cases of suspected hearing loss. This type of impedance testing is generally administered by an audiologist, a professional trained in administering and interpreting hearing tests. The ear canal is blocked with an earplug containing a transmitter and receiver. The transmitter releases sound of known frequency and intensity into the ear canal while also changing the pressure in the ear canal by pumping air into it. The receiver then measures the amount of energy reflected back. The machine analyzes the efficiency of reflection at various pressures and prints out a graph. By comparison of the graph to that from an eardrum with normal mobility, conclusions can be drawn about the degree of immobility and, consequently, about the stage of the middle-ear infection. Many pediatricians or family practice doctors have handheld versions of this instrument, which resemble an otoscope but are capable of transmitting sound and measuring reflected sound intensity.

When an ear infection has been diagnosed, the treatment is generally with antibiotics. For outer-ear infections, drops containing antibiotic or antifungal agents are prescribed. For middle-ear infections, antibiotics are prescribed that can be taken by mouth. The patient is rechecked in about three weeks to ensure that the ear has healed.

In some case, the ear does not heal or the fluid in the middle ear does not go away. This can occur if a new infection starts before the ear is fully recovered or if the infecting microorganisms are resistant to the antibiotic used for treatment. In cases of chronic or repeated otitis media, a surgical procedure called a myringotomy can be performed in which a small slit is made in the eardrum to release fluid from the middle ear. Often, a small tube is inserted into the slit. These ear tubes, or tympanostomy tubes, keep the middle ear ventilated, allowing it to dry and heal. In most cases, these tubes are spontaneously pushed out by the eardrum as healing takes place, usually within three to six months. Patients must be cautious to keep water out of their ears while the tubes are in place.

Permanently damaged eardrums—from an explosion, for example—can be replaced by a graft. This procedure is called tympanoplasty, and the tissue used for the graft is generally taken from a vein from the same person. If the ossicles are damaged, they too can be replaced, in this case by metal copies of the bones. For example, when otosclerosis has damaged the stapes (stirrup) bone, hearing can often be restored by replacing it with a metal substitute.

Tumors, osteomas in the ear canal, or cholesteatomas on the eardrum may need to be removed surgically. Surgery may also be needed if infections have spread into the surrounding bone. Bone infections or abnormalities of the inner ear are diagnosed by X rays or by computerized axial tomography (CAT) scans.

For some persons who have complete sensorineural hearing loss, some awareness of sound can be restored with a cochlear implant. This electronic device is surgically implanted and takes the place of the nonexistent hair cells in detecting sound and generating nerve impulses.

Problems of balance may sometimes be treated successfully with drugs to limit the swelling in the labyrinth. Ringing in the ears (tinnitus) is usually resolved when the underlying condition is resolved. In some cases, tinnitus is caused by drugs (large doses of aspirin, for example) and will cease when the drugs are stopped.

Doctors who specialize in diagnosis and treatment of disorders of the ear and who do these surgeries are called otorhinolaryngologists (ear, nose, and throat doctors). They are medical doctors who have several years of training beyond medical school in surgery and in problems of the ear, nose, and throat.

PERSPECTIVE AND PROSPECTS

The basic anatomy of the ear has been known for some time. Bartolommeo Eustachio (1520-1574), an Italian anatomist, first described the Eustachian tube as well as a number of the nerves and muscles involved in the functioning of the ear. An understanding of how the ear functions to discriminate the pitch of sounds, however, was not arrived at until the twentieth century. Georg von Békésy won the Nobel Prize in Physiology or Medicine in 1961 for his work on the acoustics of the ear and how it functions to analyze sounds of varying frequencies (pitch).

Treatment of diseases of the ear has been radically changed by the advent of antibiotics. Older texts describe rupture of the eardrum by middle-ear fluid as a desired outcome of middle-ear infection, one which would ensure that the infection drained and healed, rather than becoming chronic.

Chronic ear infections used to be associated with diseases such as tuberculosis, measles, and syphilis, which are themselves far less common since the widespread use of antibiotics or vaccines. In the past, chronic ear infections were much more likely to result in mastoiditis, or infection of the air spaces of the mastoid bone, requiring surgical removal of the infected portions of the mastoid bone.

Adenoids and tonsils were frequently removed from patients with recurrent ear infections, as these were thought to be the source of the reinfection. It is now known that these tissues are involved in the formation of immunity to infectious bacteria and viruses. Their removal is not advocated in most circumstances—except, for example, when they are large enough to block the opening of the Eustachian tube.

Reconstructive surgery began in the 1950's with the development by Samuel Rosen and others of the operation to free up the calcified stapes bone in cases of otosclerosis. Today virtually all the components of the middle ear can be replaced.

While ear infections used to be much more dangerous, perhaps there is an equal danger today of taking threats to the ears too lightly. Chronic ear infections can still cause permanent hearing loss and even become life-threatening infections if left untreated. Damage involving the inner ear remains untreatable, as do many cases of tinnitus and loss of balance. Because the largest source of inner ear damage is prolonged exposure to noise, the prevention of damage is far more effective than treatment.

—Pamela J. Baker, Ph.D.

See also Altitude sickness; Anatomy; Audiology; Biophysics; Dyslexia; Ear infections and disorders; Ear surgery; Hearing loss; Ménière's disease; Motion sickness; Nervous system; Neurology; Neurology, pediatric; Otorhinolaryngology; Plastic, cosmetic, and reconstructive surgery; Sense organs; Speech disorders; Systems and organs.

FOR FURTHER INFORMATION:

Clark, Randolph Lee, and Russell W. Cumley, eds. *The Book of Health: A Medical Encyclopedia for Everyone.* 2d ed. Princeton, N.J.: Van Nostrand, 1962. This edited text is interesting in historical context as a contrast to present therapies in the age of antibiotics.

Clayman, Charles B., ed. *The American Medical Association Family Medical Guide.* 3d ed. New York: Random House, 1994. Includes a nondetailed, readable descrip-

tion of the anatomy of the ear and a complete listing of common ailments, each with a section on treatment that includes "self-help" and "professional help." Good illustrations and some photographs are provided.

Davis, Hallowell, and S. Richard Silverman. *Hearing and Deafness.* 4th ed. New York: Holt, Rinehart and Winston, 1978. Contains a detailed description of the anatomy and physiology of the ear, including the physics, neurobiology, and cell biology involved in normal and abnormal hearing. Good illustrations and photographs.

Rosenthal, Richard. *The Hearing Loss Handbook.* New York: St. Martin's Press, 1975. Written in a very conversational style by a hard-of-hearing person, this book describes the anatomy of the ear and its diseases, the many ways in which people deny their hearing loss, and the ins and outs of dealing with the many professionals involved in the remediation of hearing loss. Although the section on hearing aids is outdated, this remains an excellent book for any person (or their relatives and friends) who is suffering a gradual hearing loss.

Suddarth, Doris S., ed. *The Lippincott Manual of Nursing Practice.* 5th ed. Philadelphia: J. B. Lippincott, 1991. Presents hearing problems and other problems of the ear, each in outline form, with sections including clinical manifestations, management, and patient education. Contains an extensive bibliography.

Zuckerman, Barry S., and Pamela A. M. Zuckerman. *Child Health: A Pediatrician's Guide for Parents.* New York: Hearst Books, 1986. A very readable description of the ear ailments and treatments most common to children. Includes sections on swimming, otitis media, glue ear, ear tubes, hearing tests, and other topics.

EATING DISORDERS
DISEASE/DISORDER

ANATOMY OR SYSTEM AFFECTED: Endocrine system, gastrointestinal system, glands, intestines, psychic-emotional system, reproductive system, stomach

SPECIALTIES AND RELATED FIELDS: Nutrition, psychiatry, psychology

DEFINITION: A set of emotional disorders centering on body image that lead to misuse of food in a variety of ways—through overeating, overeating and purging, or undereating—that severely threaten the physical and mental well-being of the individual.

KEY TERMS:

amenorrhea: the cessation of menstruation

anorexia nervosa: a disorder characterized by the phobic avoidance of eating, the relentless pursuit of thinness, and fear of gaining weight

arrythmia: irregularity or loss of rhythm, especially of the heartbeat

bulimia: a disorder characterized by binge eating followed by self-induced vomiting

electrolytes: ionized salts in blood, tissue fluid, and cells, including salts of potassium, sodium, and chloride

CAUSES AND SYMPTOMS

The presence of an eating disorder in a patient is defined by an abnormal mental and physical relationship between body image and eating. While obesity is considered an eating disorder, the most prominent conditions are anorexia nervosa and bulimia nervosa. Anorexia nervosa (the word "anorexia" comes from the Greek for "loss of appetite") is an illness characterized by the relentless pursuit of thinness and fear of gaining weight. Bulimia nervosa (the word "bulimia" comes from the Greek for "ox appetite") refers to binge eating followed by self-induced vomiting. These conditions are related in intimate, yet ill-defined ways.

Anorexia nervosa affects more women than men by the overwhelming ratio of nineteen to one. It most often begins in adolescence and is more common among the upper and middle classes of the Western world. According to most studies, its incidence increased severalfold from the 1970's to the 1990's. Prevalence figures vary from 0.5 to 0.8 cases per one hundred adolescent girls. A familiar pattern of anorexia nervosa is often present, and studies indicate that 16 percent of the mothers and 23 percent of the fathers of anorectic patients had a history of significantly low adolescent weight or weight phobia.

The criteria for anorexia nervosa include intense fear of becoming obese, which does not diminish with the progression of weight loss; disturbance of body image, or feeling "fat" even when emaciated; refusal to maintain body weight over a minimal weight for age and height; the loss of 25 percent of original body weight or being 25 percent below expected weight based on standard growth charts; and no known physical illness that would account for the weight loss. Anorexia nervosa is also classified into primary and secondary forms. The primary condition is the distinct constellation of behaviors described above. In secondary anorexia nervosa, the weight loss results from another emotional or organic disorder.

The most prominent symptom of anorexia nervosa is a phobic avoidance of eating that goes beyond any reasonable level of dieting in the presence of striking thinness. Attending this symptom is the characteristic distorted body image and faulty perceptions of hunger and satiety, as well as a pervasive sense of inadequacy.

The distortion of body image renders patients unable to evaluate their body weight accurately, so that they react to weight loss by intensifying their desire for thinness. Patients characteristically describe themselves as "fat" and "gross" even when totally emaciated. The degree of disturbance in body image is a useful prognostic index. Faulty perception of inner, visceral sensations, such as hunger and satiety, extends also to emotional states. The problem of nonrecognition of feelings is usually intensified with starvation.

Other cognitive distortions are also common in anorectic patients. Dichotomous reasoning—the assessment of self or others—is either idealized or degraded. Personalization of situations and a tendency to overgeneralize are common. Anorectics display an extraordinary amount of energy, directed to exercise and schoolwork in the face of starvation, but may curtail or avoid social relationships. Crying spells and complaints of depression are common findings and may persist in some anorectic patients even after weight is gained.

Sleep disturbances have also been reported in anorectics. Obsessive and/or compulsive behaviors, usually developing after the onset of the eating symptoms, abound with anorexia. Obsession with cleanliness and house cleaning, frequent handwashing, compulsive studying habits, and ritualistic behaviors are common.

As expected, the most striking compulsions involve food and eating. Anorectics' intense involvement with food belies their apparent lack of interest in it. The term "anorexia" is, in fact, a misnomer because lack of appetite is rare until late in the illness. Anorectics often carry large quantities of sweets in their purses and hide candies or cookies in various places. They frequently collect recipes and engage in elaborate meal preparation for others. Anorectics' behavior also includes refusal to eat with their families and in public places. When unable to reduce food intake openly, they may resort to such subterfuge as hiding food or disposing of it in toilets. If the restriction of food intake does not suffice for losing weight, the patient may resort to vomiting, usually at night and in secret. Self-induced vomiting then becomes associated with bulimia. Some patients also abuse laxatives and diuretics.

Commonly reported physical symptoms include constipation, abdominal pain, and cold intolerance. With severe weight loss, feelings of weakness and lethargy replace the drive to exercise. Amenorrhea (cessation of menstruation) occurs in virtually all cases, although it is not essential for a diagnosis of anorexia. Weight loss generally precedes the loss of the menstrual cycle. Other physical symptoms reveal the effects of starvation. Potassium depletion is the most frequent serious problem occurring with both anorexia and bulimia. Gastrointestinal disturbances are common, and death may occur from either infection or electrolyte imbalance.

Bulimia usually occurs between the ages of twelve and forty, with greatest frequency between the ages of fifteen and thirty. Unlike anorectics, bulimics usually are of normal weight, although some have a history of anorexia or obesity. Like anorectics, however, they are not satisfied by normal food intake. The characteristic symptom of bulimia is episodic, uncontrollable binge eating followed by vomiting or purging. The binge eating, usually preceded by a period of dieting lasting a few months or more, occurs when patients are alone at home and lasts about one hour. In the early stages of the illness, patients may need to stimulate their throat with a finger or spoon to induce vomiting, but later they can vomit at will. At times, abrasions and bruises on the back of the hand are produced during vomiting. The binge-purge cycle is usually followed by sadness, self-deprecation, and regret. Bulimic patients have troubled interpersonal relationships, poor self-concept, a high level of anxiety and depression, and poor impulse control. Alcohol and drug abuse are not uncommon with bulimia, in contrast to their infrequency with anorexia.

From the medical perspective, bulimia is nearly as damaging to its practitioners as anorexia. Dental problems, including discoloration and erosion of tooth enamel and irritation of gums by highly acidic gastric juice, are frequent. Electrolyte imbalance, such as metabolic alkalosis or hypokalemia (low potassium levels) caused by the self-induced vomiting, is a constant threat. Parotid gland enlargement, esophageal lacerations, and acute gastric dilatation may occur. Cardiac irregularities may also result. The chronic use of emetics such as ipecac to induce vomiting after eating may result in cardiomyopathy (disease of the middle layer of the walls of the heart, the myocardium), occasionally with a fatal outcome. While their menstrual periods are irregular, these patients are seldom amenorrheic.

Another eating disorder, obesity, is the most prevalent nutritional disorder of the Western world. Using the most commonly accepted definition of obesity—a body weight greater than 20 percent above an individual's normal or desirable weight—approximately 35 percent of adults in the United States were considered obese in the early 1990's. This figure represents twice the proportion of the population that was obese in 1900. Evidently, more sedentary lifestyles strongly contributed to this increase, since the average caloric intake of the population decreased by 5 percent since 1910. Although the problem affects both sexes, obesity is found in a larger portion of women than men. In the forty- to forty-nine-year-old age group, 40 percent of women, while only 30 percent of men, were found to meet the criterion for obesity. Prevalence of obesity increases with both age and lower socioeconomic status.

While results of both animal and human studies suggest that obesity is genetically influenced to some degree, most human obesity is reflective of numerous influences and conditions. Evidence indicates that the relationship between caloric intake and adipose tissue is not as straightforward as had been assumed. In the light of this evidence, the failure to lose unwanted pounds and the failure to maintain hard-won weight loss experienced by many dieters seem much more understandable. In the past, obese individuals often were viewed pejoratively by others and by themselves. They were seen as having insufficient willpower and self-discipline. It was incorrectly assumed that it is no more difficult for most obese individuals to lose fat by decreasing caloric intake than it is for individuals in a normal weight

range and that it would be just as easy for the obese to maintain normal weight as it is for those who have never been obese.

TREATMENT AND THERAPY

The management of anorectic patients, in either hospital or outpatient settings, may include individual psychotherapy, family therapy, behavior modification, and pharmacotherapy. Many anorectic patients are quite physically ill when they first consult a physician, and medical evaluation and management in a hospital may be necessary at this stage. A gastroenterologist or other medical specialist familiar with this condition may be required to evaluate electrolyte disturbance, emaciation, hypothermia, skin problems, hair loss, sensitivity to cold, fatigue, and cardiac arrhythmias. Starvation may cause cognitive and psychological disturbances that limit the patient's cooperation with treatment.

Indications for hospitalization are weight loss exceeding 30 percent of ideal body weight or the presence of serious medical complications. Most clinicians continue the hospitalization until 80 percent to 85 percent of the ideal body weight is reached. The hospitalization makes possible hyperalimentation (intravenous infusion of nutrients) when medically necessary. Furthermore, individual and family psychiatric evaluations can be performed and a therapeutic alliance established more rapidly with the patient hospitalized.

Most programs utilize behavior modification during the course of hospitalization, making increased privileges such as physical and social activities and visiting contingent on weight gain. A medically safe rate of weight gain is approximately one-quarter of a pound a day. Patients are weighed daily, after the bladder is emptied, and daily fluid intake and output are recorded. Patients with bulimic characteristics may be required to stay in the room two hours after each meal without access to the bathroom to prevent vomiting. Some behavior modification programs emphasize formal contracting, negative contingencies, the practice of avoidance behavior, relaxation techniques, role-playing, and systematic desensitization.

The goal of dynamic psychotherapy is to achieve patient autonomy and independence. The female anorectic patient often uses her body as a battleground for the separation or individuation struggle with her mother. The cognitive therapeutic approach begins with helping the patient to articulate beliefs, change her view of herself as the center of the universe, and render her expectations of the consequences of food intake less catastrophic. The therapist acknowledges the patient's beliefs as genuine, particularly the belief that her self-worth is dependent on achieving and maintaining a low weight. Through a gradual modification of self-assessment, the deficits in the patient's self-esteem are remedied. The therapist also challenges the cultural values surrounding body shape and addresses behavioral and family issues such as setting weight goals and living conditions.

The behavioral management of bulimia includes an examination of the patient's thinking and behavior toward eating and life challenges in general. The patient is made fully aware of the extent of her binging by being asked to keep a daily record of her eating and vomiting practices. A contract is then established with the patient to help her restrict her eating to three or four planned meals per day. The second stage of treatment emphasizes self-control in eating as well as in other areas of the patient's life. In the final stage of treatment, the patient is assisted in maintaining her new, more constructive eating behaviors.

Almost all clinicians work intensively with the family of anorectic patients, particularly in the initial stage of treatment. Family treatment begins with the current family structure and later addresses the early family functioning that can influence family dynamics dramatically. Multigenerational sources of conflict are also examined.

Family therapy with bulimics explores the sources of family conflicts and helps the family to resolve them. Particular attention is directed toward gender roles in the family, as well as the anxiety of the parents in allowing their children autonomy and self-sufficiency. The roots of impulsive and depressive behaviors and the role of parental satisfaction with the patients' lives and circumstances are often explored and addressed.

In the treatment of obesity, the use of a reduced-calorie diet regimen alone does not appear to be an effective treatment approach for many patients, and it is believed that clinicians may do more harm than good by prescribing it. In addition to the high number of therapeutic failures and possible exacerbation of the problem, negative emotional responses are common side effects. Depression, anxiety, irritability, and preoccupation with food appear to be associated with dieting. Such responses have been found to occur in as many as half of the general obese population while on weight-loss diets and are seen with even greater frequency in the severely obese. Some researchers conclude that some cases are better off with no treatment. Their reasoning is based not only on the ineffectiveness of past treatments and the evidence of biological bases for differences in body size but also on the fact that mild to moderate obesity does not appear to put women (or men) at significant health risk. Moreover, an increase in the incidence of serious eating disorders in women has accompanied the increasingly stringent cultural standards of thinness for women. Given the present level of knowledge, it may be that some individuals would benefit most by adjusting to a weight that is higher than the culturally determined ideal.

When an individual of twenty-five to thirty-four years of age is more than 100 percent above normal weight level, however, there is a twelvefold increase in mortality, and the

need for treatment is clear. Although much of the increased risk is related to the effects of extreme overweight on other diseases (such as diabetes, hypertension, and arthritis), these risks can decrease with weight loss. Conservative treatments have had very poor success rates with this group, both in achieving weight reduction and in maintaining any reductions accomplished. Inpatient starvation therapy has had some success in reducing weight in the severely obese but is a disruptive, expensive, and risky procedure requiring very careful medical monitoring to avoid fatality. Furthermore, for those patients who successfully reduce their weight by this method, only about half will maintain the reduction.

Severe obesity seems to be treated most effectively by surgical measures, which include wiring the jaws to make oral intake nearly impossible, reducing the size of the stomach by suturing methods, or short-circuiting a portion of the intestine so as to reduce the area available for uptake of nutrients. None of these methods, however, are without risk.

PERSPECTIVE AND PROSPECTS

The apparent increase in the incidence of anorexia and bulimia in the 1980's and the interest that they have generated both within the scientific community and among the general public have created the impression that these are new diseases. Although scientific writings on the two disorders were uncommon before the early 1960's, eating disorders are by no means recent developments.

Many early accounts of what might have been the condition of anorexia nervosa exist. The clearest and most detailed account is probably the treatise by Richard Morton, a London physician, in his *Phthisiologica: Or, A Treatise of Consumptions* (1964), first published in Latin. In the book, he described several conditions of consumption, devoting one section to the condition of "nervous consumption" in which the emaciation occurred without any remarkable fever, cough, or shortness of breath. He believed the illness to be the result of violent "passions of the mind," the intemperate drinking of alcohol, and an "unwholesome air." He then described two cases, an eighteen-year-old woman who subsequently died following a "fainting fit" and a sixteen-year-old boy who made a partial recovery.

The term "anorexia nervosa" was first used by Sir William Gull (1816-1890), a physician at Guy's Hospital in London, in a paper published in 1874 in which he described the case histories of four women, including one for whom the illness was fatal. He had first mentioned the illness, briefly calling it "apepsia hysterica," in a lengthy address on diagnosis in medicine that he delivered in Oxford, England, in 1868. By 1874, however, he believed that the term "anorexia" would be more correct, and he preferred the more general term "nervosa," since the disease occurs in males as well as females. As part of the clinical picture of the illness, he emphasized the presence of amenorrhea, constipation, bradycardia, loss of appetite, emaciation, and in some cases low body temperature, edema in the legs, and cyanotic peripheries. He commented particularly on the remarkable restlessness and "mental perversity" of the patients and was convinced that the loss of appetite was central in origin. He found the illness to occur mainly in young females between the ages of sixteen and twenty-three.

Ernest Charles Laseque (1816-1883), a professor of clinical medicine in Paris, published an article in 1873 in which he reported on eight patients. He found the illness to occur mostly in young women between the ages of fifteen and twenty, with the onset precipitated by some emotional upset. He also described the occurrence of diminished food intake, constipation, increased activity, amenorrhea, and the patient's contentment with her condition despite the entreaties and threats of family members.

Despite these promising beginnings, the concept of anorexia nervosa was not clearly established until modern times. The main reason for the conceptual confusion was the overgeneralized interpretation of the nature of the patient's refusal to eat. A second source of confusion was the erroneous view that severe emaciation was a frequent, if not primary, feature of hypopituitarism, a condition first described in 1914. That anorexia nervosa was not related to hypopituitarism was finally clarified by researchers in 1949, but the overgeneralized interpretation of the nature of the food refusal persisted into the early 1960's.

If anorexia is taken to mean a loss of the desire to eat, then there is no doubt that the term "anorexia nervosa" is a misnomer. Anorectic patients refuse to eat not because they have no appetite, but because they are afraid to eat; the food refusal or aversion to eating is the result of an implacable and distorted attitude toward weight, shape, and fatness. The idea that this characteristic attitude is the primary feature of the disorder was not clearly formulated until the early 1960's. Once the concept took hold, the illness of anorexia nervosa became distinguishable from other illnesses that led to similar malnutrition. Thus, for example, a person with hysteria may refuse to eat because of a genuine loss of appetite but does demonstrate the characteristic pursuit of thinness. In the 1980's, there was a revival of the idea that the eating disorders are merely variants of an affective illness.

After occurrences of vomiting and binge eating in a context of anorexia nervosa were described, other investigators proposed two subgroups of anorectic patients: the restrictors and the vomiters. This idea was taken further in 1980 by researchers who divided anorexia nervosa into the restrictor and the bulimic subgroups. The occurrence of binge eating in the context of obesity was described as early as 1959, and in 1970, one investigator described the condition as the "stuffing syndrome." Meanwhile, in 1977, several researchers in Japan proposed that *kibarashigui* (binge eat-

ing with an orgiastic quality) be delineated as a separate syndrome from anorexia nervosa. The confusion produced by using a symptom (bulimia) to describe a syndrome (also bulimia) is considerable, and in the English-speaking world the terms "bulimarexia," "dietary chaos syndrome," and "abnormal normal weight control syndrome" have been proposed for the binge-eating syndrome in patients with a normal or near-normal weight.

In 1980, the American Psychiatric Association (APA) distinguished bulimia as a syndrome from anorexia nervosa, and in 1987, the APA replaced the term with "bulimia nervosa." Doubts still persisted, however, regarding the identification of the eating disorders. On the one hand, the boundary between the disorders and "normal" dieting behavior seems blurred. On the other hand, the eating disorders are sometimes considered to be variants of other psychiatric illnesses, previously schizophrenia, obsessive-compulsive disorder, and in the 1980's, the mood disorders. A discussion of the eating disorders is necessary if researchers are to agree on definitions so that the disorders are distinguishable from a major depression or from each other.   —*Genevieve Slomski, Ph.D.*

See also Addiction; Amenorrhea; Anorexia nervosa; Anxiety; Depression; Malnutrition; Nutrition; Obesity; Obsessive-compulsive disorder; Psychiatric disorders; Psychiatry; Psychiatry, child and adolescent; Puberty and adolescence; Stress; Sports medicine; Vitamins and minerals; Weight loss and gain.

FOR FURTHER INFORMATION:

Brownell, Kelly D., and Christopher G. Fairburn, eds. *Eating Disorders and Obesity: A Comprehensive Handbook.* New York: Guilford Press, 1995. This text addresses all eating disorders, particularly obesity. Includes references and an index.

Bruch, Hilde. *Eating Disorders: Obesity, Anorexia Nervosa, and the Person Within.* New York: Basic Books, 1973. Intended for the general audience, this work provides useful information on eating disorders, their detection, and treatment alternatives. Contains a bibliography.

Field, Howard L., and Barbara B. Domangue, eds. *Eating Disorders Throughout the Life Span.* New York: Praeger, 1987. This collection of essays, intended for the layperson as well as the professional, offers insight into eating disorders of infancy and childhood, adolescent and adult eating disorders, and eating disturbances in the elderly. Includes a bibliography.

Garner, David M., and Paul E. Garfinkel, eds. *Handbook of Treatment for Eating Disorders.* 2d ed. New York: Guilford Press, 1997. This is an updated source on the diagnosis, assessment, and treatment of eating disorders, as well as key issues associated with developing eating disorders.

Harkaway, Jill Elka, ed. *Eating Disorders.* Rockville, Md.: Aspen, 1987. This edited volume discusses anorexia nervosa and obesity. The authors recognize the complexity of eating disorders and present several models for treatment. These excellent essays present case illustrations, descriptions of techniques, and ideas for family and therapists alike.

Hsu, L. K. George. *Eating Disorders*. New York: Guilford Press, 1990. The work provides a summary of the knowledge about the eating disorders of anorexia and bulimia, a historical development of the concepts, their clinical features, methods of diagnostic evaluation, and various treatment options.

Stunkard, Albert J., and Eliot Stellar, eds. *Eating and Its Disorders*. New York: Raven Press, 1984. This scholarly volume begins with an in-depth analysis of the brain mechanisms underlying appetite control and the signals in the brain that activate these mechanisms. The second section presents a synthesis of scientific thinking on body weight regulation. The concluding section features clinical approaches to obesity, anorexia, and bulimia.

EBOLA VIRUS

DISEASE/DISORDER

ANATOMY OR SYSTEM AFFECTED: Blood, circulatory system, gastrointestinal system, muscles, skin

SPECIALTIES AND RELATED FIELDS: Epidemiology, public health, virology

DEFINITION: A virus responsible for a severe and often fatal hemorrhagic fever.

KEY TERMS:

Filoviridae: the family to which the Ebola virus belongs
maculopapular rash: a discolored skin rash observed in patients with Ebola fever

CAUSES AND SYMPTOMS

The Ebola virus is named after the Ebola River in northern Zaire, Africa, where it was first detected in 1976 when hundreds of deaths were recorded there as well as in neighboring Sudan. A fatal disease among cynomolgus laboratory monkeys that were imported from the Philippines showed similar symptoms of the Ebola virus in 1989, but that disease is possibly attributed to the closely related Marburg virus. An equally devastating outbreak among humans took place again in early 1995 in Kirkwit, 500 kilometers east of Kinshasha, Zaire; the disease claimed the lives of 244 patients out of 315 reported cases, a 77 percent fatality rate. It is interesting to note that the epidemic ended within a few months, as suddenly as it began; this puzzled scientists, who are still unaware of the causes and nature of this so-called hot virus. Despite the dreadful speed with which the disease killed its victims, scientists were happy that they contained it with a relatively small number of fatalities. Recently obtained historical documentation suggests the possibility that the Athenian plague at the beginning of the Peloponnesian War around 430 B.C. could be attributed to the Ebola virus.

The Ebola virus appears to have an incubation period of four to sixteen days, after which time the impact is devastating. The patient develops appetite loss, increasing fever, headaches, and muscle aches. The next stage involves disseminated intravascular coagulation (DIC), a condition characterized by both blood clots and hemorrhaging. The clots usually form in vital internal organs such as the liver, spleen, and brain, with subsequent collapse of the neighboring capillaries. Other symptoms include vomiting, diarrhea with blood and mucus, and conjunctivitis. An unusual type of skin irritation known as maculopapular rash first appears in the trunk and quickly covers the rest of the body. The final stages of the disease involve a spontaneous hemorrhaging from all body outlets, coupled with shock and kidney failure and often death within eight to seventeen days.

TREATMENT AND THERAPY

The Ebola virus is classified as a ribonucleic acid (RNA) virus and is closely related to the Marburg virus, first discovered in 1967. The Marburg and the Ebola viruses make up the only two members of the Filoviridae family, which was first established in 1987. Electron microscope studies show the Ebola virus as long filaments, 650 to 14,000 nanometers in length, that are often either branched or intertwined. Its virus part, known as the virion, contains one single noninfectious minus-strand RNA molecule and an endogenous RNA polymerase. The lipoprotein envelope contains a single glycoprotein, which behaves as the type-specific antigen. Spikes are approximately 7 nanometers in length, are spaced at approximately 10 nanometer intervals, and are visible on the virion surface. It is believed that once in the body, the virus produces proteins that suppress the organism's immune system, thus allowing its uninhibited reproduction. Strong evidence indicates that the glycoprotein is the mediator of virus entry in the cell. The Ebola virus can be transmitted through contact with body fluids, such as blood, semen, mucus, saliva, and even urine and feces.

The level of infectivity of the Ebola virus is quite stable at room temperature. Its inactivation is accomplished via ultraviolet or gamma irradiation, 1 percent formalin, beta propiolactone, and an exposure to phenolic disinfectants and lipid solvents, such as deoxycholase and ether. The virus isolation is usually achieved from acute-phase serum of appropriate cell cultures, such as the Ebola-Sudan virus MA-104 cells from a fetal rhesus monkey kidney cell line. Satisfactory results have been accomplished using tissues from the liver, spleen, lymph nodes, kidneys, and heart during autopsy. The virus isolation from brain and other nervous tissues, however, has been rather unsuccessful so far. Neutralization tests have been inconsistent for all filoviruses. Ebola strains, however, show cross-reactions in tests of immunofluorescence assays.

There appears to be no known or standard treatment for

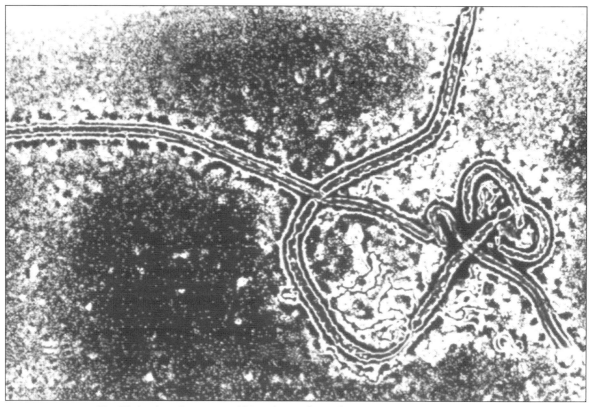

The Ebola virus that causes African hemorrhagic fever. (Larry Mulvehill/Rainbow)

Ebola fever. No chemotherapeutic or immunization strategies are available, and no antiviral drug has been shown to provide positive results, even under in vitro conditions. Human interferon, human convalescent plasma, and anticoagulation therapy have been used with unconvincing results.

At this stage, therapy involves sustaining the desired fluid and electrolyte balance by the frequent administration of fluids. Bleeding may be fought off with blood and plasma transfusion. Sanitary conditions to avoid further contact with the disease are required. Proper decontamination of medical equipment, isolation of the patients from the rest of the community, and prompt disposal of infected tissues, blood, and even corpses limit the spread of the disease.

PERSPECTIVE AND PROSPECTS

The puzzling characteristics of the Ebola virus are the location of its primary natural reservoir, its sudden eruption and the unknown reason for its quick end, and the unusual discovery of the virus in the organs of people who have survived it.

In the past, experimental work on the virus has been slow because of its high pathogenicity. The progress of recombinant deoxyribonucleic acid (DNA) technology has shed the first light on the molecular structure of this virus. It is hoped that further work using this technique as well

as the results of lower pathogenicity viruses (such as the Reston virus) will provide the desired information on replication and virus-host interactions. Finally, the improvement of the various diagnostic tools will allow more accurate virus identification and assessment of transmission modes.

In 1995, the World Health Organization (WHO) investigators and epidemiologists captured about three thousand birds, rodents, and other animals and insects that are suspected of spreading the disease in order to investigate the source of the virus. The results, however, were obscure and inconclusive, and the main facts about the disease are still a mystery, with the exception of the established link between primates and Ebola virus infection in humans. This conclusion was reached after the fatal infection of a French researcher in Ivory Coast who performed an autopsy on a chimpanzee that had died from a disease with the same symptoms as Ebola fever. Yet, the human outbreaks in Zaire and the Sudan have not been traced to monkeys. As long as these puzzling questions linger, the disease should be contained, with particular emphasis on the improvement of sanitary conditions and the control of body fluid contact.

—*Soraya Ghayourmanesh, Ph.D.*

See also Bleeding; Epidemiology; Tropical medicine; Viral infections; Zoonoses.

FOR FURTHER INFORMATION:

"Ebola." In *McGraw-Hill Encyclopedia of Science and Technology.* 8th ed. Vol. 5. New York: McGraw-Hill, 1997.

Jahrling, P. B. "Filoviruses and Arenaviruses." In *Manual of Clinical Microbiology*, edited by A. Balows. Washington, D.C.: American Society of Microbiology, 1991.

ECG OR EKG. *See* ELECTROCARDIOGRAPHY (ECG OR EKG).

ECLAMPSIA
DISEASE/DISORDER

ANATOMY OR SYSTEM AFFECTED: Blood vessels, circulatory system, nervous system

SPECIALTIES AND RELATED FIELDS: Obstetrics

DEFINITION: Hypertension induced by pregnancy is known in its convulsive form as eclampsia and in its nonconvulsive form as preeclampsia; the cause of this dangerous rise in blood pressure has not been identified. Preeclampsia may appear in the second or third trimesters and may be associated with edema (especially of the face) and sudden excessive weight gains; treatment may range from bed rest and sedatives to the induction of labor if the pregnancy is near term. If the preeclampsia worsens, life-threatening eclampsia may develop, resulting in seizures and possibly stillbirth, premature labor, renal failure, liver damage, and coma. If the seizures can be controlled, a cesarean section is usually performed. *—Jason Georges and Tracy Irons-Georges*

See also Cesarean section; Childbirth, complications of; Hypertension; Obstetrics; Pregnancy and gestation; Seizures; Stillbirth.

ECTOPIC PREGNANCY
DISEASE/DISORDER

ANATOMY OR SYSTEM AFFECTED: Reproductive system, uterus

SPECIALTIES AND RELATED FIELDS: Obstetrics

DEFINITION: An ectopic pregnancy is one in which the fertilized egg implants itself in a location other than in the uterus; these other sites may include the Fallopian tubes, the ovaries, or the internal cervical os (near the cervix). Symptoms may range from those normally associated with intrauterine pregnancy to mild abdominal pain. In rare cases, the fetus may survive if the ovum implants in the abdominal viscera, but otherwise surgical intervention may be required to save the mother, if possible leaving the Fallopian tubes and ovaries intact for future pregnancies. Ectopic pregnancy may be caused by

Ectopic pregnancy

Ectopic pregnancy results when the fertilized egg implants itself outside the uterus and begins to develop; surgical intervention is usually required.

congenital defects, sexually transmitted diseases, or the use of an intrauterine contraceptive device (IUD).

—*Jason Georges and Tracy Irons-Georges*

See also Conception; Contraception; Genital disorders, female; Miscarriage; Obstetrics; Pregnancy and gestation.

ECZEMA

DISEASE/DISORDER

ANATOMY OR SYSTEM AFFECTED: Hair, skin

SPECIALTIES AND RELATED FIELDS: Dermatology, toxicology

DEFINITION: Eczema, usually called dermatitis, is a skin disorder characterized by a general pattern of reddening, swelling, blistering, crusting, and scabbing. Chronic cases result in thickening of the skin, peeling, and changes in skin color. Both phases feature itching that may be intense. Dermatitis is associated with allergic reactions, infections, toxic reactions, and skin irritations. For example, atopic dermatitis is a genetic condition in which the patient has widespread sensitivities to certain substances and environmental factors, while contact dermatitis is caused by a reaction to a mild irritant over a long period of time or to a specific substance after sensitization to it. Treatment depends on the cause and may include corticosteroid creams.

—*Jason Georges and Tracy Irons-Georges*

See also Allergies; Dermatitis; Dermatology; Itching; Rashes; Skin; Skin disorders.

Common Sites of Eczema

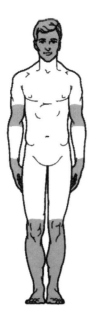

EDEMA

DISEASE/DISORDER

ANATOMY OR SYSTEM AFFECTED: Blood vessels, circulatory system, liver, lungs, lymphatic system, respiratory system, skin

SPECIALTIES AND RELATED FIELDS: Internal medicine, nephrology, pulmonary medicine

DEFINITION: Accumulation of fluid in body tissues that may indicate a variety of diseases, including cardiovascular, kidney, liver, and medication problems.

KEY TERMS:

extracellular fluid: the fluid outside cells; includes the fluid within the vascular system and the lymphatic system and the fluid surrounding individual cells

hydrostatic pressure: the physical pressure on a fluid, such as blood; it tends to push fluids across membranes toward areas of lower pressure

interstitial fluid: the fluid between the vascular system and cells; nutrients from the vascular compartment must diffuse across the interstitial compartment to enter the cells

intracellular fluid: the fluid within cells

intravascular fluid: the fluid carried within the blood vessels; it is in a constant state of motion because of the pumping action of the heart

osmotic pressure: the ability of a concentrated fluid on one side of a membrane to draw water away from a less concentrated fluid on the other side

PROCESS AND EFFECTS

Edema is not a disease, but a condition that may be caused by a number of diseases. It signals a breakdown in the body's fluid-regulating mechanisms. The body's water can be envisioned as divided into three compartments: the intracellular compartment, the interstitial compartment, and the vascular compartment. The intracellular compartment consists of the fluid contained within the individual cells. The vascular compartment consists of all the water that is contained within the heart, the arteries, the capillaries, and the veins. The last compartment, and in many ways the most important for a discussion of edema, is called the interstitial compartment. This compartment includes all the water not contained in either the cells or the blood vessels. The interstitial compartment contains all the fluids between the intracellular compartment and the vascular compartment and the fluid in the lymphatic system. The sizes of these compartments are approximately as follows: intracellular fluid at 66 percent, interstitial fluid at 25 percent, and the vascular fluid at only 8 percent of the total body water.

When the interstitial compartment becomes overloaded with fluid, edema develops. To understand the physiology of edema formation, it may be helpful to follow a molecule of water as it travels through the various compartments, beginning when the molecule enters the aorta soon after leaving the heart. The blood has just been ejected from the heart under high pressure, and it speedily begins its trip through the body. It passes from the great vessel, the aorta, into smaller and smaller arteries that divide and spread throughout the body. At each branching, the pressure and speed of the water molecule decreases. Finally, the molecule enters a capillary, a vessel so small that red blood cells must flow in a single file. The wall of this vessel is composed only of the membrane of a single capillary cell. There are small passages between adjacent capillary cells leading to the interstitial compartment, but they are normally closed.

The hydrostatic pressure on the water molecule is much lower than when it was racing through the aorta, but it is still higher than the surrounding interstitial compartment. At the arterial end of the capillary, the blood pressure is sufficient to overcome the barrier of the capillary cell's membrane. A fair number of water and other molecules are pushed through the membrane into the interstitial compartment.

In the interstitial compartment, the water molecule is essentially under no pressure, and it floats amid glucose molecules, oxygen molecules, and many other compounds. Glucose and oxygen molecules enter the cells, and when the water molecule is close to a glucose molecule it is taken inside a cell with that molecule. The water molecule is eventually expelled by the cell, which has produced extra water from the metabolic process.

Back in the interstitial compartment, the molecule floats with a very subtle flow toward the venous end of the capillary. This occurs because, as the arterial end of the capillary pushes out water molecules, it loses hydrostatic pressure, eventually equaling the pressure of the interstitial compartment. Once the pressure equalizes, another phenomenon that has been thus far overshadowed by the hydrostatic pressure takes over—osmotic pressure. Osmotic pressure is the force exercised by a concentrated fluid that is separated by a membrane from a less concentrated fluid. It draws water molecules across the membrane from the less concentrated side. The more concentrated is the fluid, the greater is the drawing power. The ratio of nonwater molecules to that of water molecules determines concentration.

The fluid that stays within the capillary remains more concentrated than the interstitial fluid for two reasons. First, the plasma proteins in the vascular compartment are too large to be forced across the capillary membrane; albumin is one such protein. These proteins stay within the vascular compartment and maintain a relatively concentrated state, compared to the interstitial compartment. At the same time, the concentration of the fluid in the interstitial compartment is being lowered constantly by the cellular compartment's actions. Cells remove molecules of substances such as glucose to metabolize, and afterward they release water—a by-product of the metabolic process. Both processes conspire

Edema

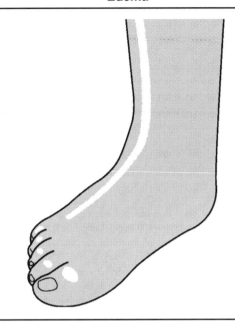

Edema may appear chronically (as seen here, in the ankles), with characteristic swelling and stretched, shiny skin; it can be a symptom of many diseases.

to lower the total concentration of the interstitial compartment. The net result of this process is that water molecules return to the capillaries at the venous end because of osmotic pressure.

The water molecule is caught by this force and is returned to the vascular compartment. Back in the capillary, the molecule's journey is not yet complete. Now in a tiny vein, it moves along with blood. On the venous side of the circulatory system, the process of branching is reversed, and small veins join to form increasingly larger ones. The water molecule rides along in these progressively larger veins. The pressure surrounding the molecule is still low, but it is now higher than the pressure at the venous end of the capillary. One may wonder how this is possible if the venous pressure at the beginning of the venous system is essentially zero, and there is only one pump, the heart, in the body. As the molecule flows through the various veins, it occasionally passes one-way valves that allow blood to flow only toward the heart. The action of these valves, combined with muscular contractions from activities such as walking or tapping the foot, force blood toward the heart. Without these valves, it would be impossible for the venous blood to flow against gravity and return to the heart; the blood would simply sit at the lowest point in the body. Fortunately, these valves and contractions move the molecule against gravity, returning it to the heart to begin a new cycle.

In certain disease states, there is marked capillary dilation and excessive capillary permeability, and excessive amounts of fluid are allowed to leave the intravascular compartment. The fluid accumulates in the interstitial space. When capillary permeability is increased, plasma proteins also tend to leave the vascular space, reducing the intravascular compartment's osmotic pressure while increasing the interstitial compartment's osmotic pressure. As a result, the rate of return of fluid from the interstitial compartment to the vascular compartment is lowered, thus increasing the interstitial fluid levels.

Another route of return of interstitial fluid to the circulation is via the lymphatic system. The lymphatic system is similar to the venous system, but it carries no red blood cells. It runs through the lymph nodes, carrying some of the interstitial fluid that has not been able to return to the vascular compartment at the capillary level. If lymphatic vessels become obstructed, water in the interstitial compartment accumulates and edema may result.

CAUSES AND SYMPTOMS

Heart failure is a major cause of edema. When the right ventricle of the heart fails, it cannot cope with all the venous blood returning to the heart. As a consequence, the veins become distended, the interstitial compartment is overloaded, and edema occurs. If the patient with heart failure is mostly upright, the edema collects in the legs; if the patient has been lying in bed for some time, the edema tends to accumulate in the lower back. Other clinical signs of right heart failure include distended neck veins, an enlarged and tender liver, and a "galloping" sound on listening to the heart with a stethoscope.

When the left ventricle of the heart fails, the congestion affects the pulmonary veins instead of the neck and leg veins. Fluid accumulates in the same fashion within the interstitial compartment of the lungs; this condition is termed pulmonary edema. Patients develop shortness of breath with minimal activity, upon lying down, and periodically through the night. They may need to sleep on several pillows to minimize this symptom. This condition can usually be diagnosed by listening to the lungs and heart through a stethoscope and by taking an X ray of the chest.

Deep vein thrombosis is another common cause of edema of the lower limbs. When a thrombus (a blood clot inside a blood vessel) develops in a large vein of the legs, the patient usually complains of pain and tenderness of the affected leg. There is usually redness and edema as well. If the thrombus affects a small vein, it may not be noticed. The diagnosis can be made by several specialized tests, such as ultrasound testing and/or impedance plethysmography. Other tests may be needed to make the diagnosis, such as injecting radiographic dye in a vein in the foot and then taking X rays to determine whether the flow in the veins is obstructed, or using radioactive agents that bind to the clot. Risks for developing venous thrombosis include immobility (even for relatively short periods of time such as a long car or plane ride), injury, a personal or family history of venous thrombosis, the use of birth control pills, and certain types of cancer. Elderly patients are at particular risk because of relative immobility and an increased frequency of minor trauma to the legs.

When repeated or large thrombi develop, the veins deep inside the thigh (the deep venous system) become blocked, and blood flow shifts toward the superficial veins. The deep veins are surrounded by muscular tissue, and venous flow is assisted by muscular contractions of the leg (the muscular pump), but the superficial veins are surrounded only by skin and subcutaneous tissue and cannot take advantage of the muscular pump. As a consequence, the superficial veins become distended and visible as varicose veins.

When vein blockage occurs, the valves inside become damaged. Hydrostatic pressure of the venous system below the blockage then rises. The venous end of the capillary is normally where the osmotic pressure of the vascular compartment pulls water from the interstitial compartment back into the vascular compartment. In a situation of increased hydrostatic pressure, however, this process is slowed or stopped. As a result, fluid accumulates in the interstitial space, leading to the formation of edema.

A dangerous complication of deep vein thrombosis occurs when part of a thrombus breaks off, enters the circulation, and reaches the lung; this is called a pulmonary embolus. It blocks the flow of blood to the lung, impairing oxygenation. Small emboli may have little or no effect on the patient, while larger emboli may cause severe shortness of breath, chest pain, or even death.

Another potential cause of edema is the presence of a mass in the pelvis or abdomen compressing the large veins passing through the area and interfering with the venous return from the lower limbs to the heart. The resulting venous congestion leads to edema of the lower limbs. The edema may affect either one or both legs, depending on the size and location of the mass. This diagnosis can usually be established by a thorough clinical examination, including rectal and vaginal examinations and X-ray studies.

Postural (or gravitational) edema of the lower limbs is the most common type of edema affecting older people; it is more pronounced toward the end of the day. It can be differentiated from the edema resulting from heart failure by the lack of signs associated with heart failure and by the presence of diseases restricting the patients' degree of mobility. These diseases include Parkinson's disease, osteoarthritis, strokes, and muscle weakness. Postural edema of the lower limbs results from a combination of factors, the most important being diminished mobility. If a person stands or sits for prolonged periods of time without moving, the muscular pump becomes ineffective. Venous compression also plays an important role in the development of this type of edema. It will occur when the veins in the thigh are compressed between the weight of the body and the surface on which the patient sits, or when the edge of a reclining chair compresses the veins in the calves. Other factors that aggravate postural edema include varicose veins, venous thrombi, heart failure, some types of medication, and low blood albumin levels.

Albumin is formed in the liver from dietary protein. It is essential to maintaining adequate osmotic pressure inside the blood vessels and ensuring the return of fluid from the interstitial space to the vascular compartment. When edema is caused by inadequate blood levels of albumin, it tends to be quite extensive. The patient's entire body and even face are often affected. There are several reasons that the liver may be unable to produce the necessary amount of albumin, including malnutrition, liver impairment, the aging process, and excessive protein loss.

In cases of malnutrition, the liver does not receive a sufficient quantity of raw material from the diet to produce albumin; this occurs when the patient does not ingest enough protein. Healthy adults need at least 0.5 gram of protein for each pound of their body weight. Two groups of people are particularly susceptible to becoming malnourished: the poor and the elderly. Infants and children of poor families who cannot afford to prepare nutritious meals often suffer from malnutrition. The elderly, especially men living on their own, are also vulnerable, regardless of their income.

A liver damaged by excessive and prolonged consumption of alcohol, diseases, or the intake of some type of medication or other chemical toxins will be unable to manufacture albumin at the necessary rate to maintain a normal concentration in the blood. Clinically, the patient shows other evidence of liver impairment in addition to edema. For example, fluid may also accumulate in the abdominal cavity, a condition known as ascites. The diagnosis of liver damage is made by clinical examination and supporting laboratory investigations. The livers of older people, even in the absence of disease, are often less efficient at producing albumin.

The albumin also can be deficient if an excessive amount of albumin is lost from the body. This condition may occur in certain types of diseases affecting the kidneys or the gastrointestinal tract. An excessive amount of protein also may be lost if a patient has large, oozing pressure ulcers, extensive burns, or chronic lung conditions that produce large amounts of sputum.

Patients with strokes and paralysis sometimes develop edema of the paralyzed limb. The mechanism of edema formation in these patients is not entirely understood. It probably results from a combination of an impairment of the nerves controlling the dilation and a constriction of the affected limb blood vessels, along with postural and gravitational factors.

Severe allergic states, toxic states, or local inflammation are associated with increased capillary permeability that results in edema. The amount of fluid flowing out to the capillaries far exceeds the amount that can be returned to the capillaries at the venous end. A number of medications can induce edema by promoting the retention of fluid, including steroids, estrogens, some arthritis medications, a few blood pressure medications, and certain antibiotics. Salt intake tends to cause a retention of fluid as well. Obstruction of the lymphatic system often leads to accumulation of fluid in the interstitial compartment. Obstruction can occur in certain types of cancer, after radiation treatment, and in certain parasitic infestations.

TREATMENT AND THERAPY

The management of edema depends on the specific reason for its presence. To determine the cause of edema, a thorough history, including current medications, dietary habits, and activity level, is of prime importance. Performing a detailed physical examination is also a vital step. It is frequently necessary to obtain laboratory, ultrasound, and/or X-ray studies before a final diagnosis is made. Once a treatable cause is found, then therapy aimed at the cause should be instituted.

If no treatable, specific disease is responsible for the edema, conservative treatment aimed at reducing the edema to manageable levels without inducing side effects should be initiated. Frequent elevation of the feet to the level of the heart, support stockings, and an avoidance of prolonged standing or sitting are the first steps. If support stockings are ineffective or are too uncomfortable, then custom-made, fitted stockings are available. A low-salt diet is important in the management of edema because a high salt intake worsens the fluid retention. If all these measures fail, then diuretics in small doses may be useful.

Diuretics work by increasing the amount of urine produced. Urine is made of fluids removed from the vascular compartment by the kidneys. The vascular compartment then replenishes itself by drawing water from the interstitial compartment. This reduction in the amount of interstitial fluid improves the edema. There are various types of diuretics, which differ in their potency, duration of action, and side effects. Potential side effects include dizziness, fatigue, sodium and potassium deficiency, excessively low blood pressure, dehydration, sexual dysfunction, the worsening of a diabetic's blood sugar control, increased uric acid levels, and increased blood cholesterol levels. Although diuretics are a convenient and effective means of treating simple edema, it is important to keep in mind that the cure should not be worse than the disease. When the potential side effects of diuretic therapy are compared to the almost total lack of complications of conservative treatment, one can see that mild edema which is not secondary to significant disease is best managed conservatively. Edema caused by more serious diseases, however, calls for more intensive measures.

PERSPECTIVE AND PROSPECTS

The prevalence of edema could decrease as people become more health-conscious and medical progress is made. Nutritious diets, avoidance of excessive salt, and an increased awareness of the dangers of excessive alcohol intake and of the benefits of regular physical exercise all contribute to decreasing the incidence of edema. Improved methods for the early detection, prevention, and management of diseases that may ultimately result in edema could also significantly reduce the scope of the problem. It is also expected that safer and more convenient methods of treating edema will become available.

—*Ronald C. Hamdy, M.D., Mark R. Doman, M.D., and Katherine Hoffman Doman*

See also Arteriosclerosis; Circulation; Embolism; Elephantiasis; Heart; Heart disease; Heart failure; Kidney disorders; Kidneys; Kwashiorkor; Liver; Liver disorders; Lungs; Malnutrition; Nutrition; Phlebitis; Pulmonary diseases; Pulmonary medicine; Pulmonary medicine, pediatric; Respiration; Thrombosis and thrombus; Varicose vein removal; Varicosis; Vascular medicine; Vascular system; Venous insufficiency.

FOR FURTHER INFORMATION:

Andreoli, Thomas, et al., eds. *Cecil Essentials of Medicine*. 4th ed. Philadelphia: W. B. Saunders, 1997. A good introductory text to internal medicine that can also be easily understood by nonscientists.

Barnhart, Edward R., ed. *Physician's Desk Reference*. 47th ed. Oradell, N.J.: Medical Economics Data, 1993. The most up-to-date listing of drugs and drug side effects that is regularly available. The information contained is required by the Food and Drug Administration to allow the marketing of medications. Includes all reported drug side effects, although it can be difficult to sort out the more frequent side effects and adverse reactions from the rare ones.

Bergan, John J., and James S. T. Yao, eds. *Venous Problems*. Chicago: Yearbook Medical Publishers, 1978. Contains the most thorough treatment of human venous problems. Causality, diagnosis (including the tests used to make a diagnosis), and the surgical treatment of venous abnormalities are discussed.

Guyton, Arthur C. *Human Physiology and Mechanisms of Disease*. 6th ed. Philadelphia: W. B. Saunders, 1997. The standard reference text in human physiology. A background in basic physiology is helpful in understanding this work.

Michaelson, Cydney, ed. *Congestive Heart Failure*. St. Louis: C. V. Mosby, 1983. An excellent basic, yet thorough, treatise on the subject of heart failure. The authors discuss the circulatory system in states of both health and disease, low-salt diets, and the drug treatment for heart failure.

Spence, Alexander P., and Elliott B. Mason. *Human Anatomy and Physiology*. 4th ed. St. Paul, Minn.: West, 1992. This text is a basic introduction to physiology and anatomy.

Staub, Norman, and Aubrey Taylor, eds. *Edema*. New York: Raven Press, 1984. A thorough and advanced treatment of edema—its many forms and causes.

EDUCATION, MEDICAL

HEALTH CARE SYSTEM

DEFINITION: In the United States, the educational process that leads to obtaining and maintaining a state license to practice medicine, a process which generally involves obtaining two academic degrees and one or more medical certifications; the entire of medical education takes a minimum of eleven years beyond high school.

KEY TERMS:

continuing medical education (CME): medical lectures given by hospitals, medical societies, specialists, and conferences that, in the United States, must be approved to meet the requirements for CME credits

generalist: a medical practitioner who belongs to one of the three largest specialties of medicine—family medicine, internal medicine, and pediatrics; sometimes, practitioners of obstetrics/gynecology (OB/GYN) and general surgery are considered to be generalists

internship: the first year of supervised, postgraduate training after receiving a Doctor of Medicine (M.D.) or Doctor of Osteopathy (D.O.) degree, which allows individuals to practice clinical medicine with a limited license; for M.D.'s, this is called year one of residency, and for D.O.'s this is called year one of internship

residency: a course of postgraduate medical education undertaken after receiving an M.D. or D.O. degree and leading to certification in a generalist or specialist branch of medicine

specialist: referring to specialties of medicine not categorized as generalist

STRUCTURE AND CURRICULUM

During the course of the twentieth century, the medical education system in the United States developed from a one-year or two-year program to the present requirement of eleven or more years of formal education and training after completion of secondary school.

College or university. A person who wishes to be licensed as a physician by one of the fifty states usually begins by completing a bachelor's degree at an accredited college or university. This is, by far, the norm, although it is not an absolute requirement. Some colleges and universities offer a premedical undergraduate program that emphasizes biology, chemistry, and other courses in scientific disciplines. In the past, medical schools preferred graduates of these premedical programs over those with liberal arts or science degrees. Today, many medical schools seek more well rounded students who have degrees in liberal arts disci-

The Requirements for Fully Licensed Physicians

Place or Event	Degree or Program	Years
College or University	B.A. or B.S.	4
Medical School	Preclinical	2
Medical School	Clinical	2
Graduation	D.O. or M.D.	–
Internship or Residency	D.O. or M.D. Limited License	1
Residency (1st)	Generalist or Specialist	2-5
Residency (2d/3d)	Subspecialist (Optional)	0-5
Continuing Education	CME (150 credits)	every 3
	TOTAL	11-19+

plines. This change has been made in response to societal pressures to graduate more physicians who have a humanistic approach to medical practice. An effort has also been made to provide educational opportunities for members of disadvantaged and minority groups. Therefore, any person with a good grade-point average may consider applying to medical school regardless of the type or the nature of the bachelor-level education.

Preparation. The first choice that an individual must make when considering a career as a physician is to ask, "What type of medical school do I wish to attend?" In the United States, two medical degrees are granted: Doctor of Medicine (M.D.) and Doctor of Osteopathy (D.O.). M.D.'s are occasionally referred to as allopathic physicians to distinguish them from osteopathic physicians. Historically, allopathic education stressed the importance of disease in causing illness. Laboratory tests and the prescription of medications are generally used in diagnosis and treatment. Osteopathic education historically looked to the musculoskeletal system with respect to health and illness. This distinction is largely a historic remnant. The curriculum of both M.D. and D.O. schools are nearly identical. Both types of physicians train in the same residencies, and both receive the same license to practice medicine and surgery.

Medical school (preclinical). The first two years of medical school are generally devoted to the study of academic medicine. This period is known as preclinical education. These years stress the need to master material from basic sciences and to understand the scientific method of research. Courses such as anatomy, biochemistry, histology, immunology, microbiology, neurology, pathology, and physiology are taught. Achievement is marked by success in test taking through memorization, the analysis of detailed information, and the integration of new material. Actual contact with practicing physicians and their patients is not stressed. As a result, this phase is sometimes criticized for teaching medical knowledge that is separated from medical practice. Some medical schools are adjusting the curriculum in the preclinical years to reduce this dichotomy. At the end of the second year, students must pass the first component of the examination to obtain licensure.

Medical school (clinical). The second two years of medical education stress the clinical knowledge needed to become a physician. Classroom education is concerned with physical diagnosis, the identification of diseases, treatments, and associated procedures and techniques. Medical schools require students to observe physicians practicing medicine with patients in both hospital and office settings. Opportunities are available for students to spend time away from their medical school learning about various specialties. The standard curriculum requires all students to study internal medicine, surgery, pediatrics, obstetrics and gynecology, and psychiatry. Other specialties are studied on an elective basis. For example, a medical student may spend a month observing family practice physicians working in hospitals and their offices and receive a grade for that month. In this manner, students gain some experience by direct exposure to several medical specialties. At the end of the fourth year, students must pass the second component of the examination to obtain licensure.

Internship. In the past, many generalist physicians, after one year of internship, entered private practice. Today, the year of internship is completed under close medical supervision. This prepares a new physician for more independent practice. All new physicians complete their first year of internship in a residency program before receiving their full medical license in the second year of residency. Physicians who receive their medical education outside of a U.S. school must pass the same test as American medical students before being eligible to complete residency training. Some internships are spent rotating through the areas of medicine, surgery, pediatrics, and obstetrics before entering specialized training in areas such as radiology, dermatology, and some surgical specialties. During the first year of residency, a physician has a limited license to practice medicine. Upon completion of the internship or first-year residency and successful passage of the third portion of the standard licensure examination, a physician is granted a full license to practice medicine and surgery.

Residency. The three generalist areas in which resident physicians learn clinical medicine, also known as primary care specialties, are family medicine, internal medicine, and pediatrics. Family medicine treats the whole family throughout life, internal medicine treats adults, and pediatrics treats children and teenagers. The end of childhood and the beginning of adulthood is not clearly defined, and there is some overlap. Most pediatricians will treat patients up to the age of twenty-two, when they typically complete college. The lowest age for patients of internists is usually sixteen. The many specialist areas of medicine are concerned with specific organ systems, disease processes, or prevention. For example, a psychiatrist has a residency in the area of mental illness, while an emergency room (ER) physician has a residency in the practice of medicine in the ER.

Residency education is the time when a physician who has been graduated from medical school first becomes responsible for patient care, under both direct and indirect supervision. Residency teaches and evaluates the skill of a new physician in applying the knowledge gained in medical school to clinical practice. Residency programs are usually three to five years in length. After each year, the resident is given more independence of practice and more responsibility to supervise newer physicians. Upon completion of a residency program, a physician becomes eligible for certification by one of the generalist or specialist boards of medicine. Most boards require one or two years of independent practice before allowing candidates to seek board certification. A physician must take and pass yet another examination concerning knowledge related to the specialty area for which certification is desired. Many board certifications must be renewed periodically (every five to seven years) as a condition of retaining board-certified status.

Second residency (subspecialization). Some physicians choose to complete additional training in their medical specialty. This subspecialty medical education is usually called a fellowship. For example, a general surgeon may complete a multiyear residency in cardiac surgery, or a psychiatrist may complete a subspecialty residency in children's mental illness. Some highly subspecialized physicians need seven to ten years after medical school to complete their subspecialty training. An example of this level of specialization is forensic pathology, which requires residency training in pathology and fellowships in forensic and chemical pathology. Pediatric neurosurgery is another example.

Continuing medical education. All states require that physicians complete a certain number of continuing medical education (CME) credits in order to maintain their medical licensure. One hundred fifty CME credits over three years is a common requirement. Some specialties also require national examinations for recertification in the specialty. For physicians in the United States, medical education is an exercise in lifelong learning.

ISSUES AND PHILOSOPHIES

American medical education is undergoing one of the greatest challenges in its history. Medical schools are being asked to teach physicians how to be effective and efficient caregivers to all persons. The corporate system of medical care demands medical care that is effective, cost-conscious or economically efficient, and delivered in a positive and caring manner. Health maintenance organizations (HMOs), preferred provider organizations (PPOs), and other organizational alliances of physicians expect the medical educational system to teach these values and skills.

The national government adds one more criterion: Physicians must be able to do the above for all citizens. In a pluralistic and democratic society, a physician must acknowledge various social, ethnic, cultural, and regional needs. Medical educators must train socially conscious physicians. Physicians must be available to practice in either rural or inner-city areas. They must be able to treat various populations, such as African Americans and Native Americans, for their specific needs. Physicians are being asked to be cognizant of and caring toward all Americans.

The medical philosophy that allows for an increase of psychological skills and social awareness in medical education is called the biopsychosocial model. As the label indicates, it conceptualizes a medical education system which teaches physicians solid medical knowledge ("bio"), an improved ability to relate to patients ("psycho"), and an awareness of different social systems and cultural attitudes as they affect medical care ("social"). The biopsychosocial model of care is a proposed revision of what the medical education system should teach physicians. It may be the medical school curriculum of the future.

PERSPECTIVE AND PROSPECTS

The history of American medical education can be understood as falling into five periods of development. Each period stressed a certain philosophy and direction unique to its times. The current philosophy of medical education has aspects of all five periods, affecting how, what, and why physicians are taught.

The British period (1750-1815). American medical education was established on the British model. The emphasis in British medical education was based on developing a physician's medical knowledge through direct observation of patient care in clinical settings. There were few formal centers for medical training. They functioned to instruct teaching physicians and to transmit new medical knowledge. In America, there were only six medical schools. Most medical education was clinical and taught by older physicians to younger physicians in an office setting. There were no formal educational requirements. Most physicians could read and write, possessing the equivalent of only two or three years of formal education.

The French period (1815-1865). French physicians, who developed the skills of classification, influenced American medical education through methods of diagnosis and the use of hospitals. In the United States, many hospitals were built, and there was a significant expansion in the number of medical schools. Large groups of patients were admitted to hospitals and grouped on wards by diagnosis. The hospital-office model of medical education began to develop.

The German period (1865-1915). Laboratory methods

and germ theory were introduced into medical education from Germany. Some medical schools began to educate physicians in the laboratory approach to medicine. Office practice was less important in medical education. The period of formal education was still relatively brief, often less than two years in total length. At the end of the German period, many medical schools that were not teaching laboratory methods were closed.

The American period (1915-1965). American medical education embraced a scientific approach to medical education, first detailed by Abraham Flexner in *Medical Education in the United States and Canada,* published in 1910 in a report on reforming American medical education. Physician-scientists were to be educated by quality medical schools to provide clinical medicine according to the scientific method. This model was successfully introduced into American medical education. It was considered the norm until the concerns of corporate interests and government interests became vital.

The corporate period (1965-   ). Medicare and Medicaid programs were created and supported by the national government in order to provide quality medical care to all Americans. Corporate interests require that medical education be effective in controlling health costs to industry. Many of the current challenges facing medical education revolve around teaching physicians the two concerns of access and cost-effectiveness.

In the early 1990's, the Council on Graduate Medical Education (COGME) suggested that certain humanistic and corporate medical education goals be reached by the year 2000. At least 50 percent of residency graduates should enter practice as generalist physicians. The number of underrepresented minority students should be doubled. Shortages of physicians in rural and urban areas should be eliminated. The purpose of these goals was to avoid a severe physician shortage for some populations, areas of specialty, and geographic centers.

With a system of managed medical care in place, COGME projected a shortage of 35,000 generalist physicians and a surplus of 115,000 specialist physicians by the year 2000. In 1990, fewer than one-third of all American physicians practiced primary care. It appears that in the future, the trend toward specialization will be reversed. Those who plan, those who pay, and those who organize the various systems to deliver medical care in the United States no longer believe that so many specialty-trained physicians will be needed. Yet, the demand by Americans for specialized health care services has not diminished. A clash between recipients and providers appears to be inevitable. The next decades in American medicine are likely to be turbulent, as various stakeholders struggle to redefine the American system of health care.

There is an acknowledged maldistribution of physicians. Most prefer to practice in suburban and medical center settings, leaving significant numbers of Americans without easy access to adequate health care. Many planners also believe that the promised efficiency of managed care will result in a decreased need for physicians. In the mid-1990's, state legislatures began to reduce the amounts of support for medical education, effectively forcing medical schools to reduce the number of physicians that they graduate. The final outcomes of these policy changes are unclear. The results of this trend, however, will be felt by American society for decades.   *—Gerald T. Terlep, Ph.D.*
updated by L. Fleming Fallon, Jr., M.D., M.P.H.

See also American Medical Association; Ethics; Hippocratic oath; Nursing; Osteopathic medicine; *specific specialties.*

FOR FURTHER INFORMATION:

Rivo, Marc L., et al. "Defining the Generalist Physician's Training." *Journal of the American Medical Association* 271 (May 18, 1994): 1499-1504. Rivo writes a clear, fact-filled article on major current issues in medical education. The article is accessible to the general reader. It also contains charts and references for further research.

Starr, Paul. "The Framework of Health Care Reform." *New England Journal of Medicine* 330, no. 15 (April 14, 1994): 1086-1088. This recent article reviews several proposals for health care reform. The author has provided commentary on the American health care system for many years.

_____. *The Social Transformation of American Medicine.* New York: Basic Books, 1982. This classic book provides an excellent history of the history of medical education in the United States. It is clearly written and easy to understand.

EEG. *See* ELECTROENCEPHALOGRAPHY (EEG).

ELECTRICAL SHOCK
DISEASE/DISORDER

ANATOMY OR SYSTEM AFFECTED: Heart, nervous system, skin

SPECIALTIES AND RELATED FIELDS: Critical care, emergency medicine, neurology

DEFINITION: The physical effect of an electrical current entering the body and the resulting damage.

CAUSES AND SYMPTOMS

Electric shock ranges from a harmless jolt of static electricity to a power line's lethal discharge. The severity of the shock depends on the current flowing through the body, and the current is determined by the skin's electrical resistance. Dry skin has a very high resistance; thus 110 volts produces a small, harmless current. The resistance for perspiring hands, however, is lower by a factor of 100, resulting in potentially fatal currents. Because of their proximity to the heart, currents traveling between bodily extremities are particularly dangerous.

Electric shock causes injury or death in one of three ways: paralysis of the breathing center in the brain, paralysis of the heart, or ventricular fibrillation (extremely rapid and uncontrolled twitching of the heart muscle).

The threshold of feeling (the minimum current detectable) ranges from 0.5 to 1.0 milliamperes. Currents up to 5.0 milliamperes, the maximum harmless current, are not hazardous, unless they trigger an accident by involuntary reaction. Currents in this range create a tingling sensation. The minimum current that causes muscular paralysis occurs between 10 and 15 milliamperes. Currents of this magnitude cause a painful jolt. Above 18 milliamperes, the current contracts chest muscles and breathing ceases. Unconsciousness and death follow within minutes unless the current is interrupted and respiration resumed. A short exposure to currents of 50 milliamperes causes severe pain, possible fainting, and complete exhaustion, while currents in the 100 to 300 milliampere range produce ventricular fibrillation, which is fatal unless quickly corrected. During ventricular fibrillation, the heart stops its rhythmic pumping and flutters uselessly. Since blood stops flowing, the victim dies from oxygen deprivation to the brain in a matter of minutes. This is the most common cause of death for victims of electric shock.

Relatively high currents (above 300 milliamperes) may produce ventricular paralysis, deep burns in the body's tissue, or irreversible damage to the central nervous system. Victims are more likely to survive a large but brief current, even through smaller, sustained currents are usually lethal. Burning or charring of the skin at the point of contact may be a contributing factor to the delayed death that often follows severe electric shock. Very high voltage discharges of short duration, such as a lightning strike, tend to disrupt the body's nervous impulses, but victims may survive. On the other hand, any electric current large enough to raise body temperature significantly produces immediate death.

TREATMENT AND THERAPY

Before medical treatment can be applied, the current must be stopped or the shock victim must be separated from the current source without being touched. Nonconducting materials such as dry, heavy blankets or pieces of wood can be used for this purpose. If the victim is not breathing, artificial respiration immediately applied provides adequate short-term life support, though the victim may become stiff or rigid in reaction to the shock. Victims of electric shock may suffer from severe burns and permanent aftereffects, including eye cataracts, angina, or disorders of the nervous system.

Electric shock can usually be prevented by strictly adhering to safety guidelines and using commonsensical precautions. Careful inspection of appliances and tools, compliance with manufacturers' safety standards, and the avoidance of unnecessary risks greatly reduce the chance of an electric shock. Electrical appliances or tools should never be used when standing in water or on damp ground, and dry gloves, shoes, and floors provide considerable protection against dangerous shocks from 110 volt circuits.

Electrical safety is also provided by isolation, guarding, insulation, grounding, and ground fault interrupters. Isolation means that high-voltage wires strung overhead are not within reach, while guarding provides a barrier around high voltage devices, such as are found in television sets.

Old wire insulation may become brittle with age and develop small cracks. Defective wires are hazardous and should be replaced immediately. Most modern power tools are double-insulated; the motor is insulated from the plastic insulating frame. These devices do not require grounding, as no exposed metal parts become electrically live if the wire insulation fails.

In a home, grounding is accomplished by a third wire in outlets, connected through a grounding circuit to a water pipe. If an appliance plug has a third prong, it will ground the frame to the grounding circuit. In the event of a short circuit, the grounding circuit provides a low resistance path, resulting in a current surge which trips the circuit breaker.

In some instances, however, the current may be inadequate to trip a circuit breaker (which usually requires 15 or 20 amperes), but current in excess of 10 milliamperes could still be lethal to humans. A ground-fault interrupter ensures nearly complete protection by detecting leakage currents as small as 5 milliamperes and breaking the circuit. This relatively inexpensive device operates very rapidly and provides an extremely high degree of safety against electrocution in the household. Many localities now have codes which require the installation of ground-fault interrupters in bathrooms, kitchens, and other areas where water is used.

—*George R. Plitnik, Ph.D.*

See also Burns and scalds; Critical care; Critical care, pediatric; Emergency medicine; Shock; Resuscitation; Unconsciousness.

FOR FURTHER INFORMATION:

Beausoliel, Robert W., and W. J. Meese. *Survey of Ground Fault Circuit Interrupter Usage for Protection Against Hazardous Shock.* Washington, D.C.: Government Printing Office, 1976. A monograph on ground-fault interrupters and their use.

Bridges, J. E., et al., eds. *International Symposium on Electrical Shock Safety Criteria.* New York: Pergamon Press, 1985. The summary of a symposium covering the physiological effects of shock, bioelectrical conditions, and safety measures.

Hewitt, Paul G. *Conceptual Physics.* 8th ed. Reading, Mass.: Addison-Wesley, 1998. Comprehensive coverage of physics for the layperson that includes detailed discussions of the laws of electricity and electrical devices.

U.S. Department of Labor. Occupational Safety and Health Administration. *Controlling Electrical Hazards.* Washington, D.C.: Government Printing Office, 1991. A report which identifies common electrical hazards and discusses their prevention.

ELECTROCARDIOGRAPHY (ECG OR EKG)

PROCEDURE

ANATOMY OR SYSTEM AFFECTED: Chest, circulatory system, heart

SPECIALTIES AND RELATED FIELDS: Biotechnology, cardiology, critical care, emergency medicine, exercise physiology, preventive medicine

DEFINITION: A noninvasive procedure that provides insight into the rate, rhythm, and general health of the heart.

KEY TERMS:

ECG waves: the repeated deflections of an electrocardiogram; one complete wave consists of a P wave, followed by a QRS complex, and then a T wave and represents one complete cardiac cycle, or heartbeat

electrocardiogram (ECG or EKG): a record of the waves produced by the rhythmically changing electrical conduction within the heart; often recorded by a strip chart recorder

INDICATIONS AND PROCEDURES

Electrocardiography is a useful medical diagnostic and evaluative procedure that reveals much information about the function or malfunction of a person's heart. ECG is a noninvasive, easy-to-use, and economical tool that is an essential part of diagnosing chest pain. It serves an important role in both cardiology and emergency medicine. ECG is also commonly used in preventive medicine to monitor heart health. For this purpose, ECG is frequently used in a format known as a stress test. Athletes often have ECG analysis performed as a part of their training and cardiovascular conditioning.

In a stress test, a person is studied for regularity of rhythm, rate, and unimpeded flow of electrical conduction within the heart. ECG recordings are first made while the person is at rest, then during light exercise, and, finally, if healthy enough, during rigorous exercise. Such exercise causes the heart to work harder and allows a physician to determine if a person has a heart that beats with a regular, repetitive rhythm and at an appropriate pace for the level of rest or exercise. The stress of exercise can also help in assessing whether the heart muscle masses contract in the

Electrocardiography

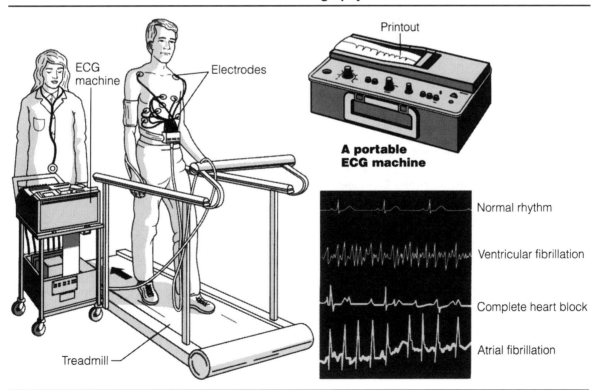

The electrical activity of the heart can be measured with an electrocardiograph (ECG or EKG) machine; characteristic patterns can be used to diagnose arrhythmias (irregular heartbeats). The patient may also be asked to walk on a treadmill while the heart is monitored in order to gauge its function during exercise.

proper sequence: atrial contraction followed by ventricular contraction. An irregularity of electrical conduction, poor muscle contraction, dead regions of the heart tissue (from a recent or old heart attack), and other maladies can be revealed.

In order to obtain an electrocardiogram, small metallic contact points are taped to the patient's skin via an electrically conductive adhesive or gel. The electric impulses travel across the skin to these contact points; from there, leads (plastic-coated wires) are attached to the recording device so that a complete circuit is made. Either a monitor screen or a strip chart recorder traces the electrical impulses. The waves are plotted in units of millivolts (on the y-axis) versus time in units of seconds (on the x-axis).

A twelve-lead ECG has replaced the original four-lead type. A twelve-lead ECG allows the physician to explore the performance of the heart from twelve different orientations, or angles, so that much more of the heart mass is evaluated. The leads (also called electrodes) are placed on the body as follows: one on the right leg, which serves as the ground electrode; one on each of the other extremities; and six on the precordium, which is the area around the sternum and on the left chest wall (over the heart). The leads are explored in different combinations.

USES AND COMPLICATIONS

Healthy people, including athletes or certain members of the armed services, may take a stress test in order to have their health and cardiovascular conditioning monitored during training. Some professionals are required to take stress tests on a regular basis, such as commercial airline pilots and astronauts. In addition, people who have a family history of cardiovascular disease, or who are concerned about their heart health for other reasons, may have a stress test performed to find early warning signs and allow intervention before a crisis occurs. Finally, it should be noted that some insurance companies require stress tests of their applicants in order to determine insurability before issuing or rejecting a policy.

Treatment for chest pain is highly dependent on the electrical patterns seen on the ECG. Drugs may be administered or withheld depending on the shape or duration reported for the P wave, QRS complex, and T-wave patterns. Left-sided versus right-sided heart disease can be discerned from the traces; infarction (heart attack) can be distinguished from angina. Although the waves in the electrocardiogram for an infarcted or anginal heart are abnormal, the patterns become abnormal in a predictable, and therefore diagnostic, manner.

Diagnostic patterns can also be seen for arrhythmias (unusual and abnormal beating patterns), such as ectopic foci, in which some part of the heart other than the sinoatrial (S-A) node (the natural pacemaker) is abnormally in control of determining when the heart contracts, or heart block, whereby electrical conduction is interrupted.

ECG is routinely used to keep close tabs on heart patients

and in the postsurgery monitoring of patients who have had open heart or thoracic surgery. Certain kinds of neonatal or infant malformations or malfunctions may also be evaluated with ECG.

Because ECG is a superficial and noninvasive technique, there are no real risks associated with having this procedure performed.

PERSPECTIVE AND PROSPECTS

Electrocardiography was once a wet, messy, and awkward procedure to perform: A patient dangled one arm in a huge jar filled with a conducting salt solution and placed the left leg in another saline-filled container. Changing the leads to include other limbs required the patient to take a good amount of soaking. Although it was a clumsy procedure, the basic premise of ECG remains unchanged: The heart exhibits regular patterns of electrical activity that can be useful diagnostically.

Recent advances in electrocardiography have involved the use of multiple electrode systems along with computers and recorders that allow rapid and simultaneous multiple-lead input and output. In addition, modern electronic instrumentation allows continuous ECG monitoring so that patients in intensive care units, coronary care units, or emergency rooms can be assessed on a second-by-second basis when seconds count. Undoubtedly, the ECG systems available today, coupled with thoughtful and informed interpretation by medical doctors and emergency medical technicians (EMTs), are responsible for saving many lives. —*Mary C. Fields*

See also Angina; Arrhythmias; Biofeedback; Cardiology; Cardiology, pediatric; Critical care; Critical care, pediatric; Emergency medicine; Exercise physiology; Heart; Heart attack; Paramedics; Stress; Stress reduction.

FOR FURTHER INFORMATION:

Conover, Mary Boudreau. *Understanding Electrocardiography.* 7th ed. St. Louis: C. V. Mosby, 1996.

Phibbs, Brendan. *The Human Heart: A Complete Text on Function and Disease.* 5th ed. St. Louis: G. W. Manning, 1992.

Rawlings, Charles A. *Electrocardiography.* Redmond, Wash.: SpaceLabs, 1991.

Wellens, Hein J. J., and Mary Boudreau Conover. *The ECG in Emergency Decision Making.* Philadelphia: W. B. Saunders, 1992.

ELECTROCAUTERIZATION

PROCEDURE

ANATOMY OR SYSTEM AFFECTED: Blood vessels, circulatory system, genitals (female), reproductive system, skin, uterus

SPECIALTIES AND RELATED FIELDS: Dermatology, general surgery, gynecology

DEFINITION: Cauterization is the destruction of tissue for therapeutic purposes; electrocauterization employs an electric current to do so. This technique is widely employed to halt bleeding from small blood vessels, especially during surgical procedures. It may be used to stop severe nosebleeds or to destroy abnormal blood vessels in the skin. Another major use of electrocauterization is in the treatment of cervicitis, an inflammation or infection of the cervix caused by common vaginal infections, sexually transmitted diseases (STDs), pelvic inflammatory disease, or breaks in cervical tissue from childbirth, intrauterine device insertion, or abortion. For severe cases of cervicitis which do not involve STDs, and when other forms of therapy have failed, electrocauterization may be prescribed to repair the damage. Such procedures are generally performed in a doctor's office without anesthesia. A long, thin electrocautery device is inserted into the vaginal canal, and short bursts of electrical activity destroy the inflamed cervical tissue. Recovery from gynecological electrocauterization may be painful and take up to six weeks, and fertility problems may be a consequence. —*Karen E. Kalumuck, Ph.D.*

See also Cervical procedures; Cryotherapy and cryosurgery; Dermatology; Dermatopathology; Genital disorders, female; Healing; Laser use in surgery; Pelvic inflammatory disease (PID); Sexually transmitted diseases; Skin; Skin disorders; Skin lesion removal; Surgery, general; Surgical procedures; Tumor removal; Tumors.

ELECTROCONVULSIVE THERAPY
PROCEDURE
ANATOMY OR SYSTEM AFFECTED: Brain, nerves, nervous system, psychic-emotional system
SPECIALTIES AND RELATED FIELDS: Neurology, psychiatry
DEFINITION: A treatment for severe mood disorders in which an electrical current is used to induce seizures in the brain, altering its chemistry and thereby relieving depression or mania.
KEY TERMS:
affective disorders: any of a number of mental conditions characterized by a primary disturbance of mood as distinct from thinking or behavior
anesthetic: any of a variety of drugs used to cause a patient to become unconscious and amnesic for a brief period of time; electroconvulsive therapy is conducted under the influence of very short-acting anesthetics, such as methohexital, thiamylal sodium, thiopental sodium, and etomidate
convulsion: an instance of high-frequency and amplitude-random electrical activity in the brain; electroconvulsive therapy causes a convulsion in the brain, which is believed to be related to its mechanism of action
electrocardiogram: a recording of the electrical activity of the heart; used during electroconvulsive therapy to monitor changes in heart rate, rhythm, and conduction, any or all of which may be temporarily affected by this procedure

electroencephalogram: a brain wave trace used to monitor the onset, termination, and duration of the convulsion or seizure
muscle relaxant: any of a number of medications used to paralyze the muscles of the patient temporarily before delivering the electrical stimulus; the main medication used for this purpose is succinylcholine
organic brain syndrome (organicity): changes in memory, orientation, and perception that occur as a side effect of electroconvulsive therapy
seizure: used interchangeably with the term "convulsion"
INDICATIONS AND PROCEDURES
Electroconvulsive therapy (ECT), formerly called electroshock or shock therapy, is a very powerful treatment for mood disorders. It is based on the idea that electrically induced convulsions change the chemistry of the brain in a way that relieves the symptoms of severe mental illness, in which depression, mania, or both become debilitating.

In most situations, electroconvulsive therapy involves the participation of the psychiatrist providing the treatment and an anesthesiologist, who anesthetizes the patient for the procedure. The patient is instructed to take nothing by mouth for eight hours prior to the treatment, so that the stomach is empty for the induction of general anesthesia. The danger of having food or liquid in the stomach is that it might be aspirated into the lungs, where it could cause pneumonia, respiratory obstruction, or death. An intravenous needle is placed in an arm vein. The patient is then connected to a number of monitors, including a blood pressure cuff, electrocardiogram, and pulse oximeter (to measure the level of tissue oxygenation). The patient is then anesthetized with a short-acting intravenous drug (usually methohexital, also known as Brevital). This is followed by the administration of a short-acting muscle relaxant (usually succinylcholine). Ventilation is controlled by mask, using 100 percent oxygen. As soon as it is determined that the muscles are paralyzed, a mild electrical current is administered to the patient's brain. The duration of the stimulus is two seconds or less. There is a brief contraction of the muscles of the face, followed by a generalized seizure, which is monitored on the electroencephalogram. Small amounts of physical movement may be seen in the face, feet, or hands. These movements are not nearly as severe as those that occurred before the advent of muscle relaxants. The anesthesiologist continues to ventilate the patient until the effects of the muscle relaxant have worn off and spontaneous respiration is reestablished (three to five minutes). There is a period of confusion and disorientation that rapidly follows the treatment; it clears quickly. With each successive treatment, the patient is left with an ongoing loss of memory which will gradually clear after the course of therapy is finished. The average patient requires between six and twelve treatments. They are administered two or three times per week.

The decision to conduct electroconvulsive therapy usually comes after there has been failure in other forms of treatment, including medication and psychotherapy. Since there are so many medications and combinations of medication that can be used, however, ECT arguably cannot be thought of as a treatment of last resort, as it was in earlier decades. The idea of administering ECT generally arises when it is critical that the patient improve as rapidly as possible. This consideration is often punctuated by frustration on the part of the patient, the family, and/or the psychiatrist with the slowness of response to current therapeutic modalities. In the 1980's, ECT began to be considered earlier rather than later in the course of treatment. It is realistic to say that if one or two medications are not successful, it is unlikely that others will be successful. Yet there are always those cases in which a sudden and complete remission in affective illness occurs without the use of ECT.

Affective illnesses tend to recur. When treating a patient for the first time, the doctor cannot know whether the effect of ECT will last for a week, months, or years. Some people need only one course of ECT in a lifetime; others will respond well and remain symptom-free for many years, requiring further ECT when symptoms recur. For many patients who develop devastating symptomatology with their illnesses, the early initiation of a course of ECT is warranted. Those who have responded well to only ECT in the past will forgo medication trials in favor of starting ECT as soon as the symptoms reappear. For those patients who respond well to ECT but who have recurrences within weeks or months, maintenance ECT may be a reasonable option. With this regime, a single treatment is given every four to twelve weeks in order to prevent a recurrence of affective symptoms. The actual frequency of treatment is based on each patient's particular clinical course and history. For many patients, maintenance ECT has been a way of preventing multiple and frequent hospitalizations. Very little cognitive impairment is associated with low-frequency maintenance ECT, and patients go on to live very productive lives while being maintained in this way.

The following case is an example of the uses of electroconvulsive therapy in clinical practice: A seventy-five-year-old white, widowed female was referred by her psychiatrist for evaluation for electroconvulsive therapy. She had been well until two years prior to this evaluation. At that time, a month following the death of her husband, she began to experience a variety of symptoms, including loss of appetite with a ten-pound weight loss, decreased interest in her friends and the ordinary activities of life which she had found enjoyable, and sleep disturbance characterized by difficulty falling asleep and early morning awakening. The sleep difficulty was responsive to the use of triazolam, a sleep-inducing drug. Additionally, she began to experience episodes of dizziness that were made worse by antidepressant medications. She was not actively suicidal, but she did experience a wish to die and join her husband, who she believed was waiting for her. She had been treated with tricyclic antidepressants (nortriptyline and desipramine) with lithium augmentation, but the side effects of constipation and dizziness made these medications intolerable. Her depression did not improve, and she began to exhibit medical signs of dehydration and malnutrition. The treating psychiatrist believed that electroconvulsive therapy was indicated and that it should be instituted as rapidly as possible as a lifesaving measure.

The patient was given a course of seven unilateral ECT treatments over the period of a month. She responded to the treatments with an elevation in her mood, an improvement in sleep and appetite, and increasing engagement with hospital staff and family. When she was discharged from the hospital, she showed evidence of mild memory impairment. In the weeks following her treatment, her memory improved, and she became brighter and resumed her normal activities with vigor. She was started on a small dose of fluoxitine (Prozac), an antidepressant known to have a milder side effect profile than the medications she had taken previously. After one year of follow-up, she was still doing well.

Electroconvulsive therapy continues to be widely practiced in the United States and abroad. There is consensus within the field of psychiatry that it is a valuable tool in the psychiatric armamentarium. Patients, patient advocates, and clinicians alike, however, continue to be concerned about its ethical and appropriate use. Practitioners support efforts of the lay community to ensure the proper and ethical use of ECT as long as it does not obstruct access to the treatment for those who require it.

USES AND COMPLICATIONS

Electroconvulsive therapy is used for a variety of psychiatric conditions, including major depressive disorder, depressed bipolar disorder, manic bipolar disorder, mixed bipolar disorder, schizophrenia, manic excitement, and catatonia. Before starting electroconvulsive therapy, all patients are screened for medical illnesses, for two reasons. First, a variety of medical illnesses are associated with depression or mania; the list is long and includes occult cancer, hypothyroidism, vitamin deficiencies, endocrine abnormalities, and brain tumors or infections, among many others. If there is a treatable cause for depression, it must be found and treated before the decision to perform electroconvulsive therapy is made. Once it is clear that the psychiatric illness is not being caused by something else, ECT may be used. It is important to note that there are certain untreatable medical causes for depression or mania in which the affective illness may respond to ECT. For example, depressed patients with Alzheimer's disease may respond to ECT, showing significant improvements in mood. Brain-injured patients with depression may, in some circumstances, respond to electroconvulsive therapy.

The second reason for screening the patient is to establish that it is safe to proceed with ECT. A routine evaluation should include a medical history and physical examination, psychiatric history, mental status examination, blood count, blood chemistries, urinalysis, and electrocardiogram. Other tests may be done if they seem important to rule out other possible illnesses. Such tests might include a computed tomography (CT) scan, a magnetic resonance imaging (MRI) scan, an electroencephalogram (EEG, or brain wave study), or tests for antidepressant drug levels.

There are no absolute reasons not to perform electroconvulsive therapy. There are certain conditions, however, that produce a significant increase in risk with ECT. Cerebral aneurysm may increase the danger of electroconvulsive therapy. An aneurysm is a balloonlike swelling of an artery, which may cause severe brain damage if it bursts. The high blood pressure associated with ECT may cause a cerebral aneurysm to burst. Patients who have recently experienced a heart attack are at increased risk of dying with ECT. Electroconvulsive therapy should be delayed for six months, if possible, following a heart attack. Other illnesses that increase risk include emphysema, multiple sclerosis, and muscular dystrophy.

Despite these risks, electroconvulsive therapy is considered by many to be the safest of the somatic treatments available in psychiatry. The death rate from ECT itself is one patient in ten thousand—much lower, for example, than the death rate for patients taking antidepressant medications; the death rate from suicide in depressed people is much higher. Electroconvulsive therapy may be done safely with patients representing a broad range of age and physical condition. For the elderly, malnourished patient, it is clearly safer and more effective than medication. Prior to the use of muscle relaxants, broken bones and vertebrae were a considerable problem with ECT. This is no longer the case. Complications such as uncontrolled hypertension, stroke, and heart attack rarely occur; they are extremely unlikely, because the patients are medically screened prior to beginning the treatment.

In each situation, the risk of doing ECT must be weighed against the risk of not doing the treatment. If the patient is imminently suicidal—so that he or she cannot be left alone—ECT may be indicated even though the risk is high. Similarly, patients who are starving to death as a result of their illness may require immediate treatment. Patients with manic excitement or delirium, who are completely out of control and require seclusion, may require ECT despite increased risk.

The most disturbing and severe side effect of ECT is memory loss. It is believed that this side effect is attributable to the electricity that is passed through the brain. The postseizure state may also have some effect. What seems to be clear is that this memory deficit is not the result of physical damage to the brain. Some memories, especially those of events that occur around the time of the treatment, may be permanently lost. Many patients will lose their memory of the periods of most severe depression or mania. The ability to learn new information may be temporarily lost. Most people return to reasonable function within the first month and to complete function after six months.

There are a number of ways to gauge the response of a patient to ECT. It is a complicated process that has to take into account and weigh three factors: the improvement of the mood of the patient, the number of treatments or total seizure seconds, and the amount of confusion and/or memory loss that is produced. Additionally, it is important to gauge the emotional response of the patient and the family to the changes being brought about by the treatment.

With each successive treatment, the patient's mood should get better. If the patient has been depressed, there should be a decrease of the depressive symptoms. Appetite and sleep patterns should improve. There should be an increased level of activity, and social engagement should get better. These changes may first be noticeable to the family and hospital staff. Very often, the improvement becomes apparent to the patient later. Occasionally, the improvement will not be obvious until there has been a chance for the confusion and memory loss to resolve. If the patient is manic, there should be an improvement in symptoms of hyperactivity, grandiosity, irritability, and inability to organize activity and behavior. The response of mania to ECT is often very rapid, and the results may be quite gratifying.

If confusion occurs too early in the course of ECT and it is clear that more treatment needs to be done, decreasing the frequency of treatment from three times a week to once or twice a week may be indicated. Ultimately the decision to stop ECT is based on balancing the above-mentioned factors in an optimal way. This determination is made by the clinician with the input of the patient and all the others (psychiatrist, family, and staff) who know the patient best. If the patient does not seem to be improving and is not having memory difficulty, ECT should be continued. Some patients may need as many as twenty treatments to achieve resolution of the mood disorder.

Electroconvulsive therapy is the most effective treatment for major affective disorders. The likelihood of success depends on the specific diagnosis as well as the accuracy of the diagnostic assessment. Patients who have not responded to adequate trials of medication are less likely to respond to ECT than are those who have not been treated with medication. This would seem to reflect the idea that treatment-resistant affective illnesses are less likely to respond to any form of treatment.

PERSPECTIVE AND PROSPECTS

Electroconvulsive therapy was discovered as a therapy of mental illness in the early 1930's. It was first used by Ugo

Cerletti and Lucio Bini in Italy. The basis of its use was the observation that patients with epilepsy did not suffer from schizophrenia. It was believed that there was something about brain seizures that either prevented or was protective against schizophrenia. While that clinical observation was not accurate, it became the impetus for research into the curative effects of electrically induced seizures.

The first electrical convulsions were induced without the benefit of general anesthesia. Patients had violent seizures and often suffered broken bones and teeth. They were held down in order to keep the seizures from causing excessive physical harm. The responses to ECT in certain patients were quite dramatic. Affective symptoms such as depression and mania could often be eliminated. Agitated behavior associated with schizophrenia could be mitigated and patients suffering from catatonia would often become animated as a result of a course of electroconvulsive therapy. The therapy was soon brought to the United States, where it enjoyed frequent use until the early 1950's.

At that time, antipsychotic and antidepressant medications for the treatment of psychiatric illnesses became available. The drugs chlorpromazine and imipramine were shown to be effective in managing the symptoms of schizophrenia and affective illness. As a result, electroconvulsive therapy was used less frequently and then only in severe, treatment-refractory cases. The political climate of the 1960's and 1970's and films such as *One Flew over the Cuckoo's Nest* (1975) portrayed ECT as a tool of the repressive and oppressing psychiatric establishment to exert behavioral and mind control over an unwitting public. Laws were passed in many jurisdictions, making it more difficult for patients to obtain ECT. There were efforts to outlaw ECT. Now, however, even the most powerful patient advocacy groups accept the appropriate use of this treatment.

Electroconvulsive therapy has been utilized with increasing frequency for a number of reasons: recognition of its efficacy, the safety of electroconvulsive therapy in medically ill patients, the increased safety of anesthetic techniques, improved diagnostic criteria, an improved process of informed consent, and disappointing efficacy and side effects of medication in certain patients.

One of the reasons for the renewed interest in ECT is the improvement in informed consent procedures. Physicians no longer adopt as authoritative an attitude toward patients as they did in the past. In the early years of ECT, patients were not informed of all the potential side effects of the treatment. They were often not told that they had alternatives and what the risks and side effects of the alternatives were. The result was that they experienced complications and side effects for which they were not prepared. They became disappointed and angry. Modern informed consent procedures allow the patient to participate as fully as possible in the decision to take any par-

ticular form of therapy. The patient is cognizant of the fact that there are choices and alternatives. The patient is also aware that he or she may decide to discontinue treatment at any time if there is no benefit and the side effects are intolerable. Accurate descriptions of side effects and complications are given to the patient. The patient is apprised of the fact that the treatment may fail and that the treatment is being done this time because it is the one that is most likely to help at this juncture. The patient learns that the choice is simply the best choice, not the only one. Both patients and doctors have benefited from such an enlightened approach to informed consent.

—*Frank Guerra, M.D.*

See also Brain; Depression; Emotions, biomedical causes and effects of; Epilepsy; Manic-depressive disorder; Memory loss; Nervous system; Neurology; Psychiatric disorders; Psychiatry; Psychiatry, child and adolescent; Psychiatry, geriatric; Schizophrenia; Seizures; Sleep disorders.

FOR FURTHER INFORMATION:

Abrams, Richard. *Electroconvulsive Therapy*. 3d ed. New York: Oxford University Press, 1997. A textbook on electroconvulsive therapy that presents a complete picture of all aspects of treatment, from the scientific to the clinical.

American Psychiatric Association. *The Practice of Electroconvulsive Therapy: Recommendations for Treatment, Training, and Privileging*. Washington, D.C.: American Psychiatric Press, 1990. This book is the result of the work of a task force on electroconvulsive therapy in the American Psychiatric Association. It shows how psychiatrists have worked to make the practice of ECT as ethical and safe as possible. Argues for the importance of this form of treatment to psychiatric patients.

Endler, Norman S. *Holiday of Darkness*. New York: John Wiley & Sons, 1982. This book documents the clinical depression of the author, a psychologist, who responded well to electroconvulsive therapy. A very important work that many patients who are contemplating the possibility of ECT may find comforting and useful.

Endler, Norman S., and Emmanuel Persad. *Electroconvulsive Therapy: The Myths and the Realities*. Toronto: Hans Huber, 1988. Another good text on electroconvulsive therapy written by a psychologist who experienced the treatment for his own depression. He has gone on to become a much-honored and internationally recognized teacher and researcher in the field of psychology.

Fink, Max. *Convulsive Therapy: Theory and Practice*. New York: Raven Press, 1979. This book continues to be an excellent introduction to electroconvulsive therapy by the leading practitioner and researcher in the United States. A classic text.

Kellner, Charles H., et al. *Handbook of ECT*. Washington, D.C.: American Psychiatric Press, 1997. This source describes the procedure, its pros and cons, and how it works and is used in contemporary medicine.

ELECTROENCEPHALOGRAPHY (EEG)

PROCEDURE

ANATOMY OR SYSTEM AFFECTED: Brain, head, nervous system, psychic-emotional system

SPECIALTIES AND RELATED FIELDS: Biotechnology, critical care, emergency medicine, neurology, pathology, psychiatry, psychology, speech pathology

DEFINITION: The tracing of the electrical potentials produced by brain cells on a graphic chart, as detected by electrodes placed on the scalp.

KEY TERMS:

brain stem: the medulla oblongata, pons, and mesencephalon portions of the brain, which perform motor, sensory, and reflex functions and contain the corticospinal and reticulospinal tracts

cerebrum: the largest and uppermost section of the brain, which integrates memory, speech, writing, and emotional responses

epilepsy: uncontrollable excessive activity in either all or part of the central nervous system

lesion: a visible local tissue abnormality such as a wound, sore, rash, or boil which can be benign, cancerous, gross, occult, or primary

neurologic: dealing with the nervous system and its disorders

seizure: a sudden, violent, and involuntary contraction of a group of muscles; may be paroxysmal and episodic

INDICATIONS AND PROCEDURES

Clinical electroencephalography (EEG) uses from eight to sixteen pairs of electrodes called derivations. The "international 10-20" system of electrode placement provides coverage of the scalp at standard locations denoted by the letters *F* (frontal), *C* (central), *P* (parietal), *T* (temporal), and *O* (occipital). Subscripts of odd for left-sided placement, even for right-sided placements and *z* for midline placement further define electrode location. During the procedure, the patient remains quiet, with eyes closed, and refrains from talking or moving. In some circumstances, however, prescribed activities such as hyperventilation may be requested. An EEG test is used to diagnose seizure disorders, brain-stem disorders, focal lesions, and impaired consciousness.

Electrical potentials caused by normal brain activity have atypical amplitude of 30 to 100 millivolts and an irregular wavelike variation in time. The main generators of the EEG are probably postsynaptic potentials, with the largest contribution arising from pyramidal cells in the third cortical layer. The ongoing rhythms on an EEG background recording are classified according to the frequencies that they produce as delta (less than 3.5 hertz), theta (4.0 to 7.5 hertz), alpha (8.0 to 13.0 hertz), and beta (greater than 13.5 hertz). In awake but relaxed normal adults, the background consists primarily of alpha activity in occipital and parietal areas and beta activity in central and frontal areas. Variations

in this activity can occur as a function of behavioral state and aging. Alpha waves disappear during sleep and are replaced by synchronous beta waves of higher frequency but lower voltage. Theta waves can occur during emotional stress, particularly during extreme disappointment and frustration. Delta waves occur in deep sleep and infancy and with serious organic brain disease.

USES AND COMPLICATIONS

During neurosurgery, electrodes can be applied directly to the surface of the brain (intracranial EEG) or placed within brain tissue (depth EEG) to detect lesions or tumors. Electrical activity of the cerebrum is detected through the skull in the same way that the electrical activity originating in the heart is detected by an electrocardiogram (ECG or EKG) through the chest wall. The amplitude of the EEG, however, is much smaller than the ECG because the EEG is generated by cells that are not synchronously activated and are not geometrically aligned, whereas the ECG is generated by cells that are synchronously activated and aligned.

Electroencephalography

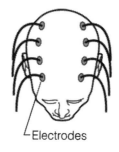
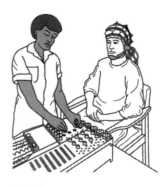

Electrodes

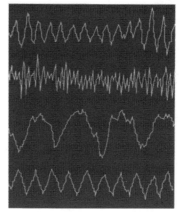

Alpha waves α

Beta waves β

Delta waves δ

Theta waves θ

The electrical activity of the brain can be measured with an electroencephalograph (EEG) machine; characteristic patterns can be used to diagnose some brain disorders and to determine levels of consciousness.

Variations in brain wave activity correlate with neurological conditions such as epilepsy, abnormal psychopathological states, and level of consciousness such as during different stages of sleep.

The two general categories of EEG abnormalities are alterations in background activity and paroxysmal activity. An EEG background with global abnormalities indicates diffuse brain dysfunction associated with developmental delay, metabolic disturbances, infections, and degenerative diseases. EEG background abnormalities are generally not specific enough to establish a diagnosis—for example, the "burst-suppression" pattern may indicate severe anoxic brain injury as well as a coma induced by barbiturates. Some disorders do have characteristic EEG features: An excess of beta activity suggests intoxication, whereas triphasic slow waves are typical of metabolic encephalopathies, particularly as a result of hepatic or renal dysfunction. Psychiatric illness is generally not associated with prominent EEG changes. Therefore, a normal EEG helps to distinguish psychogenic unresponsiveness from neurologic disease. EEG silence is an adjunctive test in the determination of brain death, but it is not a definitive one because it may be produced by reversible conditions such as hypothermia. Focal or lateralized EEG abnormalities in the background imply similarly localized disturbances in brain function and thus suggest the presence of lesions.

Paroxysmal EEG activity consisting of spikes and sharp waves reflects the pathologic synchronization of neurons. The location and character of paroxysmal activity in epileptic patients help clarify the disorder, guide rational anticonvulsant therapy, and assist in determining a prognosis. The diagnostic value of an EEG is often enhanced by activation procedures, such as hyperventilation, photic (light) stimulation, and prolonged ambulatory monitoring, or by using special recording sites, such as nasopharyngeal leads, anterior temporal leads, and surgically placed subdural and depth electrodes. During a seizure, paroxysmal EEG activity replaces normal background activity and becomes continuous and rhythmic. In partial seizures, paroxysmal activity begins in one brain region and spreads to uninvolved regions.

PERSPECTIVE AND PROSPECTS

One of the most important uses of EEGs has been to diagnose certain types of epilepsy and to pinpoint the area in the brain causing the disturbance. Epilepsy is characterized by uncontrollable excessive activity in either all or part of the central nervous system and is classified into three types: grand mal epilepsy, petit mal epilepsy, and focal epilepsy. Additionally, EEGs are often used to localize tumors or other space-occupying lesions in the brain. Such abnormalities may be so large as to cause a complete or partial block in electrical activity in a certain portion of the cerebral cortex, resulting in reduced voltage. More frequently, however, a tumor compresses the surrounding nervous tissue and thereby causes abnormal electrical excitation in these areas.

Some researchers predict new uses of EEG technology in the future, although many of these applications appear dubious. Attempts to interpret thought patterns so that an EEG could serve as a lie detector or measurement of intellectual ability, for example, have proven unsuccessful.

—Daniel G. Graetzer, Ph.D.

See also Brain; Brain disorders; Critical care; Critical care, pediatric; Emergency medicine; Epilepsy; Headaches; Neurology; Neurology, pediatric; Neurosurgery; Positron emission tomography (PET) scanning; Seizures; Tumor removal; Tumors.

FOR FURTHER INFORMATION:

Daly, David D., and Timothy A. Pedley, eds. *Current Practice of Clinical Electroencephalography.* 2d ed. New York: Raven Press, 1990.

Kooi, K. A., et al. *Fundamentals of Electroencephalography.* 2d ed. Hagerstown, Md.: Harper & Row, 1978.

Prince, D. A. "Neurophysiology of Epilepsy." *Annual Review of Neuroscience* 1 (1978): 395-415.

Regan, David. "Electrical Responses Evoked from the Human Brain." *Scientific American* 241, no. 6 (December, 1979): 134-146.

ELECTROLYTES. *See* FLUIDS AND ELECTROLYTES.

ELEPHANTIASIS
DISEASE/DISORDER

ANATOMY OR SYSTEM AFFECTED: Lymphatic system

SPECIALTIES AND RELATED FIELDS: Environmental health, epidemiology, public health

DEFINITION: A grossly disfiguring disease caused by a roundworm parasite; it is the advanced stage of the disease Bancroft's filariasis, contracted through roundworms.

KEY TERMS:

acute disease: a disease in which symptoms develop rapidly and which runs its course quickly

chronic disease: a disease that develops more slowly than an acute disease and persists for a long time

host: any organism on or in which another organism (called a parasite) lives, usually for the purpose of nourishment or protection

inflammation: a response of the body to tissue damage caused by injury or infection and characterized by redness, pain, heat, and swelling

lymph nodes: globular structures located along the routes of the lymphatic vessels that filter microorganisms from the lymph

lymphatic system: a body system consisting of lymphatic vessels and lymph nodes that transports lymph through body tissues and organs; closely associated with the cardiovascular system *lymphatic vessels:* vessels that form a system for returning lymph to the bloodstream

parasite: an organism that lives on or within another organism, called the host, from which it derives sustenance or protection at the host's expense

CAUSES AND SYMPTOMS

Elephantiasis is found worldwide, mostly in the tropics and subtropics. Most cases of elephantiasis are a result of infection with a parasitic worm called *Wuchereria bancrofti* (*W. bancrofti*). *W. bancrofti* belongs to a group of worms called filaria, or roundworms, and infection with a filarial worm is called filariasis. Filariasis caused by *W. bancrofti* is the most common and widespread type of human filarial infection and is often called Bancroft's filariasis. Elephantiasis is the advanced, chronic stage of Bancroft's filariasis, and only a small percentage of persons with Bancroft's filariasis will develop elephantiasis. During Bancroft's filariasis, adult forms of *W. bancrofti* live inside the human lymphatic system, and it is the person's reaction to the presence of the worm that causes the symptoms of the disease. The worm's life cycle is important in understanding how the disease is transmitted from one person to another, how the symptoms develop, and how to prevent and reduce the incidence of the disease.

The adult worms live in human lymphatic vessels and lymph nodes and measure about four centimeters in length for the male and nine centimeters in length for the female. Both are threadlike and about 0.3 millimeter in diameter. After mating, the female releases large numbers of embryos or microfilariae (microscopic roundworms), which are more than one hundred times smaller in length and ten times thinner than their parents. They make their way from the lymphatic system into the bloodstream, where they can circulate for two years or longer. Interestingly, most strains of microfilariae (all except those found in the South Pacific Islands) exhibit a nocturnal periodicity, in which they appear in the peripheral blood system (the outer blood vessels, such as those in the arms, legs, and skin) only at night, mostly between the hours of 10 P.M. and 2 A.M., and the remainder of the time they spend in the blood vessels of the lungs and other internal organs. This nighttime cycling into the peripheral blood is somehow related to the patient's sleeping habits, and although it is unknown exactly how or why the microfilariae do this, it is necessary for the survival of the worms. The microfilariae must develop through at least three different stages (called the first, second, and third larval stages) before they are ready to mature into adults; these stages take place not within humans, but within certain types of mosquitoes, which bite at night. Thus, the microfilariae appear in the peripheral blood just in time for the mosquitoes to bite an infected human and extract them so that they can continue their life cycle. It is important to note, therefore, that both humans and the proper type of mosquito are needed to keep a filariasis infection going in a particular area.

Female night-feeding mosquitoes of the genera *Culex*, *Aedes*, and *Anopheles* serve as intermediate hosts for *Wuchereria bancrofti*. The mosquitoes bite an infected person and ingest microfilariae from the peripheral blood. The microfilariae pass into the intestines of the mosquito, invade the intestinal wall, and within a day find their way to the thoracic muscles (the muscles in the middle part of the mosquito's body). There they develop from first-stage to third-stage larvae in about two weeks, and the new third-stage larvae move from the thoracic muscles to the head and mouth of the mosquito. Only the third-stage larvae are able to infect humans successfully, and the third stage can mature only inside humans. When the mosquito takes a blood meal, infective larvae make their way through the proboscis (the tubular sucking organ with which a mosquito bites a person) and enters the skin through the puncture wound. After they enter the skin, the larvae move by an unknown route to the lymphatic system, where they develop into adult worms. It takes about one year or longer for the larvae to grow into adults, mate, and produce more microfilariae.

A person contracts Bancroft's filariasis by being bitten by an infected mosquito. Various forms of the disease can occur, depending on the person's immune response and the number of times the person is bitten. The period of time from when a person is first infected with larvae to the time microfilariae appear in the blood can be between one and two years. Even after this time some persons, especially young people, show no symptoms at all, yet they may have numerous microfilariae in their blood. This period of being a carrier of microfilariae without showing any signs of disease may last several years, and such carriers act as reservoirs for infecting the mosquito population.

In those patients showing symptoms from the infection, there are two stages of the disease: acute and chronic. In acute disease, the most common symptoms are a recurrent fever and lymphangitis and/or lymphadenitis in the arms, legs, or genitals. These symptoms are caused by an inflammatory response to the adult worms trapped inside the lymphatic system. Lymphangitis, an inflammation of the lymph vessels, is characterized by a hard, cordlike swelling or a red superficial streak that is tender and painful. Lymphadenitis is characterized by swollen and painful lymph nodes. The attacks of fever and lymphangitis or lymphadenitis recur at irregular intervals and may last from three weeks up to three months. The attacks usually become less frequent as the disease becomes more chronic. In the absence of reinfection, there is usually a steady improvement in the victim, each relapse being milder. Thus, without specific therapy, this condition is self-limiting and presumably will not become chronic in those acquiring the infection during a brief visit to an area where the disease is endemic.

The most obvious symptoms caused as a result of *W. bancrofti* infection, such as elephantiasis, are noted in the chronic stage. Chronic disease occurs only after years of repeated infection with the worms. It is seen only in areas where the disease is endemic and only occurs in a small percentage of the infected population. The symptoms are the result of an accumulation of damage caused by inflammatory reactions to the adult worms. The inflammation causes tissue death and a buildup of scar tissue that eventually results in the blockage of the lymphatic vessels in which the worms live. One of the functions of lymphatic vessels is to carry excess fluid away from tissues and bring it back to the blood, where it enters the circulation again as the fluid portion of the blood. If the lymphatic vessels are blocked, the excess fluid stays in the tissues, and swelling occurs. When this swelling is extensive, grotesque enlargement of that part of the body occurs. Elephantiasis is characterized by gross enlargement of a body part caused by the accumulation of fluid and connective tissue. It most frequently affects the legs, but may also occur in the arms, breasts, scrotum, vulva, or any other body part. The disease starts with the slight enlargement of one leg or arm (or other body part). The limb increases in size with recurrent attacks of fever. Gradually, the affected part swells, and the swelling, which is soft at first, becomes hard following the growth of connective tissue in the area. In addition, the skin over the swollen area changes so that it becomes coarse and thickened, looking almost like elephant hide. The elephant-like skin, along with the enlarged body parts, gave the disease the name "elephantiasis."

TREATMENT AND THERAPY

One way in which doctors can tell whether a person has Bancroft's filariasis is by taking a sample of peripheral blood between 10 P.M. and 2 A.M. and looking at the blood under a microscope to try to find microfilariae. Sometimes, the ability to find microfilariae is enhanced by filtering the blood to concentrate the possible microfilariae in a smaller volume of liquid. Many persons infected with *W. bancrofti* have no detectable microfilariae in their blood, so other methods are available. In the absence of microfilariae, a diagnosis can be made on the basis of a history of exposure, symptoms of the disease, positive antibody or skin tests, or the presence of worms in a sample of lymph tissue. It is important to note that occasionally a few other filarial worms and at least one bacteria can also cause elephantiasis; therefore, if symptoms of elephantiasis are observed, it is important to discover the correct cause so that the proper treatment can be given. Since chronic infection occurs after prolonged residence in areas where the disease occurs, patients with acute disease should be removed from those areas. They also should be reassured that elephantiasis is a rare complication that is limited to persons who have had constant exposure to infected mosquitoes for years.

The best way to avoid contracting filariasis when traveling to an affected area is to avoid being bitten by mosquitoes. Insect repellent, mosquito netting, and other methods

Elephantiasis

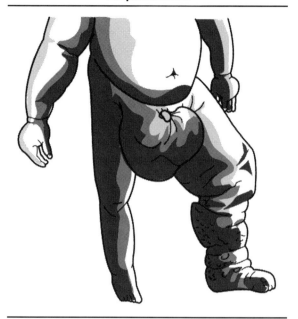

The common symptoms of acute elephantiasis are a recurrent fever and lymphangitis and/or lymphadenitis in the arms, legs, or genitals; if the conditions develop into chronic elephantiasis, the result can be layers of scar tissue that block the lymphatic vessels, leading to a buildup of fluid in the tissues. Grotesque swellings and tissue growth may result.

are helpful in this regard. No drugs or vaccines are available to prevent infection once a person is bitten.

A problem in the treatment of all parasitic diseases is finding a drug that will kill the parasite without harming the human host. The drug diethylcarbamazine (DEC) is the drug of choice in treating Bancroft's filariasis. Its advantages are that it can be taken orally, patients have a relatively high tolerance to the drug, and it has relatively rapid, beneficial, clinical effects. Generally, in the treatment of acute disease, excellent results are obtained when the proper dosage of the drug is given. There are only two relatively mild side effects of DEC. The first is nausea or vomiting. This symptom depends on the amount of the drug given; therefore, lower doses help alleviate this side effect. The second is fever and dizziness, the severity of which depends on the number of microfilariae a person has in his or her blood; the more microfilariae, the more severe the reaction. It is important to warn patients ahead of time about the fever reaction and encourage them to continue taking their doses anyway. The fever reaction is a sign that the patient is being cured, but the cure will not completely work if the patient does not finish the whole regimen of drug doses. Other drugs have been used in the treatment of filariasis (suramin, metrifonate, levamisole) but are generally less effective or more toxic than DEC. Additional treatment measures include bed rest and supportive measures, such as using hot and cold compresses to reduce swelling. The administration of antibiotics for patients with secondary bacterial infections and painkillers as well as anti-inflammatory agents during the painful, acute stage is helpful. Sometimes, swollen limbs can be wrapped in pressure bandages to force the lymph from them. If the distortion is not too great, this method is successful. It should also be noted that, although drugs such as DEC might be effective in killing *W. bancrofti*, the chronic lesions resulting from the infection are mostly incurable. Signs of chronic filariasis, such as elephantiasis of the limbs or the scrotum, are usually unaffected or only incompletely cured by medication, and it sometimes becomes necessary to apply surgical or other symptomatic treatments to relieve the suffering of the patients. Chronic obstruction in less advanced stages is sometimes improved by surgery. The surgical removal of an elephantoid breast, vulva, or scrotum is sometimes necessary.

Theoretically, it should be possible first to control and eventually to eliminate Bancroft's filariasis. Conditions that are highly favorable for continued propagation of the infection include a pool of microfilariae carriers in the human population and the right species of mosquitoes breeding near human habitations. Thus, control can be effected by treating all microfilariae carriers in an affected area and eliminating the necessary mosquitoes. Microfilariae carriers can be effectively treated with DEC. The decision usually is between giving mass drug treatment to the entire population in an affected area or only treating those persons who are microfilariae positive. Usually, if the infection is at a high rate and very widespread in an area, it is best to treat the entire population, since it would be very time consuming, difficult, and expensive to find all the microfilariae carriers. In other areas that are smaller or in which the pockets of infection are well defined, it is better to identify all the microfilariae-positive persons and treat only those persons until they are cured. The second control measure is to eliminate the mosquito population. It is important to note that eliminating the mosquitoes alone will not control the disease, especially in tropical areas, since the breeding period and season in which the disease can be transmitted is so extensive. In some temperate areas, where Bancroft's filariasis used to be endemic, measures that removed the mosquitoes alone aided in the elimination of the disease from that area, since in temperate areas the breeding period and thus the season for transmission is so short. In tropical areas, both DEC therapy and mosquito control must be applied in order to control the disease. The mosquito population can be controlled in four ways. First, general sanitation measures can be carried out in order to reduce the areas where the mosquitoes are breeding; for example, draining swamps. Second, insecticides can be used to kill

the adult mosquitoes. Third, larvacides can be applied to sources of water where mosquitoes breed in order to kill the mosquito larvae. Finally, natural mosquito predators, such as certain species of fish, can be introduced into waters where mosquitoes breed to eat the mosquito larvae. Numerous problems stand in the way of eradication, such as poor sanitation, persons who do not cooperate with medical intervention, mosquitoes that become resistant to all known insecticides, increasing technology that yields increasing water supplies and therefore places for mosquitoes to breed, large populations, ignorance of the cause of the disease, and lack of medicine and a way of distributing that medicine.

PERSPECTIVE AND PROSPECTS

Dramatic symptoms of elephantiasis, especially the enormous swelling of legs or scrotum, were recorded in much of the ancient medical literature of India, Persia, and the Far East. The embryonic form of microfilariae was first discovered and described by a Frenchman in Paris in 1863. The organism was named for O. Wucherer, who also discovered microfilariae in 1866, and Joseph Bancroft, who discovered the adult worm in 1876. Two important facts about *W. bancrofti*—namely, its development in mosquitoes and the nocturnal periodicity of the microfilariae—were discovered by Patrick Manson between 1877 and 1879. This was the first example of a disease being transmitted by a mosquito, and its discovery earned for Manson the title of Father of Tropical Medicine. These and most of the other essential facts of the disease were discovered before the end of the nineteenth century. Progress in the epidemiology and control of filariasis came after World War II. In 1947, DEC was shown to kill filariae in animals, and this result was followed by the successful use of DEC in the treatment of humans. The first promising results in the control of Bancroft's filariasis by mass administration of DEC were reported in 1957 on a small island in the South Pacific. Through subsequent studies, it has become clear that effective control of the infection can be achieved if sufficient dosages of DEC are administered to infected populations.

Filariasis is a serious health hazard and public health problem in many tropical countries. Infection with *Wuchereria bancrofti* has been recorded in nearly all countries or territories in the tropical and subtropical zones of the world. The infection occurs primarily in coastal areas and islands that experience long periods of high humidity and heat. Infections have also been noted from some temperate zone districts, such as mainland Japan, central China, and some European countries. There is more Bancroft's filariasis now than there was a hundred years ago, principally because of increases in population in affected areas and in increased resistance of mosquitoes to insecticides. In 1947, it was estimated that 189 million people were infected with *W. bancrofti*. More recently, the World Health Organization estimated that 250 million people are infected and 400 million are at risk.

Bancroft's filariasis was introduced into and became endemic to Charleston, South Carolina, until 1920. It disappeared in the United States before World War II, presumably because of a reduction of mosquitoes resulting from improved sanitation. Servicemen in the Pacific in World War II were concerned about contracting elephantiasis; although several thousand showed signs of acute filariasis, only twenty had microfilariae in their blood, and no one developed elephantiasis. In the United States today, the infection is most frequently seen in immigrants, military veterans, and missionaries. It is important for physicians to be aware of this and other tropical diseases so that they can treat the occasional patient who is suffering from one of them, since most of these diseases are more successfully treated in the early stages of the disease.

—*Vicki J. Isola, Ph.D.*

See also Arthropod-borne diseases; Bites and stings; Edema; Inflammation; Lymphadenopathy and lymphoma; Lymphatic system; Parasitic diseases; Roundworm; Tropical medicine; Worms; Zoonoses.

FOR FURTHER INFORMATION:

Beaver, Paul C., and Rodney C. Jung. *Animal Agents and Vectors of Human Disease*. 5th ed. Philadelphia, Pa.: Lea & Febiger, 1985. Discusses all major parasitic diseases. Chapter 12, "Filariae," which describes those diseases caused by filarial worms, contains helpful photographs and diagrams.

Foster, William D. *A History of Parasitology*. Edinburgh: E. & S. Livingstone, 1965. Describes the history of the discovery of the causes of parasitic diseases. Chapter 7, "*Wuchereria Bancrofti*," gives a detailed and interesting account of the history behind the discovery of the causes and nature of Bancroft's filariasis.

Ransford, Oliver. *'Bid the Sickness Cease.'* London: John Murray, 1983. Discusses the effect of disease on the development of Africa. Chapter 6, "The Father of Tropical Medicine," describes how Patrick Manson made the original discoveries of the cause of elephantiasis.

Roberts, Larry S., and John Janovy, Jr., eds. *Gerald D. Schmidt and Larry S. Roberts' Foundations of Parasitology*. Rev. 5th ed. Dubuque, Iowa: Wm. C. Brown, 1996. Gives a good general description of all parasitic diseases, their causes, effects, and treatments. Deals specifically with diseases caused by filariae, including *Wuchereria bancrofti*.

Sasa, Manabu. *Human Filariasis*. Baltimore: University Park Press, 1976. This book, though written as a field guide for the person working in some aspect of filariasis, is extremely well organized and easy to read. It describes in detail every filarial disease, including infections with *Wuchereria bancrofti*. It gives comprehensive details of the geographic distribution of the disease in every country in the world and describes the current methodology in studying filariasis and trying to control the disease.

Zinsser, Hans. *Zinsser Microbiology*. Edited by Wolfgang K. Joklik et al. 20th ed. Norwalk, Conn.: Appleton and Lange, 1992. The information presented in this textbook is thorough, logical, and supplemented by interesting diagrams, photographs, and charts. Contains a thorough description of Bancroft's filariasis.

EMBOLISM

DISEASE/DISORDER

ANATOMY OR SYSTEM AFFECTED: Blood vessels, brain, chest, circulatory system, head, heart, lungs, respiratory system

SPECIALTIES AND RELATED FIELDS: Internal medicine, vascular medicine

DEFINITION: Embolism is the obstruction of circulation through a blood vessel by an embolus, such as a blood clot, a piece of tissue, cholesterol, fat, bone marrow, or an air bubble. Pulmonary embolism, the presence of an obstruction in the lung, is the most common site because all the blood in the body must pass through the lungs with every circuit made. Emboli can form after an operation or prolonged inactivity because of illness or injury: Blood clots may form in the deep veins of the legs, and pieces of these clots break away to travel through the bloodstream. Emboli can be removed surgically, or drugs to dissolve blood clots and to prevent their formation may be administered.

—*Jason Georges and Tracy Irons-Georges*

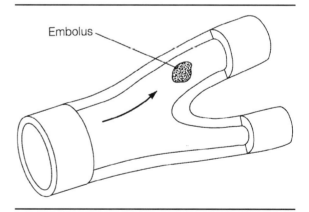

An embolus is any material that is flowing in the bloodstream that obstructs a blood vessel; it may, for example, be a piece of a fatty plaque that has broken off an arterial wall.

See also Arteriosclerosis; Blood and blood components; Cholesterol; Circulation; Elephantiasis; Embolism; Heart; Heart disease; Hypercholesterolemia; Lungs; Phlebitis; Pulmonary diseases; Pulmonary medicine; Pulmonary medicine, pediatric; Respiration; Thrombosis and thrombus; Varicose vein removal; Varicosis; Vascular medicine; Vascular system; Venous insufficiency.

EMBRYOLOGY

SPECIALTY

ANATOMY OR SYSTEM AFFECTED: All

SPECIALTIES AND RELATED FIELDS: Genetics, neonatology, obstetrics, perinatology

DEFINITION: The study of prenatal development from conception until the moment of birth.

KEY TERMS:

blastocyst: a small, hollow ball of cells which typifies one of the early embryonic stages in humans

cleavage: the process by which the fertilized egg undergoes a series of rapid cell divisions, which results in the formation of a blastocyst

congenital malformation: any anatomical defect present at birth

embryo: the developing human from conception until the end of the eighth week

fetus: the developing human from the end of the eighth week until the moment of birth

neural tube: the embryonic structure that gives rise to the central nervous system

teratogens: substances that induce congenital malformations when embryonic tissues and organs are exposed to them

zygote: the fertilized egg; the first cell of a new organism

SCIENCE AND PROFESSION

The study of human embryology is the study of human prenatal development. The three stages of development are cleavage (the first week), embryonic development (the second through eighth weeks), and fetal development (the ninth through thirty-eighth weeks).

After an egg is fertilized by sperm in the uterine, or Fallopian, tube, the resulting zygote begins to divide rapidly. This period of rapid cell division is known as cleavage. By the third day, the zygote has divided into a solid ball containing twelve to sixteen cells. The small ball of cells resembles a mulberry and is called the morula, which is Latin for "mulberry." The morula moves from the uterine tube into the uterus.

The morula develops a central cavity as spaces begin to form between the inner cells. At this stage, the developing human is called a blastocyst. The ring of cells on the outer edge of the hollow ball is called the trophoblast and will form a placenta, while the cluster of cells within becomes the inner cell mass and will form the embryo. By the end of the first week, the surface of the inner cell mass has flattened to form an embryonic disc, and the blastocyst has attached to the lining of the uterus and begun to embed itself.

During the second week of development, the trophoblast makes connections with the uterus to form the placenta. Blood vessels from the embryo link it to the placenta through the umbilical cord, through which the embryo receives food and oxygen and releases wastes. Two sacs develop around the embryo: the fluid-filled amniotic sac that surrounds and cushions the embryo and the yolk sac that hangs beneath to provide nourishment. Finally, a large chorionic sac develops around the embryo and the two smaller sacs.

During the third week, the cells of the embryo are arranged in three layers. The outer layer of cells is called the ectoderm, the middle layer is the mesoderm, and the inner layer is the endoderm. The ectoderm gives rise to the epidermis (outer layer) of the skin and to the nervous system; the mesoderm gives rise to blood, bone, cartilage, and muscle; and the endoderm gives rise to body linings and glands.

Other significant events of the third week are the development of the primitive streak and notochord. The primitive streak is a thickened line of cells on the embryonic disk indicating the future embryonic axis. Development of the primitive streak stimulates the formation of a supporting rod of tissue beneath it called the notochord. The presence of the notochord triggers the ectoderm in the primitive streak above it to thicken, and the thickened area will give rise to the brain and spinal cord. Later, when vertebrae and muscles develop around the neural tissue, the notochord will disappear.

The Development of an Embryo in the First Two Months

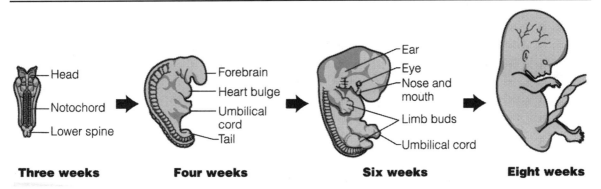

Three weeks — Head, Notochord, Lower spine

Four weeks — Forebrain, Heart bulge, Umbilical cord, Tail

Six weeks — Ear, Eye, Nose and mouth, Limb buds, Umbilical cord

Eight weeks

The important event of the fourth week is the formation of the neural tube. After the thickened neural plate tissue has formed, an upward folding forms a groove, finally closing to form a neural tube. Closure begins at the head end and proceeds backward. The neural tube then sinks beneath surrounding ectodermal surface cells, which will become the skin covering the embryo.

Blocks of mesoderm cells line up along either side of the notochord and neural tube. These blocks are called somites, and eventually forty-two to forty-four pairs will form. They give rise to muscle, to the skeleton and cartilage of the head and trunk, and to the inner layer of skin. At the same time, embryonic blood vessels develop on the yolk sac. Because the human embryo is provided little yolk, there is need for early development of a circulatory system.

The heart is formed and begins to beat in the fourth week, though it is not yet connected to many blood vessels. During the fourth through eighth weeks, all the organ systems develop, and the embryo is especially vulnerable to teratogens (environmental agents that interfere with normal development). A noticeable change in shape is seen during the fourth week because the rapidly increasing number of cells causes a folding under at the edges of the embryonic disk. The flattened disk takes on a cylindrical shape, and the folding process causes curvature of the embryo and it comes to lie on its side in a C-shaped position.

The beginnings of arms and legs are first seen in the fourth week and are called limb buds, appearing first as small bumps. The lower end of the embryo resembles a tail, and the swollen cranial part of the neural tube constricts to form three early sections of the brain. The eyes and ears begin to develop from the early brain tissue.

During the fifth through eighth weeks, the head enlarges as a result of rapid brain development. The head makes up almost half the embryo, and facial features begin to appear. Sexual differences exist but are difficult to detect. Nerves and muscles have developed enough to allow movement. By the end of the eighth week the limb buds have grown and differentiated into appendages with paddle-shaped hands and feet and short, webbed digits. The tail disappears, and the embryo begins to demonstrate human characteristics. By convention, the embryo is now called a fetus.

The fetal stage of development is the period between the ninth and thirty-eighth weeks, until birth. Organs formed during the embryonic stage grow and differentiate during the fetal stage. The body has the largest growth spurt between the ninth and twentieth weeks, but the greatest weight gain occurs during the last weeks of pregnancy.

In the third month, the difference between the sexes becomes apparent, urine begins to form and is excreted into the amniotic fluid, and the fetus can blink its eyelids. The fetus nearly doubles in length during the fourth month, and the head no longer appears to be so disproportionately large. Ossification of the skeleton begins, and by the end of the fourth month, ovaries are differentiated in the female fetus and already contain many cells destined to become eggs.

During the fifth month, fetal movements are felt by the mother, and the heartbeat can be heard with a stethoscope. Movements until this time usually go unnoticed. The average length of time that elapses between the first movement felt by the mother and delivery is twenty-one weeks.

During the sixth month, weight is gained by the fetus, but it is not until the seventh month that a baby usually can survive premature birth, when the body systems are mature enough to function. During the eighth month, the eyes develop the ability to control the amount of light that enters them. Fat accumulates under the skin and fills in wrinkles. The skin becomes pink and smooth, and the arms and legs may become chubby. In the male fetus, the testes descend into the scrotal sac. Growth slows as birth approaches. The usual gestation length is 266 days, or thirty-eight weeks after fertilization.

Diagnostic and Treatment Techniques

Knowledge of normal embryonic development is very important both in helping women provide optimal prenatal care for their children and in promoting scientific research for improved prenatal treatment, better understanding of malignant growths, and insight into the aging process.

Environmental stress to the embryo during the fourth through eighth weeks can cause abnormal development and result in congenital malformation, which may be defined as any anatomical defect present at birth. Environmental agents that cause malformations are known as teratogens. Malformations may develop from genetic or environmental factors, but most often they are caused by a combination of the two. Some of the common teratogens are viral infections, drug use, a poor diet, smoking, alcohol consumption, and irradiation.

The genetic makeup of some individuals makes them particularly sensitive to certain agents, while others are resistant. The abnormalities may be immediately apparent at birth or hidden within the body and discovered later. Embryos with severe structural abnormalities often do not survive, and such abnormalities represent an important cause of miscarriages.

Genetic birth defects are passed on from one generation to another and result from a gene mutation at some time in the past. Mutations are caused by accidental rearrangement of deoxyribonucleic acid (DNA), the material of which genes are made, and range in severity from mild to life-threatening. They may cause such conditions as extra fingers and toes, cataracts, dwarfism, albinism, and cystic fibrosis. Gene mutations on a sex chromosome are described as sex-linked and are usually passed from mother to son; these include hemophilia, hydrocephalus (an excessive amount of cerebrospinal fluid), color blindness, and a form of baldness.

Abnormalities in the embryo may result because of unequal distribution of chromosomes in the formation of eggs or sperm. This imbalance can cause a variety of problems in development, such as Down syndrome and abnormal sexual development because of variable numbers of sex chromosomes. The normal human cell contains twenty-three chromosomes, twenty-two pairs of which are nonsex chromosomes, or autosomes. The last pair consists of the two sex chromosomes. Females normally have two X chromosomes, and males have an X and a Y chromosome.

When females have only one X, a set of conditions known as Turner's syndrome results. The embryo will develop as a normal female, though ovaries will not fully form and there may be congenital heart defects. Because the single X chromosome does not cause enough estrogen to be produced, sexual maturity will not occur. If a male embryo should receive only the Y chromosome, it cannot survive. Sometimes a male will receive two (or more) X chromosomes along with a Y chromosome (XXY), producing Klinefelter's syndrome. The appearance of the child is normal, but at puberty the breasts may enlarge and the testes will not mature, causing sterility. Males receiving two Y chromosomes (XYY) develop normally, but they may be quite tall and find controlling their impulses to be difficult.

Viral infections in the mother during the embryonic stages can cause problems in organ formation by disturbing normal cell division, fetal vascularization, and the development of the immune system. The organs most vulnerable to infection will be those undergoing rapid cell division and growth at the time of infection. For example, the lens of the eye is forming during the sixth week of development, and infection at this time could cause the formation of cataracts.

While most microorganisms cannot pass through the placenta to reach the embryo or fetus, those that can are capable of causing major problems in the embryonic development. Rubella, the virus that causes German measles, often causes birth defects in children should infection occur shortly before or during the first three months of pregnancy. The developing ears, eyes, and heart are especially susceptible to damage during this time. When a rubella infection occurs during the first five weeks of pregnancy, interference with organ development is most pronounced. After the fifth week, the risks of infection are not as great, but central nervous system impairment may occur as late as the seventh month.

The most common source of fetal infection may be the cytomegalovirus (CMV), a form of herpes which causes abortion during the first three months of pregnancy. If infection occurs later, the liver and brain are especially vulnerable and impairment in vision, hearing, and mental ability may result. Evidence has also suggested that the immune system of the fetus is adversely affected.

Other viruses may affect fetal development as well. When herpes simplex infects the fetus several weeks before birth, blindness or mental retardation may result. *Toxoplasma gondii*, a parasite of animals often kept as pets, may adversely affect eye and brain development without the mother having known that she had the infection. Syphilis infection in the mother leads to death or serious fetal abnormalities unless it is treated before the sixteenth week of pregnancy; if it is untreated, the fetus may possess hearing impairment, hydrocephalus, facial abnormalities, and mental retardation. Women infected with acquired immunodeficiency syndrome (AIDS) may transmit the virus to their infants before or during birth.

Certain chemicals can cross the placenta and produce malformation of developing tissues and organs. During an embryo's first twenty-five days, damage to the primitive streak can cause malformation in bone, blood, and muscle. While bones and teeth are being formed, they may be adversely affected by antibiotics such as tetracycline.

At one time, thalidomide was widely used as an antinauseant in Great Britain and Germany and to some extent in the United States. Large numbers of congenital abnormalities began to appear in newborns, and the drug was withdrawn from the market after two years. Thalidomide caused failure of normal limb development and was especially damaging during the third to seventh weeks.

Exposure to other chemicals causes central nervous system disorders when the neural tube fails to close. When the anterior end of the tube does not close, development of the brain and spinal cord will be absent or incomplete and anencephaly results. Babies can live no more than a few days with this condition because the higher control centers of the brain are missing. If the posterior end of the tube fails to close, one or more vertebrae will not develop completely, exposing the spinal cord; this condition is called spina bifida. This condition varies in severity with the amount of neural tissue that remains exposed, because exposed tissue degenerates.

It has been long believed that neural tube disorders accompanied maternal depletion of folic acid, one of the B vitamins, and research has substantiated that relationship. Anencephaly and spina bifida rarely occur in the infants of women taking folic acid supplements. One of the harmful effects of alcohol and anticonvulsants is their depletion of the body's natural folic acid. A decrease in the mother's folic acid levels in the first through third months of pregnancy can cause abortion or growth deformities.

Maternal smoking is strongly implicated in low infant birth weights and higher fetal and infant mortality rates. Cigarette smoke may cause cardiac abnormalities, cleft lip and palate, and a missing brain. Nicotine decreases blood flow to the uterus and interferes with normal development, allowing less oxygen to reach the embryo.

Alcohol use may be the number-one cause of birth defects. Exposure of the fetus to alcohol in the blood results in fetal alcohol syndrome. Symptoms may include growth deficiencies, an abnormally small head, facial malformation, and damage to the heart and the nervous and reproductive systems. Behavioral disorders such as hyperactivity, attention deficit, and inability to relate to others may accompany fetal alcohol syndrome.

Radiation treatments given to pregnant women may cause cell death, chromosomal injury, and growth retardation in the developing embryo. The effect is proportional to the dosage of radiation. Malformations may be visible at birth, or a condition such as leukemia may develop later. Abnormalities caused by radiation include cleft palate, an abnormally small head, mental retardation, and spina bifida. Diagnostic X rays are not believed to emit enough radiation to cause abnormalities in embryonic development, but precautions should be taken.

Oxygen deficiency to the embryo or fetus occurs when mothers use cocaine. Maternal blood pressure fluctuates with the use of this drug, and the embryonic brain is deprived of oxygen, resulting in vision problems, lack of coordination, and mental retardation. Too little oxygen to the fetus may also cause death from lung collapse soon after birth.

Obvious physical malformations resulting from embryonic exposure to drugs have been recognized for a number of years, but recent investigators have found there are more subtle levels of effect that may show up later as behavioral problems. Physical abnormalities have been easily documented, but more attention is needed regarding the behavioral effects caused by teratogens.

PERSPECTIVE AND PROSPECTS

The first recorded observations of a developing embryo were performed on a chick by Hippocrates in the fifth century B.C. In the fourth century B.C., Aristotle wondered whether a preformed human unfolded in the embryo and enlarged with time, or whether a very simple embryonic structure gradually became more and more complex. This question was debated for nearly two thousand years until the early nineteenth century, when microscopic studies of chick embryos were carefully conducted and described.

Understanding human embryology is foundational for recognizing the relationships that exist between the body systems and congenital malformations in newborns. This field of study takes on new importance in the light of advances of modern technology, which have made prenatal diagnosis and treatment a reality.

The study of embryology is also making contributions toward finding the causes of malignant growth. Malignancy is a breakdown in the mechanisms for normal growth and differentiation first seen in the early embryo. Questions about uninhibited malignant growth may be answered by studying embryonic tissues and organs.

The study of old age is another area in which embryo-

logical research is valuable. Understanding the clock mechanisms of embryonic cells has led to greater understanding of the "winding down" of cells in old age. It is also important that researchers discover how environmental conditions modify rates of growth and affect the cell's clock. The degree to which the human life span can be expanded remains one of the most challenging questions in the area of aging.

In addition to the health benefits that may be derived from embryological research, this field is an important source of insight into some of the moral and ethical dilemmas facing humankind. Artificial insemination, contraception, and abortion regulations are some of the problems that will require close collaboration between ethicists and scientists, especially embryologists.

—*Katherine H. Houp, Ph.D.*

See also Abortion; Amniocentesis; Birth defects; Brain disorders; Cerebral palsy; Cesarean section; Chorionic villus sampling; Cloning; Conception; Down syndrome; Embryology; Fetal alcohol syndrome; Genetic counseling; Genetic diseases; Genetics and inheritance; Growth; Gynecology; In vitro fertilization; Miscarriage; Multiple births; Neonatology; Obstetrics; Perinatology; Pregnancy and gestation; Premature birth; Reproductive system; Rh factor; Rubella; Sexual differentiation; Spina bifida; Stillbirth; Toxoplasmosis; Ultrasonography.

FOR FURTHER INFORMATION:

Mader, Sylvia S. *Inquiry into Life.* 6th ed. Dubuque, Iowa: W. C. Brown, 1991. An introductory-level college text designed to cover the entire range of biological topics. The text is very well written, and concepts are beautifully illustrated with color diagrams, photographs, and photomicrographs. Chapter 21, "Development," gives a clear description of typical early developmental stages of all vertebrates and offers a section on human embryology and fetal development, adulthood, and aging.

Marieb, Elaine N. *Essentials of Human Anatomy and Physiology.* 5th ed. Redwood City, Calif.: Benjamin/Cummings, 1997. This introductory anatomy and physiology textbook, easily accessible to those with little science background, is richly illustrated with diagrams and photographs, which help to illuminate body systems and processes. In-depth discussions of prevalent diseases and disorders and of current areas of research make this an all-around useful reference work.

Moore, Keith L., and T. V. N. Persaud. *The Developing Human.* 5th ed. Philadelphia: W. B. Saunders, 1993. This widely used textbook gives a clear and careful description of normal human development during the entire prenatal period. Excellent illustrations and diagrams are given to help students visualize developmental sequences, and photographs are included to illustrate many congenital abnormalities. Clinically oriented problems are provided at the end of each chapter.

Oppenheimer, Steve B., and George Lefevre, Jr. *Introduction to Embryonic Development*. 2d ed. Boston: Allyn & Bacon, 1984. An intermediate-level college text which gives extensive coverage to the embryological stages in primitive chordate and vertebrate classes. The text reflects the rapid advancement of the field of embryology, describing many experiments that have led to greater understanding of the mechanics of developmental processes.

Patten, Bradley M. *Patten's Human Embryology*. Edited by Clark Edward Corliss. 4th ed. New York: McGraw-Hill, 1976. A revised version of Patten's classic text designed for clinical studies in the health professions. Gives thorough coverage to the human developmental process, using a systems approach.

Riley, Edward P., and Charles V. Vorhees, eds. *Handbook of Behavioral Teratology*. New York: Plenum Press, 1986. An informative compilation of learnings in the field of behavioral teratology. Covers historical context, general principles, and specific drugs and environmental agents that act as behavioral teratogens. Effects are listed for each agent that has been studied.

Snell, Richard S. *Clinical Embryology for Medical Students*. 3d ed. Boston: Little, Brown, 1984. A concise, well-written, and well-illustrated medical text describing the normal stages in human development from gamete formation to birth. Descriptions of the more common congenital anomalies are provided. Includes photographs of human embryos.

Tortora, Gerard J., and Sandra Reynolds Grabowski. *Principles of Anatomy and Physiology*. 8th ed. New York: HarperCollins College Publishers, 1996. An intermediate-level college text widely used in fields of allied health. Written in a very readable fashion; has excellent color diagrams and photographs on every page. Chapter 29, "Development and Inheritance," gives a thorough overview of human prenatal development from fertilization through birth.

EMERGENCY MEDICINE

SPECIALTY

ANATOMY OR SYSTEM AFFECTED: All

SPECIALTIES AND RELATED FIELDS: Cardiology, critical care, gastroenterology, geriatrics and gerontology, neurology, nursing, obstetrics, pediatrics, pharmacology, psychiatry, public health, pulmonary medicine, radiology, sports medicine, toxicology

DEFINITION: The care of patients who are experiencing immediate health crises, a field defined by twenty-four-hour availability, the management of multiple patients simultaneously, and the need for broad-based skills and interventions.

KEY TERMS:

diagnostic: relating to the determination of the nature of a disease

emergency medical services: the complete chain of human and physical resources that provides patient care in cases of sudden illness or injury

heuristics: methods used to aid and guide in the discovery of a disease process when incomplete knowledge exists

paramedic: a person trained and certified to provide prehospital emergency medical care

pathologic: pertaining to the study of disease and the development of abnormal conditions

pathophysiology: an alteration in function as seen in disease

patient assessment: the systematic gathering of information in order to determine the nature of a patient's illness

triage: the medical screening of patients to determine their relative priority for treatment

SCIENCE AND PROFESSION

The field of emergency medicine is defined as care to acutely ill and injured patients, both in the prehospital setting and in the emergency room. It is practiced as a patient-demanded and continuously accessible care and is defined by the location of its practice rather than by an anatomical concern. Emergency medicine encompasses all medical specialties and physical systems. The commitment to rapid, prudent intervention under stressful and often chaotic conditions is of paramount importance to the critically ill patient. This branch of medicine is characterized by its complexity of problems, its twenty-four-hour availability to a variety of patients, and its effective and broad-based understanding of disease and injury. These features are used to orchestrate the response of multiple hands with the ultimate goal of referring the patient to ongoing care.

The hourglass is an appropriate symbol of the nature of this medical division. It not only portrays the importance of time and the need for quick intervention, but its shape—wide at either end and narrowing in the middle—is an appropriate visualization of the pattern of emergency medical treatment. A large number of patients converge on a single area, the emergency room, where they are diagnosed, treated, and eventually released to other appropriate care, diverging on a wide range of follow-up options.

Unique to the field of emergency medicine is the importance of rapid definition and comprehension of the pathophysiology of the critically ill patient. Emergency care physicians must have a unique understanding of the practice of medicine, the nature of disease and injury, availing themselves of a host of clinical skills needed for the treatment of the variety of physical and psychological problems that require treatment. Emergency rooms are a melting pot of problems; most are medical, many are not. All of them reflect some person's perception of an emergency. Success in the emergency medical field often depends on the ability of personnel to use not only their medical knowledge but their knowledge of people as well.

Most often those seeking the assistance of emergency medical providers are people suffering from pain of illness or trauma; however, any patient may seek treatment at the emergency room. Often loneliness, disability, or homelessness serves as the motivation to seek treatment. Regardless of what brought the patient, the emergency physician strives to recognize and deal with the patient's "emergency," remembering that not all patients are as ill as they might think and that not all are as well as they might appear. Physicians of this specialty sift through a multitude of information. It is necessary to know the patient's pertinent medical history and the history of the present illness or complaint before appropriate and effective treatment can be prescribed. Patients rarely follow a preconceived plan. Emergency medicine works best, therefore, when its practitioners follow heuristics—that is, incomplete guides that lead to greater knowledge, a holistic approach.

Emergency medicine is primarily a hospital-based specialty; however, it also involves extensive prehospital responsibilities. Many times, patients seeking emergency care are first the responsibility of police, fire, or ambulance personnel. In these situations, the role of emergency medicine must be viewed under the wider context of the emergency medical system. This system—beginning with the first aid administered by bystanders leading to initial treatment and transportation by trained certified emergency medical technicians, paramedics, or flight nurses and culminating with care at an emergency room or a highly equipped trauma center—forms a uniquely structured unit. The emergency medical system is designed to provide rapid quality intervention regardless of prehospital conditions. The emergency medical physician is best viewed as a central part of a team whose knowledge and understanding of the whole allow the best possible care to patients undergoing health crises.

Emergency physicians are charged with the responsibility of providing the highest standard of care in the hospital setting. They ensure that both staff members and equipment are maintained at their utmost level of quality. Trends, breakthroughs, and recent advances are monitored via journals and other medical publications. Training of personnel must keep pace with medical advancement. Developing an overall program depends as much on its planning as its dissemination. The emergency physician often plays the role of teacher, actively influencing the overall quality of the program through education and skills development. Thus, the exercise of emergency medicine is truly a team effort, with all members acting in accordance with their training and level of competence in order to minimize further injury or discomfort.

In practice, emergency medicine encompasses any person or structure involved in the immediate decision making and/or actions necessary to prevent death or further disability of a patient in the midst of a health crisis. It represents a chain of human and physical resources brought together for the purpose of providing total patient care. In this respect, everyone has a part to play in the deliverance of emergency care. The bottom line of emergency medicine is the welfare of the patient. Thus, it is most appropriate to view the practice of emergency medicine in the context of the entire emergency medical system.

The components of the emergency medical system include recognition of the emergency, initiation of emergency medical response, treatment at the scene, transport by members of an emergency medical team to the appropriate facility, treatment in the emergency room or trauma center, and release of the patient. These components are only as strong as the weakest link.

DIAGNOSTIC AND TREATMENT TECHNIQUES

Recognition of an emergency is the first step in emergency care. Often this step is complicated by the patient's own denial and ignorance of basic symptoms. "Emergency" is in part defined by the patient's ability to identify, accept, and respond to a given situation. Regardless of the nature of the illness or injury, the sooner an emergency is defined the sooner care can be provided. The typical heart attack victim, for example, waits an average of three hours after experiencing symptoms before seeking help. In such cases, treatment by bystanders who have been trained in first aid and cardiopulmonary resuscitation (CPR) has proven effective.

In the United States, the response of emergency medical personnel has been aided by the implementation of the 911 emergency system. While not all communities have this capability, its use is increasing. It has been documented that patients who receive treatment at an appropriate facility within sixty minutes of the onset of a life-threatening emergency are more likely to survive. This "golden hour" is precious time.

Operating under protocols developed and approved by the emergency medical director and emergency medical councils of a given locale, emergency medical technicians (EMTs) and paramedics are trained and authorized to deliver care to the patient in need at the scene. EMTs and paramedics are charged with the initial assessment of the patient's condition, immediate stabilization prior to transport, and deliverance of care as far as his or her training allows, and the transport of the patient.

Unique to the field of emergency medicine is the special relationship of the paramedic with the doctor. Many people in need of emergency care are first treated outside the hospital. In these cases, emergency caregivers on the scene act as the eyes, ears, and hands of the physician. Through the EMT or paramedic, using telecommunications, an emergency doctor can speed the process of diagnosis. Signs and symptoms relayed through these trained professionals enable a doctor to make an accurate assessment of the patient's condition and to request a variety of treatments for a patient whom they cannot see or touch. Linked by telephone or radio, the medic and doctor can capitalize on the golden hour with the initiation of quality care.

Paramedics operate under the medical license of a medical command physician who has met all criteria set forth by the Department of Health and has been approved to provide medical directives to prehospital and interhospital providers. Protocols are the recognized practices that are within the training of the EMT and paramedic. They serve as standard procedures for prehospital treatment. While it is recognized that situations will arise which call for deviation from particular aspects of a given protocol, they are the standards under which the doctor and emergency personnel on the scene operate.

Treatment at the scene is followed by transport with advanced life support by members of the emergency medical system in 85 percent of all emergency cases. This requires much-needed equipment for the further treatment of patients. Deficiencies in the vehicle, equipment, or training of medical personnel can seriously endanger a patient. Thus, government agencies have been designated to grant permission for ambulance services and hospitals to engage in the practice of emergency medicine. This licensure process is designed to demand a level of competency for health care providers and ensure the public's protection.

Since only about 5 percent of all emergency department admissions constitute life-threatening situations, not all facilities stand at the same level of readiness for a given emergency. Transportation to the appropriate facility, therefore, requires a matching of patient's need to the hospital's capabilities. Hospitals are categorized according to their ability to render emergency intensive care, as well as to provide needed support services on a patient-demand basis. In general, they are viewed as emergency facilities and trauma facilities where trauma centers are designed to provide twenty-four-hour, comprehensive emergency intensive care, including operating rooms and intensive care nurses.

When the patient reaches the emergency facility, during the first five to fifteen minutes of care, many important decisions are made by the physician on duty. The process continues to overlap with needed diagnostic tests and consultations in an effort to provide quality care directed at the source of the illness or injury. The patient's immediate needs are cared for by emergency department staff until the patient is moved to a site of continued care or released to his or her own care.

Questions correctly phrased and sharply directed are effective tools for the rapid diagnosis needed in emergency medicine. The key to this field is the ability to triage, stabilize, prioritize, treat, and refer.

Triage is the system used for categorizing and sorting patients according to the severity of their problems. Emergency practitioners seek to ascertain the nature of the patient's problem and consider any life-threatening consequences of the present condition. This stage of triage allows for immediate care to the more seriously endangered person, relegating the more stable, less seriously ill or wounded patients to a waiting period. The emergency room, in other words, does not operate on a first come, first served basis.

Secondary to triage is stabilization. This term refers to any immediate treatment or intervening steps taken to alleviate conditions that would result in greater pain or defect and/or lead to irreversible or fatal consequences. Primary stabilization steps include ensuring an unobstructed airway and providing adequate ventilation and cardiovascular function.

Once patients have been stabilized, all illnesses must be looked at on the scale of their hierarchical importance. Life-threatening diseases or injuries are treated before more moderate or minor conditions. This system of prioritization can be illustrated from patient to patient: A heart attack victim, for example, is treated prior to the patient with an ankle sprain. It can also be applied for multiple conditions within the same patient. The heart attack victim with a sprained ankle receives treatment first for the life-threatening cardiovascular incident.

Treatment of the critically ill patient often poses a series of further questions. What is the primary disorder? Is there more than one active pathologic process present? How does the patient appear? Is the patient's presentation consistent with the initial diagnosis? Is a hospital stay warranted? What consultations are needed to diagnose and treat this patient?

The emergency physician's approach is to consider the most serious disease consistent with the patient's presentation and chief complaint. By rule of thumb, thinking the worst and hoping for the best is often the psychological stance of the emergency care provider. Only when more severe conditions have been ruled out are more minor processes considered. Often too, this broad view of patient assessment allows for multiple diagnosis. Through continued probing, alternate and additional conditions are often uncovered. It is not unlikely that the patient who seeks treatment for a head injury after a fall is diagnosed with a more serious condition which caused the fall. Focusing only on the immediate condition would endanger the patient. Success in this medical field therefore demands broad-based medical knowledge and diagnostic tools.

Emergency medicine is not practiced in a vacuum. Its very nature necessitates its interfacing with a variety of medical specialties. The emergency room is often only the first step in patient recovery. Initial diagnosis and stabilization must be coupled with plans for ongoing treatment and evaluation. Consultations and referrals play important roles in the overall care of a patient.

PERSPECTIVE AND PROSPECTS

Historians are unable to document specific systems for emergency patients before the 1790's. The need to provide care to the battlefield wounded is seen as the first implementation of emergency response. Early wartime treatment did not, however, include prehospital treatment. Clara Barton is credited with providing the first professional-level prehospital emergency care for the wounded as part of the American Red Cross. Ambulance services began in major cities of the United States at the beginning of the twentieth century, but it was not until 1960 that the National Academy of Sciences' National Research Council actually studied the problem of emergency care.

Emergency medicine as a specialty is relatively new. Not until 1975, when the House of Delegates of the American Medical Association defined the emergency physician, did the medical community even recognize this branch of medicine. In 1981, the American College of Emergency Physicians added further recognition through the development of the definition of emergency medicine. Since then, growth and changes have enabled this field to develop as a major specialty, evolving to accept greater responsibility in both education and practice.

The development of emergency medicine and the increasing number of health care providers in this field have been dramatic. In 1990, there were a total of 23,000 emergency physicians, 85,000 emergency nurses, and 521,734 emergency technicians. These health care providers delivered care to the nearly 87 million emergency department patients seen that year.

Emergency medicine developed at a time when both the general public and the medical community recognized the need for quality accessible care in the emergency situation. It has grown to include a gamut of services provided by a community. In addition to responding to the acutely ill or injured, emergency medicine has grown to accept responsibilities of education, administration, and advocacy.

Included in the role of today's emergency medical providers' is the administration of the entire emergency medical system within a community. This system includes the development of public education programs such as CPR instruction, poison control education, and the introduction of the 911 system. Emergency management systems and coordinators are now part of every state and local government. Disaster planning for both natural and human-made accidents also comes under the heading of emergency medicine.

Research, too, plays an important role in emergency medicine. The desire to identify, understand, and disseminate scientific rationale for basic resuscitative interventions, as well as the need to improve preventive medical techniques, are often driving forces in scientific research.

Finally, emergency medicine plays a key role in many of society's problems. Homelessness, drug use and abuse, acquired immunodeficiency syndrome (AIDS), and rising health costs have all contributed to the increase in the number of patients seen in the emergency room. In response, those administering emergency medical care have tried to communicate such problems to the general public and legislative bodies, as well as educate them regarding preventive measures. Being on the front line of medicine brings a special obligation to improve laws and services to ensure public safety and well-being.

—*Mary Beth McGranaghan*

See also Abdominal disorders; Altitude sickness; Amputation; Aneurysms; Antibiotics; Appendectomy; Appendicitis; Asphyxiation; Bites and stings; Bleeding; Botulism; Burns and scalds; Cardiology; Cardiology, pediatric; Catheterization; Cesarean section; Choking; Coma; Concussion; Critical care; Critical care, pediatric; Electrical shock; Electrocardiography (ECG or EKG); Electroencephalography (EEG); Fracture and dislocation; Fracture repair; Frostbite; Grafts and grafting; Head and neck disorders; Heart attack; Heat exhaustion and heat stroke; Hospitals; Hyperthermia and hypothermia; Intoxication; Laceration repair; Meningitis; Nursing; Obstetrics; Paramedics; Peritonitis; Pneumonia; Poisoning; Radiation sickness; Resuscitation; Reye's syndrome; Salmonella; Shock; Snakebites; Spinal disorders; Splenectomy; Sports medicine; Staphylococcal infections; Streptococcal infections; Strokes and TIAs; Thrombolytic therapy and TPA; Tracheostomy; Transfusion; Unconsciousness; Veterinary medicine; Wounds.

FOR FURTHER INFORMATION:

Bledsoe, Bryan E., Robert S. Porter, and Bruce R. Shade. *Brady Paramedic Emergency Care*. 3d ed. Upper Saddle River, N.J.: Brady Prentice Hall Education, Career & Technology, 1997. A comprehensive guide to the practice of emergency medicine as it applies to and is practiced by the paramedic. A solid overview of the basics of prehospital care. This text focuses on advanced life support practices.

Caroline, Nancy L. *Emergency Care in the Streets*. 3d ed. Boston: Little, Brown, 1987. This text provides a sophisticated understanding of the fundamental concepts of advanced life support and the underlying physiology. A focused approach written by a physician who has spent many hours in the field as a prehospital care provider. Includes new chapters on AIDS and other communicable diseases.

Grant, Harvey D., et al. *Brady Emergency Care*. Rev. 7th ed. Englewood Cliffs, N.J.: Brady Prentice Hall Education, Career, & Technology, 1995. This simple text has been acclaimed for its comprehensive, accurate, and up-to-the-minute treatment of emergency care. Easy to read, this book provides the contemporary standards on CPR from the American Heart Association and a full treatment on many emergency medical protocols for prehospital treatment.

Hamilton, Glenn C., ed. *Emergency Medicine: An Approach to Clinical Problem-Solving*. New York: W. B. Saunders, 1991. Addressed to students of medicine, this text provides a detailed, well-written script for the clinical setting. Facilitates the reader's understanding of the emergency scene. Actual medical cases are integrated into the chapters in order to reinforce concepts.

Miller, Robert H., ed. *Textbook of Basic Emergency Medicine*. 2d ed. St. Louis: C. V. Mosby, 1980. This superbly written textbook is one of the most highly regarded in the field. Each chapter provides a well-organized introduction to physical anatomy and disease processes.

Rosen, Peter, ed. *Emergency Medicine: Concepts and Clinical Practice*. 2 vols. 2d ed. St. Louis: C. V. Mosby, 1988. A logical and straightforward presentation of current standards of emergency medicine. Intended to be a reference in busy emergency rooms. The writing is clear and to the point.

Tintinalli, Judith E., ed. *Emergency Medicine: A Comprehensive Study Guide*. 4th ed. New York: McGraw-Hill, 1988. This bible of emergency medicine provides a basic understanding of the field. Describes in detail key diagnostic techniques and treatments.

EMOTIONS, BIOMEDICAL CAUSES AND EFFECTS OF
BIOLOGY

ANATOMY OR SYSTEM AFFECTED: Brain, endocrine system, gastrointestinal system, immune system, muscles, musculoskeletal system, nerves, nervous system, psychic-emotional system

SPECIALTIES AND RELATED FIELDS: Neurology, psychiatry, psychology

DEFINITION: Agitations of the passions or sensibilities and the accompanying physiological changes.

KEY TERMS:

autonomic nervous system: the division of the nervous system that regulates involuntary action; comprises the sympathetic and parasympathetic systems

bipolar disorder: a syndrome characterized by alternating periods of mania and depression; also called manic-depressive disorder

Kluver-Bucy syndrome: a series of symptoms first observed in monkeys following temporal lobe removal, such as psychic blindness, abnormal oral tendencies, and changes in sexuality

loss-of-control syndrome: a pattern of behavior characterized by violent and emotional outbursts, occasionally associated with temporal lobe seizures

major depressive syndrome: a syndrome characterized by profound sadness and loss of pleasure in normal activities

sympathetic nervous system: the division of the autonomic nervous system concerned primarily with preparing the individual to expend energy

STRUCTURE AND FUNCTIONS

A central characteristic of being human is the ability to feel and express a wide range of emotions. Just what happens in the human brain and body to generate these feelings, however, is unclear. Over the years, it has been dem-

onstrated that activity in the sympathetic nervous system is important in the expression and experience of emotional states, although the role of various regions of the brain in emotion has proved to be more elusive.

No consensus exists on how many different emotions humans are capable of experiencing, as so much depends on definitions and the type of evidence admitted. Most theorists agree, however, that emotions have a significant impact on human behavior. The term "emotion" usually means some subjectively felt effect. In addition, at least three other factors can be considered part of emotion: physiological arousal (increased heart rate, sweating palms), expressive changes of the muscles of the face and body (smiles, frowns), and behavior (striking with a fist, cringing).

The best-studied physical responses characteristic of emotional states are those produced by the sympathetic nervous system, which controls many different internal organs of the body, as well as the salivary and sweat glands. Several of the responses produced by this system occur in emotional states. These responses are recorded in an attempt to study, measure, and evaluate emotion. The most commonly used responses include changes in heart rate, blood pressure, dilation of the pupils, and sweat gland activity. Physiological arousal in emotion also includes changes in the secretion of some hormones such as adrenaline, testosterone, and cortisol, measured from their presence in such body fluids as urine, saliva, and blood plasma.

The nervous system provides for rapid communication in the body, as it is concerned with events that occur on the order of milliseconds. Its structural and functional unit is the neuron, or nerve cell. Neurons have certain distinctive regions. The dendrites, or bushy protrusions, are the part specialized in receiving excitation, whether from an external stimuli or from another cell. The axon, or elongated part of the cell, takes care of distributing excitation away from the dendrite zone. Axons can be very long and form bundles that make up nerves.

The entire nervous system is a functional unit, and an impulse arising in any receptor can be transmitted to every effector in the body. Synapses are the functional junctions where connections between neurons form. In this region, one cell comes into contact, or near contact, with another cell, thus influencing it. Nerve impulses are propagated electrochemical reactions. The neural message must jump from the axon of one neuron to the dendrite of another for transmission to occur. The most common way of achieving this is through a chemical transmitter substance, also called a neurotransmitter. Chemical transmission at a synapse involves two steps. The first is the release of the specific chemical or neurotransmitter on the arrival of a nerve impulse. The chemical is released from its storage place in the tip of the axon into the narrow space between adjacent neurons. Once this has taken place, the specific transmitter substance is attached to a specific molecular site in the dendrite of the other neuron. This attachment produces a change in the properties of its cell membrane so that a new nerve impulse is set up, and the transmission continues.

The rapidly acting neurotransmitters include norepinephrine, epinephrine, dopamine, serotonin, acetylcholine, gamma aminobutyric acid (GABA), glycine, glutamate, and probably aspartate and adenosine triphosphate (ATP). The action of these neurotransmitters depends on the chemistry of the receptor to which they bind, and there are several types of receptor for each neurotransmitter. Receptors for neurotransmitters are important targets for toxins and drugs. For example, psychoactive drugs exert their effects at synapses, mostly by binding to specific receptors, but also by interfering with the degradation or removal of the transmitter from the synaptic cleft so that it lingers longer in the system.

From research on people with spinal cord injuries, it was found that while emotions may not be caused by feedback from sympathetic activity, this activity does play an important role in reinforcing emotional feelings, making them more intense and longer lasting.

Many different regions of the brain participate in emotions. The neocortex is responsible for dealing with symbolic manipulation, and bodily responses to emotion involve circuits located in lower brain regions such as the hypothalamus. Hormonal changes bring the endocrine system into play.

Dramatic changes in personality and emotional expression often occur following damage to various areas of the brain, such as weakening of emotional control with an injury to the frontal lobes. There is controversy, however, regarding where in the brain emotion is actually experienced. Research has pointed to certain parts of the brain below the cerebral cortex, such as the hypothalamus and the amygdala, as possible key participants. Two syndromes corroborate this finding. In loss-of-control syndrome, emotional outbursts are caused by abnormal electrical discharges in the region of the temporal lobe and amygdala. These spontaneous discharges are characteristic of epilepsy and are thought to result from congenital defects, high fever, brain infection, or trauma. Epilepsy can be controlled with drugs that inhibit the electrical discharges, since uncontrolled discharges result in epileptic seizures. Violent behavior and periods of intense emotion are common prior to an epileptic attack, although in some cases the sensations that take place before the seizure are interpreted by the individual as ecstasy of the highest order. Kluver-Bucy syndrome refers to a series of symptoms first observed in monkeys following temporal lobe removal: psychic blindness, abnormal oral tendencies, changes in sexuality, tameness (a significant lack of emotion), and hypermetamorphosis (a tendency to examine and react to virtually everything in the environment). Some or all the symptoms described have been seen in human patients following strokes, brain injury,

brain infections, and other traumas, although the presence of all five in a single individual is very rare. Subsequent research has suggested that changes in emotionality and sexuality are probably caused by damage to the amygdala, while psychic blindness is more likely attributable to the removal of the neocortex of the temporal lobe.

Besides the temporal lobe and the amygdala, portions of the limbic system such as the septal area and the hypothalamus are involved in emotional responses. The pleasure centers of the brain are found in the limbic system (which includes the septal area, amygdala, cingulate cortex, and hippocampus), the hypothalamus, and the brain stem. Brain regions can be classified as positive, negative, or neutral with respect to whether animals will work to turn on or turn off electrical stimulation of these particular areas. Virtually all the cerebral neurocortex and cerebellum is neutral, much of the limbic system and hypothalamus is positive, and some regions of the brain stem and hippocampus are negative. In some cases, electrical stimulation of positive sites mimic the effects of a naturally rewarding event so well that animals prefer the electrical stimulation to the actual experience.

Some research has indicated possible differences between the brain hemispheres in the understanding and expression of emotion. Such data come from the examination of neurological patients having brain damage confined to either side of the brain. Those patients with damage to the left hemisphere are more likely to suffer catastrophic reaction, characterized by intense fear, depressions, and a generally negative outlook on life. The ones with damage on the right side show an attitude of indifference or even unusual cheerfulness. One possible interpretation is that the observed emotions are a result of dominance by the healthy hemisphere, suggesting that the right side is responsible for negative emotional states such as fear, anger, and depression and that the left side produces more positive emotional states. Another possible explanation can reverse this conclusion, simply by stating that the damaged hemisphere becomes dominant in these cases. Identifying emotions with one side of the brain or the other, however, ignores some important data. For example, some patients with frontal lobe damage in either hemisphere will display changes in personality and emotional reactions.

The relationship between behavioral and physiological response processes has long provided an important focus for both laboratory and clinical studies of emotion. For example, research concerned with shyness in children is aimed at investigating the role of sympathetic arousal in emotion. It has been shown that children who are inhibited and quiet when placed in an unfamiliar social situation show larger sympathetic responses than more relaxed, spontaneous children.

Emotions are also the focus of research in the detection of deception, especially as it relates to criminal investigations. A polygraph is a device used to measure involuntary body responses such as changes in respiration, heart rate, and blood pressure in relation to various kinds of questions. It can determine whether the individual is trying to be deceptive. The use of a polygraph is based on two main assumptions: first, that physiological responses during emotional arousal are involuntary, and second, that only individuals with guilty knowledge will display emotional arousal to certain questions asked by the tester. There are three types of questions: irrelevant questions, such as "What is your name?"; control questions, which deal with issues similar to those under consideration but not directly relevant; and relevant questions. The questions are asked in an unpredictable order, sometimes more than once. It is assumed that the person is being deceptive if the polygraph shows more arousal to relevant questions than to control ones. In a controlled laboratory setting, the polygraph is 80 to 90 percent effective in identifying guilty individuals and 90 to 95 percent effective in identifying innocent individuals. It is a process filled with interpretive problems that have to be solved.

Almost every drug found to be effective in altering affecting states in humans has also been found to exert effects upon catecholamines (such as norepinephrine and epinephrine) in the brain. These effects would suggest that catecholamines are involved in the mediation of affective states and in the action of the drugs that affect them. Drugs that are associated with depressive phenomena in humans normally cause the loss of catecholamines, while drugs that elevate the mood (antidepressants) have the opposite effect by blocking the mechanisms that destroy the compounds.

DISORDERS AND DISEASES

Mood disorders fall into one of two categories: major depressive disorder and bipolar disorder. Major depressive syndrome is characterized by profound sadness and loss of pleasure in normal activities. Bipolar (manic-depressive) disorder is characterized by alternating periods of mania and depression.

Major depressive syndrome can often be treated without drugs. In many cases, however, drugs accelerate the recovery process. Two of the main families of antidepressant drugs are the tricyclics and the monoamine oxidase inhibitors (MAOIs). The generic name for one of the major tricyclic drugs is imipramine (Tofranil or Janimine), and one example of an MAOI is isocarboxazid (Marplan). Both drugs are believed to help lift depression by increasing the availability of monoamine neurotransmitters at synapses in critical circuits in the brain. Monoamine neurotransmitters include norepinephrine, epinephrine, dopamine, and serotonin. Tricyclic compounds increase the time the neurotransmitter is available in the synapse, and thus the duration of neurotransmitter action. MAOIs inhibit the action of the enzyme that normally degrades monoamines. Although these are the most common antidepressant drugs, not all of

them belong to these families, and not all act by these mechanisms. Antidepressant drugs, like any other drugs, can have bothersome side effects that may include constipation, urinary retention, blurred vision, and weight gain. More severe side effects include abnormalities in heart function and blood pressure; this presents a problem in dealing with elderly patients, who tend to be depressed. The drugs are provided to the patient in one-week doses at a time, since a fatal dose is only ten to fifteen times the daily dose.

Electroconvulsive therapy (formerly called shock therapy) is another treatment for severe depression. It is a controversial therapy used as a last resort for severe cases, normally for patients who do not respond to other methods and who are at extreme risk for suicide. The process involves administration of a brief electric current through the head, enough to produce an electrical pattern resembling a grand mal epileptic seizure. Patients are given sedatives so that they are not aware of the current or convulsions. This treatment works for about 70 percent of the patients. Possible side effects include headaches and loss of memory for events just before the shock; sometimes this memory comes back, and sometimes it does not.

Bipolar mood disorder is much less common than major depressive syndrome. The main method of treatment is to administer lithium salts, although their mechanism of action is not known.

Anxiety disorders are the most common emotional disorders, as up to 8 percent of the population experiences them. Included in this group is panic disorder. A panic attack includes shortness of breath, dizziness, acceleration of heart rate, and sweating. It can take place by anticipation of something or for no reason at all. Although attacks last only a few minutes, they are very disturbing. These symptoms involve activation of the sympathetic division of the nervous system. Other anxiety disorders are phobias (chronic fears of certain situations) and obsessive-compulsive disorder. The benzodiazepines are drugs that are effective in the treatment of panic disorder. They include alprazolam (Xanax), chlordiazepoxide (Librium), and diazepam (Valium). These drugs enhance the inhibitory effect of GABA, a major inhibitory neurotransmitter, at synapses throughout the brain. Obsessive-compulsive disorder is characterized by stereotyped rituals or compulsions that develop in an attempt to deal with the anxiety produced by obsessions (such as the fear of germs). It has been successfully treated with some of the tricyclic drugs, such as clomipramine.

PERSPECTIVE AND PROSPECTS

The word "passion" was frequently used by early philosophers to connote roughly what is now referred to as emotion: the phenomena of anger, fear, love, jealousy, and so on. In the fourth century B.C., Aristotle made a distinction between experiences that involve concurrent activity of both soul and body (such as appetites and passions) and those that involve activity of the soul alone (thinking). In the thirteenth century, Saint Thomas Aquinas was more explicit in affirming this belief in such a distinction, placing his argument within the context of Christian theology. In the seventeenth century, René Descartes directed his attention specifically to the passions. He reiterated that every passion experienced by the soul has its physical counterpart, and he emphasized the role of environmental stimulation in the generation of a passion and proposed a mechanism by which the environment created the passions. Descartes also established conceptual distinctions among passion (of the soul), bodily commotion (activity of the visceral organs), and action (motion of the somatic musculature) and indicated close correspondence among the three.

About two centuries passed without significant development in theoretical ideas about emotion. Interest was renewed, however, as a result of the publication of Charles Darwin's *The Expression of Emotions in Man and Animals* (1872), in which he drew attention to emotional behavior as the biologically significant aspect of emotion and pointed out the causal role of stimulus events or situations in producing behavior.

The American philosopher and psychologist William James proposed the first explicit psychological theory of emotion in 1884. He claimed that emotions are the result, not the cause, of bodily arousal. According to James, bodily arousal is produced by the action of the sympathetic system. These reactions he believed to be reflexive responses to emotion-provoking situations. The emotion would then be produced by feedback from nerves bringing input from various internal organs (the heart and stomach) and blood vessels affected by the sympathetic system. This theory triggered the serious experimental study of emotion. Danish physiologist Carl Lange independently published a similar theory in 1885, and as a result, the theory is known as the James-Lange theory of emotion. Although it was frequently criticized, this theory dominated the field of emotion research for more than fifty years.

In 1915, Walter Cannon provided convincing experimental evidence of endocrine and autonomic participation in emotional response patterns. In 1927, he conducted a dramatic experiment by removing the sympathetic nervous system of a few cats. All the nerve connections between sympathetic neurons and internal organs and blood vessels were eliminated. According to the James-Lange theory, the cats should feel no emotions. They still displayed clear-cut emotional behaviors, however, and Cannon proposed that external stimuli caused emotion by simultaneously activating neural circuits in the neocortex and triggering responses in the sympathetic nervous system. Most modern theories are more closely aligned with Cannon's work than with the James-Lange hypothesis.

In 1962, Stanley Schachter and Jerome Singer followed up on Gregorio Maranon's 1924 experiment on the role of bodily responses in emotion. They proposed that people need to attribute their feelings to some emotional state and that the complete emotional experience is a joint product of cognition and feedback from sympathetic arousal. The role of sympathetic activity in emotion is still an active topic of research.

Various experiments have sought to discover the functions of certain regions of the brain, as they relate to emotional responses. In 1939, psychologist Heinrich Kluver and neurosurgeon Paul Bucy were interested in identifying the regions of the brain where drugs produce hallucinations. They speculated that the temporal lobe might be involved since brief hallucinations precede temporal lobe epileptic attacks. Both temporal lobes of monkeys were removed, and a constellation of dramatic behavioral changes was observed, proving their theory. In 1954, James Olds and Peter Milner published a report that rats would press a lever for the sole reward of passing electrical current into certain regions of their brains. This phenomenon is known as self-stimulation, and it led to the discovery of the pleasure centers of the brain. Fearlike responses have been elicited from electrical stimulation of three regions of a cat's brain: the tectum, the thalamus, and portions of the hippocampus. Such sites are called negatively reinforcing regions.

As additional information is accumulated, the complexity of the human brain becomes increasingly evident. Emotion is no exception. The biochemical aspects of emotional states have been studied extensively, and considerable information has been acquired, largely in terms of the biochemical changes that accompany and feed back into the central emotional state. Yet there are still many areas to be explored, including complete elucidation of the mechanism of action of some drugs and thus better treatment options for certain disorders.   —*Maria Pacheco, Ph.D.*

See also Addiction; Aging; Alcoholism; Anxiety; Autism; Brain; Brain disorders; Death and dying; Depression; Electroconvulsive therapy; Endocrinology; Endocrinology, pediatric; Epilepsy; Grief and guilt; Hormones; Hypochondriasis; Light therapy; Manic depressive disorder; Midlife crisis; Nervous system; Obsessive-compulsive disorder; Panic attacks; Paranoia; Phobias; Postpartum depression; Psychiatric disorders; Psychiatry; Psychiatry, child and adolescent; Psychiatry, geriatric; Psychoanalysis; Psychosis; Psychosomatic disorders; Puberty and adolescence; Schizophrenia; Sexual dysfunction; Sibling rivalry; Stress; Strokes and TIAs.

FOR FURTHER INFORMATION:

Black, Perry, ed. *Physiological Correlates of Emotion*. New York: Academic Press, 1970. Different topics are presented in terms of the research that led to their discovery or development, with a critical discussion and a summary at the end of each topic.

Cooper, J. R., F. E. Bloom, and R. H. Roth. *The Biochemical Basis of Neuropharmacology*. 7th ed. New York: Oxford University Press, 1996. A fine treatise on the drugs that affect the nervous system, such as psychotropic drugs that affect mood and behavior, sedatives, and other drugs that affect the autonomic nervous system.

Heilman, K. M., and Paul Satz, eds. *Neuropsychology of Human Emotion*. New York: Guilford Press, 1983. This book contains chapters by different authors on right-hemisphere involvement in emotion, the emotional changes associated with epilepsy, and other neurological and psychiatric diseases.

Kimble, D. P. *Biological Psychology*. 2d ed. Fort Worth, Tex.: Harcourt Brace Jovanovich, 1992. An excellent textbook which provides good suggestions for further readings of the various topics presented. A well-written, easy-to-read presentation of the topic of emotion and its causes.

Wender, P. H., and D. F. Klein. *Mind, Mood, and Medicine: A Guide to the New Biopsychiatry*. New York: Farrar, Straus & Giroux, 1981. Provides a comprehensive account of the psychopharmacological revolution that has transformed psychiatry. Written specifically for the layperson, the text also presents a brief history of twentieth century psychiatry and its consequences.

EMPHYSEMA
DISEASE/DISORDER

ANATOMY OR SYSTEM AFFECTED: Chest, lungs, respiratory system

SPECIALTIES AND RELATED FIELDS: Internal medicine, pulmonary medicine

DEFINITION: A disease of the lung characterized by enlargement of the small bronchioles or lung alveoli, the destruction of alveoli, decreased elastic recoil of these structures, and the trapping of air in the lungs, resulting in shortness of breath, reduced oxygen to the body, and a variety of serious and eventually fatal complications.

KEY TERMS:

alveoli: tiny, delicate, balloonlike air sacs composed of blood vessels that are supported by connecting tissue and enclosed in a very thin membrane; these sacs are found at the ends of the bronchioles

bronchioles: small branches of the bronchi, which are extensions of the trachea (the central duct that conducts air from the environment to the pulmonary system)

bullous emphysema: localized areas of emphysema within the lung substance

centrilobular (centriacinar) emphysema: a type of emphysema that destroys single alveoli, entering directly into the walls of terminal and respiratory bronchioles

diffusion: the passage of oxygen into the bloodstream from the alveoli and the return or exchange of carbon dioxide across the membrane between the blood vessels and the alveoli

panlobular (panacinar) emphysema: a type of emphysema

that involves weakening and enlargement of the air sacs, which are clustered at the end of respiratory bronchioles

perfusion: the flow of blood through the lungs or other vessels in the body

ventilation: the transport of air from the mouth through the bronchial tree to the air sacs and back through the nose or mouth to the outside; ventilation includes both inspiration (breathing in) and expiration (breathing out)

CAUSES AND SYMPTOMS

Emphysema is a lung disease in which damage to these organs causes shortness of breath and can lead to heart or respiratory failure. A discussion of the structure and function of the normal lung can illuminate the nature and effects of this damage.

Gases, smoke, germs, allergens, and environmental pollutants pass from the nose and mouth into a large duct called the trachea. The trachea branches into smaller ducts, the bronchi and bronchioles (small branches of the bronchi), which lead to tiny air sacs called alveoli. The respiratory system is like a tree: The trachea is the trunk, the bronchi and bronchioles are similar to the branches, and the alveoli are similar to the leaves. The blood vessels of the alveoli carry red blood cells, which pick up oxygen and transport it to the rest of the body. The cellular waste product, carbon dioxide, is released to the alveoli from the bloodstream and then exhaled. The alveoli are supported by a framework of delicate elastic fibers and give the lung a very distensible quality and the ability to "snap back," or recoil.

The lungs and bronchial tubes are surrounded by the chest wall, composed of bone and muscle and functioning like a bellows. The lung is elastic and passively increases in size to fill the chest space during inspiration and decreases in size during expiration. As the lung (including the alveoli) enlarges, air from the environment flows in to fill this space. During exhalation, the muscles relax, the elasticity of the lung returns it to a normal size, and the air is pushed out. Air must pass through the bronchial tree to the alveoli before oxygen can get into the bloodstream and carbon dioxide can get out, because it is the alveoli that are in contact with blood vessels. The bronchial tree has two kinds of special lining cells. The first type can secrete mucus as a sticky protection against injury and irritation. The second type of cell is covered with fine, hairlike structures called cilia. These cells are supported by smooth muscle cells and elastic and collagen fibers. The cilia wave in the direction of the mouth and act as a defense system by physically removing germs and irritating substances. The cilia are covered with mucus, which helps to trap irritants and germs.

When alveoli are exposed to irritants such as cigarette smoke, they produce a defensive cell called an alveolar macrophage. These cells engulf irritants and bacteria and call for white blood cells, which aid in the defense against foreign bodies, to come into the lungs. The lung tissue also becomes a target for the enzymes or chemical substances produced by the alveolar macrophages and leukocytes (white blood cells). In a healthy body, natural defense systems inhibit the enzymes released by the alveolar macrophages and leukocytes, but it seems that this inhibiting function is impaired in smokers. In some cases, an individual may inherit a deficiency in an enzyme inhibitor. The enzymes vigorously attack the elastin and collagen of the lungs, the lung loses its elastic recoil, and air is trapped.

Emphysema

In emphysema, the body releases enzymes in response to inhaling irritants in the air, such as cigarette smoke; these enzymes reduce the lung's elasticity, compromising the bronchioles' ability to expand and contract normally. Air becomes trapped in the alveoli upon inhalation (top) and cannot escape upon exhalation (bottom). Over time, breathing becomes extremely difficult.

Emphysema, and a related disease, bronchitis, often work in concert. They are often lumped under the term "chronic obstructive pulmonary disease." Chronic bronchitis weakens and narrows the bronchi. Often, bronchial walls collapse, choking off the vital flow of air. Air is also trapped within the bronchial walls. Weakened by enzymes, the walls of the alveoli rupture and blood vessels die. Lung tissue is replaced with scar tissue, leaving areas of destroyed alveoli that appear as "holes" on an X ray. Small areas of destroyed alveoli are called blebs, and larger ones are called bullae.

As emphysema progresses, a patient has a set of large, overexpanded lungs with a weakened and partially plugged bronchial tree subject to airway collapse and air trapping with blebs and bullae. Breathing, especially exhalation, becomes a slow and difficult process. The patient often develops a "barrel chest" and is known, in medical circles, as a "blue bloater." The scientific world calls the mismatching of breathing to blood distribution a ventilation-to-perfusion imbalance; that is, when air arrives in the alveolus, there are no blood vessels there to transport their vital gaseous cargo to the cells (as a result of enzymatic damage). A person with chronic obstructive pulmonary disease has a bronchial tree with a narrow, defective trunk and sparse leaves.

The loss of elasticity of the lung and alveoli is a critical problem in the emphysemic patient. About one-half of the lungs' elastic recoil force comes from surface tension. The other half comes from the elastic nature of certain fibers throughout the lungs' structure. Emphysema weakens both of these forces because it destroys the elastic fibers and interferes with the surface tension. Fluid, a saline solution, bathes all the body's cells and surfaces. In the lung, this fluid contains surfactant, a substance that interferes with water's tendency to form a spherical drop with a pull into its center (and ultimate collapse). The tissue that gives shape to the lungs is composed of specialized fibers which contain a protein called elastin. These elastic fibers are also found in the alveolar walls and in the elastic connective tissue of the airways and air sacs. The amount of elastin in lung tissue determines its behavior. Healthy lungs maintain a proper balance between destruction of elastin and renewal. (Other parts of the body, such as bones, do this as well.) If too little elastin is destroyed, the lungs have difficulty expanding. If too much is destroyed, the lungs overexpand and cannot recoil properly.

The process of elastin destruction and renewal involves complex regulation. Specialized lung cells produce new elastin protein. Others produce elastase, an enzyme that destroys elastin. The liver plays a role in the production of a special enzyme known as alpha-1-antitrypsin, which controls the amount of elastase so that too much elastin is not digested. In emphysema, these regulatory systems fail: Too much elastin is destroyed because elastase is no longer controlled, apparently because alpha-1-antitrypsin production has been reduced to a trickle.

The loss of elastin (and thus elastic recoil) means that the lungs expand beyond the normal range during inspiration and cannot resume their resting size during expiration. Thus, alveoli overinflate and rupture. This further reduces elasticity because the loss of each alveolus further impairs the surface tension contribution to the lungs' ability to recoil. Thus, a state of hyperinflation is assumed in the emphysemic patient. This leads to stretched and narrowed alveolar capillaries, loss of elastic tissue, and dissolution of alveolar walls. The lungs increase in size, the thoracic (chest) cage assumes the inspiratory position, and the diaphragm becomes low and flat instead of convex. The patient becomes short of breath with any type of exertion. As the disease worsens, the patient's skin takes on a cyanotic color, as a result of poor oxygenation and perfusion. Wheezing is often present, and coughing is difficult and tiring. In the worst cases, even talking is enough exertion to produce a spasmodic cough. The hyperinflated chest causes inspiration to become a major effort, and the entire chest cage lifts up, resulting in considerable strain. The head moves with each inspiration while the chest remains relatively fixed.

Emphysema may be diagnosed by the early symptom of dyspnea (shortness of breath) on exertion. In advanced cases, the distended chest, depressed diaphragm, increased blood carbon dioxide content, and severe dyspnea clearly point to the disease.

Treatment and Therapy

The initial step in treating emphysema is to open the airways by eliminating the causes of irritation: smoke, dry air, infection, and allergies. The second treatment is to clean out the airways. There are several techniques and medicines for loosening airway mucus and expelling it. In most chronic obstructive lung diseases, including emphysema, the mucus becomes thick and purulent; coughing up mucus of this type is difficult. In addition, in emphysema the natural cleansing action of the cilia and lung elasticity are impaired. Thus, treatment is aimed at the patient consciously taking over the function of cleaning out the lungs. Coughing is nature's way of bringing up mucus (phlegm), and the emphysemic patient is urged to cough. Since the mucus is thick, one needs to do whatever is necessary to thin it out and to lubricate the airways so that the mucus slips up easily with coughing. The cough must come from deep within the chest in order to be "productive" (to raise mucus).

Moisture is helpful in loosening up thick mucus; hence, drinking large amounts of fluid is encouraged. Adding a humidifier or a vaporizer to a home is often helpful to the emphysemic patient. There are also machines known as nebulizers and intermittent positive pressure breathing (IPPB) machines that can help to add moisture to the airway of the patient with emphysema. Nebulizers are more effective in getting moisture beyond the throat and major airways

than cold vaporizers. Nebulizers, which get their name from the Latin word for cloud or mist, create a mist that is a profusion of tiny droplets that keep themselves apart, even as they bump into one another. Nebulizers release only the smallest droplets—those which can penetrate far down into air passages, where thick mucus is likely to be. (Atomizers produce small droplets as well, but they also spray large droplets.) IPPBs have a special kind of valve that opens when one begins to breathe and allows the air to move into the lungs under mild pressure. As soon as the patient has come to the end of the inhalation, the valve closes and allows the patient to exhale freely.

When phlegm cannot be brought up by breathing mist, a technique called postural drainage is often combined with chest wall percussion or vibration. The idea is to move one's body to a position such that airways are perpendicular to the floor, or at least tilted down, so that gravity can help pull the mucus toward the larger airways, from which the phlegm can be coughed up. Percussion, or clapping the chest, is another way to loosen the mucus in the airways so that it can be coughed up.

A number of medications are useful in the treatment of emphysema. The bronchodilator drugs are xanthines, such as theophylline (Theo-Dur), that relieve bronchospasms; reduce wheezing and dyspnea, and improve respiratory muscle function. Theophylline is a drug that is similar chemically to caffeine. Whereas caffeine stimulates the skeletal muscles and the central nervous system, however, theophylline is potent as a cardiac stimulant and a smooth muscle relaxer. It has also been learned that theophylline stimulates mucociliary clearance of the airways, strengthens the diaphragm, and suppresses edema. Theophylline holds two benefits for the chronic obstructive pulmonary diseased patient: It helps get rid of mucus, and it strengthens the diaphragm, the main respiratory muscle. Common side effects are nausea, stomach pain, vomiting, insomnia, rapid heartbeat, loss of appetite, and restlessness. Another category of bronchodilator are the beta adrenergic stimulants such as metaproterenol (Alupent). Their side effects include nervousness, headache, nausea, and muscle cramps.

The antibiotics sometimes prescribed for emphysemic patients are used to combat bacterial infection. Common antibiotics include tetracycline, penicillin, cephalosporin, erythromycin, and sulfa drugs. Their side effects include a burning sensation in the stomach, vomiting, diarrhea, increased sensitivity to sunlight, rashes, itching, hives, fever, and weakness.

The steroid hormones, such as prednisone, decrease swelling, inflammation, and bronchospasms; they also relieve wheezing. Side effects include blurred vision, frequent urination, thirst, black stools, bone pain, mood changes, weight gain, swelling of the feet, muscle weakness, hoarseness, and a sore mouth.

Other drugs given for emphysema include digitalis, cardiac glycosides, diuretics, mast cell inhibitors, expectorants, and parasympatholytics. Digitalis and cardiac glycosides, such as digoxin, improve the strength of heart contractions and treat disturbances in heart rhythm. Side effects are loss of appetite, abdominal pain, nausea, slow uneven pulse, blurred vision, diarrhea, mood changes, and weakness. Diuretics, such as furosemide (Lasix), are often given to prevent excessive fluid retention. Such drugs cause loss of hearing, skin rashes, hives, bleeding, bruising, jaundice, an irregular or fast heartbeat, muscle cramps, light-headedness, dizziness, and weakness. Mast cell inhibitors are a unique category of drugs that inhibit the release of body chemicals that cause wheezing and bronchospasm; however, they also cause weakness, nosebleeds, and nasal congestion. Expectorants, such as Robitussin, are used to thin secretions and have no known side effects. The parasympatholytics are a type of bronchodilator drug that inhibits the nerves that cause bronchospasm. They are apparently free from the many side effects associated with other bronchodilator drugs.

The emphysemic patient should avoid both excessive heat and excessive cold. If body temperature rises above normal, the heart works faster, as do the lungs. Excessive cold stresses the body to maintain its normal temperature. Smog, air pollution, dusts, powders, and hairspray should be avoided. Finally, a healthy diet consisting of foods high in calcium, vitamins, complex carbohydrates, proteins, and fiber is advised for the patient with lung disease.

A healthy core diet is high in complex carbohydrates; is low in sugars, fats, and cholesterol; and has adequate protein for moderate stress. It should be high in fiber and contain approximately 1,000 milligrams of calcium, 15,000 milligrams of Vitamin A, and 250 milligrams of Vitamin C. Snack foods can include skim milk, fruit, popcorn, and fresh salads. The respiratory distress of the emphysemic patient uses vast amounts of energy, and the patient should eat several small meals a day so as not to distend the stomach and limit movement of the diaphragm. Liquids are important in keeping airways clear. Good nutrition is helpful in maintaining strength and improving the quality of life for the patient with lung disease.

PERSPECTIVE AND PROSPECTS

Chronic bronchitis and emphysema are responsible for at least fifty thousand deaths a year in the United States alone. An increase in air pollution and cigarette consumption are apparent causes for this rise. In males over forty, chronic obstructive pulmonary disease (COPD) is second to heart disease as a cause of disability. With more females and young people smoking, the incidence of lung disease is likely to increase. Aside from death, a disease such as emphysema can cause long years of disability, joblessness, loss of income, depression, hospitalization, and an inability to perform normal activities.

Smoking is, by far, the single most important risk factor for emphysema. In the United States especially, social ac-

ceptance of women smokers began after World War II and has increased the number of women being diagnosed with COPD. Socioeconomic status also influences smoking habits. In many countries in Europe, the mortality rate from lung disease for the lowest socioeconomic class has been six times higher than for the highest. In the United States, the COPD mortality rate among unskilled and semiskilled laborers is twice as high as among professionals. Families with lower incomes usually live in small, often overcrowded apartments; such overcrowding makes respiratory infections more frequent. Often, family members of the COPD patient also smoke, increasing the surrounding air pollution.

In the United States, COPD causes 3 percent of all deaths. In some cases, it causes another 100,000 Americans to be too weak to survive other, unrelated medical conditions. Therefore, an annual figure of 150,000 deaths from COPD-related diseases is more realistic. The expanding COPD population is a growing market for pharmaceutical firms. For example, greater amounts of bronchodilator medications will be needed; hence, pharmaceutical firms are anxious to find longer-acting and more effective drugs for these patients to buy.

A number of economic pressures are likely to move COPD treatment from the hospital to the home. When effectively carried out by a well-trained health team, home care can lower medical costs. The COPD patient who finds a knowledgeable doctor and who begins a comprehensive rehabilitation program is the one who can look forward to a life that is more productive and more comfortable.

—*Jane A. Slezak, Ph.D.*

See also Environmental diseases; Lungs; Pulmonary diseases; Pulmonary medicine; Pulmonary medicine, pediatric; Respiration.

FOR FURTHER INFORMATION:

Bates, David V. *Respiratory Function in Disease*. 3d ed. Philadelphia: W. B. Saunders, 1989. Summarizes the effects of disease on pulmonary function. Also discussed are some of the more sophisticated pulmonary function tests. Exercise testing, obesity, and the effects of drugs are other topics reviewed in this work.

Berland, Theodore, and Gordon L. Snider. *Living with Your Bronchitis and Emphysema*. New York: St. Martin's Press, 1972. A book for persons suffering from respiratory disease and making adjustments, both emotionally and physically, because of the disease. An invaluable source of information on healthy and unhealthy breathing in the modern world.

Decker, Caroline D. "Room to Breathe." *Saturday Evening Post* 266, no. 6 (November/December, 1994): 48-49. This article on emphysema discusses lung surgery. Illustrated with photographs.

Haas, François, and Sheila Sperber Haas. *The Chronic Bronchitis and Emphysema Handbook*. New York: John Wiley & Sons, 1990. Helps patients with COPD learn to lead full and productive lives. Provides information pertinent to their disease and describes the treatments and medications available to them in order to improve their quality of life.

Shayevitz, Myra, and Berton Shayevitz. *Living Well with Emphysema and Bronchitis.* Garden City, N.Y.: Doubleday, 1985. Provides suggestions for living a full life in spite of lung disease. It clearly explains the causes and complications of emphysema, treatment modalities, and the medications available to alleviate discomfort.

Wolff, Ronald K. "Effects of Airborne Pollutants on Mucociliary Clearance." *Environmental Health Perspectives* 66 (April, 1986): 223-237. The role of mucociliary clearance as a lung defense mechanism is described in this article. The abnormal elimination of bronchial mucus is considered a possible factor in the pathogenesis of COPD. The role of certain pollutants, which pose a challenge to the mucociliary system, are detailed.

ENCEPHALITIS

DISEASE/DISORDER

ANATOMY OR SYSTEM AFFECTED: Brain, nervous system
SPECIALTIES AND RELATED FIELDS: Neurology, virology
DEFINITION: A family of diseases resulting from viral infection or complications from another disease; inflammation of the brain resulting in a variety of usually serious symptoms and sometimes death.

KEY TERMS:

athetosis: involuntary writhing movements of limbs and/or body, face, and tongue
dementia: loss of mental ability as a result of brain deterioration
diabetes insipidus: production of copious amounts of urine
hemiplegia: paralysis of one side of the body
nuchal: having to do with the nape of the neck
pleocytosis: an increase in the number of white blood cells in the cerebrospinal fluid
postencephalitic symptoms: symptoms commencing immediately after or years after an attack of encephalitis lethargica as a direct or indirect consequence of the infection
viremia: invasion of cells by viruses

CAUSES AND SYMPTOMS

Encephalitis, a noncontagious disease, is an inflammation of the brain. It most often results from viral infection, but it may also arise as a complication of measles, chickenpox, herpes simplex virus 1, or several other diseases. A nonviral form, encephalitis lethargica (sometimes referred to as "sleeping sickness") is implicated in parkinsonism. Between one thousand and five thousand cases are reported annually to the Centers for Disease Control in Atlanta, Georgia; the highest incidence is in the summer and early fall months, and worldwide, most cases are reported in the tropics. The disease affects the sexes equally, and no age group is unaffected.

The viruses that cause most cases of encephalitis are called arboviruses, animal viruses carried by arthropods and transmitted to vertebrate hosts. In a vertebrate, one of these viruses undergoes viremia, then multiplies in an arthropod when it feeds on the vertebrate host. The arthropod then passes the virus to another vertebrate, also while feeding. Arthropods implicated in passing on the virus to humans are mosquitoes, and rarely, ticks. Mosquitoes (and ticks) pick up the virus as they feed on an infected host. There are several variables, however, that determine whether the virus will be passed on to the next host. First, each different virus has a "preferred" arthropod carrier. Second, the concentration of the virus in the vertebrate host is crucial; more than 100,000 infectious doses per millimeter may be required for infection. Third, the incubation period for replication of the virus in the arthropod must be met; four days to two weeks generally must pass before the carrier can infect a vertebrate, but the virus may remain infective for several weeks after that. The incubation period is often influenced by environmental temperature; high temperature often accelerates incubation times and frequently results in epidemics.

Symptoms of encephalitis develop one to two weeks after the bite of the mosquito and may come on gradually or quite suddenly and forcefully. Acute viral infection of the central nervous system varies from disease to disease because each virus may affect different parts of the nervous system and/or nerve cells. For example, if the meninges (outer covering of the brain and cord) are infected, symptoms may include headache, fever, stiff neck, and pleocytosis. If the fundamental tissues of the brain (parenchymal cells) are involved, loss of consciousness, seizures, focal neurological deficits, and an increased pressure within the brain (such is the case with encephalitis) may also occur. In addition to all other symptoms, if the hypothalamic-pituitary region becomes involved, sudden increases or decreases in body temperature may occur, and diabetes insipidus may result from a lack of antidiuretic hormone secretion. Swelling of the brain may lead to coma and is often followed by cardiac and respiratory arrest. In these cases, the disease may be deemed fatal. If the spinal cord becomes infected, symptoms manifested include paralysis of bowel and bladder.

The three most common symptoms of the acute state (with sudden, forceful onset) are headache, disturbances of sleep rhythm, and visual abnormalities (blurred vision or double vision). Headaches, though common, are not often severe but may accompany vomiting and other body aches. Sleep disturbances generally include lethargy during the day and insomnia at night. More severe cases suffer fever and delirium. Other common symptoms might include drowsiness, stupor, and eye muscle weakness. Because of the infrequency with which encephalitis strikes and the complete change in symptoms in the latter half of the twentieth century, the acute stage may never be observed. Still, in a study of two thousand cases, 38 percent of the patients died, all during the acute phase. These deaths occurred during the first month, most frequently on the fourteenth day. Those most likely to succumb were children under one year of age and adults over the age of seventy. Young adults between the ages of twenty and thirty were most likely to survive. Complete recovery, however, occurred in only about one-fourth of the cases. The remainder of the survivors suffered some degree of dementia.

Symptoms of the chronic stage include sleep disturbances (lethargy and/or insomnia), some dementia, depression, irritability, and anxiety in adults. Children often experience such behavior disorders as stealing, animal cruelty, and other criminal mischief. Respiratory disorders are common in chronic cases, but visual disturbances persist in only a few cases. Since the epidemic during and after World War I that brought so much attention to the disease, the symptoms have undergone remarkable changes. With the epidemic form, the symptoms came on suddenly and with force. Years later, the onset became less terrifying but the chronic stage was often more severe. The most noted symptom in current cases is not during the course of the disease but later. Such is the case with those suffering postencephalitic parkinsonism. The long-range effects may be delayed as long as forty years before onset. Other lingering aftereffects may be deterioration of mental faculties. In children who have contracted the disease, behavioral disorders may result.

Very infrequently, encephalitis has been implicated in epilepsy. This link would be likely only if the disease caused lesions in the brain. Injuries to or inflammation of a child's nervous system may be the basis for hyperactivity in as many of 80 percent of those children suffering from hyperactivity. Although there are many ways these events can happen, it is not unreasonable to expect that some children who have recovered from encephalitis will experience hyperactivity. In fact, their hyperactivity may be the only real neurological aftermath of the disease.

The encephalitis that was prevalent during World War I was usually accompanied by sleep lasting days or even weeks. (Sometimes called "sleeping sickness" or "sleepy sickness," this type of encephalitis is not to be confused with African sleeping sickness, which is caused by the parasite trypanosoma, borne by the tsetse fly.) Its scientific name is encephalitis lethargica, and it is sometimes referred to as von Economo's disease. This sleep results from lesions in the midbrain as well as the hypothalamic and subthalamic regions of the brain. The lesions also induce continual drowsiness as well as motor deficiencies. Encephalitis lethargica is a type of coma, but the patient can be easily roused with stimulation although he or she lies inert, making no sound. The patient's eyes can follow movement or watch the observer carefully. Rarely, encephalitis lethargica

may produce symptoms suggestive of chorea (characterized by involuntary movements).

Postinfection encephalitis may occur during, or as a result of, infectious diseases such as influenza or measles. It may also appear after vaccination against rabies, smallpox, or measles. Postinfection encephalitis does not occur as frequently as the other types, but neither is it affected by the sufferer's age. Because children are most often vaccinated, however, they are more susceptible to postinfection encephalitis.

In the United States, four types are commonly recognized. St. Louis encephalitis is geographically the most widespread as well as the most common type of arbovirus-induced encephalitis. It is found primarily in the South and Midwest and mostly victimizes the elderly. Affected areas of the nervous system include the basal ganglia, brainstem, and white matter of the brain and occasionally the spinal cord. The usual symptoms are fever, reduced heart rate, drowsiness, stupor, nuchal rigidity, athetoses and tremors of the hands, and sometimes seizures. Unusual symptoms may include urinary dysfunction (painful urination and pus in the urine), uncoordinated muscular movements, diabetes insipidus as a result of a lack of antidiuretic hormone, and oculomotor paralysis. Even so, recovery rates are considered to be good for St. Louis encephalitis.

Eastern equine encephalitis is very rare, but the most deadly, with 20 to 40 percent mortality. It is mostly found all along the East Coast where there are horses and pheasants. Eastern equine encephalitis produces numerous large lesions in the brain and is accompanied by high fever, drowsiness, cyanosis (lack of oxygen because of respiratory distress), twitching, seizures, and nuchal rigidity. Not only are mortality rates high, but there is likelihood of severe disabilities including speech difficulties, paralyses, and mental retardation as well.

California encephalitis, sometimes called Western encephalitis, is also rare. Found west of the Mississippi, it is not often fatal or serious. It comes on strong with headache, fever, vomiting, confusion, stupor with perhaps coma, seizures, and respiratory failure. The respiratory failure may cause death in 5 percent of the cases. Aftereffects are rare but might include parkinsonism or learning difficulties. A fourth type of encephalitis found in the United States is LaCrosse, which occurs in the north-central states and West Virginia. Its victims are most often young children.

Encephalitis may occur sporadically as a result of other viral infections such as herpes simplex virus 1, measles (it rarely follows German measles), mumps, rabies, and even during the course of human immunodeficiency virus (HIV) infection. The most common form of fatal sporadic encephalitis is caused by herpes simplex virus 1. It accounts for 5 to 10 percent of the total number of encephalitis cases in the United States each year. If untreated, it is fatal in as many as 70 percent of the cases. Herpes simplex-induced encephalitis produces fever, headache, seizures, and coma and is sometimes preceded by a span of bizarre behavior. These personality changes are likely the result of lesions in the temporal lobes and may include terror and hallucinations. The patient may suffer some paralysis, particularly of the face and arm. Deep coma with respiratory arrest may occur. Of those surviving herpes-induced encephalitis, about half continue to suffer major motor and sensory deficits, speech problems, and frequently, an amnestic syndrome (Korsakoff's psychosis). Two antiviral agents are used to combat the disease with moderate success: acyclovir (often the drug of choice) and adenosine arabinoside. Acyclovir is active only in the cells invaded by the herpes simplex virus and inhibits deoxyribonucleic acid (DNA) replication (effectively halting cell division and numerical growth). HIV-infected patients often experience herpes simplex virus 1, which means that acquired immunodeficiency syndrome (AIDS) patients with this herpes virus may develop encephalitis.

Occasionally, a child under two years of age apparently fights off a bout of measles, only to succumb to a slow invasion of encephalitis that may be fatal. The encephalitis may appear before the rash, with the rash, or after the rash. It may not make an appearance until the child is between ages four and eighteen. In these rare cases (one in every 200,000 cases), known as subacute sclerosing panencephalitis (SSPE), the initial symptoms may be mild. The child may experience poor concentration at first; then symptoms might progress through stages of erratic jerking of the limbs, blindness, severe mental retardation, and then death. There may be a sudden onset with symptoms of fever, lethargy, delirium, catatonia, or excitement. Seizures are common, and mortality rates are high. SSPE results when the measles virus persists in the brain, killing some nerve cells and destroying the myelin sheath surrounding others. SSPE is rare because of the widespread use of antimeasles vaccines.

Another disease of the nervous system that most frequently affects children is acute toxic encephalitis. The difference occurs in the changes it induces in the nervous system. There is not only brain cell degeneration but also edema of the brain and small hemorrhages. Acute toxic encephalitis may also occur in children suffering from burns because of the toxemic effects that burns have on nerve cells.

Several theories have been proposed to answer why other diseases lead to encephalitis. One of these is that the central nervous system reacts to the virus that caused the original disease. Another theory suggests that there may be poisonous substances that develop during the course of the original disease that induce encephalitis. The least popular theory is that enzymes already in the patient or enzymes produced by the original disease are activated. These enzymes destroy the myelin around the nerve cells. Still others believe that postinfection encephalitis is an autoimmune disease. Because of the rarity of postinfection encephalitis, it may be years before the answer is found.

TREATMENT AND THERAPY

Generally, in order to diagnose a patient with encephalitis (which is often indistinguishable from viral meningitis), a physician must review the patient's medical history in the light of the presence or absence of an epidemic, as well as the presence of signs and symptoms. If they indeed are indicative of the possibility, a lumbar puncture and examination of spinal fluid are performed. The amount of pressure the fluid exerts is checked; if pleocytosis and an elevated protein level are found, they too, indicate the likelihood of encephalitis. In some cases, the blood is found to contain increased numbers of neutralizing antibodies. Because the onset of fever, the aches and pains, and other symptoms characterize many infections and diseases as well as encephalitis, specific diagnosis can be made only by isolating the virus or sometimes through a blood workup. Because it is extremely difficult to isolate the virus in the blood, successful diagnosis may be made when two specific antibodies increase in the blood. Although sometimes misdiagnosed as poliomyelitis or multiple sclerosis, encephalitis can be distinguished from these diseases by the sleep disturbances it causes and by the visual disturbances that it may induce. It is unlikely to cause paralysis and only infrequently results in convulsions, unlike the other diseases. Encephalitis is also occasionally misdiagnosed as meningitis but differs from it in that the spinal fluid does not contain an excess of cells as in meningitis. An electroencephalogram (EEG) can be useful because it might show the appropriate disturbance of cerebral activity.

At one time, as many as seventy-five methods of treatment for encephalitis were reported. Yet none of these actually influences how the disease progresses. The only thing that can be treated, therefore, is the symptoms. Placement in intensive care as early as possible is desirable because of the rapid progression of the illness. Relieving the headache and reducing the fever so the sufferer can be as comfortable as possible would likely be the first course taken. Seizures can be treated with anticonvulsant drugs such as phenytoin. Intracranial pressure should be monitored, and if the pressure does rise, nasotracheal intubation (a tube placed in the nose) with hyperventilation from a ventilator might aid in decreasing pressure. During convalescence, speech and physical therapy may be necessary. The length of convalescence depends on how severe the illness has been, but it may take several months for recovery. The prognosis for those with viral encephalitis depends on the causative agent. In order to control the spread of the mosquito-borne encephalitis virus, a thorough knowledge and understanding of the mosquito population is necessary. Breeding sites must be located, and the distribution and density of the adult mosquito population must be determined, especially those in areas near human populations. This information can be used to contain the mosquito population by using larvivorous fish or chemical insecticides. If one is in an area that is experiencing an outbreak, the best prevention is to remain indoors after dark, thereby avoiding the time that mosquitoes are feeding. If one must go out, one should spray exposed areas with insect repellent and/or wear long sleeves and pants of tightly woven material. The use of window screens, residual insecticide application on and around screen doors, and mosquito netting over cribs offers other ways to retard the number of mosquitoes that can enter the house or to prevent mosquito bites.

PERSPECTIVE AND PROSPECTS

A look at history reveals numerous cases and minor epidemics of encephalitis. In 1580, Europe was inundated with a fever-causing lethargic disease resulting in parkinsonism and other long-lasting neurological effects. Other serious epidemics occurred in London between 1672 and 1673 and again between 1673 and 1675. The most common (and highly unusual) symptom of this epidemic was hiccuping. Epidemics also occurred in the German city of Tübingen from 1712 to 1713, in France and Germany in the latter half of the eighteenth century, and in Italy following a deadly influenza outbreak in 1889 and 1890. None of these epidemics, however, was nearly as widespread as the pandemic that began in the winter of 1916-1917. This major outbreak began in the European city of Vienna, and within three years it had spread worldwide. It seemed each case was different; no two patients experienced the same signs and symptoms the same way. Because of such variations, diagnosis such as epidemic delirium, epidemic schizophrenia, epidemic parkinsonism, rabies, and polio were erroneously made. Seemingly, thousands of new diseases were instantly pervading the globe. It was Constantin von Economo who, through his pathological studies on the brain tissues of many of those who died, not only found a unique pattern of damage but also isolated the virus common to all. Von Economo named this "new" disease encephalitis lethargica.

As this epidemic seized the world, more than five million people were either killed or severely affected. It lasted ten years, leaving as suddenly as it had come. Of those who died, one-third succumbed during the acute stages of the sleeping sickness (in such a deep comatose state as to preclude arousal, or in such a state of sleeplessness as to invalidate sedation). Even those who survived the coma/wakefulness attacks were so affected that they failed to recover to their predisease alertness. Many were simply conscious, unaware, speechless, motionless, and without energy, motivation, appetite, or desire. They knew what was occurring around them but were totally apathetic to the events, showing no behavior at all.

Sixty years after the epidemic of World War I, many survivors were still alive. Some had active lives despite parkinsonism, tics, and other problems. They were the lucky few; most postencephalitic patients suffered gross debilitating neurological damage, never to function independently again. Many of the survivors were bedridden and robbed of movement, speech, and perhaps memory. Most of them were banished to asylums, nursing homes, or other "special" places where they were untreated and forgotten.

—*Iona C. Baldridge*

See also Arthropod-borne diseases; Bites and stings; Brain; Brain disorders; Dementia; Hemiplegia; Nervous system; Neurology; Neurology, pediatric; Parasitic diseases; Sleeping sickness; Viral infections.

FOR FURTHER INFORMATION:

Aminoff, Michael J., ed. *Neurology and General Medicine.* New York: Churchill Livingstone, 1989. This compilation by numerous contributors relates neurological disorders that may occur as a result of or in conjunction with general medical disorders. The intended audience is medical professionals.

Bowsher, David, ed. *Neurological Emergencies in Medical Practice: A Handbook for the Non-Specialist.* London: Croom Helm, 1988. A brief book delineating the recognition and treatment of neurological emergencies written by doctors for doctors. Therefore, it is filled with medical language and is not easily read by the layperson.

Horsfall, Frank L., Jr., and Igor Tamm, eds. *Viral and Rickettsial Infections of Man.* 4th ed. Philadelphia: J. B. Lippincott, 1965. A somewhat dated but well-organized, comprehensive look at many infections caused by viruses and rickettsias. Written as an aid to medical students and graduate students, but still fairly readable.

Johnson, Richard T. *Viral Infections of the Nervous System.* New York: Raven Press, 1982. A readable volume, with a clinical audience in mind; punctuated with pictures and tables. Emphasizes the biology of nervous system infections, and references to laboratory diagnoses, prevention, and therapy are also included.

Sacks, Oliver. *Awakenings.* New York: Summit Books, 1987. An insightful and intriguing look into twenty case histories of patients suffering from postencephalitic symptoms. Traces the history of the first drug treatment of these patients and their reentry into "life."

Taylor, Joyce W., and Sally Ballenger. *Neurological Dysfunctions and Nursing Intervention.* New York: McGraw-Hill, 1980. This text is filled with medical terminology regarding the brain and its related diseases. Written for nursing students, but most readers can achieve a basic understanding of neurological diseases with this work.

Walton, John N., and W. Russell Brain. *Brain's Diseases of the Nervous System.* 10th ed. Oxford, England: Oxford University Press, 1993. A lengthy, complex volume written to educate and inform medical professionals on all aspects of neurological dysfunctions. Its completeness provides a wide range of material, but it is intended for diagnostic usage.

ENDARTERECTOMY
PROCEDURE

ANATOMY OR SYSTEM AFFECTED: Blood vessels, circulatory system, neck

SPECIALTIES AND RELATED FIELDS: General surgery, vascular medicine

DEFINITION: A surgical procedure used to remove plaque from the lining of the carotid arteries in the neck.

INDICATIONS AND PROCEDURES

The internal carotid artery lies in the side of the neck, slightly in front of and beneath the sternocleidomastoid muscle. A skin incision is made anterior to this muscle. The branches of the carotid artery, adjacent blood vessels, and nerves are freed and inspected. A clamp is applied to the common carotid artery. Two additional clamps are applied to the external and internal carotid arteries to prevent bleeding and to prevent emboli from migrating to the brain during the procedure.

A lengthwise incision is made in the internal carotid artery from a point about 3.8 centimeters (1.5 inches) above the beginning of the vessel into the common carotid artery,

Endarterectomy

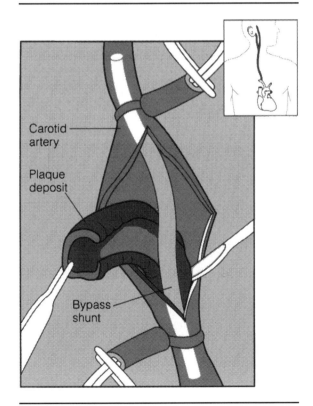

Carotid artery

Plaque deposit

Bypass shunt

The excision of plaque deposits from the carotid artery in the neck is called endarterectomy; the inset shows the location of the carotid artery.

about 2.5 centimeters (1 inch) below the beginning of the vessel. The edges of the artery are retracted, and the interior is exposed. The plaque can usually be scraped off the walls of the artery. The internal lining of the artery is carefully closed, and any tears are sutured. The carotid artery is then sewed together with fine suture material. If the underlying disease has been extensive or if the lining of the artery was damaged, a portion of the saphenous vein in the patient's leg is used to repair the arterial wall.

Restoring blood flow is crucial; it is important to avoid both leaks in the artery and the formation of emboli. The clamp on the external carotid artery is briefly released, and a small amount of blood is allowed to flow back into the repaired area to check for leaks under low pressure. This clamp is reapplied. The clamp on the common carotid artery is removed to check for leaks under high pressure. The clamp to the external carotid artery is removed next. Blood is allowed to flow, flushing any emboli from the operative site and away from the brain. If all is well, the clamp on the internal carotid artery is removed.

The structures that were pulled away from the carotid artery are released and briefly inspected to ensure that no damage has been done. The edges of the skin are then brought together and closed with sutures. The patient returns in about a week for a checkup and removal of the sutures.

USES AND COMPLICATIONS

Endarterectomy is used to restore adequate blood flow to the brain, thus preventing periods of ischemia that can result in loss of consciousness. Complications include emboli, which cause strokes by blocking important blood vessels.

Endarterectomy is successful in most patients and restores more normal circulation. It has decreased the incidence of strokes in younger patients.

—*L. Fleming Fallon, Jr., M.D., M.P.H.*

See also Angioplasty; Arteriosclerosis; Bypass surgery; Circulation; Embolism; Strokes and TIAs; Vascular medicine; Vascular system.

ENDOCARDITIS
DISEASE/DISORDER

ANATOMY OR SYSTEM AFFECTED: Circulatory system, heart

SPECIALTIES AND RELATED FIELDS: Bacteriology, cardiology, internal medicine, vascular medicine

DEFINITION: Inflammatory lesions of the endocardium, the lining of the heart.

CAUSES AND SYMPTOMS

The lesions of endocarditis may be noninfective, as in rheumatic fever, or infective. The latter are characterized by direct invasion of the endocardium by microorganisms, most often bacteria. Bacterial endocarditis may occur on normal or previously damaged heart valves and also on ar-

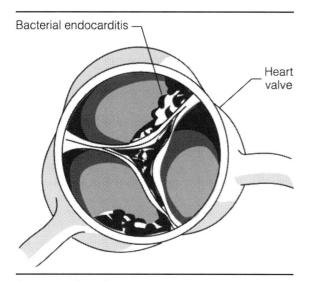

Bacterial endocarditis

Heart valve

Bacterial endocarditis of a heart valve occurs when bacteria invade and cause inflammatory lesions; untreated, the condition is usually fatal.

tificial (prosthetic) heart valves. Rarely, endocarditis may occur on the wall (mural surface) of the heart or at the site of an abnormal hole between the pumping chambers of the heart, called a ventricular septal defect.

In areas of turbulent blood flow, platelet-fibrin deposition can occur, providing a nidus for subsequent bacterial colonization. Transient bacteremia may accompany infection elsewhere in the body or some medical and dental procedures, and these circulating bacteria can adhere to the endocardium, especially at platelet-fibrin deposition sites, and produce endocarditis. Intravenous drug abusers using unsterile equipment and drugs often inject bacteria along with the drugs, which can result in endocarditis. The lesions produced by these depositions plus bacteria are called vegetations. Clinical symptoms and signs usually begin about two weeks later.

Bacterial endocarditis usually involves either the mitral or the aortic heart valve. In intravenous drug abusers, the tricuspid heart valve is more commonly affected because it is the first valve to be reached by the endocardium-damaging drugs and contaminating bacteria. The pulmonic valve is only rarely the site of endocarditis. Occasionally, more than one heart valve is infected; this occurs most often in intravenous drug abusers or patients with multiple prosthetic heart valves.

Gram-positive cocci are the most common cause of bacterial endocarditis. Different species predominate in various conditions or situations: *Streptococcus viridans* in native valves, *Staphylococcus aureus* in the valves of intravenous drug abusers, and *Staphylococcus epidermidis* in prosthetic heart valves. Gram-negative bacilli are found in association with prosthetic heart valves or intravenous drug addiction.

The clinical manifestations of endocarditis are varied and often nonspecific. Early symptoms are similar to those encountered in most infections: fever, malaise, and fatigue. As the disease progresses, more cardiovascular and renal-related symptoms may appear: dyspnea, chest pain, and stroke. Fever and heart murmurs are found in most patients. Enlargement of the spleen, skin lesions, and evidence of emboli are commonly present.

The key to the diagnosis of bacterial endocarditis is to suspect the presence of the illness and obtain blood cultures. Febrile patients who have a heart murmur, cardiac failure, a prosthetic heart valve, history of intravenous drug abuse, preexisting valvular disease, stroke (especially in young adults), multiple pulmonary emboli, sudden arterial occlusion, unexplained prolonged fever, or multiple positive blood cultures are likely to have endocarditis. The hallmark of bacterial endocarditis is continuous bacteremia; thus, nearly all blood cultures will be positive. Other nonspecific blood tests, such as an erythrocyte sedimentation rate, or specific blood tests, such as tests for teichoic acid antibodies, may be helpful in establishing a diagnosis.

TREATMENT AND THERAPY

Endocarditis may be prevented by administering prophylactic antibiotics to patients with preexisting heart abnormalities that predispose them to endocarditis when they are likely to have transient bacteremia. An example would be a patient with an artificial heart valve scheduled to have a dental cleaning.

Endocarditis is one of the few infections that is nearly always fatal if mistreated. Antibacterial therapy with agents capable of killing the offending bacteria, along with supportive medical care and cardiac surgery when indicated, cures most patients.

PERSPECTIVE AND PROSPECTS

The first demonstration of bacteria in vegetations associated with endocarditis was by Emmanuel Winge of Oslo, Norway, in 1869. Fifty years later, a fresh section was cut from the preserved heart valve described by Winge, and staining by modern methods revealed a chain of streptococci verifying his discovery. It was not until 1943, when Leo Loewe successfully treated seven cases of bacterial endocarditis with penicillin, that the era of modern therapy of this serious illness began.

Endocarditis accounts for approximately one case in every 1,000 hospital admissions in the United States. The incidence remained fairly constant between the 1960's and the 1990's, but the type of patient has changed: Heroin addicts, the elderly, and patients with prosthetic heart valves constitute an increasing percentage of endocarditis cases.

—*H. Bradford Hawley, M.D.*

See also Bacterial infections; Cardiology; Cardiology, pediatric; Circulation; Heart; Heart disease; Heart valve replacement; Mitral insufficiency; Rheumatic fever; Vascular medicine; Vascular system.

FOR FURTHER INFORMATION:

Kaye, Donald, ed. *Infective Endocarditis.* 2d ed. New York: Raven Press, 1992. An excellent text covering all the features of endocarditis in the modern era.

Kerr, Andrew. *Subacute Bacterial Endocarditis.* Springfield, Ill.: Charles C Thomas, 1955. The classic monograph describing the history and natural course of the disease.

Magilligan, Donald J., Jr., and Edward L. Quinn, eds. *Endocarditis: Medical and Surgical Management.* New York: Marcel Dekker, 1986. Discusses the treatment of endocarditis and its complications.

ENDOCRINE DISORDERS

DISEASE/DISORDER

ANATOMY OR SYSTEM AFFECTED: Endocrine system, glands

SPECIALTIES AND RELATED FIELDS: Endocrinology

DEFINITION: Breakdowns in the normal functioning of the endocrine system, which controls the metabolic processes of the body.

KEY TERMS:

cyclic AMP: a chemical that acts as a second messenger to bring about a response by the cell to the presence of some hormones at their receptors

endocrine: a secretion into the bloodstream rather than by way of a duct, such as hormones

feedback: the mechanism whereby a hormone inhibits its own production; often involves the inhibition of the hypothalamus and tropic hormones

hypothalamohypophysial: relating to the hypothalamus and the hypophysis (pituitary gland)

target cell or organ: a cell or organ possessing the specific hormone receptors needed to respond to a given hormone

tropic: hormones that feed a particular physiological state

tropin: hormones that cause a "turning toward" a particular physiological state

PROCESS AND EFFECTS

In order to understand endocrine disorders, it is necessary to review briefly the location of the principal endocrine glands, the hormones secreted, and the normal functions of the hormones. The hormones are released into the bloodstream and are carried throughout the body, where they affect target cells or organs that have receptors for the given hormone.

The pituitary gland, or hypophysis, is sometimes called the master gland because of its widespread influences on many other endocrine glands and the body as a whole. It is located in the midline on the lower part of the brain just above the posterior part of the roof of the mouth. The pituitary has three lobes: the posterior lobe, the intermediate lobe, and the anterior lobe.

The posterior lobe does not synthesize hormones, but it does have nerve fibers coming into it from the hypothalamus of the brain. The ends of these axons release two hormones that are synthesized in the hypothalamus, oxytocin and antidiuretic hormone (ADH). Oxytocin causes the contraction of the smooth muscles of the uterus during childbirth and the contraction of tissues in the mammary glands to release milk during nursing. ADH causes the kidneys to reabsorb water and thereby reduce the volume of urine to normal levels when necessary.

The intermediate lobe of the pituitary secretes melanocyte-stimulating hormone (MSH), a hormone with an uncertain role in humans but known to cause the darkening of melanocytes in animals. Sometimes, the intermediate lobe is considered to be a part of the anterior lobe.

The anterior lobe of the pituitary is under the control of releasing hormones produced by the hypothalamus and carried to the anterior lobe by special blood vessels. In response to these releasing hormones, some stimulatory and some inhibitory, the anterior lobe produces thyroid-stimulating hormone (TSH), adrenocorticotropic hormone (ACTH), follicle-stimulating hormone (FSH), luteinizing hormone (LH), prolactin, and somatotropin or growth hormone (GH). TSH stimulates the thyroid to produce thyroxine, ACTH stimulates the adrenal cortex to produce some of its hormones, FSH stimulates the growth of the cells surrounding eggs in the ovary and causes the ovary to produce estrogen, LH induces ovulation (the release of an egg from the ovary) and stimulates the secretion of progesterone by the ovary, prolactin is essential for milk production and various metabolic functions, and GH is needed for normal growth.

The pineal gland, or epiphysis, is a neuroendocrine gland attached to the roof of the diencephalon in the brain. It produces melatonin, which is released into the bloodstream during the night and has important functions related to an individual's biological clock.

The thyroid gland is located below the larynx in the front of the throat. It produces the hormones thyroxine (T_3) and triiodothyronine (T_4), which are essential for maintaining a normal level of metabolism and heat production, as well as enabling normal development of the brain in young children. C-cells in the thyroid produce calcitonin, which is involved in blood calcium regulation. This is also true for parathyroid hormone, a product of the nearby parathyroid glands. The thymus, located under the breast bone or sternum, produces the hormone thymosin that stimulates the immune system. Even the heart is an endocrine gland: It produces atrial natriuretic factor, which stimulates sodium excretion by the kidneys. The pancreas, located near the stomach and small intestine, produces digestive enzymes that pass to the duodenum, but also it produces insulin and glucagon in special cells called pancreatic islets. Insulin causes blood sugar (glucose) to be taken up from the blood into the tissues of the body, and glucagon causes stored starch (glycogen) to be broken down in the liver and thereby increases blood glucose levels.

Glands of the Endocrine System

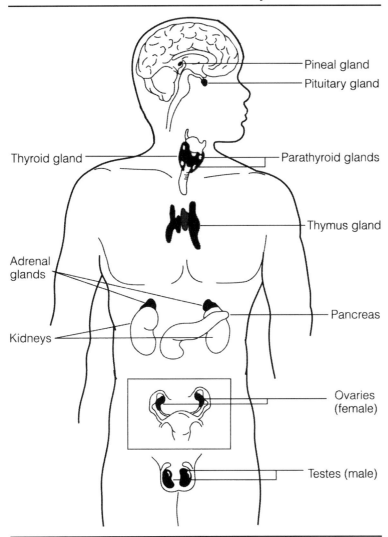

Pineal gland
Pituitary gland
Thyroid gland
Parathyroid glands
Thymus gland
Adrenal glands
Pancreas
Kidneys
Ovaries (female)
Testes (male)

The pair of adrenal glands, located on the kidneys, are made up of two components: first, a cortex that produces glucocorticoids, mineralocorticoids, and sex steroids or androgens; and second, a medulla, or inner part, that secretes adrenaline and noradrenaline. The gonads, testes or ovaries, are located in the pelvic region and produce several hormones, including the estrogen and progesterone that are essential for reproduction in females and the testosterone that is essential for reproduction in males. The kidneys and digestive tract also produce hormones that regulate red blood cell formation and the functioning of the digestive tract, respectively.

COMPLICATIONS AND DISORDERS

A wide variety of endocrine disorders can be treated successfully. In fact, the ability to restore normal endocrine function with replacement therapy has long been one of the techniques for showing the existence of hypothesized hormones.

The posterior pituitary releases both oxytocin and ADH. Chemicals similar to oxytocin are sometimes given to induce contractions in pregnant women so that birth will occur at a predetermined time. The other hormone released from the posterior pituitary, ADH, normally causes the reabsorption of water within the tubules of the kidney. A deficiency of ADH leads to diabetes insipidus, a condition in which many liters of water a day are excreted by the urinary system; this necessitates that the patient drink huge quantities of water simply to stay alive. A synthetic form of ADH, desmopressin acetate, can be given in the form of a nasal spray that diffuses into the bloodstream and thus restores the reabsorption of water by the kidneys.

The anterior lobe of the pituitary produces six known hormones. The production of these hormones is stimulated and/or inhibited by special releasing hormones secreted by the hypothalamus and carried to the anterior lobe by the hypothalamohypophysial portal system of blood vessels. Thus, the source of some anterior pituitary disorders can reside in the hypothalamus. Tumors of anterior pituitary cells can result in the overproduction of a hormone, or if the tumor is destructive, the underproduction of a hormone. Radiation or surgery can be used to destroy tumors and thereby restore normal pituitary functioning.

Anterior pituitary hormones can be the basis of a variety of disorders. As with other hormones, there may be below-normal production of the hormone (hyposecretion) or overproduction of the hormone (hypersecretion). Because the pituitary hormones are often supportive of hormone secretion by the target organ or tissue, hyposecretion or hypersecretion of the tropic or supportive hormone leads to a similar change in the production of hormones by the target organ or tissue.

For example, hyperthyroidism, or Graves' disease, can be caused by excessive secretion of TSH by the pituitary, leading to hypersecretion of thyroxine or by nodules within the thyroid that produce excessive thyroxine. In the diagnosis process, blood levels of both TSH and thyroxine are usually measured to determine the specific cause of the disorder. Similarly, hypothyroidism can be induced by deficits at several levels. The lack of iodine in the diet can prevent the production of thyroxine, which requires iodide as part of its molecular composition. The production of thyroxine usually has a negative feedback effect on the hypothalamus and pituitary, reducing TSH production. The failure to produce thyroxine causes high blood levels of TSH and an abnormal growth of the thyroid that results in a greatly enlarged thyroid, called a goiter. The addition of iodine to salt has eliminated the incidence of goiter in developed countries. Even with an adequate supply of iodine in the diet, however, hypothyroidism can still develop from other sources. The usual treatment is to ingest a dose of thyroxine daily.

Other examples of anterior pituitary disorders include those involving changes in GH secretion. Undersecretion of GH can lead to short stature or even dwarfism, in which an individual has normal body proportions but is smaller than normal. Now it is possible to obtain human GH from bacteria genetically engineered to produce it. Replacement GH can be given during the normal growth years to enhance growth. A tumor sometimes develops in the pituitary cells that produce GH, and this can cause abnormally increased growth or gigantism. If the tumor develops during the adult years, only a few areas of abnormal growth can occur, such as in the facial bones and the bones of the hands and feet. This condition is called acromegaly. Abraham Lincoln is thought to have had abnormal levels of GH that caused gigantism in his youth and then acromegaly in his later years. Acromegaly can be treated by radiation or surgery of the anterior pituitary.

Pineal gland tumors have been associated with precocious puberty, in which children become sexually developed in early childhood. It is thought that melatonin normally inhibits sexual development during this period. The pineal gland is influenced by changes in the daily photo-period, so that the highest levels of melatonin appear in the blood during the night, especially during the long nights of winter. Seasonal affective disorder (SAD), a mental depression that occurs during the late fall and winter, has been linked to seasonally high melatonin levels. Daily exposure to bright lights to mimic summer has been used to treat SAD. The pineal gland and melatonin are also being studied with regard to jet lag and disorders associated with shift work. The pineal gland thus seems to be involved in the functioning of the body's biological clock.

The pancreatic islets, also called the islets of Langerhans, produce insulin and glucagon. Diabetes mellitus is caused by insufficient insulin production (type 1 or juvenile-onset diabetes) or by the lack of functional insulin receptors on body cells (type 2 or maturity-onset diabetes). Type 1 diabetes can be treated with insulin injections, an implanted insulin pump, or even a transplant of fetal pancreatic tissue. Type 2 diabetes is treated with diet and weight loss. Weight

loss induces an increase in insulin receptors. In addition to the symptoms of high blood sugar levels in the diabetic, long-term damage to the kidneys, blood vessels to the retina, and blood vessels in the legs and feet are important concerns.

The adrenal cortex produces glucocorticoids, mineralocorticoids, and androgens, any of which can be the basis of hyposecretion or hypersecretion. Addison's disease is caused by hyposecretion, whereas Cushing's syndrome is caused by hypersecretion or more-than-sufficient replacement therapy. Similar to those of the thyroid, the adrenal cortex secretions have a negative feedback on the hypothalamus and the anterior pituitary. Addison's disease is characterized by low blood pressure and a poor physiological response to stress. The high levels of ACTH—high because of inadequate feedback of corticoids on the hypothalamus and anterior pituitary—cause a bronzing of the skin because ACTH is similar in its molecular composition to MSH. During an adrenal crisis, exogenous adrenal corticoids are essential to avoid death. Corticoids can be given to prevent inflammation, but their overuse can lead to adrenal cortex suppression by the negative feedback mechanism. The abuse of androgens by athletes wanting to buildup their muscles can also result in adrenal suppression, sterility, and damage to the heart. Tumors of androgen-producing cells in women can cause beard growth, increased muscle development, and other changes associated with sex hormones.

PERSPECTIVE AND PROSPECTS

The early history of endocrinology noted that boys who were castrated failed to undergo the changes associated with puberty. A. A. Berthold in 1849 described the effects of castration in cockerels. The birds failed to develop large combs and waddles and failed to show male behavior. He noted that these effects could be reversed if testes were transplanted back into the cockerels. W. M. Bayliss and E. H. Starling in 1902 first introduced the term "hormone" to refer to secretin. They found that secretin is produced by the small intestine in response to acid in the chyme and that secretin causes the pancreas to release digestive enzymes into the small intestine. Most important, F. G. Banting and G. H. Best in 1922 reported their extraction of insulin from the pancreas of dogs and their success in alleviating diabetes in dogs by means of injections of the insulin. Fredrick Sanger in 1953 established the amino acid sequence for insulin and later won a Nobel Prize for this achievement.

Another Nobel Prize was awarded to Earl W. Sutherland, Jr., in 1971 for his demonstration in 1962 of the role of cyclic AMP as a second messenger in the sequence involved in the stimulation of cells by many hormones. Andrew V. Schally and Roger C. L. Guillemin in 1977 received a Nobel Prize for their work in isolating and determining the structures of hypothalamic regulatory peptides.

More recent achievements in endocrinological research have centered on the identification of receptors that bind with the hormone when the hormone stimulates a cell and on the genetic engineering of bacteria to produce hormones such as human growth hormone. The use of fetal tissues in endocrinological research and therapy—the host usually does not reject fetal implants—continue to be areas for future research. —*John T. Burns, Ph.D.*

See also Addison's disease; Adrenalectomy; Amenorrhea; Cushing's syndrome; Diabetes mellitus; Dwarfism; Dysmenorrhea; Endocrinology, pediatric; Endocrinology; Endometriosis; Estrogen replacement therapy; Gigantism; Glands; Goiter; Growth; Hormone replacement therapy; Hormones; Hyperparathyroidism and hypoparathyroidism; Hypoglycemia; Infertility in females; Infertility in males; Liver; Menopause; Menorrhagia; Ovarian cysts; Pancreas; Pancreatitis; Parathyroidectomy; Pregnancy and gestation; Prostate gland; Prostate gland removal; Puberty and adolescence; Steroids; Testicular surgery; Thyroid gland; Thyroid disorders; Thyroidectomy.

FOR FURTHER INFORMATION:

Griffin, James E., and Sergio R. Ojeda, eds. *Textbook of Endocrine Physiology.* 3d ed. New York: Oxford University Press, 1996. A detailed account of normal and abnormal functioning of the endocrine system written by specialists. Intended for first year medical students.

Hadley, Mac E. *Endocrinology.* 3d ed. Englewood Cliffs, N.J.: Prentice Hall, 1992. A college-level text covering the endocrine system, primarily in humans and mammals. Recommended for a technical but understandable coverage of the field.

Jubiz, William. *Endocrinology: A Logical Approach for Clinicians.* 2d ed. New York: McGraw-Hill, 1985. An excellent source of information on specific endocrine disorders, symptoms and current treatment. Not recommended for the unmotivated reader.

Martini, Frederic. *Fundamentals of Anatomy and Physiology.* 2d ed. Englewood Cliffs, N.J.: Prentice Hall, 1992. A good place to start for a solid overview of the anatomy and physiology of the endocrine system before considering the details of disease states.

Thibodeau, Gary A., and Kevin T. Patton. *Anatomy and Physiology.* 2d ed. St. Louis: Mosby Year Book, 1993. An elementary examination of the endocrine system is provided.

Shaw, Michael, ed. *Everything You Need to Know About Diseases.* Springhouse, Pa.: Springhouse Press, 1996. This well-illustrated consumer reference, compiled by more than one hundred doctors and medical experts, describes five hundred illnesses and conditions, their causes, symptoms, diagnosis, treatment, and prevention. A valuable reference book for everyone interested in health and disease. Of particular interest is chapter 12, "Hormone and Gland Disorders."

ENDOCRINOLOGY
SPECIALTY
ANATOMY OR SYSTEM AFFECTED: Brain, endocrine system, glands, immune system, nervous system, pancreas, psychic-emotional system, reproductive system, uterus

SPECIALTIES AND RELATED FIELDS: Biochemistry, genetics, gynecology, immunology

DEFINITION: The science dealing with how the internal secretions from ductless glands in the body act both in normal physiology and in disease states.

KEY TERMS:
adrenal gland: an endocrine gland situated immediately above the upper pole of each kidney; it consists of an inner part or medulla, which produces epinephrine and norepinephrine, and an outer part or cortex, which produces steroid hormones

endocrine pancreas: specialized secretory tissue dispersed within the pancreas called islets of Langerhans, which are responsible for the secretion of glucagon and insulin

hypothalamus: the region of the brain called the diencephalon, forming the floor of the third ventricle, including neighboring associated nuclei

metabolism: the process of tissue change, which may be synthetic (anabolic) or degradative (catabolic)

parathyroid gland: one of four small endocrine glands situated underneath the thyroid gland, whose main product is parathyroid hormone, which is responsible for the regulation of serum calcium levels

pituitary gland: a small (0.5-gram), two-lobed endocrine gland that is attached by a stalk to the brain at the level of the hypothalamus

thyroid gland: a 20-gram endocrine gland that sits in front of the trachea and consists of two lateral lobes connected in the middle by an isthmus

SCIENCE AND PROFESSION

The rates of metabolic pathways in the body are controlled mainly by the endocrine system, in conjunction with the nervous system. These two systems are integrated in the neuroendocrine system, which controls the secretion of hormones by the endocrine glands. The study of endocrinology deals with the normal physiology and pathophysiology of endocrine glands. The endocrine glands that are typically the main focus of clinical endocrinologists are the hypothalamus, pituitary gland, thyroid, parathyroid, adrenal glands, endocrine pancreas, ovaries, and testes. The endocrine system regulates virtually all activities of the body, including growth and development, homeostasis, energy production, and reproduction.

The hypothalamus is a highly specialized endocrine organ that sits at the base of the brain and that functions as the master gland of the endocrine system. It is the main integrator for the endocrine and nervous systems. The hypothalamus produces a number of chemical mediators which have direct control over the pituitary gland. These chemicals are made in the cells of the hypothalamus and reach the pituitary gland, which sits just below it, by a special hypophyseoportal blood system. In adult humans, the pituitary is divided into two lobes: the anterior lobe (adenohypophysis) and the posterior lobe (neural lobe).

Vasopressin and oxytocin are the two main hormones that are made in the hypothalamus but stored in the posterior lobe of the pituitary for release when needed. Vasopressin (also known as antidiuretic hormone, or ADH) is a hormone that maintains a normal water concentration in the blood and is a regulator of circulating blood volume. Oxytocin is a hormone that is involved in lactation and obstetrical labor.

The hypothalamic-pituitary-thyroid axis is important in the control of basal metabolic rate. There are a number of releasing hormones secreted from the hypothalamus that control the release of anterior pituitary hormones, which then cause the release of hormone at the end organ. Most of these hormones have the chemical structures of peptides. Thyrotropin-releasing hormone (TRH) was the first hypothalamic releasing hormone that was synthesized and used clinically. TRH, secreted in nanogram quantities, is a cyclic tripeptide that causes release of thyrotropin-stimulating hormone (TSH) from the thyrotropic cells of the anterior pituitary gland. The release of TSH is in microgram quantities and leads to an increase in thyroid hormone release by the thyroid gland. The amount of thyroid hormone synthesized is on the order of milligrams. Therefore, the secretion of minute amounts of the TRH allows for the production of thyroid hormone that is a millionfold greater than the amount of TRH itself. This is an example of an amplifying cascade, a system by which the central nervous system can control all metabolic processes with the secretion of very small amounts of hypothalamic releasing hormones. This intricate system possesses controls to stop the production of too much hormone as well. Such negative feedback is an important concept in endocrinology. In the case of the thyroid, an increased amount of thyroid hormone produced by the thyroid gland will cause the pituitary and hypothalamus to decrease the amounts that they produce of TSH and TRH, respectively. Many hormones are subject to the laws of negative feedback control. TRH also causes potent release of the anterior pituitary hormone called prolactin. Thyroid hormone is important in determining basal metabolism and is needed for proper development in the newborn child. The thyroid gland produces both thyroxine (T_4, also called tetraiodothyronine) and triiodothyronine (T_3), both of which it synthesizes from iodine and the amino acid tyrosine.

The hypothalamic-pituitary-adrenal axis is critical in the reaction to stress, both physical and emotional. Corticotropin-releasing hormone (CRH) is a polypeptide, consisting of forty-one amino acids, that causes the production of the proopiomelanocortin molecule by the corticotropic cells of the anterior pituitary. The proopiomelanocortin molecule is cleaved by proteolytic enzymes to yield adrenocorticotropic hormone (ACTH, also called corticotropin), melanocyte-stimulating hormone, and lipotropin. It is ACTH made by the anterior pituitary which then stimulates the adrenal cortex to produce steroid hormones. The main stress hormone produced by the adrenal cortex in response to ACTH is the glucocorticoid cortisol. ACTH also has some control over the production of the mineralocorticoid aldosterone and the androgens dehydroepiandrosterone and testosterone. These steroids are synthesized from cholesterol. The production of cortisol (also known as hydrocortisone) is subject to negative feedback by CRH and ACTH.

The hypothalamic-pituitary-gonadal axis is involved in the control of reproduction. Gonadotropin-releasing hormone (GnRH), also known as luteinizing hormone-releasing hormone (LHRH), is produced by the hypothalamus and stimulates the release of luteinizing hormone (LH) and follicle-stimulating hormone (FSH) from the gonadotrophic cells of the anterior pituitary. LH and FSH have different effects in men and women. In men, LH controls the production and secretion of testosterone by the Leydig's cells of the testes. The release of LH is regulated by negative feedback from testosterone. FSH along with testosterone acts on the Sertoli cells of the seminiferous tubule of the testis at the time of puberty to start sperm production. In women, LH controls ovulation by the ovary and also the development of the corpus luteum, which produces progesterone. Progesterone is a steroid hormone that is critically important for the maintenance of pregnancy. FSH in women stimulates the development and maturation of a primary follicle and oocyte. The ovarian follicle in the nonpregnant woman is the main site of production of estradiol. Estradiol is the principal estrogen made in the reproductive years by the ovary and is responsible for the development of female secondary sexual characteristics.

Growth hormone-releasing hormone (GHRH) is a polypeptide with forty-four amino acids that stimulates the release of growth hormone (GH) from the somatotrophic cells of the anterior pituitary. The regulation of GH secretion is under dual control. While GHRH positively releases GH, somatostatin (a polypeptide with fourteen amino acids, also released from the hypothalamus) inhibits the release of GH. Somatostatin has a wide variety of functions, including the suppression of insulin, glucagon, and gastrointestinal hormones. GH released from the pituitary circulates in the bloodstream and stimulates the production of somatomedins by the liver. Several somatomedins are produced, all of which have a profound effect on growth, with the most important one in humans being somatomedin C, also called insulin-like growth factor I (IGF I). Molecular biological techniques have shown that many cells outside the liver also produce IGF I; in these cells, IGF I acts in autocrine or paracrine ways to cause the growth of the cells or to affect neighboring cells.

Prolactin is a peptide hormone that is secreted by the lactotrophs of the anterior pituitary. It is involved in the differentiation of the mammary gland cells and initiates the production of milk proteins and other constituents. Prolactin may also have other functions, as a stress hormone or growth hormone. Prolactin is under tonic negative control. The inhibition of prolactin release is caused by dopamine, which is produced by the hypothalamus. Thus, while dopamine is normally considered to be a neurotransmitter, in the case of prolactin release it acts as an inhibitory hormone. Serotonin, also classically thought of as a neurotransmitter, may cause the stimulation of prolactin release from the anterior pituitary.

DIAGNOSTIC AND TREATMENT TECHNIQUES

One of the most common medical problems seen by specialists in the field of endocrinology is a patient with type I diabetes mellitus, sometimes also called juvenile-onset or insulin-dependent diabetes mellitus. "Insulin-dependent" is probably more appropriate, as not all patients with type I diabetes mellitus develop the disease in childhood. Type I diabetes is an autoimmune disease in which antibodies to different parts of the pancreatic beta cell, the cell that normally produces insulin, are produced. Some of these antibodies are cytotoxic; that is, they actually destroy the pancreatic beta cell. The most striking characteristic of patients with type I diabetes is that they produce very little insulin. The symptoms of type I diabetes include increased thirst, increased urination, blurring of vision, and weight loss. A doctor would confirm the diagnosis by running blood tests for glucose and insulin. The glucose level would be high, and the insulin level would be low. The treatment includes controlled diet, exercise, insulin therapy and self-monitoring of blood glucose. With proper control of blood glucose, patients with type I diabetes can lead normal, productive lives.

Graves' disease is another autoimmune disease that is commonly seen by endocrinologists. Graves' disease is caused by the production of thyroid-stimulating immunoglobulin antibodies that bind to and activate TSH receptors. As a result, the thyroid gland produces too much thyroid hormone and the thyroid gland enlarges in size. The antibodies also commonly affect the eyes, causing a characteristic bulging. The clinical symptoms of hyperthyroidism include increased heart rate, anxiety, heat sensitivity, sleeplessness, diarrhea, and abdominal pain. Patients often lose considerable weight, despite having a great appetite and eating large amounts of food. Sometimes, the diagnosis is missed, leading to an extensive evaluation for a variety of other diseases. Often, a family history of thyroid disease or other endocrine disease can be found.

The usual method of screening for Graves' disease is with a simple blood test for thyroid function, which includes testing for T_4, T_3, and TSH. In patients with Graves' disease, both T_4 and T_3 will be elevated, and TSH will be very low. If the blood test reveals this pattern, the next usual step is to proceed to a radioactive iodine uptake and scan test, which involves giving a very small amount of radioactive iodine by mouth and having the patient return twenty-four hours later for a scan. The thyroid gland normally accumulates iodine and thus will accumulate the radioactive iodine as well. The radioactive iodine emits a gamma-ray energy that can be picked up by a solid-crystal scintillation counter placed over the thyroid gland. With this device, one can determine the percentage of iodine uptake and also obtain a picture of the thyroid gland. The normal radioactive iodine uptake is about 10 to 30 percent of the dose, depending somewhat on the amount of total body iodine, which is derived from the diet. Patients with Graves' disease will have high radioactive iodine uptakes.

Those who suffer from Graves' disease can be treated by three different means, depending on the circumstances. The first treatment that is often tried is antithyroid drugs, either propylthiouracil or methimazole. These drugs belong to the class of sulfonamides and inhibit the production of new thyroid hormone by blocking the attachment of iodine to the amino acid tyrosine. Another mode of therapy is the use of radioactive iodine. A dose of radioactive iodine (on the order of 5 to 10 millicuries) is used to destroy part of the thyroid gland. The gamma-ray energy emitted from the iodine molecule that has traveled to the thyroid gland is enough to kill some thyroid cells. An alternative way to destroy the thyroid gland is to remove it surgically (thyroidectomy). Endocrinologists rarely send patients for surgery, as the other therapies are often effective. The goal of all treatments is to bring the level of thyroid hormone into the normal range, as well as to shrink the thyroid gland. After treatment, the patient's level of thyroid hormone sometimes falls to levels that are below normal. The symptoms of hypothyroidism are the opposite of hyperthyroidism and include fatigue, weight gain, cold sensitivity, constipation, and dry skin. If this happens, the patient is treated with thyroid hormone replacement. The dose is adjusted for each individual to produce normal levels of T_4, T_3, and TSH.

A less common but important endocrine disorder is the existence of a pituitary tumor that secretes prolactin, called a prolactinoma. Prolactinomas are diagnosed earlier in women than in men, as women with the disorder often complain of a lack of menstrual periods and spontaneous milk production from the breasts, known as galactorrhea. These tumors, which can be quite small, are called microadenomas because they are less than 10 millimeters in size. They can affect men as well, causing decreased sex drive and impotence. Macroadenomas are tumors greater than 10 millimeters in size. When the tumors increase in size, they can cause symptoms such as headache and decreased vision. It is important to note that most microadenomas never progress to macroadenomas. Vision loss and/or decreased eye movement can be seen with a macroadenoma and are reason for immediate treatment.

Doctors screen patients for a prolactinoma by running a blood test for prolactin. There are other reasons for mild elevations in prolactin levels, including the use of certain psychiatric drugs such as phenothiazines or the antihypertensive drugs reserpine and methyldopa, primary hypothyroidism, cirrhosis, and chronic renal failure. If a pituitary tumor is suspected, then other biochemical tests of pituitary function are conducted to determine if the rest of the gland is functioning normally. At that time, imaging tests are often done to get a picture of the hypothalamic-pituitary area; this can be done with either computed tomography (CT) scanning or magnetic resonance imaging (MRI). Patients with macroadenomas will require treatment. In patients with little neurological involvement, medical therapy may be initiated. Bromocriptine, a semisynthetic ergot alkaloid which is an inhibitor of prolactin secretion, may be used. It has been shown that patients treated with this drug have reduction in tumor size. Patients can be maintained on the drug indefinitely because prolactin levels return to pretreatment levels when the drug is stopped. If there is severe neurologic involvement, with loss of vision and other eye problems, immediate surgery may be indicated. There is a very high incidence of tumor recurrence after surgery, requiring medical and/or radiation therapy.

PERSPECTIVE AND PROSPECTS

The field of endocrinology is a continuously evolving one. Advances in biomedical technology, including molecular biology and cell biology, have made it a demanding job for the clinician to keep up with all the breakthroughs in the field. The challenge for endocrinology will be to apply many of these new technologies to novel treatments for patients with endocrine diseases.

An example of the progression of the field of endocrinology can be seen in the history of pituitary diseases. The start of pituitary endocrinology is ascribed to Pierre Marie, the French neurologist who in 1886 first described pituitary enlargement in a patient with acromegaly (enlargement of the skull, jaw, hands, and feet) and linked the disease to a pituitary abnormality. During the first half of the twentieth century, many of the hypothalamic and pituitary hormones were isolated and characterized. The field of endocrinology was revolutionized by the development of the radioimmunoassay, which allows sensitive and specific measurements of hormones. The radioimmunoassay replaced bioassay techniques, which were laborious, time-consuming, and not always precise. This technique has allowed for rapid measurement of hormones and improved screening for endocrine diseases involving hormone deficiency or hormone excess.

The development of new hormone assays has been complemented by the development of noninvasive imaging techniques. Before the advent of CT scanning in the late 1970's, it was an ordeal to diagnose a pituitary tumor. Pneumoencephalography was often performed, which involved injecting air into the fluid-containing structures of the brain, with associated risk and discomfort to the patient. In the 1980's, with new generations of high-resolution CT scanners that were more sensitive than early scanners, smaller pituitary lesions could be detected and diagnosed. That decade also ushered in the use of MRI to diagnose disorders of the hypothalamic-pituitary unit. MRI has allowed doctors to evaluate the hypothalamus, pituitary, and nearby structures very precisely; it has become the method of choice for evaluating patients with pituitary disease. MRI can easily visualize the optic chiasm in the forebrain and the vascular structures surrounding the pituitary.

In patients who require surgery, advances have helped decrease mortality rates. Harvey Cushing pioneered the transsphenoidal technique in 1927 but abandoned it in favor of the transfrontal approach. This involves reaching the pituitary tumor by retracting the frontal lobes to visualize the pituitary gland sitting underneath. The modern era of transsphenoidal pituitary surgery was developed by Gérard Guiot and Jules Hardy in the late 1960's. Transsphenoidal surgery done with an operating microscope to visualize the pituitary contents allows for selective removal of the tumor, leaving the normal pituitary gland intact. The advantage of this approach from below, instead of from above, includes minimal movement of the brain and less blood loss. This technique requires a neurosurgeon with much skill and experience. There are also new drug treatments for patients with pituitary diseases, such as bromocriptine for use in patients with prolactinomas and octreotide (a somatostatin analogue) to lower growth hormone levels in patients with acromegaly. *—RoseMarie Pasmantier, M.D.*

See also Addison's disease; Adrenalectomy; Chronobiology; Cushing's syndrome; Diabetes mellitus; Dwarfism; Endocrine disorders; Endocrinology, pediatric; Enzymes; Estrogen replacement therapy; Gigantism; Glands; Goiter; Growth; Gynecology; Hair loss and baldness; Hormone replacement therapy; Hormones; Hyperparathyroidism and hypoparathyroidism; Hypoglycemia; Hysterectomy; Melatonin; Menopause; Menstruation; Obesity; Paget's disease; Pancreas; Pancreatitis; Parathyroidectomy; Pharmacology; Pharmacy; Prostate gland; Prostate gland removal; Puberty and adolescence; Sex change surgery; Sexual differentiation; Steroids; Thyroid disorders; Thyroid gland; Thyroidectomy; Weight loss and gain.

FOR FURTHER INFORMATION:

Braverman, Lewis E., and Robert D. Utiger, eds. *Werner and Ingbar's "The Thyroid."* 6th ed. Philadelphia: J. B. Lippincott, 1991. An exhaustive textbook on all aspects of the thyroid, including history, anatomy, biology, pathology, basic and clinical research, and the thyroid in development and pregnancy.

Davidson, Mayer B. *Diabetes Mellitus*. 3d ed. New York: Churchill Livingstone, 1991. A very good, practical approach to the overall management of the endocrine patient with diabetes mellitus.

Imura, Hiroo, ed. *The Pituitary Gland*. 2d ed. New York: Raven Press, 1994. Good discussion of the master gland, the hypothalamic-pituitary unit.

Lebovitz, Harold E., ed. *Therapy of Diabetes Mellitus and Related Disorders*. Alexandria, Va.: American Diabetes Association, 1991. A comprehensive treatise on the treatment of various aspects of diabetes mellitus. The different chapters are written by experts in the field.

Netter, Frank H. *The CIBA Collection of Medical Illustrations: Endocrine System*. Vol. 4. Summit, N.J.: CIBA Pharmaceutical, 1981. A beautiful color atlas depicting the anatomy of all the classic endocrine glands, by one of the most famous medical illustrators of the twentieth century. Many endocrine disorders are also shown in pictorial format.

Slaunwhite, W. Roy. *Fundamentals of Endocrinology*. New York: Marcel Dekker, 1988. This book is a good primer for people who want to know the basics of endocrinology. It is divided into seven categories: nutrition, growth, thyroid hormones, salt and water metabolism, metabolism of calcium and phosphorus, reproduction, and fuel metabolism.

Speroff, Leon, Robert H. Glass, and Nathan G. Kase, eds. *Clinical Gynecologic Endocrinology and Infertility*. 4th ed. Baltimore: Williams & Wilkins, 1989. An excellent textbook which brings together all aspects of endocrinology in women from embryology to old age. Good discussion of the problems seen in infertile couples.

Tepperman, Jay, and Helen M. Tepperman. *Metabolic and Endocrine Physiology*. Chicago: Year Book Medical Publishers, 1987. This book gives a good overview of hormonal mechanisms in health and disease.

Vaughan, E. Daracott, Jr., and Robert M. Carey, eds. *Adrenal Disorders*. New York: Thieme Medical Publishers, 1989. Comprehensive study of the anatomy, embryology, imaging, and diagnostic testing of the adrenal glands, including the cortex and the medulla.

Wilson, Jean D., and Daniel W. Foster, eds. *Williams Textbook of Endocrinology*. 8th ed. Philadelphia: W. B. Saunders, 1992. This extensive book on endocrinology covers all the different aspects of the field. It is written by recognized experts in endocrinology in a very readable style.

ENDOCRINOLOGY, PEDIATRIC

SPECIALTY

ANATOMY OR SYSTEM AFFECTED: Brain, endocrine system, glands, immune system, nervous system, pancreas, psychic-emotional system

SPECIALTIES AND RELATED FIELDS: Biochemistry, genetics, immunology, neonatology, pediatrics

DEFINITION: The study of the normal and abnormal function of the endocrine (ductless) glands in children and adolescents.

KEY TERMS:

hormone: a chemical molecule produced in either the hypothalamus or one of the endocrine glands that is secreted and travels (usually via the bloodstream) to a target organ or to specific receptor cells, causing a specific response

hypothalamus: a very small portion of the base of the brain, immediately adjacent to the pituitary gland

insulin: a hormone that is essential in regulating blood glucose, as well as in assimilating carbohydrates for growth and energy

pancreas: a large gland near the stomach which has both exocrine and endocrine functions and which produces insulin

pituitary gland: a very small gland at the base of the brain that is referred to as the master gland; with the hypothalamus, it regulates most of the endocrine systems

thyroid: a gland in the anterior neck which regulates the level of the body's metabolism and which is instrumental in normal physical and mental growth

SCIENCE AND PROFESSION

Pediatric endocrinology is a major subspecialty, limited to children and adolescents, which involves the study of normal as well as abnormal functions of the endocrine system, which involves the glands of internal or ductless secretions. These practitioners, referred to as endocrinologists or pediatric endocrinologists, are doctors of medicine or osteopathy who have completed three years of pediatric residency training and an additional two to three years of fellowship training in endocrinology.

Endocrinology is one of the most interesting and challenging fields in pediatrics because it involves a blend of basic science and technology in the clinical setting. Some of the diagnoses are very difficult, yet they are almost always completely logical. Endocrinology is tightly related to other areas of pediatrics, such as adolescent medicine, genetics, growth, development, nutrition, and metabolism. These relationships make this field even more complex and intellectually stimulating.

Pediatric endocrinology and adult endocrinology are relatively young fields, probably beginning with the discovery in 1888 that "myxedema" (hypothyroidism) could be improved by feeding the patient thyroid extract. Both fields deal with the major endocrine glands and their disorders, such as diabetes mellitus or hypothyroidism, but there are several key differences, most related to growth (both physical and mental), potential, and genetics. Some major areas of specific emphasis in pediatric endocrinology include diabetes mellitus (which presents very differently in children), disorders of growth, disorders of sexual maturation and differentiation, genetic disorders, and adolescent medicine.

DIAGNOSTIC AND TREATMENT TECHNIQUES

In pediatric endocrinology, as in all medical fields, history taking and physical examination are the starting points and usually the most useful tools for diagnosis. Endocrinology is a specialty that is particularly aided by science. Blood and urine chemistries, hormone assays, chromosomal analyses, X rays, computed tomography (CT) scans, magnetic resonance imaging (MRI), and a host of other sophisticated tests have advanced diagnosis and treatment and have made this specialty one of the favorites for physicians who like science. Virtually all the known hormones can be assayed accurately and quickly.

Since insulin was first available for injection in 1922, there have also been amazing advances in treatment. Many of the treatments in endocrinology involve hormone therapy. In 1985, recombinant growth hormone was synthesized for the first time. This development has allowed endocrinologists to treat not only pituitary dwarfism but also other kinds of growth deficiencies, such as Turner's syndrome.

Turner's syndrome is a relatively common chromosomal abnormality affecting females and resulting in short stature and lack of sexual development. While these girls will never become fertile, the combination of growth hormone for stature and other hormonal therapy for the development of secondary sexual characteristics enables them to have a normal female body. Studies have shown that normal body image and the presence of menstruation is essential for the self-esteem of these patients.

Diabetes mellitus is the most common significant endocrine disorder in both adults and children. What was commonly referred to as juvenile diabetes years ago is now called diabetes mellitus, type I. Unlike type II, which usually presents insidiously in middle-aged and older adults, type I presents rapidly, and the patient will need daily injectable insulin treatments. Diabetes in children is complex to manage not only because of the insulin treatment but also because of the patients' growth, metabolism, fluctuating activity levels, and the physiologic and psychological changes that occur, especially in adolescence.

Now small portable and quite accurate glucometers allow patients to measure blood glucose (sugar) at home, making diabetes management much simpler. Tighter control of blood glucose will decrease or delay the onset of long-term complications of the disease, such as blindness, heart disease, and kidney disease. In the United States, newborn screening, which is now done in all fifty states, has virtually eliminated cretinism, which tragically resulted when congenital hypothyroidism was not diagnosed until later in childhood. These children were irreversibly mentally retarded.

Enhanced techniques in pediatric and neurosurgery, greatly aided by scans, play a role in the treatment of some endocrine disorders. Very small tumors and masses can be identified and often removed successfully. Often, endocri-

nologists and oncologists work together in concert with the surgeon.

Although this subspecialty is one of the most scientific and laboratory-based in pediatrics, it is also a field where emotional support, counseling, and often mental health care is given. Children do not like being "different," and body image is very important in children and particularly in teenagers. Even when a child appears absolutely normal, the frustration of ongoing monitoring and treatment is resented and can result in rebellion, especially in children with diabetes. Often, a team approach is needed, which involves professionals, teachers, family, and peers.

PERSPECTIVE AND PROSPECTS

The future promises ever-advancing and dramatic tools for the diagnosis and treatment of endocrine disorders, as well as for their prevention. On the immediate horizon, an implantible glucose pump, which can serve as a substitute pancreas, can change the lives of diabetic patients dramatically. A new method for rapidly analyzing blood glucose using the surface of the skin was scheduled for release in 1995. In addition, genetic engineering may revolutionize the approaches to treating many of these diseases.

—*C. Mervyn Rasmussen, M.D.*

See also Addison's disease; Adrenalectomy; Chronobiology; Diabetes mellitus; Dwarfism; Endocrine disorders; Endocrinology; Enzymes; Gigantism; Glands; Growth; Gynecology; Hormone replacement therapy; Hormones; Hyperparathyroidism and hypoparathyroidism; Hypoglycemia; Melatonin; Menstruation; Obesity; Pancreas; Pancreatitis; Parathyroidectomy; Pediatrics; Pharmacology; Pharmacy; Puberty and adolescence; Steroids; Thyroid disorders; Thyroid gland; Thyroidectomy; Weight loss and gain.

FOR FURTHER INFORMATION:

Little, Marjorie. *Diabetes.* New York: Chelsea House, 1991. A clearly written overview directed toward a nonspecialized audience. Includes a fourteen-page chapter on type I (juvenile) diabetes.

Sperling, Mark A., ed. *Pediatric Endocrinology.* Philadelphia: W. B. Saunders, 1996. Discusses endocrine diseases in infancy and childhood. Includes a bibliography and an index.

The World Book Encyclopedia. 22 vols. Chicago: World Book, 1994. Volume G, pages 207 to 209, offers a clear and concise overview of the endocrine system.

ENDODONTIC DISEASE

DISEASE/DISORDER

ANATOMY OR SYSTEM AFFECTED: Gums, mouth, teeth
SPECIALTIES AND RELATED FIELDS: Dentistry
DEFINITION: Endodontics is the field of dentistry concerned with diseases of the dental pulp found within teeth and diseases of the surrounding tissues, the gums. Endodontic disease can be caused by damage to the nerves in the teeth and gums and resulting infection by micro-

organisms. Dental caries, commonly known as cavities, are one example of pulp decay that must be removed. If the entire pulp has died or becomes untreatable, root canal treatment may be required, in which the pulp is completely replaced with filling paste and the surface of the tooth is sealed with a cement crown.

—Jason Georges and Tracy Irons-Georges

See also Caries, dental; Dental diseases; Dentistry; Gingivitis; Periodontal surgery; Periodontitis; Root canal treatment; Teeth; Tooth extraction; Toothache.

ENDOMETRIAL BIOPSY
PROCEDURE
ANATOMY OR SYSTEM AFFECTED: Genitals, reproductive system, uterus
SPECIALTIES AND RELATED FIELDS: General surgery, gynecology
DEFINITION: A procedure designed to obtain a sample of the uterine lining (endometrium) for diagnostic analysis.

INDICATIONS AND PROCEDURES
Endometrial biopsy is a diagnostic procedure used to assess such medical disorders as female infertility and abnormal vaginal bleeding. It is an outpatient procedure performed with local anesthesia, and it takes only thirty seconds. A small plastic cylinder is placed into the uterus through the cervix. A suction device or metal scraping instrument in the cylinder removes a small sample of the endometrium. The sample is sent to a laboratory for microscopic analysis.

USES AND COMPLICATIONS
If infertility testing reveals no obvious physical problems or abnormalities in sperm number and viability of a couple, further procedures are conducted, including an endometrial biopsy. The quality of the uterine lining is distinctly different while under the influence of estrogen, just prior to ovulation, as compared to its quality while progesterone is being produced after ovulation. Endometrial tissue analysis can reveal if the woman is not ovulating or is producing inadequate progesterone to support a pregnancy after ovulation. This procedure can be performed between a week after ovulation to the first day of the woman's menstrual period.

If the cause of infertility is a lack of ovulation, a variety of drug and hormone therapies are available to induce ovulation. Inadequacies in maintaining the uterine lining after ovulation may be treated with natural progesterone or other medications.

Bleeding between menstrual periods or a heavy increase in menstrual flow may be indicative of a host of conditions. In some cases, an endometrial biopsy may be performed to analyze the uterine lining for abnormal cell growth that may be indicative of cancer or such conditions as uterine polyps and fibroids. Surgical removal of abnormal growths and/or cancer therapies are initiated when appropriate.

Possible complications of endometrial biopsy include minor cramping and spotting after the procedure. Some physicians believe that there may be a small risk to a newly implanted embryo and advise the use of birth control during the several weeks prior to the biopsy.

—Karen E. Kalumuck, Ph.D.

See also Biopsy; Cancer; Cervical, ovarian, and uterine cancers; Cervical procedures; Genital disorders, female; Gynecology; Infertility in females; Oncology; Reproductive system.

ENDOMETRIOSIS
DISEASE/DISORDER
ANATOMY OR SYSTEM AFFECTED: Reproductive system, uterus
SPECIALTIES AND RELATED FIELDS: Gynecology
DEFINITION: Growth of cells of the uterine lining at sites outside the uterus, causing severe pain and infertility.
KEY TERMS:
cervix: an oval-shaped organ that separates the uterus and the vagina
dysmenorrhea: painful menstruation
dyspareunia: painful sexual intercourse
endometrium: the tissue that lines the uterus, builds up, and sheds at the end of each menstrual cycle; when it grows outside the uterus, endometriosis occurs
Fallopian tubes: two tubes extending from the ovaries to the uterus; during ovulation, an egg travels down one of these tubes to the uterus
hysterectomy: surgery that removes part or all of the uterus
implant: an abnormal endometrial growth outside the uterus
laparoscopy: a surgical procedure in which a small incision made near the navel is used to view the uterus and other abdominal organs with a lighted tube called a laparoscope
laparotomy: a surgical procedure, often exploratory in nature, carried out through the abdominal wall; it may be used to correct endometriosis
laser: a concentrated, high-energy light beam often used to destroy abnormal tissue
oophorectomy (or *ovariectomy*): removal of the ovaries, which is often necessary in cases of severe endometriosis
prostaglandins: fatlike hormones that control the contraction and relaxation of the uterus and other smooth muscle tissue

CAUSES AND SYMPTOMS
Endometriosis, the presence of endometrial tissue outside its normal location as the lining of the uterus, is a disabling disease in women that causes severe pain and in many cases infertility. The classic symptoms of endometriosis are very painful menstruation (dysmenorrhea), painful intercourse (dyspareunia), and infertility. Some other common endometriosis symptoms include nausea, vomiting, diarrhea, and fatigue.

It has been estimated that endometriosis affects between five million and twenty-five million American women. Often, it is incorrectly stereotyped as being a disease of upwardly mobile, professional women. According to many experts, the incidence of endometriosis worldwide and across most racial groups is probably very similar. They propose that the reported occurrence rate difference for some racial groups, such as a lower incidence in African Americans, has been a socioeconomic phenomenon attributable to the social class of women who seek medical treatment for the symptoms of endometriosis and to the highly stratified responses of many health care professionals who have dealt with the disease.

The symptoms of endometriosis arise from abnormalities in the effects of the menstrual cycle on the endometrial tissue lining the uterus. The endometrium normally thickens and becomes swollen with blood (engorged) during the cycle, a process controlled by female hormones called estrogens and progestins. This engorgement is designed to prepare the uterus for conception by optimizing conditions for implantation in the endometrium of a fertilized egg, which enters the uterus via one of the Fallopian tubes leading from the ovaries.

By the middle of the menstrual cycle, the endometrial lining is normally about ten times thicker than that at its beginning. If the egg that is released into the uterus is not fertilized, pregnancy does not occur and decreases in production of the female sex hormones result in the breakdown of the endometrium. Endometrial tissue mixed with blood leaves the uterus as the menstrual flow and a new menstrual cycle begins. This series of uterine changes occurs repeatedly, as a monthly cycle, from puberty (which usually occurs between the ages of twelve and fourteen) to the menopause (which usually occurs between the ages of forty-five and fifty-five).

In women who develop endometriosis, some endometrial tissue begins to grow ectopically (in an abnormal position) at sites outside the uterus. The ectopic endometrial growths may be found attached to the ovaries, the Fallopian tubes, the urinary bladder, the rectum, other abdominal organs, and even the lungs. Regardless of body location, these implants behave as if they were still in the uterus, thickening and bleeding each month as the menstrual cycle proceeds. Like the endometrium at its normal uterine site, the ectopic tissue responds to the hormones that circulate through the body in the blood. Its inappropriate position in the body prevents this ectopic endometrial tissue from leaving the body as menstrual flow; as a result, some implants grow to be quite large.

In many cases, the endometrial growths that form between two organs become fibrous bands called adhesions. The fibrous nature of adhesions is attributable to the alternating swelling and breakdown of the ectopic tissue, which yields fibrous scar tissue. The alterations in size of living

Common Sites of Endometriosis

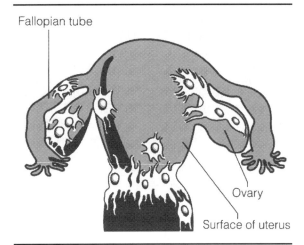

Fallopian tube

Ovary

Surface of uterus

portions of the adhesions and other endometrial implants during the monthly menstrual cycle cause many afflicted women considerable pain. Because the body location of implants varies, the site of the pain may be almost anywhere, such as the back, the chest, the rectum, or the abdomen. For example, dyspareunia occurs when adhesions hold a uterus tightly to the abdominal wall, making its movement during intercourse painful.

The presence of endometriosis is usually confirmed by laparoscopy, viewed as being the most reliable method for its diagnosis. Laparoscopy is carried out after a physician makes an initial diagnosis of probable endometriosis from a combined study including an examination of the patient's medical history and careful exploration of the patient's physical problems over a period of at least six months. During prelaparoscopy treatment, the patient is very often maintained on pain medication and other therapeutic drugs that will produce symptomatic relief.

For laparoscopy, the patient is anesthetized with a general anesthetic, a small incision is made near the navel, and a flexible lighted tube—a laparoscope—is inserted into this incision. The laparoscope, equipped with fiber optics, enables the examining physician to search the patient's abdominal organs for endometrial implants. Visibility of the abdominal organs in laparoscopic examination can be enhanced by pumping harmless carbon dioxide gas into the abdomen, causing it to distend. Women who undergo laparoscopy usually require a day of postoperative bed rest, followed by seven to ten days of curtailed physical activity. After a laparoscopic diagnosis of endometriosis is made, a variety of surgical and therapeutic drug treatments can be employed to manage the disease.

About 40 percent of all women who have endometriosis are infertile; contemporary wisdom evaluates this relationship as one of cause and effect, which should make this disease the second most common cause of fertility problems. The actual basis for this infertility is not always clear, but it is often the result of damage to the ovaries and Fallopian tubes, scar tissue produced by implants on these and other abdominal organs, and hormone imbalances.

Because the incidence of infertility accompanying endometriosis increases with the severity of the disease, all potentially afflicted women are encouraged to seek early diagnosis. Many experts advise all women with abnormal menstrual cycles, dysmenorrhea, severe menstrual bleeding, abnormal vaginal bleeding, and repeated dyspareunia to seek the advice of a physician trained in identifying and dealing with endometriosis. Because the disease can begin to present symptoms at any age, teenagers are also encouraged to seek medical attention if they experience any of these symptoms.

John Sampson coined the term "endometriosis" in the 1920's. Sampson's theory for its causation, still widely accepted, is termed retrograde menstruation. Also called menstrual backup, this theory proposes that the backing up of some menstrual flow into the Fallopian tubes, and then into the abdominal cavity, forms the endometrial implants. Evidence supporting this theory, according to many physicians, is the fact that such backup is common. Others point out, however, that the backup is often found in women who do not have the disease. A surgical experiment was performed on female monkeys to test this theory. Their uteri were turned upside down so that the menstrual flow would spill into the abdominal cavity. Sixty percent of the animals developed endometriosis postoperatively—an inconclusive result.

Complicating the issue is the fact that implants are also found in tissues (such as in the lung) that cannot be reached by menstrual backup. It has been theorized that the presence of these implants results from the entry of endometrial cells into the lymphatic system, which returns body fluid to the blood and protects the body from many other diseases. This transplantation theory is supported by the occurrence of endometriosis in various portions of the lymphatic system and in tissues that could not otherwise become sites of endometriosis.

A third theory explaining the growth of implants is the iatrogenic, or nosocomial, transmission of endometrial tissue. These terms both indicate an accidental creation of the disease through the actions of physicians. Such implant formation is viewed as occurring most often after cesarean delivery of a baby when passage through the birth canal would otherwise be fatal to mother and/or child. Another proposed cause is episiotomy—widening of the birth canal by an incision between the anus and vagina—to ease births.

Any surgical procedure that allows the spread of endometrial tissue can be implicated, including surgical procedures carried out to correct existing endometriosis, because of the ease with which endometrial tissue implants itself anywhere in the body. Abnormal endometrial tissue growth, called adenomyosis, can also occur in the uterus and is viewed as a separate disease entity.

Other theories regarding the genesis of endometriosis include an immunologic theory, which proposes that women who develop endometriosis are lacking in antibodies that normally cause the destruction of endometrial tissue at sites where it does not belong, and a hormonal theory, which suggests the existence of large imbalances in hormones such as the prostaglandins that serve as the body's messengers in controlling biological processes. Several of these theories—retrograde menstruation, the transplantation theory, and iatrogenic transmission—all have support, but none has been proved unequivocally. Future evidence will identify whether one cause is dominant, whether they all interact to produce the disease, or whether endometriosis is actually a group of diseases that simply resemble one another in the eyes of contemporary medical science.

TREATMENT AND THERAPY

Laparoscopic examination most often identifies endometriosis as chocolate-colored lumps (chocolate cysts) ranging from the size of a pinhead to several inches across or as filmy coverings over parts of abdominal organs and ligaments. Once a diagnosis of the disease is confirmed by laparoscopy, endometriosis is treated by chemotherapy, surgery, or a combination of both methods. The only permanent, contemporary cure for endometriosis, however, is the onset of the biological menopause at the end of a woman's childbearing years. As long as menstruation continues, implant development is likely to recur, regardless of its cause. Nevertheless, a temporary cure of endometriosis is better than no cure at all.

The chemotherapy that many physicians use to treat mild cases of endometriosis (and for prelaparoscopy periods) is analgesic painkillers, including aspirin, acetaminophen, and ibuprofen. The analgesics inhibit the body's production of prostaglandins, and the symptoms of the disease are merely covered up. Therefore, analgesics are of quite limited value except during a prelaparoscopy diagnostic period or with mild cases of endometriosis. In addition, the long-term administration of aspirin will often produce gastrointestinal bleeding, and excess use of acetaminophen can lead to severe liver damage. In some cases of very severe endometriosis pain, narcotic painkillers are given, such as codeine, Percodan (oxycodone and aspirin), or morphine. Narcotics are addicting and should be avoided unless absolutely necessary.

More effective for long-term management of the disease is hormone therapy. Such therapy is designed to prevent the monthly occurrence of menstruation—that is, to freeze the body in a sort of chemical menopause. The hormone types used, made by pharmaceutical companies, are chemical cousins of female hormones (estrogens and progestins), male hormones (androgens), and a brain hormone that controls ovulation (gonadotropin-releasing hormone, or GnRH). Appropriate hormone therapy is often useful for years, although each hormone class produces disadvantageous side effects in many patients.

The use of estrogens stops ovulation and menstruation, freeing many women with endometriosis from painful symptoms. Numerous estrogen preparations have been prescribed, including the birth control pills that contain them. Drawbacks of estrogen use can include weight gain, nausea, breast soreness, depression, blood-clotting abnormalities, and elevated risk of vaginal cancer. In addition, estrogen administration may cause endometrial implants to enlarge.

The use of progestins arose from the discovery that pregnancy—which is maintained by high levels of a natural progestin called progesterone—reversed the symptoms of many suffering from endometriosis. This realization led to the utilization of synthetic progestins to cause prolonged false pregnancy. The rationale is that all endometrial implants will die off and be reabsorbed during the prolonged absence of menstruation. The method works in most patients, and pain-free periods of up to five years are often observed. In some cases, however, side effects include nausea, depression, insomnia, and a very slow resumption of normal menstruation (such as lags of up to a year) when the therapy is stopped. In addition, progestins are ineffective in treating large implants; in fact, their use in such cases can lead to severe complications.

In the 1970's, studies showing the potential for heart attacks, high blood pressure, and strokes in patients receiving long-term female hormone therapy led to a search for more advantageous hormone medications. An alternative developed was the synthetic male hormone danazol (Danocrine), which is very effective. One of its advantages over female hormones is the ability to shrink large implants and restore fertility to those patients whose problems arise from nonfunctional ovaries or Fallopian tubes. Danazol has become the drug of choice for treating millions of endometriosis sufferers. Problems associated with danazol use, however, can include weight gain, masculinization (decreased bust size, facial hair growth, and deepened voice), fatigue, depression, and baldness. Those women contemplating danazol use should be aware that it can also complicate pregnancy.

Because of the side effects of these hormones, other chemotherapy was sought. Another valuable drug that has become available is GnRH, which suppresses the function of the ovaries in a fashion equivalent to surgical oophorectomy (removal of the ovaries). This hormone produces none of the side effects of the sex hormones, such as weight gain, depression, or masculinization, but some evidence indicates that it may lead to osteoporosis.

Thus, despite the fact that hormone therapy may relieve or reduce pain for years, contemporary chemotherapy is flawed by many undesirable side effects. Perhaps more serious, however, is the high recurrence rate of endometriosis that is observed after the therapy is stopped. Consequently, it appears that the best treatment of endometriosis combines chemotherapy with surgery.

The extent of the surgery carried out to combat endometriosis is variable and depends on the observations made during laparoscopy. In cases of relatively mild endometriosis, conservative laparotomy surgery removes endometriosis implants, adhesions, and lesions. This type of procedure attempts to relieve endometriosis pain, to minimize the chances of postoperative recurrence of the disease, and to allow the patient to have children. Even in the most severe cases of this type, the uterus, an ovary, and its associated Fallopian tube are retained. Such surgery will often include removal of the appendix, whether diseased or not, because it is very likely to develop implants. The surgical techniques performed are the conventional excision of diseased tissue or the use of lasers to vaporize it. Many physicians prefer lasers because it is believed that they decrease the chances of recurrent endometriosis resulting from retained implant tissue or iatrogenic causes.

In more serious cases, hysterectomy is carried out. All visible implants, adhesions, and lesions are removed from the abdominal organs, as in conservative surgery. In addition, the uterus and cervix are taken out, but one or both ovaries are retained. This allows female hormone production to continue normally until the menopause. Uterine removal makes it impossible to have children, however, and may lead to profound psychological problems that require psychiatric help. Women planning to elect for hysterectomy to treat endometriosis should be aware of such potential difficulties. In many cases of conservative surgery or hysterectomy, danazol is used, both preoperatively and postoperatively, to minimize implant size.

The most extensive surgery carried out on the women afflicted with endometriosis is radical hysterectomy, also called definitive surgery, in which the ovaries and/or the vagina are also removed. The resultant symptoms are menopausal and may include vaginal bleeding atrophy (when the vagina is retained), increased risk of heart disease, and the development of osteoporosis. To counter the occurrence of these symptoms, replacement therapy with female hormones is suggested. Paradoxically, this hormone therapy can lead to the return of endometriosis by stimulating the growth of residual implant tissue.

PERSPECTIVE AND PROSPECTS

Modern treatment of endometriosis is viewed by many physicians as beginning in the 1950's. A landmark development in this field was the accurate diagnosis of endometriosis via the laparoscope, which was invented in Europe and introduced into the United States in the 1960's. Medical science has progressed greatly since that time. Physicians and researchers have recognized the wide occurrence of the disease and accepted its symptoms as valid; realized that hysterectomy will not necessarily put an end to the disease; utilized chemotherapeutic tools, including hormones and painkillers, as treatments and as adjuncts to surgery; developed laser surgery and other techniques that decrease the occurrence of formerly ignored iatrogenic endometriosis; and understood that the disease can ravage teenagers as well and that these young women should be examined as early as possible.

As pointed out by Niels H. Lauersen and Constance De-Swaan in *The Endometriosis Answer Book* (1988), more research than ever is "exploring the intricacies of the disease." Moreover, the efforts and information base of the proactive American Endometriosis Association, founded in 1980, have been very valuable. As a result, a potentially or presently afflicted woman is much more aware of the problems associated with the disease. In addition, she has a source for obtaining objective information on topics including state-of-the-art treatment, physician and hospital choice, and both physical and psychological outcomes of treatment.

Many potentially viable avenues for better endometriosis diagnosis and treatment have become the objects of intense investigation. These include the use of ultrasonography and radiology techniques for the predictive, nonsurgical examination of the course of growth or the chemotherapeutic destruction of implants; the design of new drugs to be utilized in the battle against endometriosis; endeavors aimed at the development of diagnostic tests for the disease that will stop it before symptoms develop; and the design of dietary treatments to soften its effects.

Regrettably, because of the insidious nature of endometriosis—which has the ability to strike almost anywhere in the body—some confusion about the disease still exists. New drugs, surgical techniques, and other aids are expected to be helpful in clarifying many of these issues. Particular value is being placed on the study of the immunologic aspects of endometriosis. Scientists hope to explain why the disease strikes some women and not others, to uncover its etiologic basis, and to solve the widespread problems of iatrogenic implant formation and other types of endometriosis recurrence.   —*Sanford S. Singer, Ph.D.*

See also Amenorrhea; Cervical, ovarian, and uterine cancers; Childbirth, complications of; Dysmenorrhea; Endometrial biopsy; Genital disorders, female; Gynecology; Hysterectomy; Infertility in females; Menorrhagia; Menstruation; Pregnancy and gestation; Reproductive system.

FOR FURTHER INFORMATION:

Barnhart, Edward R., ed. *Physician's Desk Reference.* 47th ed. Oradell, N.J.: Medical Economics, 1993. This atlas of prescription drugs includes the drugs used against endometriosis, the companies that produce them, their useful dose ranges, their effects on metabolism and toxicology, and their contraindications. A useful reference work for physicians and patients that is found in most public libraries.

Breitkopf, Lyle J., and Marion Gordon Bakoulis. *Coping with Endometriosis.* New York: Prentice Hall, 1988. This book explores how patients cope with endometriosis in a clear manner. Topical coverage includes an overview of endometriosis, interactions between afflicted patients and physicians, causation theories, severity classification, treatment, infertility, and the management of endometriosis. Contains a glossary and a bibliography.

Lauersen, Niels H., and Constance DeSwaan. *The Endometriosis Answer Book: New Hope, New Help.* New York: Rawson Associates, 1988. This detailed book covers endometriosis well. Some of the main subdivisions are an explanation of the disease, the choice of a physician, medical and surgical treatment, and support groups. An extensive bibliography is included.

Older, Julia. *Endometriosis.* New York: Charles Scribner's Sons, 1984. Discusses endometriosis causation theories, diagnosis of the disease, its medical and surgical treatment, possible complications, racial and age relatedness, and prevention of the disease. The glossary and bibliography are also very useful.

Shaw, Michael, ed. *Everything You Need to Know About Diseases.* Springhouse, Pa.: Springhouse Press, 1996. This well-illustrated consumer reference, compiled by more than one hundred doctors and medical experts, describes five hundred illnesses and conditions, their causes, symptoms, diagnosis, treatment, and prevention. A valuable reference book for everyone interested in health and disease. Of particular interest is chapter 9, "Gynecologic Disorders."

Sherwood, Lauralee. *Human Physiology: From Cells to Systems.* 3d ed. Belmont, Calif.: Wadsworth, 1997. This college text contains much useful biological information. Included are details about the menstrual cycle, hormones, the endometrium, and many helpful definitions. Valuable diagrams and glossary terms also abound. Clearly written, the book is a mine of information for interested readers.

Weinstein, Kate. *Living with Endometriosis.* Reading, Mass.: Addison-Wesley, 1987. The main divisions of this handy book are medical aspects, treatments and outcomes, emotional problems, and pain and psychiatric problems. Highlights include the complete description of the female reproductive system and menstruation, the glossary, and appendices on organizations, literature, and pain management centers.

Wigfall-Williams, Wanda. *Hysterectomy: Learning the Facts, Coping with the Feelings, and Facing the Future.* New York: Michael Kesend, 1986. Explains clearly the reasons that hysterectomy may be necessary, including the presence of endometriosis. Gives solid guidelines for physician and surgery choice. Also explores the depression that may follow this procedure and how to deal with it, hormone replacement therapy, and alterations in sexual function. A glossary and many references are included.

ENDOSCOPY

PROCEDURE

ANATOMY OR SYSTEM AFFECTED: Abdomen, anus, bladder, gastrointestinal system, intestines, joints, knees, lungs, stomach, urinary system

SPECIALTIES AND RELATED FIELDS: Gastroenterology, gynecology, obstetrics, orthopedics, proctology, pulmonary medicine, urology

DEFINITION: The use of a flexible tube to look into body structures in order to inspect and sometimes correct pathologies.

KEY TERMS:

biopsy: the collection and study of body tissue, often to determine whether it is cancerous

fiber optics: the transmission of light through thin, flexible tubes

pathology: a disease condition; also the study of diseases

INDICATIONS AND PROCEDURES

Early endoscopes were simply rigid hollow tubes with a light source. They were inserted into body orifices, such as the anus or the mouth, to allow the physician to look directly at processes within. Modern instruments are more sophisticated. They use fiber optics in flexible cables to penetrate deep into body structures. For example, one form of colonoscope can be threaded though the entire lower intestine, allowing the physician to search for pathologies all the way from the anus to the cecum of the colon (large intestine).

There are eight basic types of endoscope: gastroscope, colonoscope, bronchoscope, cystoscope, laparoscope, colposcope, arthroscope, and amnioscope. Their primary uses are diagnostic; however, they can be fitted with special instruments to perform many different tasks, including taking bits of tissue for biopsy and carrying out surgical procedures.

USES AND COMPLICATIONS

The gastroscope and its variants are used to inspect structures of the gastrointestinal system. The name of one class of procedure gives an idea of how sophisticated the gastroscope has become: esophagogastroduodenoscopy. As the term implies, this technique can be used to investigate the esophagus (the tube leading to the stomach), the stomach itself, and the intestines all the way into the duodenum (the first link of the small intestine). Further, in a procedure called endoscopic retrograde cholangiopancreatography, the endoscope can be used to investigate processes in the gallbladder, the cystic duct, the common hepatic duct, and the common bile duct. By far the most common use of the gastroscope is in the diagnosis and management of esophageal and stomach problems. The gastroscope is used to con-

firm the suspicion of stomach ulcers and other gastroesophageal conditions and to monitor therapy.

The colonoscope and its variants are critical in the diagnosis of diseases in the lower intestine and in some aspects of therapy. The long, flexible fiber-optic tube can be threaded through the anus and rectum into the S-shaped sigmoid colon (flexible fiber-optic sigmoidoscopy). The tube can be made to rise up the descending colon, across the transverse colon, and down the ascending colon to the cecum. With the colonoscope, the physician can discover abnormalities such as polyps, diverticula, and blockages and the presence of cancer, Crohn's disease, ulcerative colitis, and many other diseases. The physician can also use the colonoscope to remove polyps; this is the major therapeutic use of colonoscopy.

Like most other forms of endoscopy, bronchoscopy is used for both diagnosis and treatment. The bronchoscope allows direct visualization of the trachea (the tube leading from the throat to the lungs) and the bronchi (the two main airducts leading into the lungs). It will show certain forms of lung cancer, various infectious states, and other pathologies. The bronchoscope can also be used to remove foreign objects, excise local tumors, remove mucus plugs, and improve bronchial drainage.

The cystoscope is used for visual inspection of the urethra and bladder. The bladder stores urine; the urethra is the tube through which it is eliminated. Cystoscopy discovers many of the conditions that can afflict these organs: obstruction, infection, cancer, and other disorders.

The laparoscope is used to look into the abdominal cavity for evidence of a wide variety of conditions. It can inspect the liver, help evaluate liver disease, and take tissue samples for biopsy. Laparoscopy can confirm the diagnosis of ectopic pregnancy (a condition in which a fetus develops outside the womb, usually in one of the Fallopian tubes). It can confirm the presence or absence of abdominal cancers and diagnose disease conditions in the gallbladder, spleen, peritoneum (the membrane that surrounds the abdomen), and the diaphragm, as well as give some views of the small and large intestine. In an important, relatively new development, the laparoscope is being used to remove gallbladders (cholecystectomy). This procedure is far less traumatic than the old surgery, often permitting release of the patient a day or two after the operation rather than requiring weeks of recuperation.

The colposcope is used to inspect vaginal tissue and adjacent organs. Common reasons for colposcopy include abnormal bleeding and suspicion of tumors.

Arthroscopy, the investigation of joint structures by endoscopy, is now the most common invasive technique used on patients with arthritis or joint damage. In addition to viewing the area, the arthroscope can be fitted with various instruments to perform surgical procedures.

The term "amnioscope" comes from the amnion, the

membrane that surrounds a fetus. This type of endoscope is used to enter the uterus and inspect the growing fetus in the search for any visible abnormalities.

Endoscopy is one of the most useful and most-used techniques for diagnosis because it permits the investigation of many internal body organs without surgery. It is extraordi-narily safe in the hands of experienced practitioners and is relatively free of pain and discomfort. In addition, special-ized endoscopes are assuming greater roles in therapy. Many procedures that once involved major surgery can now be conducted through the endoscope, saving the patient pain, trauma, and expense.

Endoscopy and Its Uses

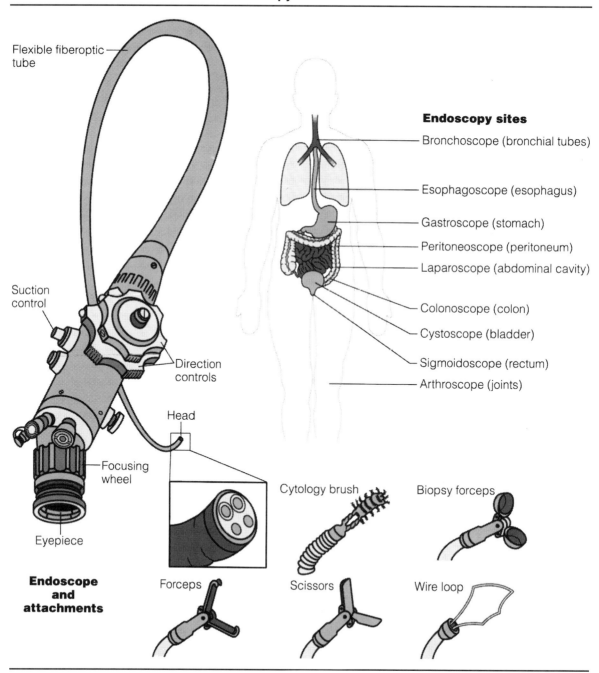

Flexible fiberoptic tube

Suction control

Direction controls

Head

Focusing wheel

Eyepiece

Endoscope and attachments

Forceps

Cytology brush

Scissors

Biopsy forceps

Wire loop

Endoscopy sites

Bronchoscope (bronchial tubes)

Esophagoscope (esophagus)

Gastroscope (stomach)

Peritoneoscope (peritoneum)

Laparoscope (abdominal cavity)

Colonoscope (colon)

Cystoscope (bladder)

Sigmoidoscope (rectum)

Arthroscope (joints)

Perspective and Prospects

Endoscopes have become highly sophisticated instruments with enormous range throughout the body and enormous potential. Colonoscopy, for example, promises to revolutionize the treatment of cancerous and precancerous polyps by helping physicians attain a clearer understanding of the polyp-to-cancer progression. The laparoscope has revolutionized gallbladder removal, as the arthroscope has revolutionized joint surgery. The gastroscope gives the physician new security and control in the management of gastrointestinal conditions and the bronchoscope facilitates many lung procedures.

Similarly throughout the entire range of endoscopy, new opportunities are opening and leading to significant improvements in therapy, and these improvements will continue. Electronic and video techniques are being introduced into endoscopy, and this new technology promises to widen the applications and therapeutic range of endoscopy still further.

—*C. Richard Falcon*

See also Abdominal disorders; Arthritis; Arthroscopy; Biopsy; Cholecystectomy; Colon and rectal polyp removal; Colon cancer; Colonoscopy; Cystoscopy; Gallbladder diseases; Gastrointestinal disorders; Invasive tests; Laparoscopy; Pulmonary diseases; Stone removal; Stones.

For Further Information:

Horton, Edward, et al. *The Marshall Cavendish Illustrated Encyclopedia of Family Health.* 24 vols. London: Marshall Cavendish, 1986.

Larson, David E., ed. *Mayo Clinic Family Health Book.* 2d ed. New York: William Morrow, 1996.

Enemas

Procedure

Anatomy or system affected: Abdomen, anus, gastrointestinal system, intestines

Specialties and related fields: Gastroenterology

Definition: A procedure to assist the body in evacuating fecal material from the bowel.

Indications and Procedures

Enemas are used primarily for two purposes: cleansing and retention. Many solutions have been used to promote cleansing. The most commonly used is made up of mild soapsuds and tap water. Commercially prepared solutions containing premeasured mild soap and water are also available.

To receive an enema, the patient should lie on the left side of the body with the upper thigh drawn up to the abdomen. The solution should be slightly above body temperature. The source of the enema fluid should be 30 to 45 centimeters (12 to 18 inches) above the anus. All air should be removed from the tubing that connects the enema reservoir and the tip. The tip is warmed in the hands, lubricated with a commercial preparation or a bit of soapy water, and gently inserted into the anus with a combination of soft pressure and a twisting motion. The tip should not be in-serted more than 10 centimeters (4 inches) into the rectum. The solution is allowed to flow slowly into the rectum to prevent cramping.

A towel may be held gently against the rectum to prevent leakage. If cramping does occur, the flow should be interrupted by pinching the tubing. For an adult, approximately 1 liter (1 quart) of solution is probably sufficient; the patient should hold the solution for two to three minutes. The enema tube is tightly clamped and slowly withdrawn; a towel is again held against the anus to catch any leakage. A readily available bedpan or toilet stool is used while the patient evacuates the bowel. Depending on the need for the enema, the procedure may be repeated.

The procedure for administering a retention enema is similar except that the solution is instilled very slowly to promote retention. Lubricants or medicines are administered in this fashion. The patient holds the instilled solution as long as possible before evacuating the bowel.

Uses and Complications

Cleansing enemas are used to promote bowel evacuation by softening fecal material and stimulating the movement by bowel walls (peristalsis). Retention enemas are used to lubricate or soothe the mucosal lining of the rectum, to apply medication to the bowel wall or for absorption by the colon, and to soften feces.

There is no physiological need to have a bowel movement every day; normality is defined as from three to ten per week. Enemas should not be used routinely for cleansing because the bowel quickly becomes dependent on them. This problem is especially common among older individuals.

—*L. Fleming Fallon, Jr., M.D., M.P.H.*

See also Colon and rectal polyp removal; Colon and rectal surgery; Colon cancer; Colonoscopy; Gastroenterology; Gastrointestinal system; Hemorrhoid banding and removal; Hemorrhoids; Internal medicine; Intestines; Peristalsis; Proctology; Surgery, general.

Enuresis. *See* Bed-wetting.

Environmental diseases

Disease/disorder

Anatomy or system affected: All

Specialties and related fields: Environmental health, epidemiology, occupational health, public health, toxicology

Definition: A wide variety of conditions and diseases resulting from largely human-mediated hazards in both the natural and humanmade (for example, home and workplace) environments; an area of special concern given rapid environmental degradation during the twentieth century.

Key terms:

emphysema: the overinflation of bronchial tubes and alveoli with air, resulting in reduced lung function *environment:* the biological, physical, cultural, and mental factors that influence health; anything external to an individual

food chain: a sequence—plant, herbivore, primary carnivore, and secondary and tertiary carnivore—in which each level depends on the stored energy from the lower level and often concentrates contaminants in the process

mutagen: a substance or event that effects a permanent, inheritable change in the genetic makeup of an organism

organic compound or waste: a chemical compound based on carbon, with or without hydrogen and other elements—in the context of environmental disease, usually a manufactured product

risk factor: a factor that increases the chances of an effect

teratogen: a substance or event that causes malformation in a developing fetus

CAUSES AND SYMPTOMS

Environmental health explores the influence of external factors on human health and disease. Technically, almost any condition except those of purely genetic origin could be considered as environmentally caused or having an environmental component, but the term "environmental disease" is usually applied to the effects of human alterations in the physical environment and excludes transmissible disease caused by pathogenic organisms, except in cases where human alteration of the environment is an important factor in epidemiology. Health hazards generally classed as environmental include air and water (including groundwater) pollution, toxic wastes, lead, asbestos, pesticides and herbicides, ionizing and nonionizing radiation, noise, and light.

In the United States, the Clean Air Act of 1970 established maximum levels for sulfur and nitrogen dioxide, particulates, hydrocarbons, ozone, and carbon monoxide—the most common air pollutants of concern in urban environments. Even with increasingly stringent controls on emissions from automobiles and industry, air quality in urban areas frequently does not meet minimum standards. Carbon monoxide lowers the oxygen-carrying capacity of the blood, nitrogen and sulfur dioxide react with water to form acids which damage lung tissue, ozone damages tissue directly, and particulates may accumulate in the lungs. The result is decreased lung capacity and function. Cigarette smoking increases susceptibility to other forms of lung damage.

Indoor air quality poses additional concerns. Emphasis on energy efficiency in building design decreases air exchange. Carpets and furniture release organic compounds, and cleaning solvents leave a volatile residue. Formaldehyde from foam stuffing and insulation inhibits liver function and is a suspected carcinogen. Breathing in an enclosed space decreases atmospheric oxygen and increases carbon dioxide. In some areas, radioactive radon gas released by the soil becomes concentrated in buildings. A ventilation system which draws its air from a polluted outdoor environment, such as a loading dock, will fail to perform its function. Secondhand cigarette smoke poses the same hazards of emphysema and lung cancer to people chronically exposed to it in an enclosed environment as to the smokers themselves. The phenomenon known as "sick building syndrome," in which large numbers of people in one building complain of respiratory illness, headaches, and impaired concentration, results from a combination of these factors.

Lead additives in gasoline were once a significant source of atmospheric lead, but they are being phased out; unfortunately, they leave a permanent residue in soils of high-traffic areas. Levels of 20 micrograms per deciliter of lead in the blood inhibit hemoglobin production, slow the transmission of nerve impulses, and are suspected of causing cognitive impairment in children; higher levels cause anemia, weakness, stomach pains, and nervous system impairment. Even levels below 5 micrograms may be hazardous to children. Because of lead in the paint and plumbing in old houses and soil contamination, blood lead levels high enough to cause developmental impairment in children occur frequently in older parts of cities; low-income residents are most likely to be at risk. Mercury, another metallic neurotoxin, is introduced into water in small amounts through industrial effluent but becomes concentrated in the food chain, where it poses a hazard to people who eat large quantities of fish. Any waterborne pollutant that is not rapidly degraded has the potential for being concentrated in the food chain. Shellfish, which filter nutrients from seawater, can concentrate toxins. The most notorious cause of shellfish poisoning is a naturally occurring neurotoxic alga, but polychlorinated biphenyls (PCBs) and pesticides have also been implicated. Some metals, including lead, arsenic, and mercury, remain toxic indefinitely and are exceedingly difficult to remove from an environment into which they have been introduced.

Inhalation of asbestos fibers carries a high risk of developing lung cancer after an interval of twenty or thirty years, a connection first established among shipyard workers. Between 1940 and 1970, asbestos was used extensively in public buildings as insulation. It is estimated that three to five million workers in the United States were exposed to unacceptably high levels of airborne fibers during this period, and millions of people continue to be exposed when building materials deteriorate. Asbestos abatement adds considerably to the cost of renovating old public buildings.

Urban drinking water in industrialized countries is monitored for hazardous contaminants; there is some question as to whether chlorine and fluoride, added for legitimate health reasons, are completely without negative effects. Well water in irrigated agricultural areas may have high levels of nitrates, which decrease blood oxygen and have been implicated in miscarriages and birth defects.

Organic chemical compounds make up 60 percent of the hazardous wastes generated by industry. This category

Asbestosis

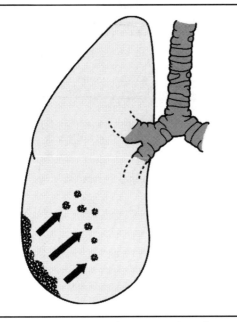

Asbestosis—the progressive destruction of respiratory tissues via inhalation of dust-sized asbestos fibers that attach to the walls of the lung and then spread outward—is often the result of prolonged exposure to asbestos-containing materials (in shipyards, office buildings, manufacturing plants); it is one of a wide variety of environmental diseases.

includes PCBs (including dioxin), chlorofluorocarbons, phthalate esters, chlorinated benzenes, and chloromethanes, solvents (such as benzene and carbon tetrachloride), plasticizers, fire retardants, pesticides, and herbicides. Many are acutely toxic—dioxin is one of the most potent toxins known—and require elaborate precautions to prevent worker exposure or accidental contamination of foodstuffs. PCBs, which are used in a wide variety of manufacturing processes, have been shown to cause cancer and reproductive disorders in laboratory animals and have been linked to these conditions in humans. The herbicide 2,4,5-T, the defoliant "Agent Orange" used during the Vietnam War, is the subject of continuing claims against the manufacturer and the Veterans Administration by soldiers who later developed neurological symptoms, immune disorders, or cancer or who had children with birth defects.

The burial of toxic by-products of manufacturing processes in landfills has created an ongoing environmental health crisis as containers rupture and chemicals leach into the surrounding soil. Underground fuel storage tanks pose a similar problem. Toxins leached from a waste dump eventually enter streams and become disseminated or, if volatile, enter the atmosphere. Residents of the infamous Love Canal

site in New York State were made ill by fumes from contaminated soil and groundwater.

High energy from X-ray sources and radioactive materials is termed "ionizing" because such radiation can cause chemical changes in molecules, including genetic material. Chronic exposure to ionizing radiation poses a high risk of cancer, inheritable mutations, and fetal malformation. Exposure may be occupational, as with workers in the nuclear power industry or hospital radiology laboratories. Some radioactive by-products of nuclear weapons testing and reactor accidents (such as strontium 90 or carbon 14) are exceptionally hazardous because they are structurally incorporated into living tissue and become concentrated in the food chain. The by-products of the nuclear reactor accident in Chernobyl, Ukraine, in 1987 were disseminated across international boundaries and will continue to endanger the health of millions of people in Belarus, Ukraine, and Eastern Europe. Whether widespread atmospheric testing of nuclear weapons in the 1950's caused radiation damage in the population at large is unknown; military personnel involved in the testing and inhabitants of the regions near test sites report increased rates of suspected radiation-induced illness.

Hazards of nonionizing radiation (visible, ultraviolet, infrared, or microwave) are less well established. Intense visible light can damage vision. Artificial lighting is known to disrupt reproductive cycles in plants and invertebrates and could have subtle effects on human biology. That the level of microwave radiation to which the public at large is inadvertently exposed is well below levels known to produce adverse effects is not completely reassuring. Ultraviolet light, principally from sunlight, is a factor in skin cancer, which is increasing both because of the popularity of sunbathing and because ozone depletion increases ultraviolet exposure.

A category of severe lung disease affects workers in environments with a high concentration of particulate matter in the air: black lung disease, from coal dust in coal mines; silicosis, from fine rock powder in mines; and byssinosis, from textile fibers in spinning and weaving mills. The result of long-term breathing of particulates is obstruction and emphysema, which may be fatal.

Electromagnetic fields produced by power lines and electrical devices are an area of increasing controversy as electricity becomes more ubiquitous. One study found a higher-than-average rate of childhood leukemia near high-tension power lines; other studies have failed to confirm this finding. Women who work constantly at video display terminals have somewhat higher miscarriage rates than other office workers.

Exposure to industrial solvents has been a significant source of workplace illness. Among the most dangerous solvents are benzene, used in a variety of processes and produced as a by-product in the coking industry; vinyl chloride, used in plastics manufacture; and formaldehyde. All of these chemicals are carcinogenic.

Repetitive motion injuries are an increasing occupational hazard. Any body part subject to constant, selective hard use, especially where tasks and workstations are poorly designed, may develop problems. The most common compensation claims arise from damage to the spinal column from lifting heavy objects and damage to nerves in the hand and forearm from repetitive, rapid hand movements (such as carpal tunnel syndrome).

SOCIETAL INTERVENTION

In order to improve environmental health, health professionals and regulatory agencies must anticipate and minimize future hazards, identify existing health problems that may have an environmental component and attempt to determine whether a connection exists, and redress the mistakes of the past. It is notoriously difficult to prove that an illness has an environmental cause. Suspicion arises when epidemiological statistics on reportable illnesses show that some condition known to be influenced by environmental factors—such as cancer, endocrine disorders, reproductive disorders, or immunodeficiency—occurs at an unusually high frequency in some subset of the population, occurs in a restricted geographical area, or is increasing throughout the general population. Even then, the cause may not be environmental; the acquired immunodeficiency syndrome (AIDS) epidemic was thought by some to be an environmental effect until the causative organism was identified.

The time interval between exposure and illness can be as long as twenty or thirty years, during which the exposed population may have dispersed and may no longer be readily identifiable. Subtle effects such as mild immunosuppression or cognitive impairment may escape detection or be dismissed as psychosomatic. Multiple environmental, behavioral, and even genetic factors are often involved, confounding efforts to pinpoint a cause. In the United States and Western Europe, high rates of exposure to pollutants are correlated with poverty and thus with higher-than-normal rates of malnutrition, alcohol and drug abuse, and inadequate access to health care. Tobacco smoking is a common confounding behavioral factor in environmental diagnosis. Where liability is involved, there are powerful financial incentives on the side of disproving the environmental or occupational linkage.

When a new technology or chemical is introduced, regulations in most countries require an assessment of health impact, which includes experimentation with animal models and risk assessment to determine the probable impact on the human population. Animal experimentation is most effective at demonstrating short-term and acute effects of toxic materials, but it is poor at demonstrating effects of long-term, low-level exposure. Risk assessment must take into consideration unusually susceptible individuals (pregnant women, for example), deliberate or accidental overexposure, and synergistic effects. In the realm of environ-

mental legislation, risk assessment is also influenced by psychology; people are more willing to accept familiar risks over which they have personal control.

PERSPECTIVE AND PROSPECTS

Concern for occupational health begins with the Industrial Revolution in the early nineteenth century, finding some of its earliest expression in the recognition that some industrial jobs were inappropriate for children. Although many occupations in preindustrial societies carried a high risk trauma, only a few involved chronic exposure to toxic substances. The combined effects of heavy physical labor and malnutrition are not infrequently seen in skeletons from archeological excavations, but injury caused by repetitive motion under assembly-line conditions is a modern phenomenon.

Concerns about the effects of pollution and toxic wastes on the general population are of even more recent origin. Sanitarians in the first half of the twentieth century directed their attention toward reducing transmissible disease through the prevention of water and food supply contamination and the control of insect vectors. Several factors increased public awareness of environmental health problems in the United States and led to creation of agencies and legislation to address the problem, beginning in 1970: Urban-industrial air pollution contributed to hundreds of deaths from respiratory disease in Pennsylvania (1948) and London (1952); there was much publicity surrounding the dangers of pesticides to wildlife in the 1960's; a variety of health problems, including increased cancer risk, were found in Love Canal, a housing development in New York State built on a toxic waste dump; and it was demonstrated that urban lead levels were high enough to impair psychomotor development in children.

The increase in the proportion of morbidity and mortality attributable to environmental factors in the late twentieth century is the result of not only the exponential increase in energy use and the output of complex synthetic chemicals but also of changing demographics. Effects of low-level exposure to toxins may take decades to produce disease and may never become apparent in populations with a low life expectancy. In developing countries, where environmental protection is rudimentary and life expectancies are increasing rapidly, the adverse health effects of environmental degradation are particularly visible.

In the United States, specific legislation addresses compensation for miners, asbestos workers, and other specific victims of exposure to hazardous materials. On a worldwide basis, monitoring of hazardous substances is a prime concern of the World Health Organization. As incidents such as the accidental release of cyanide from a fertilizer plant in Bhopal, India, indicate, provisions for industrial safety and for separating residential and industrial areas in the developing world are unsatisfactory. The former Soviet Union represents what in many ways is a worst-case scenario combing rapid, concentrated industrialization with poor environmental controls. Some of the earliest signs that the Communist regime was weakening came from the environmental movement in its agitation for better protection for human and natural resources. Safeguarding environmental health and addressing existing hazards and environmentally caused illnesses requires a major expenditure of funds and effort, which is likely to continue growing as the delayed effects of industrial practices introduced since World War II continue to become apparent.

—*Martha Sherwood-Pike, Ph.D.*

See also Allergies; Asthma; Bronchitis; Cancer; Carpal tunnel syndrome; *E. coli* infection; Emphysema; Environmental health; Epidemiology; Food poisoning; Lead poisoning; Lung cancer; Malignant melanoma removal; Occupational health; Poisoning; Pulmonary diseases; Radiation sickness; Respiration; Skin cancer; Skin lesion removal; Toxicology.

FOR FURTHER INFORMATION:

Congressional Quarterly Inc. *Environment and Health.* Washington, D.C.: Author, 1981. The focus of this report is legislation introduced between 1970 and 1980 in Congress to address environmental health problems, including the background that led to the introduction of such legislation. The table "The Regulatory Maze: Agencies Involved in Environmental and Occupational Health" and the chronology of legislation by year and type of problem are clear and informative.

Cooper, M. G., ed. *Risk: Man-Made Hazards to Man.* Oxford, England: Clarendon Press, 1985. A book about how people perceive and assess risks, factors that affect environmental legislation. In addition to a discussion of statistics and the effects of publicity, this British publication adopts a conservative view that hazards are often overstated.

Cralley, Lester V., Lewis J. Cralley, George D. Clayton, and John Jurgiel. *Industrial Environmental Health: The Worker and the Community.* New York: Academic Press, 1972. Part of the Environmental Science Interdisciplinary Monograph Series from Academic Press. A detailed catalog of known workplace hazards, including toxic materials, radiation, and noise. The emphasis is on monitoring techniques and a thorough survey of the literature. The text is rather technical.

Greenberg, Michael R., ed. *Public Health and the Environment: The United States Experience.* New York: Guilford Press, 1987. This text explores modern environmental problems from the point of view of public health. Part 1, a survey of the contribution of the environment to disease, includes sections on worker health and lifestyle as a factor in chronic disease.

Journal of Environmental Health, 1963-   . This journal published by the National Environmental Health Association offers articles on a wide variety of environmental and occupational health issues. The journal also acts as a forum for concerns of environmental health professionals and sanitarians.

National Research Council. Committee on Environmental Epidemiology. *Public Health and Hazardous Wastes.* Vol. 1 in *Environmental Epidemiology.* Washington, D.C.: National Academy Press, 1991. The report of a committee assigned to investigate the question of whether the federal hazardous waste programs in the United States actually protect human health. Reviews agencies and the methodologies of exposure assessment, the extent of the problem in the United States, and specific examples of hazardous wastes in air, groundwater, soil, and food. Includes charts and maps summarizing data and extensive bibliographies. A lengthy glossary is provided. A good factual reference on many aspects of environmental health.

Rom, William N., ed. *Environmental and Occupational Medicine.* 2d ed. Boston: Little, Brown, 1992. The emphasis in this textbook is on industrial occupational safety, with approximately a third of the work devoted to the diagnosis and pathology of occupational lung diseases, including byssinosis and black lung disease. The effects of acute and chronic exposure to heavy metals, solvents, and other toxic substances are organized by agent. Intended as a guide for medical practitioners treating patients with environmental illnesses and as a guide to the prevention of exposure for professionals concerned with workplace safety.

ENVIRONMENTAL HEALTH
SPECIALTY
ANATOMY OR SYSTEM AFFECTED: All

SPECIALTIES AND RELATED FIELDS: Epidemiology, occupational health, preventive medicine, psychology, pulmonary medicine, toxicology

DEFINITION: The control of all factors in the physical environment that exercise, or may exercise, a deleterious effect on human physical development, health, and survival.

KEY TERMS:

community: a group of people living in the same locality

hygiene: the science of health and the prevention of disease

pollution: a noxious substance that contaminates the environment

remediation: correcting an evil, fault, or error

sanitation: the application of measures designed to protect public health

SCIENCE AND PROFESSION

The environment is the sum of all external influences and conditions affecting the life and development of an organism. For humans, a healthy environment means that the surroundings in which humans live, work, and play meet some predetermined quality standard. The field of environmental health encompasses the air that humans breathe, the water that they drink, the food that they consume, and the shelter that they inhabit. The definition also includes the identification of pollutants, waste materials, and other environmental factors that adversely affect life and health. The study of environmental health encompasses the fields of environmental engineering and sanitation, public health engineering, and sanitary engineering. The majority of professionals working in the field of environmental health are trained as civil engineers, environmental engineers, toxicologists, or preventive medicine specialists. Many are also qualified in subspecialties such as hydrogeology, epidemiology, public sanitation, and occupational health.

Environmental health deals with the control of factors in the physical environment that cause (or may cause) a negative effect on the health and survival of communities. Consideration is given to the physical, economic, and social impact of the controlling measures. These measures include controlling, modifying, or adapting the physical, chemical, and biological factors of the environment in the interest of human health, comfort, and social well-being. Environmental health is concerned not only with simple survival and the prevention of disease and poisoning but also with the maintenance of an environment that is suited to efficient human performance and that preserves human comfort and enjoyment.

DIAGNOSTIC AND TREATMENT TECHNIQUES

The field of environmental health covers an extremely broad area of human living space. For practical purposes, those involved in the profession of environmental health concern themselves with the impact of humans on the environment and the impact of the environment on humans, balancing their appraisals and allocations of available resources. The scope of environmental health research and community environmental health planning usually involves the following topics: water supplies, water pollution and wastewater treatment, solid waste disposal, pest control, soil pollution, food hygiene, air pollution, radiation control, noise control, transportation control, safe housing, land use planning, public recreation, abuse of controlled substances, resource conservation, postdisaster sanitation, accident prevention, medical facilities, and occupational health, particularly the control of physical, chemical, and biological hazards.

The implementation of effective environmental health strategies must take place within the context of comprehensive regional or area-wide community planning. Planning considerations for a community's environmental health are based on individual community aspirations and goals, priorities, local resources, and the availability of outside resources required to meet projected health standards. The planning and implementation of environmental health activities directly involve engineers, sanitarians, medical specialists, planners, architects, geologists, biologists, chem-

ists, technicians, naturalists, and related personnel. The natural and physical scientists provide research necessary for communities to locate and use available resources responsibly, and they also identify potential and existing health hazards. The engineering specialties provide know-how to communities concerning the design, installation, and operation of equipment. When a problem is identified or emergency occurs, it is often the engineering professionals who direct remediation efforts. Medical specialists, with scientific backup, determine dangers to a community's physical health; if health problems arise, they concern themselves with curing disease. The implementation of any environmental health strategy is clearly a team effort.

PERSPECTIVE AND PROSPECTS

The concept of environmental health in modern society is considerably expanded from that of the past. Activities in the field of environmental health were once controlled only because they were known to be disease-related. The present concept of environmental health is to provide a high quality of living.

The field of environmental health concerns itself with the control of physical factors affecting the health of humans and is different from the prevention and control of individual illness and the preservation of human health. Most environmental health problems are the direct result of human activities and interactions with natural resources. Human manipulation of natural resources causes changes to the environment. These changes can be local or global, anticipated or unanticipated. At the present time, humans are living in a polluted environment, the result of centuries of lack of concern and appreciation of the ecologic consequences of human activities. The cumulative effects of human actions on the environment have risen steeply and continuously, while human response to mounting problems of environmental quality has been sporadic and targeted toward high-profile or emergency problems. As a result, environmental programs have been developed to preserve wildlife, manage resources, combat communicable disease, increase agricultural production, and ensure healthy and sanitary living conditions for human populations.

As a direct reflection of the public's concern about environmental degradation, environmental health has become a rapidly growing specialty in the fields of engineering, medicine, environmental science, and resource management. As public awareness of the devastating effects of pollution and resource depletion grows, the demand for qualified environmental health professionals and administrators increases. Whether these sought-after professionals are asked to offer stopgap measures for environmental problems that have already progressed to dangerous, possibly unresolvable levels or whether they are employed to foster a new, more holistic approach to the natural world will depend on the environmental conscience of modern civilization.

—*Randall L. Milstein, Ph.D.*

See also Allergies; Arthropod-borne diseases; Asthma; Bacteriology; Cholera; Environmental diseases; Environmental health; Epidemiology; Food poisoning; Frostbite; Heat exhaustion and heat stroke; Hyperthermia and hypothermia; Immune system; Immunization and vaccination; Immunology; Interstitial pulmonary fibrosis (IPF); Lead poisoning; Legionnaires' disease; Lice, mites, and ticks; Lung cancer; Lungs; Lyme disease; Malaria; Microbiology; Nasopharyngeal disorders; Occupational health; Parasitic diseases; Plague; Poisoning; Poisonous plants; Preventive medicine; Pulmonary diseases; Pulmonary medicine; Pulmonary medicine, pediatric; Salmonella; Skin cancer; Snakebites; Stress; Stress reduction; Toxicology; Tropical medicine.

FOR FURTHER INFORMATION:

Higgins, Thomas. *Hazardous Waste Minimization Handbook*. Chelsea, Mich.: Lewis, 1989.

Moeller, D. W. *Environmental Health*. Rev. ed. Cambridge, Mass.: Harvard University Press, 1997.

Raven, Peter H., Linda R. Berg, and George B. Johnson. *Environment*. Fort Worth, Tex.: Saunders College Publishing, 1995.

Steger, Will, and Jon Bowermaster. *Saving the Earth: A Citizen's Guide to Environmental Action*. New York: Alfred A. Knopf, 1990.

ENZYME THERAPY
PROCEDURE
ANATOMY OR SYSTEM AFFECTED: All

SPECIALTIES AND RELATED FIELDS: Alternative medicine, immunology, nutrition

DEFINITION: Proteins that facilitate chemical reactions are called enzymes. Proteases are enzymes that aid digestion by degrading specific types of proteins. Incomplete digestion of proteins can lead to allergies and the formation of toxins. Proteases also clear the small intestine of potentially troubling bacteria, yeast, and protozoa. In some cases, proteases may be administered to aid digestive problems. Pancreatin is an enzyme derived from fresh hog pancreas. It can help to alleviate pancreative insufficiency, the symptoms of which include impaired digestion, abdominal discomfort, and malnutrition. It is also used to treat inflammatory and autoimmune disorders such as rheumatoid arthritis. The ingestion of bromelain, an enzyme found in pineapple, can aid in digestion and pancreatic insufficiency. Papain, which is isolated from unripe papaya, is also used as a digestive aid and allows some people to tolerate wheat gluten. Another therapeutic use of enzymes is in dissolving blood clots formed by thrombophlebitis; this prevents loose clots from causing heart attacks or strokes. Some enzymes are used to treat acquired immunodeficiency syndrome (AIDS), but their success has not been documented.

—Karen E. Kalumuck, Ph.D.

See also Alternative medicine; Digestion; Enzymes; Food biochemistry; Immune system; Immunology; Metabolism; Pancreas; Pharmacology; Phlebitis; Rheumatoid arthritis; Thrombosis and thrombus; Toxicology.

ENZYMES
BIOLOGY
ANATOMY OR SYSTEM INVOLVED: Cells, immune system

SPECIALTIES AND RELATED FIELDS: Biochemistry, cytology, endocrinology, genetics, pharmacology

DEFINITION: Large molecules, produced by cells, that catalyze chemical reactions inside living organisms.

KEY TERMS:

active site: the part of an enzyme where the substrate is bound; this is the site where the reaction occurs

activity: a measure of the ability of an enzyme to catalyze its reaction

amino acid: the fundamental building blocks of proteins; there are twenty amino acids, each with a different chemistry

catalysis: increasing the speed of a chemical reaction

molecule: a collection of atoms bonded together; normally neutral because it has an equal number of protons and electrons

mutation: a substitution of one amino acid for another in the amino acid sequence of a protein

protein: large molecules made up of amino acids connected by peptide bonds; the sequence of amino acids in a protein determines its three-dimensional structure

substrates: reactants that enzymes convert into products; every enzyme is specific for one specific substrate

STRUCTURE AND FUNCTIONS

Enzymes are remarkable molecules because they increase rates of biochemical reactions. Each enzyme within a cell selectively speeds up, or catalyzes, one particular reaction or type of reaction. The vast majority of enzymes belong to the class of large molecules known as proteins. Proteins are built by combining amino acids. There are twenty amino acids, which can be divided into three classes: hydrophobic, charged, and polar. Hydrophobic amino acids behave chemically like oils, avoiding contact with water. Charged amino acids are ionic, containing one extra or one less electron than do neutral molecules. Polar amino acids are attracted to water and other polar amino acids. Each of these three classes of amino acids has a distinct chemistry. The specific order of the amino acid sequence defines the structure and function of every protein. Inside cells, enzymes catalyze reactions so that they occur millions of times faster than they would without the presence of these proteins. Each cell in the body produces many different enzymes. Different sets of enzymes are found in different tissues, reflecting the specialized function of each particular enzyme. There are thousands of different enzymes working in the body: many have yet to be discovered.

Protein enzymes work by bringing the reactants in a chemical reaction together in the most favorable geometrical arrangement, so that bonds can be easily broken and reformed. This is possible because different enzymes have different three-dimensional shapes. It is the shape of the enzyme that determines its chemistry. Each enzyme combines with a specific substrate, or reactant, and catalyzes its characteristic reaction. When the reaction is over, the substrate has been converted into products. The enzyme remains unchanged, ready to catalyze another reaction with the next substrate molecule it encounters.

Enzymes play a significant role in treating diseases. Because enzymes have specific functions, a particular enzyme that has the required function to treat the disorder can be administered. Modern methods of genetic engineering allow the production of desired enzymes. Scientists can use bacteria as factories to produce large amounts of enzyme from an organism by copying the gene from the organism of interest into bacterial cells. The bacteria are then grown in culture, producing the enzyme of interest as they grow. This procedure is a much safer method than the old procedure of isolating enzyme from animal tissues, because the enzymes produced are free of viruses and other contaminants present in animal tissues. Proteins produced by genetic engineering techniques are called recombinant proteins.

Sometimes enzymes can be used as drugs for the treatment of specific diseases. Streptokinase is an enzyme mixture that is useful in clearing blood clots that occur in the heart and the lower extremities. Another useful enzyme for dissolving blood clots that occur as a result of heart attacks is human tissue plasminogen activator (TPA). Recombinant TPA is produced by genetic engineering techniques, using bacteria cultures to produce large quantities of human TPA. The administration of TPA within an hour of the formation of a blood clot in a coronary artery dramatically increases survival rates of heart attack victims. Some types of adult leukemia are treated by intravenous administration of the asparaginase enzyme. Tumor cells require the molecule asparagine to grow, and they scavenge it from the bloodstream. Asparaginase drastically reduces the amount of asparagine in the blood, thus slowing the growth of the tumor. Because most enzymes do not last long in blood, huge amounts of enzymes are required for therapeutic effects. In classic hemophilia, the factor VIII enzyme is missing or is genetically mutated so that it has a very low activity. This enzyme is essential for inducing the formation of blood clots. In the past, it was a laborious task to collect a concentrated blood plasma sample containing factor VIII, which was administered to hemophiliacs to stop hemorrhages. This treatment carried the risk of infecting the patient with viruses that cause acquired immunodeficiency syndrome (AIDS), hepatitis, and other diseases. Purified recombinant factor VIII is now available. Because the recombinant human factor VIII is produced by bacteria, it cannot

The Function of Some Enzymes

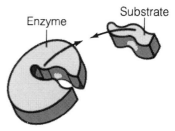

An enzyme combines with a substrate that has molecules of a complementary shape.

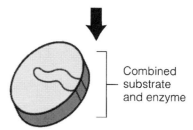

The interaction between the enzyme and substrate causes a chemical change in the substrate, splitting it in two.

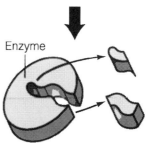

The enzyme is unchanged and can repeat the process with another substrate molecule.

be infected with the viruses that cause hepatitis and AIDS.

A classic enzyme inhibitor used as a drug is penicillin. Penicillin was discovered in 1928 by Alexander Fleming, after he noticed that bacterial growth was prevented by a contaminating mold known as *Penicillium*. Ten years later, Howard Florey and Ernst Chain performed the key experiments that led to the isolation, characterization, and clinical use of this wonder drug antibiotic. In 1957, Joshua Lederberg showed that penicillin interferes with the synthesis of the cell walls of bacteria. In 1965, James Park and Jack Strominger independently discovered that penicillin blocks the last step in cell wall synthesis. The last step is the cross-linking of different strands of the wall and is catalyzed by the enzyme glycopeptide transpeptidase. The shape of penicillin resembles that of the normal substrate of glycopeptide transpeptidase, so that penicillin binds to the active site of the transpeptidase enzyme. Once bound to the active site, penicillin forms a permanent bond with one of the amino acid residues. This chemical reaction permanently inhibits the glycopeptide transpeptidase enzyme, thus preventing the transpeptidase from cross-linking the bacterial wall.

Several anticancer drugs work by blocking the synthesis of deoxythymidylate (dTMP), as an abundant supply of dTMP is required for rapid cell division to be sustained. Drugs that inhibit the enzymes thymidylate synthase and dihydrofolate reductase are very effective agents in cancer chemotherapy. Thymidylate synthase, which makes dTMP from deoxyuridylate, is irreversibly inhibited by the drug fluorouracil. This drug is converted into fluorodeoxyuridylate (F-dUMP), which chemically reacts with thymidylate synthase so that the enzyme can no longer function in its normal role of making dTMP from deoxyuridylate. The synthesis of dTMP can also be blocked by drugs that inhibit the enzyme dihydrofolate reductase. The normal substrate for dihydrofolate reductase is the molecule dihydrofolate. Drugs such as aminopterin and methotrexate bind to the active site of the reductase enzyme, inhibiting rapid cell growth. Methotrexate is very effective at inhibiting rapidly growing tumors such as acute leukemia and choriocarcinoma. Unfortunately methotrexate kills all rapidly dividing cells, including stem cells in bone marrow, epithelial cells of the intestinal tract, and hair follicles, which explains the many toxic side effects of this drug. Computer-aided drug design has been applied to the dihydrofolate reductase enzyme, with encouraging results.

The activity of an enzyme is a measure of how efficiently a particular enzyme catalyzes its reaction. A loss in activity corresponds to a decrease in catalytic efficiency, and an increase in activity corresponds to an increase in catalytic efficiency. Many drugs increase enzyme activity (enzyme induction), and many decrease enzyme activity (enzyme inhibition). Both enzyme induction and enzyme inhibition result from the interaction of the drug with the enzyme, altering the surface of the enzyme where the substrate normally is bound during catalysis. In enzyme induction, the surface is altered such that the substrate is bound tighter than usual, while in enzyme inhibition, the surface is altered so that the substrate cannot bind to the enzyme. The structures of many enzyme inhibitors are similar to the structures of substrates. Inhibitors bind at active sites of enzymes. Drugs that are enzyme inhibitors are very powerful medical tools, as they bind to the enzyme and are not easily removed.

Universities, government agencies, and pharmaceutical companies are continually seeking to develop drugs that specifically bind and inhibit enzymes responsible for disease. Much effort is spent trying to design drugs in a rational manner, using the most powerful tools of chemistry.

Techniques such as X-ray crystallography, nuclear magnetic resonance (NMR) spectroscopy, and computational chemistry allow researchers to determine the shapes of enzymes, their substrates, and their inhibitors. These efforts allow the research team to design drugs that bind more specifically to the target enzyme, thus increasing the effectiveness and lowering the toxicity of the drug.

DISORDERS AND DISEASES

Defects in enzymes, known as mutations, can cause disease. A protein molecule is mutated when one or more of the original amino acids in the protein is replaced by a different amino acid. For example, if an enzyme consists of one hundred amino acids, and amino acid number 35 is changed from one kind of amino acid to a different kind, the protein is now a mutant. A mutated enzyme has a slightly altered shape compared to the original enzyme. If the change in shape causes the enzyme to perform its chemistry more slowly than the original enzyme, then the cell and tissue have an impaired function. In particular, if an amino acid is changed from one of the three classes (hydrophobic, charged, or polar) to a different class, then the mutation is more likely to cause a change in the structure and function of the enzyme. Not all mutations are harmful, but a single mutation in a key region of an enzyme can be fatal to a living organism.

Many diseases are diagnosed by measuring enzyme concentrations and activities in the body. Enzyme concentration refers to the amount of enzyme present, while enzyme activity refers to the ability of the enzyme to perform its chemistry. Enzyme concentrations and activities can be measured in blood or in tissue. Disease of tissues and organs can cause cellular damage, so that enzymes that are normally not present in significant quantities in blood are raised to very high levels as they flow from the damaged tissue into the blood plasma. Detection of particular enzymes in blood plasma indicates a diseased organ. The higher the concentration of enzyme in the blood, the more extensive the damage to that tissue or organ. The detection of these enzymes in the blood is a diagnostic tool, indicating a particular disorder. Genetic diseases caused by a mutation in an enzyme can be detected by laboratory tests that measure enzyme activity or enzyme shape.

Disease diagnosis is often made by measuring the concentration or activity of enzymes. Isozymes are enzymes that catalyze the same reaction but have slightly different structures. Most isozymes are enzymes consisting of two or more subunits, with different combinations of the subunits differentiating the isozymes. Isozymes of the enzymes lactate dehydrogenase, creatine kinase, and alkaline phosphatase are used for clinical applications. Monitoring of the isozyme concentrations and activities of lactate dehydrogenase and creatine kinase in the blood shows whether a patient has suffered a heart attack. Creatine kinase consists of two subunits. The two possible subunits are M, which stands for muscle type, and B, which stands for brain type. There are three possible isozymes: MM, BB, and MB. The MM isozyme consists of two M subunits and is the only isozyme found in skeletal muscle, the BB isozyme consists of two B subunits and is the only isozyme found in the brain, and the MB isozyme consists of one M and one B subunit and is found only in the heart. Lactate dehydrogenase consists of four subunits, made from five combinations of two subunits. The two subunits are the heart subunit, designated by H, and the muscle subunit, designated by M. The HHHH and HHHM isozymes are found in the heart and in red blood cells, the HHMM isozyme is found in the brain and kidney, and the MMMM isozyme is found in the liver and skeletal muscle. After a heart attack, the cellular breakup of heart tissue releases the MB isozyme of creatine kinase into the bloodstream within six to eighteen hours. Release of lactate dehydrogenase into the blood is slower than that of creatine kinase, occurring one to two days after the appearance of creatine kinase. In a healthy person, the activity of the HHHM isozyme of lactate dehydrogenase is higher than that of the HHHH isozyme. In heart attack victims, however, the activity of the HHHH isozyme becomes greater than that of the HHHM isozyme between twelve and twenty-four hours after the attack. Measurement of increased concentration of the MB isozyme a short while after a suspected heart attack, followed by the switch in lactate dehydrogenase activity between the HHHH and HHHM isozymes, indicates that a heart attack occurred. Secondary complications of a heart attack can also be followed with isozyme measurements. For example, increased activity of the MMMM isozyme of lactate dehydrogenase is an indication of liver congestion.

Certain medical conditions can be screened by using immobilized enzymes as reagents in desktop clinical analyzers. For example, screening tests for cholesterol and triglycerides can be completed in a few minutes using 0.01 milliliter of blood plasma. The enzymes cholesterol oxidase and lipase are immobilized, or fixed in place, in a detection kit. If cholesterol is present, cholesterol oxidase breaks off hydrogen peroxide from the cholesterol. The enzyme peroxidase and a colorless dye is included in the detection kit, and peroxidase catalyzes the reaction of the colorless dye and hydrogen peroxide to form a colored dye that can be easily measured from the amount of light reflected from the solution. The enzyme lipase allows the accurate determination of triglycerides in blood.

A mutation in a protein that acts as a natural inhibitor of an enzyme can cause disease. For example, emphysema is a destructive lung disease in which the alveolar walls of the lungs are destroyed by an enzyme known as elastase. A person with emphysema breathes much harder to exchange the same volume of air because the alveoli, or air pockets, have become much less efficient. Normally, the elastase enzyme is prevented from destroying lung tissue by the protein antitrypsin. Antitrypsin is made in the liver and flows to the lungs, where it binds to the active site of elastase and prevents it from digesting lung tissue. Emphysema can occur when the negatively charged amino acid at position 53 of the amino acid sequence of antitrypsin is replaced with a positively charged amino acid. This mutation changes the chemical nature of antitrypsin such that the mutant antitrypsin is released from the liver at a much slower rate. The level of this mutant antitrypsin in the lungs is 15 percent of the normal level. The net result of this one amino acid mutation in the antitrypsin protein is that most of the elastase enzyme is free to destroy lung tissue. Cigarette smoking dramatically increases the incidence of emphysema in people who have the mutant antitrypsin. Cigarette smoke reacts with the hydrophobic amino acid at position 358 of antitrypsin, adding one oxygen atom at this position in the amino acid sequence. The addition of this one extra oxygen atom at this critical place in antitrypsin changes the chemical nature of the hydrophobic amino acid so that the antitrypsin no longer can bind to elastase. Because only 15 percent of the mutant antitrypsin gets from the liver to the lungs in the first place, cigarette smoking puts people with this particular mutation at grave risk for developing emphysema.

PERSPECTIVE AND PROSPECTS

Enzymatic reactions have been used by humankind since prehistoric times. It has been known for more than six thousand years that fermentation processes transform grapes into wine, but it was not until the nineteenth century that it was understood that the conversion of grape sugar to alcohol is a process catalyzed by enzymes found in yeast. In the 1700's, Antoine Lavoisier showed that a solution of sugar could be fermented if provided with the sediment of a previous fermentation and that the sugar was converted to alcohol and carbon dioxide in this process. At this time, it was thought that there was a vital force responsible for the workings of a living cell. This notion of a vital force slowed the development of the discipline of biochemistry considerably, as many good scientists struggled to understand the fermentation process. In 1828, Friedrich Wöhler synthesized urea in a test tube, providing strong evidence against the concept of a vital force. In 1833, Anselme Payen and Jean Persoz discovered the first enzyme, diastase (now known as amylase), which converted starch into sugar. The next year, Johann Eberle showed that the presence of a stomach is not required for gastric digestion to take place. In 1836, Theodor Schwann made the very important discovery that the active ingredient in digestion, which he called pepsin, could be extracted from the stomach wall.

The next year, Jöns Jakob Berzelius developed the idea of catalysis, making the point that both living and inorganic systems had catalysts. In the late 1850's, Louis Pasteur confirmed and extended the earlier experiments of Schwann.

Despite his brilliant experimental abilities, however, Pasteur was handicapped in his research by his belief that fermentation could happen only within a living organism. In 1860, Marcelin Berthelot showed that a living being was not the ferment, but produced the ferment, in sharp contrast to Pasteur's vitalist ideas. Pasteur's response to this work was that Berthelot and he meant different things by the use of the word "ferment." Moritz Traube, a German wine merchant, realized that chemical processes and living bodies were mostly based on ferment actions, and he published these ideas in 1858 and again in 1878. In 1878, Friedrich Kühne proposed that to remove the discrepancy over the meaning of the word "ferment," the word "enzyme" should be used, as it means "in yeast." It was not until 1897 that Eduard Buchner showed that living cells are not essential for fermentation to occur, as he extracted from yeast a cell-free juice containing the entire fermentation system.

From 1894 to 1898, Emil Fischer used synthetic organic chemistry for the preparation of substrates of known structure and configuration. He showed that enzymes have a very high degree of specificity for their own particular substrate and developed the famous "lock-and-key" hypothesis. This theory, which has been only slightly modified, states that the shape of a substrate and the enzyme's active site must be complementary for catalysis to occur. Purification of enzymes remained a difficult problem, and it was not until 1926 that James Summer crystallized the first enzyme, jack bean urease. The sequence of protein enzymes could be determined experimentally after 1952, when Frederick Sanger developed his methods for amino acid sequencing. In 1965, David Phillips produced the first three-dimensional picture of an enzyme, determining the shape of lysozyme. The advent of genetic engineering techniques in the 1970's revolutionized the field of enzyme research and the use of enzymes in medical applications by enabling the production of copious amounts of recombinant proteins.

—*George C. Shields, Ph.D.*

See also Antibiotics; Bacteriology; Blood and blood components; Blood testing; Cholesterol; Digestion; Emphysema; Enzyme therapy; Food biochemistry; Genetic diseases; Genetic engineering; Genetics and inheritance; Glycolysis; Hemophilia; Laboratory tests; Leukemia; Metabolism; Mutation; Oncology; Pharmacology; Pulmonary medicine; Screening; Thrombolytic therapy and TPA.

FOR FURTHER INFORMATION:

Campbell, Neil A. *Biology*. 4th ed. Redwood City, Calif.: Benjamin/Cummings, 1997. This classic introductory textbook provides an excellent discussion of essential biological structures and mechanisms. Its extensive and detailed illustrations help to make even difficult concepts accessible to the nonspecialist. Of particular interest is the chapter on enzymes, entitled "An Introduction to Metabolism."

Fruton, Joseph S. *Molecules and Life*. New York: Wiley-

Interscience, 1972. Fruton, a Yale biochemist, has filled his book with historical essays on the interplay of chemistry and biology. The first part of the book, "From Ferments to Enzymes," is an interesting account of how science progressed from the known results of fermentation to the chemical knowledge that enzymes were the molecules responsible for this and all other biochemical processes. The essay on the nature of proteins is also of interest. An excellent book.

Kornberg, Arthur. *For the Love of Enzymes*. Cambridge, Mass.: Harvard University Press, 1989. Both an autobiography of a great biochemist and a history of the study of enzymes. Arthur Kornberg won a Nobel Prize for the laboratory synthesis of deoxyribonucleic acid (DNA). An excellent scientific biography.

Liska, Ken. *Drugs and the Human Body*. 3d ed. New York: Macmillan, 1990. An easy-to-read book about the effects of drugs on the human body. A good overview of how drugs interact with various molecules in the body, including many cases in which enzymes are drug targets.

Needham, Joseph, ed. *The Chemistry of Life*. Cambridge, England: Cambridge University Press, 1970. Contains eight lectures on the history of biochemistry. Chapter 2, by Malcolm Dixon, describes the history of enzymes. Chapter 7, by M. Teich, takes a broader view, describing the historical foundations of modern biochemistry. In chapter 8, R. Peters describes the British biochemistry pioneers of the nineteenth century. These pioneers were full-time medical doctors who did research out of compassion for their patients.

Palmer, Trevor. *Understanding Enzymes*. 4th ed. London: Prentice Hall, 1995. A standard text on enzymes and how they function. Includes a bibliography and an index.

Phillips, D. C. "The Three-Dimensional Structure of an Enzyme Molecule." *Scientific American* 215 (November, 1966): 78. The three-dimensional structure of lysozyme is analyzed. This is the story of how the shape of the first enzyme molecule was determined and of how the shape determines the function of lysozyme. Written by the leader of the research team that solved the structure of this enzyme.

EPIDEMIOLOGY

SPECIALTY

ANATOMY OR SYSTEM AFFECTED: All

SPECIALTIES AND RELATED FIELDS: Environmental health, microbiology, pathology, public health

DEFINITION: The scientific study of the distribution of disease in human populations, as well as its causes and effects.

KEY TERMS:

endemic disease: a disease which is usually present in a population and whose frequency does not fluctuate greatly

epidemic: a marked increase in the frequency of a disease in a population, compared to historical experience

infectivity: the ability of an organism to enter and reproduce within a host

pathogenicity: the ability of an organism to cause disease

virulence: a measure of the severity of disease

SCIENCE AND PROFESSION

While etiology studies the causes of disease in individuals, epidemiology studies the causes and effects of disease in populations. Historically, epidemics of contagious disease have been one of the most important causes of human mortality and have played a profound role in influencing human history; the emergence of acquired immunodeficiency syndrome (AIDS) and the resurgence of other epidemic diseases have demonstrated the continuing importance of epidemiology to medical science.

An epidemic is characterized by a large increase in the frequency of a disease within a population. Until relatively recently, the term was used primarily for outbreaks of contagious diseases caused by infectious agents, but current epidemiology also concerns itself with environmentally caused diseases, such as radiation-induced cancers, and with mental and behavioral problems, such as drug use. Outbreaks of diseases in plants and animals are also loosely termed epidemics but are more properly termed epiphytotics and epizootics, respectively.

The defining characteristic of an epidemic is not the absolute frequency of the disease or its severity, but the abrupt increase in its frequency. In contrast, an endemic disease is one whose frequency within a population does not vary markedly with time. An epidemic may be local in scope and limited in its effects; an endemic disease may be widespread and an important source of mortality within a population. The extreme case is a pandemic, an epidemic which transcends national boundaries and affects huge numbers of individuals on a worldwide basis. The most notorious pandemics in recorded history were the bubonic plague that swept Eurasia in the fourteenth century, killing an estimated one-third of the population of Europe, and the influenza epidemic of 1918-1919, which killed approximately 20 million people worldwide. The AIDS epidemic, not recognized in the United States and Europe as a major public health threat until the early 1980's, has reached pandemic status; because of its predominantly sexual mode of transmission and relatively low infectivity, however, the number of infected individuals is far lower than would be the case for a disease transmitted by casual contact.

Epidemics have played an important role in human life since the dawn of recorded history. Studies of animal populations and of primitive hunting communities, however, suggest that epidemics are more a burden of civilization than a part of the human condition, because effective spread of disease between humans requires high population densities. A virulent, easily transmitted pathogen simply cannot be sustained in a self-contained group of a few dozen or hundred individuals who have few contacts with the world at large. Even with the advent of agriculture and settled life, the inhabitants of the Americas, Australia, and Oceania enjoyed relative freedom from epidemic diseases before the coming of Europeans. Although human pathogens are derived from animal pathogens—many of them, presumably, through long coevolution with humans and their hominid ancestors, others through mutations in more recent times— the most common animal reservoirs of human disease are those animals most closely related to humans. Thus Africa and tropical Asia, home to the great apes and humankind's immediate ancestors, have always harbored the greatest diversity of human pathogens, while Australia and isolated Pacific islands had very few.

The devastating effect of the introduction of Eurasian and African diseases, chiefly of an epidemic nature, into Australia, Oceania, and the Americas eclipses even the great plague pandemic of the 1300's in its historical impact. The decimation of native populations in these areas under European influence must be ascribed first to disease and second to impoverishment and social dislocation, with direct military action as a poor, insignificant third. In the period between 1770 and 1870, the native population of Hawaii declined by 90 percent, and the native population of Tasmania became extinct. As much as 50 percent of Mexico's estimated pre-Columbian population of 25 million may have perished of smallpox and other epidemic diseases during and immediately after the Spanish Conquest; a hundred years later, the population had declined by 90 percent. In contrast, European colonial activity in West Africa and Southeast Asia did not result in precipitous native population decline.

Surveying a wide variety of historical evidence, William McNeill concluded that the historical experience of Mexico and Hawaii represented the usual result of the confluence of disease pools and the introduction of a virulent pathogen into a previously unexposed population: destruction of 30 percent to 50 percent of the population in a few years, followed by more gradual decline until the remaining human population becomes genetically resistant, the pathogen disappears because of a lack of hosts, or the human population becomes extinct. Parallels to the Amerindian experience can be found in Japan, where diseases (principally the plague) introduced from China killed half the population in the eighth century; in medieval Europe; and perhaps in late antiquity, according to McNeill's hypothesis that the depopulation of the Roman Empire between 150 and 400 was caused by measles and smallpox introduced from the Orient.

The nature and severity of an epidemic of infectious disease are influenced by the nature of the pathogen and by the physical and social makeup of the affected population. Characteristics of the pathogen include transmissibility (the ease with which a pathogen is passed from one host to another), infectivity (its ability to grow and multiply in that host), pathogenicity (its ability to produce clinical disease), and virulence (the severity of the disease produced). The worst epidemic diseases, such as smallpox, are highly transmissible, infective, pathogenic, and virulent. Chickenpox is highly transmissible and infective but not very virulent. Diseases that are not highly transmissible, such as leprosy, or are selectively pathogenic, such as tuberculosis, are more likely to be endemic than epidemic.

Each infectious disease has characteristic modes of transmission that must be understood for the purpose of disease prevention. Respiratory diseases transmitted as airborne particles—smallpox, influenza, measles, pneumonic plague—spread rapidly and are difficult to control through sanitation and quarantine. Diseases spread through fecal contamination of water and food—cholera, hepatitis, typhoid, poliomyelitis—are more easily avoided and, in industrialized countries, tend to occur in localized outbreaks with identifiable sources. Blood-borne diseases transmitted by biting arthropods—malaria, yellow fever, typhus, bubonic plague—can erupt in devastating epidemics when both host and vector populations are high. Localized outbreaks of arthropod-transmitted diseases that have natural animal reservoirs (including yellow fever, St. Louis encephalitis, bubonic plague, murine typhus, and Lyme disease) occur throughout the world, but human-to-human chains of transmission are most likely to occur in Third World countries beset by social upheaval. The spread of sexually transmitted diseases is also aided by war and social dislocation. The transmission of blood-borne viral diseases through contaminated hypodermic needles became significant in the latter part of the twentieth century.

Human resistance to disease is a function of genetic makeup, age, and general health. The impact of a measles epidemic illustrates these relationships. Europeans, through many generations of epidemics that killed the most susceptible individuals, inherit an immune system which is effective at fighting this virus. Disease resistance decreases with increasing age. Although no specific treatment for measles existed until a vaccine was developed in the 1960's, mortality rates in the United States declined dramatically between 1850 and 1950 as a result of improved nutrition and housing and better nursing care. The mortality rate of untreated measles among American children in the 1950's was one in two hundred or three hundred, among poor European slum dwellers in the nineteenth century was one in twenty or thirty, and among Amerindians and Polynesians, who were both impoverished and lacking genetic resistance, was one in two or three.

Diseases caused by behavioral and environmental factors can also be viewed as occurring in epidemics. A major explanation for the increased prominence of noninfectious diseases as causes of mortality and morbidity has been an increasing life span; the cumulative effects of environmental toxins and unhealthy behavior exhibit themselves only as

an individual ages. The age-specific frequency of Alzheimer's disease in the United States remained relatively constant in the twentieth century, but because of increasing longevity, the frequency increased dramatically.

Both longevity and changes in behavior contributed to the increase in mortality from lung cancer in industrialized countries in the twentieth century. The various lines of investigation linking this epidemic to tobacco smoking are a good example of epidemiological research. Recent increases in the incidence of skin cancer seem to be linked partly to the popularity of sunbathing and partly to increases in ultraviolet radiation caused by pollution.

Localized clusters of disease and mortality often point to a single environmental hazard. The long-term adverse effects of lead, asbestos, and herbicides have been identified and characterized based on observations of groups of peoples with high levels of exposure to these substances.

DIAGNOSTIC AND TREATMENT TECHNIQUES

Epidemiologists may be actively involved in the diagnosis and collection of field data, or they may rely on data submitted by physicians, hospitals, and public health workers. The data generated by the study of epidemiology are used for a variety of purposes: to suggest hypotheses and avenues of research in the case of a condition whose cause or causes (etiology) are unknown, to assist health care workers in diagnosis and treatment, to encourage private and public agencies to adopt policies to slow the spread of disease, and to influence public and private policy so as to reduce underlying social and environmental causes of disease.

Cultural practices that have their root in informal epidemiological observation and serve to accomplish one of the four aims outlined above can be found throughout history. For example, not eating pork is a way of preventing the transmission of trichinosis. Mongols, who avoided trapping marmots in the belief that they were the reincarnations of deceased ancestors, were less likely to contract bubonic plague than the Chinese, who had no such cultural taboo. Scientific epidemiology, which relies on a correct understanding of the causes of disease, dates from the mid-nineteenth century. The classic pioneering study is that of John Snow, who conducted a thorough investigation of cholera cases during an epidemic in London in 1854. By mapping the distribution of cases, he was able to link them to specific contaminated water sources. He recommended the boiling of drinking water, strict hygiene in the tending of infected patients, and better sanitation in food preparation; the result was real progress in reducing the severity of that and subsequent epidemics. It is interesting to note that the understanding of the etiology of certain major plant diseases (wheat stem rust, bunt, potato blight) and the epidemiological recommendations for their control antedate corresponding developments in human diseases by half a century.

The discoveries by Robert Koch, Louis Pasteur, and others linking specific microorganisms to human disease ushered in an era when the most effective method for improving human health was the prevention of infection, principally through epidemiological public health measures. Sewage treatment, water purification, and the inspection of food preparation facilities reduced the incidence of cholera, typhoid, and hepatitis; draining and channeling stagnant water to control mosquitoes made malaria and yellow fever rare diseases in the United States and southern Europe. The pesticide DDT (although subsequently condemned because of the serious environmental problems that it caused) performed a laudable service to human health in the aftermath of World War II, killing the vectors of louse-borne typhus and other diseases.

In the field of nontransmissible disease, the early twentieth century saw great progress in the understanding of nutritional deficiencies. Pellagra (a niacin deficiency) and scurvy (a vitamin C deficiency) may still occur in epidemics among institutionalized persons, but they are treated with simple dietary methods.

Today, the World Health Organization of the United Nations coordinates epidemiological efforts between nations and within poorer countries that do not have the resources to address their internal epidemiological problems. Most countries have a central agency which monitors the occurrence of disease within the country; states, provinces, and other political divisions also have epidemiological public health agencies. In countries with a national health service, the activities of primary care physicians and clinics are closely coordinated with public health administration.

Statistics are the raw material of epidemiological investigation. Death certificates record both the primary and contributing causes of death, the age and sex of the deceased, and the place of death. Census figures give a picture of the community in which epidemiological events occur, such as its racial and socioeconomic composition, age structure, and population density. Physicians and hospitals are required to notify the public health authorities of the occurrence of certain "reportable" diseases, such as AIDS, syphilis, and tuberculosis. Hospital admission records will reflect increases in conditions requiring hospitalization, while school and workplace attendance figures reflect outbreaks of milder communicable diseases.

Some outbreaks are routine and predictable, and the measures for controlling them are well established. When influenza cases increase, public health authorities identify the strain responsible and take steps to immunize those individuals who are most at risk for severe disease. Identifying the source of contaminated food or water is critical to controlling outbreaks of hepatitis A and typhoid in industrialized countries. When war or natural disaster disrupts the normal infrastructure of modern life, it is considered prudent to inoculate the affected population against a variety of infectious diseases.

The history of the discovery of Lyme disease illustrates how epidemiology works. Physician and hospital records indicated a clustering of cases diagnosed as juvenile arthritis near Lyme, Connecticut. By comparing the cases and observing their common characteristics, epidemiologists deduced that an arthropod-transmitted organism normally found on wild animals was probably responsible. Armed with this information, they surveyed microorganisms found in biting arthropods and were able to establish that the same spirochaete was found in wild deer, deer ticks, and patients exhibiting symptoms of juvenile arthritis. This organism, and the chronic disease that it causes, proved to be widespread, although not particularly common among humans. Knowing the etiology of the disease enabled physicians to diagnose the condition correctly and to treat it.

Environmentally and behaviorally caused diseases are less amenable to control by health professionals alone, and consequently can prove much more intractable. This is particularly true when there are powerful economic factors working at cross purposes to disease control measures. The epidemiologist can demonstrate that the increase in lung cancer in the twentieth century paralleled an increase in tobacco consumption and that smokers account for most cases of lung cancer. The biomedical investigator studying etiology can show that tobacco derivatives cause cancer in laboratory animals and may ultimately be able to explain how this is brought about at the molecular level. Physicians can advise patients not to smoke, and psychologists can devise therapies to help people quit smoking. None of these efforts, however, will achieve definitive success as long as there are powerful forces encouraging people to smoke and undermining the efforts of the health professionals. The difficulty is compounded, as with any addictive drug, by the active participation of the very people who are the victims of the epidemic in perpetuating the conditions that favor it.

PERSPECTIVE AND PROSPECTS

Tremendous progress was made in controlling epidemic disease over the course of the twentieth century, so much so that there was a period when epidemics of life-threatening contagious diseases were viewed as past history in industrialized countries and there was optimism that the same result could be achieved in the Third World as well. The gradual elimination of smallpox was viewed as a model. A worldwide scourge until vaccination was discovered in the eighteenth century, smallpox had become rare in Europe and the United States by the end of the nineteenth century. In the 1960's, when the World Health Organization embarked on a worldwide campaign to eliminate smallpox, it was endemic only in parts of Africa and India. Since 1980, no new cases have been reported worldwide. Poliomyelitis, the subject of a massive worldwide inoculation campaign, was declared to be absent from the Western Hemisphere in 1989. With diseases for which an effective vaccine is available, it is possible at relatively low cost to inoculate a high proportion of the population, breaking the chain of infection. Water purification and the destruction of insect vectors are also effective in reducing disease incidence.

Yet the worldwide epidemic of AIDS and the resurgence of malaria, tuberculosis, and cholera as epidemic diseases in the late twentieth century are ample evidence that the epidemiological battle against disease is far from won, and that medical science's current arsenal of weapons against infectious disease has serious inadequacies. The factors favoring an increase in epidemics of transmissible disease in the last decades of the twentieth century included an increase in the speed and frequency of international travel, the emergence of drug-resistant strains of a wide variety of pathogens, and a high level of political and social instability in developing nations. Some scientists believe that increasing exploitation of tropical rain forests is responsible for bringing humans into contact with the diseases of nonhuman primates, which then have the potential to spread throughout the world. Such is probably the case with AIDS, whose spread from a center of origin in tropical Africa was aided by the fact that infected individuals can carry and transmit the virus for years without exhibiting clinical symptoms of disease. Most methods of preventing and treating viral illnesses in humans rely on bolstering the normal human immune response, so a virus which undermines this response poses a difficult challenge to medical science.

AIDS is only one notable example of dozens of tropical diseases that have the potential for causing lethal worldwide epidemics. Commenting on Ebola virus, a virulent pathogen responsible for a 1976 epidemic in Zaire in which 90 percent of the victims died, a prominent virologist confessed to being afraid and noted that "fortunately, Ebola does not have a significant respiratory component, or the world would be a far different place today. There would be a lot fewer of us." A related virus, lethal to monkeys and infective but nonvirulent in humans, swept a primate quarantine facility in Maryland, and another member of this virus group caused a localized lethal epidemic among monkeys and laboratory workers in Marburg, Germany. Many other lethal transmissible viruses have been identified.

AIDS, the widespread use of immunosuppressant drugs, and the aging of the population have created significant numbers of individuals who have weakened immune systems and are susceptible to infection by animal pathogens. It is worth noting that the worst pandemic in recorded human history, the fourteenth century bubonic plague epidemic, occurred when an animal pathogen became established in a human population and then mutated from a moderately transmissible, arthropod-borne disease to a highly transmissible, airborne infection. The likelihood that animal pathogens will spread to humans and that they will be disseminated internationally is increasing, and the chances of a mutation toward increased transmissibility or

virulence increases with the number of infected individuals. The potential for a worldwide pandemic capable of overwhelming the efforts of modern medical science certainly exists, although its probability cannot be estimated.

—Martha Sherwood-Pike, Ph.D.

See also Acquired immunodeficiency syndrome (AIDS); Arthropod-borne diseases; Bacterial infections; Bacteriology; Biostatistics; Childhood infectious diseases; Cholera; Creutzfeldt-Jakob disease and mad cow disease; Disease; *E. coli* infection; Ebola virus; Elephantiasis; Environmental diseases; Environmental health; Food poisoning; Forensic pathology; Hanta virus; Hepatitis; Influenza; Laboratory tests; Legionnaires' disease; Leprosy; Lice, mites, and ticks; Malaria; Measles, red; Microbiology; Occupational health; Parasitic diseases; Pathology; Plague; Poisoning; Poliomyelitis; Prion diseases; Pulmonary diseases; Rabies; Salmonella; Sexually transmitted diseases; Stress; Tropical medicine; Veterinary medicine; Viral infections; World Health Organization; Yellow fever; Zoonoses.

FOR FURTHER INFORMATION:

Clegg, E. J., and J. P. Garlick, eds. *Disease and Urbanization.* London: Taylor & Francis, 1980. A series of papers discussing the impact of the growth of cities on the frequency of disease. One paper compares the relative impacts of improved living standards and urban services versus specific medical intervention in reducing disease mortality, concluding that the former is far more important.

Fox, John P., Carrie E. Hall, and Lila R. Elveback. *Epidemiology: Man and Disease.* New York: Macmillan, 1970. A textbook treating the historical development of epidemiology as a science, the factors of interest in studying the spread and fluctuations of disease in human populations, the use of vital statistics and public health data, and epidemiological research. This text treats contagious disease as a historical and Third World problem and noncontagious disease as the principal concern of epidemiologists in industrialized countries.

Goldsmid, John. *The Deadly Legacy: Australian History and Transmissible Disease.* Kensington, New South Wales, Australia: New South Wales University Press, 1988. Because of its isolation before the eighteenth century, the epidemiological history of Australia is more completely documented than that of any other continent. This book discusses the disease history of Aborigines and settlers, as well as the history of government efforts to control epidemics from the early nineteenth century to the late twentieth century, with good coverage of the control measures in effect in 1988.

McNeill, William H. *Plagues and Peoples.* Garden City, N.Y.: Doubleday, 1976. The author adopts the controversial view that epidemic diseases are the main driving force behind human history and summons an impressive array of evidence to support his claim. He views periods of social and political upheaval as the result of the confluence of disease pools and the subsequent decimation by disease of populations exposed to novel pathogens. A readable text for the layperson, full of interesting anecdotes.

Preston, Richard. "A Reporter at Large: Crisis in the Hot Zone." *The New Yorker* 68 (October 26, 1992): 58. Focusing on how U.S. government epidemiologists controlled an outbreak of deadly Ebola virus in a primate quarantine facility in Maryland, this article gives a good overview of the various "new" human diseases that have surfaced, including AIDS, and the worldwide threat that they pose.

Ranger, Terence, and Paul Slack, eds. *Epidemics and Ideas: Essays on the Historical Perception of Pestilence*. Cambridge, England: Cambridge University Press, 1992. A collection of papers describing the interplay among perceptions of the etiology of disease, social and religious attitudes, and politics in epidemics from classical antiquity to the present. For example, in sixteenth century Italy, the transmission of plague from the poor to the upper classes was viewed as punishment from God visited on the rich for their lack of charity, whereas in nineteenth century England, the high incidence of disease among the lower classes was viewed as resulting from poor constitution and moral character.

Timmreck, Thomas C. *An Introduction to Epidemiology*. Boston: Jones and Bartlett, 1994. A book in the Jones and Bartlett series in health sciences. Discusses epidemiological methods. Includes a bibliography and an index.

Epilepsy

Disease/disorder

Anatomy or system affected: Brain, head, nerves, nervous system

Specialties and related fields: Neurology

Definition: A serious neurologic disease characterized by seizures, which may involve convulsions and loss of consciousness.

Key terms:

anticonvulsant: a therapeutic drug that prevents or diminishes convulsions

aura: a sensory symptom or group of such symptoms that precedes a grand mal seizure

clonic phase: the portion of an epileptic seizure that is characterized by convulsions

electroencephalogram (EEG): a graphic recording of the electrical activity of the brain, as recorded by an electroencephalograph

grand mal: a type of epileptic seizure characterized by severe convulsions, body stiffening, and loss of consciousness during which victims fall down; also called tonic-clonic seizure

idiopathic disease: a disease of unknown origin

petit mal: a mild type of epileptic seizure characterized by a very short lapse of consciousness, usually without convulsions; the epileptic does not fall down

seizure: a sudden convulsive attack of epilepsy that can involve loss of consciousness and falling down

seizure discharges: characteristic brain waves seen in the EEGs of epileptics; their strength and frequency depend upon whether a seizure is occurring and its type

status epilepticus: a rare, life-threatening condition in which many sequential seizures occur without recovery between them

tonic-clonic seizure: another term for a grand mal seizure

tonic phase: the portion of an epileptic seizure characterized by loss of consciousness and body stiffness

Causes and Symptoms

Epilepsy is characterized by seizures, commonly called fits, which may involve convulsions and the loss or consciousness. It was called the "falling disease" or "sacred disease" in antiquity and was mentioned in 2080 B.C. in the laws of the famous Babylonian king Hamurabi. Epilepsy is a serious neurologic disease that usually appears between the ages of two and fourteen. It does not affect intelligence, as shown by the fact that the range of intelligence quotients (IQs) for epileptics is quite similar to that of the general population. In addition, many epileptics have achieved fame, such as Alexander the Great, English poet Lord Byron, Julius Caesar, Russian novelist Fyodor Dostoevski, and Dutch artist Vincent Van Gogh.

In 400 B.C., Hippocates of Cos proposed that epilepsy arose from physical problems in the brain. This origin of the disease is now known to be unequivocally true. Despite many centuries of exhaustive study and effort, however, only a small percentage (20 percent) of cases of epilepsy caused by brain injuries, brain tumors, and other diseases are curable. This type of epilepsy is called symptomatic epilepsy. In contrast, 80 percent of epileptics can be treated to control the occurrence of seizures but cannot be cured of the disease, which is therefore a lifelong affliction. In these cases, the basis of the epilepsy is not known, although the suspected cause is genetically programmed brain damage that still evades discovery. Most epilepsy is, therefore, an idiopathic disease (one of unknown origin), and such epileptics are thus said to suffer from idiopathic epilepsy.

A common denominator in idiopathic epilepsy, and also in symptomatic epilepsy, is that it is evidenced by unusual electrical discharges, brain waves, seen in the electroencephalograms (EEGs) of epileptics. These brain waves are called seizure discharges. They vary in both their strength and their frequency, depending on whether an epileptic is having a seizure and what type of seizure is occurring. Seizure discharges are almost always present and recognizable in the EEGs of epileptics, even during sleep.

There are four types of common epileptic seizures. Two

of these are partial (local) seizures called focal motor and temporal lobe seizures, respectively. The others, grand mal and petit mal, are generalized and may involve the entire body. A focal motor seizure is characterized by rhythmic jerking of the facial muscles, an arm, or a leg. As with other epileptic seizures, it is caused by abnormal electrical discharges in the portion of the brain that controls normal movement in the body part that is affected. This abnormal electrical activity is always seen as seizure discharges in the EEG of the affected part of the brain.

In contrast, temporal lobe seizures, again characterized by seizure discharges in a distinct portion of the cerebrum of the brain, are characterized by sensory hallucinations and other types of consciousness alteration, a meaningless physical action, or even a babble of some incomprehensible language. Thus, for example, temporal lobe seizures may explain some cases of people "speaking in tongues" in religious experiences or in the days of the Delphic oracles of ancient Greece.

The term "grand mal" refers to the most severe type of epileptic seizure. Also called tonic-clonic seizures, grand mal attacks are characterized by very severe EEG seizure discharges throughout the entire brain. A grand mal seizure is usually preceded by sensory symptoms called an aura (probably related to temporal lobe seizures), which warn an epileptic of an impending attack. The aura is quickly followed by the grand mal seizure itself, which involves the loss of consciousness, localized or widespread jerking and convulsions, and severe body stiffness.

Epileptics suffering a grand mal seizure usually fall to the ground, may foam at the mouth, and often bite their tongues or the inside of their cheeks unless something is placed in the mouth before they lose consciousness. In a few cases, the victim will loose bladder or bowel control. In untreated epileptics, grand mal seizures can occur weekly. Most of these attacks last for only a minute or two, followed quickly by full recovery after a brief sense of disorientation and feelings of severe exhaustion. In some cases, however, grand mal seizures may last for up to five minutes and lead to temporary amnesia or to other mental deficits of a longer duration. In rare cases, the life-threatening condition of status epilepticus occurs, in which many sequential tonic-clonic seizures occur over several hours without recovery between them.

The fourth type of epileptic seizure is petit mal, which is often called generalized nonconvulsive seizure or, more simply, absence. A petit mal seizure consists of a brief period of loss of consciousness (ten to forty seconds) without the epileptic falling down. The epileptic usually appears to be daydreaming (absent) and shows no other symptoms. Often a victim of a petit mal seizure is not even aware that the event has occurred. In some cases, a petit mal seizure is accompanied by mild jerking of hands, head, or facial features and/or rapid blinking of the eyes. Petit mal attacks

can be quite dangerous if they occur while an epileptic is driving a motor vehicle.

Diagnosing epilepsy usually requires a patient history, a careful physical examination, blood tests, and a neurologic examination. The patient history is most valuable when it includes eyewitness accounts of the symptoms, the frequency of occurrence, and the usual duration range of the seizures observed. In addition, documentation of any preceding severe trauma, infection, or episodes of addictive drug exposure provides useful information that will often differentiate between idiopathic and symptomatic epilepsy.

Evidence of trauma is quite important, as head injuries that caused unconsciousness are often the basis for later symptomatic epilepsy. Similarly, infectious diseases of the brain, including meningitis and encephalitis, can cause this type of epilepsy. Finally, excess use of alcohol or other psychoactive drugs can also be causative agents for symptomatic epilepsy.

Blood tests for serum glucose and calcium, electroencephalography, and computed tomography (CT) scanning are also useful diagnostic tools. The EEG will nearly always show seizure discharges in epileptics, and the location of the discharges in the brain may localize problem areas associated with the disease. CT scanning is most useful for identifying tumors and other serious brain damage that may cause symptomatic epilepsy. When all tests are negative except for abnormal EEGs, the epilepsy is considered idiopathic.

It is thought that the generation of epileptic symptoms occurs because of a malfunction in nerve impulse transport in some of the billions of nerve cells (neurons) that make up the brain and link it to the body organs that it innervates. This nerve impulse transport is an electrochemical process caused by the ability of the neurons to retain substances (including potassium) and to excrete substances (including sodium). This ability generates the weak electrical current that makes up a nerve impulse and that is registered by electroencephalography.

A nerve impulse leaves a given neuron via an outgoing extension (or axon), passes across a tiny synaptic gap that separates the axon from the next neuron in line, and enters an incoming extension (or dendrite) of that cell. The process is repeated until the impulse is transmitted to its site of action. The cell bodies of neurons make up the gray matter of the brain, and axons and dendrites (white matter) may be viewed as connecting wires.

Passage across synaptic gaps between neurons is mediated by chemicals called neurotransmitters, and it is now believed that epilepsy results when unknown materials cause abnormal electrical impulses by altering neurotransmitter production rates and/or the ability of sodium, potassium, and related substances to enter or leave neurons. The various nervous impulse abnormalities that cause epilepsy can be shown to occur in the portions of the gray matter of the cerebrum that control high-brain functions. For example, the frontal lobe—which controls speech, body movement, and eye movements—is associated with temporal lobe seizures.

Treatment and Therapy

Idiopathic epilepsy is viewed as the expression of a large group of different diseases, all of which present themselves clinically as seizures. This is extrapolated from the various types of symptomatic epilepsy observed, which have causes that include faulty biochemical processes (such as inappropriate calcium levels), brain tumors or severe brain injury, infectious diseases (such as encephalitis), and the chronic overuse of addictive drugs. As to why idiopathic epilepsy causes are not identifiable, the general biomedical wisdom states that present technology is too imprecise to detect its causes.

Symptomatic epilepsy is treated with medication and either by the extirpation of the tumor or other causative brain tissue abnormality that was engendered by trauma or disease or by the correction of the metabolic disorder involved. The more common, incurable idiopathic disease is usually treated entirely with medication that relieves symptoms. This treatment is essential because without it most epileptics cannot attend school successfully, maintain continued employment, or drive a motor vehicle safely.

A large number of anticonvulsant drugs are presently available for epilepsy management. It must, however, be made clear that no one therapeutic drug will control all types of seizures. In addition, some patients require several such drugs for effective therapy, and the natural history of a given case of epilepsy may often require periodic changes from drug to drug as the disease evolves. Furthermore, every therapeutic antiepilepsy drug has dangerous side effects that may occur when it is present in the body above certain levels or after it is used beyond some given time period. Therefore, each epileptic patient must be monitored at frequent intervals to ascertain that no dangerous physical symptoms are developing and that the drug levels in the body (monitored by the measurement of drug content in blood samples) are within a tolerable range.

More than twenty antiepilepsy drugs are widely used. Phenytoin (Dilantin) is very effective for grand mal seizures. Because of its slow metabolism, phenytoin can be administered relatively infrequently, but this slow metabolism also requires seven to ten days before its anticonvulsant effects occur. Side effects include cosmetically unpleasant hair overgrowth, swelling of the gums, and skin rash. These symptoms are particularly common in epileptic children. More serious are central nervous effects including ataxia (unsteadiness in walking), drowsiness, anemia, and marked thyroid deficiency. Most such symptoms are reversed by decreasing the drug doses or by discontinuing it. Phenytoin is often given, together with other antiepilepsy drugs, to produce optimum seizure prevention. In those cases, great care must be taken to prevent dangerous syn-

ergistic drug effects from occurring. High phenytoin doses also produce blood levels of the drug that are very close to toxic 25 micrograms per milliliter values.

Carbamazepine (Tegretol) is another frequently used antiepileptic drug. Chemically related to the drugs used as antidepressants, it is useful against both psychomotor epilepsy and grand mal seizures. Common carbamazepine side effects are ataxia, drowsiness, and double vision. A more dangerous, and fortunately less common, side effect is the inability of bone marrow to produce blood cells. Again, very serious and unexpected complications occur in mixed-drug therapy that includes carbamazepine, and at high doses toxic blood levels of the drug may be exceeded.

Phenobarbital, a sedative hypnotic also used as a tranquilizer by nonepileptics, is a standby for treating epilepsy. It too can have serious side effects, including a lowered attention span, hyperactivity, and learning difficulties. In addition, when given with phenytoin, phenobarbital will speed up the excretion of that drug, lowering its effective levels.

Four major lessons can be learned from these three drugs. First, individual antiepilepsy drugs have many different side effects. Second, there are concrete reasons that epileptics taking therapeutic drugs must be monitored carefully for physical symptoms. Third, at high antiepileptic drug doses, the blood levels attained may closely approximate and even exceed toxic values. Fourth, drug interactions in mixed drug therapy can be counterproductive.

About 20 percent of idiopathic epileptics do not achieve adequate seizure control after prolonged and varied drug therapy. Another option for some—but not all—such people is brain surgery. This type of brain surgery is usually elected after two conditions are met. First, often-repeated EEGs must show that most or all of the portion of the brain in which the seizures develop is very localized. Second, these affected areas must be in a brain region that the patient can lose without significant mental loss (often in the prefrontal or temporal cerebral lobes). When such surgery is carried out, it is reported that 50 to 75 percent of the patients who are treated and given chronic, postoperative antiepilepsy drugs become able to achieve seizure control.

The most frequent antiepilepsy surgery is temporal lobectomy. The brain has two temporal lobes, one of which is dominant in the control of language, memory, and thought expression. A temporal lobectomy is carried out by removing the nondominant temporal lobe, when it is the site of epilepsy. About 6 percent of temporal lobectomies lead to a partial loss of temporal lobe functions, which may include impaired vision, movement, memory, and speech.

Another common type of antiepilepsy surgery is called corpus callosotomy. This procedure involves partially disconnecting the two cerebral hemispheres by severing some of the nerves in the corpus callosum that links them. This surgery is performed when an epileptic has frequent, uncontrollable grand mal attacks that cause many dangerous falls. The procedure usually results in reduced numbers of seizures and decreases in their severity.

Physicians now believe that many cases of epilepsy may be prevented by methods aimed at avoiding head injury (especially in children) and the use of techniques such as amniocentesis to identify potential epileptics and treat them before birth. Furthermore, the prophylactic administration of antiepilepsy drugs to nonepileptic people who are afflicted with encephalitis and other diseases known to produce epilepsy is viewed as wise.

PERSPECTIVE AND PROSPECTS

A great number of advances have occurred in the treatment of epilepsy via therapeutic drugs and surgical techniques. With the exception of symptomatic epilepsy, drug therapy has been the method of choice because it is less drastic than surgery, easier to manage, and rarely has the potential for irreversible damage to patients that can be caused by the removal of a portion of the brain. The main antiepileptic drugs are phenytoin, carbamazepine, and phenobarbital, but a tremendous variety of other chemical therapies has been investigated and utilized successfully.

Such treatments include high doses of vitamins, injections of muscle relaxants, and changes in diet. The variety is unsurprising, considering the vast number of disease issues that can cause seizures. For example, the rare genetic disease phenylketonuria (PKU) can cause epilepsy. Phenylketonuric epilepsy is often treated by use of a ketogenic diet rich in fats; the clear value of this treatment is unexplained. Readers are encouraged to investigate the many epilepsy treatments that have not been noted. Such an examination may be quite valuable because there are about a million epileptics in the United States alone, and some estimates indicate that four of every thousand humans are likely to develop some epileptic symptoms during their lifetime.

Modern surgical treatment of epilepsy reportedly began in 1828, with the efforts of Benjamin Dudley, who removed epilepsy-causing blood clots and skull fragments from five patients, who all survived despite primitive and nonsterile operating rooms. The next landmark in such surgery was the removal of a brain tumor by the German physician R. J. Godlee, in 1884, without the benefit of X rays or EEG techniques, which did not then exist.

By the 1950's EEGs were used to locate epileptic brain foci, and physicians such as the Canadians Wilder Penfield and Herbert Jasper pioneered its use to locate brain regions to remove for epilepsy remission without damaging vital functions. After considerable evolution over the course of forty years, antiepilepsy surgery by the 1990's had become widespread, commonplace, and relatively safe.

Nevertheless, because of the imperfections of all available methodologies, 5 to 8 percent of epileptics cannot achieve seizure control by any method or method combination and even the "well-managed" epilepsy treatment regimen has its flaws. There is still much to be learned

about curing epilepsy. It is hoped that the efforts of ongoing biomedical research, both in basic science and in clinical settings, will eliminate epilepsy through the development of new therapeutic drugs and sophisticated advances in surgery and other nondrug methods.

—Sanford S. Singer, Ph.D.

See also Brain; Brain disorders; Computed tomography (CT) scanning; Electroencephalography (EEG); Nervous system; Neurology; Neurology, pediatric; Neurosurgery; Phenylketonuria (PKU); Seizures; Unconsciousness.

FOR FURTHER INFORMATION:

Barnhart, Edward R., ed. *Physician's Desk Reference.* 47th ed. Oradell, N.J.: Medical Economics, 1993. An atlas of all the prescription drugs available in the United States. Includes a listing of the drugs used against epilepsy, their producers, their useful dose ranges, their metabolism and toxicology, and their contraindications. Found in most public libraries, it is a valuable reference for physicians and patients.

Berkow, Robert, and Andrew J. Fletcher, eds. *The Merck Manual of Diagnosis and Therapy.* 16th ed. Rahway, N.J.: Merck Sharp & Dohme Research Laboratories, 1992. Contains a compendium of data on the characteristics, etiology, diagnosis, and treatment of adult epilepsy. Also discusses seizure disorders of children and newborns. Designed for physicians, the material is also useful to less specialized readers.

Gumnit, Robert J., ed. *Living Well with Epilepsy.* New York: Demos, 1990. Designed to give people with epilepsy the outlook necessary to live successfully with the disease. Among the topics covered are causes and treatment, high-quality care, medical and surgical options, the problems of epileptic children, sexuality and pregnancy, the workplace, rights, and resources.

Hopkins, Anthony. *Epilepsy: The Facts.* New York: Oxford University Press, 1981. The author wishes to eliminate misunderstanding about epilepsy and educate people about it. This is done nicely by clear coverage of topics including explanation of epilepsy, seizure types and causes, epilepsy treatment methods, and information on living with the disease.

Nogen, Alan G. *Epilepsy: A Medical Handbook for Physicians, Nurses, Teachers, and Parents.* Dallas, Tex.: Taylor, 1980. This comprehensive handbook provides a valuable overview for physicians, nurses, teachers, and parents of epileptics. Topical coverage includes history, epilepsy types, diagnosis and causes, treatments, life with epilepsy, and community resources for epileptics. Also contains an excellent glossary.

Scott, Donald. *About Epilepsy.* New York: International Universities Press, 1973. This book "aims to inform a wide range of people about epilepsy." Included are causation, types and diagnosis, treatment, medication, the history of epilepsy, famous and infamous epileptics, and care and familial aspects. Contains a bibliography and a glossary.

EPISIOTOMY

PROCEDURE

ANATOMY OR SYSTEM AFFECTED: Anus, genitals, reproductive system

SPECIALTIES AND RELATED FIELDS: Gynecology, obstetrics

DEFINITION: A surgical cut made in the pelvic floor to enlarge the vagina for the facilitation of childbirth.

INDICATIONS AND PROCEDURES

An episiotomy is performed to enlarge the vaginal opening and ease the delivery of a baby during childbirth. While not a routine procedure, some circumstances which indicate the need for an episiotomy include rapid delivery, breech delivery, and presentation of the baby with face to the front of the birth canal, all of which prevent the perineum (the area between the vagina and the anus) from stretching rapidly enough to prevent tearing. Scarring from vaginal surgeries also limits the ability of the vagina to expand.

During the procedure, a local anesthetic is injected into the perineum. The obstetrician uses straight-bladed blunt scissors to snip the tissue between the vagina and anus, avoiding the anal sphincter muscle. After delivery, the incision is carefully stitched together, along with any minor tears in the birth canal.

USES AND COMPLICATIONS

The birth canal has very limited space to accommodate an infant, and situations such as feet-first or face-forward presentation can lead to compression of the umbilical cord and interruption of the oxygen supply to the baby, or even to potential crushing of the infant. An episiotomy can facilitate a rapid delivery in these circumstances, thereby preventing serious injury to the infant. Failure of the perineum to stretch sufficiently to accommodate the child can result in severe, irregular tears of the vagina and even of the anal sphincter muscles. Ragged tears are very difficult to repair surgically and are much more prone to infection. Tearing of the anal sphincter could lead to permanent incontinence. The easily repaired incisions of episiotomy eliminate these potential difficulties.

Healing of the incisions is rapid and straightforward, but the area may itch and be somewhat painful for a few weeks. Painkilling drugs may be prescribed, and ice packs can be used to alleviate pain. Women who do not desire episiotomies and have controlled, problem-free deliveries may try to stretch the perineum gradually by massaging it with warm oil during the delivery.—*Karen E. Kalumuck, Ph.D.*

See also Childbirth; Childbirth, complications of; Incontinence; Obstetrics.

EPSTEIN-BARR VIRUS. *See* CHRONIC FATIGUE SYNDROME; MONONUCLEOSIS.

ESTROGEN REPLACEMENT THERAPY

PROCEDURE

ANATOMY OR SYSTEM AFFECTED: Bones, breasts, circulatory system, endocrine system, uterus

SPECIALTIES AND RELATED FIELDS: Endocrinology, geriatrics and gerontology

DEFINITION: A therapy for women going through the menopause in which estrogen, sometimes in combination with progesterone, is used to reduce menopausal symptoms and to continue protection against cardiovascular disease and osteoporosis.

KEY TERMS:

menopause: the end of the menstrual cycle in women; brought on either by surgery (the removal of the ovaries) or naturally, when the hormones that control the cycle gradually decline, usually between the ages of forty-eight and fifty-three

perimenopause: the time prior to the menopause when the hormone cycle is less efficient but there is normal secretion of follicle-stimulating hormone; usually accompanied by some menopausal symptoms

INDICATIONS AND PROCEDURES

The female menstrual cycle is controlled by four hormones. Follicle-stimulating hormone (FSH) and luteinizing hormone (LH) are released by the pituitary gland. They cause the release of estrogen and progesterone from the ovaries and uterus. In a complicated combination of positive and negative feedback, the four hormones create a very regular cycle in most women. The cycle has three phases: follicular, which starts with menstrual bleeding and usually lasts for twelve to fourteen days; ovulatory, which lasts for one to three days and results in ovulation; and luteal, which lasts for thirteen to fourteen days and ends in the onset of menstruation. As a woman ages, the ovaries become less efficient, estrogen levels decrease, the follicular phase varies, and ovulation does not always occur. The result is the perimenopause. A woman is perimenopausal when estrogen levels are lower than normal but FSH levels are still cyclical, often accompanied by some of the physical signs of the menopause such as hot flashes and night sweats.

After two to four years of the perimenopause, most women have become menopausal. This means the end of the menstrual cycle and a decrease in the controlling hormones. Because estrogen has both a positive and negative feedback function, it appears to dominate the control of the cycle. Over time, the control for FSH and LH becomes so weak that they are no longer released cyclically and instead are released together in pulses. The physical effects of the decrease of estrogen is thinning of the vaginal epithelium and loss of its secretions, a decrease in breast mass, and an accelerated loss of bone. Hot flashes, night sweats, and emotional mood swings accompany the internal changes and are usually the signs and symptoms that let a woman know that the menopause is beginning. In addition, the strong influence by estrogen as a protection against heart disease is lost at the menopause.

Once the menopause has been confirmed by a blood test, the woman and her physician need to decide on a course of treatment or if there is a need for treatment. The decision is made by balancing the benefits and risks of estrogen replacement therapy.

USES AND COMPLICATIONS

The benefits of estrogen replacement therapy include relief of the classic symptoms of the menopause, reduction of bone loss, possible prevention of osteoporosis, reduction in risk of heart disease, the possible improvement of memory and mental functioning in women with mild Alzheimer's disease, and the possible reduction of the risk for colon cancer. These benefits are balanced by an increased risk of endometrial cancer, increased risk of uterine fibroids and endometriosis, similar symptoms to premenstrual syndrome (PMS), possible menstrual discharge, increased risk of breast cancer, increased risk of gallstones and blood clots, and possible weight gain.

The way in which estrogen is given has some effect on certain risks and benefits. Estrogen alone via pill or skin patch should be considered only for a woman with no uterus or for very short duration for classic menopausal symptoms. By itself, estrogen increases the risk for uterine and breast growths, both cancerous and benign. Cyclical therapy is daily estrogen in a pill or patch combined with a progesterone pill for a certain number of days per month. This method significantly reduces the uterine problems but increases the chance of menstrual bleeding and premenstrual symptoms. Continuous therapy is estrogen and progesterone daily. This usually prevents menstrual bleeding, but the effect of progesterone on possible breast tumors is still unknown.

The best way to determine a course of treatment is to do a family health history. If osteoporosis or heart disease are prevalent, then estrogen replacement therapy or hormone replacement therapy may be recommended. The increased risk of breast cancer is greater in families with a history of breast cancer. Recent research on women using hormone replacement therapy for long-term health have demonstrated risk reduction for heart disease and osteoporosis even when the therapy is started ten years after the menopause and continued for five to ten years. This approach may thwart the increase in breast cancer risk, since this type of cancer usually takes ten to fifteen years to progress. In hormone replacement therapy, the lowest risks for endometrial cancers is achieved when progesterone is taken only ten to twenty-one days a month.

PERSPECTIVE AND PROSPECTS

In addition to the research being done on hormone combinations, there has been a small but growing push for "natural" menopause relief. Little solid research has been published on nutritional methods using foods or herbs. One area that appears to have some potential is the use of phytoestrogens, plant sources of estrogens. They come in two classes: isoflavones (soybeans) and lignans (flax seeds, whole grains, and some fruits and vegetables). The soybean research compared Asian women to white American women for osteoporosis; Asian women have a similar risk but a much lower incidence. The typical Japanese woman eats soy foods daily and also has a lower incidence of breast cancer and heart disease. Recent studies have compared the effect of phytoestrogens on cancer risk. Results suggest that a high intake of phytoestrogens reduces the incidence of both breast and endometrial cancer. A possible confounder with lignans could be the amount of fiber accompanying that form of phytoestrogen; fiber may be the source of the protection, but the strength of the protective effect warrants further study. —*Wendy E. S. Repovich, Ph.D.*

See also Breast cancer; Cancer; Cervical, ovarian, and uterine cancers; Endocrinology; Heart disease; Hormone replacement therapy; Hormones; Hysterectomy; Menopause; Menstruation; Osteoporosis; Premenstrual syndrome (PMS); Reproductive system.

FOR FURTHER INFORMATION:

Jetter, Alexis. "Should You Trust Her?" *Health* 11 (July/August, 1997): 102-113.

Margen, Sheldon, Joyce C. Lashof, and Patricia A. Buffler, eds. *Women's Health 1995.* The University of California at Berkeley Wellness Report. New York: Health Letter Associates, 1995.

Runowicz, Carolyn, ed. "Hormone Therapy: When and for How Long?" *Health News, from the publishers of The New England Journal of Medicine*, March 25, 1997, 1-2.

ETHICS

DEFINITION: A philosophical discipline that attempts to analyze systematically the way in which moral decisions are made. In the field of medicine, this involves defining appropriate patient care, humane biological research, an equitable distribution of scarce medical resources, and a just health care delivery system.

KEY TERMS:

beneficence: a principle of medical ethics which requires that actions be taken for the patient's good

casuistry: a form of moral reasoning whereby specific cases about which there is moral uncertainty are compared to other cases about which there is moral certainty

distributive justice: a principle of medical ethics dealing with the fair and equitable distribution of scarce resources

euthanasia: the taking of a life under the presumption that this act is the only means of relieving intolerable suffering

nonmaleficence: a principle of medical ethics which requires that the actions taken not harm the patient

prima facie: the concept that one ethical principle is morally binding unless the action it requires violates another equal or greater principle

respect for autonomy: a principle of medical ethics which requires that the autonomous decisions of patients be honored

wedge argument: a logically contrived argument supporting a morally acceptable action which subsequently leads to other actions that are considered morally unacceptable

THE PRINCIPLES OF MEDICAL ETHICS

In the course of their work, health care professionals are faced with many situations that have moral significance. These situations are characterized by such questions as whether or when to proceed with treatment, which therapy to administer, which patient to see first, how to conduct research using human subjects, where to assign resources that are in short supply, or how to set up an equitable health care system. The discipline of medical ethics seeks to engage in a systematic examination of these questions which is as objective as possible.

Ethical questions in general fall into two categories. A quandary is a moral question about which detailed ethical analysis yields a single, undisputed answer. A dilemma, on the other hand, is a moral question to which there are at least two ethically defensible responses, with neither one taking clear precedence over the other. Ethical analysis consists of the application of primary principles to concrete, clinical situations. It also employs comparative reasoning, in which a particular problem is compared to other situations about which a moral consensus exists. Principled reasoning rests on four fundamental principles of biomedical ethics: respect for autonomy, nonmaleficence, beneficence, and justice.

The principle of respect for autonomy requires that every person be free to take whatever autonomous action or make whatever autonomous decision he or she wishes without constraint by other individuals. An example of respect for autonomy is the doctrine of informed consent, which requires that patients or research subjects be provided with adequate information that they clearly understand before voluntarily submitting to therapy or participating in a research trial.

The principle of nonmaleficence states that one should not inflict evil or harm upon a patient. Although straightforward in its enunciation, it is clear that this principle may come into conflict with the principle of respect for autonomy in cases where a request for withdrawal of therapy is made. Similarly, this principle may come into conflict with obligations to promote the good of the patient, as many medical decisions involve the use of therapies or diagnostic procedures that have undesirable side effects. The principle of double effect in the Roman Catholic moral tradition has attempted to resolve this latter conflict by stating that if the intent of an action is to effect an overriding good, the action is defensible even if unintended but foreseen harmful consequences ensue. Some commentators suggest, however, that intent is an artificial distinction because all the conse-

quences, both good and bad, are foreseen. As a result, the potential for harm should be weighed against the potential for benefit in deciding the best course of action. A formal evaluation of this kind is commonly referred to as a risk-benefit analysis. Individual interpretation of the principle of nonmaleficence lies at the heart of debates over abortion, euthanasia, and treatment withdrawal.

The principle of beneficence expresses an obligation to promote the patient's good. This can be construed as any action that prevents harm, supplants harm, or does active good to a person. As such, this principle provides the basis for all medical practice, be it preventive, epidemiologic, acute, or chronic care. Not all actions can be considered uniformly beneficial. Certain kinds of therapy that may prove to be lifesaving can leave a patient with what he or she finds to be an unacceptable quality of life. An examination of the positive and negative consequences of successful medical treatment is commonly called a benefit-burden analysis. In this context, the principle of beneficence most frequently comes into conflict with the principle of respect for autonomy. In situations such as these, the physician's appeal to beneficence is often considered paternalistic.

The principle of justice applies primarily to the distribution of health care resources in what can be considered to be a just and fair fashion. As there are many competing theories of justice, there is no one clear statement of this principle that can be succinctly applied to all situations. Nevertheless, the principle does require careful consideration of the means by which health care is allocated under conditions of scarcity. In the United States, scarce resources may comprise such entities as transplantable organs, intensive care beds, expensive medical technologies in general, and, in some circumstances, basic medical care itself. Under conditions of scarcity, one's understanding of justice can easily come into conflict with obligations to each of the three preceding principles. In general, the more scarce the resource, the more concerns about distributive justice will influence the deployment of that resource.

Although some commentators tend to assign primacy to one of these principles, while relegating others to subordinate roles, the prevailing approach to principled reasoning interprets each one as being prima facie binding. Each principle confers a binding obligation upon the medical professional to the extent that it does not conflict with another equally binding principle. When two prima facie principles require actions that are diametrically opposed to each other, there is an appeal to proportionality which allows the requirements of each principle to be evaluated in the light of the circumstances at hand. On a case-by-case basis, one principle may be judged to be more binding than another, depending on the context of the problem.

An alternative form of ethical analysis employs the technique of casuistry, or case-based analysis. Using this method, the circumstances of a particular ethical quandary or dilemma (the "reference case") are compared to those of a case about which it is abundantly clear what the correct moral decision should be (the "paradigm case"). The degree to which the reference case resembles or differs from the paradigm case provides guidance as to what the ethically appropriate course of action might be. This particular method of analysis has the advantage of being similar to the way in which conclusions are reached both in common law and in clinical medicine. Clinical decisions are regularly made in medical practice by comparing the facts of a particular case about which the treatment may be in question to those of similar cases in which the correct treatment is known.

A problem for those who favor casuistic analysis is the wedge argument, sometimes known as the "slippery slope." Detractors suggest that the use of a particular logical argument, such as the defense for withholding or withdrawing certain kinds of therapy, will drive a wedge further and further into the fabric of society until an undesirable consequence (for example, active nonvoluntary euthanasia) ensues. Proponents of casuistry respond that the undesirable consequence is far enough removed from the paradigm case as to no longer resemble it.

Most clinical ethicists combine principle-based analysis with case-based reasoning in order to answer the specific ethical questions that arise in the practice of medicine. In addition, clinical ethicists also benefit from training in law, sociology, and psychology in addition to the study of primary medical science and philosophy.

ETHICAL DISPUTES IN MEDICAL PRACTICE

Ethical issues in medicine can be divided into macrocosmic (large-scale) and microcosmic (small-scale) concerns. Macrocosmic issues are those which apply to a broad social constituency and therefore often intersect with both statutory and common law. Microcosmic concerns, on the other hand, are those which arise in the day-to-day practice of medicine, the discussion and resolution of which generally have less of a far-reaching impact on the society as a whole.

Primary among the macrocosmic ethical debates is the question of health care allocation. This centers largely on the development of health care delivery systems in particular and health care financing in general. Proposals for reform of the U.S. health care system range from the creation of a single-payer national health insurance program, which would insure each and every citizen, to a series of proposals which would establish multiple requirements for private health insurance, often linking these requirements to employment. A problem common to all proposals for health care reform is the definition of what constitutes a basic minimum of health care to which each citizen is entitled. Even if consensus can be reached regarding such a basic minimum, questions still remain as to how and to whom scarce resources will be allocated. Scarce resources in this

setting can be divided into those which are in limited supply, such as transplantable organs, and those which may be prohibitively expensive, such as advanced medical technologies. In both cases, solutions to the problem of scarcity require an assessment of mechanisms for both increasing supply and distributing the resource in an ethically acceptable fashion.

Other issues being argued at the macrocosmic level are broad social policies regarding such concerns as euthanasia, physician-assisted suicide, voluntary abortion, and regulations governing the withholding and withdrawal of life-sustaining therapy. Biomedical research using fetal tissue from induced abortions and research aimed at precisely mapping the human genetic code have raised serious ethical questions regarding both the morality of these endeavors and the nature of life itself. The question of whether—and if so, how—to screen patients for the human immunodeficiency virus (HIV) that causes acquired immunodeficiency syndrome (AIDS) has been argued in both state and federal courts.

Public issues such as these are approached by a number of mechanisms. In the United States, blue-ribbon panels, such as the President's Commission for the Study of Ethical Problems in Medicine and Biomedical and Behavioral Research at the federal level or the New York State Task Force on Life and the Law at the state level, can study a problem and issue a consensus report with policy recommendations. These panels have the advantage of bringing together people who represent a wide range of opinions to discuss a topic in detail in a relatively quiet environment prior to subjecting their conclusions to the glare of the political process. Another avenue is the formation of grassroots organizations that attempt to generate a public consensus about ethically sensitive issues. Examples of these organizations are Oregon Health Decisions and the New York Citizen's Committee on Health Care Decisions.

In one fashion or another, issues of public concern in the United States are often argued on the floor of both federal and state legislatures. There are currently numerous state laws regarding appropriate mechanisms for withholding and withdrawing therapy. Federal legislation, such as the Patient Self Determination Act, has also been enacted, governing the disclosure of patients' rights to determine the course of their care when they lack decision-making capacity.

U.S. research involving human subjects is subjected to ethical review at both the macrocosmic and the microcosmic level. Nationally, it is regulated by agencies such as the Food and Drug Administration (FDA). At the microcosmic level, the FDA mandates and supervises the administration of institutional review boards (IRBs), which are charged with the responsibility of assuring that human subjects are involved in creditable research, are treated in a humane manner, are not subjected to undue risks, and are fully cognizant both of the nature of the project in which they are participating and of any potential risks and benefits associated with it.

Resource allocation is a problem at the microcosmic as well as the macrocosmic level; however, the issues in small-scale settings revolve around who constitutes an appropriate candidate for a limited number of intensive care beds or what are the appropriate eligibility criteria for organ transplantation at a particular institution. Perhaps the most common microcosmic problems for hospitals and nursing homes are individual decisions regarding when to terminate life-sustaining therapy. Other common microcosmic dilemmas involve maternal-fetal conflict where the autonomous requests or medical best interests of the mother do not coincide with the presumed best interests of her unborn child.

In situations such as these, both acute and chronic health care facilities often solicit the assistance of institutional ethics committees. Such committees are characteristically composed of individuals representing a broad spectrum of professional disciplines as well as community members not directly employed by the facility. A typical committee might consist of representatives from physician and nursing staffs, social service, psychiatry, pastoral care, special care services (such as intensive care, AIDS management, and neonatal intensive care) that often have a greater number of patients with ethical concerns than others, and hospital administration. Many committees also employ the services of philosophers, attorneys, designated community representatives, or representatives of special interest groups.

In situations that require an institutional response, these committees will often assist in policy development. Examples include institutional policies specifying admission and discharge criteria for intensive care, or policies governing the procedures for withholding or withdrawing therapy. Ethics committees also serve as primary educational resources for both institutional staff and members of the surrounding community.

When the care of individual patients raises ethical questions, many committees have established mechanisms for case consultation or case review. Consultations of this type involve an in-depth review of the patient's clinical condition, as well as of various other social, religious, psychological, or family matters that may be pertinent. After a complete assessment of the facts of the case, consultants then investigate the various ethical arguments that support alternative courses of action before issuing a final recommendation. Case consultation is usually performed by a subcommittee of the institutional ethics committee and is sometimes offered by individual consultants who are not members of the committee. In most cases, the recommendations of the consultants are not binding. Certain models, however, require that some limited kinds of consultative recommendations determine the outcome in specific settings.

Although intervention by an ethics committee often allows for the resolution of ethical disputes within the walls of an institution, sometimes irreconcilable differences require judicial review by a court of law. Under these circumstances, the court's decision regarding a particular case becomes a matter of public record, providing precedent for future similar cases. In this way, certain ethical dilemmas that arise as microcosmic problems end up generating a body of common law which can have profound effects at the macrocosmic level.

PERSPECTIVE AND PROSPECTS

Although the literature on biomedical ethics increased dramatically during the last half of the twentieth century, the roots of ethics in medicine are as old as the profession itself. An ethical code of behavior is central to the Hippocratic writings of the fifth century B.C. Hippocratic texts were expanded upon by medieval physicians in Western societies so that, by the fifteenth century, rules of conduct had been established in the medical schools of the time. Eighteenth century Enlightenment physicians such as Benjamin Rush, Samuel Bard, John Gregory, and Thomas Percival stressed the need for primary moral rules of medical practice and began to wrestle with questions of truth telling in the physician-patient relationship. Percival's writings in particular became the basis for the first American Medical Association Code of Ethics, issued in 1847. Nineteenth century physicians such as Worthington Hooker, Austin Flint, Sr., and Sir William Osler continued to refine a primarily beneficence-based understanding of ethical behavior on the part of the professional. Osler in particular argued that physicians should be broadly educated in the liberal arts so as to be able to practice medicine properly.

In 1949, the Nuremberg Code established the first basic ethical requirements for the conduct of medical research. This document was a direct result of the Nuremberg trials of Nazi war criminals who had engaged in human experimentation considered far outside the grounds of decency. The code was later expanded and revised to become the Declaration of Helsinki of the World Medical Association, originally issued in 1964.

In the 1950's, medical ethics began to move away from being primarily a set of internally generated rules of professional behavior. The writings of such nonphysicians as Joseph Fletcher and Paul Ramsey, both originally trained in theology, began to examine the impact of medicine and medical technology on the moral fabric of society.

The 1960's and 1970's brought an emphasis on patient autonomy to the consideration of biomedical ethics in the United States. The ascendancy of autonomy parallels a rise in the technological capabilities of modern medicine, a time of unusually pronounced affluence in the West, and the appearance of what have since become paradigm legal challenges to the notion of the physician or medical institution as the sole participant in medical decision making. Concurrent with this trend was the appearance of new institutions dedicated to the study of biomedical ethics such as the Kennedy Institute of Ethics at Georgetown University and the Hastings Center in New York. At the same time, ethical theories developed by nineteenth century philosophers such as John Stuart Mill and Immanuel Kant began to be applied to situations arising out of medical practice by a number of individuals whose primary training was in philosophy and theology rather than in clinical medicine.

In the 1980's and 1990's, the prospect of scarcity came to dominate ethical discussions in the United States, raising concern about such questions as health care rationing and public access to medical care. This emphasis on distributive justice began to temper the autonomy-driven concerns of the previous two decades. The confrontation between the demands of autonomous individuals and the obligations of social justice promises to be the primary focus of medical ethics well into the future.

—John Arthur McClung, M.D.

See also Abortion; Aging, extended care for the; Animal rights vs. research; Cesarean section; Circumcision, female, and genital mutilation; Circumcision, male; Cloning; Contraception; Electroconvulsive therapy; Euthanasia; Fetal tissue transplantation; Genetic engineering; Hippocratic oath; Hysterectomy; In vitro fertilization; Law and medicine; Malpractice; Mastectomy and lumpectomy; Resuscitation; Screening; Sterilization; Terminally ill, extended care for the; Transplantation; World Health Organization.

FOR FURTHER INFORMATION:

Beauchamp, Tom L., and James F. Childress. *Principles of Biomedical Ethics.* 3d ed. New York: Oxford University Press, 1989. A lucidly written, basic textbook of bioethics. Although some commentators are critical of a primarily principle-based approach to bioethics, this book remains the most widely recognized introductory resource in the field.

Beauchamp, Tom L., and Laurence B. McCullough. *Medical Ethics: The Moral Responsibilities of Physicians.* Englewood Cliffs, N.J.: Prentice Hall, 1984. An excellent introduction to the common problems encountered in clinical ethics. Each chapter opens with a case study that serves as the focal point for the discussion of the topic at hand. One of the best references for readers who are completely new to the field.

Beauchamp, Tom L., and LeRoy Walters, eds. *Contemporary Issues in Bioethics.* 2d ed. Belmont, Calif.: Wadsworth, 1982. A composite of readings culled from legal decisions, seminal legislation, ethical codes of conduct, and the writings of well-known ethicists. The readings are organized by topic and are preceded by a short summary of ethical theory. This work serves as a good companion volume to a basic text.

Jonsen, Albert R., Mark Siegler, and William J. Winslade. *Clinical Ethics.* 3d ed. New York: McGraw-Hill, 1992. A handbook of medical ethics aimed primarily at the physician in training. The authors present a method for evaluating the ethical dimensions of clinical cases, after which the book is organized lexically so that commonly encountered problems can be located easily. A very concise reference which concentrates on practical rather than theoretical priorities.

Jonsen, Albert R., and Stephen Toulmin. *The Abuse of Casuistry: A History of Moral Reasoning.* Berkeley: University of California Press, 1988. A well-constructed history of the technique of case-based analysis which concludes with a practical description of how this approach can be used as an alternative to principle-based analysis in clinical situations.

Reich, Warren T., ed. *Encyclopedia of Bioethics.* 2d ed. New York: Free Press, 1992. A broad look at the entire field of bioethics. Probably the most comprehensive collection of readings currently available under one title.

Veatch, Robert M. *Case Studies in Medical Ethics.* Cambridge, Mass.: Harvard University Press, 1977. A good survey of ethical issues in which each is introduced by way of 112 separate case presentations. This reference provides excellent material for group discussions and panel debates.

EUTHANASIA

ETHICS

DEFINITION: The intentional termination of a life, which may be active (resulting from specific actions causing death) or passive (resulting from the refusal or withdrawal of life-sustaining treatment), voluntary (with the patient's consent) or involuntary (on behalf of infants or others who are incapable of making this decision, such as comatose patients).

KEY TERMS:

active euthanasia: administration of a drug or some other means that directly causes death; the motivation is to relieve patient suffering

durable power of attorney: designation of a person who will have legal authority to make health care decisions if the patient becomes incapable of making decisions for himself or herself

living will: a legal document in which the patient states a preference regarding life-prolonging treatment in the event that he or she cannot choose

nonvoluntary euthanasia: a decision to terminate life made by another when the patient is incapable of making a decision for himself or herself

passive euthanasia: ending life by refusing or withdrawing life-sustaining medical treatment

voluntary euthanasia: a patient's consent to a decision which results in the shortening of his or her life

THE CONTROVERSY SURROUNDING EUTHANASIA

In the past, the role of the doctor was clear: The physician should minimize suffering and save lives whenever possible. In the present, it is possible for these two goals to be at odds. Saving lives in some situations seems to prolong the misery of the patient. In other cases, procedures or treatments may only marginally postpone the time of death. Advances in medical technology enable many to live who would have died just a few years ago, and massive amounts of money are spent each year on medical research with the goal of prolonging life. Experts in U.S. population trends indicate that by the year 2030, those over the age of sixty-five will comprise about 20 percent of the country's total population. These people will probably be healthy and alert well into their eighties; however, in the last years of their lives they will probably require significant medical care, putting financial stress on the health care system. The complex issues surrounding death, suffering, and economics create an insistency for answers to difficult ethical questions. Does all life have value? Should one fight against death even when suffering is intense? Should suffering be lessened if the time of death is brought nearer? Should a patient be given the right to refuse medical treatment if the result is death? Should others be allowed to make this decision for the patient? Should other factors such as the financial or emotional burden on the family be part of the decision-making process? Once a decision has been made to terminate suffering by death, is there any ethical difference between discontinuing medical treatment and giving a lethal dosage of painkilling medication? Should laws be put into place that offer guidelines in these situations, or should each case be decided on an individual basis? And who should decide? There is a wide range of opinion and much uncertainty involving euthanasia and what constitutes a "good" death.

Euthanasia comes from a Greek word that can be translated as "good death" and is defined in several ways, depending on the philosophical stance of the one giving the definition. Tom Beauchamp, in his book *Health and Human Values* (1983), defines euthanasia as

> putting to death or failing to prevent death in cases of terminal illness or injury; the motive is to relieve comatoseness, physical suffering, anxiety or a serious sense of burdensomeness to self and others. In euthanasia at least one other person causes or helps to cause the death of one who desires death or, in the case of an incompetent person, makes a substituted decision, either to cause death directly or to withdraw something that sustains life.

Most patients who express a wish to die more quickly are terminally ill; however, euthanasia is sometimes considered as a solution for nonterminal patients as well. An example of the latter would be seriously deformed or retarded infants whose futures are judged to have a poor "quality of life" and who would be a serious burden on their families and society.

When discussing the ethical implications of euthanasia, the types of cases have been divided into various classes.

A distinction is made between voluntary and nonvoluntary euthanasia. In voluntary euthanasia, the patient consents to a specific course of medical action in which death is hastened. Nonvoluntary euthanasia would occur in cases in which the patient is not able to make decisions about his or her death because of an inability to communicate or a lack of mental facility. Each of these classes has advocates and antagonists. Some believe that voluntary euthanasia should always be allowed, but others would limit voluntary euthanasia to only those patients who have a terminal illness. Some, although agreeing in principle that voluntary euthanasia in terminal situations is ethically permissible, nevertheless oppose euthanasia of any type because of the possibility of abuses. With nonvoluntary euthanasia, the main ethical issues deal with when such an action should be performed and who should make the decision. If a person is in an irreversible coma, most agree that that person's physical life could be ended; however, arguments based on "quality of life" can easily become widened to include persons with physical or mental disabilities. Infants with severe deformities can sometimes be saved but not fully cured with medical technology, and some individuals would advocate nonvoluntary euthanasia in these cases because of the suffering of the infants' caregivers. Some believe that family members or those who stand to gain from the decision should not be allowed to make the decision. Others point out that the family is the most likely to know what the wishes of the patient would have been. Most believe that the medical care personnel, although knowledgeable, should not have the power to decide, and many are reluctant to institute rigid laws. The possibility of misappropriated self-interest from each of these parties magnifies the difficulty of arriving at well-defined criteria.

The second type of classification is between passive and active euthanasia. Passive euthanasia occurs when sustaining medical treatment is refused or withdrawn and death is allowed to take its course. Active euthanasia involves the administration of a drug or some other means that directly causes death. Once again, there are many opinions surrounding these two types. One position is that there is no difference between active and passive euthanasia because in each the end is premeditated death with the motive of prevention of suffering. In fact, some argue that active euthanasia is more compassionate than letting death occur naturally, which may involve suffering. In opposition, others believe that there is a fundamental difference between active and passive euthanasia. A person may have the right to die, but not the right to be killed. Passive euthanasia, they argue, is merely allowing a death which is inevitable to occur. Active euthanasia, if voluntary, is equated with suicide because a human being seizes control of death; if nonvoluntary, it is considered murder.

Passive euthanasia, although generally more publicly acceptable than active euthanasia, has become a topic of controversy as the types of medical treatment that can be withdrawn are debated. A distinction is sometimes made between ordinary and extraordinary means. Defining these terms is difficult, since what may be extraordinary for one patient is not for another, depending on other medical conditions that the patient may have. In addition, what is considered an extraordinary technique today may be judged ordinary in the future. Another way to assess whether passive euthanasia should be allowed in a particular situation is to weigh the benefits against the burdens for the patient. Although most agree that there are cases in which high-tech equipment such as respirators can be withdrawn, there is a question about whether administration of food and water should ever be discontinued. Here the line between passive and active euthanasia is blurred.

RELIGIOUS AND LEGAL IMPLICATIONS

Decisions about death concern everyone because everyone will die. Eventually, each individual will be the patient who is making the decisions or for whom the decisions are being made. In the meantime, one may be called upon to make decisions for others. Even those not directly involved in the hard cases are affected, as taxpayers and subscribers to medical insurance, by the decisions made on the behalf of others. In a difficult moral issue such as this, individuals look to different institutions for guidelines. Two sources of guidance are the church and the law.

In 1971, the Roman Catholic church issued a statement entitled *Ethical and Religious Directives for Catholic Health Facilities*. Included in this directive was the statement, "[I]t is not euthanasia to give a dying person sedatives and analgesics for alleviation of pain, when such a measure is judged necessary, even though they may deprive the patient of the use of reason or shorten his life." This thinking was reaffirmed by a 1980 statement from the Vatican which considers suffering and expense for the family legitimate reasons to withdraw medical treatment when death is imminent. Bishops from The Netherlands, in a letter to a government commission, state "[B]odily deterioration alone does not have to be unworthy of a man. History shows how many people, beaten, tortured and broken in body, sometimes even grew in personality in spite of it. Dying becomes unworthy of a man, if family and friends begin to look upon the dying person as a burden, withdraw themselves from him. . . ." When speaking of passive euthanasia, the bishops state, "We see no reason to call this euthanasia. Such a person after all dies of his own illness. His death is neither intended nor caused, only nothing is done anymore to postpone it." Christians from Protestant churches may reflect a wider spectrum of positions. Joseph Fletcher, an Episcopal priest, defines a person as one having the ability to think and reason. If a patient does not meet these criteria, according to Fletcher, his or her life may be ended out of compassion for the person he or she once was. The United Church of Christ illustrates this view in its policy

statement: "When illness takes away those abilities we associate with full personhood . . . we may well feel that the mere continuance of the body by machine or drugs is a violation of their person. . . . We do not believe simply the continuance of mere physical existence is either morally defensible or socially desirable or is God's will."

These varied positions generally are derived from differing emphases on two truths concerning the nature of God and the role of suffering in the life of the believer. First is the belief that God is the giver of life and that human beings should not usurp God's authority in matters of life and death. Second, alleviation of suffering is of critical importance to God, since it is not loving one's neighbor to allow him or her to suffer. Those who give more weight to the first statement believe as well that God's will allows for suffering and that the suffering can be used for a good purpose in the life of the believer. Those who emphasize the second principle insist that a living God would not prolong the suffering of people needlessly and that one should not desperately fight to prolong a life which God has willed to die.

C. Everett Koop, former surgeon general of the United States, differentiates between the positive role of a physician in providing a patient "all the life to which he or she is entitled" and the negative role of "prolonging the act of dying." Koop has opposed euthanasia in any form, cautioning against the possibility of sliding down a slippery slope toward making choices about death that reflect the caregivers' "quality of life" more than the patient's.

Dr. Jack Kervorkian, a Michigan physician, became the most well known advocate of assisted suicide in the United States. From 1990 to 1997, Kervorkian assisted at least sixty-six people in terminating their lives. According to Kervorkian's lawyer, many other assisted suicides have not been publicized. Kervorkian believes that physician-assisted suicide is a matter of individual choice and that should be seen as a rational way to end tremendous pain and suffering. Most of the patients assisted by him spent many years suffering from extremely painful and debilitating diseases, such as multiple sclerosis, bone cancer, and brain cancer.

The American Medical Association (AMA) has criticized this view, calling it a violation of professional ethics. When faced with pain and suffering, the AMA asserts that it is a doctor's responsibility to provide adequate "comfort" care, not death. In the AMA's view, Kervorkian is "a reckless instrument of death." Three trials in Michigan for assisting in suicide failed to produce a guilty verdict for Kervorkian, and he continued to assert his right to help people end painful lives.

During the course of reevaluating the issues involved in terminating a life, the law has been in a state of flux. The decisions that are made by the courts act on the legal precedents of an individual's right to determine what is done to his or her own body and society's position against suicide. The balancing of these two premises has been handled legally by allowing refusal of treatment (passive euthanasia) but disallowing the use of poison or some other method that would cause death (active euthanasia). The latter is labeled suicide, and anyone who assists in such an act can be found guilty of assisting a suicide, or of murder. Following the Karen Ann Quinlan case in 1976, in which the family of a comatose woman secured permission to withdraw life-sustaining treatment, the courts routinely allowed family members to make decisions regarding life-sustaining treatment if the patient could not do so. The area of greatest legal controversy involves the withdrawal of food and water. Some courts have charged doctors with murder for the withdrawal of basic life support measures such as food and water. Others have ruled that invasive procedures to provide food and water (intravenously, for example) are similar to other medical procedures and may be discontinued if the benefit to the patient's quality of life is negligible.

In 1994, 51 percent of the voters in Oregon passed the world's first "death with dignity" law. It allowed physician-assisted suicide. Doctors could begin prescribing fatal overdoses of drugs to terminally ill patients. The vote was reaffirmed in 1997 by 60 percent of the state's voters, despite opposition from the Roman Catholic Church, the AMA, and various anti-abortion and right-to-life groups. The 9th United States Circuit Court of Appeals in San Francisco then lifted a lower court order blocking implementation of the law.

Doctors in Oregon became free to prescribe fatal doses of barbiturates to patients with less than six months to live. Physicians were required to file forms with the Oregon Health Division before prescribing the overdose. Then, there would be a fifteen-day waiting period between the request for suicide assistance and the approval of the prescription. Opponents of the Oregon law charged that it perverted the practice of medicine and forced many suffering people to "choose" an early death to save themselves from expensive medical care or pain that could be manageable if physicians were aware of new methods of pain control. The National Right to Life Committee indicated that it would continue to fight implementation of the law in federal courts.

Although the laws vary from state to state, most states allow residents to make their wishes known regarding terminal health care either by writing a living will or by choosing a durable power of attorney. A living will is a document in which one can state that some medical treatments should not be used in the event that one becomes incapacitated to the point where one cannot choose. Living wills allow the patient to decide in advance and protect health care providers from lawsuits. Which treatment options can be terminated and when this action can be put into effect may be

limited in some states. Most states have a specific format that should be followed when drawing up a living will and require that the document be signed in the presence of two witnesses. Often, qualifying additions can be made by the individual that specify whether food and water may be withdrawn and whether the living will should go into effect only when death is imminent or also when a person has an incurable illness but death is not imminent. A copy of the living will should be given to the patient's physician and become a part of the patient's medical records. The preparation or execution of a living will cannot affect a person's life insurance coverage or the payment of benefits. Since the medical circumstances of one's life may change and a person's ethical stance may also change, a patient may change the living will at any time by signing a written statement.

A second way in which a person can control what kind of decisions will be made regarding his or her death is to choose a decision maker in advance. This person assumes a durable power of attorney and is legally allowed to act on the patient's behalf, making medical treatment decisions. One advantage of a durable power of attorney over a living will is that the patient can choose someone who shares similar ethical and religious values. Since it is difficult to foresee every medical situation that could arise, there is more security with a durable power of attorney in knowing that the person will have similar values and will therefore probably make the same judgments as the patient. Usually a primary agent and a secondary agent are designated in the event that the primary agent is unavailable. This is especially important if the primary agent is a spouse or a close relative who could, for example, be involved in an accident at the same time as the patient.

PERSPECTIVE AND PROSPECTS

Although large numbers of court decision, articles, and books suggest that the issues involved in euthanasia are recent products of medical technology, these questions are not new. Euthanasia was widely practiced in Western classical culture. The Greeks did not believe that all humans had the right to live, and in Athens, infants with disabilities were often killed. Although in general they did not condone suicide, Pythagoras, Plato, and Aristotle believed that a person could choose to die earlier in the face of an incurable disease and that others could help that person to die. Seneca, the Roman Stoic philosopher, was an avid proponent of euthanasia, stating:

> Against all the injuries of life, I have the refuge of death. If I can choose between a death of torture and one that is simple and easy, why should I not select the latter? As I choose the ship in which I sail and the house which I shall inhabit, so I will choose the death by which I leave life.

The famous Hippocratic oath for physicians acted in opposition to the prevailing cultural bias in favor of euthanasia. Contained in this oath is the statement, "I will never give a deadly drug to anybody if asked for it . . . or make a suggestion to this effect." Interestingly, the AMA has reaffirmed this position in a policy statement:

> . . . the intentional termination of the life of one human being by another—"mercy killing"—is contrary to that for which the medical profession stands and is contrary to the policy of the American Medical Association.

Jewish and Christian theology has traditionally opposed any form of euthanasia or suicide, avowing that since God is the author of life and death, life is sacred. Therefore, a man rebels against God if he prematurely shortens his life, because he violates the Sixth Commandment, "Thou shalt not kill." Suffering was viewed not as an evil to be avoided at all costs but as a condition to be accepted. The Apostle Paul served as an example for early Christians. In 2 Corinthians, he prayed for physical healing, yet when it did not come, he accepted his weakness as a way to increase his dependence on God. This position was affirmed by Saint Augustine in his work *De Civitate Dei* (413-426; *The City of God*) when he condemned suicide as a "detestable and damnable wickedness" which was worse than murder because it left no room for repentance. These strong indictments from the Church against suicide and euthanasia were largely responsible for changing the Greco-Roman attitudes toward the value of human life. They were accepted as society's position until the advent of technologies that made it possible to extend life beyond what would have been the point of death a few years ago.

Although these issues have been debated among both physicians and philosophers for centuries, there is a heightened need for thoughtful discussion and resolution today. Clearly, the decisions surrounding the issue of euthanasia are very complicated. The choice is not simply between commitments to "sanctity of life" or "quality of life" viewpoints. No consensus has yet been reached across the spectrum of society, and instead variety of alternatives are supported by groups of individuals. A clear understanding of all positions in the debate is the best preparation for making personal decisions at the time of death.

—*Katherine B. Frederich, Ph.D.*
updated by Leslie V. Tischauser, Ph.D.

See also Aging, extended care for the; Critical care; Critical care, pediatric; Death and dying; Ethics; Hippocratic oath; Law and medicine; Pain management; Psychiatry; Psychiatry, geriatric; Suicide; Terminally ill, extended care for the.

FOR FURTHER INFORMATION:

Biomedical-Ethical Issues. Valley Forge, Pa.: United Ministries in Education, 1983. This book is a compilation of policy statements concerning the moral issues raised by developments in biomedical science. Judicial decisions, state statutes on living wills, and policy statements from religious and medical groups are included in the chapter entitled "Euthanasia and the Right to Refuse Treatment."

Gorovitz, Samuel. *Drawing the Line*. New York: Oxford University Press, 1991. This book reflects on the author's seven-week sabbatical in residence at Beth Israel Hospital. Gorovitz presents numerous insights drawn from conversations with patients and medical personnel.

Harron, Frank, John Burnside, and Tom Beauchamp. *Health and Human Values*. New Haven, Conn.: Yale University Press, 1983. Using a case-study approach, the authors consider the different types of euthanasia and report on policy statements from interested social groups.

Koop, C. Everett. *The Right to Live, the Right to Die*. Wheaton, Ill.: Tyndale House, 1980. The former surgeon general of the United States presents views on euthanasia from a physician's perspective.

Rachels, James. *The End of Life*. New York: Oxford University Press, 1986. The author presents several distinctions made between cases of euthanasia and the arguments for and against those distinctions.

Shannon, Thomas A., ed. *Bioethics*. New York: Paulist Press, 1976. A collection of writings on the ethical questions that surround the major biological problems of modern times. More than one hundred pages are devoted to issues surrounding death and dying.

Spring, Beth, and Ed Larson. *Euthanasia*. Portland: Multnomah Press, 1988. This book considers the spiritual, medical, and legal issues in terminal health care, citing numerous perspectives from the religious community. Contains two chapters detailing practical guidelines for writing living wills and durable powers of attorney.

Wennberg, Robert N. *Terminal Choices*. Grand Rapids, Mich.: Wm. B. Eerdmans, 1989. The author presents a helpful history of the euthanasia debate and also discusses possible moral distinctions between treatment refusal and treatment withdrawal.

EXERCISE PHYSIOLOGY

SPECIALTY

ANATOMY OR SYSTEM AFFECTED: Circulatory system, heart, joints, knees, lungs, muscles, musculoskeletal system, respiratory system, tendons

SPECIALTIES AND RELATED FIELDS: Cardiology, family practice, nutrition, physical therapy, preventive medicine, sports medicine

DEFINITION: The science that studies the effects on the body of various intensities and types of physical activity, including cellular metabolism, cardiovascular responses, respiratory responses, neural and hormonal adaptations, and muscular adaptations to exercise.

KEY TERMS:

adenosine triphosphate (ATP): a high-energy compound found in the cell which provides energy for all bodily functions *aerobic:* metabolism involving the breakdown of energy substrates using oxygen

anaerobic: metabolism involving the breakdown of energy substrates without using oxygen

atherosclerosis: hardening and thickening of the walls of the arteries caused by a buildup of fatty deposits

electrocardiogram (ECG): a graphic record of electrical currents of the heart

glycogen: the form that glucose takes when it is stored in the muscles and liver

heart rate: the number of times the heart contracts, or beats, per minute

maximal oxygen uptake: the maximum rate of oxygen consumption during exercise

metabolic equivalent (MET): a unit used to estimate the metabolic cost of physical activity; 1 MET is equal to 3.5 milliliters of oxygen consumed per kilogram of body weight per minute

SCIENCE AND PROFESSION

The primary focus of research in the field of exercise physiology is to gain a better understanding of the quantity and type of exercise needed for health maintenance and rehabilitation. A major goal of professionals in exercise physiology is to find ways to incorporate appropriate levels of physical activity into the lifestyles of all individuals.

Physiology is the science of physical and chemical factors and processes involved in the function of living organisms. The study of exercise physiology examines these factors and processes as they relate to physical exertion. The physical responses that occur are specific to the intensity, duration, and type of exercise performed.

Low or moderate exercise intensity relies on oxygen to release energy for work. This process is often referred to as aerobic exercise. In the muscles, carbohydrates and fats are broken down to produce adenosine triphosphate (ATP), the basic molecule used for energy. Aerobic exercise can be sustained for several minutes to several hours.

Higher-intensity exercise is predominantly fueled anaerobically (in the absence of oxygen) and can be sustained for up to two minutes only. Muscle glycogen is broken down without oxygen to produce ATP. Anaerobic metabolism is much less efficient at producing ATP than is aerobic metabolism.

During anaerobic metabolism, a by-product called lactic acid begins to accumulate in the blood as blood lactate. The point at which this accumulation begins is called the anaerobic threshold (AT), or the onset of blood lactate accumulation (OBLA). Blood lactate can cause muscle soreness and stiffness, but it also can be used as fuel during aerobic metabolism.

A third and less often used energy system is the creatine phosphate (ATP-CP) system. Utilizing the very limited supply of ATP that is stored in the muscles, phosphate molecules are exchanged between ATP and CP to provide energy. This system provides only enough fuel for a few seconds of maximum effort.

The type of muscle fiber recruited to perform a specific type of exercise is also dependent on exercise intensity. Skeletal muscle is composed of "slow-twitch" and two types of "fast-twitch" muscle fibers. Slow-twitch fibers are more suited to using oxygen than are fast-twitch fibers, and they are recruited primarily for aerobic exercise. One type of fast-twitch fiber also functions during aerobic activity. The second type of fast-twitch fiber serves to facilitate anaerobic, or high-intensity, exercise.

Exercise mode is also a factor in the physiological responses to exercise. Dynamic exercise (alternating muscular contraction and relaxation through a range of motion) using many large muscles requires more oxygen than does activity utilizing smaller and fewer muscles. The greater the oxygen requirement of the physical activity, the greater the cardiorespiratory benefits.

Many bodily adaptations occur over a training period of six to eight weeks, and other benefits are gradually manifested over several months. The positive adaptations include reduced resting and working heart rates. As the heart becomes stronger, there is a subsequent increase in stroke volume (the volume of blood the heart pumps with each beat), which allows the heart to beat less frequently while maintaining the same cardiac output (the volume of the blood pumped from the heart each minute). Another beneficial adaptation is increased metabolic efficiency. This is partially facilitated by an increase in the number of mitochondria (the organelles responsible for ATP production) in the muscle cells.

One of the most recognized representations of aerobic fitness is the maximum volume of oxygen $\dot{V}O_{2max}$ an individual can use during exercise. $\dot{V}O_{2max}$ is improved through habitual, relatively high-intensity aerobic activity. After three to six months of regular training, levels of high-density lipoproteins (HDLs) in the blood increase. HDL molecules remove cholesterol (a fatty substance) from the tissues to aid in protecting the heart from atherosclerosis.

Various internal and external factors influence the metabolic processes that take place during and after exercise. Internally, nutrition, degree of hydration, body composition, flexibility, sex, and age are some of the variables that play a role in the physiological responses. Other internal variables include medical conditions such as heart disease, diabetes, and hypertension (high blood pressure). Externally, environmental conditions such as temperature, humidity, and altitude alter how the exercising body functions.

Various modes of exercise testing and data collection are used to study the physiological responses of the body to exercise. Treadmills and cycle ergometers (instruments used to measure work and power output) are among the most common methods of evaluating maximum oxygen consumption. During these tests, special equipment and computers analyze expired air, heart rate is monitored with an electrocardiograph (ECG), and blood pressure is taken using a sphygmomanometer. Blood samples and muscle fiber samples can also be extracted to aid in identifying the fuel system and type of muscle fibers being used. Other data sometimes collected, such as skin temperatures and body core temperatures, can provide pertinent information.

Metabolic equivalent units, or METs, are often used to translate a person's capability into workloads on various pieces of exercise equipment or into everyday tasks. For every 3.5 milliliters of oxygen consumed per kilogram of body weight per minute, the subject is said to be performing at a workload of one MET. One MET is approximately equivalent to 1.5 kilocalories per minute, or the amount of energy expended per kilogram of body weight in one minute when a person is at rest.

Another factor greatly affecting the physical response to exercise is body composition. The three major structural components of the body are muscle, bone, and fat. Body composition can be evaluated using a combination of anthropometric measurements. These measurements include body weight, standard height, measurements of circumferences at various locations using a tape measure, measure-

ments of skeletal diameters using a sliding metric stick, and measurements of skinfold thicknesses using calipers.

Body fat can be estimated using several methods, the most accurate of which is based on a calculation of body density. This method is called hydrostatic weighing, which involves weighing the subject under water while taking into account the residual volume of air in the lungs. The principle underlying this measurement of body density is based on the fact that fat is less dense than water and will float, whereas bone and muscle, which are denser than water, will sink. One biochemical technique often used to determine levels of body fat is based on the relatively constant level of potassium 40 naturally existing in lean body mass. Another method utilizes ultrasound waves to measure the thickness of fat layers. X rays and computed tomography (CT) scanning can be used to provide images from which fat and bone can be measured. Bioelectrical impedance (BIA) is a method of estimating body composition based on the resistance imposed on a low voltage electrical current sent through the body. The most widely used and easily assessable method, however, involves measurement of skinfolds at various sites on the body using calipers. In all cases, mathematical formulas have been devised to interpret the

The Effects of Exercise on the Body

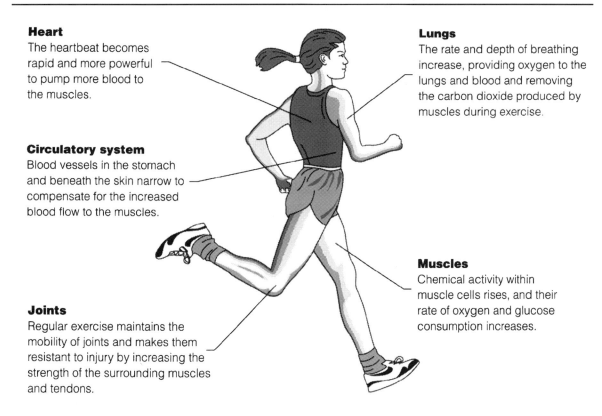

Heart
The heartbeat becomes rapid and more powerful to pump more blood to the muscles.

Circulatory system
Blood vessels in the stomach and beneath the skin narrow to compensate for the increased blood flow to the muscles.

Joints
Regular exercise maintains the mobility of joints and makes them resistant to injury by increasing the strength of the surrounding muscles and tendons.

Lungs
The rate and depth of breathing increase, providing oxygen to the lungs and blood and removing the carbon dioxide produced by muscles during exercise.

Muscles
Chemical activity within muscle cells rises, and their rate of oxygen and glucose consumption increases.

collected data and provide the best estimate of an individual's body composition.

Other tests have been developed to determine muscular strength, muscular endurance, and flexibility. Muscular strength is often measured by performance of one maximal effort produced by a selected muscle group. Muscular endurance of a muscle or muscle group is often demonstrated by the length of time or number of repetitions a particular, submaximal workload or skill can be performed.

Two major types of flexibility have been identified. One type consists of the flexibility through the range of motion of a muscle group or joint. This is called static flexibility. It can be measured using a metric stick or a protractor-type instrument called a goniometer. Dynamic flexibility is the other major identified type of flexibility. It is the torque of or resistance to movement. Methods to measure dynamic flexibility have not been developed.

Overlapping the science of exercise physiology are the studies of biomechanics or kinesiology (sciences dealing with human movement) and nutrition. Only through an understanding of efficient body mechanics and proper nutrition can the physiological responses of the body to exercise be identified correctly.

DIAGNOSTIC AND TREATMENT TECHNIQUES

Exercise prescription is the primary focus in the application of exercise physiology. General health maintenance, cardiac rehabilitation, and competitive athletics are three major areas of exercise prescription.

Before making recommendations for an exercise program, an exercise physiologist must evaluate the physical limitations of the exerciser. In a normal, health maintenance setting—often called a "wellness" program—a health-related questionnaire can reveal relevant information. Such a questionnaire should include questions about family medical history and the subject's history of heart trouble or chest pain, bone or joint problems, and high blood pressure. The presence of any of these problems suggests the need for a physician's consent prior to exercising. After the individual has been deemed eligible to participate, an assessment of the level of physical fitness should be performed. Determining or estimating $\dot{V}O_{2max}$, muscular strength, muscular endurance, flexibility, and body composition is usually included in this assessment. It is then possible to design a program best suited to the needs of the individual.

For the healthy adult participant, the American College of Sports Medicine (ACSM), a widely recognized authoritative body on exercise prescription, recommends three to five sessions of aerobic exercise weekly. Each session should include a five- to ten-minute warm-up period, twenty to sixty minutes of aerobic exercise at a predetermined exercise intensity, and a five- to ten-minute cooldown period.

In order to recommend an appropriate aerobic exercise intensity, the exercise physiologist must determine an individual's maximum heart rate. The best way to obtain this maximum heart rate is to administer a maximal exercise test. Such a test can be supervised by an exercise physiologist or an exercise test technician; it is advisable, especially for the older participant, that a cardiologist also be in attendance. An ECG is monitored for irregularities as the subject walks, runs, cycles, or performs some dynamic exercise to exhaustion or until the onset of irregular symptoms or discomfort.

Exercise prescription using heart rate as a measure can be achieved by various methods. A direct correlation exists between exercise intensity, in terms of oxygen consumption, and heart rate. From data collected during a maximal exercise test, a target heart rate range of 40 percent to 85 percent of functional capacity can be calculated. Another method used to determine an appropriate heart rate range is based on the difference between an individual's resting heart rate and maximum heart rate, called the heart rate reserve (HRR). Values representing 60 percent and 80 percent of the heart rate reserve are calculated and added to the resting heart rate, yielding the individual's target heart rate range. A third method involves calculating 70 percent and 85 percent of the maximum heart rate. Although this method is less accurate than the other two methods, it is the simplest way to estimate a target heart rate range.

Intensity of exercise can also be prescribed using METs. This method relies on the predetermined metabolic equivalents required to perform activities at various intensities. Activity levels reflecting 40 percent to 85 percent of functional capacity can be calculated.

The rating of perceived exertion (RPE) is another method of prescribing exercise intensity. Verbal responses by the participant describing how an exercise feels at various intensities are assigned to a numerical scale, which is then correlated to heart rate. Through practice, the participant can correlate heart rate with the RPE, reducing the necessity of frequent pulse monitoring in the healthy individual.

Adequate physical fitness can be defined as the ability to perform daily tasks with enough reserve for emergency situations. All aspects of health-related fitness direct attention toward this goal. Aerobic exercise often provides some conditioning for muscular endurance, but muscular strength and flexibility need to be addressed separately.

The ACSM recommends resistance training using the "overload principle," which involves placing habitual stress on a system, causing it to adapt and respond. For this training, it is suggested that eight to twelve repetitions of eight to ten strengthening exercises of the major muscle groups be performed a minimum of two days per week.

Flexibility of connective tissue and muscle tissue is essential to maximize physical performance and to limit musculoskeletal injuries. At least one stretching exercise for each major muscle group should be executed three to four times per week while the muscles are warm. Three methods of stretching that have been designed to improve flexibility are ballistic stretching, static stretching, and proprioceptive neuromuscular facilitation (PNF). Ballistic stretching incorporates a bouncing motion and is generally prescribed only in sports that replicate this type of movement. During a static stretch, the muscles and connective tissue are passively stretched to their maximum lengths. PNF involves a contract-relax sequence of the muscle.

In addition to exercise prescription for cardiorespiratory fitness, muscular fitness, and flexibility, it is appropriate for the exercise physiologist to make recommendations concerning body composition. Exercise is an effective tool in fat loss. Dietary caloric restriction without exercise results in a greater loss of muscle mass along with fat loss than if exercise is part of a weight loss program.

For persons with special health concerns, such as diabetes mellitus or high blood pressure, the exercise physiologist works with the participant's physician. The physician is responsible for prescribing necessary medications and often decides which modes of exercise are contraindicated (those that should be avoided).

A second application, cardiac rehabilitation, takes exercise prescription a step further. Participation of the heart patient is more individualized than in wellness programs. The condition of the circulatory system, pulmonary system, and joints are only a few of the special concerns. Secondary conditions such as obesity, diabetes, and hypertension must also be considered. The responsibilities of cardiac rehabilitation specialists include monitoring blood sugar in diabetic patients and blood pressure in all patients, especially those with hypertension. Many drugs affect heart rate or blood pressure, and most of these participants are taking more than one type of medication. Patients with heart damage caused by a heart attack may display atypical heart rhythms, which can be seen on an ECG monitor. Furthermore, the stage of recovery of the postsurgical patient is a major factor in recommending the type, frequency, intensity, and duration of exercise.

Patient education is also important. Lifestyle is usually the main factor in the development of heart disease. Cardiac patients often have never participated in a regular exercise program. Frequently, they are smokers, are overweight, and have poor eating habits. Helping them to identify and correct destructive health-related behaviors is the focus of education for the heart patient.

A third application of the study of exercise physiology involves dealing with the competitive athlete. In this case, findings from the most recent research are constantly applied to yield the best athletic performance possible. A delicate balance of aerobic training, anaerobic training, strength training, endurance training, and flexibility exercises are combined with the optimum percentage of body fat, proper nutrition, and adequate sleep. The program that is designed must enhance the athletic qualities that are most beneficial to the sport in which the athlete participates.

The competitive athlete usually pushes beyond the boundaries of general exercise prescription in terms of intensity, duration, and frequency of exercise performance. As a result, the athlete risks suffering more injuries than the individual who exercises for health benefits. If the athlete sustains an injury, the exercise physiologist may work in conjunction with an athletic trainer or sports physician to return the athlete to competition as soon as possible.

PERSPECTIVE AND PROSPECTS

The modern study of exercise physiology developed out of an interest in physical fitness. In the United States, and possibly much of the world, that interest was primarily driven by a desire to prepare soldiers for war adequately.

In the United States, the concern for development and maintenance of physical fitness was well established by the end of the twentieth century. As early as 1819, Stanford and Harvard universities offered professional physical education programs. At least one textbook on the physiology of exercise was published by that time.

Much of the pioneer work in this field, however, was done in Europe. Nobel Prize-winning European research on muscular exercise, oxygen utilization as it relates to the upper limits of physical performance, and production of lactic acid during glucose metabolism dates back to the 1920's.

In the early 1950's, poor performance by children in the United States on a minimal muscular fitness test helped lead to the formation of what is now known as the President's Council on Physical Fitness and Sport. Concurrently, a significant number of deaths of middle-aged American males were found to be caused by poor health habits associated with coronary artery disease. A need for more research in the areas of health and physical activity was recognized by the mid-1960's. The subsequent research was facilitated by the existence of fifty-eight exercise physiology research laboratories in colleges and universities throughout the country.

Organizations such as the American Physiological Society (APS), the American Alliance of Health, Physical Education, and Recreation (AAHPER), and the American College of Sports Medicine (ACSM) were established by the mid-1950's. In an effort to ensure that well-trained professionals were involved in cardiac rehabilitation programs, the ASCM developed a certification program in 1975. Certifications for fitness personnel were added later.

A better understanding of fundamental physiological mechanisms should stem from increasingly more sophisticated testing equipment, allowing practitioners to be more effective in measuring physical fitness and in prescribing exercise programs. Health maintenance has become a priority as the number of adults over the age of fifty continues to increase. Advances in medical techniques also increase the survival rate of victims of heart attacks, creating a need for more cardiac rehabilitation programs and practitioners. Health care professionals and the general population need to be made more aware of the benefits of exercise in the maintenance of good health and in the rehabilitation of individuals with medical problems.

—*Kathleen O'Boyle*

See also Biofeedback; Bones and the skeleton; Cardiac rehabilitation; Cardiology; Electrocardiography (ECG or EKG); Glycolysis; Heart; Kinesiology; Lungs; Metabolism; Muscle sprains, spasms, and disorders; Muscles; Nutrition; Orthopedics; Orthopedics, pediatric; Oxygen therapy; Physical rehabilitation; Physiology; Preventive medicine; Pulmonary medicine; Respiration; Sports medicine; Vascular system.

FOR FURTHER INFORMATION:

American College of Sports Medicine. *Guidelines for Exercise Testing and Prescription*. 4th ed. Philadelphia: Lea & Febiger, 1991. This manual provides guidelines for the professional working in preventive exercise programs or in cardiac rehabilitation. The recommendations are based on the most-up-to-date research available at the time of publication. Requirements for certification through the ACSM are also explained in detail.

_____. *Resource Manual for Guidelines for Exercise Testing and Prescription*. Philadelphia: Lea & Febiger, 1988. Based on the objective of providing safe and effective exercise programs for all individuals, this publication provides an excellent overview of many of the topics of concern to the exercise physiologist. Specific recommendations regarding stress testing and exercise prescription are included in the text.

Brooks, George A., and Thomas D. Fahey. *Fundamentals of Human Performance*. New York: Macmillan, 1987. This textbook was written for students of physical education, nursing, nutrition, and physical therapy who need a practical introduction to exercise physiology. The theoretical basis and practical application of physical activity are explained through a discussion of metabolic phenomena.

Costill, David L. *Inside Running: Basics of Sports Physiology*. Indianapolis: Benchmark, 1986. Provides a description of the body's responses to exercise and training in terms that can be understood by individuals who are unfamiliar with exercise physiology. Promotes a greater appreciation for the roles that heredity and nutrition play in athletic success. Written for the athlete and the athletic trainer.

McArdle, William D., Frank I. Katch, and Victor L. Katch. *Exercise Physiology: Energy, Nutrition, and Human Performance*. 4th ed. Baltimore: Williams & Wilkins, 1996. This textbook is designed for the serious student of exercise physiology. Provides relatively detailed explanations of various energy systems in the body.

Powers, Scott K., and Edward T. Howley. *Exercise Physiology: Theory and Application to Fitness and Performance*. Dubuque: Wm. C. Brown, 1990. The upper-level undergraduate or beginning graduate student will find detailed information concerning exercise physiology in this useful textbook. Designed for students who are serious about the study of exercise science.

Sharkey, Brian J. *Physiology of Fitness*. 3d ed. Champaign, Ill.: Human Kinetics Books, 1990. Provides an excellent learning opportunity for the junior college student. Offers a guide to the prescription of exercise for health, fitness, and performance, but takes things a step further by explaining the scientific basis for these guidelines.

EXTENDED CARE FOR THE AGING. *See* AGING, EXTENDED CARE FOR THE.

EXTENDED CARE FOR THE TERMINALLY ILL. *See* TERMINALLY ILL, EXTENDED CARE FOR THE.

EXTREMITIES. *See* FEET; FOOT DISORDERS; LOWER EXTREMITIES; UPPER EXTREMITIES.

EYE DISORDERS. *See* CATARACTS; EYES; GLAUCOMA; VISUAL DISORDERS.

EYE SURGERY

PROCEDURES

ANATOMY OR SYSTEM AFFECTED: Eyes

SPECIALTIES AND RELATED FIELDS: General surgery, ophthalmology

DEFINITION: The surgical treatment of diseases, injuries, or deformities of the eyes.

KEY TERMS:

cryosurgery: the destruction of tissue by the application of extreme cold

diathermy: the heating of body tissues because of the resistance to the passage of high-frequency electromagnetic radiation, electric current, or ultrasonic waves; also known as electrocoagulation

photocoagulation: the condensation of protein material by the controlled use of an intense beam of light (such as a xenon arc light or argon laser)

INDICATIONS AND PROCEDURES

In addition to cataract surgery, corneal transplantation, and radial keratotomy, ophthalmic (or eye) surgeries include pterygium removal, retinal detachment repair, and tear duct surgery. A pterygium is a yellow nodule of elastic tissue on the surface of the eye that most commonly occurs on the nasal side. It may extend from the conjunctiva onto the cornea. Pterygium formation is most common in the elderly and thought to be secondary to ultraviolet (UV) light ex-

posure and dry wind. Commonly, anti-inflammatory drugs such as weak ophthalmic steroids are effective. The lesion may interfere with vision, however, sometimes simply by limiting ocular motility. Most patients decide to have a pterygium removed because of cosmetic reasons. Since recurrence is common, prevention by wearing UV-blocking sunglasses is recommended. During pterygium removal, the surgeon will cut 0.5 millimeter beyond the attached edges of the pterygium. If the attached ends extend into the cornea, part of it will be removed as well.

Normally, an intact sensory retina remains in contact with the pigmented epithelium layer by suction. A retinal tear can be caused by extremely rapid eye movements or sudden rotation (as in trauma), usually in one eye only. These tears are the result of movement sufficient to generate a large inertial force. The result is vitreous fluid flow into the space between the retina and epithelium and the loss of retinal function. Some patients experience small detachments that may be self-limiting and may not require surgery unless they become progressive. With more severe tears, the condition usually progresses until the detachment is total. The patient may experience sudden visual change or loss. The most common procedures to correct retinal detachment are laser photocoagulation, cryotherapy, scleral buckle procedures, and diathermy. Since laser photocoagulation has several advantages, the other procedures are used less frequently. The goal is to form a scar, making the retina adhere to the pigmented epithelial layer and reestablishing a watertight seal in the intraretinal space. The adjacent cells and their function are destroyed, but fibrous connective (scar) tissue remains. With lasers, the resultant scar formation is instantaneous, and eye immobilization is not critical. The treatment is easier to gauge than other therapies, which result in much more widespread tissue destruction.

Tear duct surgery mainly serves to correct conditions leading to abnormalities in the tear (lacrimal) ducts and gland function. Infection or irritation of the lacrimal system is termed dacryocystitis. This condition may be attributable to narrowing or blockage of the lacrimal duct system, a dacryolith (stone), or a dacryoma (tumor). In most cases, lacrimal system problems result in dry, scratchy eyes. These patients are usually treated with ophthalmic lubricants. For cases in which infection or a foreign body (such as a dacryolith) are the cause, topical antibiotics are usually effective. In acute cases, drainage is enhanced by insertion of a tube into the nasolacrimal duct, which will control the swelling. Later, the infected area can be removed. In all cases of tear duct surgery, the goal is to reopen the lacrimal system to allow normal function of tear formation, eye lubrication, and tear removal and drainage.

USES AND COMPLICATIONS

The range of ophthalmic surgeries is vast. They are usually described by anatomical site: the eyelid, iris, conjunctiva, cornea, lens, retina, extraocular muscles, lacrimal system, and structures around the eye (orbit). The instruments used are similar to those used in any other surgery except that they are usually smaller in order to allow for great surgical precision and minute manipulations within the eye. Any sutures must be delicate yet strong. Technological advances are allowing increasing use of noninvasive (incisionless) surgical procedures using lasers.

The most common minor eye surgeries have varying success rates. For example, unless the area is aggressively excised, a pterygium tends to reform after surgery; recurrences are far more problematic and more difficult to remove. With proper care, 90 percent of retinal detachments can be repaired with only one operation. If the retina remains reattached for at least six months, it is unlikely that it will detach again. Despite this success rate, however, many patients will experience scotomas (holes in the visual field) after retinal detachment repair. Tear duct surgery is reserved for patients who fail to respond to antibiotic treatment or patients who experience chronic problems secondary to a stone. Surgery and postoperative antibiotics usually resolve the problem.

PERSPECTIVE AND PROSPECTS

Eye surgery in its crudest form has been in existence since ancient Babylon. Practitioners of the time treated cataracts by stabbing the eye with a sharp stick. This procedure would displace the cataract, allowing the patient to distinguish shapes that could not be recognized previously. This type of procedure was used until modern surgery made possible the removal of the entire cataract.

In the late 1970's, microscopic surgical technology advanced to the point that cloudy sections of the cataract could be removed. Reduction in instrument sizes meant smaller incisions and less tissue damage resulting from surgery. Artificial lens technology advanced to allow the surgeon to correct visual defects with little or no surgery. The advent of intraocular lens implantation with the removal of the diseased lens further improved patient outcomes. The future will see even smaller incisions, more laser surgery, and further enhancement of lens material to allow greater correction and less eye surgery.

—*Charles C. Marsh, Pharm.D.*

See also Blindness; Cataract surgery; Cataracts; Corneal transplantation; Eyes; Glaucoma; Laser use in surgery; Macular degeneration; Myopia; Ophthalmology; Radial keratotomy; Sense organs; Visual disorders.

FOR FURTHER INFORMATION:

Dorland, W. A. Newman. *Dorland's Illustrated Medical Dictionary.* 28th ed. Philadelphia: W. B. Saunders, 1994.

King, John Harry, and Joseph A. C. Wadsworth, eds. *An Atlas of Ophthalmic Surgery.* Philadelphia: J. B. Lippincott, 1970.

Vaughan, Daniel, Taylor Asbury, and Paul Riordan-Eva, eds. *General Ophthalmology.* 14th ed. Norwalk, Conn.: Appleton and Lange, 1995.

EYES

ANATOMY

ANATOMY OR SYSTEM AFFECTED: Nervous system

SPECIALTIES AND RELATED FIELDS: Ophthalmology, optometry

DEFINITION: The body structures that receive and transform information about objects into neural impulses that can be translated by the brain into visual images.

KEY TERMS:

accommodation: adjustments of the crystalline lens that are necessary for clear vision at various distances

cornea: the transparent structure forming the anterior part of the fibrous tunic of the eye; light must pass through this structure to reach the retina

crystalline lens: the transparent focusing mechanism of the eye; it is a biconvex structure situated between the posterior chamber and the vitreous body of the eye

diopter: a unit of power of a lens equal to the reciprocal of the focal length of the lens in meters

iris: the circular pigmented membrane behind the cornea, perforated by the pupil; the most anterior portion of the vascular tunic of the eye

photoreceptor: a light-responsive nerve cell or receptor which is located in the retina of the eye

pupil: the opening at the center of the iris through which light passes

retina: the innermost of the three tunics of the eyeball, which is situated around the vitreous body and is continuous posteriorly with the optic nerve; it contains the photoreceptors

sclera: the tough outer coat or fibrous tunic of the eyeball, which covers the posterior five-sixths of its surface and is continuous anteriorly with the cornea

visual acuity: clarity or clearness in vision

STRUCTURE AND FUNCTIONS

The eye captures pictures from the environment and transforms them into neural impulses that are processed by the brain into visual images. The retina, with its light-sensitive cells, acts as a camera to "put the picture on film," while neural processing in the brain "develops the film" and forms a visual image that is meaningful and informative for the individual.

The human eye originates during development, that is, while the individual is being formed as an embryo in the uterus. Eye formation begins during the end of the third week of development when outgrowths of brain neural tissue, called the optic vesicles, form at the sides of the forebrain region. The optic vesicle induces overlying embryonic tissue to thicken in one region, forming a primitive lens structure called the lens placode. The lens placode, in turn, induces the optic vesicles to form a cuplike structure, the optic cup, while the brain's connection of the vesicles narrows into a slender stalk that forms the optic nerve. The inner part of the optic cup forms the neural or sensory retina, with its photoreceptors, while the outer part of the optic cup develops into the layers of tissues, or tunics, that make up the wall of the eyeball. The lens placode further condenses and solidifies by forming lens fibers that become transparent. The function of the lens will eventually be to focus light onto the retina. The major structures of the eye—the retina, lens, and eyeball coats—are initially formed by the fifth month of fetal development. During the remainder of the prenatal period, eye structures continue to enlarge, mature, and form increasingly complex neural networks with the visual processing regions of the brain.

At birth, an infant's eyes are about two-thirds the size of adult eyes. Until after their first month of life, most newborns lack complete retinal development, especially in the area that is responsible for visual acuity. As a result, infants cannot focus their eyes properly and typically have a vacant stare during their first weeks of life. Most of the subsequent eye growth occurs rapidly during the remainder of the first year of life. From the second year of life until puberty, the rate of eye growth progressively slows. After puberty, eye growth is negligible.

The adult human eye weighs approximately 7.5 grams and measures approximately 24.5 millimeters in its anterior-to-posterior diameter. All movement of the eyeball, or globe, is accomplished by six voluntary muscles attached anteriorly by ligaments to the outer coat of the globe and posteriorly to a tendinous ring located behind the globe. One voluntary muscle elevates the upper lid.

Three concentric tunics form the globe itself. The outermost fibrous tunic consists of two portions. In the small, anterior portion, the tunic fibrils are arranged in a regular pattern, forming the transparent cornea. Posteriorly, the tunic fibrils are irregularly spaced, forming the opaque, white sclera. The innermost tunic, or nervous tunic, consists of two parts: the pars optica, or retina, containing photoreceptor cells, and the pars ceca lining the iris and ciliary body. Tucked between the outer and inner tunics lies the vascular tunic consisting of the pigmented iris, which gives the eye its distinctive color; the ciliary body, which forms the aqueous humor to provide nourishment for the anterior structures of the globe; and the highly vascular choroid, which provides nourishment for the retina and also acts as a cooling system by regulating blood flow to the chemically active retina. In the center of the circular, pigmented iris lies the pupil, which is a small opening into the posterior parts of the eyeball.

The cavity that contains the globe, circumscribed by the concentric tunics, is filled with a clear, jellylike substance called the vitreous body. This substance is anteriorly bounded in the vitreous cavity by the transparent crystalline lens that lies just posterior to the pupil. The crystalline lens is elastic in structure, allowing for variations in thickness that change the focusing power of the eye.

The eye can refract, or bend, light rays because of the

curved surfaces of two transparent structures, the cornea and the crystalline lens, through which light rays must pass to reach the retina. Any curved surface, or lens, will refract light rays to a greater or lesser degree depending on the steepness or flatness of the surface curve. The steeper the curve, the greater the refracting power. If a curved surface refracts light rays to an intersection point one meter away from the refracting lens, this lens is defined as having 1 diopter of power. The human eye has approximately 59 diopters of power in its constituent parts, including the cornea and crystalline lens.

Light rays emitted from a distant point of light enter the eye in a basically parallel pattern and are bent to intersect perfectly at the retina, forming an image of the distant point of light. If the point of light is near the eye, the rays that are emitted are divergent in pattern. These divergent rays must also be refracted to meet at a point on the retina, but these rays require more bending—hence, a steeper curved surface is needed. By a process called accommodation, the human eye automatically adjusts the thickness of the crystalline lens, forming a steeper curve on its surface and thereby creating a perfect image on the retina. Variations from the normal in either the length of an eyeball or the

curves of the cornea and crystalline lens will result in a refractive error or blurred image on the retina.

The major task of the eye is to focus environmental light rays on the photoreceptor cell, the rods and cones of the retina. These photoreceptors absorb the light energy, transforming it into electrical signals that are carried to the visual center of the brain. Cones are specialized for color or daylight vision and have greater visual discrimination or acuity than the rods, which are specialized for black-and-white or nighttime vision.

The fovea is a pin-sized depression in the center of the retina that contains only cone cells in high concentrations. This makes the fovea the point of the most distinct vision, or greatest visual acuity. When the eye focuses on an object, the object's image falls on the retina in the area of the fovea. Immediately surrounding the fovea is a larger area called the macula lutea that contains a relatively high concentration of cones. Macula lutea acuity, while not as great as in the fovea, is much greater than in the retina's periphery, which contains fewer cones. The concentration of cones is greatest in the fovea and declines toward the periphery of the retina. Conversely, the concentration of the rods is greater at the more peripheral areas of the retina than in

The Anatomy of the Human Eye

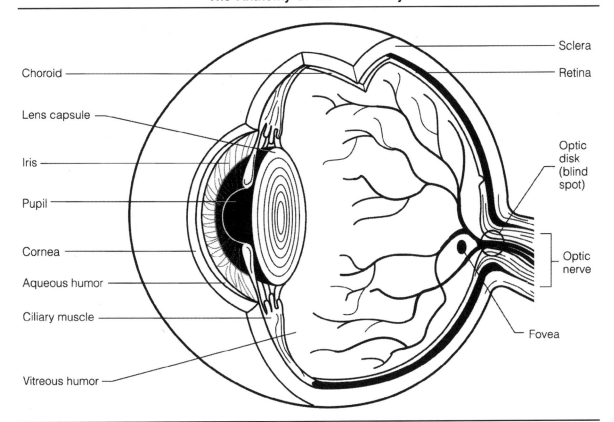

the macula luteal area. The retina of each eye contains about 100 million rod cells and about 300 million cone cells.

The optic nerve carries impulses from the photoreceptors to the brain. This nerve exits the retina in a central location called the blind spot. No image can be detected in this area because it contains neither rods nor cones. Normally, an individual is not aware of the retinal blind spot because the brain's neural processing compensates for the missing information when some portion of a peripheral image falls across this part of the retina.

On a cellular level, rod and cone photoreceptors consist of three parts: an outer segment that detects the light stimulus, an inner segment that provides the metabolic energy for the cell, and a synaptic terminal that transmits the visual signal to the next nerve cell in the visual pathway leading to the brain. The outer segment is rod-shaped in the rods and cone-shaped in the cones (hence their names). This segment is made of a stack of flattened membranes containing photopigment molecules that undergo chemical changes when activated by light.

The rod photopigment, called rhodopsin, cannot discriminate between various colors of light. Thus rods provide vision only in shades of grey by detecting different intensities of light. Rhodopsin is a purple pigment (a combination of blue and red colors), and it transmits light in the blue and red regions of the visual spectrum while absorbing energy from the green region of the spectrum. The light that is absorbed best by a photopigment is called its absorption maximum. Thus at night, when rods are used for vision, a green car is seen far more easily than a red car, because red light is poorly absorbed by rhodopsin. Only absorbed light produces the photochemical reaction that results in vision.

When rhodopsin absorbs light, the photopigment dissociates or separates into two parts: retinene, which is derived from vitamin A, and opsin, a protein. This separation of retinene from opsin, called the bleaching reaction, causes the production of nerve impulses in the photoreceptors. In the presence of bright light, practically all the rhodopsin undergoes the bleaching reaction and the person is in a light-adapted state. When a light-adapted person initially enters a darkened room, vision is poor since the light sensitivity of the rod photoreceptors is very low. After some time in the dark, however, a gradual increase in light sensitivity, called dark adaptation, occurs as increased amounts of retinene and opsin are recombined by the rods to form rhodopsin. The increased level of rhodopsin occurs after a few minutes in the dark and reaches a maximum sensitivity in about twenty minutes.

Each kind of cone—red, green, and blue—is distinguished by its unique photopigment, which responds to a particular wavelength or color of light. Combinations of cone colors provide the basis for color vision. While each type of cone is most sensitive to the particular wavelength of light indicated by its color—red, green, or blue—cones can respond to other colors with varying degrees. One's perception of color rests on the differential response of each cone type to a particular wavelength of light. The extent that each cone type is activated is coded and sent in separate parallel pathways to the brain. A color vision center in the brain combines and processes these parallel inputs to create the perception of color. Color is thus a concept in the mind of the viewer.

The intricacies of the human visual system require various methods to assess eye structure and function. Visual acuity is a measure of central cone function. Clinically, the most common method for testing visual acuity is by the use of a Snellen chart, consisting of a white background with black letters. All symbols on the chart create, or subtend, a visual angle at the approximate center of the eye. The smaller the symbol, the smaller the angle and the more difficult cone recognition becomes. At the standard distance of twenty feet, the smallest letters on the Snellen chart subtend an angle of five minutes of arc at the eye's center. The larger letters on the chart are calibrated such that each consecutively larger letter subtends a multiple unit of five minutes of arc. If the eye can detect the smallest letters on the chart, the patient is said to have normal (20/20) vision. The numerator of the clinical fraction designates the test distance of twenty feet. The denominator varies with the patient's visual function, identifying the distance at which the smallest letter recognized by the patient subtends an angle of five minutes of arc. For example, if the smallest letter recognized is fifty minutes of arc in size, the fraction used to record this visual acuity is 20/200 because the letter with fifty minutes of arc is ten times bigger than the smallest letters on the chart. Therefore, the distance needed for this letter to create five minutes of arc at the eye is ten times further than the normal twenty feet. In this example, the patient is said to have a refractive error.

DISORDERS AND DISEASES

Commonly existing refractive errors are astigmatism, myopia, hyperopia, and presbyopia. Presbyopia is an anomaly that occurs with aging when the crystalline lens loses its ability to accommodate. Causes include thickening of the lens and changes in the attachment fibers that anchor the lens. Because of these alterations, the lens is not able to change its shape and the eye remains focused at a specific distance. To compensate for this problem, bifocal spectacles are normally prescribed, with the upper region of the lens focused for distant vision and the lower lens focused for near vision. Hyperopia, also called farsightedness, results when an eyeball is too short. Because light rays are not bent sufficiently by the lens system, the image is focused not on the retina but behind the retina. To compensate for this problem, spectacles with convex lenses are prescribed, which bring the focus point back on the retina. Conversely, myopia, or nearsightedness, results from an abnormally long eyeball. In this case, the lens system focuses in front of the retina. This abnormal vision can be corrected by spectacles with a concave lens. Astigmatism results from a refractive error of the lens system usually caused by an irregular shape in the cornea or less frequently by an irregular shape in the lens. The consequence of this anomaly is that some light rays are focused in front of the retina and some behind the retina, creating a blurred image. To correct the focusing error, a special irregular spectacle must be made to correct the abnormal irregularity of the eye's lens system.

An examiner can assess the amount of refractive error based on a patient's verbal choice as to which of a given series of lenses sharpens the retinal image of the letters on the Snellen chart. Refractive error can also be determined when a patient is not capable of response. A retinoscope is often used to shine a light through the pupil onto the retina. An image of the light is reflected back out to the examiner who, in turn, can assess refractive error by the movement and shape of the image.

Visual field testing is a measure of the integrity of the neural pathways to the vision center in the brain. To test visual fields clinically, the patient focuses on a central target. While continuing to focus centrally, test targets are serially brought into the patient's peripheral vision, or visual field. The smaller and dimmer the test target, the more sensitive the test. The simplest visual field test technique is by confrontation. The patient and examiner sit facing each other one meter apart. If both patient and examiner cover their right eyes, the patient's left visual field is being tested. Since the patient's left visual field is congruent to the examiner's left visual field, the examiner can detect visual field defects when the patient is not responsive to a test target brought into view from the side. Lesions to some portion of the visual pathway to the brain will result in a scotoma, or blind area, in the corresponding visual field.

A biomicroscope, or slitlamp microscope, is commonly used to assess external eye structures, including the eyelids, lashes, conjunctiva, cornea, sclera, and one internal structure, the crystalline lens. The white part of the eye, or sclera, is covered with a thin, transparent covering called the conjunctiva. Infections and tumors often invade this external structure. Though the normally transparent crystalline lens is essentially free of infections and tumors, it can become cloudy or opaque and develop a cataract. Causes for cataract formation are multiple, the most common being the aging process; less frequently, trauma to the lens or a secondary symptom of systemic disease can result in cataracts. When the cataract is so dense that it obstructs vision, the crystalline lens is surgically removed and replaced with an artificial, plastic lens.

To view internal eye structures, the pupil is dilated to allow more light to be introduced into the interior and posterior regions of the eyeball. Two commonly used instruments are the handheld ophthalmoscope and the head-mounted indirect ophthalmoscope. Diseases of the retina include retinal tears, detachments, artery or vein occlusions, degenerations, and retinopathies secondary to systemic disease.

Glaucoma is an eye disease characterized by raised pressure inside the eye. Normal eye pressure is stabilized by the balance between the production and removal of the aqueous humor, the solution that bathes the internal, anterior structures of the eye. Abnormal pressures are often associated with defects in the visual, or optic, nerve and in the visual field. Approximately 300 people per 100,000 are affected by glaucoma. Clinically, intraocular pressure is assessed by numerous methods in a process called tonometry.

Abnormalities of the eye muscles constitute a significant portion of visual problems. Binocular vision and good depth perception are present when both eyes are aligned properly toward an object. A weakness in any of the six rotatory eye muscles will result in a tendency for that eye to deviate away from the object, resulting in an obvious or latent eye turn called strabismus. Associated signs are eye fatigue, abnormal head postures, and double vision. To alleviate objectionable double vision, a patient often suppresses the retinal image at the brain level, resulting in functional amblyopia (often called lazy eye), in which visual acuity is deficient.

Color blindness, a trait that occurs more frequently in men than in women, is caused by a hereditary lack of one or more types of cones. For example, if the green-sensitive cones are not functioning, the colors in the visual spectral range from green to red can stimulate only red-sensitive cones. This person can perceive only one color in this range, since the ratio of stimulation of the green-red cones is constant for the colors in this range. Thus this individual is considered to be green-red color-blind and will have difficulty distinguishing green from red.

PERSPECTIVE AND PROSPECTS

Early physicians recognized the importance of good eyesight, but because of limited understanding they had minimal means to treat major eye disorders. During the Middle Ages, surgeons performed eye operations, including ones for cataracts in which the lens was pushed down and out of the way with a needle inserted into the eyeball. In the 1700's, this operation was improved when cataract lenses were extracted from the eye. In the early 1600's, Johannes Kepler described how light was focused by the lens of the eye on the retina, thus providing insight into why spectacles are valuable in cases of poor eyesight. In 1801, Thomas Young published a foundational text entitled *On the Mechanics of the Eye*. Hermann von Helmholtz in the 1800's invented the first ophthalmoscope, which allowed inspection of the interior structures of the eye. Young and Helmholtz also developed theories to explain the phenomenon of color vision. From the invention of the ophthalmoscope, the range of clinical observation was extended to the inside of the eyeball, allowing the diagnosis of eye disorders. The modern understanding of eyesight and vision is increasing with contributions from ongoing research.

Ophthalmology is the study of the structure, function, and diseases of the eye. An ophthalmologist is a physician who specializes in the diagnosis and treatment of eye disorders and diseases with surgery, drugs, and corrective lenses. An optometrist is a specialist with a doctorate in optometry who is trained to examine and test the eyes and treats defects in vision by prescribing corrective lenses. An optician is a technician who fits, adjusts, and dispenses corrective lenses that are based on the prescription of an ophthalmologist or optometrist.

Vision care personnel are vital to industry, public health, recreation, highway safety, education, and the community. Since 85 percent of learning is visual-based, good vision is extremely important in education, work, and play. Good vision enhances the production and morale of workers, and athletic performance is improved when vision problems are corrected. Vision care specialists work to promote the prevention of eye injuries and diseases while supporting practices that enhance good health and vision. Vision therapy may be used to correct many disorders of the eye such as amblyopia, reduced visual perception, reading disorders, poor eye coordination, and reduced visual acuity.

—Elva B. Miller, O.D., and Roman J. Miller, Ph.D.

See also Albinism; Astigmatism; Blindness; Cataract surgery; Cataracts; Chlamydia; Color blindness; Conjunctivitis; Corneal transplantation; Diabetes mellitus; Dyslexia; Eye surgery; Face lift and blepharoplasty; Glaucoma; Gonorrhea; Jaundice; Laser use in surgery; Macular degeneration; Microscopy, slitlamp; Myopia; Ophthalmology; Optometry; Pigmentation; Radial keratotomy; Sense organs; Systems and organs; Transplantation; Visual disorders.

For Further Information:

Guyton, Arthur C. *Human Physiology and Mechanisms of Disease.* 6th ed. Philadelphia: W. B. Saunders, 1997. Guyton is a nationally recognized authority on medical physiology, having written and edited numerous college-level and medical school textbooks on the subject. His writing style is understandable to the nonmedical specialist and student. This college-level text contains two chapters on the eye: The first deals with the optics of vision and the function of the retina; the second emphasizes the neurophysiology of vision. Highly recommended for its accuracy and readability.

Moore, Keith L. *Before We Are Born.* 3d ed. Philadelphia: W. B. Saunders, 1989. This popularized volume on basic human embryology and development contains a well-written chapter that details the development of the eye. A major strength of this work are the numerous, clearly labeled diagrams that illustrate developmental processes and formations.

Tortora, Gerard J., and Sandra Reynolds Grabowski. *Principles of Anatomy and Physiology.* 8th ed. New York: HarperCollins College, 1996. This popular college-level undergraduate anatomy and physiology text contains a well-written chapter on the special senses, emphasizing eyesight and vision. A variety of tables, diagrams, pictures, and charts complement the text, enabling the reader to visualize clearly the various parts of the eye and their functions.

Vaughan, Daniel, Taylor Asbury, and Paul Riordan-Eva, eds. *General Ophthalmology.* 14th ed. Norwalk, Conn.: Appleton and Lange, 1995. This well-illustrated textbook is an excellent reference for the serious student who desires more in-depth information on any aspect of the eye or its diseases. While the information is technical and detailed, it is written in a very readable style and format.

Zeki, Semir. "The Visual Image in Mind and Brain." *Scientific American* 267, no. 3 (September, 1992): 68-76. This excellent review article summarizes the role of the brain in processing the neural information that comes from the eyes. By analyzing retinal images, the brain develops visual images that are recognizable to the individual. Describes the types of blindness that occur as a consequence of malformations in various parts of the brain's visual processing areas even though the various parts of the eye are functioning normally.

FACE LIFT AND BLEPHAROPLASTY

PROCEDURE

ANATOMY OR SYSTEM AFFECTED: Eyes, skin

SPECIALTIES AND RELATED FIELDS: General surgery; plastic, cosmetic, and reconstructive surgery

DEFINITION: Techniques used to remove unwanted wrinkles and other indicators of aging from the face.

INDICATIONS AND PROCEDURES

Aging may create serious problems among individuals for whom success in their occupations depends on appearance. Premature wrinkling of skin on the face and eyelids or premature looseness of these tissues can create an insurmountable psychological barrier. In these situations, cosmetic surgery such as face lift (rhytidectomy) and/or blepharoplasty (the removal of excess tissue around the eyelids) is indicated.

Fine wrinkles and lines in skin are best removed by chemical peeling or dermabrasion. In chemical peeling, a mildly irritating solution is applied to the areas of concern. The mixture also contains a bonding agent, similar to adhesive. When this becomes firm, it is removed. The upper layers of skin are simultaneously peeled away, removing fine lines and grooves. The process of dermabrasion is similar in concept to sandblasting: A stream of air containing tiny particles of plastic is directed toward the skin to be treated. The particles remove cells from the surface of the skin. In the process, fine wrinkles and grooves are erased. In time, these lines and wrinkles will return. Both treatments can be repeated a few times without harm. Surgical remedies may ultimately be required.

Surgical face lifting involves making an incision at the hairline and extending it downward in front of the ear toward the angle of the jaw; the length of the incision is dependent on the amount of skin sagging that is present.

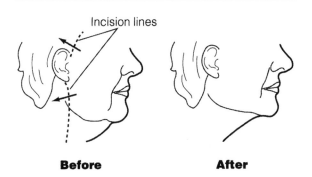

Before   **After**

A "face lift" is the term used for the excision and pulling upward of sagging skin on the face. This cosmetic procedure can smooth wrinkles and provide a more attractive profile, but there are drawbacks: The patient's appearance may be changed too dramatically, and the procedure must be repeated periodically to maintain the desired results.

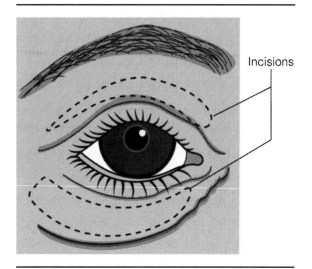

Incisions

Blepharoplasty is the removal of excess, baggy skin around the eyes.

The skin is gently separated from the underlying fascia and is pulled back and tightened until the desired degree of wrinkle elimination is achieved. Excess skin at the posterior (back) margins is removed. The edges are carefully brought together and secured with fine sutures or adhesive closures. The patient returns to the plastic surgeon in seven to ten days for follow-up evaluation.

Blepharoplasty refers to the surgical alteration of the eyelids. The surgery is similar to that described for a total face lift. An incision is made along the lower margin of the eyebrow. Skin is separated from the fascia. Sometimes, small amounts of fat are also removed. The skin of the upper eyelid is tightened. After excess tissue is removed, the free edges are attached with fine sutures. Cosmetic alteration of the lower eyelid can also be accomplished surgically. The incision is made along a natural crease in the skin just below the lower eyelid. The skin above the incision is separated from its underlying fascia. Some fat may be removed. Typically, excess skin is removed before the edges are reattached, again using very fine sutures. The patient returns to the plastic surgeon in approximately one week for removal of the sutures.

USES AND COMPLICATIONS

A face lift is a form of cosmetic surgery and is usually undertaken for aesthetic reasons. Short-term problems include bruising and swelling. Possible long-term complications include infection, scarring, and insufficient removal of unwanted wrinkles. Proper techniques can reduce the first two problems. Realistic expectations can minimize disappointment.

PERSPECTIVE AND PROSPECTS

At birth, human skin contains relatively large amounts of a molecule called collagen. Collagen provides strength to the skin; this is technically called turgor. The function of collagen is similar to the fibers in fiberglass or steel reinforcement in concrete: strength. Living on Earth, people are constantly subjected to the effects of gravity and ultraviolet radiation, which over time cause slight damage to the collagen in skin. The turgor is slowly lost. Without sufficient collagen, the skin starts to sag under the influence of gravity. Excessive exposure to the sun accelerates this process. The use of tanning beds in salons can increase the amount of harmful ultraviolet radiation, which also accelerates the aging process. With sufficient time and exposure, the typical appearance of skin in old age is seen.

There is no way to stop the human body from aging; accepting this inevitable reality can reduce both stress and anxiety. Cosmetic surgical procedures such as blepharoplasty and face lifts are temporary and only enable an individual to maintain an approximation of youthfulness. Over time, the skin will continue to change, necessitating repeat procedures. Each time the procedure is repeated, the result is diminished in comparison to an earlier procedure. Cosmetic surgery can thus only retard the appearance of aging rather than re-creating youth.

—*L. Fleming Fallon, Jr., M.D., M.P.H.*

See also Aging; Eye surgery; Plastic, cosmetic, and reconstructive surgery; Skin; Skin disorders.

FACIAL PALSY. *See* BELL'S PALSY.

FACTITIOUS DISORDERS
DISEASE/DISORDER

ANATOMY OR SYSTEM AFFECTED: Psychic-emotional system, most bodily systems

SPECIALTIES AND RELATED FIELDS: Family practice, internal medicine, psychiatry, psychology

DEFINITION: Psychophysiological disorders in which individuals intentionally produce their symptoms in order to play the role of patient.

CAUSES AND SYMPTOMS

Although factitious disorders cover a wide array of physical symptoms and are believed to be closely related to a subset of psychophysiological disorders (somatoform disorders), they are unique in all of medicine for two reasons. The first distinguishing factor is that whatever the physical disease for which treatment is sought and regardless of how serious, the patients who seek its treatment have deliberately and intentionally produced the condition. They may have done so in one of three ways, or in any combination of these three ways. First, patients fabricate, invent, lie about, and make up symptoms that they do not have; for example, they claim to have fever and night sweats or severe back pain that they actually do not have. Second, patients have the actual symptoms that they describe, but they intentionally caused them; for example, they might inject human saliva into their own skin to pro-

duce an abscess or ingest a known allergic food to cause the predictable reaction. Third, someone with a known condition such as pancreatitis has a pain episode but exaggerates its severity, or someone else with a history of migraines claims his or her headache to be yet another migraine when it is not.

The second element that makes these disorders unique (and at the same time both fascinating to study and frustrating to treat) is that the sole motivation for causing or claiming the symptoms is for these patients to become and remain patients, to assume the sick role wherein little can be expected from them. These patients are not malingerers, individuals who consciously use actual or feigned symptoms for some other gain (such as claiming a fever so one does not have to go to work or school, or insisting that one's post-traumatic stress is worse than it is to enhance the judgment in a lawsuit). In fact, it is the absence of any discernible external benefit that makes these disorders so intriguing.

Technically, psychiatrists and psychologists understand factitious disorders as having three subtypes. In the first, patients claim to have predominantly psychological symptoms such as memory loss, depression, contemplation of suicide, the hearing of voices, or false memory of childhood molestation. Characteristically, the symptoms worsen whenever the patients know themselves to be under observation. In the second, patients have predominantly physical symptoms that at least superficially suggest some general medical condition. In a more extreme form called Münchausen's syndrome, individuals will have spent much of their lives getting admitted to medical facilities and, once there, remaining as long as possible. While common complaints include vomiting, dizziness, blacking out, generalized rashes, and bleeding, the symptoms can involve any organ and seem limited only to the individuals' medical knowledge and experience with the medical system. The third subtype combines both psychological and physical complaints in such a way that neither predominates.

Regardless of subtype, factitious disorders are difficult to diagnose. Usually, the diagnosis is considered when the course of treating either a medical or a mental illness becomes atypical and protracted. Often, the person with a factitious disorder will present in a way which seems odd to the experienced clinician. The person may have an unusually extensive history of traveling, much familiarity with medical procedures and terminology, a complex medical and surgical history, few visitors during the hospitalization, behavioral disruptions and disturbances while hospitalized, exacerbation of symptoms while under observation, and/or fluctuating illness with new symptoms and complications arising as the workup proceeds. When present, these traits along with others make suspicion of factitious disorders reasonable.

No one knows how many people suffer with factitious

disorders, but the condition is generally regarded as uncommon. It is certainly rarely reported, but this in part may be attributable to the difficulties in determining the diagnosis. While brief episodes of the condition occur, most people who claim a factitious disorder have it chronically, and they usually move on to another physician or facility when they are confronted with the true nature of their illness. It is therefore likely that some individuals are reported more than once by different hospitals and providers.

There is little certainty about what causes factitious disorders. This is true in large measure because those who know the most about the subject—patients with the disorder—are notoriously unreliable in providing information about their psychological state and often seem only dimly aware of what they are doing to themselves. It may be that they are generally incapable of putting their feelings into words. They are unaware of having inner feelings and may not know, for example, that they are sad or angry. It is possible that they experience emotions more physically, behaviorally, and concretely than do most others.

Another view suggests that people learn to distinguish their primitive emotional states through the responsivity of their primary caretaker. A normal, healthy, average mother responds appropriately to her infant's differing affective states, thereby helping the infant, as he or she develops, to distinguish, define, and eventually name what he or she is feeling. When a primary caretaker is, for any of several reasons, incapable of responding in consistently appropriate ways, the infant's emotional awareness remains undifferentiated and the child experiences confusion and emotional chaos.

It is possible, too, that factitious disorder patients are motivated to assume what sociology defines as a sick role wherein people are required to acknowledge that they are ill and are required to relinquish adult responsibilities as they place themselves in the hands of designated caretakers.

TREATMENT AND THERAPY

Internists, family practitioners, and surgeons are the specialists most likely to encounter patients with factitious disorder, although psychiatrists and psychologists are often consulted in the management of these patients. These patients pose a special challenge because in a real sense they do not wish to become well even as they present themselves for treatment. They are not ill in the usual sense, and their indirect communication and manipulation often make them frustrating to treat using standard goals and expectations.

Sometimes mental and medical specialists' joint, supportive confrontation of these patients results in a disappearance of the troubling and troublesome behavior. During these confrontations, the health professionals are acknowledging that such extreme behavior evidences extreme distress in these patients, and as such is its own reason for psychotherapeutic intervention. These patients are not psychologically minded, however; they also have trouble form-

ing relationships that foster genuine self-disclosure, and they rarely accept the recommendation for psychotherapeutic treatment. Because they believe that their problems are physical, not psychological, they often become irate at the suggestion that their problems are not what they believe them to be. —*Paul Moglia, Ph.D.*

See also Hypochondriasis; Psychiatric disorders; Psychiatry; Psychiatry, child and adolescent; Psychiatry, geriatric; Psychoanalysis; Psychosomatic disorders.

FOR FURTHER INFORMATION:

American Psychiatric Association. *Diagnostic and Statistical Manual of Mental Disorders.* 4th ed. Washington, D.C.: Author, 1994.

Feldman, Marc D., and Charles V. Ford. *Patient or Pretender?: Inside the Strange World of Factitious Disorders.* New York: John Wiley & Sons, 1994.

Ford, Charles V. *The Somatizing Disorders: Illness as a Way of Life.* New York: Elsevier Biomedical, 1983.

Kenyon, F. E. "Hypochondriacal States." *The British Journal of Psychiatry* 129 (July, 1976): 1-14.

Viederman, M. "Somatoform and Factitious Disorders." In *The Personality Disorders and Neuroses*, edited by Arnold M. Cooper, Allen J. Frances, and Michael H. Sacks. New York: Basic Books, 1986.

FAINTING. *See* DIZZINESS AND FAINTING.

FAMILY PRACTICE
SPECIALTY

ANATOMY OR SYSTEM AFFECTED: All

SPECIALTIES AND RELATED FIELDS: Geriatrics and gerontology, internal medicine, obstetrics, osteopathic medicine, pediatrics, preventive medicine, psychiatry, psychology

DEFINITION: The specialty concerned with the primary health maintenance and medical care of an undifferentiated patient population, in the context of family and community.

KEY TERMS:

ambulatory care: health care provided outside the hospital, usually in a clinic or office and sometimes in the patient's home

biopsychosocial model: a model that examines the effects of illness on all spheres in which the patient functions—the biological sphere, the psychological sphere, and the social sphere

general practice: a primary care field with care provided by physicians who usually have completed less than three years of residency training; the organization from which family practice evolved

generalism: a medical and political movement concerned with primary care, often associated with the medical specialties of family practice, general internal medicine, general pediatrics, and sometimes obstetrics and gynecology

health maintenance: the practice of anticipating, finding, preventing, and/or dealing with potential or established medical problems at the earliest possible stage to minimize adverse effects on the patient

internship: a synonym for the first year of residency training

patient advocacy: the representation of the patient's interest in medical diagnosis and treatment decisions, in which the physician acts as an information source and counselor for the patient

primary care: first-line or entry-level care; the health care that most people receive for most illnesses

residency training: medical training provided in a specialty after graduation from medical school; similar to an apprenticeship and designed to mimic real-life practice as closely as possible

specialist: any physician who practices in a specialty other than the generalist areas of family practice, general internal medicine, general pediatrics, and obstetrics and gynecology

undifferentiated patient population: patients seen by family physicians regardless of age, sex, or type of problem

SCIENCE AND PROFESSION

Family practice is the direct descendant of general practice. For many years, most physicians were general practitioners. In the mid- to late twentieth century, however, the explosion of medical knowledge led to the specialization of medicine. For example, increased knowledge of the function and diseases of the heart seemed to demand creation of the specialty of cardiology. The model of the country doctor or jack-of-all-trades physician taking care of a wide range of medical problems seemed doomed to sink in the sea of subspecialization in medicine. The general practitioner, the venerable physician who hung out his or her shingle after medical school and one or more years of internship or residency training, appeared to be headed for extinction. Indeed, in their then-existent forms, the general practitioner and general practice would not have survived. Several forces came into play which did result in the passing of general practice but which also changed general practice into family practice.

The primary force pushing for general practice to survive and improve was the desire of the general public to retain the family doctor. The services that these physicians rendered and the relationships developed between physician and patients were held in high esteem. Through such voices as the American Medical Association's (AMA's) appointed Citizen Commission on Graduate Medical Education, the public requested the rescue of the family doctor.

Other major players in the movement to revive and reshape general practice included the AMA itself and the American Academy of General Practice. On February 8, 1969, approval was granted for the creation of family practice as medicine's twentieth official specialty. The American Academy of General Practice became the American Acad-

emy of Family Physicians (AAFP) and a certifying board, the American Board of Family Practice (ABFP), was established. After these steps were completed, three-year training programs (residencies) in family practice were established in medical universities and larger community hospitals to provide the necessary training for family physicians.

Family physicians are trained to provide comprehensive ongoing medical care and health maintenance for their patients. Those people who choose to become family physicians tend to value relationships over technology and service over high financial rewards. Many family physicians find themselves providing service to underserved populations and in mission work both inside and outside the United States. Family physicians often become advocates, providing counseling and advice to patients who are trying to sort out medical treatment options. They generally enjoy close relationships with their patients, who often hold them in high esteem.

Following graduation from medical school, students interested in a career in family practice begin a three-year residency in the specialty. During the residency, these physicians train in actual practice settings under the supervision of faculty physicians. Family practice residency training consists of three years of rotations with other medical specialties, such as internal medicine, pediatrics, surgery, and psychiatry. The unifying thread in family practice residency training is the continuity clinic. Throughout their training, the residents see their own patients several days a week under the supervision of family practice faculty physicians. Every effort is made to make this training as close as possible to experiences in the real world. Family practice residents will deliver their patients' babies, hospitalize their patients, and deal with the emotional issues of death and dying, chronic illness, and disability.

Family practice residents receive intensive training in behavioral and psychosocial issues, as well as "bedside manner" training. Scientific research has shown that many patients who seek care from family physicians have problems that require the physician to be a good listener and a skilled counselor. Family practice residency training emphasizes these skills. It also emphasizes the functioning (or malfunctioning) of the family as a system and the effect of major changes (such as the birth of a child or retirement) on the health and functioning of the family members.

The length of training (three years versus one year) and this emphasis on psychosocial and family systems training are two of the major differences in the training of a family physician and the training of a general practitioner. Moreover, family physicians spend up to 30 percent of their training time outside the hospital in a clinic. Family practice was the first medical specialty to emphasize this type of training, and family physicians spend more time in ambulatory (clinic) training than virtually any other specialist.

Following the successful completion of a residency program, a family physician may take a competency examination devised and administered by the American Board of Family Practice. Passing this examination allows the physician to assume the title of Diplomate of the American Board of Family Practice and makes him or her eligible to join the American Academy of Family Physicians, the advocacy and educational organization of family practice.

If family physicians wish to retain their diplomate status, they must take at least fifty hours per year of medical education. After a family physician fulfill's all educational and other requirements of the American Board of Family Practice, that physician must then retake the certifying examination every seven years or the certification will lapse. This periodic retesting is required by the American Board of Family Practice to make sure that family physicians keep up their medical education and maintain their knowledge level and clinical skills. Family practice was the first specialty to require periodic reexamination of its physicians. In fact, since family practice has mandated reexaminations, many other medical specialty organizations now require periodic reexamination of their members or are considering such a move. Many former general practitioners who did not have a chance to do a three-year family practice residency took the American Board of Family Practice certifying examination and became diplomates based on their years of practice experience and successful completion of the certifying examination. This option was closed to general practitioners in 1988.

Currently, the American Academy of Family Physicians requires new active physician members to be residency-trained in family practice. Diplomate status reflects only an educational effort by the physician and does not directly affect medical licensure. Medical licensure is based on a different testing mechanism, and license requirements vary from state to state. There are more than fifty thousand family physicians providing health care in the United States, the District of Columbia, the Virgin Islands, Guam, and Puerto Rico. Family practice residency programs are approximately four hundred in number and usually have about seven thousand residents in training.

DIAGNOSTIC AND TREATMENT TECHNIQUES

Service to patients is the primary concern of family practice and all those who practice, teach, administer, or foster the specialty. Of all the family physicians in practice, more than 93 percent are involved in direct patient care. While family physicians by no means constitute a majority of physicians, they are among the busiest when measured in terms of ambulatory patient visits. Family physicians see 30 percent of all ambulatory patients in the United States, which is more than the number of ambulatory visits to the next two specialty groups combined. Because of their training, family physicians can successfully care for more than 85 percent of all patient problems they encounter. Consultation

with other specialty physicians is sought for the problems that are outside the scope of the family physician's knowledge or abilities. This level of consultation is not unique to family physicians, as other specialty physicians find it necessary to seek consultation for 10 to 15 percent of their patients as well.

Family physicians can be found in all areas of the United States and in virtually all types of practice situations, providing a wide range of medical services. Family physicians can successfully practice in metropolitan areas or rural communities of one thousand people (or less), and they can be found teaching or doing research in medical colleges. Because of their training and the fact that they see a truly undifferentiated patient population, family physicians deliver a wide range of medical services. Besides seeing many patients in their offices, family physicians care for patients in nursing homes, make house calls, and admit patients to the hospital. Within the hospital, many family physicians care for patients in intensive care and other special care units and assist in surgery when their patients have operations. A small number perform extensive surgical procedures in the hospital setting. A sizable minority of family physicians take care of pregnant women and deliver their children; some of these physicians also perform cesarean sections. Because family physicians see anyone that walks through the door, it is not unheard of for a family physician to deliver a child in the morning, see the siblings in the office in the afternoon, and make a house call to the grandparents in the evening.

The thing that makes family physicians different from other physicians is their attention to the physician-patient relationship. The family physician has first contact with the patient and is in a position to bond with the patient. The family physician evaluates the patient's complete health needs and provides personal care in one or more areas of medicine. Such care is not limited to any particular type of problem, be it biological, behavioral, or social, and the patients seen are not screened according to age, sex, or illness. The family physician utilizes knowledge of the patient's functioning in the family and community and maintains continuity of care for the patient in a hospital, clinic, or nursing home or in the patient's own home. Thus, in family practice, the patient-physician relationship is initiated, established, and nurtured for both sexes, for all ages, and across time for many types of problems.

Because of their training, family physicians are highly sought-after care providers. Small rural communities, insurance companies, and government agencies at all levels actively seek family physicians to care for patients in a wide variety of settings. In this respect, family practice is the most versatile medical specialty. Family physicians are able to practice and live in communities that are too small to support any other types of physicians. In the early 1990's, 28.4 percent of family physicians were practicing in towns with a population of ten thousand or less. As a result, family physicians, along with general pediatricians, are the lowest paid of all physicians.

While the vast majority of family physicians find themselves providing care for patients, there is a minority of family physicians who serve in other, equally important roles. Roughly 3.5 percent of family physicians serve as administrators and educators. They can be found working in state, federal, and local governments; in the insurance industry; and in residency programs and medical schools. Family physicians in residency programs provide instruction and role modeling for family practice residents in community-based and university-based residency programs. Family physicians in medical colleges design, implement, administer, and evaluate educational programs for medical students during the four years of medical school. The Society of Teachers of Family Medicine (STFM) is the organization that supports family physicians in their teaching role. A major problem facing the United States, particularly acute for family physician faculty, is the shortage of family physicians. In 1993, it was estimated that, if every medical school graduate went into family practice, there would be just enough family physicians by the year 2003. In reality, only about 10 to 13 percent of U.S. medical students choose family practice, which is barely enough to keep up with the loss of family physicians through death and retirement. This problem can be addressed through a variety of initiatives by family physicians, government entities, foundations, and the medical insurance industry.

One problem facing the specialty of family practice is the very small percentage who are dedicated to research: only 0.3 percent of all family physicians. There is a large need for research in family practice to determine the natural course of illnesses, how best to treat them, and the effects of illness on the functioning of the family unit. The need for research in the ambulatory setting is especially acute because, while most medical research is done in the hospital setting, most medical care in the United States is provided in clinics and offices. This problem will not be easily solved because of the service focus of family practice training and the small number of family physicians dedicated to research.

The organizations representing family physicians are also concerned about providing service to the American people. The American Academy of Family Physicians has worked since its founding to increase the numbers and improve the quality of family physicians, and it proposed a plan to improve health care access for those Americans who are underserved because of financial or other barriers. Another organization of family physicians is Doctors Oughta Care (DOC). DOC is a medical activist organization that works against the number-one and number-two killers in American society: tobacco and alcohol. DOC takes a tongue-in-cheek approach and ridicules the tobacco and alcohol industries.

Its members were in large part responsible for bringing a lawsuit against the tobacco industry alleging that it actively markets cigarettes to children.

PERSPECTIVE AND PROSPECTS

Family practice developed as a medical specialty because of the demands of the citizens of the United States; it is the only medical specialty with that claim. The ancestor of family practice was general practice, and there is a direct link from the family physician to the general practitioner. Family practice has grown and evolved into the specialty best suited to provide for the primary health care needs of most patients. Because of their broad scope of practice, cost-effective methods, and versatility, family physicians are found in virtually every type of medical and administrative setting. Family physicians provide a large portion of all ambulatory health care in the United States, and in some settings they are the sole providers of health care. General practice has been around as long as there have been physicians—Hippocrates was a general practitioner—but family practice has a definite point of origin. It was created from general practice on February 8, 1969.

The present role of the family physician is and will continue to be to seek to improve the health of the people of the United States at all levels. Major problems exist for family practice, including attrition as older family physicians retire or die, lack of medical student interest in family practice as a career choice, and the lack of a solid cadre of researchers to advance medical knowledge in family practice. The major strengths supporting family practice are its service ethic, attention to the physician-patient relationship, and cost-effectiveness.

After their near demise as a recognizable group in the mid-twentieth century, family physicians have a number of reasons to expect that they will have expanded opportunities to provide for the health care needs of their patients in the future. As the United States, for example, examines its system of health care, which is the most costly and the least effective of any health care system in the developed world, many medical and political leaders look to generalism, and particularly family practice, to provide answers. Research has shown that, for many medical problems, family physicians can provide outcomes very similar to those provided by specialists. When one couples that fact with the versatility and cost-effectiveness of generalist physicians, it can be argued that to save health care dollars the nation must reverse the 30 percent to 70 percent ratio of generalist to specialist physicians. A ratio of 50 percent to 50 percent generalist to specialist physicians has been proposed at many levels in medicine and government.

Those who champion family practice can be heartened by several developments. First, it is hoped that changes in legislation will soon enhance payment for family physicians for the services they provide. Also, family physicians have formed alliances with medical specialties and other organizations concerned with the promotion of generalism. Finally, the field's solid organizational structure, which is highly regarded and very effective in its areas of operation, has made tremendous strides in promoting and nurturing family practice.

There has been a growing acceptance of family practice since its inception. Building on its long history of enjoying the respect and admiration of patients, family practice is finding itself more and more popular. Government agencies and medical insurance companies look to family physicians to meet their needs, and family practice is now found in most U.S. medical schools. For these and other reasons, it appears that the United States may be coming full circle back to the days of the country doctor.

—*Paul M. Paulman, M.D.*

See also Allergies; Anemia; Athlete's foot; Bacterial infections; Bronchitis; Chickenpox; Childhood infectious diseases; Cholesterol; Common cold; Constipation; Coughing; Cytomegalovirus (CMV); Death and dying; Diarrhea and dysentery; Digestion; Dizziness and fainting; Domestic violence; Exercise physiology; Fatigue; Fever; Fungal infections; Geriatrics and gerontology; Grief and guilt; Halitosis; Headaches; Healing; Heartburn; Hypercholesterolemia; Hyperlipidemia; Hypertension; Hypoglycemia; Indigestion; Infection; Inflammation; Influenza; Laryngitis; Measles, red; Mononucleosis; Mumps; Muscle sprains, spasms, and disorders; Nutrition; Obesity; Osteopathic medicine; Pain, types of; Pediatrics; Pertussis; Pharmacology; Pharmacy; Physical examination; Pneumonia; Poisonous plants; Preventive medicine; Psychology; Puberty and adolescence; Rashes; Rheumatic fever; Rubella; Rubeola; Scabies; Scarlet fever; Sciatica; Shingles; Shock; Sinusitis; Sore throat; Strep throat; Stress; Tetanus; Tonsillitis; Toxicology; Ulcers; Viral infections; Vitamins and minerals; Wounds.

FOR FURTHER INFORMATION:

American Academy of Family Physicians. *Facts About Family Practice 1995.* Kansas City, Mo.: American Academy of Family Physicians, 1995. This reference guide provides a list of facts about family practice physicians. Included in this publication are statistics about the location of family physicians and the scope of their practice.

_____. *Family Practice: Creation of a Specialty.* Kansas City, Mo.: American Academy of Family Physicians, 1980. This document outlines the historical events and individuals associated with the birth of family practice. Describes in great detail the steps taken in the various groups, including the American Medical Association, and some of the debate and controversy surrounding the advent of family practice. The information in this paper is based largely on conversations with individuals who were active in the process of creating this medical specialty.

American Academy of Family Physicians' Membership Directory, 1973-   . Available from the American Academy of Family Physicians, this annual publication provides a state-by-state, city-by-city listing of family physicians by name.

Rakel, Robert E. *Essentials of Family Practice.* Philadelphia: W. B. Saunders, 1993. This book outlines the core content essentials for family practice training.

Scherger, Joseph E., et al. "Responses to Questions by Medical Students About Family Practice." *The Journal of Family Practice* 26, no. 2 (1988): 169-176. Although aimed at medical students, this popular medical article provides good background information about the scope and socioeconomic aspects of family practice.

Stephens, G. Gayle. *The Intellectual Basis of Family Practice.* Kansas City, Mo.: Society of Teachers of Family Medicine Foundation, 1982. This book outlines the scientific principles that demanded the creation and continuing existence of family practice.

FATIGUE

DISEASE/DISORDER

ANATOMY OR SYSTEM AFFECTED: All

SPECIALTIES AND RELATED FIELDS: Family practice, geriatrics and gerontology, internal medicine, psychiatry

DEFINITION: A general symptom of tiredness, malaise, depression, and sometimes anxiety associated with many diseases and disorders; in some cases, no specific cause can be found.

KEY TERMS:

physical deconditioning: a condition that results when a person who has previously been exercising (has become conditioned) stops exercising

psychogenic fatigue: fatigue caused by mental factors, such as anxiety, and not attributable to any physical cause

sleep apnea: cessation of breathing during sleep, which may result from either an inhibition of the respiratory center (central apnea) or an obstruction to the flow of air (obstructive apnea)

sleep disorders: conditions resulting in sleep interruption, interfering with the restorative functions of sleep

syndrome: a collection of complaints (symptoms) and signs (abnormal findings on clinical examination) which do not match any specific disease

CAUSES AND SYMPTOMS

Almost all people suffer form fatigue at some point in their lives. It is a nonspecific complaint including tiredness, lack of energy, listlessness, or malaise. Patients often confuse fatigue with weakness, breathlessness, or dizziness, which indicate the existence of other physical disorders. Rest or a change in the daily routine ordinarily alleviates fatigue in healthy individuals. Though normally short in duration, fatigue occasionally lasts for weeks, months, or even years in some individuals. In such cases, it limits the amount of physical and mental activity in which the person can participate.

Long-term fatigue can have serious consequences. Often,

patients begin to withdraw from their normal activities. They may withdraw from society in general and may gradually become more apathetic and depressed. As a result of this progression, a patient's physical and mental capabilities may begin to deteriorate. Fatigue may be aggravated further by a reduced appetite and inadequate nutritional intake. Ultimately, these symptoms lead to malnutrition and multiple vitamin deficiencies, which intensify the fatigue state and trigger a vicious circle.

This fatigue cycle ends with a person who lacks interest and energy. Such patients may lose interest in daily events and social contacts. In later stages of fatigue, they may neglect themselves and lose track of their goals in life. The will to live and fight decreases, making them prime targets for accidents and repeated infections. They may also become potential candidates for suicide.

Physical and/or mental overactivity commonly cause recent-onset fatigue. Management of such fatigue is simple: Adequate physical and/or mental relaxation typically relieve it. Fortunately, many persistent fatigue states can be easily diagnosed and successfully treated. In some cases, however, fatigue does not respond to simple measures.

Fatigue can stem from depression. Depressed individuals often reflect boredom and a lack of interest, and frequently express uncertainty and/or anxiety about the future. These people usually appear "down." They may walk slowly with their head down, slump their shoulders, and sigh frequently. They often take unusually long to respond to questions or requests. They also show little motivation. Depressed individuals typically relate feelings of dejection, sadness, worthlessness, or helplessness. Often, they complain of feeling tired when they wake up in the morning, and no amount of sleep or rest improves their condition. In fact, they feel weary all day and frequently complain of feeling weak. They often have poor appetites and sometimes lose weight. Once these patients are questioned by a physician, however, it may become apparent that their state of fatigue actually fluctuates. At times they feel exhausted, while at other times (sometimes only minutes later) they feel refreshed and full of energy.

Other manifestations of depression include sleep disorders (particularly early morning waking), reduced appetite, altered bowel habits, and difficulty concentrating. Depressed individuals sometimes fail to recognize their condition. They may channel their depression into physical complaints such as abdominal pain, headaches, joint pain, or vaguely defined aches and pains. In older people, depression sometimes manifests itself as impaired memory.

Anxiety, another major cause of fatigue, interferes with the patient's ability to achieve adequate mental and physical rest. Anxious individuals often appear scared, worried, or fearful. They frequently report multiple physical complaints, including neck muscle tension, headaches, palpitations, difficulty in breathing, chest tightness, intestinal cramping, and trouble falling asleep. In some cases, both depression and anxiety may be present simultaneously.

Medications also constitute a major cause of fatigue. All drugs—prescription, over-the-counter, or recreational—can cause fatigue. Sleeping medications, antidepressants, antianxiety medications, muscle relaxants, allergy medications, cold medications, and certain blood pressure medications can lead to problems with fatigue.

An excessive intake of stimulants, paradoxically, sometimes leads to easy fatigability. Stimulants can interfere with proper sleeping habits and relaxation. Common culprits include caffeine and medications (such as some diet pills and nasal decongestants) that can be purchased without a prescription. So-called recreational drugs can also contribute to chronic fatigue. Depending on their tendencies, they function to cause fatigue in much the same way as the prescription and over-the-counter drugs already discussed. Cocaine and amphetamines, for example, act as stimulants. Narcotics such as heroin and barbiturates (downers) possess strong sedative qualities. Alcohol consumption in an attempt to escape loneliness, depression, or boredom may further exacerbate a sense of fatigue. Alcohol produces fatigue in two ways. It has sedative qualities, and it also intensifies the sedative effects of other medications, if taken with them.

Other drugs that may induce fatigue include diuretics and those that lower blood pressure. These medications increase the excretions of many substances through the kidneys. If inappropriately given or regulated, these drugs may alter the blood concentration of other medications taken concurrently.

Painkillers can lead to fatigue in a different way. In some individuals, they irritate the lining of the stomach and cause it to bleed. Such bleeding usually occurs in small amounts and goes unnoticed by the patient. This slight blood loss can gradually lead to anemia and fatigue.

Medications are particularly likely to cause fatigue in elderly individuals. With many drugs, their elimination from the body through metabolism or excretion may decrease with age. This often leads to higher drug concentrations in the blood than intended, resulting in a state of constant sedation and lethargy. Also, elderly individuals' brains may be more sensitive to sedation than those of younger individuals. Finally, the elderly tend to take more medication for more illnesses than younger adults. The additive side effects of multiple medicines can add to fatigue problems.

Sleep deprivation or frequent sleep interruptions lead to fatigue. A change in environment can induce sleep disorders, especially if accompanied by unfamiliar noises, excessive lighting, uncomfortable temperatures, or an excessive degree of humidity or dryness. Total sleep time may be adequate under such conditions, but quality of sleep is usually poor. Nightmares can also interrupt sleep, and if numerous and recurring, they also cause fatigue.

Some sleep interruptions are not so readily apparent. In

sleep apnea, a specific and increasingly diagnosed sleep disorder, the patient temporarily stops breathing while sleeping. This results in reduced oxygen levels and increased carbon dioxide levels in the blood. When a critical level is reached, the patient awakens briefly, takes a few deep breaths, and then falls asleep again. Many episodes of sleep apnea may occur during the night, making the sleep interrupted and less refreshing than it should be. The next day, the patient often feels tired and fatigued, but may not recognize the source of the problem. Obstructive sleep apnea normally develops in grossly overweight patients or in those with large tonsils or adenoids. Patients with obstructive sleep apnea usually snore while sleeping, and typically they are unaware of their snoring and/or sleep disturbance.

A number of diseases can lead to easy fatigability. In most illnesses, rest relieves fatigue and individuals awake refreshed after a nap or a good night's sleep. Unfortunately, they also tire quickly. Unlike psychogenic fatigue or fatigue induced by drugs, disease-related fatigue is not usually the patient's main symptom. Other symptoms and signs frequently reveal the underlying diagnosis. Individuals who suffer from severe malnutrition, anemia, endocrine system malfunction, chronic infections, tuberculosis, Lyme disease, bacterial endocarditis (a bacterial infection of the valves of the heart), chronic sinusitis, mononucleosis, hepatitis, parasitic infections, and fungal infections may all experience chronic fatigue.

In early stages of acquired immunodeficiency syndrome (AIDS), fatigue may be the only symptom. Persons at high risk for contracting the human immunodeficiency virus (HIV)—those with multiple sexual partners, homosexual men, those with a history of blood transfusion, or intravenous drug users—who complain of persistent fatigue should be tested for HIV infection.

Abnormalities of mineral or electrolyte concentrations—potassium, sodium, chloride, and calcium are the most important of these—may also cause fatigue. Such abnormalities may result from medications (diuretics are frequently responsible), diarrhea, vomiting, dietary fads, and endocrine or bone disorders.

Some less common medical causes of chronic fatigue include dysfunction of specific organs such as kidney failure or liver failure. Allergies can also produce chronic fatigue. Cancer can cause fatigue, but other symptoms usually surface and lead to a diagnosis before the patient begins to notice chronic weariness.

TREATMENT AND THERAPY

When an individual's fatigue persists in spite of adequate rest, medical help becomes necessary in order to determine the cause. Common diseases known to be associated with fatigue should be considered. Initially, the physician makes detailed inquiries about the severity of the fatigue and how long ago it started. Other important questions include whether it is progressive, whether there are any factors that make it worse or relieve it, or whether it is worse during specific times of the day. An examination of the patient's psychological state may also be necessary.

The physician should ask about the presence of any symptoms that occur along with the general sense of fatigue. For example, breathlessness may indicate a cardiovascular or respiratory disease. Abdominal pain might arouse the suspicion of a gastrointestinal disease. Weakness may point to a neuromuscular collagen disease. Excessive thirst and increased urine output may suggest diabetes mellitus, and weight loss may accompany metabolic or endocrinal abnormalities, chronic infections, or cancer.

Whether they have been prescribed by a physician or purchased over-the-counter, the medications taken regularly by a patient should be reviewed. The doctor should also inquire about alcohol and tobacco use and dietary fads. A thorough physical examination may be required. During an examination, the doctor sometimes uncovers physical signs of fatigue-inducing diseases. Blood tests and other laboratory investigations may also be needed, especially because a physical examination does not always reveal the cause.

Often, however, despite an extensive workup, no specific cause for the persistent fatigue appears. At this stage, the diagnosis of chronic fatigue syndrome should be considered. In order to fit this diagnosis, patients must have several of the symptoms associated with this syndrome. They must have complained of fatigue for at least six months, and the fatigue should be of such an extent that it interferes with normal daily activities. Since many of the symptoms associated with chronic fatigue syndrome overlap with other disorders, these other fatigue-inducing conditions must be considered and ruled out.

In order to fit the diagnosis of chronic fatigue syndrome, patients must have at least six of the classic symptoms. These include a mild fever and/or sore throat, painful lymph nodes in the neck or axilla, unexplained generalized weakness, and muscle pain or discomfort. Patients may describe marked fatigue lasting for more than twenty-four hours that is induced by levels of exercise that would have been easily tolerated before the onset of fatigue. They may suffer from generalized headaches of a type, severity, or pattern that is different from headaches experienced before the onset of chronic fatigue. Patients may also have joint pain without swelling or redness and/or neuropsychologic complaints such as a bad memory and excessive irritability. Confusion, difficulty in thinking, inability to concentrate, depression, and sleep disturbances are also on the list of associated symptoms.

No one knows the exact cause of chronic fatigue syndrome. Researchers continue to study the disease and come up with hypotheses, though none have proven entirely satisfactory. One theory argues that since patients with chronic fatigue syndrome appear to have a reduced aerobic work capacity, defects in the muscles may cause the condition.

This, however, constitutes only one of many theories concerning the syndrome and its origin.

Many patients with chronic fatigue syndrome relate that they suffered from an infectious illness immediately preceding the onset of fatigue. This pattern causes some scientists to suspect a viral origin. Typically, the illness that precedes the patient's problems with fatigue is not severe, and resembles other upper respiratory tract infections experienced previously. The implicated viruses include the Epstein-Barr virus, Coxsackie B virus, herpes simplex virus, cytomegalovirus, human herpesvirus 6, and the measles virus. It should be mentioned, however, that some patients with long-term fatigue do not have a history of a triggering infectious disease before the onset of fatigue.

Patients with chronic fatigue syndrome sometimes have a number of immune system abnormalities. Laboratory evidence exists of immune dysfunction in many patients with this syndrome, and there have been reports of improvement when immunoglobulin (antibody) therapy was given. The significance of immunological abnormalities in chronic fatigue syndrome, however, remains uncertain. Most of these abnormalities do not occur in all patients with this syndrome. Furthermore, the degree of immunologic abnormality does not always correspond with the severity of the symptoms.

Some researchers believe that the acute infectious disease that often precedes the onset of chronic fatigue syndrome forces the patient to become physically inactive. This inactivity leads to physical deconditioning, and the progression ends in chronic fatigue syndrome. Experiments in which patients with chronic fatigue syndrome were given exercise testing, however, do not support this theory completely. In the case of physical deconditioning, the heart rates of patients with chronic fatigue syndrome should have risen more rapidly with exercise than those without the syndrome. The exact opposite was found. The data were not determined consistent with the suggestion that physical deconditioning causes chronic fatigue syndrome.

A high prevalence of unrecognized psychiatric disorders exists in patients with chronic fatigue, especially depression. Depression affects about half of chronic fatigue syndrome patients and precedes other symptoms in about half of them as well. Yet a critical question remains unanswered concerning chronic fatigue syndrome: Are patients with this syndrome fatigued because they have a primary mood disorder, or has the mood disorder developed as a secondary component of the chronic fatigue syndrome?

No completely satisfactory treatment exists for chronic fatigue syndrome, since the cause remains a mystery. A group of researchers using intravenous immunoglobulin therapy met with varying degrees of success, but other investigators could not reproduce these results. Other therapeutic trials used high doses of medications such as acyclovir, liver extract, folic acid, and cyanocobalamine. A mixture of evening primrose oil and fish oil was also administered with some degree of success. Claims have also been made that patients administered magnesium sulfate improved to a larger extent than those receiving a placebo. Other therapeutic options include cognitive behavioral therapy, programs of gradually increasing physical activity, analgesics, nonsteroidal anti-inflammatory drugs (NSAIDs), and antidepressants. Finally, a number of self-help groups exist for chronic fatigue sufferers.

The prognosis and natural history of chronic fatigue syndrome are still poorly defined. Chronic fatigue syndrome does not kill patients, but it does significantly decrease the quality of life for sufferers. For the physician, management of this syndrome remains challenging. In addition to correcting any physical abnormalities present, the physician should attempt to find an activity that interests the patient and encourage him or her to become involved in it.

PERSPECTIVE AND PROSPECTS

Fatigue is generally considered a normal bodily response, protecting the individual from excessive physical and/or mental activity. After all, the normal levels of performance for individuals who do not rest usually decline. In the case of overactivity, fatigue should be viewed as a positive warning sign. Using relaxation and rest (mental and/or physical), the individual can often alleviate weariness and optimize performance.

In some cases, however, fatigue does not derive from physical or mental overactivity, nor does it respond adequately to relaxation and rest. In these instances, it interferes with an individual's ability to cope with everyday life and enjoy usual activities. The patient begins referring to fatigue as the reason for not participating in normal physical, mental, and social activities.

Unfortunately, physicians, health care professionals, society, and even the patients themselves dismiss fatigue as a trivial complaint. As a result, sufferers seek medical help only after the condition becomes advanced. This dangerous, negative attitude can delay the correct diagnosis of the underlying pathology and threaten the patient's chances for a quick recovery.

The diagnosis and management of chronic fatigue syndrome prove challenging for both physician and patient. It is important to note that chronic fatigue syndrome often stems from nonmedical causes. While the possibility of a serious medical illness should be addressed, illness-related fatigue usually occurs along with other, more prominent symptoms. The causes of chronic fatigue syndrome are numerous and can take time to define. Patients need to answer all questions related to their complaints as thoroughly and accurately as possible, so that their physicians can reach accurate diagnoses using the minimum number of tests. Extensive testing for rare medical causes of fatigue can become extraordinarily expensive and uncomfortable, so doctors select the tests that they are ordering cautiously. They must balance the benefit, the cost, and the risk of each test to the patient. Such decisions should be based on their own experience and on the available data.

Open communication between the patient and doctor is of paramount importance. It ensures a correct diagnosis, followed by the most effective treatment. Follow-up visits and reassurance may be the best therapy in many cases. Professional counselors can offer assistance with fatigue-inducing psychological disorders. Examination of sleep and relaxation habits can reveal potential problems, and steps can be taken to ensure adequate rest.

Persistent fatigue should not be discarded lightly, and serious attempts should be made to determine its underlying causes. In this respect, it may be appropriate to recall one of Hippocrates' aphorisms, "Unprovoked fatigue means disease." —*Ronald C. Hamdy, M.D., Mark R. Doman, M.D., and Katherine Hoffman Doman*

See also Aging; Anemia; Anxiety; Apnea; Chronic fatigue syndrome; Depression; Dizziness and fainting; Malnutrition; Narcolepsy; Sleep disorders; Sleeping sickness; Stress; Stress reduction.

FOR FURTHER INFORMATION:

Archer, James, Jr. *Managing Anxiety and Stress*. Muncie, Ind.: Excellerated Development, 1982. Anxiety is a common cause of persistent fatigue. This text examines the nature of anxiety. Contains several methods to combat anxiety and stress, ranging from management skills, personal relations, nutrition, and exercise to meditation and relaxation techniques. Arranged so that it can be used as a step-by-step guide to decreasing an individual's anxiety.

Feiden, Karyn. *Hope and Help for Chronic Fatigue Syndrome: The Official CFS-CFIDS Network*. New York: Prentice Hall, 1990. A complete review of chronic fatigue syndrome, presenting the many aspects of this disease. The history of this syndrome, symptomatology, theories of causation, and experimental therapies are addressed. Includes a section on surviving with this syndrome, recommending the use of support groups, social services, and self-help.

Goroll, Allan H., Lawrence A. May, and Albert G. Mulley, Jr., eds. *Primary Care Medicine*. Rev. 3d ed. Philadelphia: J. B. Lippincott, 1995. The essential text for the medical office practice of adult medicine. It is problem-oriented and easily read even by individuals without medical training. The section on the causes of fatigue is the best available.

Pembrook, Linda. *How to Beat Fatigue*. Garden City, N.Y.: Doubleday, 1975. In this book, many aspects of fatigue are presented simply and thoroughly, including sleep, drugs and alcohol, nutrition, depression, and anxiety. Covers many of the causes of fatigue, with the exception of some of the physical causes.

Talley, Joseph. *Family Practitioner's Guide to Treating Depressive Illness*. Chicago: Precept Press, 1987. Depres-

sion is probably the most common cause of persistent fatigue. This well-written text examines the multiple facets of depression. It also reviews the various therapies available, different philosophies of depressive treatments, and the use of psychotherapy.

Trubo, Richard. *How to Get a Good Night's Sleep*. Boston: Little, Brown, 1978. An easy-to-read book that examines most facets of sleep, from the physiology of sleep to such sleep disorders as sleep apnea and nightmares. The text also includes an interesting section on dreams and dreaming.

FEET

ANATOMY

ANATOMY OR SYSTEM INVOLVED: Bones, musculoskeletal system

SPECIALTIES AND RELATED FIELDS: Orthopedics, podiatry

DEFINITION: The lowest extremities, composed of a complex system of muscles and bones, that act as levers to propel the body and that must support the weight of the body in standing, walking, or running.

KEY TERMS:

distal: referring to a particular body part that is farther from the point of attachment or farther from the trunk than another part

extension: movement that increases the angle between the bones, causing them to move farther apart; straightening or extension of the ankle occurs when the toes point away from the shin

flexion: a bending movement that decreases the angle of the joint and brings two bones closer together; flexion of the ankle pulls the foot closer to the shin

hallucis: a term referring to the big toe; the flexor hallucis longus is a muscle which flexes the big toe

inferior: situated below another part; the ankle bones are inferior to the bones of the lower leg

lateral: toward the side with respect to the body's imaginary midline; away from the midline of the body, a limb, or any understood point of reference

medial: closer to an imaginary midline dividing the body into equal right and left halves than another part

plantar: having to do with the sole of the foot (for example, a plantar wart)

podiatry: the branch of medicine that deals with the study, examination, diagnosis, treatment, and prevention of diseases and malfunctions of the foot

proximal: referring to a particular body part that is closer to a point of attachment than another part

superior: above another part or closer to the head; the ankle bones are superior to the bones of the feet

STRUCTURE AND FUNCTIONS

The anatomy of the foot is very similar to that of the hand; however, the foot is adapted to perform very different functions. The human hand has the ability to perform fine

The Bones of the Foot

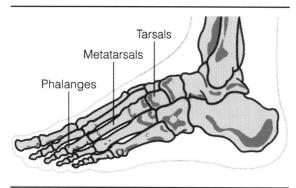

Tarsals
Metatarsals
Phalanges

movements such as grasping and writing, while the foot is involved mainly in support and movement. Therefore, the bones and muscles of the foot tend to be heavier and function without the same dexterity as the hand.

The twenty-six bones of the foot include the tarsals, metatarsals, and phalanges. The proximal portion of the foot next to the ankle is composed of seven tarsal bones: the calcaneus, talus, navicular, cuboid, medial cuneiform, intermediate cuneiform, and lateral cuneiform. The bones are rather irregular in shape and form gliding joints; these joints allow only a limited movement when compared to other joints in the body. The calcaneus forms the large heel bone, which serves as a major attachment for the muscles that are located in the back of the lower leg. Just above the calcaneus is another large foot bone called the talus. The talus rests between the tibia and the fibula, the two lower leg bones. Interestingly, the talus is the single bone that receives the entire weight of the body when an individual is standing; it must then transmit this weight to the rest of the foot below. The cuboid and the three cuneiform bones meet the proximal end of the long foot bones, the metatarsals.

The five separate metatarsal bones are relatively long and thin when compared to the tarsal bones. Anatomists distinguish between the five metatarsals by number. If one begins numbering from the medial (or inside) part of the foot, that metatarsal is number one and the lateral (or outside) metatarsal is number five. The distal portion of each metatarsal articulates (meets) with the toe bones, or phalanges.

Humans have toes that are very similar to their fingers. In fact, the numbers and names of the toe and finger bones, phalanges, are identical. The major differences lie in the fact that the finger phalanges are longer than the phalanges that make up toes. Hinge joints are located between each phalanx and allow for flexion and extension movements only. Human toes (or fingers) are made up of fourteen different phalanges. Each toe (or finger) has three phalanges except for the big toe (or thumb), which has only two. The toes are named in a similar way as the metatarsals; that is, the big toe is number one and the little toe is number five.

The three phalanges that make up each toe (except for the big toe) are named according to location. The phalanx meeting the metatarsal is referred to as the proximal phalanx. The bone at the tip of the toe is the distal phalanx, and the one in between is the middle phalanx. Since the big toe only has two phalanges, they are called proximal and distal phalanges.

Although it seems that there is only a single arch in each foot, podiatrists and anatomists identify three arches: the medial and lateral longitudinal arches and the transverse, or metatarsal, arch. The medial longitudinal arch, as the name implies, is located on the medial surface of the foot and follows the long axis from the calcaneus to the big toe. Likewise, the lateral longitudinal arch is on the lateral surface and runs from the heel to the little toe. The transverse, or metatarsal, arch crosses the width of the foot near the proximal end of the metatarsals. The bones are only one factor that maintains arches in the feet and prevents them from flattening under the weight of the body. Ligaments (which connect bones), muscles, and tendons (which attach muscles to bones) are primarily responsible for the support of the arches. The arches function to distribute body weight between the calcaneus and the distal end of the metatarsals (the balls of the feet). They also are flexible enough to absorb some of the shock to the feet from walking, running, and jumping.

While the feet seem to be composed of only bones, tendons, and ligaments, the movements of the toes and feet require an extensive system of muscles. Most of the larger muscles that act on the foot and toes are actually located in the lower leg. Anatomists divide these muscles into separate compartments: anterior, posterior, and lateral.

The muscles of the anterior compartment move the foot upward (dorsiflex) and extend the toes. These muscles include the tibialis anterior, extensor digitorum longus, extensor hallucis longus, and peroneus tertius. The tibialis anterior is attached to the top of the first metatarsal and pulls the medial part of the foot upward and slightly lateral. All the toes except the big toe are pulled up (extended) by the extensor digitorum longus. The extensor hallucis longus moves only the big toe upward, while the peroneus tertius is attached to the fifth metatarsal and moves the foot upward.

The muscles of the lateral compartment act to move the foot in a lateral or outward direction. The peroneus longus and peroneus brevis are attached to the first and fifth metatarsal, respectively. Using these attachments, the muscles can pull the foot laterally.

The muscles of the posterior compartment are the largest group and act to flex the foot and toes. All these muscles share a common tendon, the calcaneus (or Achilles) tendon. As the name suggests, this large tendon attaches to the calcaneus bone. The larger, more superficial muscles include the gastrocnemius, soleus, and plantaris; these powerful muscles are commonly called the calf muscles. Also in the posterior compartment are four smaller muscles located beneath the calf muscles: the popliteus (located directly behind the knee joint), flexor hallucis longus, flexor digitorum longus, and tibialis posterior. The popliteus rotates the lower leg medially. The flexor hallucis longus flexes the big toe. The remaining toes are flexed by the flexor digitorum longus, while the tibialis posterior acts opposite tibialis anterior to flex the foot.

Within the foot itself are some muscles known as the intrinsic foot muscles. All but one of these muscles are located on the bottom surface of the foot. This one muscle extends all the toes except the little toe. The remaining intrinsic muscles are on the plantar (bottom) surface and serve to flex the toes.

The major vessels that provide blood to the foot include branches from the anterior tibial artery. This relatively large artery is located along the anterior surface of the lower leg and branches into the dorsalis pedis artery, which serves the ankle and upper part of the foot. Physicians often check for a pulse in this foot artery to provide information about circulation to the foot and circulation in general, as this is the point furthest from the heart. The bottom part of the feet are supplied with blood by branches of the peroneal artery. At the ankle, this artery branches into plantar arteries, which supply the structures on the sole of the foot. The human toes receive most of their blood from branches of the plantar arteries called the digital arteries.

DISORDERS AND DISEASES

Even though the anatomy of the foot is resistant to the tremendous amount of force that the body places on it, it can be injured. Force injuries to the foot commonly result in fractures or breaks of the metatarsals and phalanges. Occasionally, the calcaneus may fracture from a fall on a hard surface. More commonly, patients complain of painful heel syndrome.

Because the shock-absorbing pads of tissue on the heel become thinner with age, repeated pressure on the heel can cause pain. Prolonged standing, walking, or running can add to the pressure, as can being overweight. One cause of pain is plantar fasciitis, an inflammation of the tough band of connective tissue on the sole. The inflammation occurs when the muscles located on the back of the lower leg that are attached to the connective tissue at the calcaneus pull under stress. This may even be associated with small fractures. X rays may show small spurs of bone near the site of stress; however, these spurs are not believed to be the cause of pain.

Deformities of the foot at birth are fairly common and include clubfoot, flat foot, and clawfoot. The cause of these anomalies is abnormal development. The foot of the fetus normally goes through stages where it is turned outward and inward but gradually assumes a normal position by about the seventh month of gestation. In the case of clubfoot, arrested development in the stage when the foot is turned inward causes the muscles, bones, and joints to develop in this abnormal anatomical position. At the time of birth, the deformity is readily observable and the foot immobile. Treatment includes splints, casting, and surgery. If treatment is begun at birth, the foot may look relatively normal after approximately one year.

Almost everyone is born with feet that are flat because the arches do not begin to develop until the ligaments and muscles function normally. In most people, the arches are fully formed by the age of six. In some individuals, however, the ligaments and muscles remain weak and the feet do not develop a normal arch. Flat feet can also develop in adult life, at which time they are called "fallen arches." Body weight moves along a precise path during walking or running, beginning with the heel touching the ground. Then, as the foot steps, the arch receives the forces pushing down on the foot. Because the bones, muscles, and ligaments form an arch in the foot, the arch can deform slightly and absorb some of the downward force. With further movement, the weight passes to the ball of the foot (the distal metatarsals). A fallen arch has lost this flexibility and shock-absorbing capability. The arch "falls" because of improper weight distribution along the foot, causing the arch to stretch excessively and to weaken with time. Without proper arch support, the foot begins to twist inward, or medially, causing the body weight to be transmitted to the inside of the foot rather than in a straight line toward the toes. This problem often occurs in runners who have improperly fitted shoes or a poor running style (although anyone can suffer from fallen longitudinal arches, regardless of the individual's level of physical activity). As a runner increases distance and speed without correcting his or her shoes or running form, the force applied to the feet increases. Fallen arches appear to occur particularly in runners or joggers who exercise on hard surfaces without proper technique or arch support.

A number of disorders can affect the skin of the foot. Corns are small areas of thickened skin on a toe that are usually caused by tight-fitting shoes. People with high arches are affected most because the arch increases the pressure applied to the toes during walking. If the corn becomes painful, the easiest treatment is for the person to wear better-fitting shoes. If the pain persists, a clinician can pare down the growth with a scalpel.

Plantar warts appear on the skin of the sole and are caused by a Papillomavirus. Because of pressure from the weight of the body, the plantar wart is often flattened and forced into the skin of the sole. The wart may disappear without treatment. If it persists, surgery or chemical therapy can be used to relieve the discomfort.

Athlete's foot is a common fungal infection which causes the foot to become itchy, sore, and cracked. It is usually treated with antifungal agents such as miconazole. Preventive measures including keeping the feet dry and disinfecting areas where the fungus may live, such as shower stalls.

Another common deformity is a bunion, which is a bursa (fluid-filled pad) overlying the joint at the base of the big toe. Normal structure of the first metatarsal, first phalange, and their joint is necessary to withstand the force applied to them in everyday activities. A bunion is caused by an abnormal outward projection of the joint and an inward projection of the big toe. Treatment involves correcting the position of the big toe and keeping it in a normal position. Sometimes surgery is necessary if the tissues become too swollen. In fact, some severe cases of bunions have required complete reconstruction of the toe. Unless treated, a bunion will get progressively worse.

Gout is a metabolic disorder, mainly found in men, which causes uric acid crystals to form in joints. Even though any joint can be affected, the big toe joint is likely the major site for gout because it is under chronic stress from walking. The joint is usually red, swollen, and very tender and painful. The first attack usually involves only one joint and lasts a few days. Some patients never experience another attack, but most have a second episode between six months and two years after the first. After the second attack, more joints may become involved. Treatment includes anti-inflammatory drugs and colchicine. These drugs help reduce the pain by decreasing the amount of inflammation around the joint. Physicians may also prescribe allopurinol to reduce the amount of uric acid that the body produces. Drugs are also available that increase the kidney's ability to excrete uric acid; examples of these agents are probenecid and sulfinpyrazone.

PERSPECTIVE AND PROSPECTS

Even though the feet constitute a relatively small area of the body, ailments of the feet afflict more than half the world's population. For a long time, disorders of the foot were not taken as seriously as those found in other parts of the body. It is now known, however, that poor foot health can have serious effects. For example, in children a painful foot condition not properly diagnosed and treated can result in lost school days and decreased participation in other activities. More important, an uncorrected congenital abnormality, if neglected, could have irreversible consequences. For the elderly, foot problems hinder or prevent normal activities such as taking care of personal needs, exercising, and socializing. Anything that affects the feet affects that individual's overall health and well-being.

Because of the potentially devastating problems of improper foot care, a branch of medicine developed that specifically addresses problems of the feet. Physicians known as podiatrists practice a specialized branch of medicine called podiatry. It is the job of the podiatrist to assess the cause of the foot problem and the patient's general medical condition in determining the need for and the course of treatment. This assessment often calls for contact with the patient's primary care physician for access to the patient's

medical records, as many diseases affect the whole body but present signs and symptoms in the feet. The podiatrist or other physician, such as an orthopedist, will evaluate a disorder through physical exams, laboratory tests, and anatomical tests to examine the internal structures; the latter may include X rays, computed tomography (CT) scans, or magnetic resonance imaging (MRI). The physician will then diagnose and begin treating the disorder using surgery, medical therapy, or physical therapy.

As more individuals become physically active throughout their lives, clinicians who practice sports medicine are paying closer attention to problems of the foot. Many people seek to improve their health by walking, jogging, and bicycling. All these activities have proven to be excellent for maintaining cardiovascular health, but all place additional stress on the foot. Physicians who counsel patients on physical fitness programs attempt to identify individuals who may be injury-prone. Failure to recognize an anatomical anomaly of the feet could lead to an injury or series of injuries that restrict certain activities or even cause permanent damage. Occasionally, individuals are too enthusiastic about their exercise program and experience overuse injuries involving the feet. Such injuries may cause a sudden cessation of the physical activity and may have a significant demoralizing effect on individuals who finally decide to take steps to improve their health and well-being.

People commonly neglect their feet and underemphasize the importance of the normal functional anatomy of the foot. Individuals who experience a foot injury, however, begin to appreciate the absolute importance of this rather complex but often overlooked structure.

—Matthew Berria, Ph.D.

See also Anatomy; Athlete's foot; Bones and the skeleton; Bunion removal; Cysts and ganglions; Foot disorders; Frostbite; Ganglion removal; Gout; Hammertoe correction; Heel spur removal; Lower extremities; Nail removal; Orthopedic surgery; Orthopedics; Orthopedics, pediatric; Podiatry; Sports medicine; Tendon repair; Warts.

FOR FURTHER INFORMATION:

Hales, Dianne. *An Invitation to Health*. 5th ed. Redwood City, Calif.: Benjamin/Cummings, 1992. This text should be read by anyone who wishes an overview of health topics. Chapter 7 deals with exercise and contains a section on the importance of wearing the correct shoes for a given activity.

Hole, John W., Jr., and Karen A. Koos. *Human Anatomy*. Dubuque, Iowa: Wm. C. Brown, 1991. The authors do an excellent job of describing the rather complex anatomy of the foot and lower leg in chapters 6, 7, and 8. Several views of the internal and external anatomy of the foot are given.

Mader, Sylvia S. *Human Biology*. 3d ed. Dubuque, Iowa: Wm. C. Brown, 1992. Chapter 11 provides an excellent overview of lower limb anatomy and physiology. It also addresses common medical terminology relating to foot movement.

Marieb, Elaine N. *Human Anatomy and Physiology.* 3d ed. Redwood City, Calif.: Benjamin/Cummings, 1995. This text discusses the functional significance of various anatomical structures, including the foot. Readers will enjoy the excellent pictures and diagrams of the foot and associated body parts.

Van De Graaff, Kent M. *Human Anatomy.* 4th ed. Dubuque, Iowa: Wm. C. Brown, 1992. An outstanding anatomy text which provides clinically important information in an easy-to-understand manner. Van De Graaff has taught human anatomy for years, and anyone would appreciate the approach that he has taken in presenting human structures. Chapters 7, 9, and 10 cover the anatomy of the foot and some problems that can occur if the anatomy is abnormal. Chapter 10 includes the surface anatomy of the lower leg and foot.

FETAL ALCOHOL SYNDROME
DISEASE/DISORDER

ANATOMY OR SYSTEM AFFECTED: Brain, musculoskeletal system, nervous system, reproductive system

SPECIALTIES AND RELATED FIELDS: Embryology, neonatology, obstetrics, perinatology, public health

DEFINITION: Growth retardation and mental or physical abnormalities in a child resulting from alcohol consumption by the mother during pregnancy.

Fetal alcohol syndrome was first identified in the early 1970's. Whether consumed as beer, wine, or hard liquor, alcohol is a teratogen, a toxic substance that can cause abnormalities in unborn children. The damage ranges from subtle to severe, depending on the quantity consumed and the stage of pregnancy when the exposure occurs. A critical period is in early pregnancy, when a woman may not know that she is pregnant. Even one or two drinks a day by the mother may have an effect on her child.

There are three diagnostic criteria for fetal alcohol syndrome: growth retardation, certain facial anomalies, and central nervous system impairment. Growth retardation begins in utero, causing low birth weight. Babies with low birth weight are at risk for delayed growth and development and even death. Growth impairment affects not only the skeleton but also the brain and face. The resulting head and facial abnormalities are characterized by thin lips; small, wide-set eyes; a short, upturned nose; a receding chin; and low-set ears. Fetal alcohol syndrome children have intelligence quotients (IQs) well below the mean of the population because of impaired brain growth that results in irreversible mental retardation. Fetal alcohol syndrome is a leading cause of mental retardation. Abnormalities often originate during the first trimester, when bones and organs are forming. Major organ systems such as the heart, kidney, liver, and skeleton can be impaired.

Less specific problems that result from alcohol damage are clumsiness, behavioral problems, a brief attention span, poor judgment, impaired memory, and a diminished capacity to learn from experience. These symptoms are often labeled "fetal alcohol effects."

Alcohol enters the fetal bloodstream as soon as the mother has a drink. It not only can damage the brain but also may impair the function of the placenta, which is the organ interface between maternal and fetal circulation. The exact mechanism for this damage is not completely understood. The most probable cause is that alcohol creates a glucose or oxygen deficit for the fetus. Because it is not known what dose of alcohol is safe, the best preventive measure is to abstain from alcohol during pregnancy and even when planning a pregnancy.

—*Wendy L. Stuhldreher, Ph.D., R.D.*

See also Addiction; Alcoholism; Birth defects; Childbirth; Childbirth, complications of; Embryology; Genetic diseases; Neonatology; Obstetrics; Perinatology; Pregnancy and gestation.

FETAL TISSUE TRANSPLANTATION
PROCEDURE

ANATOMY OR SYSTEM AFFECTED: Blood, brain, nervous system, pancreas, spine

SPECIALTIES AND RELATED FIELDS: Ethics, neurology

DEFINITION: The controversial use of tissue from aborted human fetuses to replace damaged tissue in patients with diseases in which the patient's own tissue has been destroyed (such as parkinsonism or diabetes mellitus).

KEY TERMS:

cannula: a narrow tube used in surgery to drain fluid or to deliver cell suspensions for a transplant

fetal: in humans, a term normally referring to the developmental period following eight weeks of gestation; in fetal tissue transplantation, refers to tissue from earlier developmental stages as well

in utero: a Latin term meaning "in the womb"

parkinsonism: a disease in which the dopamine-secreting cells of the midbrain degenerate, resulting in uncontrolled movement and rigidity

stereotaxic computed tomography: a method of imaging using a series of X rays that are compiled by a computer to give a three-dimensional image of internal structures

INDICATIONS AND PROCEDURES

Advances in technology sometimes catapult a society into ethical arenas that are not yet circumscribed by laws and clear moral boundaries. Fetal tissue transplantation is one of these advances. It is a technology that carries the hope of curing a diverse array of severe, often tragic, ailments but one that raises many difficult questions. Tissues from aborted fetuses have been shown in experimental trials to be an excellent source of replacement tissue for patients whose diseases have destroyed their own vital tissues. Parkinson's, Huntington's, and Alzheimer's diseases (in which regions of the brain deteriorate) or juvenile-onset diabetes mellitus (in which insulin-secreting cells of the pancreas degenerate) theoretically could be cured with suitable tissue replacement.

The two sources of tissue used in transplantations, donations from cadavers and from aborted fetuses, differ significantly in their suitability. Tissues from cadavers have the severe disadvantage of being immunologically rejected when grafted into anyone who is not an identical twin. The body's surveillance system that protects against infection is designed to attack and destroy any cells that carry molecular markers identifying them as foreign. Patients receiving tissue transplants from other individuals, therefore, will tolerate the tissue graft only if their immune systems are first suppressed with a battery of potent drugs, leaving the patient dangerously unarmed against infection. Fetal tissues, however, do not induce a full-scale immune response when transplanted. Fetal cells are said to be immunologically naïve since they have not yet acquired the cell surface molecular markers that are recognized by the immune system. When transplanted into a patient, they seem to be invisible to the patient's immune system and are tolerated without the use of immunosuppression.

Other properties add to the suitability of fetal tissue for transplantation. Because it is not yet fully differentiated, fetal tissue is said to be very plastic in its abilities to adapt to new locations. Moreover, once placed in a patient, it secretes factors that promote its own growth and those of the new blood vessels at the site. Tissue from an adult source does not have these properties, and consequently is slow-growing and poorly vascularized. Though growth factors can be added along with the graft, adult tissue is less responsive to these hormones than is fetal tissue.

It is the source of fetal tissue that has fired such debate over its use for transplantation. Though there has been general acceptance of using tissue from spontaneous abortions or from ectopic pregnancies which, because of their location outside of the womb, endanger the life of the mother and must be terminated, these sources are not well suited to transplantation. Spontaneous abortions rarely produce viable tissue, since in most cases the fetus has died two to three weeks before it is expelled. In addition, there are usually major genetic defects in the aborted fetus. In ectopic pregnancies as well, more than 50 percent of the fetuses are genetically abnormal, and most resolve themselves in spontaneous abortion outside a clinic setting. These types of abortions are almost always accompanied by a sense of tragic loss felt by the parents. Many researchers find it unacceptable to request permission from these parents to transplant tissue from the lost fetus.

The alternative source of fetal tissue is elected abortions. One-and-a-half million of these abortions occur in the United States every year. The debate over the ethical correctness of elected abortions has left a cloud of confusion over the issue of using this tissue for transplantation.

When an abortion is performed in a clinic, the tissue is removed by suction through a narrow tube. Normally, the tissue would be thrown away. If it is to be used for transplantation, written permission must be obtained from the woman after the abortion is completed. No discussion of transplantation is to take place prior to the abortion, and no alteration in the abortion procedure, except to keep the tissue sterile during collection, is to be made. The donor may not be paid for the tissue, and both the donor and the recipient of the tissue must remain anonymous to each other.

Once collected, the tissue is searched through to locate suitable tissue for transplantation. Normally only a small block of tissue is used, about eight cubic millimeters (the size of a thin slice of pencil eraser). The tissue is screened for infectious diseases such as hepatitis B and human immunodeficiency virus (HIV). Tissue that is collected is washed a number of times in a sterile solution to ensure that there is no bacterial contamination, and then it is maintained in a sterile, buffered salt solution until it is used. In order to increase the amount of usable tissue, the tissue may be grown in culture on a nutritive medium under carefully controlled conditions of humidity (95 percent), temperature (37 degrees Celsius), and gas (5 percent carbon dioxide in air) to stimulate normal growing conditions. Preservation of the tissue for long-term storage has been made possible by the highly refined technique of freezing the tissue in liquid nitrogen. Fetal tissue has been kept for as long as ten months in this manner before being used successfully in a transplantation. The technique should provide methods of maintaining tissue indefinitely.

The actual transplantation of the tissue is usually relatively quick and noninvasive. Often the tissue is injected into the patient as a suspension of individual cells. This permits the use of a small-bore tube called a cannula to deliver the cells to the target organ, thereby avoiding large surgical incisions. Because of modern stereotaxic imaging equipment such as computed tomography (CT) scanning and ultrasound, the physician is able to determine with extreme precision exactly where the cells are to be delivered and can visualize the position of the needle as the cells are injected. In this way, an entire region of an organ can be seeded with fetal cells. Often the patient is under only a local anesthetic. This aspect of the surgery is especially important when fetal cells are being inserted into the brain, since the physicians can then monitor the patient's ability to speak and move, to ensure that no major damage to the brain is occurring. Usually, antibiotics are given on the day of the transplantation procedure and for two additional days to avoid infection. The procedure is not dangerous, recovery is quick, and patients often go home in less than three days.

Fetal tissue transplantation is still considered an experimental procedure, and further trials are needed to fine-tune the techniques. For example, the precise age of fetal tissue that would be most effective in various cases is uncertain, though it is generally agreed that tissue from a first-trimester fetus is optimal, and it is not known which patients would respond best to the therapy. Researchers are also uncertain about whether immunosuppressive drugs should be administered. In animal trials using rats and monkeys, fetal transplants even of human tissue have been well tolerated in the absence of immunosuppression. In humans as well, fetal tissue appears to be readily accepted, with no signs of rejection, and in one study, patients did better without immunosuppression. Some surgeons, however, unwilling to risk tissue rejection, routinely give the transplant patient immunosuppressive drugs, such as cyclosporine and prednisone.

USES AND COMPLICATIONS

The major focus for fetal tissue transplantation has been the treatment of patients with Parkinson's disease, and results have been encouraging. Parkinsonism is caused by a deterioration of dopamine-secreting regions of the brain, primarily in the putamen and caudate nucleus of the midbrain. There is an accompanying loss of motor control causing tremors, rigidity, and finally paralysis, which is eventually fatal. The drugs used to treat the disorder, dopamine precursors such as L-dopa, produce side effects that cause unrelenting and uncontrolled movement of the limbs, periods in which the patient is completely frozen, and hallucinations.

Patients with parkinsonism who have received fetal tissue transplants have shown remarkable improvement and diminished requirements for drug treatment. The first case in the United States to be treated was a man with a twenty-year history of parkinsonism symptoms. He had frequent freezing spells, could not walk without a cane, and suffered from chronic constipation. He also was unable to whistle, a beloved hobby of his. He was operated on by Dr. Curt R. Freed and his associates in 1988. Following the operation, initial improvement was slow, but within a year, he was walking without a cane, his speed of movement had considerably improved, and his constipation had resolved itself. He also had regained his ability to whistle. Even after four years, improvements continued. Such results have occurred with many parkinsonism patients receiving fetal tissue transplants.

Even better results have been obtained in patients with induced Parkinson-like symptoms. In 1982, some intravenous drug users developed Parkinson-like symptoms after using a homemade preparation of "synthetic heroin" that was contaminated with 1-methyl-4-phenyl-1,2,5,6-tetrahydropyridine (MPTP). MPTP destroys dopamine-secreting cells of the substantia nigra, a region of the midbrain which communicates with the caudate nucleus and putamen. Though the region of the brain destroyed by the drug is slightly different from that of patients with parkinsonism, the manifestations of the destruction are the same. Some of these patients received fetal tissue transplants.

Within a year after their operation, they were able to walk with a normal gait, resume chores, and be virtually free of their previously uncontrollable movements.

Because no patient with parkinsonism or Parkinson-like symptoms has yet been cured by a fetal tissue transplant, some have considered the results of such experiments to be disappointing. The expectation of complete cures from a technique that is still in its early experimental phase, however, is overly optimistic. Many parkinsonism patients themselves are encouraged, and many have resumed driving and the other tasks of normal daily life.

That transplanted fetal brain tissue can replace damaged brain tissue to any extent has opened the doors of hope for many diseases. For example, Huntington's disease, a genetic disorder that destroys a different set of neurons but in the same region as that affected by parkinsonism, brings a slow death to those carrying the dominant trait. Its severe dementia and uncontrollable jerking and writhing that steadily progress have had no treatment and no cure. In animal studies in which fetal brain tissue was transplanted into rats with symptoms mimicking Huntington's disease, results have been encouraging enough to warrant human trials, and one human trial, reported by a surgeon in Mexico, has shown limited success. Researchers are hopeful, though less optimistic, that Alzheimer's disease, a form of dementia that is characterized by neuronal death within the brain, also may be treatable with fetal tissue transplants. Because the destruction is so widespread, however, it is difficult to determine where the transplants should be placed.

Type I insulin-dependent diabetes, often called juvenile-onset diabetes, also has been treated with fetal tissue transplants. More than a million people in the United States suffer from this disease caused by the destruction of pancreatic beta cells, the insulin-secreting cells that regulate sugar metabolism. Though the disease can be controlled with regular insulin shots, the long-term effects of diabetes can lead to blindness, premature aging, and renal and circulatory problems. After animal tests showed a complete reversal of the disease when fetal pancreatic tissue was transplanted into diabetic rats, human trials were initiated with great expectations. Though complete success has not been achieved, the sixteen diabetic patients who were given fetal pancreatic tissue transplants by Dr. Kevin Lafferty between 1987 and 1992 all showed significant drops in the amount of insulin needed to manage their disease. The transplanted tissue continued to pump out insulin.

An unusual variation of such procedures has been to transplant fetal tissue into fetuses diagnosed with severe metabolic diseases. It is more effective to treat the condition while the fetus is still in the womb than to wait until after birth, when damage from the disease may already be extensive. Fetuses with Hurler's syndrome and similar "storage" diseases have been treated in this way. Hurler's syndrome is a lethal condition in which tissues become clogged with stored mucupolysaccharides, long-chain sugars that the body is unable to break down because it lacks the appropriate enzyme. One of the fetuses to receive this treatment was the child of a couple who had lost two children to the disease. With the transplanted tissue, the child lived and by one year of age was producing therapeutic levels of the enzyme. It has been estimated that there are at least 155 other genetic disorders that could be similarly treated by fetal tissue transplants in utero.

The list of ailments that fetal tissue transplants may alleviate includes some of the major concerns of modern medicine. In addition to those already mentioned are sickle-cell anemia, thalassemias, metabolic disorders, immune deficiencies, myelin disorders, and spinal cord injuries. In interpreting the value of these applications, however, it is important to separate the politics of abortion from the medical issue of fetal tissue transplantation.

PERSPECTIVE AND PROSPECTS

Though controversy surrounds the use of fetal tissue for transplantation, such controversy has not included all facets of fetal tissue research. Indeed, fetal cells were used in the 1950's to develop the Salk polio vaccine and later the vaccine against rubella (German measles). With the scourge of acquired immunodeficiency syndrome (AIDS), in the 1990's fetal cells were first used to help design treatments against the AIDS virus. Even the early attempts at fetal tissue transplantation occurred quietly. Reports date as far back as 1928, when Italian surgeons attempted unsuccessfully to cure a patient with diabetes using fetal pancreatic tissue, a procedure repeated, again unsuccessfully, in the United States in 1939. In 1959, American physicians tried to cure leukemia with fetal tissue transplants, but again without success. The first real indicator that such techniques might work came in 1968, when fetal liver cells were used to treat a patient with DiGeorge syndrome. The success of this procedure resulted in its becoming the accepted treatment for this usually fatal genetic disorder.

It was not until 1987 that ethical issues over fetal tissue transplants truly surfaced in the United States. Debate was precipitated when the director of the National Institutes of Health (NIH) submitted a request to the Department of Health and Human Services to transplant fetal tissue into patients with parkinsonism. Rather than receiving approval, the request was tabled, pending a thorough study of the issue by an NIH panel on fetal tissue transplantation. The panel made a detailed report on the ethical, legal, and scientific implications of fetal tissue transplantation, concluding that it was acceptable public policy. Despite the report, however, the Secretary of Health and Human Services instituted a ban against the use of government funds for transplanting fetal tissue derived from elected abortions. While in effect, the ban influenced private funding as well. Physicians who performed fetal tissue transplants, unable to obtain grant money, were forced to charge their patients—

a bill that could reach as high as forty thousand dollars per transplant. President Bill Clinton's lifting of the ban in 1993, on his third day in office, renewed hope that rapid advances would be made in this field.

The debates over fetal tissue transplantation are far from over. Though a strict set of guidelines are in place concerning the procurement of fetal tissue, ensuring that the needs never influence decisions concerning abortion, other issues have not been addressed. Some ask whether a fetal tissue bank should be established, and if so, whether it should be government-funded to avoid commercialization. As technology continues to create increasingly complicated ethical issues, society's responsibility increases, as does its need to be scientifically informed.   —*Mary S. Tyler, Ph.D.*

See also Abortion; Alzheimer's disease; Brain; Brain disorders; Diabetes mellitus; Ethics; Genetic diseases; Genetic engineering; Neurology; Pancreas; Parkinson's disease; Transplantation.

FOR FURTHER INFORMATION:

Beardsley, Tim. "Aborting Research." *Scientific American* 267, no. 2 (August, 1992): 17-18. An excellent encapsulation of the debate over fetal tissue transplantation and the instances in which it has been used.

Freed, Curt R., Robert Breeze, and Neil Rosenberg. "Transplantation of Human Fetal Dopamine Cells for Parkinson's Disease." *Archives of Neurology* 47, no. 5 (May 1, 1990): 505-512. A historically important paper describing the techniques used by Freed, an American doctor who has been a pioneer in the technique of fetal tissue transplantation. Though written for a medical audience, most of the paper is readily understandable to a lay audience.

Lindvall, Olle, Patrik Brundin, and Håkan Widner. "Grafts of Fetal Dopamine Neurons Survive and Improve Motor Function in Parkinson's Disease." *Science* 247 (February 2, 1990): 574-577. A landmark reference describing the technique of a group of physicians led by Lindvall of Sweden. This and the paper by Freed's group (above) encompass the extent of variation in the technique, and the degrees of success.

Singer, Peter, H. Kuhse, S. Buckle, K. Dawson, and P. Kasimba, eds. *Embryo Experimentation.* Cambridge, England: Cambridge University Press, 1990. This text provides an excellent discussion of the moral questions raised by the use of fetal tissue for transplantation.

U.S. Congress. Senate. Committee on Labor and Human Resources. *Finding Medical Cures: The Promise of Fetal Tissue Transplantation Research.* 102d Congress, 1st session, 1992. Senate Report 1902. A surprisingly readable and gripping set of testimonies from physicians, interest groups, and citizens concerning the debate over the use of fetal tissue for transplantations. Interested readers can also purchase a copy from the U.S. Government Publications Office, Superintendent of Documents, Congressional Sales Office.

MAGILL'S
MEDICAL
GUIDE

ALPHABETICAL LIST OF CONTENTS

Entries by Specialties and Related Fields

Microscopy
Mutation
Oncology
Pathology
Pharmacology
Pharmacy
Sarcoma
Serology
Toxicology

DENTISTRY
Abscess drainage
Abscesses
Aging, extended care for the
Anesthesia
Anesthesiology
Caries, dental
Dental diseases
Dentistry
Endodontic disease
Forensic pathology
Fracture and dislocation
Fracture repair
Gastrointestinal system
Gingivitis
Halitosis
Head and neck disorders
Jaw wiring
Orthodontics
Periodontal surgery
Periodontitis
Plastic, cosmetic, and reconstructive
    surgery
Root canal treatment
Sense organs
Teeth
Temporomandibular joint (TMJ)
    syndrome
Tooth extraction
Toothache

DERMATOLOGY
Abscess drainage
Abscesses
Acne
Albinism
Athlete's foot
Biopsy
Burns and scalds
Carcinoma
Chickenpox
Cryotherapy and cryosurgery
Cyst removal
Cysts and ganglions

Dermatitis
Dermatology
Dermatopathology
Eczema
Electrocauterization
Fungal infections
Ganglion removal
Glands
Grafts and grafting
Hair loss and baldness
Hair transplantation
Healing
Histology
Itching
Keratoses
Laser use in surgery
Lice, mites, and ticks
Light therapy
Lupus erythematosus
Malignant melanoma removal
Nail removal
Neurofibromatosis
Pigmentation
Pimples
Plastic, cosmetic, and reconstructive
    surgery
Podiatry
Poisonous plants
Psoriasis
Puberty and adolescence
Rashes
Rosacea
Scabies
Sense organs
Skin
Skin cancer
Skin disorders
Skin lesion removal
Tattoo removal
Touch
Warts

EMBRYOLOGY
Abortion
Amniocentesis
Birth defects
Brain disorders
Cerebral palsy
Chorionic villus sampling
Cloning
Conception
Down syndrome
Embryology
Fetal alcohol syndrome

Genetic counseling
Genetic diseases
Genetics and inheritance
Growth
In vitro fertilization
Miscarriage
Multiple births
Obstetrics
Pregnancy and gestation
Reproductive system
Rh factor
Rubella
Sexual differentiation
Spina bifida
Toxoplasmosis
Ultrasonography

EMERGENCY MEDICINE
Abdominal disorders
Abscess drainage
Aging
Altitude sickness
Amputation
Anesthesia
Anesthesiology
Aneurysms
Angiography
Appendectomy
Appendicitis
Asphyxiation
Bites and stings
Bleeding
Botulism
Burns and scalds
Cardiology
Cardiology, pediatric
Catheterization
Cesarean section
Choking
Coma
Computed tomography (CT) scanning
Concussion
Critical care
Critical care, pediatric
Diphtheria
Dizziness and fainting
Domestic violence
Electrical shock
Electrocardiography (ECG or EKG)
Electroencephalography (EEG)
Emergency medicine
Food poisoning
Fracture and dislocation
Frostbite

Influenza
Intestinal disorders
Laryngitis
Measles, red
Mitral insufficiency
Mononucleosis
Motion sickness
Mumps
Muscle sprains, spasms, and disorders
Nasal polyp removal
Nasopharyngeal disorders
Nutrition
Obesity
Osgood-Schlatter disease
Osteopathic medicine
Pain, types of
Parasitic diseases
Pediatrics
Pertussis
Pharmacology
Pharmacy
Pharyngitis
Physical examination
Physician assistants
Pimples
Pneumonia
Poisonous plants
Psychiatry
Psychiatry, child and adolescent
Psychiatry, geriatric
Puberty and adolescence
Rashes
Rheumatic fever
Rubella
Rubeola
Scabies
Scarlet fever
Sciatica
Sexuality
Shingles
Shock
Sibling rivalry
Sinusitis
Skin disorders
Sore throat
Sports medicine
Sterilization
Strep throat
Stress
Temporomandibular joint (TMJ)
   syndrome
Tetanus
Tonsillitis
Toxicology

Ulcers
Urology
Vascular medicine
Vasectomy
Viral infections
Vitamins and minerals
Wounds

FORENSIC MEDICINE
Autopsy
Blood and blood components
Blood testing
Bones and the skeleton
Cytopathology
Dermatopathology
DNA and RNA
Forensic pathology
Genetics and inheritance
Hematology
Histology
Immunopathology
Laboratory tests
Law and medicine
Pathology

GASTROENTEROLOGY
Abdomen
Abdominal disorders
Appendectomy
Appendicitis
Bulimia
Bypass surgery
Cholecystectomy
Cholecystitis
Cholera
Colitis
Colon and rectal polyp removal
Colon and rectal surgery
Colon cancer
Colonoscopy
Computed tomography (CT) scanning
Constipation
Crohn's disease
Critical care
Critical care, pediatric
Cytomegalovirus (CMV)
Diarrhea and dysentery
Digestion
Diverticulitis and diverticulosis
E. coli infection
Emergency medicine
Endoscopy
Enemas
Enzymes

Fistula repair
Food biochemistry
Food poisoning
Gallbladder diseases
Gastrectomy
Gastroenterology
Gastroenterology, pediatric
Gastrointestinal disorders
Gastrointestinal system
Gastrostomy
Glands
Heartburn
Hemorrhoid banding and removal
Hemorrhoids
Hernia
Hernia repair
Ileostomy and colostomy
Indigestion
Internal medicine
Intestinal disorders
Intestines
Lactose intolerance
Laparoscopy
Liver
Liver cancer
Liver disorders
Liver transplantation
Malnutrition
Metabolism
Nausea and vomiting
Nutrition
Obstruction
Pancreas
Pancreatitis
Peristalsis
Poisonous plants
Proctology
Roundworm
Salmonella
Shigellosis
Stomach, intestinal, and pancreatic
   cancers
Stone removal
Stones
Tapeworm
Taste
Trichinosis
Ulcer surgery
Ulcers
Vagotomy
Weight loss and gain
Worms

GENERAL SURGERY

Abscess drainage
Adrenalectomy
Amputation
Anesthesia
Anesthesiology
Aneurysmectomy
Appendectomy
Biopsy
Bone marrow transplantation
Breast augmentation, reduction, and
  reconstruction
Breast biopsy
Bunion removal
Bypass surgery
Cataract surgery
Catheterization
Cervical procedures
Cesarean section
Cholecystectomy
Circumcision, female, and genital
  mutilation
Circumcision, male
Cleft lip and palate repair
Colon and rectal polyp removal
Colon and rectal surgery
Corneal transplantation
Craniotomy
Cryotherapy and cryosurgery
Cyst removal
Cystectomy
Disk removal
Ear surgery
Electrocauterization
Endarterectomy
Endometrial biopsy
Eye surgery
Face lift and blepharoplasty
Fistula repair
Ganglion removal
Gastrectomy
Grafts and grafting
Hair transplantation
Hammertoe correction
Heart transplantation
Heart valve replacement
Heel spur removal
Hemorrhoid banding and removal
Hernia repair
Hydrocelectomy
Hypospadias repair and urethroplasty
Hysterectomy
Kidney transplantation
Kneecap removal

Laceration repair
Laminectomy and spinal fusion
Laparoscopy
Laryngectomy
Laser use in surgery
Liposuction
Liver transplantation
Lung surgery
Malignant melanoma removal
Mastectomy and lumpectomy
Myomectomy
Nail removal
Nasal polyp removal
Nephrectomy
Neurosurgery
Oncology
Ophthalmology
Orthopedic surgery
Parathyroidectomy
Penile implant surgery
Periodontal surgery
Phlebitis
Plastic, cosmetic, and reconstructive
  surgery
Prostate gland removal
Rhinoplasty and submucous resection
Sex change surgery
Shunts
Skin lesion removal
Sphincterectomy
Splenectomy
Sterilization
Stone removal
Surgery, general
Surgery, pediatric
Surgical procedures
Surgical technologists
Sympathectomy
Tattoo removal
Tendon repair
Testicular surgery
Thoracic surgery
Thyroidectomy
Tonsillectomy and adenoid removal
Tracheostomy
Transfusion
Transplantation
Tumor removal
Ulcer surgery
Vagotomy
Varicose vein removal
Vasectomy

GENETICS

Aging
Albinism
Alzheimer's disease
Amniocentesis
Attention-deficit disorder (ADD)
Autoimmune disorders
Bionics and biotechnology
Birth defects
Bone marrow transplantation
Breast cancer
Breast disorders
Chorionic villus sampling
Cloning
Color blindness
Colon cancer
Cystic fibrosis
Diabetes mellitus
DNA and RNA
Down syndrome
Dwarfism
Embryology
Endocrinology
Endocrinology, pediatric
Enzymes
Gene therapy
Genetic counseling
Genetic diseases
Genetic engineering
Genetics and inheritance
Grafts and grafting
Hematology
Hematology, pediatric
Hemophilia
Immunodeficiency disorders
In vitro fertilization
Laboratory tests
Mental retardation
Muscular dystrophy
Mutation
Neonatology
Nephrology
Nephrology, pediatric
Neurofibromatosis
Neurology
Neurology, pediatric
Obstetrics
Oncology
Pediatrics
Phenylketonuria (PKU)
Porphyria
Reproductive system
Rh factor
Screening

Sexual differentiation
Sexuality
Tay-Sachs disease
Transplantation

**GERIATRICS AND
    GERONTOLOGY**
Aging
Aging, extended care for the
Alzheimer's disease
Arthritis
Bed-wetting
Blindness
Bone disorders
Bones and the skeleton
Brain disorders
Cataract surgery
Cataracts
Critical care
Death and dying
Dementia
Depression
Domestic violence
Emergency medicine
Endocrinology
Estrogen replacement therapy
Euthanasia
Family practice
Fatigue
Fracture and dislocation
Fracture repair
Hearing loss
Hip fracture repair
Hormone replacement therapy
Hormones
Hospitals
Incontinence
Memory loss
Nursing
Nutrition
Ophthalmology
Orthopedics
Osteoporosis
Pain management
Paramedics
Parkinson's disease
Pharmacology
Physician assistants
Psychiatry
Psychiatry, geriatric
Rheumatology
Sleep disorders
Spinal disorders
Spine, vertebrae, and disks

Suicide
Visual disorders

GYNECOLOGY
Abortion
Amenorrhea
Amniocentesis
Biopsy
Breast biopsy
Breast cancer
Breast disorders
Breast-feeding
Breasts, female
Cervical, ovarian, and uterine cancers
Cervical procedures
Cesarean section
Childbirth
Childbirth, complications of
Chlamydia
Circumcision, female, and genital
    mutilation
Conception
Contraception
Culdocentesis
Cyst removal
Cystectomy
Cystitis
Cysts and ganglions
Dysmenorrhea
Electrocauterization
Endocrinology
Endometrial biopsy
Endometriosis
Endoscopy
Episiotomy
Genital disorders, female
Glands
Gonorrhea
Gynecology
Herpes
Hormone replacement therapy
Hormones
Hysterectomy
In vitro fertilization
Incontinence
Infertility in females
Internal medicine
Laparoscopy
Mammography
Mastectomy and lumpectomy
Mastitis
Menopause
Menorrhagia
Menstruation

Myomectomy
Nutrition
Obstetrics
Ovarian cysts
Pelvic inflammatory disease (PID)
Peritonitis
Postpartum depression
Pregnancy and gestation
Premenstrual syndrome (PMS)
Reproductive system
Sex change surgery
Sexual differentiation
Sexual dysfunction
Sexuality
Sexually transmitted diseases
Sterilization
Syphilis
Tubal ligation
Ultrasonography
Urethritis
Urinary disorders
Urology
Warts

HEMATOLOGY
Acid-base chemistry
Acquired immunodeficiency syndrome
    (AIDS)
Anemia
Bleeding
Blood and blood components
Blood testing
Bone grafting
Bone marrow transplantation
Cholesterol
Circulation
Cytology
Cytomegalovirus (CMV)
Cytopathology
Dialysis
Fluids and electrolytes
Forensic pathology
Healing
Hematology
Hematology, pediatric
Hemophilia
Histology
Hodgkin's disease
Host-defense mechanisms
Hypercholesterolemia
Hyperlipidemia
Hypoglycemia
Immune system
Immunology

Infection
Ischemia
Jaundice
Kidneys
Laboratory tests
Leukemia
Liver
Lymphadenopathy and lymphoma
Lymphatic system
Malaria
Nephrology
Nephrology, pediatric
Rh factor
Septicemia
Serology
Sickle-cell anemia
Thalassemia
Thrombolytic therapy and TPA
Thrombosis and thrombus
Toxemia
Transfusion
Vascular medicine
Vascular system

HISTOLOGY
Autopsy
Biopsy
Cancer
Carcinoma
Cells
Cytology
Cytopathology
Dermatology
Dermatopathology
Fluids and electrolytes
Forensic pathology
Healing
Histology
Laboratory tests
Malignant melanoma removal
Microscopy
Pathology
Tumor removal
Tumors

IMMUNOLOGY
Acquired immunodeficiency syndrome
  (AIDS)
Allergies
Antibiotics
Asthma
Autoimmune disorders
Bacterial infections
Bionics and biotechnology

Bites and stings
Blood and blood components
Bone cancer
Bone grafting
Bone marrow transplantation
Breast cancer
Cancer
Carcinoma
Candidiasis
Cervical, ovarian, and uterine cancers
Childhood infectious diseases
Chronic fatigue syndrome
Colon cancer
Cytology
Cytomegalovirus (CMV)
Dermatology
Dermatopathology
Endocrinology
Endocrinology, pediatric
Enzyme therapy
Fungal infections
Grafts and grafting
Healing
Hematology
Hematology, pediatric
Homeopathy
Host-defense mechanisms
Human immunodeficiency virus (HIV)
Hypnosis
Immune system
Immunization and vaccination
Immunodeficiency disorders
Immunology
Immunopathology
Laboratory tests
Leprosy
Liver cancer
Lung cancer
Lupus erythematosus
Lymphatic system
Microbiology
Oncology
Oxygen therapy
Pancreas
Prostate cancer
Pulmonary diseases
Pulmonary medicine
Pulmonary medicine, pediatric
Rheumatology
Sarcoma
Serology
Skin cancer
Stomach, intestinal, and pancreatic
  cancers

Stress
Stress reduction
Transfusion
Transplantation
Tropical medicine

INTERNAL MEDICINE
Abdomen
Abdominal disorders
Anatomy
Anemia
Angina
Anxiety
Arrhythmias
Arteriosclerosis
Autoimmune disorders
Bacterial infections
Beriberi
Biofeedback
Bleeding
Bronchitis
Bursitis
Candidiasis
Chickenpox
Childhood infectious diseases
Cholecystitis
Cholesterol
Chronic fatigue syndrome
Cirrhosis
Claudication
Cluster headaches
Colitis
Colonoscopy
Common cold
Constipation
Coughing
Crohn's disease
Diabetes mellitus
Dialysis
Diarrhea and dysentery
Digestion
Diverticulitis and diverticulosis
Dizziness and fainting
Domestic violence
E. coli infection
Edema
Embolism
Emphysema
Endocarditis
Endoscopy
Factitious disorders
Family practice
Fatigue
Fever

Fungal infections
Gallbladder diseases
Gangrene
Gastroenterology
Gastroenterology, pediatric
Gastrointestinal disorders
Gastrointestinal system
Genetic diseases
Geriatrics and gerontology
Glomerulonephritis
Goiter
Gout
Guillain-Barré syndrome
Hanta virus
Headaches
Heart
Heart attack
Heart disease
Heart failure
Heartburn
Heat exhaustion and heat stroke
Hepatitis
Hernia
Histology
Hodgkin's disease
Human immunodeficiency virus (HIV)
Hypercholesterolemia
Hyperlipidemia
Hypertension
Hyperthermia and hypothermia
Hypertrophy
Hypoglycemia
Incontinence
Indigestion
Infection
Inflammation
Influenza
Internal medicine
Intestinal disorders
Intestines
Ischemia
Itching
Jaundice
Kaposi's sarcoma
Kidney disorders
Kidneys
Legionnaires' disease
Leprosy
Leukemia
Liver
Liver disorders
Lupus erythematosus
Lyme disease
Lymphadenopathy and lymphoma

Malignancy and metastasis
Mitral insufficiency
Mononucleosis
Motion sickness
Multiple sclerosis
Nephritis
Nephrology
Nephrology, pediatric
Nuclear medicine
Nutrition
Obesity
Occupational health
Osteopathic medicine
Paget's disease
Pain, types of
Palpitations
Pancreas
Pancreatitis
Parasitic diseases
Parkinson's disease
Peristalsis
Peritonitis
Pertussis
Pharyngitis
Phlebitis
Physical examination
Physician assistants
Physiology
Pneumonia
Proctology
Psoriasis
Puberty and adolescence
Pulmonary medicine
Pulmonary medicine, pediatric
Radiopharmaceuticals, use of
Rashes
Renal failure
Reye's syndrome
Rheumatic fever
Rheumatoid arthritis
Roundworm
Rubella
Rubeola
Scarlet fever
Schistosomiasis
Sciatica
Scurvy
Septicemia
Sexuality
Sexually transmitted diseases
Shingles
Shock
Sickle-cell anemia
Sports medicine

Staphylococcal infections
Stone removal
Stones
Streptococcal infections
Stress
Tapeworm
Tetanus
Thrombosis and thrombus
Toxemia
Tumor removal
Tumors
Ulcer surgery
Ulcers
Ultrasonography
Viral infections
Vitamins and minerals
Worms
Wounds

MICROBIOLOGY
Abscesses
Antibiotics
Autopsy
Bacterial infections
Bacteriology
Bionics and biotechnology
Drug resistance
E. coli infection
Epidemiology
Fungal infections
Gangrene
Gastroenterology
Gastroenterology, pediatric
Gastrointestinal disorders
Gastrointestinal system
Genetic engineering
Gram staining
Immune system
Immunization and vaccination
Immunology
Laboratory tests
Microbiology
Microscopy
Pathology
Pharmacology
Pharmacy
Protozoan diseases
Serology
Smallpox
Toxicology
Tropical medicine
Tuberculosis
Urinalysis
Urology

Urology, pediatric
Viral infections

NEONATOLOGY
Birth defects
Cardiology, pediatric
Cesarean section
Childbirth
Childbirth, complications of
Chlamydia
Cleft lip and palate repair
Cleft palate
Congenital heart disease
Critical care, pediatric
Cystic fibrosis
Down syndrome
E. coli infection
Endocrinology, pediatric
Fetal alcohol syndrome
Gastroenterology, pediatric
Genetic diseases
Genetics and inheritance
Hematology, pediatric
Hydrocephalus
Jaundice
Multiple births
Neonatology
Nephrology, pediatric
Neurology, pediatric
Nursing
Obstetrics
Orthopedics, pediatric
Pediatrics
Perinatology
Phenylketonuria (PKU)
Physician assistants
Premature birth
Pulmonary medicine, pediatric
Rh factor
Shunts
Sudden infant death syndrome (SIDS)
Surgery, pediatric
Tay-Sachs disease
Toxoplasmosis
Transfusion
Tropical medicine
Urology, pediatric

NEPHROLOGY
Abdomen
Cysts and ganglions
Diabetes mellitus
Dialysis
E. coli infection

Edema
Glomerulonephritis
Internal medicine
Kidney disorders
Kidney transplantation
Kidneys
Lithotripsy
Nephrectomy
Nephritis
Nephrology
Nephrology, pediatric
Renal failure
Stone removal
Stones
Transplantation
Urinalysis
Urinary disorders
Urinary system
Urology
Urology, pediatric

NEUROLOGY
Altitude sickness
Alzheimer's disease
Amnesia
Anesthesia
Anesthesiology
Aneurysmectomy
Aneurysms
Aphasia and dysphasia
Apnea
Ataxia
Attention-deficit disorder (ADD)
Audiology
Bell's palsy
Biofeedback
Biophysics
Brain
Brain disorders
Carpal tunnel syndrome
Cerebral palsy
Chiropractic
Chronobiology
Claudication
Cluster headaches
Concussion
Craniotomy
Creutzfeldt-Jakob disease and mad cow disease
Critical care
Critical care, pediatric
Cysts and ganglions
Dementia
Disk removal

Dizziness and fainting
Dyslexia
Ear infections and disorders
Ears
Electrical shock
Electroconvulsive therapy
Electroencephalography (EEG)
Emergency medicine
Emotions, biomedical causes and effects of
Encephalitis
Epilepsy
Fetal tissue transplantation
Grafts and grafting
Guillain-Barré syndrome
Hallucinations
Head and neck disorders
Headaches
Hearing loss
Hemiplegia
Learning disabilities
Lower extremities
Lumbar puncture
Melatonin
Memory loss
Ménière's disease
Meningitis
Migraine headaches
Motor neuron diseases
Multiple sclerosis
Narcolepsy
Nervous system
Neuralgia, neuritis, and neuropathy
Neurofibromatosis
Neurology
Neurology, pediatric
Neurosurgery
Numbness and tingling
Otorhinolaryngology
Pain, types of
Palsy
Paralysis
Paraplegia
Parkinson's disease
Phenylketonuria (PKU)
Physical examination
Poliomyelitis
Porphyria
Prion diseases
Psychiatry
Psychiatry, child and adolescent
Psychiatry, geriatric
Quadriplegia
Rabies

Reye's syndrome
Sciatica
Seizures
Sense organs
Skin
Sleep disorders
Smell
Snakebites
Spina bifida
Spinal disorders
Spine, vertebrae, and disks
Strokes and TIAs
Stuttering
Sympathectomy
Taste
Tay-Sachs disease
Tetanus
Tics
Touch
Trembling and shaking
Unconsciousness
Upper extremities
Vagotomy

NUCLEAR MEDICINE
Biophysics
Imaging and radiology
Invasive tests
Magnetic resonance imaging (MRI)
Noninvasive tests
Nuclear medicine
Nuclear radiology
Positron emission tomography (PET)
    scanning
Radiation therapy
Radiopharmaceuticals, use of

NURSING
Aging, extended care for the
Allied health
Anesthesiology
Cardiac rehabilitation
Critical care
Critical care, pediatric
Emergency medicine
Geriatrics and gerontology
Holistic medicine
Hospitals
Immunization and vaccination
Neonatology
Noninvasive tests
Nursing
Nutrition
Pediatrics

Physical examination
Physician assistants
Surgery, general
Surgery, pediatric
Surgical procedures
Surgical technologists

NUTRITION
Aging, extended care for the
Anorexia nervosa
Beriberi
Breast-feeding
Bulimia
Cardiac rehabilitation
Cholesterol
Digestion
Eating disorders
Enzyme therapy
Exercise physiology
Food biochemistry
Gastroenterology
Gastroenterology, pediatric
Gastrointestinal disorders
Gastrointestinal system
Geriatrics and gerontology
Hypercholesterolemia
Jaw wiring
Kwashiorkor
Lactose intolerance
Lipids
Malnutrition
Metabolism
Nursing
Nutrition
Obesity
Osteoporosis
Scurvy
Sports medicine
Taste
Tropical medicine
Ulcers
Vagotomy
Vitamins and minerals
Weight loss and gain

OBSTETRICS
Amniocentesis
Birth defects
Breast-feeding
Breasts, female
Cervical, ovarian, and uterine cancers
Cesarean section
Childbirth
Childbirth, complications of

Chorionic villus sampling
Conception
Cytomegalovirus (CMV)
Down syndrome
Eclampsia
Ectopic pregnancy
Embryology
Emergency medicine
Episiotomy
Family practice
Fetal alcohol syndrome
Genetic counseling
Genetic diseases
Genetics and inheritance
Genital disorders, female
Gonorrhea
Growth
Gynecology
In vitro fertilization
Incontinence
Invasive tests
Miscarriage
Multiple births
Neonatology
Noninvasive tests
Obstetrics
Perinatology
Postpartum depression
Pregnancy and gestation
Premature birth
Reproductive system
Rh factor
Rubella
Sexuality
Spina bifida
Stillbirth
Toxoplasmosis
Ultrasonography
Urology

OCCUPATIONAL HEALTH
Altitude sickness
Asphyxiation
Biofeedback
Cardiac rehabilitation
Carpal tunnel syndrome
Environmental diseases
Environmental health
Hearing loss
Interstitial pulmonary fibrosis (IPF)
Lead poisoning
Lung cancer
Lungs
Nasopharyngeal disorders

ORTHOPEDICS

Amputation
Arthritis
Arthroplasty
Arthroscopy
Bone cancer
Bone disorders
Bone grafting
Bones and the skeleton
Bunion removal
Bursitis
Cancer
Chiropractic
Disk removal
Dwarfism
Feet
Foot disorders
Fracture and dislocation
Fracture repair
Geriatrics and gerontology
Growth
Hammertoe correction
Heel spur removal
Hip fracture repair
Jaw wiring
Kinesiology
Kneecap removal
Laminectomy and spinal fusion
Lower extremities
Muscle sprains, spasms, and disorders
Muscles
Neurofibromatosis
Orthopedic surgery
Orthopedics
Orthopedics, pediatric
Osgood-Schlatter disease
Osteopathic medicine
Osteoarthritis
Osteoporosis
Paget's disease
Physical examination
Physical rehabilitation
Podiatry
Rheumatoid arthritis
Rheumatology
Scoliosis
Slipped disk
Spina bifida
Spinal disorders
Spine, vertebrae, and disks
Sports medicine
Tendon disorders
Tendon repair
Upper extremities

OSTEOPATHIC MEDICINE

Alternative medicine
Bones and the skeleton
Exercise physiology
Family practice
Holistic medicine
Muscle sprains, spasms, and disorders
Muscles
Nutrition
Osteopathic medicine
Physical rehabilitation

OTORHINOLARYNGOLOGY

Aromatherapy
Audiology
Cleft lip and palate repair
Cleft palate
Common cold
Ear infections and disorders
Ear surgery
Ears
Gastrointestinal system
Halitosis
Head and neck disorders
Hearing loss
Laryngectomy
Laryngitis
Ménière's disease
Motion sickness
Nasal polyp removal
Nasopharyngeal disorders
Nausea and vomiting
Otorhinolaryngology
Pharyngitis
Pulmonary diseases
Pulmonary medicine
Pulmonary medicine, pediatric
Respiration
Rhinitis
Rhinoplasty and submucous resection
Sinusitis
Sore throat
Strep throat
Sense organs
Smell
Taste
Tonsillectomy and adenoid removal
Tonsillitis
Voice and vocal cord disorders

PATHOLOGY

Autopsy
Bacteriology
Biopsy

Blood testing
Cancer
Cytology
Cytopathology
Dermatopathology
Disease
Electroencephalography (EEG)
Epidemiology
Forensic pathology
Hematology
Hematology, pediatric
Histology
Homeopathy
Immunopathology
Inflammation
Laboratory tests
Malignancy and metastasis
Microbiology
Microscopy
Mutation
Noninvasive tests
Oncology
Pathology
Prion diseases
Serology
Toxicology

PEDIATRICS

Acne
Amenorrhea
Appendectomy
Appendicitis
Attention-deficit disorder (ADD)
Bed-wetting
Birth defects
Bulimia
Cardiology, pediatric
Chickenpox
Childhood infectious diseases
Cholera
Circumcision, female, and genital
  mutilation
Circumcision, male
Cleft lip and palate repair
Cleft palate
Congenital heart disease
Critical care, pediatric
Cystic fibrosis
Cytomegalovirus (CMV)
Diabetes mellitus
Diarrhea and dysentery
Domestic violence
Down syndrome
Dwarfism

Emergency medicine
Endocrinology, pediatric
Family practice
Fever
Fistula repair
Gastroenterology, pediatric
Genetic diseases
Genetics and inheritance
Gigantism
Growth
Hematology, pediatric
Hormones
Hydrocephalus
Hypospadias repair and urethroplasty
Kwashiorkor
Learning disabilities
Malnutrition
Measles, red
Menstruation
Multiple births
Multiple sclerosis
Mumps
Muscular dystrophy
Neonatology
Nephrology, pediatric
Neurology, pediatric
Nursing
Nutrition
Orthopedics, pediatric
Osgood-Schlatter disease
Otorhinolaryngology
Pediatrics
Perinatology
Pertussis
Phenylketonuria (PKU)
Pimples
Poliomyelitis
Porphyria
Premature birth
Psychiatry, child and adolescent
Puberty and adolescence
Pulmonary medicine, pediatric
Reye's syndrome
Rheumatic fever
Rickets
Roseola
Roundworm
Rubella
Rubeola
Scarlet fever
Seizures
Sexuality
Sibling rivalry
Sore throat

Stammering
Steroids
Strep throat
Streptococcal infections
Sudden infant death syndrome (SIDS)
Surgery, pediatric
Tapeworm
Tay-Sachs disease
Tonsillectomy and adenoid removal
Tropical medicine
Urology, pediatric
Worms

PERINATOLOGY
Amniocentesis
Birth defects
Breast-feeding
Cesarean section
Childbirth
Childbirth, complications of
Chorionic villus sampling
Critical care, pediatric
Embryology
Fetal alcohol syndrome
Hematology, pediatric
Hydrocephalus
Neonatology
Neurology, pediatric
Nursing
Obstetrics
Pediatrics
Perinatology
Pregnancy and gestation
Premature birth
Shunts
Stillbirth
Sudden infant death syndrome (SIDS)

PHARMACOLOGY
Acid-base chemistry
Aging, extended care for the
Anesthesia
Anesthesiology
Antibiotics
Bacteriology
Chemotherapy
Critical care
Critical care, pediatric
Digestion
Drug resistance
Emergency medicine
Enzymes
Fluids and electrolytes
Food biochemistry

Genetic engineering
Geriatrics and gerontology
Glycolysis
Herbal medicine
Homeopathy
Hormones
Laboratory tests
Melatonin
Metabolism
Narcotics
Oncology
Pain management
Pharmacology
Pharmacy
Psychiatry
Psychiatry, child and adolescent
Psychiatry, geriatric
Rheumatology
Sports medicine
Steroids
Thrombolytic therapy and TPA
Toxicology
Tropical medicine

PHYSICAL THERAPY
Aging, extended care for the
Amputation
Arthritis
Bell's palsy
Biofeedback
Burns and scalds
Cardiac rehabilitation
Cerebral palsy
Disk removal
Exercise physiology
Grafts and grafting
Hemiplegia
Hydrotherapy
Kinesiology
Lower extremities
Muscle sprains, spasms, and disorders
Muscles
Muscular dystrophy
Neurology
Neurology, pediatric
Numbness and tingling
Orthopedic surgery
Orthopedics
Orthopedics, pediatric
Osteopathic medicine
Osteoporosis
Pain management
Palsy
Paralysis

Paraplegia
Parkinson's disease
Physical examination
Physical rehabilitation
Plastic, cosmetic, and reconstructive
  surgery
Quadriplegia
Rickets
Scoliosis
Slipped disk
Spina bifida
Spinal disorders
Spine, vertebrae, and disks
Sports medicine
Tendon disorders
Upper extremities

**PLASTIC, COSMETIC, AND
  RECONSTRUCTIVE SURGERY**
Aging
Amputation
Breast augmentation, reduction, and
  reconstruction
Breast cancer
Breast disorders
Breasts, female
Burns and scalds
Cancer
Carcinoma
Circumcision, female, and genital
  mutilation
Circumcision, male
Cleft lip and palate repair
Cleft palate
Cyst removal
Cysts and ganglions
Face lift and blepharoplasty
Grafts and grafting
Hair loss and baldness
Hair transplantation
Healing
Jaw wiring
Laceration repair
Liposuction
Malignancy and metastasis
Malignant melanoma removal
Neurofibromatosis
Obesity
Otorhinolaryngology
Plastic, cosmetic, and reconstructive
  surgery
Rhinoplasty and submucous resection
Sex change surgery
Skin

Skin lesion removal
Surgical procedures
Varicose vein removal
Varicosis

PODIATRY
Athlete's foot
Bone disorders
Bones and the skeleton
Bunion removal
Feet
Foot disorders
Fungal infections
Hammertoe correction
Heel spur removal
Lower extremities
Nail removal
Orthopedic surgery
Orthopedics
Physical examination
Podiatry
Tendon disorders
Tendon repair
Warts

PREVENTIVE MEDICINE
Acupuncture
Acupressure
Aging, extended care for the
Alternative medicine
Aromatherapy
Biofeedback
Cardiology
Chiropractic
Cholesterol
Chronobiology
Disease
Electrocardiography (ECG or EKG)
Environmental health
Exercise physiology
Family practice
Genetic counseling
Geriatrics and gerontology
Holistic medicine
Host-defense mechanisms
Hypercholesterolemia
Immune system
Immunization and vaccination
Immunology
Mammography
Meditation
Melatonin
Noninvasive tests
Nursing

Nutrition
Occupational health
Osteopathic medicine
Pharmacology
Pharmacy
Physical examination
Preventive medicine
Psychiatry
Psychiatry, child and adolescent
Psychiatry, geriatric
Qi gong
Screening
Serology
Spine, vertebrae, and disks
Sports medicine
Stress
Stress reduction
Tai Chi Chuan
Tropical medicine
Yoga

PROCTOLOGY
Colon and rectal polyp removal
Colon and rectal surgery
Colon cancer
Colonoscopy
Crohn's disease
Cystectomy
Diverticulitis and diverticulosis
Endoscopy
Fistula repair
Gastroenterology
Gastrointestinal disorders
Gastrointestinal system
Genital disorders, male
Geriatrics and gerontology
Hemorrhoid banding and removal
Hemorrhoids
Internal medicine
Intestinal disorders
Intestines
Physical examination
Proctology
Prostate cancer
Prostate gland
Prostate gland removal
Reproductive system
Urology

PSYCHIATRY
Addiction
Aging
Aging, extended care for the
Alcoholism

Alzheimer's disease
Amnesia
Anorexia nervosa
Anxiety
Attention-deficit disorder (ADD)
Autism
Brain
Brain disorders
Breast augmentation, reduction, and
    reconstruction
Bulimia
Chronic fatigue syndrome
Circumcision, female, and genital
    mutilation
Dementia
Depression
Domestic violence
Eating disorders
Electroconvulsive therapy
Electroencephalography (EEG)
Emergency medicine
Emotions, biomedical causes and
    effects of
Factitious disorders
Family practice
Fatigue
Grief and guilt
Gynecology
Hallucinations
Hypnosis
Hypochondriasis
Incontinence
Intoxication
Light therapy
Manic-depressive disorder
Memory loss
Mental retardation
Midlife crisis
Neurosis
Neurosurgery
Obesity
Obsessive-compulsive disorder
Pain management
Pain, types of
Panic attacks
Paranoia
Penile implant surgery
Phobias
Postpartum depression
Psychiatric disorders
Psychiatry
Psychiatry, child and adolescent
Psychiatry, geriatric
Psychoanalysis

Psychosis
Psychosomatic disorders
Schizophrenia
Sex change surgery
Sexual dysfunction
Sexuality
Sleep disorders
Speech disorders
Stress
Stress reduction
Sudden infant death syndrome (SIDS)
Suicide

PSYCHOLOGY
Addiction
Aging
Aging, extended care for the
Alcoholism
Amnesia
Anorexia nervosa
Anxiety
Aromatherapy
Attention-deficit disorder (ADD)
Bed-wetting
Biofeedback
Brain
Bulimia
Cardiac rehabilitation
Cirrhosis
Death and dying
Depression
Domestic violence
Dyslexia
Eating disorders
Electroencephalography (EEG)
Emotions, biomedical causes and
    effects of
Environmental health
Factitious disorders
Family practice
Forensic pathology
Genetic counseling
Grief and guilt
Gynecology
Hallucinations
Holistic medicine
Hormone replacement therapy
Hypnosis
Hypochondriasis
Kinesiology
Learning disabilities
Light therapy
Manic-depressive disorder
Meditation

Memory loss
Mental retardation
Midlife crisis
Neurosis
Nutrition
Obesity
Obsessive-compulsive disorder
Occupational health
Pain management
Panic attacks
Paranoia
Phobias
Plastic, cosmetic, and reconstructive
    surgery
Postpartum depression
Psychosomatic disorders
Puberty and adolescence
Sex change surgery
Sexual dysfunction
Sexuality
Sibling rivalry
Sleep disorders
Speech disorders
Sports medicine
Stammering
Stillbirth
Stress
Stress reduction
Stuttering
Sudden infant death syndrome (SIDS)
Suicide
Temporomandibular joint (TMJ)
    syndrome
Tics
Weight loss and gain
Yoga

PUBLIC HEALTH
Acquired immunodeficiency syndrome
    (AIDS)
Aging, extended care for the
Allied health
Alternative medicine
Arthropod-borne diseases
Bacteriology
Beriberi
Biostatistics
Blood bank
Blood testing
Botulism
Chickenpox
Childhood infectious diseases
Chlamydia
Cholera

Common cold
Creutzfeldt-Jakob disease and
    mad cow disease
Dermatology
Diarrhea and dysentery
Diphtheria
Domestic violence
Drug resistance
E. coli infection
Ebola virus
Elephantiasis
Emergency medicine
Environmental diseases
Epidemiology
Fetal alcohol syndrome
Food poisoning
Forensic pathology
Gonorrhea
Hanta virus
Hepatitis
Hospitals
Human immunodeficiency virus (HIV)
Immunization and vaccination
Influenza
Kwashiorkor
Lead poisoning
Legionnaires' disease
Leishmaniasis
Leprosy
Lice, mites, and ticks
Lyme disease
Malaria
Malnutrition
Measles, red
Medicare
Meningitis
Microbiology
Mumps
Nursing
Nutrition
Occupational health
Osteopathic medicine
Parasitic diseases
Pertussis
Pharmacology
Pharmacy
Physical examination
Physician assistants
Plague
Pneumonia
Poliomyelitis
Prion diseases
Protozoan diseases
Psychiatry

Psychiatry, child and adolescent
Psychiatry, geriatric
Rabies
Radiation sickness
Roundworm
Rubella
Rubeola
Salmonella
Schistosomiasis
Screening
Serology
Sexually transmitted diseases
Shigellosis
Sleeping sickness
Smallpox
Syphilis
Tapeworm
Tetanus
Toxicology
Toxoplasmosis
Trichinosis
Tropical medicine
Tuberculosis
Typhoid fever and typhus
World Health Organization
Worms
Yellow fever
Zoonoses

PULMONARY MEDICINE
Asthma
Bronchitis
Catheterization
Chest
Coughing
Critical care
Critical care, pediatric
Cystic fibrosis
Edema
Embolism
Emergency medicine
Emphysema
Endoscopy
Environmental health
Fluids and electrolytes
Forensic pathology
Fungal infections
Gene therapy
Geriatrics and gerontology
Hanta virus
Internal medicine
Interstitial pulmonary fibrosis (IPF)
Lung cancer
Lung surgery

Lungs
Occupational health
Oxygen therapy
Paramedics
Pediatrics
Physical examination
Pleurisy
Pneumonia
Pulmonary diseases
Pulmonary medicine
Pulmonary medicine, pediatric
Respiration
Thoracic surgery
Thrombolytic therapy and TPA
Tuberculosis
Tumor removal
Tumors

RADIOLOGY
Angiography
Biophysics
Biopsy
Bone cancer
Bone disorders
Bones and the skeleton
Cancer
Catheterization
Computed tomography (CT)
    scanning
Critical care
Critical care, pediatric
Emergency medicine
Imaging and radiology
Liver cancer
Lung cancer
Magnetic resonance imaging (MRI)
Mammography
Noninvasive tests
Nuclear medicine
Nuclear radiology
Oncology
Positron emission tomography (PET)
    scanning
Prostate cancer
Radiation sickness
Radiation therapy
Radiopharmaceuticals, use of
Sarcoma
Surgery, general
Ultrasonography

RHEUMATOLOGY
Aging
Aging, extended care for the

Arthritis
Arthroplasty
Arthroscopy
Autoimmune disorders
Bone disorders
Bones and the skeleton
Bursitis
Geriatrics and gerontology
Gout
Hydrotherapy
Inflammation
Lyme disease
Orthopedic surgery
Orthopedics
Orthopedics, pediatric
Osteoarthritis
Physical examination
Rheumatic fever
Rheumatoid arthritis
Rheumatology
Spondylitis
Sports medicine

SEROLOGY
Anemia
Blood and blood components
Blood testing
Cholesterol
Cytology
Cytopathology
Dialysis
Fluids and electrolytes
Forensic pathology
Hematology
Hematology, pediatric
Hemophilia
Hodgkin's disease
Host-defense mechanisms
Hypercholesterolemia
Hyperlipidemia
Hypoglycemia
Immune system
Immunology
Immunopathology
Jaundice
Laboratory tests
Leukemia
Malaria
Pathology
Rh factor
Septicemia
Serology
Sickle-cell anemia
Thalassemia

Toxemia
Transfusion

SPEECH PATHOLOGY
Alzheimer's disease
Aphasia and dysphasia
Audiology
Autism
Cerebral palsy
Cleft lip and palate repair
Cleft palate
Dyslexia
Ear surgery
Ears
Electroencephalography (EEG)
Jaw wiring
Laryngitis
Learning disabilities
Paralysis
Speech disorders
Stammering
Strokes and TIAs
Stuttering
Voice and vocal cord disorders

SPORTS MEDICINE
Acupressure
Anorexia nervosa
Arthroplasty
Arthroscopy
Athlete's foot
Biofeedback
Bones and the skeleton
Cardiology
Critical care
Eating disorders
Emergency medicine
Exercise physiology
Fracture and dislocation
Fracture repair
Glycolysis
Head and neck disorders
Heat exhaustion and heat stroke
Hydrotherapy
Kinesiology
Muscle sprains, spasms, and disorders
Muscles
Nutrition
Orthopedic surgery
Orthopedics
Orthopedics, pediatric
Oxygen therapy
Physical examination
Physical rehabilitation

Physiology
Psychiatry
Psychiatry, child and adolescent
Spine, vertebrae, and disks
Sports medicine
Steroids
Tendon disorders
Tendon repair

TOXICOLOGY
Bites and stings
Blood testing
Botulism
Critical care
Critical care, pediatric
Dermatitis
Eczema
Emergency medicine
Environmental diseases
Environmental health
Enzyme therapy
Food poisoning
Forensic pathology
Hepatitis
Herbal medicine
Homeopathy
Intoxication
Itching
Laboratory tests
Lead poisoning
Liver
Occupational health
Pathology
Pharmacology
Pharmacy
Poisoning
Poisonous plants
Rashes
Snakebites
Toxemia
Toxicology
Toxoplasmosis
Urinalysis

UROLOGY
Abdomen
Abdominal disorders
Bed-wetting
Catheterization
Chlamydia
Circumcision, male
Cystectomy
Cystitis
Cystoscopy

Dialysis
E. coli infection
Endoscopy
Fluids and electrolytes
Genital disorders, female
Genital disorders, male
Geriatrics and gerontology
Gonorrhea
Hydrocelectomy
Hypospadias repair and urethroplasty
Incontinence
Infertility in males
Kidney disorders
Kidney transplantation
Kidneys
Lithotripsy
Nephrectomy
Nephritis
Nephrology
Nephrology, pediatric
Pediatrics
Pelvic inflammatory disease (PID)
Penile implant surgery
Prostate cancer
Prostate gland
Prostate gland removal
Reproductive system
Schistosomiasis
Sex change surgery
Sexual differentiation
Sexual dysfunction
Sexually transmitted diseases
Sterilization
Stone removal
Stones
Syphilis
Testicular surgery
Transplantation
Ultrasonography
Urethritis
Urinalysis
Urinary disorders
Urinary system
Urology
Urology, pediatric
Vasectomy

VASCULAR MEDICINE
Amputation
Aneurysmectomy
Aneurysms
Angiography
Angioplasty
Arteriosclerosis
Biofeedback
Bleeding
Blood and blood components
Bypass surgery
Catheterization
Cholesterol
Circulation
Claudication
Diabetes mellitus
Dialysis
Embolism
Endarterectomy
Exercise physiology
Glands
Healing
Hematology
Hematology, pediatric
Hemorrhoid banding and removal
Hemorrhoids
Histology
Hypercholesterolemia
Hyperlipidemia
Ischemia
Lipids
Lymphatic system
Mitral insufficiency
Phlebitis
Podiatry
Shunts
Strokes and TIAs
Systems and organs
Thrombolytic therapy and TPA
Thrombosis and thrombus
Transfusion
Varicose vein removal
Varicosis
Vascular medicine
Vascular system
Venous insufficiency

VIROLOGY
Acquired immunodeficiency syndrome (AIDS)
Chickenpox
Childhood infectious diseases
Chlamydia
Chronic fatigue syndrome
Common cold
Creutzfeldt-Jakob disease and mad cow disease
Cytomegalovirus (CMV)
Drug resistance
Ebola virus
Encephalitis
Fever
Glomerulonephritis
Hanta virus
Hepatitis
Herpes
Human immunodeficiency virus (HIV)
Infection
Influenza
Laboratory tests
Measles, red
Microbiology
Microscopy
Mononucleosis
Mumps
Parasitic diseases
Pelvic inflammatory disease (PID)
Poliomyelitis
Pulmonary diseases
Rabies
Rheumatic fever
Rhinitis
Roseola
Rubella
Rubeola
Serology
Sexually transmitted diseases
Shingles
Smallpox
Tonsillitis
Tropical medicine
Viral infections
Warts
Yellow fever
Zoonoses

Entries by Anatomy or System Affected

Indigestion
Internal medicine
Intestinal disorders
Intestines
Kidney transplantation
Kidneys
Laparoscopy
Liposuction
Lithotripsy
Liver
Liver transplantation
Nephrectomy
Nephritis
Nephrology
Nephrology, pediatric
Obstruction
Pancreas
Pancreatitis
Peristalsis
Peritonitis
Pregnancy and gestation
Prostate cancer
Reproductive system
Roundworm
Shunts
Splenectomy
Sterilization
Stomach, intestinal, and pancreatic
  cancers
Stone removal
Stones
Syphilis
Tubal ligation
Ultrasonography
Urethritis
Urinary disorders
Urinary system
Urology
Urology, pediatric
Worms

ANUS
Colon and rectal polyp removal
Colon and rectal surgery
Colon cancer
Colon therapy
Colonoscopy
Endoscopy
Enemas
Episiotomy
Fistula repair
Hemorrhoid banding and removal
Hemorrhoids
Intestinal disorders

Intestines
Sphincterectomy

ARMS
Amputation
Bones and the skeleton
Carpal tunnel syndrome
Fracture and dislocation
Fracture repair
Liposuction
Muscles
Skin lesion removal
Tendon disorders
Tendon repair
Upper extremities

BACK
Bone disorders
Bone marrow transplantation
Bones and the skeleton
Cerebral palsy
Chiropractic
Disk removal
Dwarfism
Gigantism
Laminectomy and spinal fusion
Lumbar puncture
Muscle sprains, spasms, and disorders
Muscles
Osteoporosis
Sciatica
Scoliosis
Slipped disk
Spinal disorders
Spine, vertebrae, and disks
Spondylitis
Sympathectomy
Tendon disorders

BLADDER
Abdomen
Bed-wetting
Candidiasis
Catheterization
Cystectomy
Cystitis
Cystoscopy
Endoscopy
Fistula repair
Incontinence
Internal medicine
Lithotripsy
Schistosomiasis
Sphincterectomy

Stone removal
Stones
Ultrasonography
Urethritis
Urinalysis
Urinary disorders
Urinary system
Urology
Urology, pediatric

BLOOD
Anemia
Angiography
Arthropod-borne diseases
Bleeding
Blood and blood components
Blood testing
Bone marrow transplantation
Candidiasis
Circulation
Cytomegalovirus (CMV)
Dialysis
E. coli infection
Ebola virus
Fluids and electrolytes
Heart
Hematology
Hematology, pediatric
Hemophilia
Host-defense mechanisms
Hyperlipidemia
Hypoglycemia
Immunization and vaccination
Immunology
Ischemia
Jaundice
Laboratory tests
Leukemia
Liver
Malaria
Nephrology
Nephrology, pediatric
Pharmacology
Pharmacy
Rh factor
Scurvy
Septicemia
Serology
Sickle-cell anemia
Thalassemia
Thrombolytic therapy and TPA
Thrombosis and thrombus
Toxemia
Toxicology

Transfusion
Transplantation
Ultrasonography
Yellow fever

BLOOD VESSELS
Aneurysmectomy
Aneurysms
Angiography
Angioplasty
Arteriosclerosis
Bleeding
Blood and blood components
Blood testing
Bypass surgery
Catheterization
Cholesterol
Circulation
Claudication
Diabetes mellitus
Dizziness and fainting
Eclampsia
Edema
Electrocauterization
Embolism
Endarterectomy
Hammertoe correction
Heart
Heart disease
Heat exhaustion and heat stroke
Hemorrhoid banding and removal
Hemorrhoids
Hypercholesterolemia
Hypertension
Ischemia
Phlebitis
Shock
Strokes and TIAs
Thrombosis and thrombus
Varicose vein removal
Varicosis
Vascular medicine
Vascular system
Venous insufficiency

BONES
Amputation
Arthritis
Bone cancer
Bone disorders
Bone grafting
Bone marrow transplantation
Bones and the skeleton
Bunion removal

Cells
Cerebral palsy
Chiropractic
Cleft lip and palate repair
Cleft palate
Craniotomy
Disk removal
Dwarfism
Ear surgery
Ears
Estrogen replacement therapy
Feet
Foot disorders
Fracture and dislocation
Fracture repair
Gigantism
Hammertoe correction
Head and neck disorders
Heel spur removal
Hematology
Hematology, pediatric
Hip fracture repair
Jaw wiring
Kneecap removal
Laminectomy and spinal fusion
Lower extremities
Neurofibromatosis
Nuclear medicine
Nuclear radiology
Orthopedic surgery
Orthopedics
Orthopedics, pediatric
Osgood-Schlatter disease
Osteopathic medicine
Osteoporosis
Paget's disease
Periodontitis
Physical rehabilitation
Podiatry
Rheumatology
Rickets
Sarcoma
Scoliosis
Slipped disk
Spinal disorders
Spine, vertebrae, and disks
Sports medicine
Teeth
Temporomandibular joint (TMJ)
   syndrome
Tendon disorders
Tendon repair
Upper extremities

BRAIN
Abscess drainage
Abscesses
Addiction
Alcoholism
Altitude sickness
Alzheimer's disease
Amnesia
Anesthesia
Anesthesiology
Aneurysmectomy
Aneurysms
Angiography
Aphasia and dysphasia
Aromatherapy
Attention-deficit disorder (ADD)
Biofeedback
Brain
Brain disorders
Cluster headaches
Coma
Computed tomography (CT) scanning
Concussion
Craniotomy
Creutzfeldt-Jakob disease and mad
   cow disease
Cytomegalovirus (CMV)
Dementia
Dizziness and fainting
Down syndrome
Dwarfism
Dyslexia
Electroconvulsive therapy
Electroencephalography (EEG)
Embolism
Emotions, biomedical causes and
   effects of
Encephalitis
Endocrinology
Endocrinology, pediatric
Epilepsy
Fetal alcohol syndrome
Fetal tissue transplantation
Gigantism
Hallucinations
Head and neck disorders
Headaches
Hydrocephalus
Hypertension
Hypnosis
Kinesiology
Lead poisoning
Learning disabilities
Light therapy

Lower extremities
Nail removal
Orthopedic surgery
Orthopedics
Orthopedics, pediatric
Osteoarthritis
Podiatry
Sports medicine
Tendon repair
Warts

GALLBLADDER
Abscess drainage
Abscesses
Cholecystectomy
Cholecystitis
Fistula repair
Gallbladder diseases
Gastroenterology
Gastroenterology, pediatric
Gastrointestinal disorders
Gastrointestinal system
Internal medicine
Laparoscopy
Liver transplantation
Nuclear medicine
Stone removal
Stones
Ultrasonography

GASTROINTESTINAL SYSTEM
Abdomen
Abdominal disorders
Allergies
Appendectomy
Appendicitis
Bacterial infections
Botulism
Bulimia
Bypass surgery
Candidiasis
Childhood infectious diseases
Cholera
Cholesterol
Colitis
Colon and rectal polyp removal
Colon and rectal surgery
Colon cancer
Colon therapy
Colonoscopy
Constipation
Crohn's disease
Cytomegalovirus (CMV)
Diabetes mellitus

Diarrhea and dysentery
Digestion
Diverticulitis and diverticulosis
E. coli infection
Eating disorders
Ebola virus
Emotions, biomedical causes and
  effects of
Endoscopy
Enemas
Fistula repair
Food biochemistry
Food poisoning
Gallbladder diseases
Gastrectomy
Gastroenterology
Gastroenterology, pediatric
Gastrointestinal disorders
Gastrointestinal system
Gastrostomy
Glands
Halitosis
Heartburn
Hemorrhoid banding and removal
Hemorrhoids
Hernia
Hernia repair
Host-defense mechanisms
Ileostomy and colostomy
Incontinence
Indigestion
Internal medicine
Intestinal disorders
Intestines
Kwashiorkor
Lactose intolerance
Laparoscopy
Lipids
Liver
Malnutrition
Metabolism
Motion sickness
Muscles
Nausea and vomiting
Nutrition
Obesity
Obstruction
Pancreas
Pancreatitis
Peristalsis
Poisoning
Poisonous plants
Premenstrual syndrome (PMS)
Proctology

Protozoan diseases
Radiation sickness
Roundworm
Salmonella
Sense organs
Shigellosis
Shunts
Stomach, intestinal, and pancreatic
  cancers
Tapeworm
Taste
Teeth
Trichinosis
Tumor removal
Tumors
Typhoid fever and typhus
Ulcer surgery
Ulcers
Vagotomy
Vitamins and minerals
Weight loss and gain
Worms

GENITALS
Candidiasis
Catheterization
Cervical, ovarian, and uterine cancers
Cervical procedures
Chlamydia
Circumcision, female, and genital
  mutilation
Circumcision, male
Contraception
Culdocentesis
Cyst removal
Cysts and ganglions
Electrocauterization
Endometrial biopsy
Episiotomy
Genital disorders, female
Genital disorders, male
Glands
Gonorrhea
Gynecology
Herpes
Hydrocelectomy
Hypospadias repair and urethroplasty
Infertility in females
Infertility in males
Pelvic inflammatory disease (PID)
Penile implant surgery
Reproductive system
Sex change surgery
Sexual differentiation

Sexual dysfunction
Sexuality
Sexually transmitted diseases
Sterilization
Syphilis
Testicular surgery
Urology
Urology, pediatric
Vasectomy
Warts

GLANDS
Abscess drainage
Abscesses
Addison's disease
Adrenalectomy
Biofeedback
Breasts, female
Contraception
Cyst removal
Cysts and ganglions
Diabetes mellitus
Dwarfism
Eating disorders
Endocrine disorders
Endocrinology
Endocrinology, pediatric
Gigantism
Glands
Goiter
Hormone replacement therapy
Hormones
Hyperparathyroidism and
    hypoparathyroidism
Hypoglycemia
Internal medicine
Liver
Mastectomy and lumpectomy
Melatonin
Metabolism
Mumps
Neurosurgery
Nuclear medicine
Nuclear radiology
Obesity
Pancreas
Parathyroidectomy
Prostate gland
Prostate gland removal
Sex change surgery
Sexual differentiation
Steroids
Testicular surgery
Thyroid disorders

Thyroid gland
Thyroidectomy

GUMS
Abscess drainage
Abscesses
Caries, dental
Cleft lip and palate repair
Dental diseases
Dentistry
Endodontic disease
Gingivitis
Jaw wiring
Nutrition
Orthodontics
Periodontal surgery
Periodontitis
Root canal treatment
Scurvy
Teeth
Tooth extraction
Toothache

HAIR
Albinism
Dermatitis
Dermatology
Eczema
Hair loss and baldness
Hair transplantation
Lice, mites, and ticks
Nutrition
Pigmentation
Radiation sickness
Radiation therapy

HANDS
Amputation
Arthritis
Bones and the skeleton
Bursitis
Carpal tunnel syndrome
Cerebral palsy
Cysts and ganglions
Fracture and dislocation
Fracture repair
Frostbite
Ganglion removal
Nail removal
Neurology
Neurology, pediatric
Orthopedic surgery
Orthopedics
Orthopedics, pediatric

Osteoarthritis
Rheumatoid arthritis
Rheumatology
Skin lesion removal
Sports medicine
Tendon disorders
Tendon repair
Upper extremities
Warts

HEAD
Altitude sickness
Aneurysmectomy
Aneurysms
Angiography
Brain
Brain disorders
Cluster headaches
Coma
Computed tomography (CT) scanning
Concussion
Craniotomy
Dizziness and fainting
Electroencephalography (EEG)
Embolism
Epilepsy
Fetal tissue transplantation
Hair loss and baldness
Hair transplantation
Head and neck disorders
Headaches
Hydrocephalus
Lice, mites, and ticks
Meningitis
Migraine headaches
Nasal polyp removal
Nasopharyngeal disorders
Neurology
Neurology, pediatric
Neurosurgery
Rhinoplasty and submucous resection
Seizures
Shunts
Sports medicine
Strokes and TIAs
Temporomandibular joint (TMJ)
    syndrome
Thrombosis and thrombus
Unconsciousness

HEART
Aneurysmectomy
Aneurysms
Angina

Angiography
Angioplasty
Anxiety
Arrhythmias
Arteriosclerosis
Biofeedback
Bites and stings
Bypass surgery
Cardiac rehabilitation
Cardiology
Cardiology, pediatric
Catheterization
Circulation
Congenital heart disease
Electrical shock
Electrocardiography (ECG or EKG)
Embolism
Endocarditis
Exercise physiology
Heart
Heart attack
Heart disease
Heart failure
Heart transplantation
Heart valve replacement
Hypertension
Internal medicine
Kinesiology
Lyme disease
Mitral insufficiency
Pacemaker implantation
Palpitations
Resuscitation
Reye's syndrome
Rheumatic fever
Shock
Sports medicine
Strokes and TIAs
Thoracic surgery
Thrombolytic therapy and TPA
Thrombosis and thrombus
Toxoplasmosis
Transplantation
Ultrasonography
Yellow fever

HIPS
Aging
Arthritis
Arthroplasty
Arthroscopy
Bone disorders
Bones and the skeleton
Chiropractic

Dwarfism
Fracture and dislocation
Fracture repair
Hip fracture repair
Liposuction
Lower extremities
Orthopedic surgery
Orthopedics
Orthopedics, pediatric
Osteoarthritis
Osteoporosis
Physical rehabilitation
Rheumatoid arthritis
Rheumatology
Sciatica

IMMUNE SYSTEM
Acquired immunodeficiency syndrome
  (AIDS)
Allergies
Antibiotics
Arthritis
Asthma
Autoimmune disorders
Bacterial infections
Bacteriology
Bites and stings
Blood and blood components
Bone grafting
Bone marrow transplantation
Candidiasis
Cell therapy
Cells
Childhood infectious diseases
Chronic fatigue syndrome
Cytology
Cytomegalovirus (CMV)
Cytopathology
Dermatology
Dermatopathology
E. coli infection
Emotions, biomedical causes and
  effects of
Endocrinology
Endocrinology, pediatric
Enzyme therapy
Enzymes
Fungal infections
Grafts and grafting
Gram staining
Guillain-Barré syndrome
Healing
Hematology
Hematology, pediatric

Homeopathy
Host-defense mechanisms
Human immunodeficiency virus (HIV)
Immune system
Immunization and vaccination
Immunodeficiency disorders
Immunology
Immunopathology
Leprosy
Lupus erythematosus
Lymphatic system
Magnetic field therapy
Measles, red
Microbiology
Mumps
Mutation
Oncology
Pancreas
Pharmacology
Poisoning
Poisonous plants
Pulmonary diseases
Pulmonary medicine
Pulmonary medicine, pediatric
Rh factor
Rheumatology
Rubella
Rubeola
Sarcoma
Scarlet fever
Serology
Smallpox
Stress
Stress reduction
Toxicology
Transfusion
Transplantation

INTESTINES
Abdomen
Abdominal disorders
Appendectomy
Appendicitis
Bacterial infections
Bypass surgery
Colitis
Colon and rectal polyp removal
Colon and rectal surgery
Colon cancer
Colon therapy
Colonoscopy
Constipation
Crohn's disease
Diarrhea and dysentery

Digestion
Diverticulitis and diverticulosis
E. coli infection
Eating disorders
Endoscopy
Enemas
Fistula repair
Food poisoning
Gastroenterology
Gastroenterology, pediatric
Gastrointestinal disorders
Gastrointestinal system
Hemorrhoid banding and removal
Hemorrhoids
Hernia
Hernia repair
Ileostomy and colostomy
Indigestion
Internal medicine
Intestinal disorders
Intestines
Kaposi's sarcoma
Kwashiorkor
Lactose intolerance
Laparoscopy
Malnutrition
Metabolism
Nutrition
Obesity
Obstruction
Peristalsis
Proctology
Roundworm
Salmonella
Sphincterectomy
Stomach, intestinal, and pancreatic
  cancers
Tapeworm
Trichinosis
Tumor removal
Tumors
Ulcer surgery
Ulcers
Worms

JOINTS
Amputation
Arthritis
Arthroplasty
Arthroscopy
Bursitis
Carpal tunnel syndrome
Cell therapy
Chlamydia

Cyst removal
Cysts and ganglions
Endoscopy
Exercise physiology
Fracture and dislocation
Gout
Hip fracture repair
Kneecap removal
Lupus erythematosus
Lyme disease
Orthopedic surgery
Orthopedics
Orthopedics, pediatric
Osteoarthritis
Physical rehabilitation
Rheumatoid arthritis
Rheumatology
Spondylitis
Sports medicine
Temporomandibular joint (TMJ)
  syndrome
Tendon disorders
Tendon repair

KIDNEYS
Abdomen
Abscess drainage
Abscesses
Adrenalectomy
Cysts and ganglions
Dialysis
Glomerulonephritis
Hanta virus
Hypertension
Internal medicine
Kidney disorders
Kidney transplantation
Kidneys
Laparoscopy
Lithotripsy
Metabolism
Nephrectomy
Nephritis
Nephrology
Nephrology, pediatric
Nuclear medicine
Nuclear radiology
Renal failure
Reye's syndrome
Stone removal
Stones
Transplantation
Ultrasonography
Urinalysis

Urinary disorders
Urinary system
Urology
Urology, pediatric

KNEES
Amputation
Arthritis
Arthroplasty
Arthroscopy
Bones and the skeleton
Bursitis
Endoscopy
Exercise physiology
Fracture and dislocation
Kneecap removal
Liposuction
Lower extremities
Orthopedic surgery
Orthopedics
Orthopedics, pediatric
Osgood-Schlatter disease
Osteoarthritis
Physical rehabilitation
Rheumatoid arthritis
Rheumatology
Sports medicine
Tendon disorders
Tendon repair

LEGS
Amputation
Arthritis
Arthroplasty
Arthroscopy
Bone disorders
Bones and the skeleton
Bursitis
Cerebral palsy
Dwarfism
Fracture and dislocation
Fracture repair
Gigantism
Hemiplegia
Hip fracture repair
Kneecap removal
Liposuction
Lower extremities
Muscle sprains, spasms, and disorders
Muscles
Muscular dystrophy
Numbness and tingling
Orthopedic surgery
Orthopedics

Orthopedics, pediatric
Osteoarthritis
Osteoporosis
Paralysis
Paraplegia
Physical rehabilitation
Poliomyelitis
Quadriplegia
Rheumatoid arthritis
Rheumatology
Rickets
Sciatica
Sports medicine
Tendon disorders
Tendon repair
Varicose vein removal
Varicosis
Venous insufficiency

LIGAMENTS
Muscle sprains, spasms, and disorders
Muscles
Orthopedic surgery
Orthopedics
Orthopedics, pediatric
Physical rehabilitation
Slipped disk
Sports medicine
Tendon disorders
Tendon repair

LIVER
Abdomen
Abdominal disorders
Abscess drainage
Abscesses
Alcoholism
Blood and blood components
Circulation
Cirrhosis
Cytomegalovirus (CMV)
Edema
Gastroenterology
Gastroenterology, pediatric
Gastrointestinal disorders
Gastrointestinal system
Hematology
Hematology, pediatric
Hepatitis
Internal medicine
Jaundice
Kaposi's sarcoma
Liver
Liver cancer

Liver disorders
Liver transplantation
Malaria
Metabolism
Reye's syndrome
Schistosomiasis
Shunts
Transplantation
Yellow fever

LUNGS
Abscess drainage
Abscesses
Allergies
Altitude sickness
Apnea
Asphyxiation
Asthma
Bacterial infections
Bronchitis
Chest
Childhood infectious diseases
Choking
Common cold
Coughing
Cystic fibrosis
Cytomegalovirus (CMV)
Diphtheria
Edema
Embolism
Emphysema
Endoscopy
Exercise physiology
Hanta virus
Heart transplantation
Influenza
Internal medicine
Interstitial pulmonary fibrosis (IPF)
Kaposi's sarcoma
Kinesiology
Legionnaires' disease
Lung cancer
Lung surgery
Lungs
Measles, red
Oxygen therapy
Pertussis
Plague
Pleurisy
Pneumonia
Pulmonary diseases
Pulmonary medicine
Pulmonary medicine, pediatric
Respiration

Resuscitation
Rubeola
Thoracic surgery
Thrombolytic therapy and TPA
Thrombosis and thrombus
Toxoplasmosis
Transplantation
Tuberculosis
Tumor removal
Tumors

LYMPHATIC SYSTEM
Angiography
Circulation
Bacterial infections
Blood and blood components
Breast cancer
Breast disorders
Cancer
Cervical, ovarian, and uterine cancers
Chemotherapy
Colon cancer
Edema
Elephantiasis
Histology
Hodgkin's disease
Immune system
Immunology
Immunopathology
Liver cancer
Lower extremities
Lung cancer
Lymphadenopathy and lymphoma
Lymphatic system
Malignancy and metastasis
Mononucleosis
Oncology
Prostate cancer
Skin cancer
Sleeping sickness
Splenectomy
Stomach, intestinal, and pancreatic
    cancers
Tonsillectomy and adenoid removal
Tonsillitis
Tumor removal
Tumors
Upper extremities
Vascular medicine
Vascular system

MOUTH
Candidiasis
Caries, dental

Cleft lip and palate repair
Dental diseases
Dentistry
Endodontic disease
Gingivitis
Halitosis
Herpes
Jaw wiring
Nutrition
Orthodontics
Periodontal surgery
Periodontitis
Root canal treatment
Sense organs
Taste
Temporomandibular joint (TMJ)
    syndrome
Tooth extraction
Toothache
Ulcers

MUSCLES
Acupressure
Amputation
Anesthesia
Anesthesiology
Ataxia
Bed-wetting
Bell's palsy
Beriberi
Biofeedback
Botulism
Breasts, female
Cerebral palsy
Chest
Childhood infectious diseases
Chronic fatigue syndrome
Claudication
Creutzfeldt-Jakob disease and mad
    cow disease
Cysts and ganglions
Ebola virus
Emotions, biomedical causes and
    effects of
Exercise physiology
Feet
Foot disorders
Glycolysis
Guillain-Barré syndrome
Head and neck disorders
Hemiplegia
Kinesiology
Lower extremities
Mastectomy and lumpectomy

Motor neuron diseases
Multiple sclerosis
Muscle sprains, spasms, and disorders
Muscles
Muscular dystrophy
Neurology
Neurology, pediatric
Numbness and tingling
Orthopedic surgery
Orthopedics
Orthopedics, pediatric
Osgood-Schlatter disease
Osteopathic medicine
Palsy
Paralysis
Paraplegia
Parkinson's disease
Physical rehabilitation
Poisoning
Poliomyelitis
Quadriplegia
Rabies
Respiration
Rheumatoid arthritis
Seizures
Speech disorders
Sphincterectomy
Sports medicine
Temporomandibular joint (TMJ)
    syndrome
Tendon disorders
Tendon repair
Tetanus
Tics
Trembling and shaking
Trichinosis
Upper extremities
Weight loss and gain
Yellow fever

MUSCULOSKELETAL SYSTEM
Acupressure
Amputation
Anatomy
Anesthesia
Anesthesiology
Arthritis
Ataxia
Bed-wetting
Bell's palsy
Beriberi
Biofeedback
Bone cancer
Bone disorders

Bone grafting
Bone marrow transplantation
Bones and the skeleton
Botulism
Breasts, female
Cells
Cerebral palsy
Chest
Childhood infectious diseases
Chiropractic
Chronic fatigue syndrome
Claudication
Cleft lip and palate repair
Cleft palate
Cysts and ganglions
Depression
Dwarfism
Ear surgery
Ears
Emotions, biomedical causes and
    effects of
Exercise physiology
Feet
Fetal alcohol syndrome
Foot disorders
Fracture and dislocation
Fracture repair
Gigantism
Glycolysis
Guillain-Barré syndrome
Hammertoe correction
Head and neck disorders
Heel spur removal
Hematology
Hematology, pediatric
Hemiplegia
Hip fracture repair
Hyperparathyroidism and
    hypoparathyroidism
Jaw wiring
Kinesiology
Kneecap removal
Lower extremities
Lupus erythematosus
Mastectomy and lumpectomy
Motor neuron diseases
Multiple sclerosis
Muscle sprains, spasms, and disorders
Muscles
Muscular dystrophy
Neurology
Neurology, pediatric
Nuclear medicine
Nuclear radiology

Diabetes mellitus
Diphtheria
Disk removal
Dizziness and fainting
Down syndrome
Dwarfism
Dyslexia
E. coli infection
Ear surgery
Ears
Eclampsia
Electrical shock
Electroconvulsive therapy
Electroencephalography (EEG)
Emotions, biomedical causes and
    effects of
Encephalitis
Endocrinology
Endocrinology, pediatric
Epilepsy
Eyes
Fetal alcohol syndrome
Fetal tissue transplantation
Gigantism
Glands
Guillain-Barré syndrome
Hallucinations
Hammertoe correction
Head and neck disorders
Headaches
Hearing loss
Heart transplantation
Hemiplegia
Hydrocephalus
Hypnosis
Kinesiology
Learning disabilities
Lead poisoning
Leprosy
Light therapy
Lower extremities
Lyme disease
Malaria
Memory loss
Meningitis
Mental retardation
Migraine headaches
Motor neuron diseases
Multiple sclerosis
Narcolepsy
Narcotics
Nausea and vomiting
Nervous system
Neuralgia, neuritis, and neuropathy

Neurofibromatosis
Neurology
Neurology, pediatric
Neurosurgery
Nuclear radiology
Numbness and tingling
Orthopedic surgery
Orthopedics
Orthopedics, pediatric
Paget's disease
Palsy
Paralysis
Paraplegia
Parkinson's disease
Pharmacology
Pharmacy
Phenylketonuria (PKU)
Physical rehabilitation
Poisoning
Poliomyelitis
Porphyria
Premenstrual syndrome (PMS)
Prion diseases
Quadriplegia
Rabies
Reye's syndrome
Sciatica
Seizures
Sense organs
Shingles
Shunts
Skin
Sleep disorders
Sleeping sickness
Smell
Snakebites
Spina bifida
Spinal disorders
Spine, vertebrae, and disks
Sports medicine
Stammering
Strokes and TIAs
Stuttering
Sympathectomy
Syphilis
Taste
Tay-Sachs disease
Teeth
Tetanus
Thrombolytic therapy and TPA
Tics
Touch
Toxicology
Toxoplasmosis

Trembling and shaking
Unconsciousness
Upper extremities
Vagotomy
Yellow fever

NOSE
Allergies
Aromatherapy
Childhood infectious diseases
Common cold
Halitosis
Nasal polyp removal
Nasopharyngeal disorders
Otorhinolaryngology
Plastic, cosmetic, and reconstructive
    surgery
Pulmonary medicine
Pulmonary medicine, pediatric
Respiration
Rhinitis
Rhinoplasty and submucous resection
Rosacea
Sense organs
Sinusitis
Skin lesion removal
Smell
Sore throat
Taste
Viral infections

PANCREAS
Abscess drainage
Abscesses
Diabetes mellitus
Digestion
Endocrinology
Endocrinology, pediatric
Fetal tissue transplantation
Food biochemistry
Gastroenterology
Gastroenterology, pediatric
Gastrointestinal disorders
Gastrointestinal system
Glands
Hormones
Internal medicine
Metabolism
Pancreas
Pancreatitis
Stomach, intestinal, and pancreatic
    cancers
Transplantation

PSYCHIC-EMOTIONAL SYSTEM
Addiction
Aging
Alcoholism
Alzheimer's disease
Amnesia
Anesthesia
Anesthesiology
Anorexia nervosa
Anxiety
Aphasia and dysphasia
Aromatherapy
Attention-deficit disorder (ADD)
Autism
Biofeedback
Brain
Brain disorders
Bulimia
Chronic fatigue syndrome
Cluster headaches
Coma
Concussion
Death and dying
Dementia
Depression
Dizziness and fainting
Domestic violence
Down syndrome
Dyslexia
Eating disorders
Electroconvulsive therapy
Electroencephalography (EEG)
Emotions, biomedical causes and
    effects of
Endocrinology
Endocrinology, pediatric
Factitious disorders
Grief and guilt
Hallucinations
Headaches
Hormone replacement therapy
Hormones
Hydrocephalus
Hypnosis
Hypochondriasis
Kinesiology
Lead poisoning
Learning disabilities
Light therapy
Manic-depressive disorder
Memory loss
Menopause
Mental retardation
Midlife crisis

Migraine headaches
Miscarriage
Narcolepsy
Narcotics
Neurology
Neurology, pediatric
Neurosis
Neurosurgery
Obesity
Obsessive-compulsive disorder
Palpitations
Panic attacks
Paranoia
Pharmacology
Pharmacy
Phobias
Postpartum depression
Psychiatric disorders
Psychiatry
Psychiatry, child and adolescent
Psychiatry, geriatric
Psychoanalysis
Psychosis
Psychosomatic disorders
Puberty and adolescence
Rabies
Schizophrenia
Sexual dysfunction
Sexuality
Sibling rivalry
Sleep disorders
Speech disorders
Stammering
Stillbirth
Stress
Strokes and TIAs
Stuttering
Suicide
Tics
Weight loss and gain

REPRODUCTIVE SYSTEM
Abdomen
Abdominal disorders
Abortion
Acquired immunodeficiency syndrome
    (AIDS)
Amenorrhea
Amniocentesis
Anatomy
Anorexia nervosa
Breast-feeding
Breasts, female
Candidiasis

Catheterization
Cervical, ovarian, and uterine cancers
Cervical procedures
Cesarean section
Childbirth
Childbirth, complications of
Chlamydia
Chorionic villus sampling
Circumcision, female, and genital
    mutilation
Circumcision, male
Conception
Contraception
Culdocentesis
Cyst removal
Cysts and ganglions
Dysmenorrhea
Eating disorders
Ectopic pregnancy
Electrocauterization
Endocrinology
Endometrial biopsy
Endometriosis
Episiotomy
Fetal alcohol syndrome
Fistula repair
Genetic counseling
Genital disorders, female
Genital disorders, male
Glands
Gonorrhea
Gynecology
Hernia
Herpes
Hormone replacement therapy
Hormones
Human immunodeficiency virus (HIV)
Hydrocelectomy
Hypospadias repair and urethroplasty
Hysterectomy
In vitro fertilization
Infertility in females
Infertility in males
Internal medicine
Laparoscopy
Menopause
Menorrhagia
Menstruation
Miscarriage
Multiple births
Mumps
Myomectomy
Obstetrics
Ovarian cysts

Pelvic inflammatory disease (PID)
Penile implant surgery
Pregnancy and gestation
Premature birth
Premenstrual syndrome (PMS)
Prostate cancer
Prostate gland
Puberty and adolescence
Reproductive system
Sex change surgery
Sexual differentiation
Sexual dysfunction
Sexuality
Sexually transmitted diseases
Sterilization
Stillbirth
Syphilis
Testicular surgery
Tubal ligation
Ultrasonography
Urology
Urology, pediatric
Vasectomy
Warts

RESPIRATORY SYSTEM

Abscess drainage
Abscesses
Altitude sickness
Apnea
Asphyxiation
Asthma
Bacterial infections
Bronchitis
Chest
Chickenpox
Childhood infectious diseases
Choking
Common cold
Coughing
Cystic fibrosis
Diphtheria
Edema
Embolism
Emphysema
Exercise physiology
Fluids and electrolytes
Fungal infections
Halitosis
Hanta virus
Head and neck disorders
Heart transplantation
Influenza
Internal medicine

Interstitial pulmonary fibrosis (IPF)
Kinesiology
Laryngectomy
Laryngitis
Legionnaires' disease
Lung cancer
Lung surgery
Lungs
Measles, red
Mononucleosis
Nasopharyngeal disorders
Otorhinolaryngology
Oxygen therapy
Pertussis
Pharyngitis
Plague
Pleurisy
Pneumonia
Poisoning
Pulmonary diseases
Pulmonary medicine
Pulmonary medicine, pediatric
Respiration
Resuscitation
Rheumatic fever
Rhinitis
Roundworm
Rubeola
Sinusitis
Smallpox
Sore throat
Strep throat
Thoracic surgery
Thrombolytic therapy and TPA
Thrombosis and thrombus
Tonsillectomy and adenoid removal
Tonsillitis
Toxoplasmosis
Tracheostomy
Transplantation
Tuberculosis
Tumor removal
Tumors
Voice and vocal cord disorders
Worms

SKIN

Abscess drainage
Abscesses
Acne
Acupressure
Acupuncture
Albinism
Allergies

Amputation
Anesthesia
Anesthesiology
Anxiety
Arthropod-borne diseases
Athlete's foot
Biopsy
Bites and stings
Blood testing
Burns and scalds
Candidiasis
Cell therapy
Cells
Chickenpox
Cleft lip and palate repair
Cryotherapy and cryosurgery
Cyst removal
Cysts and ganglions
Dermatitis
Dermatology
Dermatopathology
Ebola virus
Eczema
Edema
Electrical shock
Electrocauterization
Face lift and blepharoplasty
Frostbite
Fungal infections
Glands
Grafts and grafting
Hair loss and baldness
Hair transplantation
Heat exhaustion and heat stroke
Host-defense mechanisms
Itching
Jaundice
Kaposi's sarcoma
Keratoses
Laceration repair
Laser use in surgery
Leishmaniasis
Leprosy
Lice, mites, and ticks
Light therapy
Lower extremities
Lupus erythematosus
Lyme disease
Malignant melanoma removal
Measles, red
Neurofibromatosis
Numbness and tingling
Obesity
Pigmentation

Pimples
Plastic, cosmetic, and reconstructive
  surgery
Poisonous plants
Porphyria
Psoriasis
Radiation sickness
Rashes
Rosacea
Roseola
Rubella
Rubeola
Scabies
Scarlet fever
Scurvy
Sense organs
Shingles
Skin
Skin cancer
Skin disorders
Skin lesion removal
Smallpox
Tattoo removal
Touch
Upper extremities
Warts

SPINE
Anesthesia
Anesthesiology
Bone cancer
Bone disorders
Bones and the skeleton
Cerebral palsy
Chiropractic
Disk removal
Dystrophy
Fracture and dislocation
Head and neck disorders
Kinesiology
Laminectomy and spinal fusion
Lumbar puncture
Meningitis
Motor neuron diseases
Multiple sclerosis
Muscle sprains, spasms, and disorders
Muscular dystrophy
Nervous system
Neuralgia, neuritis, and neuropathy
Neurology
Neurology, pediatric
Neurosurgery
Numbness and tingling
Orthopedic surgery

Orthopedics
Orthopedics, pediatric
Osteoarthritis
Osteoporosis
Paget's disease
Paralysis
Paraplegia
Physical rehabilitation
Poliomyelitis
Quadriplegia
Sciatica
Scoliosis
Slipped disk
Spina bifida
Spinal disorders
Spine, vertebrae, and disks
Spondylitis
Sports medicine
Sympathectomy

SPLEEN
Abdomen
Abdominal disorders
Abscess drainage
Abscesses
Anemia
Bleeding
Hematology
Hematology, pediatric
Immune system
Internal medicine
Lymphatic system
Metabolism
Splenectomy
Transplantation

STOMACH
Abdomen
Abdominal disorders
Abscess drainage
Abscesses
Allergies
Botulism
Bulimia
Bypass surgery
Colitis
Crohn's disease
Digestion
Eating disorders
Endoscopy
Food biochemistry
Food poisoning
Gastrectomy
Gastroenterology

Gastroenterology, pediatric
Gastrointestinal disorders
Gastrointestinal system
Gastrostomy
Halitosis
Heartburn
Hernia
Hernia repair
Indigestion
Influenza
Internal medicine
Kwashiorkor
Lactose intolerance
Malnutrition
Metabolism
Motion sickness
Nausea and vomiting
Nutrition
Obesity
Peristalsis
Poisoning
Poisonous plants
Radiation sickness
Roundworm
Salmonella
Stomach, intestinal, and pancreatic
  cancers
Ulcer surgery
Ulcers
Vagotomy
Vitamins and minerals
Weight loss and gain

TEETH
Caries, dental
Dental diseases
Dentistry
Endodontic disease
Forensic pathology
Fracture repair
Gastrointestinal system
Gingivitis
Jaw wiring
Nutrition
Orthodontics
Periodontal surgery
Periodontitis
Root canal treatment
Teeth
Temporomandibular joint (TMJ)
  syndrome
Tooth extraction
Toothache
Veterinary medicine